Textbook of Human Nutrition

Textbook of Human Nutrition

SECOND EDITION

(Late) Anjana Agarwal MSc PhD
Visiting Faculty
Department of Food Science and Nutrition Consultant
SNDT Women's University
Mumbai, Maharashtra, India

Shobha A Udipi MSc PhD
Research Director and Head
Hon Director, Integrative Nutrition and Ayurceuticals
Kasturba Health Society-Medical Research Centre
Mumbai, Maharashtra, India
Professor Emeritus
Transdisciplinary University of Health Sciences and Technology
Bengaluru, Karnataka, India
Former Professor and Head,
Department of Food Science and Nutrition
SNDT Women's University
Mumbai, Maharashtra, India

Foreword
Poonam Agrawal

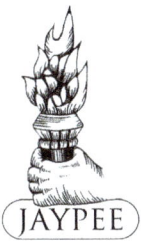

JAYPEE BROTHERS MEDICAL PUBLISHERS
The Health Sciences Publisher
New Delhi | London

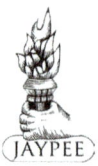

Jaypee Brothers Medical Publishers (P) Ltd

Headquarters
Jaypee Brothers Medical Publishers (P) Ltd
EMCA House, 23/23-B
Ansari Road, Daryaganj
New Delhi 110 002, India
Landline: +91-11-23272143, +91-11-23272703
+91-11-23282021, +91-11-23245672
Email: jaypee@jaypeebrothers.com

Corporate Office
Jaypee Brothers Medical Publishers (P) Ltd
4838/24, Ansari Road, Daryaganj
New Delhi 110 002, India
Phone: +91-11-43574357
Fax: +91-11-43574314
Email: jaypee@jaypeebrothers.com

Overseas Office
J.P. Medical Ltd
83 Victoria Street, London
SW1H 0HW (UK)
Phone: +44 20 3170 8910
Fax: +44 (0)20 3008 6180
Email: info@jpmedpub.com

Website: www.jaypeebrothers.com
Website: www.jaypeedigital.com

© 2022, Jaypee Brothers Medical Publishers

The views and opinions expressed in this book are solely those of the original contributor(s)/author(s) and do not necessarily represent those of editor(s) of the book.

All rights reserved. No part of this publication may be reproduced, stored or transmitted in any form or by any means, electronic, mechanical, photocopying, recording or otherwise, without the prior permission in writing of the publishers.

All brand names and product names used in this book are trade names, service marks, trademarks or registered trademarks of their respective owners. The publisher is not associated with any product or vendor mentioned in this book.

Medical knowledge and practice change constantly. This book is designed to provide accurate, authoritative information about the subject matter in question. However, readers are advised to check the most current information available on procedures included and check information from the manufacturer of each product to be administered, to verify the recommended dose, formula, method and duration of administration, adverse effects and contraindications. It is the responsibility of the practitioner to take all appropriate safety precautions. Neither the publisher nor the author(s)/editor(s) assume any liability for any injury and/or damage to persons or property arising from or related to use of material in this book.

This book is sold on the understanding that the publisher is not engaged in providing professional medical services. If such advice or services are required, the services of a competent medical professional should be sought.

Every effort has been made where necessary to contact holders of copyright to obtain permission to reproduce copyright material. If any have been inadvertently overlooked, the publisher will be pleased to make the necessary arrangements at the first opportunity.

Inquiries for bulk sales may be solicited at: jaypee@jaypeebrothers.com

Textbook of Human Nutrition

First Edition: 2014

Second Edition: **2022**

ISBN: 978-93-89587-86-9

Dedicated to

Our revered parents
Ravindra Kumar Garg and Sushila Rani Garg
— ***(Late)* Anjana Agarwal**
Anand Padmanabh Udipi and Durga Anand Udipi
—**Shobha A Udipi**

Dedicated to

Our revered parents
Ravindra Kumar Garg and Sushila Rani Garg
— *(Late)* **Anjana Agarwal**
Anand Padmanabh Udipi and Durga Anand Udipi
—**Shobha A Udipi**

Foreword

It gives me immense pleasure and satisfaction to introduce the second edition of highly well received book on Food and Nutrition, '*Textbook of Human Nutrition*'. The unique features of the first edition, inter alia, the laboratory laurels, coverage of wide spectrum of related topics, in depth description supported by suitable latest data and apt expression made the first edition almost a 'must read' book for students, teachers/faculty, professionals alike. The high demand of the book coupled with latest developments in this rapidly updating domain necessitated bringing out of the next edition. The authors and the publisher both must be applauded for realizing this and accomplishing the task timely in most appropriate manner.

This edition of the book, besides updated research laurels and the newest knowledge/data in the domain, has an *added chapter on nutritional assessment*. Special feature of the book is that it places knowledge/information before the learner backed by evidence, thus satisfying the analytical and critical minds! Needless to say that it leads to sound understanding and better retention of concepts. The book keeps an eye on the future, thus will stay relevant for times to come, facilitate research and planning.

The book is a balanced combination of foundation knowledge in the area of food and nutrition as well as that of its application aspect. The first chapter has the capacity to generate interest in the book of anyone who reads it, from the domain or otherwise, when it relates Food and Nutrition with Health as never before every individual was as health conscious as today and seeks to stay fit living on suitable diet. The latter will also probably jump to Chapter 5, the Energy Metabolism, Energy Balance and Body Weight! The students of nutrition will go on systematically to know about the specific nutrients, the Carbohydrates; Proteins and Amino Acids; Lipids, Fats and Fatty Acids; Vitamins; Minerals; and Water, Electrolytes and Acid-Base Balance presented in Chapters 2–4 and 6–8. The next three chapters, titled Recommended Dietary Allowances and Dietary Guidelines; Food Exchanges; and Nutrition and Dietary Considerations at Different Life Stages are devoted to equipping the learner in dietary planning. The chapter that follows relates to the clinical aspect on nutrition and is again of interest to just everyone as it deals with Nutrition in Deficiency Disorders and Some Diet Related Diseases. And thereafter the added chapter of the new edition, i.e., the Assessment of Nutritional Status, many aspects of which are of every day application to all in general. One chapter is specifically devoted to Food and Nutritional Security interweaving new technologies facilitating its assurance. The last two chapters, Nutrition and Health Significance of Food Ingredients and Nutritional Implications of Food Processing and Packaging again have a high general appeal for all those who seek to remain healthy and fit by adopting good eating practices; are conscious of what they eat or drink and whether it is healthful. Chapter 15 needs a special mention as it throws light on New Horizons in Nutrition with innovative lenses. This chapter includes Functional Foods, Nutraceuticals, Probiotics, Health Supplements, Food Supplements, Nutrition for Sportspersons, Astronauts; for climbers at high altitude and Nutrigenomics; thus has enough to keep the learner updated with futuristic orientation.

This book has been written keeping in mind the syllabi of Food and Nutrition subject at the undergraduate and postgraduate level for the students of Home Science, Nutrition and related Sciences, Nursing and Medicine domains but I am convinced that it will continue to be very useful for research scholars, health professionals, planners and administrators and the knowledge lovers, in general.

Poonam Agrawal
PhD Post Doctorate (Germany)
Former Dean, Faculty of Home Science
GB Pant University of Agriculture and Technology
Pantnagar, Uttarakhand, India
Professor, Vocational Education
NCERT, New Delhi, India
profdrpoonam@gmail.com

Preface to the Second Edition

The gigantic problem of human malnutrition has affected large sections of the population in the world especially south Asian countries. The most vulnerable groups include children, adolescent girls, pregnant women, lactating mothers, elderly, sick, disabled and malnourished. There are millions of people for whom availability and affordability of nutritious foods is beyond reach and millions of people are at risk of undernutrition, and micronutrient deficiency disorders, lower immunity resulting in infectious diseases that ultimately compromised human capital and productivity. Thus, low birth weight, underweight, stunting and anemia and many unprecedented events have been found to shake the economy of the developing countries. Also, in these populations millions are overweight/obese and are at risk of suffering from the associated non-communicable diseases such as diabetes, cardiovascular problems, hypertension, inflammatory conditions, and neurological disorders. Evidence supports the linkage of nutrition with pathogenesis, and progression of many diseases.

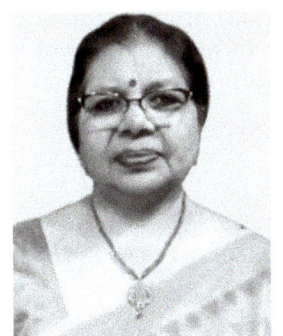 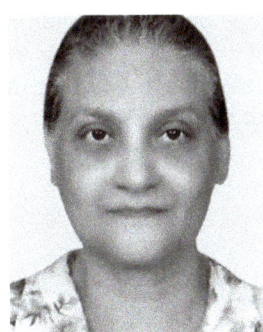

(Late) **Anjana Agarwal**   **Shobha A Udipi**

In recent years large sections of the population including health professionals are realizing the role of nutrition in promotion and maintenance of good health and prevention of diseases. Good nutrition is pivotal for good health and that can be achieved by selecting the right kinds of food and food combinations in adequate amounts at the right time in synergy with circadian rhythms and body constitution of the individual.

Nature is undeniably the Ultimate Power.

This prompted us to revise our book and bring out the second edition of "*Textbook of Human Nutrition*". The reader of this new edition will also get acquainted in Chapter 1 with sustainability, climate change, and the impact of pollution, pesticides, gas emission, marketing and social media on nutrition, health, and dietary patterns.

This book is dedicated to explain each nutrient in terms of its discovery, digestion, absorption, detailed functions, food sources, causes and consequences of deficient or excess intake in the next six chapters. Explanation on energy metabolism, water and electrolyte balance and body weight regulation as well as the latest Recommended Dietary Allowances for Indian population given by ICMR-NIN in 2020. These topics and meal planning using food exchanges have been covered in the next four chapters to help our readers particularly students, nutrition and medical practitioners to be well-versed in these areas. The book highlights the significance of various nutrients in each life stage/epoch (pregnancy, lactation, infancy, childhood, adolescence, adulthood, and old age); diet related diseases like obesity, diabetes, hypertension, and osteoporosis.

One new chapter is added in this second edition of the book on "*Assessment of Nutritional Status*". This chapter explains the use of nutrition screening, anthropometric, biochemical, clinical, and dietary intake methods for the individual as well as in pediatric and geriatric population in different settings. New digital technologies used for the purpose are also discussed.

Since India's rank on the hunger index is quite low, issues such food insecurity, malnutrition, anemia, iodine deficiency disorders, protein-energy malnutrition and vitamin A deficiency that are public health problems have been covered. The Government of India is taking several steps to combat food insecurity and malnutrition with several public nutrition programs. One full chapter is assigned to discuss these including the possible solutions through Integrated Child Development Services (ICDS), Mid-day meal, Public Distribution System (PDS) and Anemia Mukt Bharat and Poshan Abhiyan (National Nutrition Mission). In addition, the NFHS-V (2020) data has been given in brief for malnutrition as well as non-communicable diseases that are now public health problems that the country has to tackle. Updated guidelines for physical activity, diabetes, hypertension by national and international agencies such as WHO, IDF, etc., are included.

Two chapters focus on the information on emerging technologies such as food fortification, biofortification, genetic modification, biotechnology nanotechnology, food irradiation. Special nutrient and dietary modifications and guidelines are suggested for sports persons, astronauts, travelers at high altitudes.

Upcoming areas of prebiotics, probiotics, functional foods, nutraceuticals, bioactive compounds, and nutrigenomics are well explored in this book. Further advancement in the field of food processing, food packaging including Nova classification of processed foods is dealt along with nutritional and health significance of different reactions during cooking. Wide range of food ingredients are consumed in India and other parts of the world. Some people would like to know something about these food ingredients; hence their quest may be satisfied in Chapter 16. Some new foods are added to the previous list of 275 ingredients.

This book has special boxes labeled as 'Laboratory Laurel' or 'Research Glimpse' in each chapter to acquaint the reader with research involved in different concepts and to motivate them to understand the research perspective. Laboratory Laurel signifies the experimental work and Research Glimpse generally gives a brief summary of the review of research studies.

The target audiences for this book are the undergraduate and postgraduate students who have Nutrition as part of their syllabus. It caters to those who have not been exposed much to the subject but need to have knowledge about Nutrition in their own fields including nursing and medical students. It can also serve as a reference book for professionals and members of a health-conscious general public. This book attempts to bring updated and recent information in as simple a manner as possible. Attempts are made to enable understanding and improve readability through use of tables, boxes, figures, flowcharts, and illustrations.

(Late) **Anjana Agarwal**
Shobha A Udipi

Preface to the First Edition

The gigantic problem of human malnutrition has affected large sections of the population in the world especially South Asian countries. The most vulnerable sections of society who face or are likely to face these problems include children, pregnant women, lactating mothers and those persons for whom availability and affordability of nutritious foods are beyond reach. Both undernutrition and overnutrition increase the risk of chronic, degenerative diseases such as childhood and adult obesity, diabetes, cardiovascular problems and hypertension.

The above-mentioned issues motivated us to write this book that deals with important aspects of nutrition to help the reader to be aware of the importance of nutrients and measures to maintain good health through consumption of appropriate quantity and quality of food as well as modifying diet patterns to prevent nutrition and diet-related problems.

The target audiences for this book are the undergraduate and postgraduate students who have Nutrition as part of their syllabus. It caters to those who have not been exposed much to the subject but need to have knowledge about nutrition in their own fields including nursing and medical students. It can also serve as a reference book for professionals and members of a health conscious general public. This book attempts to bring updated and recent information in as simple manner as possible.

The book consists of sixteen chapters. It helps the reader to understand basics of nutrition in the first 10 chapters that deal with various nutrients. These chapters present the fundamentals and give brief insights into important recent concepts. Undoubtedly, every book on nutrition deals with basics of nutrition, the functions of different nutrients such as carbohydrates, proteins, fats and lipids, vitamins and minerals, water, meal planning issues, and nutrition in different life stages. This book has also covered the same to help the student understand the role of each nutrient at biochemical and physiological levels. New classification of nutrients given by expert groups, role of non-starch polysaccharides, glycemic index and glycemic load, artificial sweeteners, bioactive peptides, individual amino acids, fatty acids particularly omega-3 and other essential fatty acids have been included. How much food and individual nutrients are required by the body based on age, sex, activity level and physiological status with the latest Recommended Dietary Allowances (RDA, 2010) given by National Institute of Nutrition (NIN), India, are dealt with.

The remaining chapters deal with issues that are important for nutritionists and relevant to the problems faced by this country. Chapter 11 deals with nutrition during the life cycle, with adequate information about the crucial role of maternal, fetal and child nutrition. The role of breastfeeding and complementary feeding has been explained in detail. Important issues such as maternal malnutrition, low birth weight and preterm babies are included. This chapter also deals with how food behavior can affect the nutritional status of children, adolescents, adults and elders. Guidelines are provided to help improve food habits and ensure good nutritional status. The Government of India has taken several concrete steps to eradicate the problems of hunger and malnutrition including anemia, iodine deficiency disorders, protein-energy malnutrition and vitamin A deficiency through various programs. These programs and schemes such as the Integrated community development services (ICDS), Public distribution system (PDS) and the most recent efforts to improve food and nutrition security are dealt with in Chapter 12.

The book also covers use of food-based approaches through dietary diversification, the role of food fortification, supplementation, biotechnology and various new technologies such as biofortification, genetic modification, nanotechnology, food irradiation to enable students to widen their knowledge and realize the potential of these technologies for improving food and nutrition security as well as preventing spoilage of grains, enhancing the shelf-life of foods including fruits and vegetables, enhancing functionality and health benefits of foods, nutritional quality and bioavailability of nutrients among others.

In addition, the role of nutrition in physical fitness, sports and space travel, at high altitudes as well as nutrigenomics has been dealt with. These topics may not be in most syllabi, but there is a need for students to be aware about these important areas and be updated with recent information and guidelines.

The role of food beyond the functions of nutrients has been known for more than 5,000 years. Scientific and evidence-base researches throw light on valuable compounds—phytochemicals, probiotics, nutraceuticals in foods. Functional foods and nutraceuticals are important areas not only for research but also from industrial perspective. These topics are also dealt with to introduce students to these important areas and enable the reader to make informed choices for good health.

During our teaching and personal experience, we have found that many persons are interested in the health benefits of various food ingredients and their uses. Hence, Chapter 15 covers the nutritional and health implications of more than 275 food items. Food is consumed after it is processed by various techniques and undergoes various physicochemical changes under the influence of oxygen, heat, light, pH, organism and several other varietal factors. These factors tend to alter the nutritional quality of edible foods. The understanding of these changes may help the reader to take care to prevent nutrient loss and to make best food choices by using different combinations of food ingredients.

"Laboratory Laurels" and "Research Glimpses" are included in each chapter, to bring to light the vast scientific research underlying the knowledge presented and to motivate readers to understand the research perspective. Attempts have been made to enable understanding and improve readability through use of diagrams, flow charts, illustrations and photographs.

Anjana Agarwal
Shobha A Udipi

Acknowledgments

"Aum saha navavatu saha nau bhunaktu
Saha veeryam karavavahay
Tejasvinavadheetamastu
Maa viddvishavhay
Aum Shanti Shanti Shanti"

First and foremost, we thank the Almighty for inspiring us, giving us the insights and the strength to keep working and bringing out the second edition of the *"Textbook of Human Nutrition"* that will hopefully be useful to people who study nutrition science and care for their health and wellbeing. Writing has never been an easy task and now revising also seems to be a herculean task in order to retain the original, but also update and embellish the content of the book with new and updated concepts. Many individuals and groups of people deserve the heartfelt gratitude from both the authors.

We extend our heartfelt thanks to all those students whose queries in the class and all those people whose food behaviors have made us think deeply and take decisions to share subject knowledge and experience with them. The due credit also goes to all those authors, researchers and expert committee members in national and international organizations to recommend the guidelines, and present their documents in print as well as on-line in the field of nutrition and associated topics whose works has handsomely enriched content of this book.

The first author takes the opportunity to express her sincere gratitude to an eminent nutrition scientist, Prof (Dr) Shobha A Udipi, Professor and Head (Retd) in the Department of Food Science and Nutrition, Postgraduate Studies Research, SNDT Women's University, Mumbai, for sharing the authorship and ever ready support to integrate the updated information in this book. Without her this book could never get this flavor.

I sincerely express my silent admiration to those dignitaries who have always been the instrument and inspirational model in shaping my career in nutrition and always given me unbiased support in every hour of the need. These include Dr KK Kapur, Reader (Retd) Lady Irwin College, New Delhi; Prof (Dr) Poonam Agrawal, Head Division of Educational Research, NCERT, New Delhi; Dr Poonam Sikka, Principal Scientist, CIRB, Hissar; Dr Rita Raghuvanshi, Dean, College of Home Science, GB Pant University of Agriculture and Technology, Pantnagar, Dr G Subbulakshmi, distinguished Expert in Nutrition and Food technology and the recipient of Lifetime Achievement Award and Prof (Dr) KS Ray (Retd), SNDT Women's University, Mumbai, Dr Padmini Ghugre, Associate Professor (Retd), Food Science and Nutrition, SNDT Women's University and Mrs Rajalakshmi Nair, Nutrition Specialist, UNICEF, Maharashtra. Both authors thank Dr Shweta Khandelwal, Head, Nutrition Research and Additional Professor, Public Health Foundation of India, Dr Sheryl Salis Founder and Director Nurture Health Solutions and a certified Diabetes Educator and Dr Jai Ghanekar, Consultant Nutritionist, and Visiting Faculty SNDT Women's University.

Dr Udipi is overwhelmed with the moral support and encouragement given by her sister Mrs Pratibha Anand Kulkarni and her junior colleague Mrs Varsha Thakkar at every stage of this venture. She is also greatly appreciative of the guidance and the motivation received from her mentors Dr Ashok Vaidya, Prof Emeritus and Dr Rama Vaidya, Research Director and Hon Director, Division of Metabolic and Endocrine Disorders at Kasturba Health Society's, Medical Research Centre, Maharashtra, to which she is also attached as Hon Director, Integrative Nutrition and Ayurceuticals. She is also grateful for all the encouragement and moral support given to her by Dr Deepak Dave, Medical Director.

The key author deeply expresses her admiration and obligation to her husband, Mr Ramesh Chandra for his unstinted support throughout writing of the first as well as second edition of this book. Both the authors appreciate him for his silent encouragement and proofreading of the manuscript. The first author appreciates the consistent encouragement given by Mr Anil Garg, Founder and CEO of Doodle Powel with a broad product line in health and wellness, Ghaziabad. Mr Sunil Garg, Managing Director of Sunmitra Education Technologies, Lucknow, and his family always stood with her in all thick and thins of her dream project of book writing and provided timely and diligent inputs. Further my young team of Animesh-Aditi, Anukriti-Virat, Sonakshi and Shivam, always kept her in high spirits. Moral support of her maternal uncles Mr Ramesh (late), Rakesh, Rajendra and Gopesh Goyals and all members of their families guided her like a mentor in all times of need. Without the blessings role of parent in-laws (late) and affectionate appreciation of each family member of she could never have jumped into this venture of book writing.

Constant upgradation of guidelines and newer concepts in the field of nutrition and health forced us to rethink and rewrite this book in new edition. To proceed in this task our publisher Jaypee Brothers Medical Publishers, New Delhi, India and the concerned team particularly Shri Jitendar P Vij (Group Chairman), Mr Ankit Vij (Managing Director), Mr MS Mani (Group President), Dr Madhu Choudhary (Publishing Head -Education), Ms Samina Khan (Executive Assistant to Publishing Head-Education), Dr Astha Sawhney (Development Editor) deserve special thanks from deep core of our hearts for constant coordination and guidance.

Mrs Maneesha Gaur is owed special thanks for designing and development of the graphs and illustrations in this book. All those persons who may not have been named but have silently contributed in shaping this book deserve a big round of applause.

The people who deserve the special expression of gratitude are Dr J Chhibber and Dr L Tripathi and Shri Anand P Udipi, whose prophetic blessings has kept our morale up through the venture.

Contents

1. FOOD, NUTRITION, AND HEALTH — 1
What is Food? 2
What is Nutrition? 2
What are Nutrients? 3
Phytochemicals 5
Food Choices 5
Good Nutrition and Malnutrition 11
Strategies to Combat Malnutrition 17
Health 18

2. CARBOHYDRATES — 21
What are Carbohydrates? 21
Functions of Carbohydrates 21
Classification of Carbohydrates 22
Recommended Dietary Allowance for Carbohydrates 33
Food Sources of Carbohydrates 34
Consequences of Inadequate Carbohydrate Intake 34
Consequences of Excessive Intake of Carbohydrates 35
Glycemic Index 40
Sugar Substitutes/Sweeteners 43
Digestion and Absorption of Carbohydrates 43

3. PROTEIN AND AMINO ACIDS — 46
Proteins 46
Amino Acids: The Basic Building Blocks 52
Proteins in Food 53
Recommended Dietary Allowances for Protein 55
Food Sources of Protein 56
Deficiency of Protein: Its Causes and Consequences 57
Consequences of Excessive Intake of Protein 59
Protein Homeostasis 60
Nitrogen Balance 61
Evaluation of Protein Quality 61
Peptides 63
Roles of Individual Amino Acids or Functions of Amino Acids 66
Digestion of Proteins 72

4. FATS, OILS, AND LIPIDS — 77
Introduction 77
Functions of Fats and Lipids 78
Classification of Fats, Oils, and Lipids 79
Lipids and Adipose Tissue 86
Derived Lipids 86
Fatty Acids 91
Essential Fatty Acids 98
Recommended Dietary Allowance of Fats and Oils 105
Food Sources of Fats and Oils 107
Consequences of Insufficient Intake of Fats and Oils 108
Consequences of Excessive Consumption of Fats and Oils 108
Ways to Reduce Fat Intake 109
Adverse Effects of Using Rancid or Reheated Oils 109
Fat Replacers 110
Digestion and Absorption of Fat 113
Absorption 113

5. ENERGY METABOLISM, ENERGY BALANCE AND BODY WEIGHT — 116
What Is Energy? 116
Energy Metabolism 117
Energy Balance 120
Energy Expenditure 120
Energy Requirements 127
Energy Intake 129
Eating Disorders 133
Body Composition 134
Body Weight 141
Body Types 143

6. VITAMINS — 149
Classification of Vitamins 149
Functions of Vitamin A 152
Vitamin K 164
Water-Soluble Vitamins 166
Vitamin-Like Compounds 184

7. MINERALS — 192
Classification of Minerals 192
Trace Elements 208

8. WATER, ELECTROLYTES AND ACID-BASE BALANCE — 240
Components of Body Fluids 241
Water Balance 243
Water Imbalance 247
Water Intoxication 250
Electrolytes and Electrolyte Balance 250
Acid–Base Balance 258
Role of Lungs and Kidneys in Maintenance of Acid–Base Balance 261

9. RECOMMENDED DIETARY ALLOWANCES AND DIETARY GUIDELINES — 265
Recommended Dietary Allowances (RDA) 267
Dietary Guidelines 273
Food Guide for Indians 276
Food Groups 279

Use of Food Composition Tables   281
Meal Planning for Nutritionally Adequate Diets   282
Daily Meals   284
Percentage of Contribution of Different Nutrients   286
Daily Value (DV)   287
Nutrient Density   288

10. FOOD EXCHANGES   293

Food Exchanges   293
Food Exchange Lists   294

11. NUTRITION AND DIETARY CONSIDERATIONS AT DIFFERENT LIFE STAGES   304

Growth   305
Development   305
The First 1000 Days   306
Pregnancy and Fetal Development   307
Lactation   319
Breastfeeding   321
Childhood Years   323
Adults   340
Old age   342

12. NUTRITION IN DEFICIENCY DISORDERS AND SOME DIET-RELATED DISEASES   348

Protein–Energy Malnutrition (PEM)   349
Assessment of Nutritional Status   353
Moderate Acute Malnutrition (MAM)   353
Severe Acute Malnutrition (SAM)   353
Prevention and Control of Protein-Energy Malnutrition (PEM)   354
Vitamin A Deficiency   355
Iodine Deficiency Disorders   358
Nutritional Anemia   361
Overweight and Obesity   367
Diabetes   373
Hypertension   380
Osteoporosis   382

13. ASSESSMENT OF NUTRITIONAL STATUS   389

Nutritional Status   389
Anthropometric Measurements   394
Skinfold Measurement   398
Protein Status   402
Clinical Assessment   409
Dietary Assessment   411
Innovative Methodologies for Dietary Intake   413
Nutritional Assessment of Hospitalized Patients   415
Nutritional Assessment in Pediatric Population   417
Nutritional Screening and Assessment in Geriatric Population   418

14. ENSURING FOOD AND NUTRITIONAL SECURITY: NEW TECHNOLOGIES   420

Dimensions of Food Security   423
Nutrition Security   424
Technologies for Food and Nutrition Security   426
National Programs to Ensure Food and Nutrition Security   440

15. NEW HORIZONS IN NUTRITION   447

Functional Foods   447
Nutraceuticals   448
Sports Nutrition   457
Ergogenic Aids   469
Nutrition at High Altitude   469
Nutrition in Space   471
Nanotechnology   474
Nutrigenomics and Nutrigenetics   476

16. NUTRITION AND HEALTH SIGNIFICANCE OF FOOD INGREDIENTS   481

Cereals, Millets, and their Products   482
Lesser Known Cereals or Pseudocereals   487
Ready-to-Use Cereal Products   488
Pulses, Legumes, Beans, and Peas   489
Vegetables   492
Fruits   499
Milk and Milk Products   506
Eggs   509
Fish and Seafoods   509
Meat and Poultry   510
Sugars and Sweeteners   511
Fats and Oils   512
Spices, Herbs, and Condiments   516

17. NUTRITIONAL IMPLICATIONS OF FOOD PROCESSING AND PACKAGING   523

Browning   524
Nutrition Aspects of Different Methods of Food Processing   529
Novel Food Processing Technologies   548
Packaging   549
Packaging Materials and their Impact on Nutrition and Safety   550
Bio-based Packaging and Edible Films   551
Types of Food Packaging   551
Packaging for Different Types of Foods   552

APPENDICES   557

Appendix 1: *Food Sources of Energy (100 g edible portion)*   557
Appendix 2: *Dietary Fiber in Common Foods (100 g edible portion)*   560
Appendix 3: *Energy Requirements of Indian Men and Women at Different Ages and Body Weights*   562
Appendix 4: *Summary of Estimated Average Requirements (EAR) for Indians–2020*   563
Appendix 5: *Glycemic Index and Glycemic Load of Some Commonly Consumed Foods and Food Preparations*   564

Index 567

CHAPTER 1

Food, Nutrition, and Health

> **KEY CONCERNS**
> - What is the role of food and nutrition in my life?
> - What are the different nutrients and phytochemicals?
> - Can food choices affect my health?
> - What are malnutrition and its major causes?
> - How does food and nutrition influence my health?
>
> **KEY CONCEPTS**
> - Food and its functions
> - Nutrition, nutrients, and phytochemicals
> - What affects our food choices?
> - What are good nutrition and malnutrition?
> - Nutrition, health, and well-being

Food is a necessity of life and its use is a skill and science.

INTRODUCTION

Since the dawn of civilization, man has harnessed natural resources for survival. Over the centuries, man evolved from being a hunter-gatherer to a cultivator of several food crops and domesticated animals to ensure regular food supply throughout the year. With progress of time, industrial development and mechanization has changed the scenario of food production. Further, scientific advances in molecular biology, genetics, plant breeding, nutrition science, and biotechnology brought sea changes in accessibility to food and health services. **From** the **"green revolution"** in the 1960s, the world is now sailing rapidly toward **"gene revolution"**. In India, the green revolution made remarkable contributions toward meeting the growing demands of the continually increasing population. After decades of research, there has been a paradigm shift from a focus largely on food security to now encompass nutrition and health security. Many technologies like food irradiation, biofortification, food fortification, and approaches such as dietary diversification and nutrition awareness through various forms of media have not only helped to achieve adequate food supplies but supported efforts for ensuring good nutrition and health of the population.

Despite this tremendous improvement in food production, accessibility to nutritional and health services seemingly lag behind. There are 800 million people hungry in the world indicating one in every nine people according to the State of Food Security and Nutrition in the World, 2018, making the Sustainable Development Goal (SDG) of hunger eradication difficult to achieve (*www.fao.org*). In spite of the economic progress in our country, a substantial proportion of the population suffers from one or more nutritional problems and malnutrition still looms large on India's horizon.

Maternal nutrition plays a critical role in the unresolved problem of malnutrition. Low birth weight babies are born of undernourished, underweight, and anemic mothers. Such infants are at high risk of morbidity and mortality. Mortality among infants and children under 5 years of age is primarily due to the deficiency of energy, protein, and other important nutrients.

Survival, however, does not guarantee good health and productivity. Undernourished children continue to have impaired growth, maturation, and poor adjustments with self and the environment. In adulthood, they may tend to become victims of noncommunicable diseases. Genes for these metabolic conditions may be programmed during intrauterine life and further unhealthy lifestyle, poor dietary habits, and vocational demands set the stage for chronic poor health conditions.

Simultaneously, the prevalence of overweight and obesity in India is increasing, making India face the double burden of malnutrition. Overweight and obesity among pregnant mothers also program the developing fetus, making them susceptible to noncommunicable diseases in adolescence and adulthood. Thus, nutrition has tremendous intergenerational impact and poor nutrition, qualitative and quantitative, at both ends of the continuum, has tremendous implications for the health and well-being of the individual, the family, community, and the nation. There are enough indications that people are deficient in some or the other vitamin or mineral whether overnourished or undernourished. Hence, triple burden of malnutrition is another scenario in public nutrition.

Where is the real crisis? Health indicators for India including hunger index, malnutrition, poverty, morbidity, and mortality, indicate that there is a need for serious concern. Innumerable studies and surveys at various levels reveal that one important factor is the poor availability of food to people from low socioeconomic background as well as distribution within the family. Sociocultural biases play a strong role in dietary patterns. Inadequate knowledge with regard to nutrition and health among both educated and uneducated people is another contributory factor.

At the turn of this century, increasing globalization, improvements in transportation, and technological development have changed dietary practices and lifestyles especially in cities. A wide variety of foods like bread/chapatti/rice, milk, fruits, and vegetables are commonly consumed. Besides this, pulses and legumes/beans, nuts or egg/meat/fish, etc. are also a part of the daily meals. However, many foods are manufactured or modified in the food industry such as soy nuggets, nondairy cream, instant noodles, beverages, ready-to-eat snacks, breakfast cereals, etc. A wide array of processed foods is available, some of which are good for health but some may have unfavorable effects. Globalization, especially, has exposed Indians to a tremendous variety of cuisines, and ready-to-eat food items provided by food chains that sell pizzas, burgers, etc. Interestingly, many unhealthy foods are more attractive, palatable, and irresistible. Many of them are produced by street vendors and help in satisfying appetite. Also, there are many mobile apps which help persons to order ready-to-eat food at the doorstep. Frequent indulgence in such foods, due to ignorance about their health consequences, may have adverse effects on health and nutritional status. Globalization and industrialization have further amplified prevalence of degenerative diseases like obesity, diabetes, hypertension, heart disease, and cancer.

Since the early 1900s, the arena of nutrition knowledge has widened through exhaustive research in nutrition science and it is recognized that nutrition is one of the core contributing factors to health and well-being. Scientific investigations on the sociocultural effects on diet and lifestyle have further changed the face of nutrition science. Renaissance of ancient health systems has highlighted the tremendous potential of hidden valuable components in food which are beneficial for health and healing. These components are functional foods, phytochemicals/phytoactives, nutraceuticals, and dietary supplements. Many health conscious people are looking forward to naturally occurring food components in food products, to protect them from harmful effects of processing, use of chemical fertilizers and pesticides, occupational challenges, environmental fluctuations, and thereby improve their health status.

Food is one of the basic needs to sustain life. It is a reservoir of nutrients and other beneficial compounds. The health of a person is strongly interlinked with the quantity as well as the quality of food eaten. Every person, irrespective of age, race, religion, and culture, eats food. There an innumerable number of cuisines and dishes in every region, community, and religion to satisfy biological and sensory requirements. A considerable proportion of every person's life revolves around food—from thinking about it, procuring it, preparing, and serving it to family/friends and for special occasions. Many people have to work hard to earn their daily "bread", whereas for others, it is a matter of pleasure and enjoyment. Food is also a topic for discourse, discussion, research, and development. Most industries are connected directly or indirectly with food. It is an integral part of our value system, which is associated with power and status, and is used as a symbol of hospitality and for pursuit of pleasure and happiness. Some parents may use food as a reward or punishment.

WHAT IS FOOD?

Food is an edible substance obtained from plant, animal or marine sources. It nourishes the body and sustains life. Food must satisfy hunger and fulfill physiological, psychological, social, and sensory needs. It also protects the body from diseases. Food contains the substances called nutrients that are necessary for growth, survival, and different processes of the body. Food is a key element to good health and well-being.

> **Food Safety and Standards Authority of India (2006)** defines food as "any article manufactured, sold or represented for use as food or drink including alcoholic drinks and chewing gum" and "foods for special dietary uses or functional foods or nutraceuticals" are the ones that provide particular dietary requirement, may contain minerals, vitamins, plant or botanicals, may be in the form of powders, granules, tablets, capsules, liquids, gel, and other dosage forms but not parenteral, no claims of cure or mitigating any specific diseases, disorder permitted and only claims on health benefit permitted."

Nutritious Food

Nutritious food is that which can fulfill the primary functions of the food. It provides sufficient energy and all essential nutrients, helps in maintaining all biological processes of the body, maintains body weight, and protects us from invasion of any harmful microorganisms and onset of any disease.

Functions of Food

Food is a consumable commodity and its functions vary widely. From the nutritional point of view, food must provide nourishment for:
- Maintenance of life
- Growth and development
- Functioning of vital organs
- Production of energy
- Protection of body from infection, inflammation, and diseases.

Food also fulfills psychological and social functions which are listed in Figure 1.1.

WHAT IS NUTRITION?

Nutrition is the process of utilizing the food within the body. It includes ingestion, digestion, absorption, and utilization of food for a wide range of biological functions in the body. Nutrition is directly associated with the nutrient composition of food and the methods of food processing, food handling,

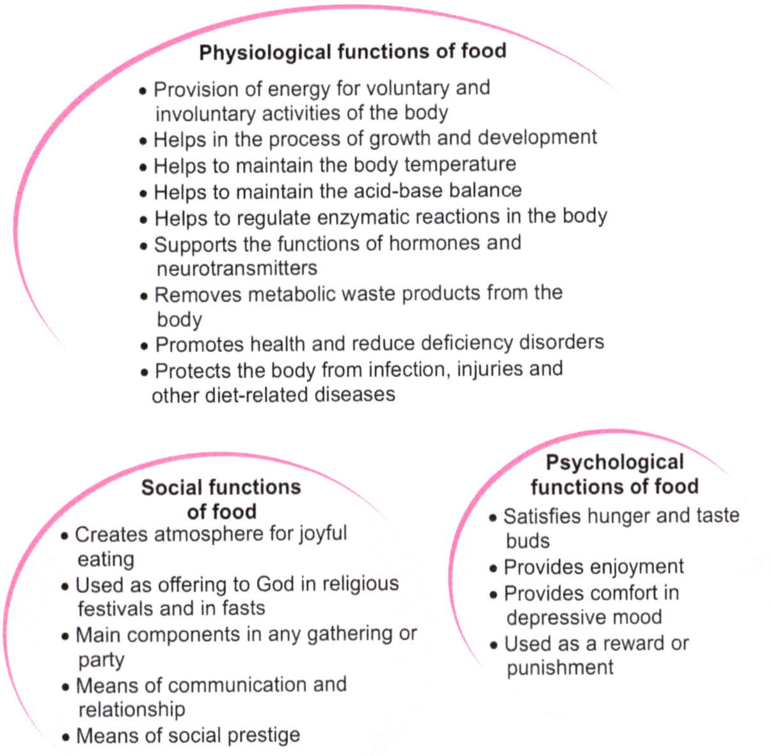

Physiological functions of food
- Provision of energy for voluntary and involuntary activities of the body
- Helps in the process of growth and development
- Helps to maintain the body temperature
- Helps to maintain the acid-base balance
- Helps to regulate enzymatic reactions in the body
- Supports the functions of hormones and neurotransmitters
- Removes metabolic waste products from the body
- Promotes health and reduce deficiency disorders
- Protects the body from infection, injuries and other diet-related diseases

Social functions of food
- Creates atmosphere for joyful eating
- Used as offering to God in religious festivals and in fasts
- Main components in any gathering or party
- Means of communication and relationship
- Means of social prestige

Psychological functions of food
- Satisfies hunger and taste buds
- Provides enjoyment
- Provides comfort in depressive mood
- Used as a reward or punishment

Fig. 1.1: Functions of food.

and food storage. It is also linked with the body's ability to digest, absorb, metabolize, and store nutrients or their products of metabolism as well to excrete them. All of these are influenced by our state of health, age, and physiological state.

Nutrition is the science of food and its components, their actions, interactions, and balance within the body. It includes the study of processing of food within the body (digestion, absorption, transport, function, and disposal of end-products) for its utilization for (i) provision of energy, (ii) building of body tissues and their repair, and (iii) protection from microorganisms, heat, and other stressors.

"**Human nutrition** describes the processes whereby cellular organelles, cells, tissues, organs, systems, and the body as a whole, obtain and use necessary substances obtained from food to maintain structural and functional integrity" (Vorster, 2009). It also includes the influence of social, cultural, environmental, political, and economic factors on food intake and thereby on nutrition and health.

> **Nutrition** is the science that links food to health and disease.
> **Dietetics** is the application of nutrition science to use food judiciously to maintain good nutritional status in health and disease conditions.

Nutrition is a multidisciplinary science that includes combined knowledge of the physical (physics and chemistry), biological sciences (physiology, molecular biology, biochemistry, genetics, microbiology, food science, pathology, and immunology) and social sciences (psychology, sociology, anthropology, economics, communication, and marketing). Physical, social, psychological, and economic factors greatly influence the nutritional and health status of an individual, society as well as the nation. Therefore, a nutritionist is required to integrate the relevant concepts from the varied disciplines.

The study of nutrition helps to make healthy food choices by understanding the following:
- The role of different nutrients in our body
- The nutritive value of foods
- Which foods are nutritious and healthy?
- The recommended dietary allowances (RDA) for different life stages
- What can happen if the right kind and right amount of food is not eaten?
- How to design nutritious recipes?
- How different processing methods can alter the nutritional quality of food
- Role of food and nutrition in health and disease.

WHAT ARE NUTRIENTS?

Foods contain various chemical components called nutrients each having distinct functions. Our body needs more than 40 nutrients to work in unison. Based on their chemical structures, nutrients are classified as carbohydrates, proteins, fats, minerals, vitamins, and water.

A nutrient is a chemical substance inherently present in numerous food sources, which the body uses to obtain energy, build tissues, and regulate biological functions. Nutrients play a critical role in health, nutrition, and disease.

The presence of nutrients in the diet is quite essential because their deficiencies can have adverse effects on health. The deficiency disorder can be reversed by putting the specific nutrient back into the diet. Thus, the significance of nutrients lies not only in promoting health but also in maintaining and bringing back the body into optimal health, e.g., severe deficiency of vitamin A can cause blindness, and excess intake causes hypervitaminosis.

Functions of Nutrients

Nutrients are required for:
- Regulation of body processes like temperature control, blood pressure, metabolism, and waste disposal.
- Structural integrity of bones, muscles and other tissues, and cell membranes.
- Energy production for physical activity, muscle contraction, and other cellular functions.
- Growth, development, and repair.
- Resistance to infection and protection from disease.

Classification of Nutrients

There are six classes of nutrients, namely carbohydrates, proteins, lipids, vitamins, minerals, and water (Fig. 1.2). In each class, there are a number of nutrients. More than 40 nutrients are involved in performing specific functions in relation to growth, development, and maintenance of the human body. Nutrients have largely been divided into two categories based on the amount required by the body.

Macronutrients

Macronutrients are organic nutrients needed in a large quantity, generally in grams. They are indispensable sources of energy that humans and other living organisms require for performing all physical, physiological, and metabolic activities. Their structures range from simple small molecules to large complex ones. Each of the large complex compounds consists of smaller building blocks which are eventually broken down in the body to perform metabolic functions. There are three macronutrients namely carbohydrates, proteins, and fat. The basic building block of carbohydrates is glucose; that of proteins are amino acids and fat is made from fatty acids.

Carbohydrates: Carbohydrates literally mean "hydrates of carbon" and are composed of carbon, hydrogen, and oxygen. Carbohydrates are a major source of energy, 1 g of it provides 4 kcal. Dietary carbohydrates are broken down into smaller units, generally "glucose" in the alimentary canal. Glucose circulates through blood and reaches cells and tissues to release energy, which is used for physical and metabolic activities. Carbohydrates occur in abundance in nature, particularly in plant foods. Cereals, pulses, sugar, and certain fruits are rich sources of carbohydrates, whereas animal foods contain negligible amount of it. Complex carbohydrates also contain dietary fibers in varying quantities and are good for health. Simple carbohydrates like sugar are not advisable to consume in large amounts in order to avoid risk of onset of several diseases, particularly noncommunicable diseases like diabetes mellitus.

Proteins: Proteins are made up of small molecules called amino acids. They contain nitrogen in addition to carbon, hydrogen, and oxygen. The human body requires approximately 20 amino acids. Amino acids are obtained after protein is digested by the gastrointestinal tract. Protein and amino acids are required to form new molecules like some proteins, hormones, enzymes, cells, tissues, and organs. A wide variety of protein molecules are used to build and maintain the body structure and to regulate body processes. Protein also provides energy (4 kcal/g). Meat, fish, poultry, egg, milk and milk products, pulses, legumes, and nuts as well as cereals are sources of protein. Vegetables and fruits are, in general, poor sources of protein. Lack of protein may compromise growth and development, immunity and many biological processes.

Lipids: Lipids are present in food and in the body. They include substances such as triglycerides, cholesterol, phospholipids, and fatty acids. The terms "lipids" and "fats" are often synonymously used in nutrition science. Fats and oils are obtained from the dietary sources like butter, ghee, and vegetable oils. Lipids and dietary fats are composed of different types of saturated and unsaturated fatty acids. Dietary fats supply 9 kcal/g that is two and a half times more energy than the energy provided by carbohydrates or protein. Besides supplying energy, lipids are carriers of fat-soluble vitamins; are precursors for synthesis of hormones and structural material for cell membranes and nerves. The amount of fat intake and the fatty acid composition of each dietary source of fat determine the health status. Excessive intake of fat and poor processing of fat-containing foods may increase the risk of obesity and associated disorders and noncommunicable diseases.

Micronutrients

Micronutrients: They are required in very small amounts, generally in milligrams or micrograms. Micronutrients are comprised of vitamins and minerals. Vitamins are organic compounds having elaborate chemical structures. They participate as coenzymes in varied biochemical reactions. They do not provide energy but some of them help in regulation of energy production and other functions. Minerals are inorganic elements, generally found in the earth's crust and water. They are important for structural components and the metabolic activities in the body.

Vitamins: Vitamins are comprised of a large group of organic compounds, some of which are soluble in fats and oils and others in water. The fat-soluble vitamins are four,

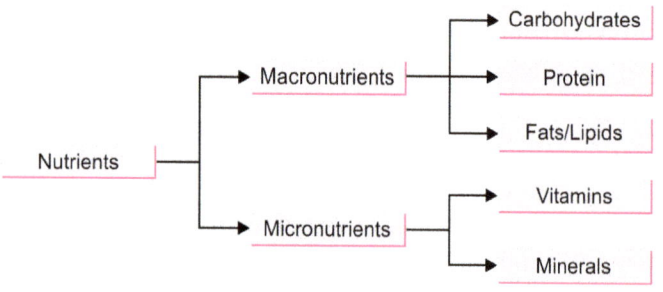

Fig. 1.2: Classification of nutrients.

i.e., vitamins A, D, E, and K. Water-soluble vitamins include vitamin B complex (thiamine, riboflavin, niacin, pantothenic acid, pyridoxine, folic acid, and vitamin B12) and vitamin C. Vitamins play a vital role in energy release from carbohydrates, lipids, and proteins; blood clotting, formation of collagen, and numerous metabolic processes.

Minerals: Minerals are inorganic elements and perform structural, metabolic, and regulatory functions in the body. Calcium, phosphorus, and magnesium are major minerals; zinc, iron, iodine, and selenium are trace elements, and boron, etc. are ultratrace elements. Sodium and potassium are also major minerals but behave like electrolytes and support electrolyte and acid–base balance. Many minerals are cofactors for enzymes. Each mineral has a specific role in the body and their deficiencies can cause disorders in the body.

Water

Water is one of the most important nutrients for survival. The human body contains approximately 45–70% which varies with age, gender, and other physiological factors. Water content of the human body is relatively higher in infancy, i.e., 70% of the total body weight and keeps decreasing with age, i.e., healthy adults carry 60% water of their total body weight and elders about 45–50% of total body weight. Water content is higher in males as compared to females. Water is present in many vital organs such as brain, liver, muscles, connective tissues, bones, kidney, and skin in varying amounts. There are various body fluids such as gastrointestinal, cerebrospinal, peritoneal, ocular, extracellular, and intracellular fluids. Water present outside as well as inside cells helps in transporting the nutrients and metabolic products in and out of the cell. Acid-base balance, temperature regulation, and lubrication of joints and others are major functions of water. Body must maintain water balance.

PHYTOCHEMICALS

Most dietary guidelines advocate the consumption of whole grains, fruits, and vegetables owing to their nutritional and health benefits. Many health professionals prescribe herbs, spices, and specific plants for healing various ailments ranging from cold, cough, and fever to diabetes, cancer, and cardiovascular and neurodegenerative diseases. Plants are rich in color, texture, and flavor and that richness usually comes from a wide array of naturally occurring compounds called "phytochemicals".

Phyto is a Greek word meaning "plant". Phytochemicals are non-nutrient, bioactive, chemical compounds found in different parts of plants. They are also referred to as phytonutrients, and are found in fruits, vegetables, whole grains, herbs, spices, nuts, and seeds. Thousands of phytochemicals have been identified in the plant kingdom. Different plants may contain different phytochemicals. One type of phytochemical may be found in more than one food item, e.g., quercetin is present in apple, red onion, grapes, pepper, black tea, and broccoli. Also, one food may contain more than one phytochemical, e.g., orange contains many phytochemicals namely β-carotene, α-carotene, β-cryptoxanthin, lutein, zeaxanthin, limonene, hesperidin, naringenin, ferulic acid, etc. There is a little confusion in using the term phytochemical and flavonoids, flavanol, proanthocyanidin, etc. Flavonoids are a group of phytochemicals. Phytochemicals are individual compounds such as resveratrol, sulforaphane, curcumin, quercetin, genistein, etc.

Phytochemicals act as antioxidants and behave like anti-inflammatory, antiviral, and antibacterial agents. They help in boosting immunity and some delay the aging process. They also help in detoxification of environmental pollutants and toxins. Therefore, it is advisable to consume enough phytochemicals from adequate amounts of whole grains, richly colored fruits, vegetables, nuts, spices and herbs, etc. Some plants may also contain some antinutrients, which can have harmful effects and hence should be consumed with caution. Foods exhibiting health benefits due to the presence of phytochemicals are called **functional foods**. These ingredients have also been incorporated in many health foods which are similar in appearance to popular foods like energy bars, nutribars, chyawanprash, etc. Nutraceuticals and dietary supplements are also sources of ingestible bioactive compounds in the form of powders, capsules and gels. Bioactive compounds can also be obtained from marine and other animal sources.

Nature has gifted man with innumerable food sources. Thus, man has access to a very wide range of foods. Yet human beings do not always choose foods from the health point of view. Invariably, people choose food for many other reasons. Let us briefly look into the factors influencing food choices.

FOOD CHOICES

Food choices begin early in life and develop under the influence of environmental exposures and experiences. Initially, food choices are often guided by parents and people surrounding the child. Thus, the child develops certain food choices/food preferences by imitating them. From the beginning, taste, texture, and gestures of people in relation to food contribute the most in shaping food choices. Food habits formed during childhood are difficult to change later in life, especially in adulthood and old age. Individuals might adapt to new foods in different situations, but still relish most of the foods they liked and ate in their childhood.

Food choice is a process of decision-making and sets a pattern of selection of food items for consumption. A wide range of determinants strongly influence food choices. These include age, gender, marital status, family composition, vocational demands, socioeconomic status, culture beliefs, climate, personality traits, and attitudes toward food.

Over a period of time, remarkable changes have occurred in food choices. Traditionally, people used to choose food on the basis of social and cultural beliefs which were mainly governed by religion and agriculture. In modern times, media and migration played important roles in food selection and consumption patterns. Further social media, facilities for food preparation, food industry, and time left after outside work (study or job or travel), and the health status of the individual

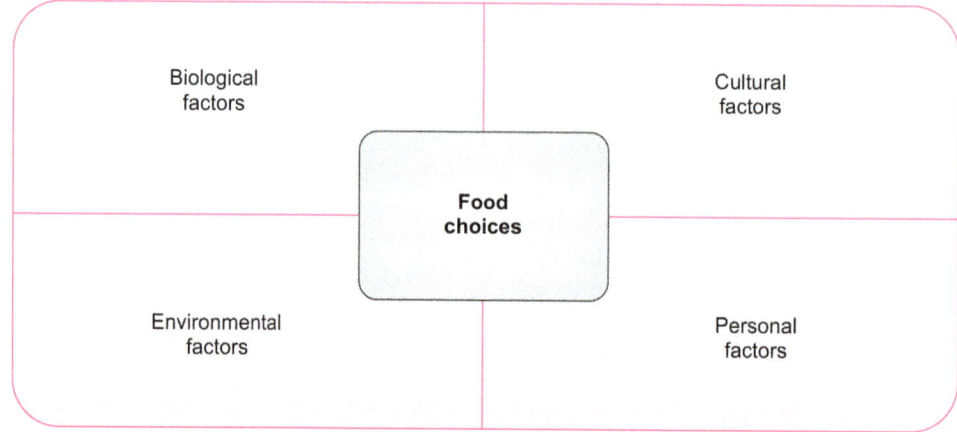

Fig. 1.3: Factors of food choices.

Various factors affecting the food choices are broadly categorized and depicted in Figure 1.3.

Biological Factors

Biological factors determine individual variations in food choices. Hunger, appetite, and taste are biological determinants of food choices, which vary widely in different age groups. Choices are influenced by physiological conditions and gender. Biological factors influencing food choices are as follows:

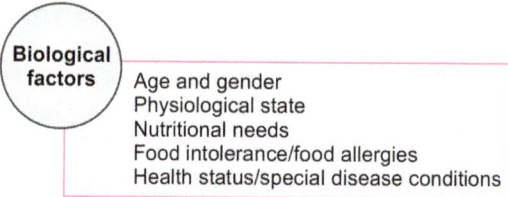

and/or family members influence the food choice. Since food emerges from environment, hence choice of food also affects environment. It results in the generation of **Greenhouse Gases** (GHG) followed by climate change in turn influence the nutritional status, health, and well-being of people at large. Regions where people sustain themselves on plant-based foods have lesser GHG as compared to places where people indulge in animal-based foods. This is relationship with the carbon footprint. Animal foods have more carbon footprint as compared to plant-based foods. Choice of food can have a big impact on emission of greenhouse gases. Fruits and vegetables have much lower carbon then lamb, cheese, egg, etc.

Research glimpse: Food production contributes to the emission of greenhouse gas (GHG). These gases along with dietary habits have made paradigm shifts in occurrence of noncommunicable diseases. The authors have systematically reviewed the evidence on changes in GHG emissions, land use, and water use for such serious impact. They have advocated the adoption of sustainable dietary patterns which can reduce 70–80% of GHG emissions of land use and 50% of water. This reduction is generally proportional to the magnitude of animal-based food restriction. Dietary shifts (shifting current Western diets to a variety of more sustainable dietary patterns) yielded modest benefits in all-cause mortality risk.

Aleksandrowicz L, Green R, Joy EJM, Smith P, Haines A. The impacts of dietary change on greenhouse gas emissions, land use, water use, and health: A systematic review. PLoS ONE. 2016;11(11):e0165797.

Carbon footprint: Carbon footprint is a measure of the amount of greenhouse gases (GHG) produced by our activities in relation to carbon dioxide (CO_2) or carbon. The activities include farming, rearing animals, building homes, using cars, aeroplanes, food manufacturing, food delivery and disposal of waste.

Greenhouse gases: Burning forest and coal, mining, industrial gases, and many human activities like agriculture, using electricity, traveling, etc. release many gases in the atmosphere raising the temperature of the earth. These gases include carbon dioxide, methane, water vapor, and nitrous oxide, while others are synthetic and are categorized as **greenhouse gases.** Among them carbon dioxide is released maximally. Carbon from solid state is converted into gaseous state, thereby increasing its atmospheric concentrations. Changes in the concentration of GHS are associated with climate changes followed by unfavorable environmental consequences such as heat waves, rising sea levels, floods and droughts, and health problems such as cancers, cardiovascular diseases, asthma, and neurogenerative diseases.

Age and Gender: Age and gender determine food preferences. With age, taste and nutritional needs may vary. Many young children like sweets and elders may prefer bitter and bland foods. Girls may choose lighter fancy delicacies while boys may go for rich sumptuous meals. There is a huge difference in food choices in each life stage. Accessibility, easy availability, advertisements, and relatively low costs tremendously influence the food choices particularly among children and adolescents. Many times, these food choices take their toll on health and put the person at risk of disease. In some cases, adults and elders are also adapting and adjusting their food choices according to the affordability and accessibility. Sometimes adults and elderly also modify their food choices with the aim of maintaining or improving their health. Children and adolescents also try new foods. Their choices are often influenced by body image, their peer group, and media. Food choices of the elderly are largely determined by the health condition(s), socioeconomic conditions as well as availability of food. Eating problems may stem from loneliness, a lack of desire or ability to cook, financial worries or physical problems.

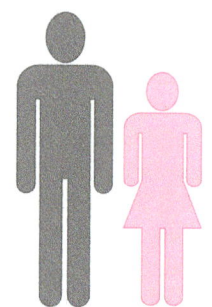

Social support from within the household and from coworkers has been found to be positively associated with improvements in fruit and vegetable consumption and with the preparative stage of shaping eating habits in childhood. Gender differences were observed in health beliefs and dietary behaviors.

> **Laboratory Laurel:** Factors that influence food choices of adolescents were studied from the perspective of parents, school staff, and adolescents. Individual factors identified were financial autonomy, food safety perceptions, lack of self-control, habit strength, taste preferences, and perceived peer norms. Barriers to eating healthy food were examined from the perspective of the environment and home. Environmental factors were poor nutritional quality of food and easy access at school. Factors in the home and family environment were time, convenience, socioeconomic status of the family. Also, eating patterns were reported to be influenced by the changing sociocultural environment.
>
> *Verstraeten R, Van Royen K, Ochoa-Avilés A, Penafiel D, Holdsworth M, Donoso S, Maes S, Kolsteren P. A conceptual framework for healthy eating behavior in Ecuadorian adolescents: A qualitative study. PLoS ONE. 2014;9(1):e87183. doi:10.1371/journal.pone.0087183.*

Physiological State: As the person passes through different stages of the life cycle, food choices vary and tend to change temporarily under certain physiological conditions like pregnancy and lactation as well as during illness. These are vulnerable periods of life when requirements for nutrients are greater, thus food choices may be influenced by the body's needs. Pregnant woman should be given more amount of nutritious food to cater to the needs of the growing fetus as well as her own and in some cultures, lactating mothers are given galactogogues to increase milk output. A pregnant woman, if feeling nauseated, may not like to eat the complete balanced meal. In many cultures, she is given specific foods and her food choices are respected during pregnancy and lactation.

Health Status: There are people who may be allergic to some foods and others who may not be able to tolerate specific foods. For example, some babies may have lactose intolerance and cannot digest milk or milk products. Often during illness, there is lack of appetite and taste is affected, which in turn may alter food choices. Even presence/absence of teeth determines the choice of foods in terms of texture. Similar things can happen in sickness. Food choices may be permanently changed as soon as a person is diagnosed with diabetes and temporarily changed when a person has indigestion or toothache.

Our physiological needs are the basic determinants of food choices that can make or mar health. Sickness often necessitates modifications in food and those who do not alter their selection of food can delay healing. In some health conditions, certain foods are restricted or specifically included, e.g., a diabetic person is asked to refrain from sweets and a person with hypertension (high blood pressure) is asked to avoid pickles/papads/sauces due to their high sodium content. A hungry person may make a different food choice than a person who has finished his/her meal. Hunger or loss of appetite can affect the choice of food.

During depression, stress, and anxiety, some individuals may experience cravings for certain foods whereas some others may not eat or dislike certain foods. Cravings for sweets, alcoholic beverages, chocolates, and junk food can lead to obesity and other health problems.

Environmental Factors

People living in different geographical locations have different food choices. Their food choices are largely governed by agroclimatic conditions and availability of food in that location. Climate not only affects the cultivation of food crops, but also postharvest handling and storage. Several environmental factors work together.

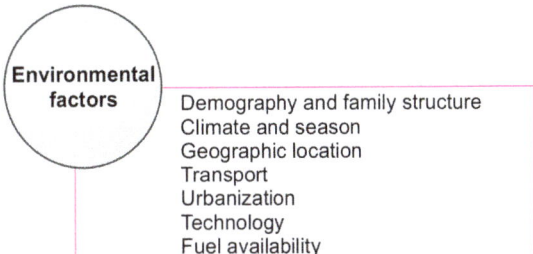

Environmental factors
- Demography and family structure
- Climate and season
- Geographic location
- Transport
- Urbanization
- Technology
- Fuel availability

Demography and Family Structure: Demography is the scientific study of the population in terms of its size and composition, pattern of living, fertility, migration, literacy rate, mortality, and morbidity in a given geographical location. Nuclear families may have different kinds of food choices compared with traditional joint families where more than one generation may live together. Family structure and daily living habits play a significant role in food selection. 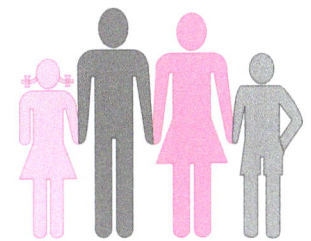 Older persons may like to have simple basic meals, whereas youngsters prefer more zesty foods like noodles, pizza, carbonated soft drinks, and cakes, etc. People living alone often compromise with one-dish meals like sandwiches or roti.

Besides family composition, the type of dwelling also determines the food choice. People staying in concrete houses may have elaborate, varied cuisines owing to better cooking and storage facilities. Consumption of processed, ready-to-eat foods is also common and they can also store drinking water, food, and beverages for later use. In contrast, for people living in temporary dwellings such as in rural and slums areas and refugee shelters, limited resources may limit the food choices.

Climate and Season: Climate determines the season and crop cultivation, which varies with season. In India, there are mainly two crops depending upon the season, i.e., "*rabi*" crop and "*kharif*" crop. In *Rabi* or "winter crop", the seeds are sown in October/November and the crops are harvested in March/April. Rabi crops include wheat, grams, barley, potato, etc. "*Kharif*" or summer season crops starts from June/July and lasts until September/October. Rice, maize, groundnut, cotton, pulses, and jowar, etc. are cultivated in this season.

Staple food crops are usually cultivated seasonally or once a year but are used throughout the year. Sometimes a third crop called "*zaid*" is also considered, in which fruits and vegetables are generally grown in summer. It has been suggested that foods contain maximum nutrients when freshly harvested. Traditionally, in India, foods are chosen in accordance with the season. It is believed that consumption of off-season foods may harm the body and increase risk of diseases, whereas consuming seasonal foods confer maximum health benefits.

"Eat fresh, seasonal, and local foods including fruits and vegetables for maximum nutrition and health benefits".

Crops undergo various environmental stresses like rain, humidity, drought, and attack by insects and pests as well as microbial contamination. Further, dramatic changes in climate may seriously affect food security and modify food choices. Droughts, famines, and heavy rainfall may sweep away the crop and affect food supplies, compromising food availability and choice. 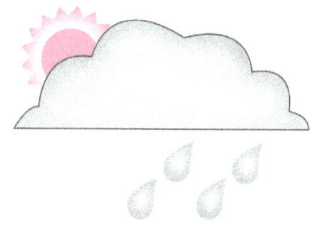 On the other hand, seasonal surpluses increase availability, influence the cost, and hence consumption pattern. Cottage industries and food industries can transform the raw food material into totally new products which can help increase food availability and variety even during off-season. However, accessibility to food in cities is not largely dependent on seasons, as it is in rural areas.

> **Research Glimpse:** Dietary deficiencies of zinc and iron are major public health problems. When CO_2 concentration in the atmosphere is elevated, then grains and legumes contain lesser amount of these two nutrients.
>
> Myers SS, Zanobetti A, Kloog I, et al. Increasing CO_2 threatens human nutrition. Nature. 2014:51:139-42.

Geographic Location: On a daily basis, people depend on locally available foods. Food choices of people residing in hilly areas are different from people from coastal areas. Foods grown in forests, hills, valleys, land pastures, dry land, and coastal areas are different, which naturally affects the food choices of the residents and their cuisines. People in hilly areas usually select specific berries, fruits, leaves, and spices, whereas people from coastal areas may prefer fish and seafoods. Kashmiris may select "*yakhini*" and Goans may like fish curry. Walnuts are cultivated in Jammu and Kashmir and cashew nuts in Goa. Coconut, banana, and tamarind may be integral ingredients of food in southern India as they are cultivated there, whereas rajma, black gram (*urad*), "*makki ki roti*", "*chhole bhature*", "*kachori*", "*samosa*", etc. are popular in North India.

Transport: Transport, geographical location, availability of vehicles, and fuel determine the accessibility and cost of food and hence the food choice. Food is transported from one place to another, from region to region and now from nation to nation. Transport facilities have increased the accessibility of wide variety of foods for most people. However, even today, 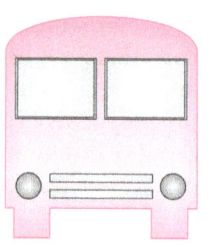 people living in remote areas have limited food choices as they do not have means of transport. Periodically, they go to nearby markets and procure food materials for several days or months. Women, children, elders, and handicapped or sick persons may not be able to go out alone due to their age, gender, social, and physical limitations. Hence, they are dependent on others for transport and their food choices may be limited. Food choice for some people is determined by the food available at home or in nearby shops or markets. Famines, droughts, heavy rainfall, cyclones, and road blockages due to bad weather and transport strikes greatly affect transport and hence the food supply. If such conditions continue for a prolonged period of time, food choices may be considerably limited. On the contrary, in large cities and metros, those who own a vehicle or know driving, may frequently go to restaurants or food courts and tend to consume snacks or meals whether they are hungry or not, sometimes just for fun. The latter practice is not desirable since it can adversely affect health.

Technology: There has been tremendous advancement in cultivation practices, postharvest systems, food product development, food preservation techniques, food packaging, food delivery systems, and the equipment used in food processing like microwaves, pulsed electric fields, use of sound waves, and solar energy. Such technologies have influenced every aspect of our life including our food choices. Food manufacturers use them to allure and satisfy the consumers. Fast-paced lifestyle and lack of time for cooking has gradually led to a shift-from consumption of primarily home-cooked foods to convenient ready-to-eat, ready-to-cook, processed foods. Food science and technology has also made it possible to prolong shelf life of foods, making it easier to obtain seasonal fruits and vegetables to reach food to far-off, distant places. The market is also flooded with ready-to-eat, ready-to-cook, health foods, dietetic foods, microwaveable meals, chilled and frozen foods, and fast foods to fulfill the needs and desires of consumers. (Also cooked food is available online or on single phone call or message).

Urbanization: Urbanization implies more concrete buildings, better transport and communication, better opportunities for education and earning and to avail wide variety of food and food products even outside the home. However, there is less agricultural land to grow fresh foods locally and urban people depend on market supply of food. Urbanization tends to change the socioeconomic status and food 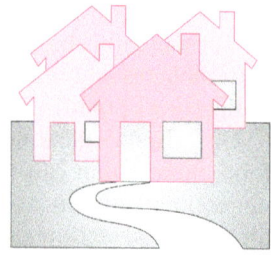 availability, accessibility and affordability, and thereby food choices. It has brought sea changes in interest, aptitude, and attitude of the people toward cooking and eating. The availability of food processing, food storage appliances, and food delivery systems has changed selection of food preparations.

Women who were primarily responsible for providing (cooking, etc.) food to the family members, now also go out to work. There are more nuclear families and persons living alone. People face time constraints and sometimes lack the desire to cook, thus use of convenience foods and eating out is increasing. Canteens in schools, workplaces, and vending machines have influenced people's choices. People tend to select food items that do not require much processing/cooking without compromising the taste.

Cultural Factors

Food culture is based on traditional beliefs, folklore associated with food and religious rituals. In every culture and religion, some foods are forbidden and some foods are specifically prescribed at certain stages of life such as pregnancy and lactation. Many foods are specially linked with festive occasions like Diwali, Holi, Christmas, Eid, Sankranti or Lohri or Christmas or during pujas. Culture shapes our food choices, pattern of cooking, eating, and serving. People can easily change their speech or dress code and imitate other cultures, but a food choice that is born out of culture and tradition is more difficult to change. Culture regulates the food habits which tend to remain stable through generations. The following factors affect food selection:

Cultural factors
- Culture, religion, community, family
- Social values snd social status
- Social interaction
- Traditions and beliefs
- Properties attached to food, e.g. 'hot'/'cold', 'light/heavy'
- Communication and information (Media, marketing and advertising)

Food cultures evolved out of agriculture practices and production, religious practices, type of family structure, and socioeconomic status. In the past, people blindly followed them out of fear of God's fury or ignorance, often without a rational basis. Friends, neighbors, and older women in the family often dictated food choices to be followed in one's life and by the entire family.

Man has an inherent desire to be accepted and appreciated in a given social group. Food is a means of communication, a symbol of status and pride. There is hardly any social meeting or gathering or any occasion, where food and drinks are not used to indicate hospitality and served as a token of friendliness and social warmth. Conversation about food also adds knowledge about several issues and can influence eating habits, sometimes favorably but not always. During childhood and adolescence, most food choices are influenced by peer groups.

Jains and many Hindus frown at meat consumption, which is permitted in Islam and Christianity. Some religions permit occasional consumption of fish, poultry, and mutton but forbid beef because the cow is considered sacred. Milk and milk products are also animal products but they are consumed as they do not involve killing and support growth of the human body rather than causing harm. Most vegetarians also favor "ahimsa" and from the nutritional perspective, research data suggest that animal foods may not be always healthy. Today, there are different eating patterns ranging from vegan (no dairy products including milk or milk products are consumed), lacto-vegetarian (milk is allowed but the person is vegetarian), lacto-ovo vegetarian (milk and eggs are included in the diet but other non-vegetarian foods are not eaten) and non-vegetarian (meat, poultry, fish, and eggs are consumed). In some places, vegetarians also consume fish. Serving good food and serving the head of the family first is customary in many cultures without looking into the needs of others in the family or considering whether they are hungry.

Culture determines the approved pattern of selection, preparation, and serving of food. In South India, the main course consists of rice, sambar, vegetable, and pickle, and butter milk, served on a plantain leaf and eaten by hand. Also, the sweet or *payasam* is served first. However, in North India, people prefer to eat chapatis or rotis with dal and "sabji" and sweets may be eaten with the meal. The new generation is undergoing a phase of changing food habits out of necessity or desire to try new foods and be innovative and to be westernized. Often people of one culture migrate from one place to another, where the culture is different. Migration and the need for survival and/or social acceptance have made people modify their dietary habits.

Media, Marketing, and Advertisements: Food choice is remarkably influenced by advertisements. Television is a strong medium that influences food choices. Many foods are promoted through print and electronic media, exhibitions, home visits, and distribution of free samples, etc. People, particularly children, may blindly trust the information that is given and select a particular brand without knowing its true worth. Even adults may choose some foods that are not necessarily healthy when they are endorsed by popular film stars or sportspersons. Diverse messages, tall health claims, and nutritional labels are meant for consumers but some of these can be fads or quackery. However, media and marketing are very powerful tools if they are used for promoting health education and creating awareness about "healthier" food choices. Simple, actionable, and accurate messages that the public can readily understand and incorporate into everyday lives, can help people have a clear idea about the quality, cost, and use so that they can make informed and healthier choices about foods.

> **Laboratory Laurel:** In order to assess the influence of media characters on children's food choices, two experiments were done. In the first experiment, self-reported food choices were noted; and in the second, the actual choices were recorded. Popular characters could encourage children in selecting one food instead of another. In the first experiment, children reported that they liked a particular food, especially sugary or salty snacks if it was associated with or branded by media characters they like and with whom they were familiar. When they were given a choice between a healthy food and a sugary or salty snack, branding the healthy food with a favorite media character did not influence the children's preference. However, children were willing to try more of a healthy food if a favorite character promoted that food.
>
> Kotler J, Schiffman JM, Hanson K. *The influence of media characters on children's food choices. Journal of Health Communication.* 2012;17(8):886–98.

Personal Factors

Personal factors have strong influences on eating habits and eating behavior of the individual. It relates to the attitudes, beliefs, food preferences, self-efficacy, and biological issues, e.g., when sad people either indulge in gluttony or refrain from food. Family friends, peer network, easily accessible and numerous eating outlets, and street vendors all affect food choice, e.g., if an ice cream parlor is situated next to or on the corner of the road near your residence, then your frequency of choosing ice cream could be higher as compared with if that facility is absent. Personal choice wins over all sociocultural and environmental barriers. A person may travel long distance just to eat food of his/her desired choice to satisfy the sensory appeal. Quite often, a person is not aware of his own nutritional needs and makes wrong food choices that are based on taste, appearance, cravings, availability, and easily get swayed by peer pressure and media. Literacy level and occupational needs also affect food choices. The following factors affect personal food choices.

Personal factors
- Education and knowledge
- Household income and financial resources (purchasing power)
- Experience with foods
- Conditioning and learning preferences
- Response to stress, anxiety and emotions
- Sensory appeal
- Living alone vs with family
- Availability of social support systems

Laboratory Laurel: A validated questionnaire was administered to examine the food choices and food fads among school-going adolescents (n = 564) in Puducherry and Trichy, South India. It was found that adolescents prefer to take their own decisions regarding choice of food items and 50% of them agreed that they eat too much during socializing events. Hence, researchers advocated that such events can be planned and used to evolve interest in healthy food habits. Only two-thirds (65%) ate breakfast regularly. 82% chose snacks based on taste over nutrition. They preferred salty, crunchy foods over healthier alternatives but they expressed their desires that all healthy foods should be tasteful. Hence 18% of them could control their desire to eat chocolates, sweets, and savories. With regard to frequency, 18% ate snacks every 3 hours. Researchers observed that these subjects are under stress of higher secondary syllabus and predisposed to overweight or obesity.

Thiruselvakumar D, Sinuvasan K, Chakravarthy RS, Venkatesh E. Factors affecting food choice and attitude of choosing food items among adolescents in South India. International Journal of Scientific and Research Publications. 2014;4(4):2250-3153.

Education and Knowledge: Education has been found to influence dietary behavior during adulthood. In young persons, nutrition knowledge may not influence dietary habits much but among adults and older individuals, it has shown an impact. Loads of information available through multiple sources on food and health has made food selection rather more complex. Knowledge of nutrition and culinary skills can help the individual to navigate and make healthy food choices. Nutrition education interventions are definitely helpful in improving food choices. Since education starts early in life, early education in schools can make a great difference in attitudes of children regarding food choices and help to shape appropriate healthy food habits among them.

Laboratory Laurel: A quantitative, cross-sectional study, with a descriptive design was done to examine college students' eating habits and knowledge of nutritional requirements for health. It is concluded that about one-third of college student participants (n = 121) were overweight. Though they have the knowledge that consuming fast food, soda, and processed food are unhealthy and they contain additives, yet they choose processed and fast food for taste and convenience.

Abraham S, Noriega Brooke R, Shin JY. College students eating habits and knowledge of nutritional requirements. Journal of Nutrition and Human Health. 2018;2(1):13–17

Purchasing Power: Household/family income, family size, and cost of food have always been important determinants of food choices in almost every household. Low income limits the ability to purchase sufficient amount of staple foods and, further, variety of foods in the diet is limited. Thus, their diets may be imbalanced and inadequate in several important nutrients due to noninclusion of valuable nutritious foods like milk and milk products, eggs, meat, vegetables, and fruits.

Factors affecting food economics
- Cost of raw material
- Cost of processing from basic preparation to final product
- Quality worth of food value
- Difference in food cost at various markets
- Cost of ready to eat foods
- Cost of eating out
- Mode of payment

Food prices determine food selection and rise in prices of commonly used food commodities like pulses and legumes, cereals, flour, sugar, milk, vegetables, and oils seriously affects the food budget. It especially affects the poor and even the rich today. On the other hand, people from higher income group can afford and may consume foods like aerated soft drinks, ice creams, chocolates, imported foods, etc. Many of these foods contain too much fat and/or sugar and less of valuable nutrients. Eating too much of these can have adverse influence on health. Availability of financial resources does not guarantee healthy food choices. Pricing strategies such as discounts, taxes, price fluctuations; offers like "buy one, get two" strategy, and bonus systems are seen as a promising approach for sales promotions. At the same time, factors like sensory appeals and health reasons are also important influences on food choice in many cases. There is a strong link between purchasing power and social status, e.g., an individual may purchase costly food items to showcase his/her social strata. Sometimes one is forced to buy high-priced food during an emergency (e.g., sickness and inaccessibility).

Sensory Appeal: People are more often concerned about satisfying their senses. "Taste" is a major factor which determines whether a person accepts or rejects the food. Smell, appearance, flavor, and texture of food also influence food choices significantly. From an early age itself, taste and familiarity are important. The pleasure someone experiences with a particular food is proportional to palatability and determines preference. Sweet and high-fat foods have an undeniable sensory appeal and hence may often be preferred over the nutritious food stuffs.

Eating Away from Home: Eating behaviors and dietary quality are influenced by the places where food is consumed—at home, school, or away from home at restaurants and fast food establishments. It is largely influenced by the purchasing power of the individual, growth of food industry, and the facilities available. Frequent eating out may negatively affect the nutritional quality of the diet as well as increase the risk of food infection/poisoning and related diseases. Eating out is often practiced either for pleasure or due to lack of time or culinary skills or interest in cooking. The food items eaten out usually are rich in energy, fat, sugar, and salt. Such practices need rethinking from other perspectives as well.

> **Laboratory Laurel:** Dining out has become a part of lifestyle in youngsters for multiple reasons and that has propelled the growth of restaurant industry. In this regard, a study was carried on dining out behavior of students of the university in Lucknow using a questionnaire. Reasons identified were pleasant aroma, good lighting, soothing music inside the restaurant, consistent service, convenient location of the restaurant, availability of fast food along with free soft drink, discounts, coupons, and schemes announcements on Facebook and other social media for students, reasonable price, availability of specific food on special occasion, and good quality food. Other reasons include lack of cooking skill, lack of knowledge of recipe befitting tastes and dietary requirements. The cooking novices who do not enjoy cooking prefer to dine outside and socialization is another major reason for dining outside home.
>
> Verma VC, Gupta DD. An investigative study of factors influencing dining out in casual restaurants among young consumers. European Business & Management. 2018;4(1):39-43.

Emotions and Stress: Emotions are deep-seated in the brain. One can recall events/incidents or experiences associated with a particular food even after 20–30 years. Stress is a common feature of modern urban life and can modify behavior that affects lifestyle such as physical activity, smoking as well as consumption of alcohol. Generally happy mood and happy events call for eating food, preferably sweets and other rich foods. However, some people indulge in eating anything available when they are anxious/stressed/in a sad mood or feeling lonely. Certain foods may contain some specific chemical substances which may trigger mood-regulating hormones. Chocolates and coffee may elevate the mood and people tend to crave such foods.

Food choices and food intake are influenced by myriad factors which critically affect the nutrition of the person. When the diet supplies adequate amounts of all necessary nutrients and the individual is healthy, the person is well-nourished. A well-nourished person is able to obtain and utilize foods at all levels and conditions and still maintains health in different phases of life. However, intakes that do not match the body's requirements result in poor nutrition and health.

As per the dietary guidelines issued by the National Institute of Nutrition (2011) "the shift from traditional to "modern" foods, changing cooking practices, has increased intake of processed and ready-to-eat foods, intensive marketing of High Fat Sugar and Salt (HFSS) foods and "health" beverages have affected people's perception of foods and their dietary behaviors. Irrational preference for such foods poses a serious health risk to the people, especially children."

GOOD NUTRITION AND MALNUTRITION

Good nutrition implies optimal intake of energy and other nutrients in accordance with the individual's requirements. Such a person is said to be well-nourished. The person is healthy, cheerful, has good immunity/resistance to infection, and can perform to a satisfactory level. Good nutrition helps to achieve good health. It is one of least expensive and most effective methods to decrease the burden of diseases and increase the chances of recovery during and after illness. Poor nutrition, on the contrary, indicates low dietary intake and a diet deficient in many nutrients in required quantity or an excess of nutrients like energy, fat, and carbohydrate that also compromises health. It is also referred to as malnutrition. It increases the risk of numerous diseases and delays recovery from illness. Table 1.1 indicates the characteristics associated with good and poor nutrition.

Good Nutrition

Good nutrition has a preventive role and promotes good health and well-being in multidimensional ways. It helps to:

- Maintain body weight for appropriate for height, age, and sex
- Maintain muscle mass
- Remain mentally alert and active
- Provide resistance to infection
- Help cope with stress
- Decrease risk of disability
- Prevent illness
- Alter the course of illness (reduces the duration and severity)
- Increase longevity
- Perform better and increase productivity
- Improve the social and economic status
- Improve the quality of life

Malnutrition

Malnutrition is rampant throughout the world. It inflicts avoidable suffering on millions of people, particularly children and women resulting in poor health and quality of life of the malnourished and hungry population. Despite sufficient food production and improvement in economic conditions of most people in different countries including India, there is a widespread malnutrition. There can be myriad of reasons for the same. Let us understand the term better. Malnutrition is an undesirable state of health resulting from imbalance in nutrient intakes (deficient or excess amount) and/or nutrient utilization in relation to the requirements of the individuals. It can be considered to be a pathological problem which adversely affects metabolic and cellular functioning and causes clinical symptoms.

The World Health Organization (WHO) defines malnutrition as "the cellular imbalance between the supply of nutrients and energy and the body's demand for them to ensure growth, maintenance, and specific functions". The term "malnutrition" is often used interchangeably with the term "undernutrition". However, in reality, it refers not only to deficiencies, but also to excess or imbalance of energy,

Table 1.1: Characteristics of good nutrition and poor nutrition.

Characteristics	Good nutrition	Poor nutrition
Physical features		
General appearance	Alert and healthy	Listless and apathetic, especially if food and nutrient intake (s) are inadequate
Weight	Normal for height/stature and frame size	Underweight or overweight/obese
Posture	Erect	Sagging shoulders
Muscles	Firm and good tone	Wasted muscles
Skeleton	Well-proportioned Strong bones	Bowed legs and beaded ribs Knock knees Increased risk of bone pain/ fracture
Eyes	Bright and good vision	Dull, poor eyesight, and blindness in extreme cases
Hair	Shiny and lustrous	Brittle, discoloration of hair, dull, and limp hair
Nails	Rounded and pink	Spoon-shaped and brittle
Skin	Healthy and smooth skin	Dry or greasy, and discoloration
Physiological features		
Brain and nerves	Good attention span, cheerful, lack of irritability, normal IQ and reflexes, and sound sleep	Lack of concentration, poor attention span, irritability, mental confusion. IQ and reflexes may be affected. Insomnia or feels sleepy
Gastrointestinal function	Good appetite, digestion, and regular elimination	Anorexia, indigestion, constipation, and diarrhea
Activity	Physically active Person is vigorous and has endurance, and not easily fatigued	Easily fatigued Tired Apathetic
Health status and quality of life		
Immunity	Resistance to infection and disease Frequency, duration, and severity of illness is less Fast recovery	High risk of infection Frequent episodes of infections More severe illness Prolonged period of illness Slow recovery
Productivity and economic status	Ability to work efficiently and effectively good work capacity High productivity, better income, and good purchasing power	Inefficient, low work capacity, and low productivity Low salaries/wages Poor purchasing power
Mental and emotional health	Ability to cope with stress, and well-adjusted individual	Inability to cope with stresses of day-to-day living Poorly adjusted

protein, and other essential nutrients. It is not only the lack of dietary intake, but people having enough food intakes or who are obese are also deficient in micronutrients. "The term malnutrition addresses three broad groups of conditions" (World Health Organization, 2018).

Undernutrition: This is due to deficiency of energy and nutrients and includes wasting, stunting, and underweight.

Overnutrition: This is due to excessive intake or overconsumption of food, especially energy rich foods. The consequences of these include overweight, obesity, and noncommunicable diseases like diabetes mellitus, heart disease, stroke, and some cancers.

Micronutrient-related Malnutrition: This is due to deficiency of micronutrients or even excess of micronutrients.

Undernutrition

Undernutrition implies the deficiency of more than one nutrient mainly due to low intake of food for a long duration may be months or even years. Dietary and nutritional requirements of the individual who is undernourished, are not met as per age, sex, activity level, and physiological status, largely due to lack of food security. In some cases, food intake may be sufficient, but a person can have problems with digestion and/or absorption of food or utilization/metabolism in the body. Whatever be the cause, the result is low body weight for age and deficiency disease (s) of minerals and vitamins. In children, undernutrition is measured in terms of underweight, stunting, and wasting are shown in Figure 1.4.

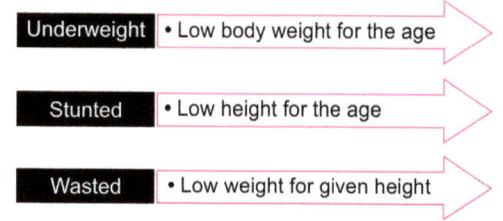

Fig. 1.4: Indicators of undernutrition.

Underweight: Underweight implies low body weight for a given age compared to reference standards. It indicates the body size and body weight. It reflects the level of food and nutrient intake as well as the possible presence of infection and disease. It is a sensitive measure and reflects changes in body weight over a short duration, e.g., the person may weigh less as per his/her age and gender even if he or she has not eaten enough food for few days, for any reason.

Stunting: Stunted means low height for age compared with reference standards. It signifies deprivation of adequate energy and nutrients over a long period of time, i.e., chronic undernutrition. In developing countries like India, stunting can be a result of undernutrition from fetal stage or intrauterine life. It is not affected by immediate circumstances related to food intake or sickness. The chronic lack of nutrients during the growing years may compromise brain development and this can influence cognitive functions. The first 1,000 days of life are especially vulnerable and this period starting from pregnancy until the end of the first 2 years of postnatal life is critical.

Wasting: Wasting implies low body weight for a given height as compared with reference standards. There can be failure to thrive or growth faltering. It reflects short-term undernutrition. Wasting is a strong predictor of mortality.

> **Research glimpse:** Wasting and stunting are closely related and often occur together in the same populations and some children may suffer from both. Both can increase the risk of morbidity and mortality, especially when both are present in the same child. Understanding their pathophysiology can help in designing better intervention programs. While planning interventions for young infants and children, use of mid-upper arm circumference (MUAC) can be used to identify children in need of treatment. In wasting, both muscle mass as well as fat mass are decreased, resulting in an increase in risk for morbidity and mortality. Similar effects are seen in stunting, however, decrease in fat mass is inconsistent in stunting. Interventions should be done for children who exhibit both wasting and stunting, who are likely to have deficits in muscle mass instead of focusing on either wasting or stunting.
>
> *Briend A, Khara T, Dolan C. Wasting and stunting—similarities and differences: policy and programmatic implications. Food Nutrition Bulletin. 2015;36(91 suppl):S15–23.*

For adults, undernutrition or overnutrition is assessed by using body mass index (BMI). A BMI below 18.5 indicates undernourishment and if the BMI is below 16, the individual is said to be severely undernourished. Another term used is **chronic energy deficiency (CED)**. CED weakens the immune system, increases susceptibility to infections, and worsens the disease impact.

> **Chronic energy deficiency (CED)** is defined as a "steady state" where an individual is in energy balance, i.e., the energy intake equals the energy expenditure, despite the low body weight and low body energy stores. Thus, by never growing to a normal size or having experienced one or more stages of energy deficiency, the individual has arrived at a reduced body weight with possibly limited physical activity, which have allowed the energy demands of a lower basal metabolic rate (BMR) and reduced amounts of activity to balance the lower intake.
>
> http://www.fao.org/docrep/t1970e/t1970e02.htm#P45_10041

Prevalence of Undernutrition

According to the most recent National Family Health Survey (NFHS-IV, 2016), 35.7% of Indian children less than 5 years of age were underweight; 38.4% were stunted and 21.0% wasted. In adults, BMI below 18.0 is an indicator of undernutrition. The percentage of undernourished men was 20.2% and 22.9% women had a BMI below 18.0.

In 21 out of 92 countries, about 10% of wasting among children requires immediate attention because they are at high risk of death. In South Asia, wasting is about 19%, which is alarmingly high. Stunting is a much bigger problem because nearly one-third of the under-5 children in developing countries are stunted. There is hardly any gender difference for underweight, but a higher percentage of undernourished children are from rural areas, urban slums, and economically poor households (UNICEF, 2012). According to the WHO (2018), 1.9 billion adults are overweight or obese, while 462 million are underweight. About 52 million children under 5 years of age are wasted, 17 million are severely wasted, and 155 million are stunted, while 41 million are overweight or obese. A recent Comprehensive National Nutrition Survey (CNNS) report of 2019 showed some rays of hope to curb malnutrition. Accordingly 32.5/34.4% (male/female) children (0-4years) were underweight; 35.4/34.0% were stunted and 18.3/16.3% were wasted.

Vulnerable Groups

Young children (0–6 months–6 years) and aged population are visible victims of undernutrition. Adolescent girls, pregnant, and lactating women are at high risk of undernutrition due to high nutritional demands of the body. However, persons from other sections of the society are also vulnerable due to various personal, economical, vocational, social, cultural and political reasons and those who are sick. The first 1,000 days of life from conception to 2 years make pregnant and lactating mothers and young children are highly vulnerable groups. Undernutrition in this period can have lifetime impact on the health of the person.

> **Research glimpse:** About one-third of the world's stunted preschool children hail from India. It is vital to understand the determinants of stunting in this diverse country if one is to address undernutrition. District-level data from the National and Family Health Survey–IV (2015–16) was examined covering about 601,509 households in 640 districts along with use of mapping and descriptive analysis to examine spatial differences in distribution of stunting. Prevalence of stunting varied from 12.4% to 65.1%. 239 of the 640 districts had stunting levels exceeding 40% and in 202 districts, the prevalence was 30–40%. More districts with high levels of stunting are located in the north and central part of the country. Statistical analysis was applied for comparing districts with high prevalence of stunting with those having low prevalence. Causes of stunting that were identified were low body mass index of women, education level, adequacy of children's diets, open defecation, age at marriage, antenatal care, and household size. The analysis highlighted that multiple factors are responsible for stunting which can be summarized as economic, health, hygiene, and demographic factors.
>
> *Menon P, Headey D, Avula R, Nguyen PH. Understanding the geographical burden of stunting in India: A regression decomposition analysis of district level data from 2015–16. Maternal and Child Nutrition. 2018;14:e12620.*

Reasons for Undernutrition

Inadequate supply of food compared to the requirements is one of the main reasons for undernutrition. Another reason is illness/infection. A person can become undernourished due to myriad reasons which may vary in different communities,

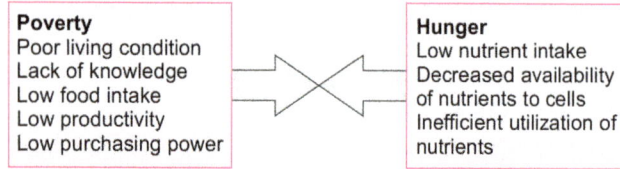

Fig. 1.5: Reasons for undernutrition.

e.g., poverty and inability to purchase food, young age at marriage, household food insecurity, inadequate dietary intake, and time to fetch water and food and meal frequency. Some of them are shown in Figure 1.5.

Undernutrition signifies inadequate supply of nutrients to the cells for optimal functioning of the body. Poverty and hunger (lack of nutrition, not just food alone) are leading causes of undernutrition which result in low intake of food, inefficient utilization of nutrients or loss of nutrients from the body. In case of infections like diarrhea, vomiting, and fever, there is depletion of nutrients from the body which further reduces the ability of the body to utilize the nutrients for their diverse functions. A sick person often lacks appetite and eats less amount of food. This ultimately becomes a vicious cycle of undernutrition and illness. Some families tend to restrict foods during infectious illness.

Various biological, social, cultural, ecological, environmental, economic, and political factors are directly or indirectly responsible for malnutrition which are indicated in Table 1.2.

Some of the factors are specific for different life stages. Infants, children, and adolescents are undernourished due to low birth weight, poor sanitation and hygiene, inadequate availability of safe drinking water, infections and illness, inadequate parenting (care) and poor feeding practices particularly during weaning after 6 months of age and lack of availability and/or utilization of health services. During pregnancy, increased nutrient demands vis-à-vis requirements increase risk of undernutrition. Adults and elders are at risk of being undernourished due to inadequate food and nutrient intake for various social, economic, and personal reasons. Many global reports indicate exposure to climate extremes such as heavy rainfall, and temperature variability can continue to cause undernourishment in many geographical regions. UNICEF has summarized these factors into a conceptual framework. This framework was first proposed in the early 1990s recent one is shown in Figure 1.6.

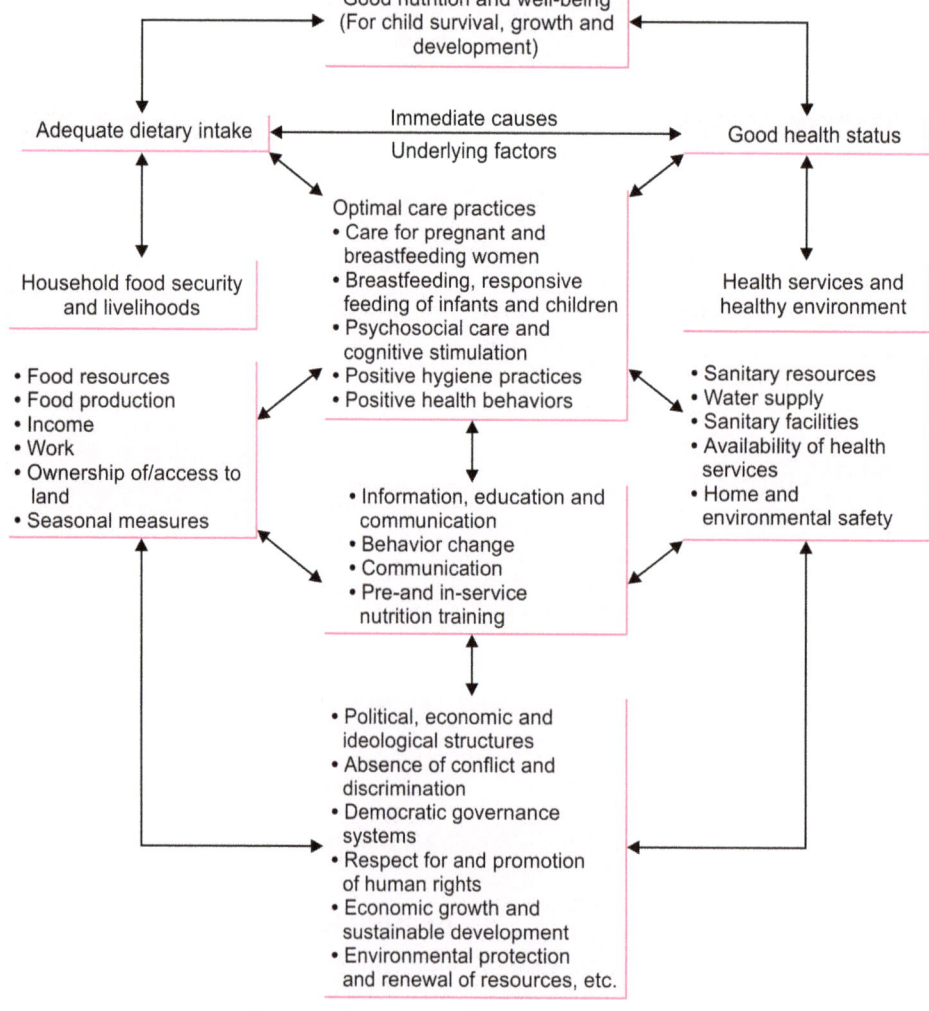

Fig. 1.6: ACF conceptual framework for nutrition.

Source: Adopted from UNICEF Conceptual Framework (1990) and ACF Framework of Causality (2004).

Table 1.2: Factors influencing malnutrition.

Major factors	Main features
Food availability and food accessibility	Food production Geographic conditions Agricultural techniques—use of hybrid seeds, fertilizers, and pesticides Insufficient amount of food Poverty and hunger Shops and market nearby living area Transportation facilities Food industries Access to and availability of nutrient-poor processed foods, snacks, and beverages Government programs for food distribution
Ecological factors	Agroclimatic conditions Geographical area—coastal, hill, plain, etc. Rainfall Type of soil Natural disasters—drought, floods, cyclone, and earthquakes
Environmental factors	Population density Housing Environmental sanitation Personal hygiene Availability of water for domestic, toilet use, irrigation, industry, etc. Safe drinking water Electricity Heavy traffic and pollution Pesticides Terrorist attacks and communal violence Use of radioactive substances, electromagnetic waves, and radiowaves like microwave Industrial affluents Unhealthy food habits due to family culture, peer group or mass media exposure, especially when endorsed by popular/cult figures
Sociocultural factors	Family size and age composition Trend of food preparation and distribution Cultural taboos and beliefs Religion Illiteracy and ignorance about nutrition Care capacity of caregivers and household Gender bias
Economic factors	Poverty Poor purchasing power and high prices of nutrient-rich foods Chronic illness, alcoholism, and addictions in one or more members of the family Using money on luxuries rather than on nutritious foods
Pathological conditions	Disease of the gastrointestinal tract Infectious diseases like diarrhea, vomiting, fever, respiratory infections, malaria, etc. Chronic degenerative diseases like diabetes, high blood pressure, etc. Malabsorption syndromes Infestations with hookworm, roundworm, etc. Accidents, injury, operation, and trauma Depression or any other psychiatric illness Eating disorders
Personal factors	Appetite and hunger Lifestyle that is not conducive to eating meals at appropriate times Irregular meal times—leads to compromised food intake Tension and violence in house especially at meal time Poor food habits *Ad libitum* snacking and drinking soft drinks Wrong examples of dietary habits by elders and influential people Poor selection and combination of food Poor skill in food preparation Inadequate or delayed weaning Unavailability of the desired food within the reach Inadequate rest Excessive working hours, odd hours shift duties, and traveling Lack of time or intention to cook food for self or family

Consequences of Undernutrition

Undernourished persons will show some signs and symptoms such as unintentional weight loss, low body weight, lack of interest in daily activities, lack of appetite (which occurs during illness also), feeling of weakness, and tiredness/fatigue. Illness and infections tend to last longer and recovery is delayed. Undernutrition increases susceptibility to infections, particularly frequent respiratory and gastrointestinal infections, e.g., pneumonia, diarrhea, and measles. Young children are especially vulnerable. Children will not grow in weight and height as they should for their age. They may also show delayed motor, social, emotional, and cognitive and language development indices. Stunting adversely impacts the brain and cognitive development which may be more prominent and harmful in later life stages.

Malnutrition affects every facet of life and people of all age groups living in all geographic areas. Millions of newborns, young and old children, youth, adults, pregnant and lactating women, and senior citizens, even sick and hospitalized persons, are victims of malnutrition. Malnutrition adversely influences individuals, families, communities, and nations. There is perhaps no harm in being lean or short, if one is healthy. These characteristics in many are genetically determined. Underweight during childhood reduces the chances of normal physical and mental development. Worldwide, deficiencies of vitamin A, iodine, iron, and zinc are prevalent and contribute to the high rates of morbidity and mortality particularly among infants and young children. Micronutrient deficiencies are also termed as "hidden hunger". The effects of undernutrition/malnutrition are shown in Figure 1.7.

Overnutrition

Excessive intake of energy and nutrients vis-à-vis the energy expenditure, for a prolonged period of time may result in overnutrition and the risk of overnutrition is much higher when the physical activity is also less. Overnutrition is characterized by overweight and poor body stature, lack of stamina, and impaired functioning of body. BMI or body mass index is used to determine the level of overweight and obesity (See Chapter 5).

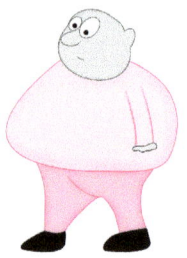

Overweight and obesity are associated with excess accumulation of fat in the body. Fat deposition varies with age, gender, and different areas in the body. In some persons, excess fat is deposited in the abdominal region that is referred to as abdominal obesity. Obesity is known to alter metabolic functions and increases risk of various morbidities such as dyslipidemia, hypertension, metabolic syndrome, hyperglycemia and diabetes mellitus. Obesity is discussed in detail in Chapter 12. Vulnerable age groups for overweight and obesity include school-age children, adolescents, and adults. NFHS–IV (2016) indicated that 18.6% adult men and 20.7% women have BMI more than 25.0.

> Adult obesity is worsening, and more than one in eight adults in the world is obese. Poor access to nutritious food due to its higher cost, the stress of living with food insecurity, and physiological adaptations to food deprivation help explain why food-insecure families may have a higher risk of overweight and obesity.
> www.fao.org, 2018

India, like some other countries, is undergoing nutrition transition that occurs when individuals and families which previously had inadequate access to food, now have access to cheap and highly palatable energy-dense foods that do not contain much micronutrients (ultraprocessed foods). Such foods are classified under NOVA classification (see box).

> **NOVA System of Food Classification:** The United Nations has designated **2016 to 2025 as the Decade of Nutrition**. As part of these efforts, the NOVA classification is now applied worldwide. The NOVA system of food classification has been developed based on the nature, extent, and purpose of industrial food processing that food products undergo. The foods are grouped into the following categories:
>
> **Group 1–Unprocessed or minimally processed foods:** These include unprocessed/raw edible seeds, fruits, leaves, stems, roots or meat, eggs, milk, algae, and water. Minimally processed foods

Contd...

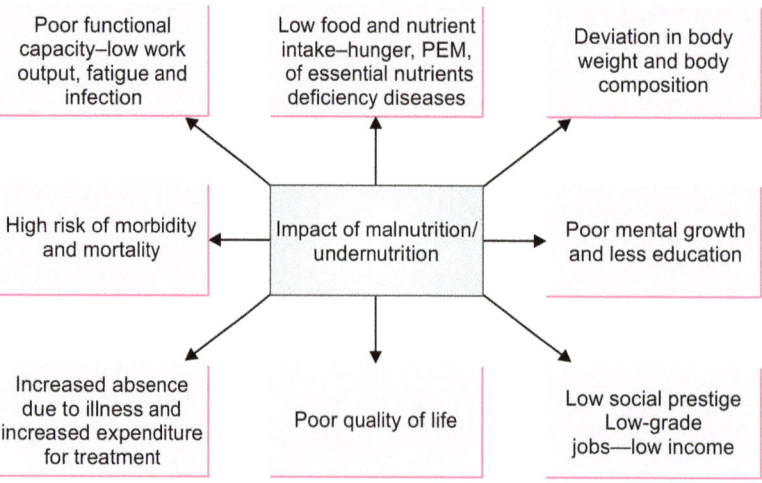

Fig. 1.7: Impact of malnutrition.

Contd...

have been processed to a relatively small extent such as removal of inedible/unwanted parts or have been dried, crushed, ground, filtered, roasted, boiled, fermented (excludes alcoholic fermentation), pasteurized, refrigerated, chilled, or frozen or put into containers, and vacuum packed. In essence, the foods have been subjected to these processes to improve their storage life, enhance their safety as well as to make them edible. Hence, most things prepared in our homes or in a restaurant or even a street food outlets are included in this food category.

Group 2–Processed culinary ingredients: These include foods like oils, butter, sugar or salt, and foods derived from Group 1 foods by using processes such as pressing, refining, grinding, milling, and drying to make a variety of food products including preserves, soups, breads, beverages, and desserts. They are generally not consumed by themselves but are eaten along with foods from Group 1.

Group 3–Processed foods: These include preserved fruits and vegetables, fish, or cheese—essentially those prepared by addition of salt, oil, sugar, etc. using foods that are part of either Group 1 or 2. Foods such as cheese are also included. These foods are essentially processed to improve their shelf-life and/or to make them more tasty and acceptable.

Group 4–Ultraprocessed foods: These are foods made from ingredients derived from foods that are classified as Group 1 foods, but not much of the food is left intact. When the food is formulated, additives are most often also used. Examples of these foods are soft drinks, packaged sweet and savory snacks, reconstituted meat products, and preprepared frozen dishes. They will usually include ingredients such as sugar, oils, fats, and salt, but also use ingredients that are not generally used in food preparations in the home or restaurants. Some ingredients can be extracts like gluten, whey, lactose, casein, etc. Many ingredients are those where foods have been subjected to more processing like hydrogenated or interesterified oils, hydrolyzed proteins, soya protein isolate, maltodextrin, invert sugar, high-fructose corn syrup, etc. Such foods generally contain preservatives, antioxidants, and stabilizers as well as ingredients that can be used to imitate natural flavors and colors or enhance the sensory qualities of foods or to mask what might be unpalatable/unacceptable to the consumer. Such additives are dyes, pigments, color stabilizers, flavors, flavor enhancers, nonsugar sweeteners, and processing aids such as carbonating, firming, bulking and antibulking, anticaking agents, emulsifiers, defoaming or foaming agents, etc.

These foods are said to be ultraprocessed because a sequence of processes can be used to combine/incorporate the ingredients for making the final product. Many of these may not be used at domestic level such as hydrolysis, extrusion, etc. Ultraprocessed foods are convenient, ready to consume, highly palatable, attractive, and have good shelf-life. The concern of health professionals is that such foods are intensively marketed in attractive forms at relatively low cost and displace other more nutritious foods in the diet and may be overconsumed, displacing Group 1 foods that are nutritious. These foods are energy dense, contain refined starches, free sugars, and salt, but are poor sources of protein and fiber.

Monteiro CA, Cannon G, Moubarac J-C, Levy RB, Louzada MLC, Jaime PC. The UN Decade of Nutrition, the NOVA food classification and the trouble with ultraprocessing. Public Health Nutrition. 2017;21(1):5-17. doi:10.1017/S1368980017000234.

According to the Global Nutrition Report (GNR, 2017), the 2030 Agenda for Sustainable Development—stunting, anemia, and overweight are serious threats for health of people. Food and Agriculture Organization (FAO) (2018) focuses on the strategies to overcome the multiple burdens of malnutrition, i.e., stunting, wasting, micronutrient deficiencies, overweight and obesity, and diet-related noncommunicable diseases by governments and policy makers of different countries. These strategies may influence the food chain system and ensure availability of healthy diets and equitable distribution of food to all. The 2020 Global Nutrition Report emphasizes on nutritional well-being for all, particularly the most population. The need for more equitable, resilient and sustainable food and health systems has never been more urgent.

STRATEGIES TO COMBAT MALNUTRITION

All human beings wish to be healthy and well-nourished. Man tries the best possible ways to achieve good health and well-being within the given resources. Since the country's population is increasing, the number of malnourished persons in this country is also escalating. Although the national food production database reflects increased and sufficient food production for the masses and there is some reduction of malnutrition, but the picture is still dismal. Malnutrition is not restricted to India. It is a global problem hence for the last many decades, it has been tackled at all levels but "no one size fits all". World Health Organization (WHO), UNICEF, World Bank, the Bill and Melinda Gates Foundation, Global Agricultural Information Network (GAIN), Consultative Group for International Agricultural Research (CGIAR) and Harvest Plus, and the Government of India, through its various programs and institutes like the Indian Council of Medical Research-National Institute of Nutrition (ICMR-NIN), nobel laureates, professors, scientists, nutritionists, economists, and policy makers are trying hard to tackle the problem of malnutrition. Overcoming malnutrition requires tackling the following challenges:

- **Hunger and food insecurity**
- **Poor health and disease**
- **Conflicts**—domestic violence to political conflicts and terrorism
- **Inequality** in gender, socioeconomic status, and intra-household food distribution
- **Education** and **status of women** in society
- **Climate change**—natural resources for food and safe drinking water, pollution, damaging land for cultivation thereby reducing the nutrient composition of soil, thus nutrient composition of food
- **Easy availability and access to processed foods**
- **Food prices and affordability of micronutrient-rich foods.**

Interventions are required from the micro level (family and individual levels) to the macro level (national level).

Interventions at the Family and Individual Levels

- Improving purchasing power
- Increasing knowledge through nutrition and health education
- Bringing about behavior change in key areas including dietary diversification
- Exclusive breastfeeding from 0–6 months of age
- Adequate and timely complementary feeding from 6–24 months

- Adequate hygiene practices at every stage of food handling and eating
- Extra care for infants, adolescent girls, pregnant and lactating women, and elders with regard to food behavior
- Improving antenatal care
- Deworming.

Interventions at National Level in India

- Green revolution was one of the major strategies to reduce hunger and death due to grain shortage. After this, there has been the White Revolution, Yellow Revolution, and Blue Revolution to increase production of milk, oilseeds and seafoods for organic farming.
- Brown revolution improving production of pulses and legumes and making them available at affordable prices.
- Several nutrition programs and health schemes were launched after independence and in the last 2-3 years, important programs have been launched.
- Establishment of agriculture universities and other universities for higher education, medicine, and technology, and subsidies to farmers for seeds, fertilizers and pesticides, attention to horticulture, dairy, and fish culture.
- Improved access to healthcare services through primary healthcare centers, hospitals, and ICDS anganwadi centers.
- Increased number of healthcare facilities and improved quality of health services—doctors, trained paramedical staff, and availability of medicine and needed infrastructure.
- Better sanitation facilities
- Access to safe drinking water
- Improvement in food access and enhancement in household food security through public distribution system and fair price shops.

> **Research glimpse:** A sustainable diet is one that is the least harmful to the environment and supports and sustains long-term ecological balance. The United Nations Food and Agriculture Organization (UNFAO) defines sustainable diets as:
> *"Those diets with low environmental impacts contribute to food and nutrition security and to healthy life for present and future generations. Sustainable diets are protective and respectful of biodiversity and ecosystems, culturally acceptable, accessible, economically fair and affordable; nutritionally adequate, safe and healthy; while optimizing natural and human resources."*
> It is a way to rethink about environment and health and now take action by reducing the food waste, buying humanely raised animal products, and purchasing food mindfully and that can be using organic, local, and seasonal food.
> http://www.fao.org/nutrition/education/food-dietary-guidelines/background/sustainable-dietary-guidelines/en/

HEALTH

The World Health Organization **(WHO)**, the apex body on health, states *"Health is a state of complete physical, mental and social well-being and not merely the absence of disease or infirmity"*. Over the years, several definitions have been given to reflect different concepts about health.

> Health is a fundamental human right, as per the Universal Declaration of Human Rights (1948) in Article 25. It states "Everyone has the right to a standard of living adequate for the health and well-being of himself and his family". This fundamental right is irrespective of race, religion, and political belief, economic, and social conditions.
> **Convention of Rights of the Child states that nutrition is a fundamental human right**

Health is the sum total of the supply and utilization of food and nutrients for the soul, mind, and body. **Health is a self-promised, self-regulatory, and self-practiced phenomenon.** "Swastha" in Sanskrit indicates the "swa" and "astha". "Swa" means self and "astha" denotes faith or commitment. It is a promise given to self to take charge of one's own health. Health resides within one's body, mind, and soul and is reflected through physical, physiological, emotional, mental, and spiritual attributes. It is one of the highest pursuits of life and a way of life to achieve its goal. Health can be viewed as an active process used by persons to adapt to his or her environment which is always dynamic and changing. Good health is critical for wellness.

According to Ayurveda, nourishment of physical, emotional, and spiritual aspects of human life is essential. According to the **Charaka Samhitā:**

"Nityamhitahara-vihara-sevisamikshyakarivishayeshvasaktah Data samahsatyaparahkshamavanaptopasevi cha bhavatiarogah"

"A person who practices regularly a wholesome lifestyle, eats wholesome food, is deliberate in all his actions, not involved in the objects of the mind (i.e., overindulgence in sense pleasures), who is generous, just, truthful, forgiving in nature, who is service-minded and helpful to one's own kin will remain unaffected by diseases".

Wellness is defined as a dynamic state of health in which a person progresses toward a higher level of functioning, achieving an optimum balance between internal and external environments. In simpler terms, it is a condition of good physical, mental, and emotional health, especially when maintained by an appropriate diet, exercise, and other lifestyle modifications. Lifestyle includes the way of living self-designed and determined daily habits related to eating, exercise, occupation, social life, managing emergencies, and still smiling while coping with stresses.

Health is influenced by numerous factors.

- **Heredity or genetics:** Phenylketonuria is an in-born error of metabolism. Sickle cell anemia is a genetic disorder. Mental retardation and congenital abnormalities in some cases are also inherent problems.
- **Age and gender:** Youth suffers less health problems while elders are more likely to have health problems, especially chronic ones like arthritis.
- **Physical condition of the individual:** Stature, physical disability, work capacity, and body weight are related to health and nutritional status. Disability, smaller body size, and reduced work capacity can be caused by poor nutrition during fetal life or later in life.
- **Nutrition and food habits:** Consuming nutritious, well-balanced diets as per the individual's requirements is important for promoting and maintaining good health

as well as preventing problems. Nutrition knowledge, interest, and motivation for skillful cooking, support promoting and maintaining good health.

- **Personality characteristics:** Calmness and confidence are usually observed in healthy persons. Healthy persons are able to cope with everyday stresses of life. Persons who do not enjoy good health may feel stressed, some may be depressed, and some may respond with anger and aggression.
- **Environment:** Housing, soil, climate, waste and sewage disposal, environmental pollution presence of plants, trees, animals, and the sociocultural features of the region where a person lives are important factors. Market transport and storage facilities for food also affect health.
- **Lifestyle:** Cultural and behavioral pattern, sleep, physical activity, smoking and use and abuse of alcohol, and narcotic drugs all influence health.
- **Economic status:** Food prices, income, literacy, occupation, purchasing power play important roles in health promotion and protection.
- **Social status:** Residence and country of origin and social network and social integration are some issues.
- **Access to and availability of health services:** Availability of and access to provision of safe water and other preventive measures, primary healthcare, immunization services, and hospitals are important for preventing disease as well as maintaining and promoting health.
- **Use of pesticides:** Pesticides are being used since long to protect the agriculture from pests, weeds or plant diseases, and humans from vector-borne diseases such as malaria, dengue fever, and schistosomiasis. Pesticides themselves are considered a pollutants as they can be inhaled, touched or ingested. They are found in air, water, and soil. In spite of numerous warnings about toxicity of pesticides, these are being used unscrupulously even today. Toxicity caused by these substances does not spare any living beings and creates havoc to health and environment both. Short-term effects can be abdominal pain, dizziness, headaches, nausea, vomiting, skin and eye problems and long-term effects can be cancer, neurological, and reproductive problems.
- **Pollution:** With increase in urbanization, industrialization, and population, increase in waste material is also inevitable to certain extent. This waste can be present in air, water, and soil. Excessive and inappropriate amount of waste generates toxic fumes and pollutes the environment making the people difficult to breathe. It results in multitudes of illnesses and diseases all around the world. Air pollution, water pollution, soil pollution and even noise pollution seriously affect the health of human beings and also other living beings.

> **Research glimpse:** Air pollution, particularly from outdoor air pollution resulting in emission from industrial activities and some vehicles, have caused millions of deaths and diseases globally. It has also resulted in increased incidence and progression of some diseases such as asthma, lung cancer, ventricular hypertrophy, Alzheimer's and Parkinson's diseases, psychological complications, autism, retinopathy, fetal growth, and low birth weight.
>
> *Contd...*

Contd...

> *Ghorani-Azam A, Riahi-Zanjani B, Balali-Mood. Effects of air pollution on human health and practical measures for prevention in Iran. Journal of Research in Medical Sciences. 2016;21:65.*
>
> According to the Lancet Commission on Pollution and Health, "Pollution is the largest environmental cause of disease and premature death in the world today. Diseases caused by pollution were responsible for an estimated 9 million premature deaths in 2015—16% of all deaths worldwide—three times more deaths than from AIDS, tuberculosis, and malaria combined and 15 times more than from all wars and other forms of violence. In the most severely affected countries, pollution-related disease is responsible for more than one death in four".
>
> https://www.thelancet.com/journals/lancet/article/PIIS0140-6736(17)32345-0/fulltext
>
> Such statistical information may vary from time to time in different countries.
>
> Devastating effects definitely call for intensive action at all levels.

- **Use of radiation:** Now most of us are exposed to radiation through wide range of gadgets like computers, mobile phones, television, microwaves, and many other types of equipment; diagnostic tool like X-ray and radiotherapy treatment. Radiation tends to increase the risk of health hazards from mild to acute and that depends upon the dose of radiation.

RAPID FIRE

1. Define food as per FSSAI (2006).
2. Name three functions of food.
3. Which three other areas of science are linked with nutrition.
4. What is difference between macro and micronutrients?
5. How do you perceive health and wellness?
6. What is malnutrition?
7. Name four major factors that affect malnutrition.
8. What is the current status of overnutrition and undernutrition in India?
9. Suggest three ways to combat malnutrition in your local area.
10. What do you understand by micronutrient malnutrition?
11. How do food choices affect health?
12. What is the impact of radiation on health?

EXERCISE

1. Observe the current food choice in your neighboring area and which factors affect their choices.
2. Observe 10 undernourished and 10 obese persons in your neighboring area, identify their characteristics and differentiate between them.
3. Design some strategies and make a presentation (verbal/PPT, etc.) to improve their health and of any one vulnerable section of society.

SUGGESTED READING

1. ACF international (2010). Taking Action-Nutrition for Survival, Growth and Development- Action for Hunger White Paper: 16.
2. Barbieri R, Coppo E, Marchese A, et al. Phytochemicals for human disease: An update on plant-derived compounds antibacterial activity. Microbiol Res. 2017;196:44-68.

3. Behrman JR, Alderman H, Hoddinott J. Hunger and Malnutrition – Challenges and Opportunities – Perspective Paper, Copenhagen Consensus, 2004.
4. Meskin MS, Bidlack WR, Davies AJ, Omaye ST (Eds). Phytochemicals in nutrition and health. CRC Press; 2002.
5. Ministry of Health and Family Welfare (MoHFW), Government of India, UNICEF and Population Council. 2019. Comprehensive National Nutrition Survey (CNNS) National Report. New Delhi.
6. National Family Heath Survey in collaboration with International Institute of Population Sciences and Ministry of Health and Family Welfare, Government of India, 2016.
7. Shridhar G, Rajendra N, Murigendra H, et al. Modern Diet and Its Impact on Human Health. J Nutr Food Sci. 2015;5:430.
8. Swaminathan MS. Mission 2007: A nutrition-secure India. Paper presentation at Silver Jubilee Symposium (Nov 2004) Towards National Nutrition Security.
9. The 2020 Global Nutrition Report in the Context of Covid-19. Development Initiatives Poverty Research Ltd.
10. Vorster HH. Introduction to Human Nutrition: A Global Perspective on Food and Nutrition (2009). In: Introduction to Human Nutrition eds Gibney MJ, Lanham - New SA, Cassidy A, Vorster HH. Wiley-Blackwell. The Nutrition Society pp 1-11.
11. WHO 2018. http://www.who.int/news-room/fact-sheets/detail/MALNUTRITion.
12. www.nhp.gov.in/healthyliving/healthy-diet.

2

CHAPTER

Carbohydrates

KEY CONCERNS
- What are the different types of carbohydrates?
- Will carbohydrate from different sources affect my health?
- What is dietary fiber and what is its role in health and disease?
- How much carbohydrate is present in various foods?
- What are sugar alcohols and artificial sweeteners?
- Why are glycemic index and glycemic load important?

KEY CONCEPTS
- Classification of carbohydrates
- Function of carbohydrates, their sources, and nutritional value
- Role of starch and dietary fiber in health and disease
- Causes and consequences of deficiency and excess
- Role of sugar alcohols and artificial sweeteners
- Significance of glycemic index and glycemic load.

Carbohydrates are the most abundant and relatively less expensive sources of energy. Across the globe, regardless of religion and race, carbohydrates supply almost half to three-fourths of the energy intake of individuals. This is because staple foods like cereals are good sources of carbohydrates. Carbohydrates form the building blocks of plants. Most plant foods contain a variety of carbohydrates in varying amounts whereas animal food sources contain only small amounts. Carbohydrates are sugars, starches, pectin, cellulose, and other compounds. Animals store some carbohydrate in the form of glycogen.

WHAT ARE CARBOHYDRATES?

- Carbohydrates are organic compounds. They are composed of carbon, hydrogen, and oxygen in a ratio of 1:2:1. Carbohydrates are hydrates of carbon because the general formula is $(CH_2O)_n$.
- In plants, carbohydrates are synthesized by **photosynthesis** in the presence of sunlight using carbon dioxide and water.

$$6CO_2 + 6H_2O + \text{Sun Energy} \xrightarrow{\text{Photosynthesis}} C_6H_{12}O_6 + 6O_2$$

Carbon dioxide + Water (+ Light Energy) = Glucose + Oxygen

- They are based on a common unit with varying linkages and chain lengths. Thus glucose is $C_6(H_2O)_6$.
- Some carbohydrates also contain other elements like nitrogen. The unit (monomer) of carbohydrates is generally **"Glucose"**, which is the major source of energy for all vital activities in the body and also for the brain.

FUNCTIONS OF CARBOHYDRATES

Most carbohydrates are sweet in taste and improve palatability of the food. In most cultures, sweets are served on special occasions. Foods rich in sugar are a mark of respect and prosperity. Most staple foods are good sources of carbohydrates and are consumed to satisfy hunger. Carbohydrates perform several important functions in the body:

- **Provide energy**: One gram of carbohydrate provides 4 kcal. Carbohydrates are metabolized in the body (in the cell) in the presence of oxygen to give adenosine triphosphate (ATP).
- **Determine the sensory qualities**: Carbohydrates greatly influence the flavor, texture, and acceptability of the food.
- **Storage form of energy**: Carbohydrates are stored in the body in the form of glycogen in liver and muscles.
- **Source of carbon**: Carbohydrates supply carbon for the synthesis of cell components like DNA and RNA. Ribose is a five-carbon unit present in DNA (deoxyribonucleic acid) and RNA (ribonucleic acid). Some carbon units from carbohydrates are used to synthesize nonessential amino acids. They are intermediates in the synthesis of the biochemical compounds such as lipids and proteins. Also, carbohydrates are part of free nucleotides, i.e., ATP and ADP, as well as coenzymes, i.e., nicotinamide adenine dinucleotide (NAD) and flavine adenine dinucleotide (FAD).
- **Cellular functions**: They participate in biological transport, cell-cell recognition, activation of growth factors, modulation of the immune system, as well as gene expression.
- **Carbohydrates are present as glycans on the cell surface**: Oligosaccharides, glycoproteins, and glycolipids are present and this diverse mixture of glycans contains a wealth of information, modulating a wide range of processes such as cell migration, proliferation, transcriptional regulation, and differentiation.
- **Formation of adipose tissue**: Excess carbohydrate is converted into fat and deposited in adipose tissue. Adipose tissue provides insulation and protects the various organs.

However, excess of adipose tissue can result in overweight and obesity, diabetes, heart problems, and many other chronic diseases.
- **Protein sparing action**: Protein also provides 4 kcal/g; however, it is required for more important functions. When our diet supplies sufficient carbohydrates to meet the body's energy needs, it spares protein for its main functions. But if our intake is inadequate, then the body obtains the required energy from protein.
- **Health benefits**: Some indigestible carbohydrates are fermented by intestinal microorganisms. The products of fermentation have health benefits such as improving gastrointestinal health, immunity, and control diabetes and other metabolic diseases. They are useful in gut motility. They also have a role in blood clotting.
- **Prevent formation of ketone bodies/antiketogenic effect**: Carbohydrate is necessary for metabolism of fat. When there is insufficient carbohydrate, fat is utilized by the body for obtaining energy. However, a small amount of carbohydrate is required to break down fat completely. In the absence of carbohydrate, fat cannot be completely broken down and small compounds called ketones are formed. Most cells can utilize ketones for energy; however, excessive formation of ketone bodies is harmful.
- **Structural role**: They form structural tissues in plants (cellulose and lignin) and microorganisms. They are also constituents of cellular organelles and in combination with lipids and proteins; they provide structural integrity as well as mechanical strength. In cell membranes and membrane receptors, carbohydrates are part of glycoproteins and glycolipids.
- **Detoxification**: Many drugs and toxic molecules are metabolized in the body and converted into a form that can be excreted easily. Some of these molecules are not soluble in water and glucuronic acid is conjugated with these molecules to convert them to a more soluble form.

CLASSIFICATION OF CARBOHYDRATES

In chemistry, carbohydrates are also referred to as "**saccharides**". Saccharide is a Greek word which means "sugar". There is a wide variety of carbohydrates, ranging from simple compounds or sugars called monosaccharides to large complex molecules (polymers) called polysaccharides.

> Monosaccharides are the basic units. Monosaccharides, i.e. glucose, fructose, and galactose are the building blocks of naturally occurring di-, oligo-, and polysaccharides.
> When two monosaccharides are linked together, we get a disaccharide; three monosaccharides together give a trisaccharide. Oligosaccharides contain 3–10 monosaccharides and polysaccharides are large compounds or polymers containing numerous (>10) monosaccharides. The number of monosaccharides linked together is expressed as degree of polymerization (DP).
> - Monosaccharides: Glucose, fructose, mannose, and galactose
> - Disaccharides: Sucrose, maltose, and lactose
> - Oligosaccharides: Raffinose, stachyose, verbascose, and fructo-oligosaccharides
> - Polysaccharides: Starch, glycogen, cellulose, pectin, and non-starch polysaccharides.

Carbohydrates contain hydroxyl groups. In addition, they also contain either an aldehyde group or a ketone group. Therefore, carbohydrates are also either polyhydroxyaldehydes or polyhydroxyketones. Monosaccharides cannot be hydrolyzed further to simpler units.

In 1998, the Food and Agriculture Organization of the United Nations/World Health Organization (FAO/WHO) had classified carbohydrates based on the molecular size, which is determined by degree of polymerization (DP, i.e., the number of monosaccharides present in a carbohydrate), the type of linkages (α and β) and character of individual monomers (monosaccharides). This classification divides carbohydrates into three main groups, namely (1) sugars (also called simple sugars) **(DP 1–2)**, (2) **oligosaccharides (short-chain carbohydrates) (DP 3–9)** and (3) **polysaccharides (DP ≥ 10)**. The main categories of food carbohydrates are given in Table 2.1.

In 2006, a review commissioned by the FAO/WHO recommended the classification of carbohydrates that was based on their digestion and absorption in the small intestine rather than on their chemical characteristics. In 2007, FAO/WHO revised the classification of carbohydrates and recommended that it be based on degree of polymerization and the physiological and health effects. It has been recommended that carbohydrates as metabolizable substrate for energy be considered in terms of their gastrointestinal and metabolic fates. Nutritionally, carbohydrates are classified as:
- Digestible carbohydrates or available carbohydrates
- Nondigestible carbohydrates or unavailable carbohydrates

Table 2.1: Classification of carbohydrates based on degree of polymerization.

Class	Degree of Polymerization (DP)	Subgroups	Examples
Sugars	1	Monosaccharides	Glucose, fructose, and galactose
	2	Disaccharides	Sucrose, maltose, lactose, and trehalose
	1–2	Polyols (sugar alcohols)	Sorbitol, mannitol, lactitol, xylitol, maltitol, erythritol isomalt, and polyglycol
Oligosaccharides	3–9	Maltooligosaccharides	Maltodextrins
		Other oligosaccharides	Raffinose, stachyose, and fructooligosaccharides
Polysaccharides	>9	Starch (α-glucans)	Amylose, amylopectin, and modified starches
		Non-starch polysaccharide (NSP)	Cellulose (insoluble), hemicellulose (soluble and insoluble forms), pectin, gums, mucilages, and hydrocolloids

Scapin T, Fernandes AC, Proenca RPC. Added sugars: Definitions, classifications, metabolism and health implications. Rev Nutr. 2017;30(5):663–77.

Table 2.2: Nutritional groupings of dietary carbohydrates based on physiological properties.

Nutritional groups based on physiological aspects	Dietary carbohydrate
Glycemic	Glucose, fructose, mannose, galactose, sucrose, maltose, lactose, trehalose, starch, and maltodextrins
Nonglycemic	Polyols (sugar alcohols), oligosaccharides (α-glucans), resistant and modified starches, and non-starch polysaccharides
Increase stool output	Polyols (except erythritol), some starches, NSP, lactose (in some populations), fructose (if taken in large amounts)
No effect on stool weight	Glucose, galactose, sucrose, maltose, trehalose, maltodextrins, oligosaccharides, most starches

Available carbohydrates: Available carbohydrates are those that are digested and absorbed in the small intestine. They include soluble sugars (mono- and disaccharides), maltodextrin, and starch (amylose and amylopectin). Those that have a glycemic effect whereas resistant carbohydrates are generally nonglycemic. Besides this, some of them will have positive effect on stool weight (Table 2.2).

Unavailable resistant carbohydrates: Unavailable resistant carbohydrates are the ones that resist digestion in the small intestine. Hence they are poorly absorbed in the intestines. They reach the human large intestine where they are partially fermented by the bacteria present in the colon. They include polyols (sugar alcohols), nondigestible oligosaccharides, fructans, non-starch polysaccharides (NSP), and resistant starch.

Carbohydrates vary in their source of supply, chemical structure, chemical reactions, chemical composition, and physical and physiological behavior. The properties of carbohydrates and how they are utilized in the body depends on the monosaccharide composition and how they are linked.

> When one consumes carbohydrate, it raises the blood sugar/glucose levels after digestion and absorption. However, some carbohydrates or carbohydrate-containing foods will lead to a spike in blood sugar faster or earlier than others. Pure sugar, sweets, and white rice can raise sugar quickly, whereas pulses have a slower and smaller effect on blood sugar. Foods that contain disaccharides like sucrose and monosaccharides like glucose will raise blood sugar faster than those that contain complex carbohydrates. The amount of carbohydrate consumed also influences the extent to which blood sugar rises. Carbohydrates that raise blood sugar levels are known as **glycemic carbohydrates** and those that do not influence blood sugar levels are called **nonglycemic carbohydrates**. Nonglycemic carbohydrates generally remain unchanged in the small intestine and pass to the large intestines where they may be fermented to different extents by the microorganisms present.

Monosaccharides

Monosaccharides are the simplest form of carbohydrate. Monosaccharides are relatively small molecules, have low molecular weight, and are soluble in water. They are simple sugars. Most common monosaccharides contain 6-carbon units called hexoses and 5-carbon units called pentoses. Glucose, fructose, and galactose are examples of hexoses, and xylose and arabinose are examples of pentosans/pentoses. Since each monosaccharide is a primary form, they are seldom broken down by hydrolysis in the intestines. They are metabolized through metabolic pathways, e.g., glucose is metabolized through glycolysis to give ATP (energy) and pyruvic acid. Fructose can be converted into glucose.

They are commonly found in our regular diet and provide varying degrees of sweetness to the food such as ripe fruits like banana, grapes, fruit juices, and also some seaweeds, yeast, fungi, etc.

They are major sources of fuel/energy and are required for biosynthesis of many molecules. Monosaccharides and disaccharides are easily absorbed and thus, rapidly raise blood sugar level. People having diabetes, obesity, and many other chronic diseases should avoid consumption of foods rich in simple sugars. It is recommended that only about 10% of dietary energy should come from simple sugars.

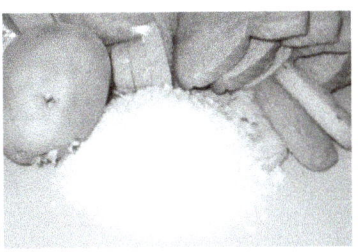

Glucose: Glucose is the principal form or basic building block of many carbohydrates such as starch, sucrose, glycogen, lactose, and maltose. Glucose is also formed during food processing or ripening of fruits. It is available in foods like fruits, sweet corn syrup, honey, and roots. It is an important monosaccharide because every other energy-yielding compound (except fat) must be converted into glucose first to obtain energy. It is a general precursor for many complex organic compounds in the body. Glucose is important for functioning of all tissues and is the prime fuel for brain, nerve cells, and red blood cells.

Excess of glucose is stored in the liver and muscles in the form of glycogen, and in adipose tissues in the form of triglycerides (fat). Glucose can enter cells with the help of the hormone "insulin", which is produced by the pancreas. The level of glucose in blood is used to indicate blood sugar level. Glucose is also required for synthesis of glycolipids, nucleic acids, and mucopolysaccharides.

Glucose in the blood is taken up by the body's cells and used to produce a fuel molecule called ATP through a series of complex processes known as cellular respiration. Cells can then use ATP to power a variety of metabolic tasks. Glucose is the form of carbohydrate that is utilized to produce energy by all cells but some organs must be supplied with glucose—these are brain, the medulla of the kidney, and red blood cells. The brain's requirement for glucose is about 140 g/day and that of anerobic tissues is approximately 40 g/day.

Fructose: It is also called fruit sugar because it is abundantly found in fruits, honey, and root vegetables. It is a component of sucrose (common or table sugar). Unlike glucose, fructose does not require insulin to be transported into muscles and fat cells. It is also part of fructooligosaccharides (FOS) and high-fructose corn syrup (HFCS). Relative sweetness of fructose (sweetest of all carbohydrates) is highest compared with other sugars. Fructose does not easily crystallize but absorbs moisture even at low relative humidity. Some fruits like dried fig and pear juice contain higher amounts of free fructose, which may cause some digestive disorders particularly among young children. In some cases, even in adults, fructose is not completely absorbed in the small intestine and reaches the large intestine intact, where it is fermented by microorganisms. The action of microorganisms results in gas formation causing bloating, and other digestive problems. Fructose is converted to glucose in the body through different biochemical pathway. Its excessive consumption may play a role in the emerging epidemic of obesity and associated disorders. Like glucose, fructose is also a source of energy.

Cells extract energy (in the form of ATP) from fructose only in the presence of oxygen that is called aerobic respiration. Although fructose gives the same amount of kilocalories as glucose, it is metabolized quite differently in the human body. After fructose is absorbed from the small intestines into blood, it is quickly taken up by the liver where a sizeable fraction (about one-third to one-half) is metabolized to glucose.

Fructose is first converted to fructose-1-phosphate, and further converted to glyceraldehyde and dihydroxyacetone phosphate. Both these products called triose phosphates are further metabolized by glycolysis. These triose phosphates may also condense together to form fructose-1,6-diphosphate, which is then converted through a series of steps to glucose-1-phosphate that is then used for producing glycogen (glycogenesis). Glycogen is the storage form of carbohydrate in mammals. Also, glucose can be produced from fructose but it does not contribute to the postprandial rise in blood sugar levels. Excess of fructose consumption leads to de novo lipogenesis (synthesis of fat molecules in the body), especially when it is consumed in liquid form. Hence it is a high risk for fatty liver and insulin resistance. There is no reverse mechanism for the fat that is synthesized from fructose to be converted back. Hence, it stays in the hepatocytes.

High-fructose corn syrup: This is a liquid sweetener used as an alternative to sucrose. It is manufactured from corn by chemical and enzymatic hydrolysis. The syrup that is obtained contains mostly glucose that then isomerizes to fructose, yielding HFCS. Three categories of HFCS are made—HFCS-90 contains 90% fructose and 10% glucose and is used in specialty applications. This is blended with glucose syrup to yield HFCS-42, containing 42% fructose and 58% glucose, and HFCS-55 that contains 55% fructose and 45% glucose. HFCS cost is relatively less than sugar. It is easy to use in soft drinks being in liquid form. It is slightly acidic so it has some preservative property. However, it is associated with increased incidence of obesity, diabetes, and other cardiovascular diseases, metabolic syndrome, and nonalcoholic fatty liver disease as well as high uric acid, it is associated health problems.

> **Research glimpse:** High intake of added sugar (table sugar or sucrose) and high-fructose corn syrup have been found to result in obesity, metabolic syndrome, and diabetes. Such sugars usually come from sugar-laden beverages, fruit juices, etc. Fructose has the ability to cause intracellular ATP depletion and increased production of uric acid and has lipogenic effects at high concentrations. Fructose-induced uric acid generation causes mitochondrial oxidative stress that stimulates fat accumulation independent of excessive caloric intake.
>
> *Johnson RJ, Nakagawa T, Sanchez-Lozada LG, et al. Sugar, uric acid, and the etiology of diabetes and obesity. Diabetes. 2013;62(10):3307-15*

> **Laboratory laurel:** Abdominal adiposity and visceral adipose tissue (VAT) have been reported to be independent factors for the increased risk for diabetes and cardiovascular diseases. In a cross-sectional study with 2,596 middle-aged individuals, habitual consumption of sugar-sweetened beverages and diet soda (carbonated beverages) was recorded by Food Frequency Questionnaire and VAT was assessed using computed tomography. An inverse association was observed between consumption of sugar-sweetened beverages and abdominal subcutaneous adipose tissue (SAT), whereas it was positively associated with VAT after adjusting for SAT. Diet soda consumption was positively associated with SAT but not with VAT or the VAT to SAT ratio.
>
> *Ma J, Sloan M, Fox CS, et al. Sugar-sweetened beverage consumption is associated with abdominal fat partitioning in healthy adults. J Nut. 2014;144(8):1283-90*

Mannose: Mannose, another monosaccharide, occurs freely in nature and is found in cranberries, red currants, black currants, peaches, gooseberries, aloe vera, soybeans, cabbage, beans, brinjal, capsicum, turnip, tomatoes, and broccoli. Fenugreek seeds contain a high amount of galactomannan, a polysaccharide, comprised of galactose and mannose. Mannose is absorbed eight times more slowly than glucose but reaches directly into the bloodstream and is distributed throughout the body tissues and fluids. Mannose is part of compounds called acute-phase proteins such as mannose-binding lectin (MBL) and mannose-binding protein (MBP). These are produced by the liver in response to infection and are important for innate immunity. During infection, bacteria tend to adhere to the epithelial lining of the target cells. However, in presence of mannose, bacteria attach themselves to the mannose molecules instead of adhering to the lining. Both bacteria and the mannose molecules are then expelled from the body, eliminating or reducing the chances of infection.

> **Laboratory laurel:** The mannose-binding lectin (MBL) belongs to the innate immunity system and recognizes and binds a variety of pathogens and thus protects the host. The genetic, biologic, and clinical properties of MBL have been studied intensively, although many aspects of its clinical relevance still remain to be discovered. MBL may serve as the first line of defence in the neonate whose own immune system is compromised. It may also be involved in neuronal migration, interneuronal recognition, and myelinization. Thus low MBL levels may increase risk of infections. However, given that MBL production is uncontrolled in some disorders, replacement therapy of MBL needs to be studied thoroughly and intensively before it is used especially for critically ill infants.
>
> *Auriti C, Prencipe G, Moriondo M, et al. Mannose-binding lectin: Biological characteristics and role in the susceptibility to infections and ischemia-reperfusion related injury in critically ill neonates. J Immunol Res. 2017:7045630.*

Galactose: Galactose is a component of lactose (milk sugar), but it is not available freely in nature. It is found not only in dairy products (all milks) and some hard cheeses, but also in some plant-based foods such as beans, lentils, sugar beet, avocado, bell pepper, papaya, watermelon, dates, mushrooms, olives, peanuts, as well as organ meats like liver, brain, and kidneys. All food items made from milk will contain galactose in small or relatively larger amounts. Galactose content ranges from less than 0.1 mg per 100 g of tissue in artichoke, mushroom, olive, and peanut to 35.4 mg per 100 g in persimmon. Fruits and vegetables like date, papaya, bell pepper, tomato, and watermelon contain more than 10 mg per 100 g. Galactose is a part of glycolipids and glycoproteins, which are present in cell membranes. Galactose in glycolipids is an essential component of the antigen that determines the blood groups (A, B, AB, and O). In liver, it is converted into glucose to release energy. It also supports the synthesis of gangliosides, which are primarily found in the myelin sheath around nerve fibers. Galactose has an important role in mitigating the growth of tumor cells and facilitating the immune process. In some body cells and connective tissues, it is present as galactosamine, glycoprotein, and mucopolysaccharides. Galactosemia is an inborn error of metabolism in which the individual lacks the galactose-1-phosphate uridyltransferase enzyme. This enzyme is necessary to break down the galactose into the glucose. Deficiency of this enzyme can cause galactosemia, an inborn error of galactose metabolism. Hence, there is a buildup of galactose in the blood which subsequently damages the liver, eyes, kidney, and brain. A person suffering from galactosemia needs to essentially live on a lactose-free and galactose-free diet throughout life.

Disaccharides

Disaccharides are composed of two monosaccharides linked together by *O*-glycosidic bond in which the oxygen from a hydroxyl group becomes linked to the carbonyl carbon. Different monosaccharides in varied combinations give different disaccharides. Three disaccharides are commonly known, namely sucrose, lactose, and maltose. Others are lactulose, trehalose, cellobiose, and chitobiose. These two types of disaccharide, e.g., lactose and lactulose contain same monosaccharides but differ in their basic structure, solubility and digestibility. Lactose is a milk sugar while lactulose is used as medicine in the treatment of constipation. Some uncommon disaccharides are isomaltose, turanose, melibiose, mannobiose, xylobiose and sophorose. Sucrose is composed of glucose and fructose; lactose is made up of glucose and galactose while maltose is a mix of two units of glucose only. In all three disaccharides, glucose is present. Disaccharides are soluble in water and sweet to taste, although they differ in their sweetness. They are freely found in nature (food). During digestion, disaccharides are hydrolyzed into their constituent monosaccharides, by the action of specific enzymes. Before they release energy, they need to be converted into glucose through metabolic reactions.

Sucrose: Sucrose, the most commonly used sugar, is also called table sugar. It is basically obtained from sugarcane and sugar beet. The white sugar crystals, we are familiar with, are obtained after processing and refining the juice. It is also found in many other foods like banana, dates, pineapple, peas, and sweet potato. Besides being used as a sweetener, sucrose is used as a preservative at high concentrations (>50%) in jams, jellies, and squashes. Sugar keeps things moist as it absorbs moisture easily (substances that are used to keep foods or other things moist are called humectants). It can easily be crystallized and caramelized and hence is used to make a wide variety of sweets and candies. However, sucrose is the main culprit in development of several health problems like tooth decay, skin problems, obesity, insulin resistance, diabetes, heart disease, etc. Since sucrose adds taste and flavor to food, persons of all ages tend to overconsume sugar-containing foods, gradually gain weight, and their risk for developing diabetes and/or heart disease increases.

Maltose: Maltose contains two molecules of glucose. It is not freely present in raw foods; rather it is produced when grains are malted or when foods are fermented. Malting is the process in which cereal/millet grains or pulses are sprouted and dried. During sprouting (germination), the cereal starch is converted into maltose by the action of the enzyme, α-amylase and gives rise to a typical flavor. Maltose is easily digestible. Malting is a process used to develop infant foods and amylase-rich foods (ARF) as well as to produce beer from barley.

Lactose: Lactose is composed of glucose and galactose. Lactose is not found in plant foods. It is synthesized in mammary glands where glucose is converted into galactose and then combined with glucose to produce lactose in the milk. Thus lactose is also called milk sugar. Mother's milk contains significant amount of lactose which is a major source of energy for infants. Lactose also helps in the absorption of calcium. Lactase, an enzyme present in the intestines, breaks down lactose into glucose and galactose, which are then absorbed. In the early years of life, lactase is present in sufficient amounts. However, as a person grows older, the synthesis of this enzyme by the intestines decreases. Thus for some people, digestion of milk becomes difficult as age progresses, due to lower amount or lack of lactase enzyme. Persons who cannot digest lactose (milk) are called lactose intolerant. For such persons, there are enzyme preparations available in the market. For lactose-intolerant infants, special formulas without lactose can be used.

> **Lactose intolerance:** Lactose intolerance is a clinical syndrome, which occurs in absence of the enzyme lactase, in the small intestine. Lactase helps to digest lactose present in milk. If lactase is deficient, digestion of lactose and milk is hampered. The symptoms are abdominal distension, cramps, and diarrhea. Lactose deficiency can be overcome by:
> 1. Removal of dairy products from the diet
> 2. Use of fermented dairy products like curd, where lactose is converted into lactic acid.
> 3. Addition of *Lactobacillus* or probiotics in the diet which help in digestion of lactose. They act in the large intestine in presence of gut flora.
> 4. Commercial preparations that are lactose free.

Dairy products like curd can be considered for persons having lactose intolerance. Such products are prepared by fermentation using starter culture of *Lactobacillus* sp., which converts lactose into lactic acid (due to which curd is sour). Such products are better digested than milk and beneficial for health in other ways. There is a probiotic effect of curd or yoghurt. Plant-based milk like soy milk, nut milk, and wheat milk can be suggested to lactose-intolerant people.

Sugar Alcohols or Polyols

Sugar alcohols are also known as "polyols" and have a Degree of Polymerization (DP) of 2. Sugar alcohols are derived from simple carbohydrates by substitution of the aldehyde group by a hydroxyl group. Some of them are naturally present in some fruits, e.g., sorbitol in plums. They are also synthesized commercially and are used in foods, beverages, and by the pharmaceutical industry. They are slowly or not completely absorbed by the human body. Therefore, they are used as alternative sweeteners as they do not raise blood sugar to the same extent that table sugar does, do not require insulin in order to be metabolized, and they provide less or negligible calories (0–3 kcal per gram). Their sweetness varies from 25% to 100% of the sweetness of sugar, i.e., sucrose. Thus they are good for diabetics and those who want to restrict sugar consumption. They are often used in combination with other sweeteners to obtain the desired flavor and sweetness.

Sugar alcohols
- Sorbitol
- Mannitol
- Xylitol
- Lactitol
- Maltitol
- Isomalt
- Erythritol
- Hydrogenated starch hydrolysate or polyglucitol

In the food industry, they are being substituted for sugar or corn syrup in development of many dietetic foods. This is because they have a mild sweet taste which can be used in the same volume as sugar and can add bulk to the food while giving almost half the amount of calories compared with sugar. Besides adding bulk, they also provide mouthfeel. Substitution for sugar or corn syrup can be done in a 1:1 ratio. They can be used to replace part or all the sugar in a food product giving low-sugar or sugar-free products. They decrease water activity in "intermediate moisture foods" and depending on the specific alcohol are used as softeners, glazing agents, humectants, stabilizers, thickeners, sequestrants, emulsifiers, anticaking agent, and rehydration of dehydrated food.

Polyols can also serve as prebiotics. However, their slow digestibility can also cause some gastric disturbances (gas and bloating) and have laxative effect if used in excess (more than 50 g a day). Therefore, these sweeteners need to be used in moderation and under guidance. They generally do not cause dental caries. Some of the sugar alcohols are discussed below:

Sorbitol: It is naturally present in fruits like pears, apples, peaches, apricots, and nectarines and plums as well as in dried fruits, such as prunes, dates, and raisins, and in some vegetables. Industrially, it is produced from either glucose or sucrose either in liquid or crystalline form. It is 60% as sweet as sucrose and provides 2.6 kcal/g. It is hygroscopic, chemically inert and stable and unlike sugar or glucose does not undergo Maillard reaction. Its glycemic index is 9. It gives a cooling sensation in the mouth and has a sweet and cooling taste. It is the most commonly used polyol that is derived from glucose.

Its digestion is rather slow; it is not well absorbed in infants, small children, and many adults. It ferments in the large intestine, producing gas, bloating and cramps or osmotic diarrhea or laxative effect on excessive intake (>10–30 g/day). Sorbitol is converted to fructose in the body. It is commonly used to make sugar-free food products such as hard candies, chewing gums, frozen desserts, baked goods, and other delicacies. It is used as a humectant to prevent loss of moisture from the food product in which it is used. It is also used to prevent crystallization.

Mannitol: Mannitol is present in pineapple, olive, sweet potato, and carrot. It is an isomer of sorbitol and is commercially manufactured by hydrogenation of specialty glucose syrups or glucose and fructose in a 1:1 mixture. In nature, mannitol is present in the exudates of some trees, and is present in some edible fungi and seaweed. Mannitol has about 50% of the sweetness of sugar; it is also converted to fructose but yields 2.1–2.4 kcal/g. Mannitol is not absorbed and hence does not cause much increase in blood glucose. Its glycemic index value is 0. Orally it has a cooling effect (but this is much less than that of other polyols) and helps to mask bitter taste.

It is not hygroscopic and is stable at high temperatures, therefore, used as a dusting powder for chewing gum to prevent sticking to wrappers or to the manufacturing equipment. It is also used in sugar-free hard candies, chocolates, and ice-cream, as well as in pharmaceuticals and nutrient tablets. Beisdes being used as a sugar substitute, it can be used as a fat substitute because it imparts a creamy texture to foods especially for preparation of low sugar and low-fat bakery foods. However, consumption of more than 10–20 g/day mannitol may cause gastric disturbances, diarrhea. Mannitol is an osmotic diuretic and is used clinically to reduce intracranial pressure and treat oliguric renal failure. Large doses of mannitol may increases excretion of sodium and potassium.

Xylitol: Xylitol is a five-carbon alchohol, produced from D-xylose and yields 2.4 kcal/g. Since its discovery in 1960s, it has been used as a sweetener. Its glycemic index is 13. It has very cooling sensation in mouth. Its major advantage is that it is not attacked by cariogenic bacteria, thus it inhibits tooth decay and formation of plaque. It is naturally found in plums, cherries, and berries as well as in some vegetables and oats. It is absorbed 50% in the small intestine, has the same sweetness as sucrose as well as bulk. It is the sweetest among the sugar alcohols. Use of xylitol is common in chewing gum and many dietetic products. Insulin is not required for its metabolism.

> **Laboratory laurel:** Xylitol has been used as a sugar substitute and is well known for its ability to prevent tooth decay. Hence, it has been used as an ingredient in chewing gum, because organisms such as *Streptococcus mutans* that cause cavities and dental caries cannot use xylitol as a source of energy. In this study, the effect of dietary xylitol was studied on influenza A virus infection (H1N1) in a mouse model. It was observed that survival of mice was enhanced when xylitol was administered with red ginseng, suggesting that there is a synergistic effect. Also with increasing dose of xylitol, the effect increased. Further, dietary xylitol together with the water-soluble fraction of red ginseng significantly reduced the lung virus titers after infection.
>
> Yin SY, Kim HJ, Kim HJ. *Protective effect of dietary xylitol on influenza a virus infection.* PLoS One. 2014;9(1):e84633.

Lactitol: It is 40% sweet as sucrose and yields 2.0 kcal/g. It is obtained from hydrogenation of lactose from milk. Its glycemic index is 6. It has a clean and mild sweet taste but has no aftertaste and cooling effect. Hence, it is often mixed with other sweeteners and is used as a thickener and emulsifier. Therapeutically, it is used for treating constipation in adults and older persons. Lactitol is observed to be more efficacious than lactulose. It is fermented by colonic bacteria and has a prebiotic effect. Common uses are as an ingredient in candies, chocolates, cookies, and cakes especially for diabetics as well as in low-calorie, low-fat and/or sugar-free foods including ice-creams, reduced-sugar preserves, and chewing gums.

Maltitol: Its sweetness is about 90% of the sweetness of sucrose/sugar but provides only 2.1 kcal/g. It is a disaccharide polyol consisting of glucose and sorbitol in equal part. It is produced by hydrogenation of high-maltose corn syrup or from starch. Its glycemic index is 35. Compared with the other polyols, it resembles sucrose the most in terms of characteristics. It is used with short-chain fructooligosaccharides (FOS) in production of sugar-free foods. Maltitol is used in coatings, chewing gum, jam, gelatin, and jelly. However, maltitol has a laxative effect; therefore, consumption should be limited. It may also be used to replace fat as it gives a creamy texture to food. Hence, it is suitable for making varied bakery products, especially because it is stable at high temperatures and has low hygroscopicity.

Isomalt: Isomalt is a bulk sweetener made from sucrose and can be used as replacement for sucrose. Its glycemic index is 9. It is a mixture of gluco-mannitol and gluco-sorbitol. Its sweetness is 45–65% of sucrose but does not crystallize as easily as sucrose. Therefore, it is used in sugar sculptures and decorative edible products. It has a low glycemic effect. Toffees, lollipops, fudge, chocolates, wafers, and cough drops may have this low sugar/calories ingredient. Isomalt absorbs very little water. Therefore, products made with it tend not to become sticky but have a longer shelf-life. Isomalt enhances flavor transfer in foods. It dissolves more slowly in the mouth so that candies with isomalt have a longer-lasting taste. It is stable to heat, but unlike other alcohols does not give a cooling sensation in the mouth. It is also used as a bulking agent, anti-caking agent, and for glazing purposes. It is anticariogenic and it has been found in toothpastes containing isomalt, enhanced remineralization of teeth. Very small amount of this sugar alcohol is absorbed and about 90% is fermented in the large intestine. It is a good prebiotic because its fermentation yields the short-chain fatty acid—butyric acid. However, consumption of large amounts may lead to laxation.

Erythritol: It is regarded as a next-generation sweetener. It is a natural-occurring component of some vegetables, fruits like pears, melons, and peaches, mushrooms, fermented beverages like wine, beer, and soya sauce. It is also a bulk sweetener, its glycemic index value is 0, and it can easily be mixed with other sugar alcohols. It is almost completely absorbed but is minimally metabolized in the human body, is poorly reabsorbed by the kidney, and is excreted in urine.

This characteristic is attributed to its high stability in acid and alkali and hot environment/high temperatures typically used in food production, thus it is suitable for use in baked products. Its sweetness is close to sucrose, making and is useful in low-calorie foods. It gives negligible calories (0.2 kcal/g) and is 70% sweet as sucrose. It is safe, has no aftertaste, and has the mouthfeel of sugar. It provides good gloss and melting characteristics. It gives baking stability and shelf-life stability, and is used in cakes, cookies, and other baked goods. It provides good texture to foods like ice-cream.

It is rapidly absorbed and rapidly eliminated by the digestive system. It is also present in some tissues of the human body such as lens, cerebrospinal fluid, and serum. It has been shown to have radical scavenging properties. Unlike other polyols, it has a laxative effect only at very high dose of about 1,000 mg/kg of body weight.

Polyglycitol (hydrogenated starch hydrolysate): The names polyglycitol or hydrogenated starch hydrolysate or polyglucitol are used interchangeably. This is a large group of hydrogenated glucose syrups, maltitol syrups, and sorbitol syrups that are manufactured using corn, wheat or potato starch. When the product contains more than 50% maltitol on a dry basis, they are called maltitol syrups whereas polyglycitols are those that contain less than 50% maltitol. They provide approximately 90% of the sweetness of sugar. They are used for a variety of purposes such as imparting desired viscosity, as bulk sweeteners, humectants, and to prevent recrystallization (because they do not crystallize). Calorie content depends on the composition of the final product and it is often used to replace corn syrup; but in general, it does not give more than 3 kcal/g, usually 2.4 kcal/g.

The advantage of using these is that they are nonreactive with other ingredients and colorless and odorless, used in food formulations such as colors, flavors or enzymes. They also improve freeze-thaw stability of frozen foods. In the human body, these products are acted upon by enzymes and hydrolyzed to sorbitol, glucose, and maltitol and only about one-tenth is converted to monosaccharides that are absorbed. The undigested part is fermented by the colonic microorganisms. If these products are consumed on an empty stomach, many times a day, there can be a laxative effect. They also exert an osmotic effect. However, doses of up to 45–90 g/day have been found to be well tolerated and did not exhibit a glycemic effect, indicating that these are useful as sweeteners for diabetics.

> **A Note of Caution:** Sugar alcohols are readily converted to glucose in the liver, especially when blood sugar is already high and carbohydrate intolerance is out-of-control. They can also be converted to fat, and may contribute to high triglycerides (a heart disease risk) and weight gain. In addition, sugar alcohols are becoming better known for their potent laxative effect and digestive upsets. Also, new researches signal the association of polyols with peripheral neuropathy in diabetics.

Oligosaccharides

Oligosaccharides contain 3–9 monosaccharide molecules. Thus, their degree of polymerization is in between that of simple sugars and polysaccharides. Raffinose, stachyose, gentiobiose, and verbascose are naturally occurring oligosaccharides found in some plant foods like legumes and soybeans, and dairy products such as yoghurt. In general, they are much less sweet (0.3–0.6 times) than sucrose. Sweetness of oligosaccharides decreases with an increase in the chain length. They are not easily digested in the human small intestine because the enzymes necessary for their hydrolysis are not present. Hence, they enter the large intestine in undigested or partially digested state. They are fermented by the gut (colonic) microorganisms/flora, and often produce flatus (gas) which gives rise to a feeling of bloating, e.g., after consuming pulses or drinking milk in some people. Also oligosaccharides do not require insulin and thus can be used in dietetic foods. Thus they are used as bulking agents, humectants and as anticariogenic substances. Because they are not digestible, they possess properties like that of dietary fiber and prebiotics. There are a numerous functional oligosaccharides in the food industry as well as pharmaceutical industries such as fructooligosaccharides, glucooligosaccharides, isomalt-oligosaccharides, soybean-meal oligosaccharides, mannan oligosaccharides, galacto-oligosaccharides, gentio-oligosaccharides, isomaltulose, lactosucrose, maltooligosaccharides, xylooligosaccharides, pectin-derived acidic oligosaccharides, and cyclodextrins. In nature, a variety of plant sources contain oligosaccharides such as wheat, rye, barley, soybean, pulses, mustard, milk, honey, sugarcane juice as well as some fruits, and vegetables like onion, asparagus, sugar beet, artichoke, chicory, leek, garlic, tomato, banana, yacón, and bamboo shoots.

> **Research glimpse:** Oligosaccharides are found in many types of bacteria, algae, fungi, and higher plants. They are not only used as food ingredients but also as pharmacological supplements. They possess functional properties of dietary fiber hence are beneficial in weight control. They behave as humectants so are useful in confectionery and baked goods. Being prebiotics they are effective in promoting the growth of normal intestinal flora/microorganisms and suppress pathogens. Other benefits include prevention of dental caries, facilitating mineral absorption, immunomodulatory action, and other potential therapeutic benefits such as anti-allergic, anti-inflammatory, antioxidant, and antiviral. These compounds are also being researched for their role in maintaining bone mass and density, apoptosis, antitumor/anticancer activity, and anti-obesity. In animal feed, oligosaccharides could serve as alternatives to antibiotics.
>
> *Patel S, Goyal A. Functional oligosaccharides: production, properties and applications. World J Microbiol and Biotechnol. 2011;27(5):1119–28.*

Fructooligosaccharides: They are nondigestible oligosaccharides that occur naturally in various edible plant foods such as grains, fruits, and vegetables such as wheat, banana, sugar beet, onion, tomato, and garlic, although the amount is relatively small. FOS is mainly composed of fructose units and provides sweet taste and good flavor. Fructooliogosaccharides is a subgroup of inulin with the degree of polymerization ranging from 2 to 10. They are not digested in the small intestine and thus provide only 1 kcal/g. Because of their low caloric density, they have the potential to be used in a variety of products such as artificial sweetener/sugar replacement in pastries, chocolates, ice-creams, etc. Its viscosity and stability in refrigeration widen its scope in many other products. The added advantage is that they are not cariogenic.

They reach the colon intact, where they are fermented by the colonic microflora and promote growth of microorganisms in the colon. Thus, they promote growth of microorganisms in the large intestine thus exhibit prebiotic effect. The colonic organisms ferment the FOS, and one of the end products of fermentation is short-chain fatty acids, which in turn confer some health benefits by reducing the risk of inflammatory diseases such as type 2 diabetes, obesity, heart disease, by reducing the cholesterol, triglyceride and blood glucose levels. FOS also provides some protection against pathogens like *Salmonella* and other organisms causing foodborne illness and other digestive disorders.

> **Laboratory laurel:** A randomized double blind crossover study was conducted to evaluate the impact of fructooligosaccharides (FOS) and galactooligosaccharides (GOS) on glycemic response on 35 adults. They were given FOS and GOS for 14 days (16 g/day) and tested for anthropometric measurements, oral glucose tolerance test (OGTT), and intestinal microbiota in feces samples. Short-term intake of high dose of FOS had adverse effect on glucose metabolism, as demonstrated by OGTT. With both FOS and GOS, significant increase in *Bifidobacterium*, and the butyrate-producing bacteria, *Phascolarctobacterium* in FOS group was observed while *Ruminococcus* in GOS group were decreased.
>
> *Liu F, Li P, Chen M, et al. Fructooligosaccharide (FOS) and Galactooligosaccharide (GOS) Increase Bifidobacterium but Reduce Butyrate Producing Bacteria with Adverse Glycemic Metabolism in healthy young population. Scientific Reports. 2017;7:11789.*

Maltooligosaccharides (Maltodextrin): Maltodextrin, a polysaccharide, is manufactured by partial hydrolysis of any starch using water, enzymes, and acid obtained from natural sources like potato, wheat, corn, rice, and tapioca. Maltodextrin is an easily digestible carbohydrate consisting of D-glucose units. It may be moderately sweet or without any distinct flavor, hence it is generally not used as a sweetener but can help in incorporating spices into foods/recipes. It has good texturizing, gelling, emulsifying, and noncrystallizing properties. It is used in a wide variety of food products and beverages such as pasta, baked foods, desserts, and energy and sports drinks, including gluten-free, baby foods and dietetic food products. It is also used in pharmaceutical industry. They provide 4 kcal/g. Since it is a highly refined form of carbohydrate, it tends to raise the blood sugar level faster. Hence foods containing maltodextrin are not good for diabetes. In food industry instead of degree of polymerization (DP) use of maltodextin is taken on the basis of a different parameter known as dextrose equivalent (DE). It is a measure of the percentage of reducing sugars in the maltodextrin relative to the percentage in glucose (100%). DE can also be calculated as 100/DP. Higher DE have lower DP. For example DE values in the range of 18–22 are often used successfully in making of gluten-free breads that is high in baked volume and long shelf-life by slowing starch retrogradation.

> **Research glimpse:** Human milk contains abundance of oligosaccharides (more than 100 different oligosaccharides) but newborns or infants cannot use them for energy purposes. However, human milk oligosaccharides (HMO) are very important because they support a healthy gut microbiome by stimulating the growth of beneficial microbes such as *Bifidobacterium*.
>
> *Thompson P, Garrido D. Chapter 5: Human Milk Oligosaccharides and health promotion through the gut microbiome. Dairy in Human Health and Disease Across the Lifespan. 2017:73-86.*

Polysaccharides

Polysaccharides are also known as complex carbohydrates. Polysaccharides contain numerous monosaccharide units linked together by glycosidic linkage. They are naturally found in plants, algae, seaweeds, and animals. Majority of the carbohydrates in our diets are polysaccharides. Different polysaccharides occurring in nature are shown in Table 2.3.

Some polysaccharides are digested in the human gastrointestinal tract, whereas others are not. Starch is digested whereas cellulose, hemicelluloses, beta-glucans, pectins, lignin, gums are not digested, hence they are referred to as non-starch polysaccharides (NSP). Different polysaccharides are shown in Figure 2.1.

Non-starch polysaccharides do not provide energy because they cannot be digested in the small intestine due to lack of the necessary enzymes. These indigestible polysaccharides are important prebiotics because, like FOS, they are utilized by the intestinal microflora. Their action generates short-chain fatty acids namely acetic acid, butyric acid, and propionic acid, which have health benefits.

Polysaccharides vary in their solubility, digestibility, and physical and physiological impact. In natural form, most of them (except pectin and agar) are insoluble in water. Temperature, pH, moisture, and combination with other molecules bring drastic changes in these polysaccharides. These properties are extensively exploited in cookery for preparation of various food products. Many of them are valued for their nutritional significance.

Starch: Starch is the storage form of energy in plants. It consists of only glucose units linked by α-(alpha) glycosidic linkage in linear or branched chains. Starch is generally present as granules in the form of mainly two components namely amylose and amylopectin. Amylose is a straight (linear) chain (polymer) of glucose molecules and amylopectin is a branched chain of glucose units.

Amylopectin is branched with 1, 6 linkages as well as 1, 4 linkages and may comprise more than 100,000 glucose residues. Starches from different food sources differ in their physiochemical properties and behavior due to differences in the amount of amylose and amylopectin present. This difference is exploited in making a wide variety of food products. The difference in the structure of starch molecules can easily be seen under a microscope. Amylose and amylopectin content of different foods are shown in Table 2.4. Most starches consist of 20–30% amylose and 70–80% amylopectin but pseudocereals like amaranth and quinoa contain about 8–12% amylose. The proportion of amylose to amylopectin in most starches is 1:3, but some starches like waxy varieties of maize or rice contain amylopectin and little or no amylose (ranging from 0–30%). Basmati rice has intermediate value. Amylose content is significantly variable by variety of the grain and tubers, milling and cooking characteristics.

Table 2.3: Different polysaccharides in plants and animals.

Polysaccharides in plants	Polysaccharides in animals	Functions
Starch, dextrin, and inulin	Glycogen	Storage or reserve substances
Cellulose, hemicellulose, and pectin	Chitin in shells of crustaceans	Structure-forming substances
Pectin, agar, and alginate	Mucopolysaccharides in connective tissues	Water-binding substances

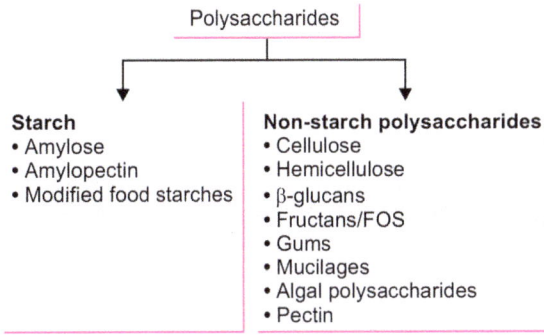

Fig. 2.1: Starch and non-starch based polysaccharides.

Table 2.4: Amylose and amylopectin in different sources of starch.

Source of starch	Amylopectin (%)	Amylose (%)
Rice	25	75
Wheat	24	76
Corn	28	72
Sorghum	22	78
Tapioca	17	83
Potato	22	78
Banana	21	79
Arrowroot	20	80
Sweet Potato	18	82
Waxy rice/corn	-	97–99

Source: Swaminathan M. Advanced Textbook on Food and Nutrition, Volume I. Bangalore: BAPPCO; 2002. p. 12

All grains, i.e., cereals and millets, pulses/legumes, and roots and tubers like potato, sweet potato, yam and tapioca are rich in starch. Starch is hydrolyzed by digestive enzymes in the intestines. Digestibility of high-amylopectin foods is better than those foods that contain amylopectin and amylose. Hence foods having high amylopectin and/or less amylose raise the blood sugar level (higher glycemic index) faster than foods that are high in amylose, and the proportion of amylose to amylopectin has an impact on insulin response to a food item. Basmati rice has higher amylose content as compared with other local rice varieties.

Starch-rich foods are classified based on amylose content, e.g., normal barley contains 25–27% amylose; waxy type (non-detectable and below 5% amylose), and high-amylose type contain more than 35% amylose. The ratio of amylose and amylopectin is an indicator of glycemic index. Amylose content also determines the texture of final product. Hence amylose can be used as a thickener, bulking agent, gelling agent, and water absorbent in preparations of puddings, cookies, and drinks.

Carbohydrates but more specifically starch is categorized as slowly digestible starch (SDS), rapidly digestible starch (RDS), and resistant starch (RS) based on how rapidly digestion by intestinal amylase takes place and will influence or determine the rise in plasma glucose. This classification also reflects the impact on postprandial blood glucose homeostasis and the associated metabolic as well as endocrine responses. Table 2.5 summarizes the characteristics of SDS, RDS, and RS.

Dextrin: Dextrin is a polymer of glucose units and is a byproduct of starch hydrolysis, which can be achieved by enzymatic degradation (salivary amylase in the mouth). Also treatment with dry heat like toasting, results in breakdown of starch to dextrin. This process is called dextrinization, which produces brown color and gives a distinct aroma to the food. This generally occurs in foods containing starch, like bread or chapati. Dextrin occurs naturally in potato, corn, wheat, etc. Dextrin is sweet in taste and easy to digest. Therefore, mastication in the mouth produces sweet taste and supports digestion. Toasted bread also tastes sweet upon chewing.

Resistant dextrin is a glucose polysaccharide that is not digestible. It is formed when starch is heated and treated with enzymes. It is fermented by the colonic microflora. In overweight adults, it has been found to have beneficial effects by reducing body weight and body mass index. It is possible that it may enhance satiety, which needs to be verified by further research.

Inulin: Inulin is a polymer of fructose units, naturally found in substantial amounts in Jerusalem artichoke and chicory tuber, although it is widely present in about 3,000 plants. Inulin, which is extracted from chicory root, is an oligosaccharide. It is used as a sucrose replacer as well as fat substitute. It gives only 25–35% of the energy obtained from digestible carbohydrates. Its sweetness is only one-tenth of the sweetness of sucrose. It gives about 1.5 kcal/g. It is not digested by human small intestines and can be used as a prebiotic. Inulin has been shown to increase *Bifidobacteria* in the colon. It helps in growth of healthy bacteria and reduces toxins and carcinogens. It has been shown to reduce lipid levels, i.e., triglycerides and cholesterol in blood. It also improves mineral absorption and activates the immune system and is useful in diabetes and weight management. It is also used in bakery products and ice-creams.

Modified starches: Starch has limited use in its native form. Therefore, its functional properties are modified by several physical and chemical methods, mainly to provide specific functional properties. The native starch that is modified and produced by various processes is called modified starch, e.g., pregelatinized starch and extruded starches. Different processes are used such as oxidation, esterification, hydroxymethylation, dextrinization, cross-linking, etc. By subjecting the native starch to the process, the stability of the starch to severe heat, shearing, freezing, etc. is improved significantly. Modified starches have a significant role in food industry for developing food products. Modified starches are used as thickeners, emulsifiers, binders, and stabilizers for bakery products and confectionery. They are polymers that are used in microencapsulation for oil-based flavors, micronutrients, fragrances, agrichemicals, and pharmaceuticals. Modified starches also have non-food applications such as in the textiles industry.

> **Modified starch** is also used in making edible films and the functionality of films is based on the ratio of amylose to amylopectin in the starch. High amylose content produces elastic films whereas high-amylopectin starch leads to films exhibiting poor mechanical properties. Chemical modifications of starch including acetylation and oxidation may be used to improve edible films properties.

Table 2.5: Characteristics of the three types of starch.

Rapidly digestible starch (RDS)	Slowly digestible starch (SDS)	Resistant starch (RS)
• Present in freshly cooked starchy foods • Rapidly digested • Absorbed in the duodenum and proximal regions of the small intestine leading to a rapid elevation of blood glucose and usually a subsequent episode of hypoglycemia. • Glucose is released within 20 minutes after digestion • These rapid and large increase in blood glucose levels can further lead to cell, tissue, and organ damage • *Sources:* Cooked starchy cereals or cooked potato still warm.	• Present in most raw cereals, legumes, and pasta • Digested slowly throughout the small intestine to provide sustained glucose release with a low initial glycemia and subsequently a slow and prolonged release of glucose, leading to prolonged energy availability, compared with more rapidly digestible starch • Glucose is released between 20 minutes and 120 minutes after digestion • *Sources:* Raw cereals, pasta, and legumes.	• It is not digested in the upper gastrointestinal tract, but is fermented by the colonic microflora, producing short-chain fatty acids that provides additional energy to the body along with butyrate that is beneficial to colonic health • Starch is not hydrolyzed even after 120 minutes • *Sources:* Unripened banana or plantain, partially milled cereals.

Non-starch Polysaccharides (NSP)

Plant substances, especially plant cell wall, contain a variety of polysaccharides, which differ in their chemical composition. Although they are polysaccharides, their structures are different from amylose and amylopectin, and they have a high molecular weight. NSPs are made up of the hexose sugars like glucose, galactose, and mannose, deoxyhexoses such as rhamnose and fucose, and glucuronic and galacturonic acids, and pentose sugars like arabinose and xylose. These complex carbohydrates are generally part of the cell wall in plants. They are not digested or absorbed in the small intestine. Examples of NSPs include cellulose, hemicelluloses, and pentosans. Hemicellulose (e.g., arabinoxylan) contains a mixture of hexose and pentose sugars, often in highly branched chains. Pectin is present in all cell walls. It is primarily a galacturonic acid polymer, although 10–25% other sugars such as rhamnose, galactose, and arabinose, may also be present as side chains.

Some polysaccharides are obtained from microorganisms and some are now industrially synthesized. These physical properties confer important physiological benefits. NSPs can be classified based on their solubility as:
- *Cellulose*: It is not soluble in water, alkali or dilute acids.
- *Non-cellulosic polymers:* These are partially soluble in water. Examples are arabinoxylans mixed linked beta-glucans, mannans, galactans, xyloglucan, and fructan.
- *Pectic polysaccharides:* These are polygalacturonic acids, which may be substituted with arabinan, galactan, and arabinogalactan.

Non-starch polysaccharides share some important physical properties such as water-holding capacity, gelling capacity, viscosity, susceptibility to fermentation, inhibiting digestive enzymes, and the capacity to bind bile acids. Thus, they confer several health benefits such as being fermented by colonic microflora resulting in increased fecal bulk and production of short-chain fatty acids, and reducing blood cholesterol levels as they reabsorb bile acids.

Cellulose: In plants, cellulose gives rigidity and strength to plant cell walls. Cellulose consists of long-straight chains of glucose units (may contain up to around 15,000 glucose units). Though both cellulose and starch contain glucose as the monomer, the difference in the linkage makes these two macromolecules different. In cellulose, the glucose units are linked by a different bond (β1-4) that cannot be cleaved by digestive enzymes in the human gastrointestinal tract, hence it does not provide energy. Cellulose is present in bran of cereals, millets, and pulses as well as nuts, vegetables, and fruits. It provides bulk to the food and gives satiety. It is one of the major sources of insoluble fiber. Cellulose is considered as dietary fiber which has several health benefits. In food industry, modified or semisynthetic polysaccharides are used such as carboxymethylcellulose (CMC), methyl cellulose, hydroxypropyl methylcellulose, hydroxypropyl cellulose, and ethyl hydroxyethyl cellulose.

Hemicelluloses: Hemicelluloses are also polymers but unlike starch and cellulose, they are a diverse group containing several monosaccharides such as xylose, arabinose and glucuronic acid in a branched structure. They are present along with cellulose in plant cell walls. Hemicelluloses are present in the outer bran layer of cereals, and legumes such as rolled oats and oat bran, as well as in vegetables. Wheat and rye contain arabinoxylans, which are formed from "pentosans" like xylose and arabinose. Arabinoxylans, which are generally found in cell walls of monocotyledons, influence intestinal fermentation, utilization of minerals (calcium and magnesium), and reduce cholesterol. They have water-holding capacity and therefore have an effect on viscosity. They also bind heavy metals. Hemicellulose helps to bind heavy metals like lead, copper, and cadmium.

> **Laboratory laurel**: Xylan, a hemicellulose, has immunomodulatory effects. It has been combined with chitosan to form a composite hydrogel to improve the healing of bone fractures. This gel is thermally responsive, and injectable form is liquid at room temperature and gels at physiological temperature. Xylan has shown a better response on animal host tissue than do pure chitosan hydrogels in tissue-engineered models. In the present study, a composite hydrogel was replaced by host tissue within a week, much before replacement occurred when chitosan hydrogels were used. In mice, when it was tested in a tibia fracture model, major remodeling of the fracture callus occurred within 4 weeks. The composite hydrogel supported healing of bone regeneration. The study revealed that the xylan/chitosan composite hydrogel can serve as a suitable bone graft substitute for helping in repair of large bones defects.
>
> *Bush JR, Liang H, Dickinson M, et al. Xylan hemicellulose improves chitosan hydrogel for bone tissue regeneration. Polym Adv Technol. 2016;27(8):1050–55.*
>
> **Laboratory laurel**: A modified rice bran hemicellulose (MRBH) was prepared from rice bran treated with shiitake enzymes. The effect of this water-soluble MRBH- and vascular endothelial growth factor (VEGF)-induced angiogenesis was studied. MRBH was found to inhibit VEGF-induced tube formation in human umbilical vein endothelial cells co-cultured with human dermal fibroblasts and there was a dose-dependent suppression of VEGF-induced proliferation and migration of these cells. It appears that MRBH reduces activation of VEGF receptor 2 by VEGF as well as some downstream signaling proteins. Thus in vitro findings indicated that MRBH has antiangiogenic effects. This has implications for diseases where angiogenesis is implicated such as cancer, rheumatoid arthritis, psoriasis, atherosclerosis, and retinal neovascularization.
>
> *Zhu X, Okubo A, Igari N, et al. Modified rice bran hemicellulose inhibits vascular endothelial growth factor-induced angiogenesis in vitro via VEGFR2 and its downstream signaling pathways. Biosci of Microbiota Food Health. 2017;36 (2):45–53.*

Pectins: Pectins (pectic substances) consist of galacturonic acid (a sugar acid) and other sugars such as arabinose, rhamnose, and galactose. Pectin is a part of the cell wall of all plants. It acts like a cementing substance to hold the cells together and helps to maintain the shape of the fruit or vegetable. Many fruits like guava, apple, strawberries, and citrus peel are good sources of pectin. Pectic substances are water soluble and when mixed with sugar, form a network in the interstices of which water is trapped, thus forming a gel. The characteristic texture of jam, marmalade, and fruit jellies is because of the pectin. In immature fruits, pectin is present in the form of protopectin, which is converted to pectin during ripening. When fruits become overripe, pectin is converted into pectic acid which no longer has the gelling capacity and the overripe fruit becomes soft and mushy. In food industry, pectins are also used as thickener in sauces and salad dressings.

Gums: Gum is a generic name for polysaccharides that have great affinity for water. Gums occur naturally in some foods like oatmeal, barley, and legumes. Some gums are also synthesized by microorganisms. Gums are also of animal origin such as chitin and chitosan, chondroitin sulfate, and hyaluronic acid. Seed gums are colored amorphous products characterized by forming viscous or clear solutions when dispersed or dissolved in cold or hot water.

There are three major categories of gums—natural gums, modified gums, and synthetic gums.
- Natural gums are a group of substances secreted by plants at the site of injury, i.e., tree exudates. Several trees are tapped for their gums. Many of these belong to the *Acacia* family. For example, gum arabic is obtained from *Acacia senegal* or *Acacia seyal*. Besides this, gums can be extracted from some legumes and are called extractive gums such as guar gum or locust bean gum. Seaweeds are also a source of gum, i.e., hydrocolloids.
- Modified gums are natural gums that have been chemically modified or produced from either cellulose or starch.
- Synthetic gums are synthetized gums, e.g., polyvinylpyrrolidone (PVP) and ethylene oxide polymers.

When mixed with water, they form a viscous solution. These have been exploited by man for years. In India, edible gum is valued for its health benefits. Gums are composed of a variety of sugars and their derivatives. Some of the commonly occurring sugars in gums are galactose, arabinose, mannose, and glucuronic acid. Gums are important for their gel-forming properties and are used extensively in the food industry as thickeners, stabilizers, and to add texture to the foods. Examples are given in Table 2.6.

Industrially, different gums are used for different purposes/in different food products. For example, guar gum and locust bean gum are used for water retention and stabilizing the products, whereas carrageenan is used as a stabilizer in ice-creams, meat products, and instant pudding. Agar is used in dairy products, confectionery, and meat products. Gums like gum arabic, tragacanth, pectins, alginates, and xanthan gum are used in confectionery, beverages, baked goods, as well as in sauces.

Gums are also used in pharmaceutical industry in a wide variety of products ranging from products used for cough suppression, as bulk laxatives, tablet binders, emulsifiers, suspending agents, stabilizing agents, thickening agents, for forming transdermal and periodontal films, as well as coating material for microcapsules.

As the name suggests gums bind the substances. They are being used as healing agents such as chondroitin sulfate, and hyaluronic acid are popularly being used to cartilage repairing as in arthritis. Supplementation of gum arabic (10 g/day) have beneficial effects on fat metabolism and fasting plasma glucose. At the same time it require culinary experience as it may give unfavorable viscous sensation in the mouth. Excess is not advisable.

Mucilages: Mucilage is a slimy substance synthesized by plants to protect the endosperm of the seed. Mucilage is composed of arabinose, rhamnose, and galacturonic acid. Black gram contains mucilages thus making the pulse slimy. The same components produce better results during fermentation of dal with rice for idli/dosa preparation. Ladies finger and colocasia root also contain mucilages. Mucilages are gel-forming that bind plant cells together. A good example of mucilage is psyllium that has been used traditionally in India to relieve constipation. Industrial uses of mucilages are similar to the applications for which gums are used.

Beta-glucans: β-glucans are non-starch polysachharides, a branched polymer of D-glucose, with different linkages, i.e., β-linkage. Due to this, the property and behavior of carbohydrate molecules change. They are mainly present in the cell walls of cereal grains especially in oats and barley, with the content ranging from 5.5 g to 9.0 g in oat bran to 4.0 g to 8.5 g in barley. They are also found in yeast but the type of linkage differs. It imparts smooth creamy mouthfeel and hence, it is used commercially as a fat substitute in foods. They are well recognized for lowering blood cholesterol and lowering glycemic index of the food. The functional properties of β-glucan make it suitable for use as a thickening, stabilizing, emulsification, and gelation agent. Thus, this is a functional ingredient that can be used in soups, sauces, beverages, and other food products, giving not only a smooth mouthfeel to these beverages but also a good source of dietary fiber. Incorporation into bread has been shown to improve the loaf volume.

> **Laboratory laurels**: Beta-glucans are present in the bran of cereal brans like that of barley and oats, and in smaller amounts in rye and wheat. They are also present in the cell wall of baker's yeast, some of fungi, and mushrooms. Beta-glucans have been shown to have hypocholesterolemic effect. The mechanisms for the effect are threefold which include binding cholesterol and bile acids, thereby reducing their absorption in the intestines; enhancing bile acid production which results in a net reduction in cholesterol that is the precursor molecule for bile acids. Also they are fermented by colonic microflora, generating short-chain fatty acids that are absorbed and inhibit synthesis of cholesterol. Other benefits conferred with include lower rise in blood sugar levels postprandially, as well as insulin responses. They (beta-1,3-glucans) are also involved in immune modulation, enhancing the immune capacity, and prevention of hepatic damage. However, soluble and insoluble beta-glucans differ in their mode of action and overall biological activity, and thus applications of these are different. These natural molecules are valuable for their therapeutic effects.
>
> *Ahmad A, Anjum FM, Zahoor T, et al. Beta glucan: a valuable functional ingredient in foods. Crit Rev Food Sci Nutr. 2012;52(3):201–12.*
>
> *Sofi S, Singh J, Rafiq S et al. β-glucan and functionality: A Review. EC Nutrition. 2017;10.2:67–74.*
>
> *Šíma P, Vetvicka V, Vannucci L. β-glucans and cholesterol (Review). Int J Mol Med. 2018;41(4):1799–1808.*

Table 2.6: Types of gums.

Types of gums	Examples
Seed/root gums	Locust bean gum, and guar gum
Exudate gum (tree extract)	Gum arabic, gum ghatti, gum karaya, and gum tragacanth
Microbial polysaccharides	Xanthan gum, gellan gum, curdlan, dextran, and pullulan

Glycogen: Glycogen is another polysaccharide found only in animals, including humans and hence, is also called animal starch. Glycogen like starch consists of several hundreds of glucose units linked together (its structure is similar to amylopectin but it is more branched than amylopectin). Glycogen is not an important dietary source of carbohydrate but is an important "reserve" energy for the body, since excess glucose is converted into glycogen (the process is called glyconeogenesis) and stored in the skeletal muscles and liver of the mammalian body. Whenever body requires extra energy, glycogen is broken down into glucose to produce energy. This process is called glycogenolysis. The human body can store about 200–500 g of glucose which can sustain the body for approximately 12 hours. However, athletes are able to increase their glycogen stores to improve performance by adopting a "carbohydrate-loading" regime.

Mucopolysaccharides: Mucopolysaccharides or glycosaminoglycans are heteropolysaccharides that are long unbranched polysaccharides consisting of long chains of repeating units of disaccharides, hexosamines (sugar-containing nitrogen), and non-nitrogenous sugars. As the name suggests, they are mucus-like substances, naturally found in extracellular cavities and connective tissue, although the pattern of distribution in the same tissue changes with maturation and aging. They provide lubrication and protection from pressure and injury by behaving like a shock absorber.

Hyaluronic acid (HA) is one such mucopolysaccharide consisting of repeating units of D-glucuronic acid (sugar) and N-acetyl-D-glucosamine. It is found in abundance in mucus membranes and fluids like synovial fluid surrounding load-bearing joints and virtually in every part of the body such as the vitreous fluid of the eye, as well as in cartilage, heart, intervertebral disks of the spine and in the fluids of the middle and inner ear, and support maintenance of structure of the eyeball and other organs. Hyaluronic acid has diverse biological functions such as control of tissue hydration and water transport. Because it binds water (it is hydrophilic), it lubricates movable parts of the body, e.g., bones, cartilages, skins, and tendons. It is also involved in many receptor-mediated roles in cell detachment, mitosis, migration, tumor development and metastasis, and inflammation. It has antibacterial activity and maintains skin elasticity.

Many nutrients like magnesium, zinc, sulfur, iron, and vitamin C are required for its synthesis. The production of HA is slowed down with age, resulting in joint problems but supply of these nutrients in sufficient amounts can retard the degradation of joints associated with age. Besides lubrication and strengthening of joints, HA supports elasticity and moisture of skin and eyes. Hyaluronic acid is found in animals, and in foods like soy. Foods that are good sources of nutrients required for synthesis of hyaluronic acid would support synthesis of hyaluronic acid.

Lipopolysaccharides: These are also known as lipoglycans or endotoxins. Lipopolysaccharide (LPS) is a major component of the outer membrane of some bacteria, especially gram-negative bacteria. When gram-negative bacteria die, lipopolysaccharide is released. LPS is a potent stimulant of innate immunity. It has many undesirable effects such as causing fever, leukocytosis, iron deficiency, platelet aggregation, thrombocytopenia (deficiency of platelets in the blood), and disorders in blood clotting. It is implicated in the pathogenesis of many inflammatory diseases. LPS can increase permeability of the gastrointestinal tract leading to "leaky gut". They are used in supplements as for immunomodulatory effect.

RECOMMENDED DIETARY ALLOWANCE FOR CARBOHYDRATES

In 2020, The Expert group of the Indian Council of Medical Research (ICMR) and National Institute of Nutrition (NIN) have issued RDA for carbohydrates for Indian population. The minimum amount of total carbohydrate (CHO) required, either from endogenous or exogenous sources, is determined by the brain's requirement for glucose. Studies have revealed that the brain can function under prolonged starvation by utilizing keto acids obtained from the breakdown of fats and proteins in the body (*in vitro*). It has been established that the utilization of glucose after the age of 1 year is the same as in childhood or adulthood. Hence the Recommended Dietary Allowance (RDA) for carbohydrates is set at 130 g/day after the age of one year which is given in Table 9.1A in Chapter 9. However, there is an increase in CHO requirement during pregnancy and lactation, i. e. 175 g and 200g/day respectively. Considering the high prevalence of obesity and associated diseases, cultural and dietary practices and physical activity patterns as well as socio-economic factors, scientific communities are advocating that we should obtain 55–60 of energy (En%) from CHO ; proteins should provide 10–15 En% and 20–30% of En should come from fats. Since carbohydrate intake should be provided mainly by complex carbohydrates, it is necessary to know the percentage of simple carbohydrate or free sugar or added sugar that can be consumed. The World Health Organization (2015) has provisionally recommended a further reduction of free sugars to less than 5%. Thus, in view of the rising trend of diseases including weight gain and overweight/obesity, dental caries etc in which free sugar plays harmful role, it is good to restrict dietary free sugars to 5–7 En%. The upper limit for the same has not been suggested yet in India.

A minimum of 30% calories should come from carbohydrates every day to prevent exhaustion and ketosis. Ketone bodies can have an adverse effect on fetal development. In lactation, fasting should not be undertaken nor should the carbohydrate intake be too low such that the mother goes into a ketotic state.

Very low-carbohydrate diets have been advocated for weight loss. However, some studies have shown that such diets in the long term are not more effective in terms of promoting weight loss as compared to low-fat diets or low-glycemic diets. Long-term adherence to a very low-carbohydrate diet that inevitably entails increasing the fat intake is difficult. Also, there is not much information on the safety of such high-fat, and low-carbohydrate diets.

Research glimpse: Added sugars consist of monosaccharides and disaccharides that are added during the production and preparation of foods and beverages and do not include sugars naturally found in milk, fruit, and fruit juice. These include sucrose, fructose, glucose, starch hydrolysates, syrups like glucose syrup, and other isolated sugar preparations.

Erickson J, Sadeghirad B, Lytvyn L, et al. The scientific basis of guideline recommendations on sugar intake: A Systematic Review. Ann intern Med. 2017;166(4):257–67.

FOOD SOURCES OF CARBOHYDRATES

Table sugar or sucrose is a pure simple carbohydrate. Major carbohydrate sources in Indian diets are cereals, pulses, roots, sugar, sweetened foods, and beverages as well as fruits. Many of these foods are our staple foods. Cereals like rice, wheat, and millets like jowar, ragi, bajra, and maize, and pulses like moong, urad, and chana provide 50–60 g of carbohydrate per 100 g of raw food. In today's world, however, ultraprocessed foods and beverages are contributing considerable amount of added sugars. Processing like milling wheat to make refined flour like maida, further increases the carbohydrate content because the dietary fiber, some protein, and fat is lost when the bran is removed. Potato, beetroot, sweet potato, yam, and banana are often blamed for high carbohydrate but contain much less than cereals and pulses, because they have a higher moisture content. Surprisingly potato, sweet potato, tapioca, yam, beet root, carrot, banana contain 14.9, 24.2, 17.8, 17.6, 6.18, 6.71 and 23.4 grams of carbohydrates per 100g raw food (IFCT, 2017). In general vegetables including green leafy vegetables and many fruits including sapota (chikoo) and watermelon are low in carbohydrates. Dried form of fruits like dried dates and dried apricot contain 72 and 70% carbohydrates. Animal foods including milk and curd are low in carbohydrates but sweets made from *khoa* contain very high in it because of concentrated form of milk and addition of sugar. Since carbohydrates particularly sugar provide sweetness and also cause high glycemic response and harmful to the body. White sugar can be replaced with jaggery, palm sugar, raisins, dates or naturally sweet food in limited amount. Carbohydrate content of several commonly consumed food items are given in Appendix 1.

The carbohydrate content of food was calculated very simply by difference, i.e., by subtracting the amount of protein, fat, fiber, ash, and moisture or water present in the food.

Carbohydrate = 100 – [crude protein + crude fat + crude fiber + ash (total minerals) + moisture content].

Added-sugar: 'Refers to sugars and syrups added to foods and drinks during processing and preparation.

Free sugars: Refers both to added sugars, like sucrose or table sugar, and sugars naturally present in honey, syrups, fruit juices and fruit concentrates. Most free sugars consumed are added to foods and drinks. Free sugars do not include sugar that is naturally present in milk and milk products.

Report of the Expert group on Consumption of fat sugar and salt and its health effects on Indian Population (FSSAI, 2017)

Contd...

Contd...

Free sugars include monosaccharides and disaccharides added to foods and beverages by the manufacturer, cook or consumer, and sugars naturally present in honey, syrups, fruit juices and fruit juice concentrates.
Guideline: Sugars intake for adults and children. WHO (2015).

CONSEQUENCES OF INADEQUATE CARBOHYDRATE INTAKE

In order to survive and provide energy for vital activities, a minimum of 100–130 g carbohydrates is needed by healthy adults. However, in certain conditions like illness, starvation or dieting, some individuals may not consume even this small amount. There are some dietary regimes that advocate low intake of carbohydrates. In low-carbohydrate diets, the meal plans focus on consumption of high amount of protein including meats and other animal-based foods resulting in high consumption of protein and fat.

In general, the body does not store much carbohydrate, except for some limited amount being stored in the liver and muscle. In absence of carbohydrates and glucose, first the body utilizes its limited glycogen stores. Then the body utilizes muscle tissue/lean body mass, using the protein for energy, resulting in loss of muscle tissue. In addition, the body utilizes either the fat in the diet and/or from the body fat stores (adipose tissue). The liver starts synthesizing ketone bodies by partial breakdown of free fatty acids. The formation of ketone bodies (ketones) is known as ketosis. Acetoacetic acid, beta-hydroxybutyric acid, and acetone are the ketone bodies. These are used to provide energy for vital activities in absence of sufficient carbohydrates. Among these three ketones, acetone is produced in smallest amounts and being volatile, it is excreted through the lungs, making the breath "fruity" in odor. Acetoacetic acid and beta-hydroxybutyric acid are negatively charged (H^+) ions. Presence of these negatively charged H^+ ions in blood, leads to changes in blood pH making it more acidic. Continued production of ketones can overwhelm the body leading to a state of acidosis.

In order to neutralize these ions, Na^+ is used and ketone bodies are then excreted in urine. Thus, if ketone bodies are produced in large amounts, loss of sodium (Na^+) from the body also occurs. Also, such low-carbohydrate diets have been found to lead to increased urinary loss of calcium and cause micronutrient deficiencies. Concomitantly, the H^+ ions can be buffered by bicarbonate ions (HCO_3^-) and other buffer systems. This can lead to a drop in blood bicarbonate, leading to more labored breathing (the person may gasp for breath). Thus, ketone bodies alter normal pH of blood and have harmful effects on health, leading to dizziness, vertigo, and coma. Ketones in the blood often rise during starvation, and with intakes of high-protein diet and low-carbohydrate diet.

Brain needs constant supply of glucose but during fasting or very low-carbohydrate intake (<20 g per day) brain has insufficient supply of glucose. There is altered mechanism to support constant supply to the central nervous system or brain. Then ketogenesis plays vital role via production of oxaloacetate. Brain cannot use fatty acids as an energy source (because they cannot cross the blood-brain barrier). They tend to have high body fat. Restriction of carbohydrate by them tends to improve glycemic control, HbA1c, lipid markers especially triglycerides, and also support weight loss. However, it should be noted that diabetic persons should monitor their blood glucose when they decide to consume very low-carbohydrate diets in order to prevent hypoglycemia. Whatever amount of carbohydrates is consumed, whole-grain cereals are to be preferred and intakes of red meat, processed meats, and refined cereals, sugar-containing foods and beverages should be reduced.

CONSEQUENCES OF EXCESSIVE INTAKE OF CARBOHYDRATES

Excessive intake of carbohydrate is common because our daily staple foods like rice, dal, and chapati, and pleasure foods like sweets, sweet beverages, soft drinks, ice-creams, and beverages are rich in carbohydrates. In addition, some of these foods also contain high amount of fat. Further people are now accustomed to rely on or overconsume ultraprocessed foods and beverages, which contain good amount of added sugars and fewer amounts of important nutrients like protein, fiber, vitamins, and minerals, and engage in less physical activity to utilize the energy. There are many such factors which result in negative consequences of excessive carbohydrate intake. It leads to overweight, obesity, diabetes, heart disease, high cholesterol level, high triglycerides, tooth decay, and other associated health problems. Ultraprocessed foods and beverages are energy-dense or contain "empty" calories and often tasty and accessible resulting in overconsumption. Sometimes carbohydrate-rich foods like sweets and chocolates become part of social prestige and acceptance.

Reasons for Excessive Carbohydrate Intake
- Staple foods like cereals and pulses are rich in carbohydrates
- High palatability and irresistible instinct towards sweet food
- Ignorance of carbohydrate content of food
- Ignorance of consequences which occur after many months and years
- Convenient lifestyle
- Easy accessibility and affordability of such foods.

Sugar promotes growth of bacteria in the dental plaque. Bacteria ferment sugar, and produce acid which eats up the tooth enamel, and expand the surface for further bacterial growth. Gargling and brushing teeth after meals and before sleep is good way to prevent tooth decay.
Sugar craving is an irresistible desire to eat something sweet. It stimulates the dopamine in the pleasure center of the brain and exerts satiation.

Simple sugars, when consumed in excess can easily be converted into fat and stored in adipose tissues. They can also raise the triglyceride and cholesterol levels in the blood. They can raise blood sugar level rapidly followed by a quick fall in blood sugar, which results in frequent episodes of hunger and overeating, eventually resulting in weight gain. Hence reducing consumption of simple sugars including high-fructose corn syrup, refined flours through various processed foods can help prevent weight gain and other maladies such as:
- Overweight and obesity
- Elevated blood triglyceride levels
- Increase in LDL cholesterol (especially caused by simple sugars)
- Decrease in HDL cholesterol levels
- Tooth decay and dental caries
- Autoimmune diseases
- Inflammation and inflammatory diseases
- Insulin resistance—predictor of diabetes II
- Polycystic ovary syndrome (PCOS)
- Depression
- Poor bone health
- Stiffness and acidity in the body
- Increased craving for sweet food.

Dietary Fiber

Dietary fiber (DF) (commonly called roughage or bulk) is a term that refers to food material, particularly plant material that is not hydrolyzed by enzymes secreted by the human digestive tract but that may be digested by microflora in the gut. The key characteristic of dietary fiber is nondigestibility. The undigested food constituents, which reach the colon, include non-starch polysaccharides such as cellulose and hemicelluloses. Dietary fiber also includes gums and mucilages, pectin, lignin, resistant dextrins, and resistant starch, polyols, and nondigestible oligosaccharides. Dietary fibers include both storage and structural polysaccharides. Pectin, gums and mucilages, cellulose, and hemicelluloses are present in plant cell walls and chitin and chitosan present in animals. Although most of the dietary fiber is constituted by carbohydrates, it also contains some waxes and indigestible cell wall proteins present in the plant cell wall.

Various definitions have been given by expert groups such as the American Association of Cereal Chemists, US Institute of Medicine, and Codex Alimentarius Commission.

The Codex Alimentarius Commission (2010) has defined dietary fiber as carbohydrate polymers derived from a plant origin, which may include fractions of lignin and/or other compounds associated with polysaccharides in the plant cell walls with ten or more monomeric units, which are not hydrolyzed by the endogenous enzymes in the small intestine (SI) of humans and belong to the following categories:
- Edible carbohydrate polymers naturally occurring in the food as consumed
- Carbohydrate polymers, which have been obtained from food raw material by physical, enzymatic or chemical means and which have been shown to have a physiological effect of benefit to health as demonstrated by generally accepted scientific evidence by competent authorities.
- Edible synthetic carbohydrate polymers the beneficial physiological effect of which is proven by generally acknowledged scientific evidence.

However, such compounds are not included in the definition of dietary fiber if extracted and reintroduced into a food. It is left to each national authority competent authorities to decide whether carbohydrates with 3-9 monomeric units should be considered as dietary fiber.

Dietary fiber means carbohydrate polymers with a degree of polymerization not lower than 3, which are neither digested nor absorbed in the small intestine. A degree of polymerization not lower than 3 is intended to exclude mono- and disaccharides. It is not intended to reflect the average degree of polymerization of a mixture. These include nondigestible soluble and insoluble carbohydrates, and lignin that are intrinsic and intact in plants, isolated or synthetic nondigestible carbohydrates.

When extracted chemically, physically, and/or enzymatically, modified or synthetically, generally accepted scientific evidence of benefits for health must be demonstrated to consider the polymer as DF. Fiber is classified as soluble and insoluble fiber. As the names denote, soluble fibers are those that dissolve easily in water and form a gel-like substance, whereas insoluble does not dissolve in water, remains intact or relatively unchanged in the digestive tract.

Each fiber differs from others in its structure. These are involved in bringing functional changes in cooking and digestion. Every dietary fiber source has different action(s) on physiology because each has different a particle size and water-holding capacity. The US Food and Drug Administration (FDA, 2016) has suggested seven isolated or synthetic nondigestible carbohydrates (NDCs) which are as follows:

Beta-glucan soluble fiber, Psyllium husk, Cellulose, Guar gum, Pectin, Locust bean gum, Hydroxypropyl methylcellulose.

> On 14 June, 2018, FDA the issued *Guidance for Industry—the Declaration of Certain Isolated or Synthetic Non-digestible Carbohydrates as Dietary Fiber on Nutrition and Supplement Facts Labels* (New Guidance). The guidance identified eight additional nondigestible carbohydrates (NDCs), the agency intends to add to the regulatory definition of dietary fiber, including mixed plant cell wall fibers, arabinoxylan, alginate, inulin and inulin-type fructans, high-amylose starch (resistant starch 2), galactooligosaccharide, polydextrose, and resistant maltodextrin.
>
> *Food Labeling: Revision of the Nutrition and Supplement Facts Labels.* Federal Register website. https://www.regulations.gov/document?D=FDA-2012-N-1210-0875. Accessed 27 June 2018.

The term "functional fiber" refers to isolated nondigestible carbohydrates that have beneficial physiological effects in humans and "total fiber" refers to the sum of dietary fiber and functional fiber.

Thus, dietary fiber is made up of carbohydrate polymers with three or more monomeric units (MU), that are neither digested nor absorbed in the human intestine and it includes:
- Non-starch polysaccharides from fruits, vegetables, cereals, and tubers whether intrinsic or extracted, chemically, physically and/or enzymatically modified or synthetic (MU≥10)
- Resistant (nondigestible) oligosaccharides (RO) (MU 3–9)
- Resistant starch (MU≥10)

Functions of Dietary Fiber

Dietary fiber has been found to exert many physiological health benefits. These constituents have been found to provide 2 kcal/g. These are also used for labeling purposes, especially for dietetic foods. Three physiological effects are well recognized as beneficial to human health. These are attenuation of postprandial blood glucose concentrations, attenuation of blood cholesterol concentration, and improved laxation. Fiber may help with weight management since it can lend bulk to the food. The benefits conferred by dietary fiber are related to the properties such as solubility, viscosity, fermentability, etc.

> **Health Benefits of Dietary Fiber**
> - Provides bulk to the diet
> - Provides better satiety and delayed hunger thus good for weight control
> - Improves bowel function—reduces constipation, i.e. improves laxation
> - Attenuates blood glucose level
> - Lowers blood cholesterol
> - Provides food for gut bacteria for fermentation—prebiotic effect
> - Helpful in reducing the risk of certain cancers
> - May enhance insulin sensitivity
> - May help reduce risk of type 2 diabetes mellitus
> - Mechanisms for CVD risk reduction are thought to be due to lowering of serum cholesterol, delayed nutrient absorption, increased insulin sensitivity, and decreased triglycerides
> - Decreased hypertension, and effects of phytochemicals that travel with fiber
> - Higher dietary fiber intakes are linked to lower blood pressure, less diabetes, and improved gut health
> - Mechanisms for impact on body weight are less clear but may be a complex interaction of hormonal effects including lower postprandial glycemia, decreased insulin secretion, effects of the food itself (mastication and satiation), and colonic effects (e.g. fermentation).

- **Improves large bowel function**: Dietary fibers that have high water-holding capacity, increase fecal bulk and improve its movement through the colon. Thus it helps in prevention and management of constipation and other related maladies such as abdominal distention (gas), diverticulosis, hemorrhoids (piles), and appendicitis. This effect on laxation and preventing constipation is attributable to insoluble fiber. Soluble dietary fibers also have been shown to improve bowel movement and chronic idiopathic constipation. Soluble fiber may also increase stool frequency.
- **Modifies blood glucose levels**: Fiber delays stomach emptying and starch digestion, slows down glucose absorption and delays rise in blood sugar levels (BGL) or helps in its stabilization. Soluble fiber provides viscosity and slows down the absorption of carbohydrate and presents rise in BGL. Addition of fiber-rich foods in the diet prevents postprandial rise in blood glucose and highly beneficial in management of diabetes mellitus.
- **Lowers cholesterol in blood and improves lipid profile**: Most sources of soluble dietary fibers are viscous in nature and the viscosity is an important property of fiber for lowering plasma cholesterol. Fibers possessing viscosity include oat bran and barley, psyllium, guar gum, locust

bean gum, and modified celluloses. However, cellulose and lignin (insoluble fibers) are not effective in reducing cholesterol because they are not viscous in nature. Total dietary fiber intake has been found to be inversely associated with not only total cholesterol but also LDL cholesterol and triglycerides, and is positively associated with HDL cholesterol, which is favorable. Water-soluble fibers are effective in reducing LDL cholesterol but do not greatly influence the HDL cholesterol.

- **Helps in weight control**: High body mass index has been found to be associated with low fiber intake. Including adequate amount of fiber in the diet improves feeling of satiety; higher fiber in food products helps to dilute the energy content and also could slow down gastric emptying thus delaying the next meal.
- **May help reduce inflammatory markers**: Increased intake of both soluble and insoluble fibers has been found to be associated with lower levels of inflammatory markers like C-reactive protein. Inflammation is linked to noncommunicable diseases.

One of the important properties of dietary fibers is their susceptibility to fermentation in the colon by microorganisms. Fibers vary in the extent to which they can be fermented depending upon the type of fiber, whether they are isolated or are present as part of the food. In general, larger particle-size fibers will tend to be fermented less and slowly, hence soluble fibers are fermented more than are insoluble fibers. The examples of soluble fibers are psyllium, oats, xanthan gum, and the examples of insoluble fibers are corn and wheat. Synthetically modified celluloses that are used as food additives are not susceptible to fermentation.

Fermentation of soluble fiber by gut flora results in the production of short-chain fatty acids (SCFA) such as butyric acid, acetic acid, and gases like carbon dioxide and hydrogen. SCFAs help reduce blood glucose levels possibly through multiple mechanisms. In some persons, SCFA are taken up by the large intestine, with butyric acid possibly being used as a source of energy by the epithelial cells. Hence, it is estimated that dietary fiber may provide about 1.5–2.5 kcal per gram of fiber. Animal studies have shown that the presence of SCFA promotes wound healing, and butyrate decreases growth of colon cancer cells.

Other benefits of fermentation of dietary fiber include increased mineral absorption, stimulation of beneficial microbes in the gut, decreased survival of pathogens, and nourishment of the colonocytes by the SCFAs as well as influencing immunity.

Types of Fiber

Lignins: Lignin is derived from the Latin word *Lignum* meaning wood and is an integral part of the secondary cell wall of plants. Lignins are not carbohydrates. They are large biopolymers consisting of phenols and other molecules. Lignins are natural polymers, insoluble in water, found in vessels and secondary tissues of all higher plants and give mechanical strength to the cell wall and to the entire plant. They form three-dimensional polymers consisting of phenylpropane units. Unlike other NSPs, lignins are not digested, they are fermented by the colonic microflora. Plants contain 15–25% lignin. In the plant cell wall, a considerable portion of lignins are linked to hemicelluloses and pectins. Lignin is found in a variety of foods such as flaxseed, strawberries, root vegetables like carrots and cereal bran, seeds like tomato seeds, vegetables with edible stems like broccoli, green beans, apples, peas, peaches, and Brazil nuts. Lignins are insoluble in water but are able to absorb water and give bulk to stools. Lignin from flaxseed also has antioxidant property. Lignin is often a waste material from the pulp and paper industry. It has shown good potential for the development of some pharmacological products including vanillin (a flavoring substance) due to the presence of phenolic and aliphatic hydroxyl groups in its structure.

> **Research glimpse:** Lignin structure is heterogeneous. Many of the effects of lignin are attributable to its antioxidant property as it has several phenolic groups. Newer methodologies have shown that lignins or their derivatives have the potential for improvement of human health. There is potential for use in treatment of obesity (lignophenols), diabetes (lignins and lignosulfonic acid), thrombosis, viral infections (lignosulfonic acid, and lignin–carbohydrate complexes), anticoagulants (low molecular-weight lignins), and cancer. Lignins may also be used to prepare nanoparticles for controlled release of herbicides and pesticides and need to be explored for applications in human medicine.
>
> *Vinardell MP, Mitjans M. Lignins and their derivatives with beneficial effects on human health. Int J Mol Sci. 2019;18(6):1219.*

Chitin and chitosan: Chitin is the second most abundant natural biopolymer (an amino polysaccharide) after cellulose. It is the principal component of the exoskeleton of invertebrates (crustaceans such as shrimp, crab, and insects) as well as cell walls of fungi. Chitosan is the deacteylated form of chitin. Both chitin and chitosan are natural antimicrobials and also have antibacterial and fungicidal activity. They are produced commercially and used industrially for several purposes such as clarification and deacidification of fruits and beverages, as a natural flavor extender, texture controlling agent, emulsifying agent, and thickening and stabilizing agent as well as humectant and stabilizers in dairy products, baked foods, confectionery, beverages etc. They are also used for purification of water, i.e., to recover metal ions, pesticides, phenols, and other chemicals and dyes. Other applications include use as analytical reagents, for color stabilization, and as livestock and fish-feed additive. They also serve as a source of dietary fiber and may be used as "added fiber".

Chitin is now used in food coatings and food additives due to its emulsifying property. It produces elastic and transparent films. The US FDA has approved its use in specific applications, and given GRAS (generally recognized as safe) status. Thus, it is also been approved for dietary use in Italy, Japan, and Finland. Although no serious side effects have been reported, some persons may have mild nausea and constipation. Individuals who are allergic to crustaceans are advised to avoid chitin and chitosan.

Caution should be exerted when taking over-the-counter products that are advertised for health benefits of chitosan. For example, a chitosan preparation is available for laxation but constipation is a reported side effect of chitosan. Studies with humans have not shown much benefit on weight loss or intestinal fat absorption, cholesterol, and triglyceride levels or the absorption of minerals like calcium.

Chitin and chitosan are used in many biomedical applications like tissue engineering, drug delivery, wound healing, and in stem cell technology and gene delivery. This is because they have good porosity, are biodegradable, have a predictable degradation rate, structural integrity, and are biocompatible besides not being toxic to cells.

Polydextrose: Polydextrose is a highly-branched glucose oligosaccharide that contains small amounts of sorbitol resistant to digestion. It is a synthetically produced food ingredient and is widely used in the food industry. It reaches the large intestine without being digested in the small intestine because it has a complex structure. It behaves like soluble fiber in terms of reducing intestinal transit time, increasing fecal bulk, and slowing down glucose absorption. In the large intestines, about 40% is fermented by the gut microbiota (hence it is considered to be a prebiotic) and the remaining 60% is excreted in feces. It does not interfere with nutrients like amino acid, potassium, and calcium. It provides about 1 kcal/g which is attributable to the SCFA produced by it being fermented in the large intestines.

It is neutral in taste, highly soluble in water, and is used as a bulking agent in a variety of foods including baked food products, dairy products, confectionery, and in functional beverages. It is approved in about 60 countries and about 20 countries recognize it as a dietary fiber. Daily intakes of 4–12 g have demonstrated physiological benefits without any accompanying side effects.

Resistant Starch

Resistant starch, as the name suggests, is the portion of starch that escapes the digestive enzymes (α-amylases) in the small intestines (resistant to digestion) and passes further into the colon. Resistant starch (RS) is considered as part of dietary fiber. Like other dietary fibers, it may be fermented by microorganisms in the colon. It may occur naturally and is found in many cereal grains, fruits, and vegetables or it can be formed during processing of foods. RS can increase the fiber intake without compromising the taste and texture as it can be incorporated into the food. RS is of four types—(1) RS1, (2) RS2, (3) RS3, and (4) RS4. Another type of resistant starch is now recognized called type 5.

Resistant starch 1: These are starch granules that are physically enclosed within cell structures in cell walls of plants (surrounded by protein matrix and cell wall materials) and therefore, not physically accessible to the digestive enzymes. Hence RS1 resists digestion due to large particle size or compact nature of food, or starch entrapment by dietary fiber.

Consequently the glycemic response is reduced. It is found in seeds, legumes, and unprocessed whole grains. Coarser milling or increasing particle size of cereal grains such as whole-grain bread or bulgur wheat can produce RS1. When either the coarse grain or the whole grain is cooked, water cannot penetrate the physical barrier provided by the thick cell wall in legumes or the protein matrix in cereals. As a result, the starch cannot be fully gelatinized and hence cannot be hydrolyzed by the intestinal enzymes readily.

Resistant starch 2: Raw starch granules are known as RS2. This is granular starch with B or C polymorph. RS 2 resists digestion because of its crystalline structure. This starch is essentially ungelatinized starch. RS2 is found in uncooked/raw potato, green banana/plantain, and high-amylose starches like high-amylose maize starch, and some legumes like peas and beans. Cooking decreases the amount of RS2 because it gets gelatinized and the starch loses its crystallinity.

Resistant starch 3: RS3 does not occur naturally (in contrast to RS1 and RS2) but is formed during food processing when starch-containing foods are cooked and cooled, e.g., rice, potato, extruded foods like noodles and pasta. It is retrograded amylose and starch. It resists digestion because after cooking, the starch molecules associate together again and form double helices. Cooking, cooling, and storage of foods without prior drying cause recrystallization (retrogradation) of gelatinized starch and increase RS 2,.e.g., when cooked rice is refrigerated, the grains become dry and tough, because it loses its water-binding capacity.

Retrograded amylose has a high gelatinization temperature (up to 170°C) and by ordinary cooking processes, it is not dissociated. However, shorter retrograded amylose chain lengths have lower gelatinization temperature. Generally amylose retrogradation contributes more to RS3 content but retrograded amylopectin may also occur. RS3 is also produced commercially from cornstarch by enzymatic treatment. RS3 is present in ready-to-eat breakfast cereals. Repeated heating and cooling has been shown to increase in RS3 in potato.

Resistant starch 4: These starches are chemically modified either by cross-linking or by adding chemical derivatives to decrease their digestibility. Such starch is not able to swell during cooking and is not susceptible to intestinal enzymes, nor can it be fermented by the intestinal microorganisms. These starches are normally not found in nature. The amount of RS4 formed depends on the type of starch and the type and level of modification. RS4 is used in food products for imparting desired properties such as color, stability to temperature, altering viscosity, and texture in baked goods such as cakes and cookies. It can also be used to impart crispiness.

Resistant starch type 5 is formed when starch interacts with lipids and the amylose and long-chain branched amylopectin form complexes with fatty acids and fatty alcohols. The complex entangles the amylopectin and so the swelling of starch granules is prevented. These complexes are not easily hydrolyzed by amylase. RS 5 is thermally stable. RS 5 is also created/synthesized, e.g., resistant maltodextrin which consists of purposefully rearranged starch molecules.

Resistant starch has several health benefits which can be explained by the physiological effects of RS as shown in Table 2.7. It is fermented in the colon by the microorganisms and short-chain fatty acids are produced. Compared with other dietary fibers, RS produces a higher proportion of butyric acid which is considered to be important for suppressing tumor cells and the proliferation of cancer cells.

Table 2.7: Physiological effects of resistant starch.

Physiological effect	Conditions for which RS may confer health benefits
Improved glycemic and insulin responses	Metabolic syndrome, impaired glucose tolerance, and diabetes
Improved gut/bowel health	Colorectal cancer, ulcerative colitis, inflammatory bowel disease, and constipation
Improved blood lipid profile, i.e. lowering of blood cholesterol	Cardiovascular disease and metabolic syndrome
Prebiotic effects	Colonic health
Increased satiety and reduced energy intake	Obesity and diabetes
Increased micronutrient absorption	General health and osteoporosis
Adjunct to oral rehydration therapy	Enhanced mineral absorption and osteoporosis
Synergistic interactions with other dietary components, e.g., dietary fiber, proteins, and lipids	Improved metabolic control and better bowel health
Thermogenesis	Obesity and diabetes

Nugent AP. Health properties of resistant starch. Nutrition Bulletin. 2005:30:27–54.

Laboratory laurel: Resistant starch (RS) is a type of dietary fiber and is categorized into five types. It provides better glycemic control as compared to other digestible carbohydrates. A health claim in this regard has been approved by the European Union. However, there is not much information about the effect of RS on blood pressure or plasma lipids. The effect of RS on gut health is encouraging and further work needs to be done in order to determine whether RS can be classified as a prebiotic. When RS is fermented by the colonic microbes, SCFA are produced. It enhances satiety but no significant effect has been observed on body weight with long-term RS consumption. RS is also being researched for its potential as an ingredient in oral rehydration solutions and treatment of chronic kidney disease.

Lockyer S, Nugent AP. Health effects of resistant starch. British Nutrition Foundation Bulletin. 2017;42:10-41.

Effects of Excess Dietary Fiber

Although there are no negative effects of dietary fiber, it tends to cause abdominal discomfort because of flatus formation. This may occur initially when a person consumes large amounts in the beginning. Flatulence (gas production) is caused by fermentation of the fiber by the anaerobic organisms in the intestines. Flatulence and abdominal fullness has been seen with intakes of about 75–80 g of dietary fiber per day. It may cause diarrhea and could temporarily obstruct the gastrointestinal tract. Hence a person interested in increasing the fiber intake should gradually and progressively increase intake to give the body time to adapt. **Drinking plenty of fluids is advisable along with consumption of high-fiber diet in order to** soften the fiber. In individuals whose food intakes are inadequate, like the elderly or young undernourished children, fiber may reduce intake of the essential nutrients, especially among those who eat small amounts of food. It also binds some minerals like calcium, iron, magnesium, copper, and zinc, and thus interferes with their bioavailability in the body. This will occur when foods which have components like phytate that binds with minerals like iron, zinc, calcium, and magnesium are consumed in high amounts. Intakes exceeding 60 g of fiber per day may reduce mineral absorption. It also hampers the absorption of fat-soluble vitamins. Diets that contain very large amount of fiber will be bulky, more satiating, and have reduced energy density. This may compromise nutrient intakes in persons whose appetite and food intakes tend to be limited, e.g., young children and elderly persons. Therefore, very high-fiber intakes are not recommended.

Research glimpse: It is well established that dietary fiber can solve the problem of constipation. However, there can be some exceptions, e.g., aggravating problem indicating idiopathic constipation. Sixty-three cases (16 males and 47 females ranging from 20 years to 80 years) of idiopathic constipation were enrolled into the study after colonoscopy and after excluding an organic cause of the constipation. All patients were explained the role of fiber in the gastrointestinal tract and asked to limit their fiber intake for 2 weeks. Symptoms of constipation noted were difficulty in evacuation of stools, anal bleeding, abdominal bloating or abdominal pain were recorded at 1 and 6 months. At the end of the study, 41 patients remained on a no-fiber diet, 16 on a reduced-fiber diet, and 6 resumed their high-fiber diet for religious or personal reasons. Patients who stopped or reduced dietary fiber had significant improvement in their symptoms such as increased bowel frequency. For no fiber, reduced fiber, and high fiber groups, respectively, symptoms of bloating were present in 0%, 31.3%, and 100% and straining to pass stools occurred in 0%, 43.8%, and 100%. Hence idiopathic constipation and its associated symptoms can be effectively reduced by stopping or even lowering the intake of dietary fiber.

Ho KS, Tan CYM, Daud MAM. Stopping or reducing dietary fiber intake reduces constipation and its associated symptoms. World J Gastroenterol. 2012;18(33):4593-6.

Recommended Dietary Allowances for Dietary Fiber

Dietary fiber (DF) requirement is assessed by considering the amount that will maintain the normal function of the large bowel in terms of providing sufficient bulk to the diet and also whether it will provide the substrates that will be fermented by the gut microorganisms. Further, low DF intakes have been associated with higher risk of non-communicable diseases (NCDs). The United States and other international organizations recommend that for long-term good health, at least 25–30 g of DF should be consumed. Further, the WHO recommends consumption of >25 g of total dietary fiber to be obtained from whole grain cereals, fruits and vegetables, to prevent NCDs. Also, excessive fiber (>60g/day) is not advisable because it may interfere with absorption of some minerals and may result in diarrhea.

However, in India, dietary fiber requirements have not been studied in depth. Therefore, the requirements for DF are assessed based on data on dietary intake obtained from dietary surveys conducted by the National Nutrition Monitoring Bureau (NNMB). The population living in western part of the country was found to consume about 30-40g fiber per day whereas northern counterparts consume higher amounts i.e., about 52 g/day. It also corresponds to the energy intake and vary with age and gender as shown in nutrient requirement RDA data given by ICMR-NIN (2020) as shown in Table 9.1 in Chapter 9. When calculating total intakes, the dietary fiber content needs to deducted. This is because soluble fiber will be fermented by the gut organisms and the fermentation products will provide about 2 kcal/g of fiber. Therefore, we cannot afford to forget the soluble fiber content in our diets when we calculate the energy derived from the food ingested. When expressed on the basis of energy intakes, 40g/2000kcal is considered safe. Intakes are generally higher with wheat-based diets than with rice-based diets.

Children should eat less than adults because the bulk and the feeling of fullness that fiber provides could cause their diet to be low in energy, if excessive amounts are eaten. For children under 2 years of age, excess amount of dietary fiber should not be given especially at the expense of nutritious foods as these children require energy and all nutrients for their growth and development.

Food Sources of Dietary Fiber

Any food containing 2.5 g fiber/serving is considered a good source. Animal foods do not contain any fiber. Rich sources of dietary fiber are found in fruits (sapota, pears, and oranges), vegetable (corn, peas, jackfruits, and broccoli), whole pulses (lentils, chickpeas and beans), and whole grains (whole- and mixed-grain food products). Though spices are consumed in lesser amounts but contain high amount of dietary fiber. Some important dietary sources of fiber are presented in the Figure 2.2 and Appendix 2.

GLYCEMIC INDEX

Carbohydrates are classified on the basis of their physiological effect as glycemic and nonglycemic. Glycemic carbohydrates are those that have an effect on blood glucose level. According to the American Diabetic Association, the glycemic index (or GI) measures how a carbohydrate-containing food raises the blood sugar level. Glycemic index is a relative indicator of blood glucose response to the carbohydrate present in foods. GI refers to the glycemic effect of available CHO (usually 50 g) in a food relative to the effect of an equal amount of available carbohydrate (usually from white bread or glucose), which is defined as having a GI of 100.

This was introduced in the early 1980s to enable assessment of the relative effect of various carbohydrates on the rise in blood sugar levels, after these carbohydrates are consumed. Some carbohydrates break down faster than others in the gastrointestinal tract, and are absorbed rapidly into the bloodstream, raising blood sugar quickly. Such carbohydrates are said to have a high GI, e.g., foods like rice or sugars like sucrose and glucose. In comparison, there are carbohydrates that are digested relatively slowly, hence the glucose is released more gradually into the bloodstream and blood sugar levels will not be raised very quickly. Such foods and carbohydrates are said to have a low glycemic index.

Although, GI does not indicate the carbohydrate content of the food or the type of carbohydrate, it signifies the physiological impact of the carbohydrate. Therefore, it is helpful in meal planning particularly for people having diabetes, insulin resistance, hyperlipidemia, polycystic ovary syndrome (PCOS), and weight problem. Glycemic index is useful in the dietary management of diabetes mellitus. GI values are given for plant foods only and not for animal foods except milk, because meat, fish, etc. do not contain enough carbohydrate. It is determined by comparing the rise in blood sugar after consuming 50 g of carbohydrate from the food being tested, with the rise in blood sugar after eating enough white bread to obtain 50 g of carbohydrate. Alternatively, 50 g glucose can also be used as the reference. The response that is obtained is expressed as a percentage of the response to the standard, i.e., the value is multiplied by 100. Glycemic index and glycemic load of several commonly consumed food items are given in Appendix 5.

The highest possible GI is 100 indicating that the test food will raise blood sugar to the same extent that the reference food or glucose do. Foods are categorized into three groups as follows:

Low-glycemic foods are those with a glycemic index of 55 or less. Examples are non-starchy fruits, whole unprocessed unrefined grains, pulses, and vegetables. Foods rich in fiber generally have low GI, e.g., green leafy vegetables, whole pulses, beans, and sweet potato, fruits like papaya, apple, pear, and orange, milk and milk products (no sugar and

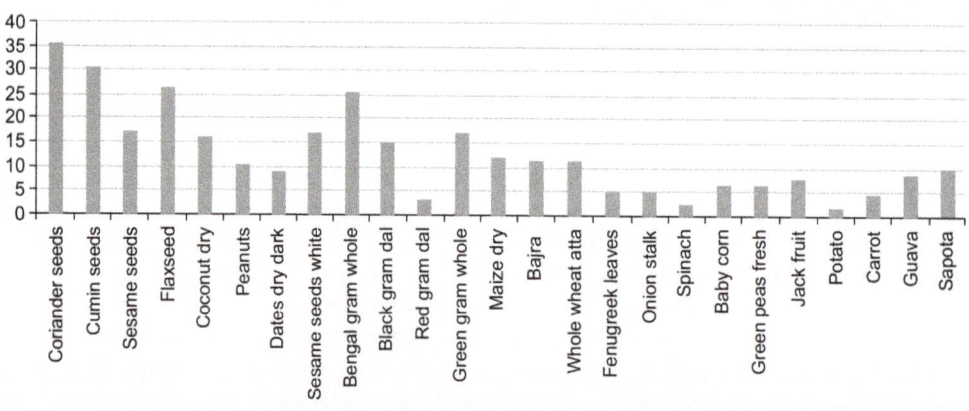

Fig. 2.2: Total dietary fiber (g/100g).

fat added), pasta, bulgur wheat, and rolled oats. Low-glycemic foods have a slower rate of carbohydrate absorption and slow rise in blood glucose level. These foods generally contain more complex carbohydrates and are valuable to manage diabetes and weight.

- Low (<55)
- Medium (55–69)
- High GI (≥70)

Medium-GI foods are those with a GI between 56 and 69, e.g., brown rice, basmati rice, whole wheat, and oats.

High-glycemic foods are usually foods with a GI of > 70%. These foods show higher potential for rapid rise in blood sugar. With the consumption of high-GI foods for a prolonged period, more insulin is frequently produced to manage the intake and cells receptors are frequently bombarded and eventually the insulin secretion or the sensitivity of the insulin receptors on the cells are either insensitive or dysfunctional, leading to insulin resistance and diabetes. High-GI foods contain large amount of starches that are easily digested, e.g., potato, rice, refined cereals like white bread, large amounts of disaccharides that will be rapidly broken down into glucose, all candies, sugar-rich food products like sweets, confectionery, bakery, refined flour, fried foods, pineapple, and fruit juices (carrot juice and beet juice). GI can be determined for individual foods as well as mixed meals.

> **Laboratory laurel**: A secondary analysis of 621 women who participated in a randomized control trial of low-glycemic index (GI) diet in pregnancy was done. Serum samples were analyzed in early pregnancy and at 28 weeks, for insulin, leptin, and markers of inflammation. Cord blood was also analyzed for the same biomarkers. There was no difference between women received advice to consume a low-GI diet and those who did not. However, rise in insulin concentrations among women who received advice was less from early pregnancy to 28 weeks of pregnancy.
>
> The dietary glycemic index and glycemic load were estimated using a food frequency questionnaire for 27,769 men and 36,684 women aged 45–75 years and who took part in the second survey of the Japan Public Health Center-based Prospective study. Development of diabetes was recorded 5 years later. Data analysis was undertaken and the possible influence of several variables was controlled for, including age, area, total energy intake, smoking habit, family history of diabetes, occupation, and physical activity, hypertension, body mass index, intakes of alcohol, calcium, dietary fiber, and coffee. Dietary glycemic load was found to be positively associated with the risk of diabetes among women. The association was stronger among women with BMI below 25 years compared with those with a higher BMI. Among women, the dietary glycemic index was positively associated with higher risk of diabetes; among men, whose fat intake was high, suggesting that total fat intake may modify the association between dietary glycemic index and the risk of type 2 diabetes.
>
> *Walsh JM, Mahony RM, Culliton M, et al. Impact of a low glycemic index diet in pregnancy on markers of maternal and fetal metabolism and inflammation. Reprod Sci.2014;21(11):1378-81.*
>
> *Oba S, Nanri A, Kurotani K, et al. Dietary glycemic index, glycemic load and incidence of type 2 diabetes in Japanese men and women: The Japan public health center-based Prospective Study. Nutr J. 2013;12(1):165.*

Glycemic Load

One limitation of glycemic index is that it compares 50 g of carbohydrate. Each food is given a numeric score based on how much the blood sugar rises. At first glance, the values for some foods appear high, e.g., many fruits have a high GI. A typical example is watermelon that has a GI of 80 but in order to get 50 g of carbohydrates the amount of watermelon that would be needed to be consumed is in several portions.

In contrast, only relatively smaller number and/or portions of cereal-based foods and desserts would give 50 g of carbohydrate, e.g., one serving of watermelon gives only 11 g of available carbohydrate compared with a medium-sized doughnut gives about 23 g of available carbohydrate. The limitation of GI is overcome by using glycemic load which describes the quantity and quality of carbohydrate, be it in a food or meal.

Glycemic load is a mathematical concept in which along with glycemic index the amount of carbohydrate in the foods is considered. "Glycemic Load" is calculated by multiplying the GI by the amount of carbohydrate. This concept was introduced in 1997 by the Harvard School of Public Health. Glycemic load quantifies the overall glycemic effect of a portion of food. It takes into account the amount of carbohydrate present in a portion of any food that is eaten and the glycemic response to that food. Higher glycemic load values indicate that a greater elevation in blood glucose response is to be expected. Glycemic Load per 100 grams of a food is calculated as:

$$GL = \frac{\text{Glycemic index of a food} \times \text{Carbohydrate content of food (net carbohydrates) in g}}{100}$$

(Net carbohydrate is equal to the total carbohydrate minus dietary fiber).

One can calculate the glycemic load of different foods consumed in the diet. By summing up the glycemic load contributed by the various foods, the overall glycemic load of the whole diet can be estimated.

Dietary GL = [GI × (carbohydrate content of food) × (servings of food/day)]

Therefore, one can control blood sugars by consuming low-GI foods and/or by restricting your intake of carbohydrates. For example, potato has high glycemic index 85/100 × 33. Glycemic load will be 27. It is advisable that low-glycemic index foods like whole grains, fruits, and vegetables should be included and intake of refined and minimally processed foods should be minimized to improve the blood sugar and blood lipid levels, hence reducing the risk of diabetes and heart diseases.

> Glycemic load is relevant since many fruits appear to have a relatively higher GI but they do not contain much carbohydrate. Hence, their GL may be lower. Apple for example has a GI of 38, whereas its GL is only 6. Similarly, the GI of banana is 51 and its GL is 13.

> **Laboratory laurels**: The PREDIMED (Prevencion con dieta mediterrnanea) study is a randomized nutrition intervention (a Mediterranean diet) for preventing primary cardiovascular disease. It is being conducted on community-dwelling men and women (55–80 years of age) who are at high risk of cardiovascular disease. This study estimated the association between dietary glycemic index and glycemic load with the risk of all-cause mortality in the PREDIMED study.

Contd...

Contd...

> At baseline and during yearly follow-ups, a validated food frequency questionnaire was filled up by each subject and each of the 137 foods in the questionnaire was assigned GI values. A total of 3,583 nondiabetics were followed up for an average of 4.7 years, during which 123 deaths occurred. Quartiles of baseline dietary GI were compared. Those who were in the lowest quartile of dietary GI and those in the highest quartile had increased risk for all-cause mortality. Yearly exposure data showed similar trends. The association between all-cause mortality and dietary glycemic load was observed only for subjects below 75 years of age. Thus the study indicated that consuming high-glycemic index foods, increased risk of all-cause mortality among elderly persons.
>
> Castro-Quezada I, Sanchez-Villegas A, Estruch R, et al. High dietary glycemic index increases total mortality in a Mediterranean population at high cardiovascular risk. PLoS ONE. 2014;9(9):e107968.

> **Laboratory laurel**: The aim of this study was to determine whether glycemic index (GI) or glycemic load (GL) of the food consumed in the morning or evening, and whether consuming low- or higher-GI/GL carbohydrates in the morning/evening during adolescence were associated with increased risk of type 2 diabetes in young adults. Subjects were selected from Dortmund Nutritional and Anthropometric Longitudinally Designed (DONALD). Two 3-day diet records had been collected during adolescence and one blood sample was taken from the same subjects when they were young adults. Statistical analysis indicated that the GI, GL, low-GI carbohydrate and higher-GI carbohydrate were related to insulin sensitivity, hepatic steatosis index, fatty liver index, and a proinflammatory score. This was not seen with the morning intake, but a higher GI and a higher-GI carbohydrate for the evening intake was associated with increased hepatic steatosis index, whereas lower GI intakes were associated with a more favorable profile. The authors recommended that the large intake of carbohydrates having high GI should be avoided to prevent development of type 2 diabetes in adulthood.
>
> Diederichs T, Herder C, Roßbach S, et al. Carbohydrates from sources with a higher glycemic index during adolescence: Is Evening Rather than Morning Intake Relevant for Risk Markers of Type 2 Diabetes in Young Adulthood? Nutrients. 2017;9(6):591.

> Another way of measuring relative **glycemic impact** is **Glycemic Glucose Equivalents (GGEs)**. GGE is based on the glycemic index and the quantity of food eaten (specific amount of a food that is consumed, typically a serving and compared with the glycemic response to a specific amount of glucose.
>
> RGI=GGE intake
>
> GGE intake = food intake (g) x (% available carbohydrate/100) x GI of a food/GI glucose (g)
>
> OR
>
> GGE intake = food intake (g) x (% available carbohydrate/100) x GI of a food/10,000

Factors affecting Glycemic Responses

Foods having similar energy values can have different GI values because they differ in the rates of their digestion, their effects on blood glucose levels, in their carbohydrate content, the type of carbohydrate especially simple sugars, the fiber content, and fat content. Processing, i.e., refining or milling can turn a medium- or low-GI food into a high-GI food, and addition of fiber and resistant starch can also reduce the GI. Similarly, fruit juices may have a higher GI than the whole fruit. Stone-ground wheat chapati will have lower GI than whole-wheat bread. Cooking, parboiling, extrusion, flaking, grinding, canning, and popping increase the GI values. There are many other factors which influence GI values, which include:

Composition of the food: The amount of fat, protein, fiber, and the type of carbohydrate influence the GI. Foods containing more amounts of protein and fat have relatively low GI. Foods containing fiber and resistant starch are also likely to have a lower GI. The nature of the monosaccharide component and also the amylose and amylopectin content, and interaction between starch and other nutrients can influence glycemic response. High amount of amylose, galactose, and fructose in food increases GI, and presence of phytates, tannins, and lectins decreases the GI.

Presence of fat is another important factor. Fat in the recipe tends to lower the GI.

Acidity level of food influences glycemic response because it affects gastric emptying and therefore the GI of a food. Addition of citric acid or fruits tends to lower the GI.

Ripeness of the fruit: More ripe the fruit, the higher the GI as more sugar is produced during ripening and this sugar will be rapidly absorbed.

Storage: Old potatoes have a higher GI than new ones; as the potatoes mature, the degree of amylopectin branching increases, rendering the starch in more mature potatoes more readily digestible than that in newer potatoes.

Prolonged cooking: Overcooked food will have more GI than stir-fry crispy or steamed vegetables.

Processing techniques: Mashed potato has a higher GI than a whole-baked potato. Food processing techniques that reduce the particle size of starch granules and make carbohydrate more accessible to digestive enzymes will increase the GI. Besides particle size, the degree of starch gelatinization, the cellular structure, and form of food influence the glycemic impact. The more refined the carbohydrate, i.e., the less the amount of bran and fiber (because the natural fiber is removed), the higher the GI. The physical structure of the carbohydrate also influences GI. The smaller the particle size, the greater the surface area exposed to intestinal enzymes, and GI is likely to be higher when particle size is larger. The longer the carbohydrate food is cooked, the higher will be the GI, as more amount of starch will be gelatinized. Fermenting foods, e.g., in sourdough bread is likely to lower the GI.

Varietal difference: Long grain rice has a higher GI than short grain. Basmati has a low GI, however, easy-to-cook basmati or other rice products are likely to have a higher GI.

Many foods that are popular including traditional foods may have a high GI. Addition of low-GI foods like beans, green leafy vegetables, and fruits in the same meal is beneficial but consuming high-GI food in one meal and low GI in another may not provide the same benefits. Although GI is a popular reference value, the proportion of carbohydrate varies considerably among different foods. Hence glycemic load has been proposed as a more accurate indicator of the glycemic response (blood glucose response).

SUGAR SUBSTITUTES/SWEETENERS

Sugar substitutes as the name suggests are used to replace sugar for its sweet taste but provide negligible calories. Since these sweeteners possess little or no nutritional value, they are also referred as "nonnutritive sweeteners". These can be obtained from natural sources or synthesized chemically. These are used in small amounts since they are many times sweeter than commonly used sugars. These are commercially available in powder or tablet form in sealed packets in various sizes. They are often mixed with beverages and sweets particularly to reduce the calorie content of the food hence preferred by diabetic people, weight watchers, and other health freaks.

> **Review glimpse:** More than 400 articles were reviewed and 14 were selected. In one study, high amount of consumption of artificially sweetened soft drinks by pregnant women was associated with risk of prematurity/preterm delivery. In another study, it was found that consumption of artificially sweetened beverages during pregnancy was linked with allergic rhinitis and asthma in the children.
>
> *Bernardo WM, Simões RS, Buzzini RF, et al. Adverse effects of the consumption of artificial sweeteners—systematic review. Rev Assoc Med Bras (1992). 2016;62(2):120–2.*
>
> Many persons use non-caloric artificial sweeteners instead of sugar either to lose or maintain weight, because sugar is rapidly absorbed, contributes to excess energy intake and weight gain, as well as increases risk of metabolic syndrome. However, epidemiological data from many large cohort studies indicate a positive correlation between artificial sweetener use and weight gain, in adults as well as children. Also interventional studies suggest that artificial sweeteners when used alone do not help in weight reduction. Because artificial sweeteners are sweet in taste, they tend to encourage sugar craving and sugar dependence.
>
> *Yang Q. Gain weight by "going diet?" Artificial sweeteners and the neurobiology of sugar cravings. Yale J Biol Med. 2010;83(2):101–8.*

These sugar substitutes are metabolized without the influence of insulin. Some of them can modify the taste and texture of the product. Some may leave a metallic aftertaste. The bulk which is provided by the common sugar is difficult to obtain from artificial sweeteners. Some commonly used sugar substitutes are aspartame, saccharin, sucralose, etc. The relative sweetness of the commonly used sweeteners in comparison to sucrose (sugar) is listed in Table 2.8. Sweetness is influenced by temperature, acidity, and the composition of the food including use of other flavoring substances.

Carbohydrate occupies an important place in the human diet. In general, it is said that 95% of the carbohydrate (excluding fiber) is digested by the human gastrointestinal tract.

DIGESTION AND ABSORPTION OF CARBOHYDRATES

The extent to which different carbohydrates are digested depends on their structure, and chemical nature, as well as the food of which carbohydrate is a part. The body utilizes mainly glucose as a source of energy. Hence, it is absolutely

Table 2.8: Commonly used sweeteners in comparison to sucrose.

Sweetener	Number of times sweeter than sugar	Uses
Non-nutritive sweeteners		
Saccharin	300–350	First artificial sweetener was synthesized in 1879. It is 300–400 times sweeter than sucrose. To minimize the bitterness (aftertaste), it is mixed with other sweeteners. It has been banned by some countries since it has been found to be carcinogenic. It should be avoided in pregnancy and in gestational diabetes. ~ 20 mg = 1 tsp sugar. ADI is 5 mg/kg of body weight and maximum daily intake is 1g/day. Used in beverages, dietetic foods, and toothpaste
Cyclamates	30	More acceptable in flavor than saccharin. No bitter aftertaste. Banned by the US FDA since it was found to be carcinogenic in animals
Aspartame	200	It is a combination of 2 amino acids namely phenylalanine and aspartic acid. It is one of the most popular artificial sweeteners available in the brand name of "Equal" and "NutraSweet". It cannot be used by persons having phenylketonuria. Some individuals may be sensitive to aspartame. Its use may pose problems related to nervous system. It should also be avoided in hot beverages, like tea and coffee as it is not heat-stable. It is also used in soft drinks, all sweet foods, and confectionery. Contains glucose or lactose as a carrier. Provides 4 kcal/gram. Maximum ADI 50 mg/kg body weight
Acesulfame-K	200	ADI 15 mg/kg body weight. No lingering aftertaste. Excellent shelf-life. Stable to temperatures used for cooking and baking. Stable in food products that are pasteurized or sterilized. Approved in more than 60 countries
Sucralose	600	It is chlorinated sugar. It can sustain heat, therefore is safe to use in hot beverages, bakery and fried items. It is minimally absorbed by the body. ADI 5 mg/kg of body weight. It can be used in beverages, baked, and Indian sweets
Stevioside		Naturally occurring sweetener obtained from Stevia, an herb, and approved by FDA as a flavor enhancer. It is rich in calcium, iron, and potassium but also contains oxalic acid. It helps in better digestion, reduction of food cravings, and increase in alertness and energy levels. Not enough information available about its safety. May be safe, if it is used sparingly
Polydextrose		Gives ~ 1kcal/g

ADI: Accepted daily intake; FDA: Food and Drug Administration.

essential for disaccharides and polysaccharides that are large complex molecules, to be broken down to monosaccharides. The human gastrointestinal tract has a well-designed system for splitting the bonds and converting them into the monosaccharides using different hydrolytic enzymes.

Digestive enzymes
Starch:
- α-amylase (salivary)
- α-amylase (pancreatic)

Disaccharides:
- Sucrase
- Isomaltase
- Maltase
- Lactase

Only monosaccharides are absorbed by the gastrointestinal tract. Monosaccharides do not require any digestive enzymes to reach the small intestine intact.

In the mouth: Digestion of carbohydrates begins in the mouth itself. When a person chews the food, it is mixed with saliva. Also chewing stimulates saliva secretion. Saliva contains the enzyme called salivary amylase (ptyalin) which acts on the starch and hydrolyzes it to smaller polysaccharides like dextrin and maltose. Disaccharides are not digested in the mouth. Digestion occurs only to a limited extent in mouth because food is held in the mouth only for a short period.

In stomach: There is no digestion of carbohydrates because there is no digestive enzyme which acts on carbohydrates and the highly acidic pH of the stomach halts the action of salivary amylase. Amylase is a protein, which denatures in presence of gastric juices and acid and stops the digestion of carbohydrates. Certain fibers provide feeling of fullness by delaying emptying of stomach.

In the small intestine: When starch reaches the **duodenum**, pancreatic or alpha (α) amylase produced by the pancreas acts on starch, further hydrolyzes it into shorter glucose chains and disaccharides. Digestibility of starch is influenced by many factors such as the ratio of amylose to amylopectin, particle size which determines bioaccessibility, whether the plant cell wall is present and constitutes a barrier to the enzymes acting upon the starch, the processing treatment that the starch has undergone, e.g., extrusion, whether the food has been cooled after cooking and further undergone heating–cooling–heating cycles (affects RS formation) and consistency of the food (liquids are digested faster than semisolids or cellular structures).

Since it takes a longer time for galactose or fructose to be converted to glucose, foods containing these sugars will not raise blood glucose (sugar) as rapidly as will glucose or sucrose-containing foods.

The disaccharides are hydrolyzed into their respective constituent monosaccharides by a separate set of enzymes. There are specific enzymes in the brush border cells of the intestinal wall for different disaccharides. Sucrase will act on sucrose and cleave it into glucose and fructose. Maltase will cleave maltose into glucose units and lactase will work upon lactose to break it into galactose and glucose. Lactase converts lactose to galactose and glucose. These monosaccharides are absorbed through the intestinal mucosa (lining) and are absorbed into portal blood through microvilli present in the small intestine. As blood from the intestines circulates through the liver, these sugars also reach the liver. Hepatocytes (liver cells) convert galactose to glucose and fructose is metabolized to yield other metabolic products or to glucose which will ultimately enter the pathways for energy production. Some amount of glucose is removed by the liver from portal blood but most of it is transported in the peripheral circulation to muscle, adipose tissue, and other tissues to provide metabolic energy.

Excess glucose is stored in the liver and muscles in the form of glycogen. Glycogen is stored in the hepatocytes only in limited amounts. Hence, any further excess amount of sugar coming into the liver is converted into lipid which is deposited in the adipose tissue. During fasting, exercise or

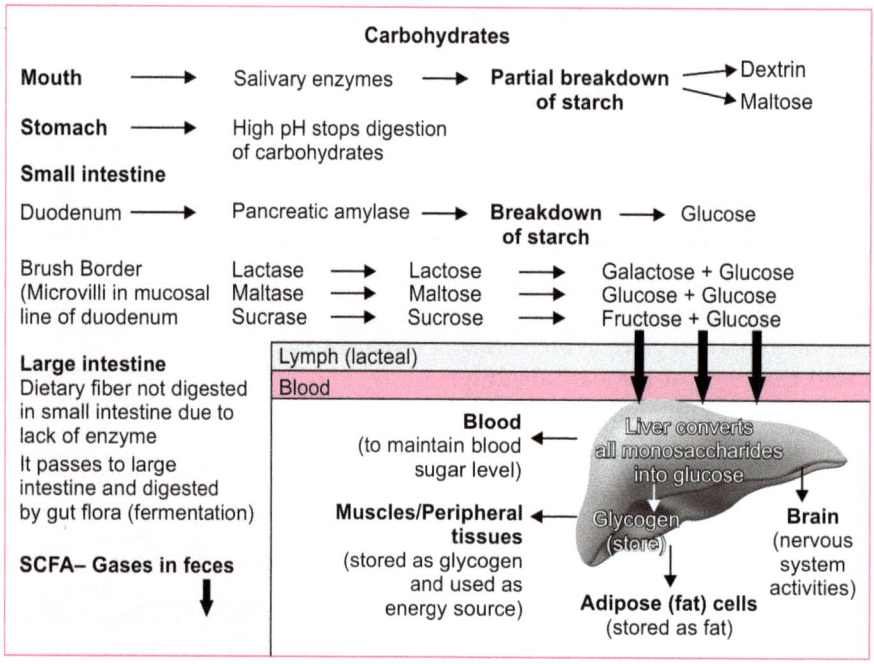

Fig. 2.3: Digestion and absorption of carbohydrates.

starvation, liver glycogen is used to provide glucose. Liver glycogen is converted back to glucose whenever blood glucose level falls below 60–80 mg/dL.

The small intestine does not contain any enzyme to digest some complex carbohydrates like resistant starch and fiber. Therefore, these directly pass into the large intestine. Here, intestinal microflora ferment the undigested carbohydrate leading to the production of short-chain fatty acids (butyrate, propionate, and acetate), and some gases (methane and carbon dioxide), and the remaining unused material is excreted out of the body as feces.

RAPID FIRE

1. Classify the carbohydrates based on degree of polysaccharides.
2. What is the difference between oligosaccharides and fructooliogosaccharides?
3. What is the difference in starch and resistance starch?
4. Name sugar alcohols and write its significance.
5. What are three main physiological effects of dietary fiber?
6. What can happen in the body in case of very low-carbohydrate diet?
7. Why refined flours are harmful over whole grains and fruit sugars?
8. What is role of amylose and amylopectin in management of blood sugar level?
9. What is glycemic index and glycemic load?
10. Name any three artificial sweeteners and the differences among them.

EXERCISE

1. Record your 1 day's diet and identify the carbohydrate. Classify the different types of carbohydrates consumed.
2. Record all the foods and beverages you have eaten in last 1 week. Calculate the carbohydrate and dietary fiber content in them.
3. Conduct a market survey for bakery and confectionery items (25) and identify the carbohydrate ingredients in them.

SUGGESTED READING

1. AACC Report. The Definition of Dietary Fiber 1. USA: Report of the Dietary Fiber Definition Committee to the Board of Directors of the American Association Of Cereal Chemists, 2001.
2. Craig SAS, Holden JF, Troup JP, et al. Polydextrose as soluble fibre and Complex carbohydrates. In: Cho SS, Prosky L, Dreher M (Eds). Complex carbohydrate in Foods. New York: Marcel Dekker Inc. 1999. pp. 229-48.
3. Cummings JH, Stephen AM. Carbohydrate terminology and classification. Eur J of Clin Nutrition. 2007;61 Suppl 1:S5-18.
4. Elia M, Cummings JH. Physiological aspects of energy metabolism and gastrointestinal effect of carbohydrate. Eur J Clin Nutr. 2007;61Suppl 1:S40-74.
5. Englyst KN, Liu SN, Englyst HN. Nutritional characterization and measurement of dietary carbohydrates. Eur J Clin Nutr. 2007;61(Suppl 1):S19-39.
6. FAO Food and Nutrition Paper No. 66. Carbohydrates in Human Nutrition, 1998, Report of joint FAO/WHO Expert consultation.
7. Food and Agriculture Organization of United Nations Dietary carbohydrate composition. [online]. Available from. http://www.fao.org/3/w8079e/w8079e0h.htm [Last accessed July 2019].
8. Joshi S, Bayer Zydus Pharma. STARCH: Recent study reveals that the Indian diabetes population consumes high amounts of carbohydrates, similar to that of the non-diabetes population. BMJ Open International Journal on November 3, 2014. [online]. Available from https://www.bayerzyduspharma.com/media/press-releases/news_68.php. [Last Accessed July, 2019].
9. King JC, Slavin JL White Potatoes, Human Health, and Dietary Guidance. Advances in Nutrition. 2013;4 (3):393S-401S.
10. Lineback DR. The Chemistry of complex carbohydrates. In: Cho SS, Prosky L, Dreher M (Eds) Complex carbohydrate in foods. New York: Marcel Dekker Inc.;1999. pp 115-30.
11. Mahan LK, and Escott-Stump S. Krause's Food & Nutrition Therapy, 12th edition. Philadelphia: WB Saunders Company; 2007.
12. Murugadass G, Dipnaik K. Preliminary study of ratio of amylose and amylopectin as indicators of glycemic index and in vitro enzymatic hydrolysis of rice and wheat starches. International Journal of Research in Medical Sciences. 2018;6(9):3095-8.
13. Nantel G. (1998). Carbohydrates in human nutrition, food and nutrition [online] Division of FAO. Available from http://www.fao.org/3/x2650T/x2650t02.htm. [Last accessed July 2019].
14. Nelsons AL. High Fiber Ingredients. USA: Eagan Press Handbook series; 2007.
15. Nishida C, Martinez NF. FAO/WHO scientific updates on carbohydrates in human nutrition: introduction. Eur J Clin Nutr. 2007; 61(Suppl 1):S1-4.
16. Rizkalla SW. Health implication of fructose consumption: A review of recent data. Nutr Metab (Lond). 2010;7:82.
17. Scapin T, Fernandes AC, Proenca RPC. Added sugars: Definitions, classifications, metabolism and health implications. Rev Nutr. 2017; 30(5):663-77.
18. Shills ME, Shike M. Modern Nutrition in Health and Disease, 10th edition. Baltimore, Maryland: Lippincott Williams & Wilkins, 2006.
19. Srilakshmi B. Nutrition Science, 2nd edition. New Delhi: New Age International Publishers, 2006.
20. Tappy L. Basics in clinical nutrition: Carbohydrate metabolism. e-SPEN, the European e-Journal of Clinical Nutrition and Metabolism. 2008;3:e192-5.
21. Te Morenga L, Mallard S, Mann J. Dietary sugars and body weight: systematic review and meta-analyses of randomised controlled trials and cohort studies. BMJ. 2012; 346:e7492.
22. Temple NJ. Fat, Sugar, Whole Grains and Heart Disease: 50 Years of Confusion Nutrients. 2018;10(1):39.
23. World Health Organization (2015). Guideline: Sugars intake for adults and children. Geneva: WHO; 2015.
24. World Health Organization, Food and Agriculture Organization of the United Nations. (1998). Carbohydrates in Human Nutrition, Report of a Joint FAO/ WHO Expert Consultation. [online]. Available from https://www.who.int/nutrition/publications/nutrientrequirements/9251041148/en/ [Last accessed July 2019].

CHAPTER 3

Protein and Amino Acids

KEY CONCERNS
- What is protein and how does it affect my strength and immunity?
- What are different types of amino acids and their functions?
- What can happen, if I eat more or if I eat less amount of protein?
- How do different sources of protein and their quality impact my body?
- How much of protein should I eat and how much is present in each food?
- What is the biological significance of peptides?

KEY CONCEPTS
- Classification of protein and amino acids
- Function of each type, their sources, and nutritional value
- Vegetable and animal sources of protein
- Role of different peptides and amino acids in relation to health
- Causes and consequences of deficiency and excess of protein
- Protein quality and protein homeostasis
- Digestion of protein

PROTEINS

Proteins are life-sustaining complex biomolecules found in all living cells and tissues. They are the basis for major structural components of animal and human tissues. They are the "building blocks" of the body along with carbohydrates, lipids, and nucleic acids. Proteins are composed of carbon, hydrogen, oxygen, nitrogen, and sometimes sulfur. No other compound in the body contains as much nitrogen as protein. The basic building blocks of all proteins are amino acids.

The body of a healthy young adult male contains approximately 14% protein, most of which is present in muscle tissues. Formation of every part of the body including teeth and bones requires protein and amino acids. Proteins perform many structural, protective, and regulatory functions in the body. The human body needs protein to function normally and without proteins, the most basic functions of life such as respiration and muscle contraction could not be carried out.

Proteins are made up of amino acids. When two amino acids bind together (L-α amino acids polymerize), the amine group of one amino acid reacts with the carboxylic acid group (-COOH) of another amino acid to form a peptide bond, also called amide linkage. Two amino acids bonded together produce a dipeptide. Similarly, three amino acids bonded together give a tripeptide. Many amino acids bonded together give a polypeptide. Peptides and polypeptides have important roles in the human body.

Dipeptide: A molecule consisting of two amino acids joined by a peptide bond.
Tripeptide: A molecule containing three amino acids joined by peptide bonds.
Oligopeptide: It consists of 4–20 amino acids.

Contd...

Contd...

Polypeptide: A macromolecule (large molecule) consisting of several (>20) amino acids linked together by peptide bonds to form a chain.
Protein: A macromolecule consisting of >30–50 amino acids joined together by peptide bonds. Proteins present in food and in the body consist of long chains of polypeptides consisting of hundreds of amino acids.

The number of amino acids and the sequence, i.e., order of the linkage of amino acids is the basis of the structure of proteins. The amino acids are linked together based on a sequence that is encoded in the DNA (the genome). There are hundreds of thousands of proteins and no two proteins are the same in terms of structure and function. Even if the same amino acids are present in different proteins, the sequence of amino acids in the polypeptide differs. This makes proteins chemically diverse. Some proteins contain relatively small number of amino acids whereas others contain thousands. Each protein performs a highly specific function. In fact, it is because of these differences that each of our bodies is unique. It is estimated that there are about 10,000 different proteins in the human body. Table 3.1 indicates the number of amino acids present in some important proteins in the human body.

The largest protein known to date is ***titin***, found in skeletal and cardiac muscle. It is estimated to contain 34,350 amino acids in a single chain.

Table 3.1: Number of amino acids present in some common proteins.

Protein	Number of amino acids	Functions
Insulin	51	Required for glucose metabolism
Hemoglobin	574	Present in red blood cells (RBCs) and is important for transporting oxygen to all tissues and cells of body
Keratin	584	Protein present in hair
Ferritin	183	Stores iron in body

Functions of Protein

Proteins perform a wide range of vital functions in the body that are important in everyday activities in the human body as well as growth and development. The functions are as follows:

Growth: Life starts with cell division. Trillions of cells divide, multiply, and join together to make different vital organs, tissues, skeleton, and the human body. Growth implies cell division or multiplication of cells for synthesis of new tissues, which entails high protein requirements during different phases of growth like in pregnancy, lactation, infancy, childhood, and adolescence.

Maintenance: Numerous voluntary and involuntary activities constantly occur in the living bodies which are governed by proteins in the form of enzymes, hormones, and antibodies. Many cells die and new cells replace them (also known as wear and tear) and for their synthesis, protein is required.

Protein is required for the synthesis of the following:

Enzymes: Enzymes are protein in nature and the body contains innumerable number of enzymes. Enzymes are involved in about 4,000 different reactions that are carried out in the body. They are biological catalysts which speed up the rate of biochemical reactions in the body. They participate in various vital processes of digestion, metabolism, DNA replication, etc. In absence of certain enzymes, many biological functions are hampered, e.g., in absence of lactase enzymes, milk is not digested well and the person suffers from lactose intolerance.

Hormones: Most hormones are peptides or polypeptides made up of several amino acids, e.g., growth hormone (GH) contains 191 amino acids, while glucagon and insulin contain 29 and 51 amino acids respectively. Hormones play a significant role in coordinating/regulating body functions, e.g., insulin controls blood sugar levels by regulating uptake of glucose into cells.

Neurotransmitters: Neurotransmitters are the biological secretions in the nervous system which transmit nerve signals in the body on biological demand. They are usually peptides but different amino acids are involved in synthesis of different neurotransmitters. For example, serotonin is a relaxing neurotransmitter which is synthesized from tryptophan. Different neurotransmitters regulate different vital functions like appetite, mood, craving, addictive behavior, sleep, etc.

Antibodies: All antibodies are proteins and are also called immunoglobulins (Ig) which play a significant role in one's ability to fight infection or develop immunity. Immunoglobulins have the capacity to fight with pathogens by binding with specific antigens. Mother's milk contains crucial immunoglobulins and thus provides immunity to the child. Low protein status can lower immunity and increase the risk of infections, illness and malnutrition. Chemokines and cytokines, special types of proteins, also participate in immune/inflammatory responses in the body.

Musculoskeletal structure: Many proteins are structural proteins providing support to the body's structure. Collagen and elastin are proteins present in connective tissue, cartilage, ligaments, tendons, bones, and skin. Collagen imparts strength to the musculoskeletal structure and elastin elasticity and resilience in muscles and tissues. Actin and myosin are also proteins present in muscle. These proteins govern contraction and expansion of muscles and are thus responsible for muscular motion. Approximately, half of the protein in our bodies is present in muscle, hence it is important to have adequate protein intake to maintain this muscle mass.

Transport proteins: Transport proteins are used by the body to transport numerous substances and specifically for substances to cross the cell membrane. Many nutrients require transport proteins. Transport proteins are very specific. For example, glucose transporter (GLUT) will transport only glucose and lipoprotein will transport fat and cholesterol and not otherwise. The cell membrane contains specific ligands which are transport proteins for entry and exit of electrolytes and other biomolecules. In the cell membrane, there are specific proteins which pick up a compound from outside the cell and deposit it inside the cell or vice versa. These are known as "pumps". For example, entry and exit of the electrolytes is dependent on the Na^+-K^+ ATPase pump. Also, proteins transport vitamins, minerals, lipids, etc. in circulation. Transferrin is a transport protein which transports iron. Hemoglobin, a protein in red blood cells (RBCs), performs the vital function of carrying oxygen from the blood to all body cells and tissues. Heme is a protein which also contains iron and participates in oxygen transport via hemoglobin from blood to cells.

> Transport occurs in biological fluids like blood and urine, and from blood to within the cell (influx) and from inside to the outside (efflux) put.
>
> Cell membrane plays a very crucial role for diverse functions occurring in the cell. Some proteins are present in extracellular membrane (surface), some are buried within the membrane, while others are present on inner side of the membrane. Proteins are an important component of the lipid bilayer of the cell membrane and are vital for the integrity of the cell. Proteins on the extracellular membrane are exposed to the outside environment of the cell and they are important for:
> - Cell to cell communication (cell signaling)
> - Carrying receptors for hormones and other signaling molecules
> - Identification of proteins like antigen.

Plasma proteins: Major plasma proteins include serum albumin or albumin (60%), globulins (35%), and fibrinogen (4–5%). All plasma proteins are synthesized in liver, except the globulins. Albumin is largely responsible for oncotic pressure of plasma which assists in the transport of ions, lipids (lipoproteins), and steroid hormones. Low albumin level (<3.5 g/dL) indicates protein deficiency characterized by edema in the peripheral tissues of the body. Globulins (immunoglobulins) participate in immune functions indicating close association between nutrition and infection. Fibrinogen plays a prime role in blood clotting by converting it into insoluble fibrin (blood clot).

Binding proteins: Many of the compounds after digestion are absorbed after first binding to a protein or are transported through blood after binding to a protein, e.g., retinol is bound to a binding protein known as Retinol-binding Protein (RBP). Other examples are B12 binding proteins (transcobalamin and haptocorrin). Some binding proteins are highly selective and bind specific substrates whereas others like albumin may bind several substrates.

Lipoproteins: As the name suggests, lipoproteins consist of lipid and protein molecules. There are several lipoproteins and the percentage of protein in them varies. Blood carries the low density lipoprotein (LDL) and high density lipoprotein (HDL). The percentage of protein in LDL is 25% and 55% in HDL.

Regulation of body fluid balance: Albumin and globulin are proteins that attract and retain water in the body. The body contains considerable amount of fluid in extracellular fluid (ECF) and intracellular fluid (ICF). Fluid cannot easily flow across the cell membrane or between two compartments. Proteins play an important role in maintaining the volume and composition of body fluids. Albumin plays significant role in regulating fluid balance and oncotic pressure between blood and surrounding tissue spaces. The oncotic pressure is an important force that is involved in fluid movement across capillaries and fluid exchange between body compartments.

> **Oncotic pressure** or colloidal osmotic pressure is generated by large molecules in solution, especially proteins. This is osmotic pressure that is the result of the difference within the ECF between the protein contents of plasma and interstitial fluid. In plasma, the oncotic pressure is only about 0.5% of the total osmotic pressure, but plays a very important role in fluid dynamics. The normal value for oncotic pressure exerted by proteins in human plasma is 26–28 mm Hg which is approximately equivalent to 1.4 mOsm/kg of water. Albumin contributes 75% to the oncotic pressure of plasma. Plasma colloidal osmotic pressure has an important role in edema. **Edema** develops when plasma oncotic pressure is below 11 mm Hg which is equivalent to albumin level of approximately 20 g/L.

Maintenance of pH or acid-base balance: Optimal functioning of the body requires a specific pH in different tissues or organs. Normal pH of blood is 7.35–7.45. Proteins present in the blood act as buffers, thus maintain the pH. This is possible because the R groups in amino acids carry charges which enable proteins to either accept or donate hydrogen (H^+) ions. When the pH is low, i.e., acidic, (H^+) ion concentration is high, proteins are able to bind the excess ions, and conversely when the pH is basic, i.e., the (H^+) ion concentration is low, proteins will donate (H^+) and restore the pH (Fig. 3.1). Hence, when there is protein deficiency, the body's ability to maintain pH is affected.

Coagulation of blood: Blood contains a protein called prothrombin. During clotting process, prothrombin is converted into thrombin. Plasma also contains another soluble protein known as fibrinogen. **Thrombin** acts on fibrinogen and forms a network called fibrin. Other proteins essential for blood clotting are factors VIII, XIII, and protein Z. Tissue plasminogen activator is a protein involved in breakdown of blood clots.

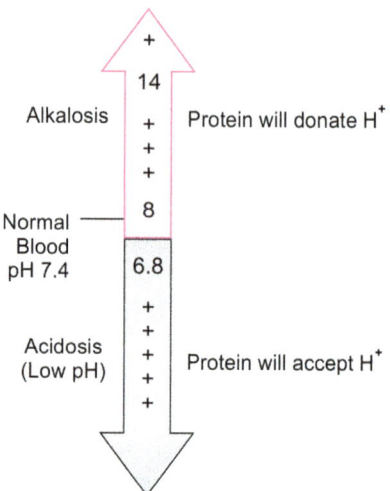

Fig. 3.1: Effect of protein on pH.

Transmission of nerve impulses: A nerve impulse is an electrical charge that travels along the membrane of neurons. Nerve cells are able to respond to specific stimuli due to the action of specific receptor proteins.

Proteins within the cell membrane act as ion channels. They facilitate movement of ions across the cell membrane. Na/K ATPase pump is such a protein.

> Tissues maintain a reservoir of undifferentiated cells, i.e. stem cells which have the ability/capacity to mature and differentiate into different types of cells. Each cell characteristically produces different types of proteins.

Cell differentiation and gene expression: Cell differentiation is a process in which the cells of the same source undergo cell division and gradually change into different cell groups that uniquely differ in morphology, structure, physiological, biochemical, and functional stability. Through cell differentiation, multicellular organs develop tissues and organs each having specific and different functions. Selective expression of specific proteins by cells is required for these differences in morphology, etc. to occur. Thus, different specific proteins are synthesized in different cells. The function of muscle cell is contraction and that of neurons is cell to cell communication. Myocytes, i.e., muscle cells synthesize actin and myosin, whereas beta cells of pancreas secrete insulin. This difference is based on their shape, size, metabolic activity or function giving each differentiated cell a different identity and function(s). Thus, different types of cells emerge such as muscle, nerve, skin, and fat cells. The functions of muscle cells differ from the cells of the skin. These differentiated cells have achieved a stable terminal state. There is unique and strictly regulated gene expression in each cell.

Only genes of specialized function will remain active and rest will remain silent in the cell. Each cell contains basic DNA or gene and transcriptor factors. The process of making genes active or silent occurs through transcriptor factors. Transcription factors regulate which genes are transcribed in a cell and are apparently essential to determine the pathway that stem cells will take during the differentiation process.

After different transcriptional programs result in the same stem cells differentiating into different types of cells that are present.

Orderly growth requires coordination of genetic expression in a sequential manner. Also, in order to live/survive, cells are constantly challenged to respond or adapt to changes in their environment. This is enabled by two important regulatory processes—transcription and translation which are crucial for synthesis of proteins. Cells can control which genes are transcribed as well as which transcripts are translated in order to regulate their activities. Proteins have a role in regulating gene expression and in cell differentiation. The human body contains about 25,000–30,000 genes, which encode for proteins and expression of these genes determines the cell functions. Control of the crucial steps transcription and translation for protein synthesis influences which proteins are synthesized and the amount of proteins present in a cell. In eukaryotic cells, gene expression is regulated by several regulatory proteins together. Thousands of transcripts are produced every second in every cell, but at any one point in time, only a fraction of the genes in a cell are expressed. Differences in gene expression profiles are due to cells having distinct sets of transcription regulators—some of which increase transcription whereas some others may either suppress or prevent transcription. Some proteins may even regulate multiple genes.

Cell signaling: Cells signal to one another for numerous reasons, one major reason being coordination of cellular activities, e.g., contraction of heart muscle. Cells also need to receive and process signals from outside their borders, in order to be able to respond to changes in their environment. Often, a cell may receive more than one signal and so the cell must integrate this information and respond in a unified manner. Cells also send messages to other cells, i.e., communicate with other cells located nearby as well as at a distance. For signaling, a protein produced by one cell may bind to a molecule produced by another cell, generating chemical signals. These signaling molecules can be hormones, growth factors, neurotransmitters or extracellular matrix components. Neurotransmitters exert their effect as signaling molecules over a short range, i.e., between adjacent neurons or neurons and muscle cells. However, for some signaling molecules, the target organ or tissue is located at quite a distance, e.g., follicle-stimulating hormone (FSH) travels from the brain to the ovary. Cells have proteins called receptors. Signaling molecules bind to these receptors and initiate a physiological response. Receptors are specific and are different for different molecules. A cell can have numerous receptors (hundreds) and the receptors differ by cell type. These receptors are generally transmembrane proteins, which bind to the signaling molecule (both extracellular signals and molecules within the cell and they influence cell function without actually entering the cell), following which the signal is transmitted to internal signaling pathways. Receptors are mainly classified into three types based on the mechanism by which the external signals are transformed into internal signals via protein action (G protein-coupled receptors), ion channel opening (ion channel receptors) or by enzyme activation (enzyme-linked receptors). There are receptors that also respond to light or pressure which means that cells are sensitive to the environment. Some receptors are also present deep inside the cell or even in the nucleus.

Provide energy: 1 g protein provides 4 kcal. Body uses protein as a source of energy, especially when it does not meet its requirements from carbohydrate and fat.

Role in food: Proteins in food directly contribute to the flavor of food. Proteins act as precursors for aroma compounds and colors formed during thermal or enzymatic reactions in production, processing, and storage of food. They also contribute significantly to the physical properties of food through their ability to build or stabilize gels, foams, emulsions, and fibrillar structure.

Classification of Proteins

Proteins can be classified in different ways based on:
- Functions
- Size, shape, and solubility of different proteins
- Location and appearance in the cell
- Molecular structure.

Based on Functions

Proteins can be classified based on their functions as shown in Table 3.2.

Table 3.2: Classification of proteins based on functions.

Type of protein	Function	Example of proteins
Structural	Providing structural materials in body	Collagen is supporting material in bones, teeth, ligaments, and tendons
Contractile	Important for movement which occurs through contraction and relaxation of muscles	Actin and myosin are muscle proteins
Transport	Important for transporting or transferring substances including nutrients from one site to another in the body	Lipoproteins transport lipids. Transferrin transports iron
Storage	Stores nutrients	Ferritin and hemosiderin store iron
Hormones	Regulators of body functions such as metabolism and the nervous system	Growth hormone—important for growth, insulin, and oxytocin is important for milk secretion
Enzymes	Act as a catalyst and speed up the rate of biochemical reactions	Pepsin, trypsin, chymotrypsin hydrolyze/break down proteins, amylase breaks down starch, and disaccharidases hydrolyze disaccharides
Protection	Provide immunity	Immunoglobulins

Based on their Size, Shape, and Solubility

Classification of protein is also based on the size, shape, and solubility of different proteins. From the biological point of view, three main categories of proteins are:
1. Simple proteins
2. Conjugated proteins
3. Derived proteins.

1. **Simple proteins:** Simple proteins are pure proteins or homo proteins and made up of only amino acids and yield only amino acids on hydrolysis. They are commonly found in animal and vegetable sources of food, e.g., egg albumin and glutelin in wheat. Enzymes like trypsin and chymotrypsin and hormones like insulin are also examples of simple proteins. The following are different types of simple proteins that differ in their size, shape, and solubility.

   Globular protein or spheroprotein: These are polypeptide chain(s) which are folded into compact globular (spherical) shape and participate in regulatory, maintenance, and catalytic roles in living organisms. They either dissolve or form colloidal suspensions in water. These proteins act as enzymes, hormones, membrane transporters and receptors, transporters of triglycerides, fatty acids and oxygen in the blood, immunoglobulins or antibodies, and grain storage proteins. Globular proteins are relatively more soluble and are present in biological fluids and participate in a wide range of biological functions, i.e., antibodies in immune system. Such proteins are generally more sensitive to temperature and pH. Hemoglobin, myoglobin, and cytochrome C are globular proteins.

   Albumin: Albumin is soluble in water and dilute salt solutions; and is precipitated by ammonium sulfate, is coagulated by heat, and found in plant and animal tissues. Examples are egg white (ovalbumin), lentils (legumelin), kidney beans (phaseolin), and wheat (leucosin).

   Globulin: Globulins are also globular proteins; insoluble in water and weak salt solution; soluble in neutral solutions of salts of strong bases with strong acids; precipitated by dilute ammonium sulfate and coagulated by heat; distributed in both plant and animal tissues. They are found in blood (serum globulins), muscle (myosin), lactoglobulin in milk, potato (tuberin), glycinin in soybean, and lentils (legumin).

   Glutelins: Glutelins are commonly found in cereals such as wheat (glutenin) and rice (oryzenin). They are insoluble in water and weak salt solution, but soluble in alkalis and acids.

   Histones: Histones are low molecular weight basic or alkaline proteins with more amounts of basic amino acids, soluble in water, salt solutions, and dilute acids, but insoluble in ammonium hydroxide. They are present in eukaryotic cell nuclei that package and order the DNA into structural units called nucleosomes. On hydrolysis, they yield large number of amino acids, particularly lysine and arginine. Because of their positive charge, they can interact with DNA which is negatively charged. Nucleoproteins are histones combined with nucleic acids. Some histones function as spools for the thread-like DNA to wrap around and help the DNA to be condensed (nuclear DNA is not in free linear strands, but is highly condensed) into chromatin so that it can fit inside the nucleus. DNA takes part in formation of chromosomes and histones play a role in gene regulation.

   Protamines: Protamines are high in arginine and are associated with DNA. They are found in fish such as mackerel (scombrine), salmon (salmine), and herring (clapeine). They are soluble in water, but not coagulated by heat.

   Prolamins: Prolamins are high in amide nitrogen and proline; insoluble in water and soluble in 70% alcohol. They occur in grain seeds like wheat and rye (gliadin), corn (zein), and barley (hordein).

   Scleroproteins: They are fibrous proteins made up of polypeptide chain(s) extended along one axis and form structural proteins like collagen, elastin, and keratins. They are insoluble in all solvents, resistant to enzymes, and unaffected by moderate changes in temperature and pH.

   Collagen: Collagen is the main constituent of connective tissues, bones, cartilage, and gelatin. It is a structural protein which forms a supporting matrix for these tissues and strengthens them. It is high in hydroxyproline. It is resistant to digestive enzymes. It is converted to gelatin when it is digested in boiling water, acid, or alkali.

   Elastin: Elastin is present in softer and flexible tissues like ligaments, tendons, and arteries. It is similar to collagen but cannot be converted to gelatin.

   Keratin: Keratin is the structural element in hair, nails, horns, and feathers. It is an important protein in the epidermis. It contains large amount of sulfur, in the form of the sulfur-containing amino acid, cystiene. It consists of four amino acids— arginine, cysteine, methionine, and lysine. Keratins are filament-forming proteins present in the epidermis having important structural and protective functions in the epithelium. Its two main functions are: (a) to adhere cells to each other and (b) to form a protective layer outside the skin. Some keratins have also been found to regulate key cellular activities, such as cell growth and protein synthesis. It is partially resistant to digestive enzymes.

   Fibrin: Fibrin is a protein formed during blood clot formation.

2. **Conjugated proteins:** Conjugated proteins contain one prosthetic group along with the protein molecule. Prosthetic group implies that a nonprotein molecule is linked to another biomolecule through covalent, noncovalent or hydrophobic bond. On hydrolysis, both protein and nonprotein molecules are separated.

> **Conjugated proteins = Protein molecule + Prosthetic group (nonprotein molecule)**

Conjugated proteins are further classified depending upon the prosthetic groups:

Nucleoproteins: Nucleoproteins are simple proteins (histones) combined with a nucleic acid (structurally associated with DNA or RNA). They are the main constituents of genes and are necessary for synthesis of protein.

Mucoproteins: Mucoprotein is a protein conjugated with polysaccharide. Such proteins occur mostly in mucus secretions, e.g., mucin (saliva) and ovomucoid (egg white). Mucoproteins are present in secretions from the gastric mucus membrane.

Glycoproteins: Glycoproteins contain carbohydrate molecules (sugars) conjugated with protein. The branches of polypeptide chain have not more than 15-20 carbohydrate units. The sugars are arabinose, glucose, mannose, N-acetyl glucosamine, N-acetyl galactosamine, galactose, fucose, and sialic acid. These proteins are present in bones, tendons, and cartilage as well as egg white and also in blood plasma.

Phosphoproteins: These proteins contain a phosphate group esterified to the amino acids serine, threonine or tyrosine. The phosphate group regulates the function of the protein. They are present in milk (casein) and egg yolk (ovovitellin).

Chromoproteins: These are colored proteins which are proteins along with nonprotein pigments, e.g., hemoglobin, myoglobin, and cytochromes.

Lipoproteins: These are proteins conjugated with lipids. The protein is called apoprotein or apolipoprotein. Conjugation of the lipid (which is insoluble in aqueous medium of plasma) with protein makes it possible for transport of lipids. LDL and HDL are lipoproteins that transport lipids in blood. Lipoproteins are important constituents of biological membranes and myelin. Lipoproteins are present in brain, nerve tissues, milk, and eggs. Besides facilitating transport of lipids, some apoproteins play a role in enzyme activation.

Metalloproteins: These are proteins that have one or more tightly bound metal ions forming part of their structure, e.g., ferritin which contains iron and ceruloplasmin which contains copper.

Flavoprotein: These proteins contain flavin nucleotides. Flavoprotein is involved in the transfer of hydrogen atoms in oxidation-reduction reactions and therefore plays an important role in energy metabolism. They serve as electron acceptors for a variety of dehydrogenases. An example of a flavin nucleotide is FAD (flavin adenosine dinucleotide).

3. **Derived proteins:** These are derivatives of simple or conjugated natural proteins (the proteins are modified) which result from the action of heat, enzymes, and/or chemicals on the protein. They are formed at various stages of hydrolysis of protein molecules. These are of two types:
   i. *Primary derived proteins* are slightly modified and are insoluble in water, e.g., casein that is coagulated by using the substance called rennet in the process of cheese manufacture.
   ii. *Secondary derived proteins* are more extensively charged. Products formed are proteoses, peptones, and peptides.

Based on Location and Appearance in the Cell

Another classification of proteins is by their location and appearance in the living cell. Based on these, proteins are categorized into four main groups:
1. **Membrane or transmembrane proteins**—these proteins are located within the cell membrane lipid bilayer.
2. **Internal proteins**—these proteins are located within the living cell and all functions are related with intercellular needs.
3. **External or secreted proteins**—these proteins function outside the cell which produces them. Such type of proteins is more common in multicellular organisms.
4. **Virus proteins**—these proteins are present only in viruses and are usually a coat for viral particles.

Based on Molecular Structure of Protein

Molecular structure of protein often forms the basis for their biological functions. The structure provides protection and support to the cells, organs, and other biological molecules. There are four levels of structures commonly found in different proteins which are of biological importance:
- **Primary structure:** Primary structure of a polypeptide or protein is the sequence of amino acids bonded together by peptide bonds. The protein sequence or amino acid sequence in the polypeptide chain defines the protein primary structure, specified by genetic information. DNA codes the primary protein structure and this is comprehensive information for the protein structure and functions. In case of viruses, RNA codes the protein structure. Each protein differs on the basis of its primary structure; therefore no two proteins are similar. The primary structure determines the chemical and physical characteristics of the protein and is very important since it determines the function of the protein. Very minor changes in the primary structure, e.g., substitution of one amino acid for another can have devastating effects since it affects protein function. A classic example is the disease, sickle cell anemia caused by one single error in the amino acid sequence in hemoglobin. Due to this error, the RBCs are sickle-shaped (hence the name of the disease) and become rigid and sticky. Consequently, they block blood flow and there can be serious damage to organs.

> **Research glimpse:** The major proteins in cow milk are caseins, with beta casein being the second most abundant protein. Different mutations in bovine beta casein gene have resulted in 12 genetic variants. Among these mutations, A1 and A2 are very common. Due to a single nucleotide difference, the A1 and A2 variants of beta casein differ at amino acid position 67 with histidine (CAT) in A1 and proline (CCT) in A2 milk. This polymorphism leads to a key conformational change in the secondary structure of expressed β-casein protein.

Contd...

Contd...

> When the A1 variant of β-casein (raw/processed milk) undergoes proteolytic digestion in the gastrointestinal tract, a bioactive peptide, beta casomorphin 7 (BCM7) is generated. Infants may absorb BCM-7 due to an immature gastrointestinal tract, whereas adults gather the biological activity locally on the intestinal brush border. Hydrolyzed milk with variant A1 of beta-casein, BCM-7 level contains four times more of this peptide than A2 milk. Buffalo milk and native Indian cows have only the A2 allele, whereas the Jersey and Holstein cows have mostly the A1 allele.
>
> Numerous studies in the literature indicate that risk of various diseases is higher with consumption of A1 type milk, and the BCM7 that is generated in the human gut, is a risk factor because it can potentially affect numerous opioid receptors in the nervous, endocrine, and immune system. BCM7 oxidizes LDL, increases risk for type 1 diabetes, heart disease, autism, schizophrenia, and sudden infant death syndrome. Decreased intake of A1 milk has been found to be associated with reduction in autistic and schizophrenic symptoms.
>
> *Sodhi M, Mukesh M, Kataria RS, Mishra BP, Joshi BK. Milk proteins and human health: A1/A2 milk hypothesis. Indian J Endocrinol Metab. 2012;16(5); PMC3475924.*

- **Secondary structure:** Secondary structure involves the way the amino acid chain twists or folds back upon it. It is a folded structure wherein the amino acid chain folds into a helix or a pleated sheet due to the interaction between the positive and negative charges of the different amino acids in the polypeptide chain.
- **Tertiary structures:** Tertiary (also called ternary) structure refers to the three-dimensional shape (3D) of the protein. It refers to a higher level of folding in which the helices and sheets of the secondary structure fold upon themselves. One example is myoglobin (muscle protein).
- **Quaternary structure:** Quaternary structure involves protein—protein interaction in which two or more polypeptides are linked to form protein complexes with subunits. Most proteins with a molecular weight of 50,000 or more are made of such units. For example, hemoglobin has four subunits.

AMINO ACIDS: THE BASIC BUILDING BLOCKS

Amino acids are the basic building blocks of proteins. Amino acids are organic compounds that contain an amine group ($-NH_2$). Each amino acid has a central carbon atom to which is bonded hydrogen, a carboxylic acid, an amino group, and an additional side group (R) (Fig. 3.2).

All amino acids except proline share the same central structure. The side group (R) is unique to each amino acid, making it different. The R may be a simple hydrogen atom whereas in some amino acids, the R group may be a complex ring structure. Some R groups may contain sulfur atoms.

Some R groups are positively charged, some have a negative charge whereas others do not have any charge. Because the R group is different for each amino acid, amino acids differ in structure, shape, size, composition, electrical charge, pH, and importantly its functions. For example, the methyl group of methionine has an important role in one-carbon metabolism, the amide group of glutamine is important in pyrimidine synthesis and the sulfhydryl group in cysteine has a role in formation of disulfide bonds that are important for cross-linking.

Classification of Amino Acids

Amino acids are also categorized according to their metabolic fate. The carbon skeletons of some amino acids are converted into precursors that are used for glucose synthesis and are known as glucogenic amino acids, whereas for others, the carbon skeleton gives rise to a precursor that is either converted into ketone bodies or fatty acids and hence they are known as ketogenic amino acids.

Glucogenic amino acids	Ketogenic amino acids
Alanine, proline, valine, phenylalanine, isoleucine, tyrosine, tryptophan, methionine, cysteine, serine, aspartic acid, and glutamic acid	Leucine, phenylalanine, isoleucine, tyrosine, tryptophan, and lysine

Some amino acids and nitrogen compounds are derived from other amino acids. For example, creatine is derived from a number of amino acids like glycine, arginine, and methionine. Dopamine, a neurotransmitter, is derived from tyrosine. Ornithine which participates in the urea cycle can be obtained from glutamate.

Basically, 20 amino acids appear to be constituents of all proteins. From the nutritional perspective, all 20 amino acids are required in the body for numerous functions in varying amounts. On the basis of the ability to synthesize in the body, these 20 amino acids are divided into two categories as shown in Figure 3.3. Out of the 20, 8 amino acids are indispensable (or essential) and 12 are dispensable (or nonessential) amino acids.

Indispensable or essential amino acids: Essential amino acids cannot be synthesized by the body in the amounts needed by the body; hence, they need to be supplied from the diet. Foods differ in their composition of essential amino acids which may be present in varying amounts in different foods. This can also be termed as obligatory dietary requirement.

Dispensable or nonessential amino acids: Dispensable amino acids are also essential for body functions but can be synthesized by a healthy body in the desired amounts under normal conditions. They are also present in foods. They are

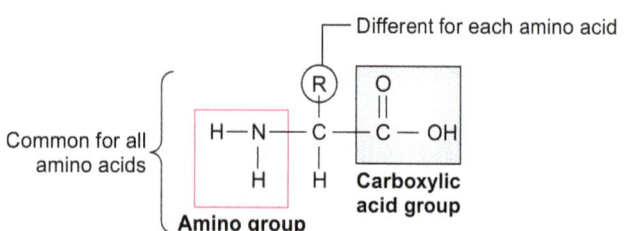

Fig. 3.2: Basic structure of amino acid.

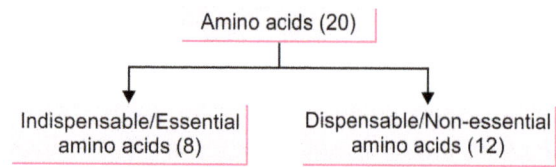

Fig. 3.3: Classification of amino acids.

Table 3.3: Different categories of amino acids.

Essential amino acids	Nonessential amino acids	Conditionally indispensable amino acids	Nonproteinogenic amino acids
Lysine	Glycine	Arginine	Taurine
Phenylalanine	Alanine	Cysteine	Ornithine
Tryptophan	Serine	Glycine	Citrulline
Methionine	Cystine	Proline	
Leucine	Tyrosine	Tyrosine	
Isoleucine	Aspartic acid	Glutamine	
Valine	Glutamic acid	Arginine	
Threonine	Proline	Cystine	
Histidine (for infants and children)	Hydroxyproline Citrulline		

important because they participate in metabolic reactions and many of them are precursors of other important biological compounds.

Limiting amino acids: During protein synthesis, the body requires specific amount of each amino acid. If any amino acid is present in too small a quantity or absent, the other amino acids can be used only to the extent that the amino acid is available, which "limits" the protein synthesis. Limiting amino acids are the essential amino acids which are short in supply in relation to the amount required by the body for protein synthesis. Lysine, methionine, and tryptophan are the most common limiting amino acids. In plant proteins, lysine is the major limiting amino acids. However, plant proteins also have lesser amounts of indispensable amino acids such as methionine, cysteine, tryptophan, threonine, and glycine.

Conditionally indispensable amino acids: Amino acids are no longer classified into only two groups—indispensable and dispensable. Experts have now added a third group of amino acids called "conditionally indispensable amino acids". These amino acids are normally synthesized by the body, but under certain physiological or pathological conditions, their rate of synthesis is not sufficient to meet cellular needs. Hence, they become essential under those "conditions". Such amino acids are called "conditionally essential/indispensable amino acids" and need to be supplied in the diet. These amino acids are listed in Table 3.3.

Preterm infants are not physiologically mature enough to produce some amino acids. Similarly, during stress or illness, when metabolic demands are higher than the amounts our diets can supply, one or more of these amino acids become conditionally essential. In order to synthesize a conditionally essential amino acid, the body requires other amino acids. For example, citrulline is needed for synthesis of arginine and methionine is required for cysteine synthesis.

Nonproteinogenic amino acids: Three amino acids, namely taurine, ornithine, and citrulline are not present in protein but are important under special circumstances, e.g., taurine in preterm infants.

PROTEINS IN FOOD

From the dietary and nutritional perspective, proteins are categorized into two, based on their essential amino acid content. This classification signifies the quality of protein and helps us in better selection of food. The two types of protein are:
1. Complete protein
2. Incomplete protein.

Complete protein: Such a protein contains all the essential amino acids (EAA) in amounts that are required by the body for protein synthesis specifically in growth. These proteins are said to be "good quality" proteins, have high biological value and are used and **"reference protein"**. Egg protein contains all the essential amino acids, hence it is considered to be a reference protein and protein quality of all other foods is compared with the reference protein. Usually, proteins from animal sources foods like milk, egg, and meat contain all essential amino acids.

> **Reference protein:** Egg is considered as a reference protein and it has highest biological value and has been assigned a value of 100. Reference protein or egg protein is used as a standard with which the quality of other proteins is compared.

Incomplete protein: These are proteins in which one or more essential amino acid is present in low or insufficient amounts (as per the body's requirements). Proteins from plant sources such as cereals, pulses, nuts, and oil seeds are not complete, because some amino acid is "limiting", e.g., zein from maize is incomplete due to low amounts of lysine and tryptophan. Wheat contains low amounts of lysine. Protein quality of incomplete protein can be improved by combining them with protein sources that will supply the limiting amino acid. Gelatin is an is an incomplete protein in contrast to other animal proteins.

When two proteins are combined in a way that one protein makes up for the lack of an amino acid that is missing in the other protein, so that together the food contains all the essential amino acids in required amounts, it improves the protein quality. The proteins are termed as "complementary protein". This is known as "mutual supplementation" or "protein complementation". Generally, plant proteins are incomplete; hence they should be consumed with animal proteins or with another plant protein which is able to complement the first. Example: Methionine is the amino acid limiting in pulses and lysine amino acid is limiting in cereals. When cereal and pulse are consumed together, they complement each other. The common food sources of complete and incomplete proteins are shown in Table 3.4.

It is noteworthy that Indian diets have evolved to ensure that complementation of protein occurs because generally Indians consume the staple cereal with a pulse or animal source of protein. Hence, in many parts of the country, rice is eaten with dal or milk/curd, buttermilk or fish or mutton or chicken. Wheat chapati or roti or bhakri made from jowar/bajra/corn/ragi is eaten with dal or whole pulses like chana, mung, rajma, etc. Idli and dosa are made from a combination of urad dal with rice. Ready-to-eat cereals like cornflakes or oats or dalia are combined with milk. Bread is eaten with egg, milk, cheese, or other sources. Such complementations improve the protein quality. Recommendations by the ICMR-NIN (2020) are that the ratios of cereals to legumes/pulses to

Table 3.4: Food sources for different types of protein.

Complete protein	Incomplete protein	Complementary protein
Milk and milk products	Cereals and millets—wheat rice, maize, and bread	Wheat chapati + curd
		Bread + milk
		Rice + milk
		Breakfast cereal + milk
		Rice + curd
		Pasta + cheese
		Bread + cheese
Egg		Bread + egg
		Wheat chapati + egg
		Rice + egg
Fish		Fish + rice
Meat/Chicken		Meat + rice
More protein combinations	Pulses	Rice + dal
		Corn + beans
		Wheat chapati + dal
		Toast + pulse soup

milk in the diet for moderately active male is 3:1:2.5, to meet the daily protein requirements. The earlier RDA (ICMR, 2010) had recommended the ratio to be 1:1:1:3.

Food proteins can be obtained from different sources:
- Muscle proteins
- Milk proteins
- Egg proteins
- Cereal proteins
- Pulse proteins.

Muscle proteins: These are obtained from red meat, fish, and poultry. They are divided into three groups based on solubility as: sarcoplasmic (e.g., myoglobin), myofibrillar (e.g., myosin and actin) and stromal proteins (e.g., collagen and elastin). Some proteins derived from muscle and other animal tissues are also used as functional (technological) ingredients in food processing (e.g., collagen and gelatin, and beef plasma protein). In addition to traditional sources of meat, there are many prepared meat products that include muscle proteins from a variety of sources. The best known product of this group is Surimi, a crude myofibrillar protein concentrate prepared by washing minced, mechanically deboned fish muscle from underutilized marine fish, or mechanically separated chicken meat or animal byproducts (e.g., beef heart muscle).

Milk proteins: They are heterogeneous and complex, and have distinct biological and physicochemical properties. Therefore, they provide a wide spectrum in their application as bioactive functional ingredients to regulate food intake and metabolism. Cow milk contains about 80% caseins and 20% whey proteins. Caseins are phosphoproteins and exist in milk as large colloidal aggregates, comprised by $\alpha s1$-, $\alpha s2$-, β- and κ-caseins and known as casein micelles. Whey proteins are represented by β-lactoglobulin, α-lactalbumin, serum albumin, immunoglobulins, lactoferrin, and proteose-peptone fractions, all of these are molecularly dispersed in the liquid fraction of milk, i.e., whey. Among milk proteins, only κ-casein contains about 5% of carbohydrates (tri- or tetrasaccharides), consisting of N-acetylneuraminic acid (sialic acid), galactose, and N-Acetylglucosamine (GlcNAc).

Egg proteins comprise about 13% of the content of whole egg. Morphologically, egg proteins can be divided into those present in egg white and in the yolk. Egg white contains mostly ovalbumin, ovotransferrin or conalbumin and ovomucoid, and some minor proteins, e.g., lysozyme, G2- and G3-globulins, ovoinhibitor, cystatin, avidin, and others. Although egg white is an excellent source of high-quality protein, it contains ovoinhibitor, a serine proteinase inhibitor that can inhibit digestive enzymes such as trypsin and chymotrypsin. This might be an important factor influencing the regulatory functions of the gastrointestinal (GI) tract, especially when raw egg whites are consumed or used for some food applications without thermal processing. Egg yolk contains α- and β-lipoproteins, phosvitin, and low-density lipoprotein (LDL), as well as minor proteins such as lipovitellin, phosvitin and vitellogenin, livetins, yolk riboflavin-binding protein, and biotin-binding protein.

Cereal proteins: Protein content of cereals and millets is 8–12%. Cereals are composed of heterogeneous groups of proteins, which based on their biological functions, are divided into two classes: metabolically active (cytoplasmic) proteins and storage proteins. Metabolically active proteins include mostly enzymes including protease inhibitors. They contain less glutamic acid and proline, and more lysine and arginine. They have a higher nutritive value than storage proteins. Storage proteins are albumins and the globulins, prolamins and glutelins, mostly representing endosperm protein, which is the main protein in cereal flours. They contain large proportion of glutamic acid and proline, and only a small proportion of lysine, arginine, threonine, and tryptophan. Even though the amino acid content varies among species of grains, lysine is the first and tryptophan is the second limiting amino acid among all grains.

Pulses protein: Protein content of pulses range from 17–30%. The major pulse/legume proteins are globulins (legumin and vicilin) and albumins (enzymatic proteins, protease inhibitors, amylase inhibitors, and lectins). Unprocessed pulses contain antinutritional factors (e.g., trypsin and chymotrypsin inhibitors), which decrease the protein digestibility, if not properly inactivated during processing. The exception is soybean that has higher protein content, i.e., 35–40%.

Proteins are also obtained from oilseeds and nuts. Examples are cruciferin or 12S protein in canola or rapeseed, 11S protein in cottonseed, 12S protein in flax and hemp, arachin in peanut, carmin in safflower, α-globulin in sesame, and helianthin in sunflower.

Fast and Slow Proteins

The concept of "fast" and "slow" proteins has been proposed. They are food proteins that are characterized by either a rapid and transient increase in plasma amino acids or a lower but more sustained response pattern of amino acid delivery into the plasma after ingestion of a protein-rich food. This is dependent on the amino acid composition of the food and the rate of its digestion. Rate of protein digestion is an important factor that regulates the postprandial rise/gain in protein. This concept is linked to the fact that an increase in plasma amino acid concentrations is a potent stimulator of muscle protein synthesis. Acute and chronic feeding after resistance exercise, show different outcomes according to the type and timing of consumption of high-quality protein sources, even when the same amount of protein is consumed. This is because the plasma amino acid levels differ according to the time of protein intake in relation to the exercise.

Whey protein is considered to be a fast protein because it quickly releases amino acids postprandially resulting in more synthesis or muscle protein as compared with the same amount of protein from casein which is considered a slow protein because it is more slowly digested and induces a smaller but prolonged increase.

RECOMMENDED DIETARY ALLOWANCES FOR PROTEIN

Dietary requirement is "the amount of protein or its constituent amino acids, or both, that must be supplied in the diet in order to satisfy the metabolic demand and achieve nitrogen equilibrium" (FAO, 2004). Dietary protein must meet physiological and metabolic demands of the body for supplying essential amino acids in adequate amounts as well as to provide additional nitrogen for synthesis of nonessential amino acids and other nitrogen-containing biological compounds. Hence recommended dietary allowances (RDA) are given in order to ensure dietary supply of adequate protein. The efficiency of utilization of dietary protein is taken into account, i.e., the quality of dietary protein is considered.

During infancy, childhood and adolescence, protein requirements are increased since there is increased cell division, synthesis of new tissue, formation of muscles and bones. During pregnancy, mothers need additional protein for development of the placenta, growth and development of the fetus as well as for synthesis of maternal proteins. During lactation, additional protein is required for synthesis of proteins that are secreted in breast milk, which is the sole source of nourishment for the young infant.

The RDA for protein is generally expressed per kilogram of body weight (BW) for normal, healthy individuals. Therefore, requirements are calculated by multiplying the per kilogram value for different age groups by the standard and normal body weight for the specific age group. On an average, an adult can maintain health with an intake of at least 0.8 g of protein/kg of body weight. However, Indians consume predominantly vegetarian diets consisting mostly of cereal-pulse or/and milk. The protein quality of such diets is lower compared with animal protein. Hence, the Expert Committee of Indian Council of Medical Research and National Nutrition (ICMR-NIN, 2020) has recommended 0.83 g/kg/day for maintenance of body weight as the safe requirement for adults, irrespective of the activity level. A healthy man requires 54 g/day and woman needs 45.7 g/day (see Table 9.1A in Chapter 9). Protein requirement for men is higher than that of women because males have more muscle mass and body weight. However, protein requirement has been reported to be higher for bodybuilders and endurance trained athletes compared to sedentary young men.

The following factors influence the requirement for amino acids and protein:
- **Dietary factors,** i.e., amino acid content, relative proportions of the amino acids, energy intake, food processing, and presence of substances that could reduce digestibility.
- **Physiological characteristics**—age particularly during periods of growth and development including pregnancy and lactation when protein accretion occurs (accumulation through synthesis of proteins in the body, and recycling of amino acids), sex, genetic background, hormones, and in response to exercise.
- **Health status** and presence of infection, trauma, neoplasia, diabetes, obesity, and cardiovascular disease. For example, gut parasites increase the need for lysine.
- **Environmental factors** such as temperature, toxic agents, air pollution, sanitation, and personal hygiene.

Protein requirement is also expressed as a percentage of the energy intake and should contribute about 10–15% of total dietary energy intake of normal healthy individuals.

Although the RDA represents a minimum amino acid requirement for most healthy individuals, higher intakes of essential or indispensable amino acids may impart metabolic benefits, including:
- Improved body composition (e.g., maintenance, growth or function of lean mass)
- Enhanced satiety
- Increased thermogenesis
- Improved glycemic regulation
- May aid in recovery after trauma, surgery, or prolonged bedrest

---

Dietary protein requirement relates to the needs of the organism. These needs are *metabolic demand,* i.e., the needs of the person *and efficiency of utilization.* Thus:

$$\text{Dietary requirement} = \frac{\text{Metabolic demand}}{\text{Efficiency of utilization}}$$

A protein source with high biological value may be required in lesser amount to fulfill requirements than the protein sources having low biological value.

Metabolic demand: It entails the demand for those amino acids and proteins which are involved in the pathways linked with maintenance of the structure and functions of the body including synthesis of hair, skin, and secretions of the body as well as urinary, fecal, and other losses. This demand greatly varies from individual to individual and within the same individual at different stages of life. When growth occurs, body synthesizes more protein and utilization of amino acids and protein by the body is high. It is difficult to precisely assess the metabolic demand, but it implies the protein requirement for the following purposes:

Obligatory demands: Even when no protein is consumed, the body continues to lose some amount of nitrogen through feces, urine, and sweat/perspiration. This is "obligatory nitrogen loss" and is the sum of all nitrogenous losses through all routes from the body.

Contd...

Contd...

> The *efficiency of utilization* is a crucial factor in determining requirements. Metabolic demand is influenced by the following factors:
>
> **Energy:** Adequacy of energy intake influence nitrogen balance. If activity level and energy expenditure remain unchanged, increased energy intake tends to improve nitrogen balance. Although why this occurs is not fully clear. It is speculated that hormonal responses to the higher energy intake may minimize net protein loss, inhibit proteolysis, and oxidation of amino acids. Low energy consumption adversely affects utilization of protein.
>
> **Micronutrients:** Micronutrients play an important role in amino acid metabolism. Vitamin B_6 is crucial in protein metabolism. B vitamins or zinc also influence the biological value of the protein. Inadequate or excess intakes of micronutrients can place metabolic demand or stress. For example, if excess iron is consumed, ferritin has to be synthesized, which may occur at the cost of synthesis of other important proteins for growth.
>
> **Lifestyle and environmental influences:** Lifestyle entails food consumption pattern and the level of physical activity which in turn affects body composition and metabolic demands. Smoking and alcohol consumption may alter the demand for different amino acids. High protein intake among athletes may increase the oxidation of amino acids. Immune responses to infections also increase metabolic demand.
>
> **Digestibility of dietary proteins:** Most proteins are digested yielding amino acids or peptides which are later absorbed. Excess is excreted to maintain nitrogen balance. Fecal nitrogen may increase when large amounts of nondigestible carbohydrate are fermented in the gut and tend to increase the bacterial biomass and soluble nitrogen-containing compounds. The digestibility of protein in Indian diets is about 85% (rice with milk or beans).
>
> **Protein Energy (PE) Ratio:** Adequate energy intake is required so that the dietary protein is utilized and deposited. It is necessary that sufficient amount of carbohydrate and fat are consumed (nonprotein energy sources) in order that dietary amino acids are utilized for protein synthesis and for the other functions that amino acids perform. If energy from CHO and fat is not enough, the body will break down protein for energy rather than for synthesis, thus compromising utilization of protein. PE ratio changes with level of energy intake. PE ratio for sedentary men and women is 10.4 and 11.1% respectively and among children and adolescents ranges from 4.8-6.7%. It should not be more than 15%.

FOOD SOURCES OF PROTEIN

Dietary proteins are obtained from plant, animal, and marine sources. Among plant foods, pulses, and nuts are rich sources and soybean is exceptionally rich as it has much higher protein content than other pulses. In typical Indian diets, cereals contribute more amount of protein. They do not have as high protein content as do pulses, but they are consumed in larger amounts and thus significantly contribute toward fulfilling the daily protein requirement. Protein content of some commonly consumed foods is given in Appendix 1.

Animal and Vegetable Proteins

Animal protein comes from meat, egg, fish, and milk. They are considered of good quality because they contain all the indispensable amino acids, the exception being gelatin. Animal proteins contain more amounts of sulfur-containing amino acids (methionine and cysteine) that on oxidation increases acid load in the body which is detrimental to health. This increased acid load stimulates resorption (removal) of bone mineral. It is also related to the increased urinary excretion of calcium and oxalate which can increase risk of formation of kidney/renal stones.

The protein in the diets of vegetarians comes from various plant sources such as pulses, nuts, seeds, and vegetables. Since cereals are not so rich in protein, but are consumed in large quantity, cereals' contribution of protein in the Indian diet is high. Vegetarian foods contain fewer amounts of sulfur amino acids, lysine, and threonine contributing low renal acid loads. Plant sources are also rich in many phytochemicals which confer additional health benefits.

In most plant proteins, i.e., legumes, nuts, oil seeds and cereals/millets (grains), the essential/indispensable amino acid content is about 62–81% as compared with hen's egg protein especially the methionine content is lower and lysine is a limiting amino acid in grains and nuts. On the other hand, nonessential/dispensable amino acid content, especially that of arginine and glycine, is 111–129% of that in egg which is the reference protein. In pulses, grains and most nuts, alanine content is higher compared with milk. Serine content in legumes, grain products, and hazelnuts is higher than in meat. In plant proteins, the major limiting amino acids are methionine, lysine, and tryptophan. Plant foods also contain relatively low amounts of leucine, an important branched chain amino acid. Generally, leucine content is less than 8% of the total protein in plant proteins, whereas in animal proteins, its content is about 8–14% of the total protein. There are a few plant protein sources that have a better content than others, e.g., dried seaweed, soybean, pumpkin seeds, and peanuts, but they need to be consumed in relatively large amounts.

Although having less amount or no animal protein in the diet limits protein synthesis, there is a need to examine other perspectives and health implications. There are feeding studies suggesting that ketogenic amino acids (present in more amounts in animal proteins) increase serum cholesterol as do a combination of lysine and methionine and that the lower levels of lysine and methionine provided by vegetarian diets may give some protection against cardiovascular disease and perhaps cancer.

Besides this, insulin is secreted by the pancreas in response to the postprandial increase in circulating amino acids. For this, essential amino acids are more effective. In contrast, dispensable amino acids especially arginine and precursors of pyruvate preferentially release glucagon. This suggests that vegetarian diets will promote glucagon activity that will in turn stimulate gluconeogenesis and downregulate insulin.

Among the animal proteins, dairy products, i.e., milk, curds/yogurt, cheese, and whey proteins are important. They have more potent effects on insulin secretion than do other commonly consumed animal proteins. The advantage of consuming these foods is that they contain bioactive peptides, that are good sources of minerals like calcium, magnesium, potassium, and low glycemic index sugars—all of these are helpful for glycemic control. Benefits can be derived therefore by persons at high risk of cardiovascular disease by increasing their intake of plant proteins, as part of a complete diet. These proteins as part of a whole diet could also help lower blood pressure.

Animal protein consumption means livestock rearing that requires large areas of land, water, nitrogen, and fossil energy. Also large amounts of greenhouse gases are transmitted. The water and nitrogen footprints of plant protein production are estimated to be much less than livestock rearing and animal protein food production. However, animal protein foods have better protein quality, with a high digestibility (more than 90%), good bioavailability and they are likely to have better efficiency than plant proteins in muscle anabolic processes.

Animal protein foods (except dairy foods) are good sources of heme iron, cholecalciferol, docosahexaenoic acid (in case of fish), vitamin B_{12} and conjugated linoleic acid, substances that are not found in most plant-based protein foods. Therefore, moderate amounts of non-vegetarian food items and dairy products should be made part of the regular diet.

DEFICIENCY OF PROTEIN: ITS CAUSES AND CONSEQUENCES

Protein and amino acids are not stored in the body, in contrast to fat which is stored in adipocytes and glucose (carbohydrate) which is stored as glycogen in muscles and liver. Skeletal muscle mass is the largest reservoir of protein. Therefore, muscle mass is a good indicator of protein homeostasis and if protein and energy intakes are inadequate (regardless of the cause, i.e., either catabolism is greater, e.g., during anorexia or starvation or anabolic stimuli are reduced), the consequence is muscle wasting. This is reflected by unintentional weight loss of about 5–10% which is the result of a combination of accelerated muscle protein degradation and reduced protein synthesis. Such a situation occurs in many chronic diseases. Thus, a marginal-to-low protein intake results in less body cell mass, compromised muscle mass, muscle size, and function although the person may be in nitrogen balance or nitrogen equilibrium may be near zero.

Optimal protein intake is necessary to avoid its deficiency. This protein should be of good quality. High quality protein such as animal protein requires less energy intake to meet the essential amino acid needs than lower quality proteins such as plant proteins. Three aspects are important in quality—the balance of amino acids in the diet, the digestibility of the proteins to release amino acids for absorption, and availability of the amino acids for protein synthesis.

The protein requirement of 0.83 g/kg/day is based on adequate energy intakes, i.e., at least 10% energy of total dietary energy should come from protein. Metabolism of protein is closely related to energy metabolism since all aspects of protein metabolism ranging from amino acid transport to synthesis of various nitrogen-containing compounds and excretion require energy. When there is inadequate energy intake, amino acids are used as metabolic fuel but their energetic efficiency is lower than that of glucose and fatty acids.

Low protein intake (<0.4–0.6 g/kg body weight per day), especially if the quality of protein is poor, having limiting amino acid (s) will have adverse effects on the body. Therefore, inadequate intake of protein even if it is of good quality or intake of poor quality proteins (even if it appears to be in fairly adequate amounts) will result in reduced synthesis of all proteins including transport proteins, enzymes, and hormones. Protein deficiency adversely affects both digestion and absorption functions of the gastrointestinal tract. Growth and turnover of the intestinal mucosa is inhibited by malnutrition or starvation, protein depletion, as well as deficiencies of specific nutrients. Dietary quality may also be important as good quality proteins stimulate amino acid utilization in the gut and therefore induce more gut amino acid retention. Anorexia is also present. Protein deficiency occurs during starvation, fasting, illness, and poor dietary habits. Fever, infection, injury, burns and surgery, and in some gastrointestinal diseases like protein losing enteropathy also can increase risk of protein deficiency, especially if dietary intake is low. Protein deficiency affects all organs. The deficiency is of great concern in young infants and children as it can severely retard the growth and development. It may also occur in adults who have highly inadequate intakes, those who may have chronic blood loss or protein malabsorption due to gastrointestinal disorders and cancer. The elderly are also at risk of protein deficiency and its consequences. Severe protein deficiency in children results in a disease Kwashiorkor. Marasmus is the consequence of severe deficiency of both protein and energy. Marasmic kwashiorkor is characterized by severe wasting and there is edema. Characteristics of kwashiorkor and marasmus are given in Chapter 12 which deals with protein-energy malnutrition.

Less severe deficiency can occur in elderly persons (with those who are homebound likely to be more vulnerable) that increases their susceptibility to metabolic and infectious diseases. Protein deficiency results in the following:

- Decreased protein synthesis and increased breakdown of skeletal muscle and proteins, due to which serum albumin is low and amino acid concentrations in blood are also low.
- Reduced levels of many hormones like insulin, growth hormone, insulin-like growth factor-1, thyroid hormones, and reduced synthesis of neurotransmitters.
- Antioxidant enzymes are reduced, resulting in greater oxidative stress.
- Compromised function of gastrointestinal tract leading to impairment in absorption, transport, and storage of several nutrients.
- Impairment in immune function and increased susceptibility to infections.
- Reduced hemoglobin resulting anemia.
- Loss of calcium, bone loss, and dental abnormalities.
- Hair changes—become brittle, break easily, and changes in color due to less production of pigments.

Signs and symptoms of deficiency depend on the severity and duration of the protein (and nutritional) deprivation, age, and whether there is any infection.

Edema: In case of protein deficiency, albumin and globulin levels in the blood (plasma) fall. Blood and fluids are forced to come out of the cells. Accumulation of fluid in interstitial spaces in tissues and organs is a condition called edema. Albumin plays an important role in regulating fluid balance. In protein deficiency, the body is unable to synthesize enough albumin, resulting in edema. Under normal circumstances, plasma fluid remains inside the blood vessel under the influence of colloidal pressure maintained by albumin. When the amount of fluid in blood is lowered, albumin is able to draw some of the interstitial fluid back into blood. With each heartbeat, some fluid along with nutrients is pushed out of the capillaries into the interstitial space but albumin does not move out along with the fluid. Edema due to protein deficiency is characterized by swelling on the ankles, hands, and face giving the person a swollen appearance, and the person becomes lethargic and depressed. It is commonly seen in children suffering from protein undernutrition, elders, and in people having very low protein diets.

Muscle wasting: Muscle wasting is the loss of muscle mass due to weakened muscles or shrinkage of it (muscle atrophy). It may be due to lack of physical activity or lack of protein intake and protein utilization in the body. The body does not store protein. However, muscle mass is a reservoir of protein. Proteolysis, i.e., protein breakdown or catabolism is accelerated in many disease conditions, such as diabetes mellitus, renal and liver failure, HIV infection and AIDS, and cancer, and this is the major cause of muscle wasting in such conditions.

When dietary protein intake is inadequate or during fasting, starvation, and in fever, infection, injury, burns and surgery, there is tissue breakdown (catabolic state). If this occurs for a long period, there can be considerable loss of muscle mass and loss of body weight. Muscle atrophy may also occur when protein degradation rates exceed protein synthesis, which occurs in fasting states, e.g., anorexia and starvation. Under such conditions, protein breakdown increases while protein synthesis declines resulting in negative muscle protein balance. Muscle protein breakdown is accelerated when there is insulin resistance, when catabolic hormone levels are high, e.g., glucocorticoid levels are high or in thyrotoxicity, or when there is inflammation. Resistance exercise training can suppress muscle proteolysis.

Sarcopenia: Sarcopenia is age-related loss of muscle mass and muscle strength which contributes substantially to physical frailty, reduces mobility in the elderly, and increase in the risk of falls and fractures. It is related to reduced independence, disability, and increased dependence on others for care of self. Sarcopenia is caused by several factors such as alterations in metabolism, neuromuscular deterioration, marginal nutrient intakes, and absorption. It can be caused by nutritional deficiency, i.e., chronic undernutrition with inadequate intakes of protein, energy, and micronutrients. The severity of muscle reduction varies considerably among persons and is generally seen in persons who are 60 years or older, with the incidence increasing with age. Institutionalized elderly are at risk.

> **Research Glimpse:** Sarcopenia is characterized by the gradual and progressive loss of muscle mass, along with reduction in strength, and physical endurance. It is a common condition in sedentary adults particularly in aging. Sarcopenia can be mitigated by regular aerobic and resistance exercise along with good nutrition with inclusion of adequate protein and energy and other lifestyle changes. The European Society for Clinical Nutrition and Metabolism (ESPEN) in 2014 has given certain recommendations for healthcare professionals to help older adults sustain muscle strength and function which are as follows:
> a. The diet should provide at least 1.0–1.2 g protein/kg body weight/day for healthy older people.
> b. The diet should provide at least 1.2–1.5 g protein/kg body weight/day for healthy older people who are malnourished or at risk of malnutrition or suffering from acute or chronic illness.
> c. All older people should undertake daily physical activity or exercise (resistance training and aerobic exercise) as long as possible.
> *Deutz NEP, Bauer JM, Barazzoni R, Biolo G, Boirie Y, Bosy-Westphal A, Cederholm T, Cruz-Jentoft A, Krznariçi Z, Nair KS, Singer P, Teta D, Tiptonm K, Calder PC. Protein intake and exercise for optimal muscle function with aging: Recommendations from the ESPEN Expert Group. Clinical Nutrition. 2014;33(6):929-36.*

Low immunity and poor resistance to infection: Antibodies are made up of protein and in protein deficiency; antibody synthesis is reduced, which increases the risk of low immunity. This leads to frequent infections which are reflected in various symptoms such as cold, cough, fever, and many infectious diseases. The immune system has many components. There are different types of cells like phagocytes, natural killer cells, dendritic cells, many proteins like lysozymes, C-reactive proteins (CRP), complement system, and interferon. T and B lymphocytes play an important role in immunity (they secrete cytokines, and chemokines that have an important role in stimulating immune cells, regulating immune, and inflammatory reactions), that may be compromised by the lack of adequate protein.

For all these, proteins and amino acids are essential. In protein deficiency, the ability to synthesize many of these is reduced. Hence, the lack of proteins tends to lower the immune capacity and makes the person vulnerable to repeated infections including respiratory infection, diarrhea, and others. Also the severity and duration of infections may increase. It is common in children who are undernourished. Most children who have severe protein–energy malnutrition have infections but they may be asymptomatic because their immune system is not functioning well; so much so that they may not even have the fever that typically occurs with inflammation.

> Neutrophils are important for engulfing invading bacteria.
> Eosinophils are important for conferring protection against viruses and parasites.

In newborn children and infants, with severe protein malnutrition, there is atrophy of the thymus and bone marrow, both of which are important for immunity because B and T cells are synthesized in them.

Delayed wound healing: Wounds can occur from either accidental injuries or surgical intervention. Wound healing comprises highly integrated and overlapping events or phases namely rapid hemostasis followed by inflammation, then cell differentiation, proliferation and migration to the site of the wound, angiogenesis (formation of new blood vessels), and tissue remodeling which is essentially regrowth of epithelial tissue over the wound surface. Optimal and appropriate wound healing also requires synthesis, crosslinking, and alignment of collagen so that the healing tissue has appropriate strength as well as the activity of a network of blood cells, different tissues, cytokines, and growth factors. All of these activities increase the demand for several nutrients including protein, vitamin C, vitamin A, zinc, energy, etc. However, in protein deficiency, the process of replacing the damaged tissue is slowed down.

Anemia: Low protein intake reduces metabolic activity resulting in impaired production of erythropoietin (EPO) hormone following by decreased production of RBCs resulting in anemia. This type of anemia is referred as macrocytic hypochromic anemia. RBCs contain hemoglobin that is also a protein. It reduces the oxygen supply to the tissues and hampers their functioning.

Growth retardation: Protein deficiency diminishes the synthesis of all proteins and tissue deposition including skeletal tissues. It adversely influences the vital functioning of cells, tissues, and organs, and eventually results in growth retardation. Thus, protein deficiency is of concern during critical periods of growth that includes pregnancy, and postnatally throughout infancy and childhood until the end of adolescence.

Poor mental development: In children, protein deficiency has negative effects on brain growth and mental performance. Brain development is a finely tuned controlled process that involves cell division, differentiation, migration, and synaptic connectivity. In the first 1,000 days of life starting in pregnancy, i.e., intrauterine life through the first 2 years of postnatal life, there are five critical neurodevelopmental processes that can be influenced by nutrition—proliferation of neurons, growth of axons and dendrites, formation of synapses and their functioning, myelination, and programmed cell death or apoptosis. Protein (as well as energy) is required for cell proliferation and differentiation and hence protein deficiency can have global effects on brain development, besides adversely affecting synaptogenesis (reduction in synapse number) and the development of the hippocampus.

Cognitive ability: It has been shown to reduce the DNA and RNA content in neurons as well as alter fatty acid profiles. This means that the number of neurons is less, less myelination (hypomyelination) occurs as well as protein synthesis is reduced, there are changes in structural proteins and production of neurotransmitters and growth factors. Further, dendritic arbor complexity is also reduced. All of these can contribute to reduced brain size (as seen in animal models). This can ultimately compromise the cognitive functions in the child, although motor development may not be affected.

Thus, protein-energy malnutrition results in a wide range of cognitive deficits. Children with protein energy malnutrition have been found to perform poorly on tests of attention, memory, learning, and visuospatial ability, and their performance unfortunately did not improve with age. However, performance on tests of attention, visual perception, and verbal comprehension improved with age although malnourished children did not perform as well as did well-nourished children.

Neurotransmitters: Acetylcholine, glutamate, gamma-aminobutyric acid (GABA), glycine, serotonin, dopamine, norepinephrine, epinephrine, and histamine are the most common neurotransmitters. Many neurotransmitters are synthesized from amino acids, e.g., serotonin is formed from tryptophan and norepinephrine and epinephrine from tyrosine. Deficiencies in these neurotransmitters can affect mood, aggressiveness, appetite or cognition.

Fatty liver: The liver plays a very important role in the metabolism and homeostasis of all macronutrients including lipids. Protein deficiency and malnutrition are known to predispose persons to nonalcoholic hepatic steatosis. One theory is that since there are no carrier proteins to carry lipid out of the liver, it accumulates thereby leading to "fatty liver" or hepatic steatosis. Protein deficiency results in a reduction in plasma triglycerides and phospholipids and rise in free fatty acids. In case of fatty liver, there is accumulation of triglycerides at the cost of hepatic phospholipids. There is also a change in glutathione peroxidase (GPX), superoxide dismutase (SOD), and other antioxidative systems, leading to an increase in lipid peroxidation which happens in development and progression of nonalcoholic liver cirrhosis particularly protein undernutrition.

CONSEQUENCES OF EXCESSIVE INTAKE OF PROTEIN

ICMR-NIN (2020) has recommended that the consumption of protein more than 2-3 times the RDA and particularly if the PE ratio of the diet is more than 34%, it may be harmful as it may increase the nitrogenous substances (urea) in the blood and urine. The Expert Group of FAO/WHO/UN (2007) has recommended 2.0 g of protein/kg of body weight as the safe limit for adults or, in general, twice the recommended level. Excess protein intake may be from the consumption of dietary sources as well as from protein supplements. A high protein intake (>2 g per kg BW per day for adults) increases the nitrogen load on the gastrointestinal tract, liver, and kidneys. In case of many individuals, a protein intake greater than its safe upper limits in different age groups can exceed the ability of the liver, intestine, and kidneys to detoxify ammonia and should be avoided. High protein intakes can have adverse effects such as intestinal discomfort, hyperaminoacidemia, hyperammonemia, hyperinsulinemia, dehydration, irritation, nausea, diarrhea, liver and kidney injuries, fatigue, headache, seizures, high risk of cardiovascular disease, or even death.

Also, problems of high protein intake can be exacerbated if carbohydrate intake is low because it will place additional burden on the liver and kidney to produce large amounts of glucose from amino acids besides the roles of these organs in disposing of excessive ammonia and urea. However, when protein intake is ≤2 g per kg per day, there is little evidence of intestinal, hepatic, renal or cardiovascular dysfunction in healthy people. In some cases, it has been observed that a dietary protein intake of 1.6 g per kg BW per day for 6 months increased the glomerular filtration rate (GFR) by 5% and the kidney mass by 2.5% in healthy adults. In adults, the GFR reaches a maximum value at a dietary protein intake of 2 g per kg BW per day. Therefore, it is important to determine that there is no preexisting kidney disease when a person is considering consuming a high protein diet. This is especially advisable for persons who are interested in high protein diets for weight loss. Persons who have renal dysfunction or gout are advised to consume an adequate amount of high-quality protein but not an excessive amount of protein. Overconsumption of dietary amino acids and protein from meals and excessive supplementation, are of concern because they can also compromise the health of humans, particularly those with hepatic or renal dysfunction.

Of special concern is when protein from animal sources is largely consumed. Excessive intake of animal protein increases uric acid level in blood. Animal protein contains purines which are broken down by the body to uric acid. Excess of uric acid in blood is deposited in joints, tendons, kidneys, and other organs and may cause gout. There is also risk of uric acid stone formation in the kidney (Fig. 3.4). Urea is an end-product of protein metabolism that is excreted through urine via kidneys. When higher amount of protein is consumed, more urea is produced. Hence, high protein intake can increase the renal load. If the kidneys are immature or are not functioning well, consuming high amount of protein beyond the safe limit of 2 g/kg body weight should be done cautiously taking care not to disturb kidney function or aggravate a pre-existing renal problem.

Studies reveal that high protein increases calcium excretion thereby depleting calcium from bones and increases the risk of osteoporosis. Since protein-rich foods are also rich in fat, judicious selection of food is essential. Animal foods are rich in protein but also contain higher amount of saturated fats and cholesterol and are low in fiber content. This combination increases risk for heart disease and obesity. Also, people who consume high protein diets may not consume enough vegetables and fruits. This can increase their risk for micronutrient deficiencies.

Many processed meat products contain nitrites that are used for preservation and color fixation. These nitrites can have adverse effect on RBC particularly among children. They can be converted into nitrosamines which are carcinogenic. Eating red meat has also been associated with colon cancer.

Excess protein intake may result in buildup of amino acids and poses a risk for brain damage and mental retardation, particularly if a person is sensitive to a particular amino acid, e.g., buildup of phenylalanine in the individuals having phenylketonuria can seriously affect brain development.

Excess protein intake often comes from the use of protein supplements and often due to its use for avoiding protein deficiency or to build extra muscles and muscle strength for the gym or otherwise. These powders generally contain protein isolates of soya, pea or whey protein concentrates along with other ingredients including sugar. Evidence has shown that prolonged use of supplements increases the risk of digestive complaints, poor appetite and allergies as well as weight gain and decline in kidney functions.

PROTEIN HOMEOSTASIS

Protein homeostasis is critical. Homeostasis is essentially maintenance of a constant internal environment within the body and is the process by which the body constantly monitors and ensures that the internal environment is stable, by making adjustments when it is subjected or exposed to different environmental conditions including diet. It is a complex phenomenon. Protein homeostasis occurs at the level of the body and also at cellular level. It is a system that governs different processes occurring inside the cell using different proteins.

> Protein homeostasis is fundamental for cell function and survival, because proteins are involved in all aspects of cellular function, ranging from cell metabolism and cell division to the cell's response to environmental challenges. Protein homeostasis is tightly regulated by the synthesis, folding, trafficking, and clearance of proteins, all of which act in an orchestrated manner to ensure proteome stability.
>
> The **proteome** is defined as the entire set or complement of proteins that is or can be expressed by a cell, tissue, or organism. This term encompasses the two words protein and genome.

Protein homeostasis at body level: It involves maintenance of body protein and amino acid homeostasis. The systems that are involved are:

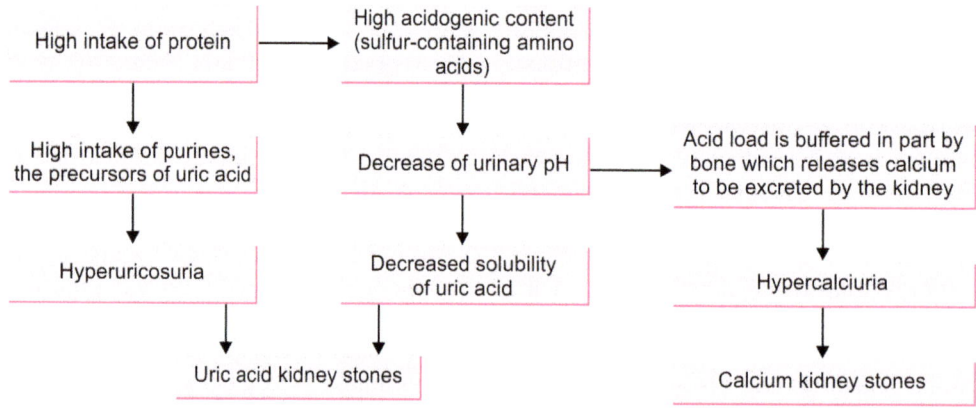

Fig. 3.4: Pathobiochemical mechanisms of animal protein-induced nephrolithiasis.

- Synthesis of proteins
- Degradation of proteins or their breakdown
- Interconversions of amino acids
- Transformation of amino acids and ultimately their oxidation with production of the waste product urea and carbon dioxide
- Synthesis of dispensable amino acids.

Protein homeostasis at cellular level: At the cellular level, homeostasis is achieved by rigorously involving mechanisms such as protein folding and protein degradation. Protein homeostasis requires the coordinated action of important systems within the cell—translation, folding, assembly or clearance of proteins for the purpose of maintaining the stability of the proteome and ensuring that renewal goes on under normal conditions. When proteins emerge from the ribosome, the newly emerging polypeptide must fold properly and it then has to be translocated to the appropriate intracellular compartment and get assembled into a stable, functional complex. Within the cell, activities of protein synthesis and assembly, disassembly, trafficking, and translocation to different intracellular compartments maintain the structural, qualitative, and functional stability of intracellular proteins. However, the proteins are many times subjected to stress. Stress can lead to partial unfolding resulting in misfolded, aggregated molecules that are capable of damaging the cell in which they are present as well as causing damaging to other cells. Disturbance in protein homeostasis therefore represents disturbances in protein translation, protein degradation, and is typically associated with aging. Alterations in protein homeostasis underlie the etiology of many diseases such as diabetes, cancer, and diseases of the nervous system.

Amino acids come from dietary sources and they are also synthesized in the body. Both together form the "**amino acid pool**" within the cells and circulating blood. Although a person's protein intake in terms of both quantity and quality (type and amount of different amino acids) varies from day-to-day and the rate of protein degradation also differs; the pattern of amino acids in the amino acid pool is maintained. This pool is important for synthesis of body proteins and other nitrogenous substances.

Several organs play an important role in homeostasis. The liver plays a very important role in metabolism of amino acids. It is the only organ capable of catabolizing (breakdown) all amino acids. It removes approximately two-thirds of the amino acids that are absorbed. A major fraction is metabolized and about one-third is used for protein synthesis. For most essential amino acids, hepatic degradation is regulated in relation to adequacy of intake and rises sharply when intake exceeds requirements. Some amino acids like isoleucine, leucine, and valine are sent into circulation to other tissues. The liver plays a key role in converting NH_3, the end product of protein and amino acid metabolism, to urea. Ammonia is harmful and by converting it to urea, liver protects the entire body. This urea is then excreted by kidneys through urine (Fig. 3.5).

Protein intake and excretion also ultimately determine protein balance. Two aspects are important in determining

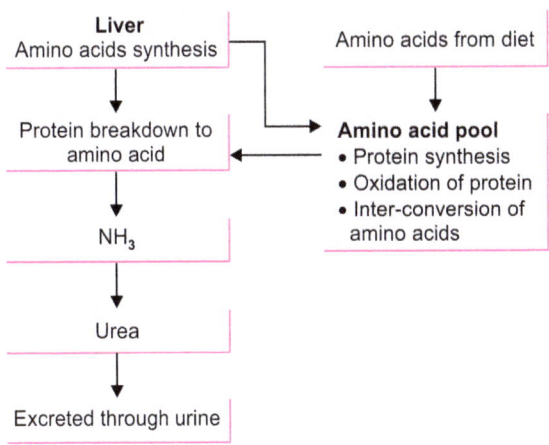

Fig. 3.5: Protein homeostasis and amino acid pool.

protein balance—balance between protein intake and excretion and balance between protein synthesis and breakdown. "**Protein turnover**" is the overall process of protein synthesis (anabolism) and breakdown (catabolism). In a healthy adult, approximately 30 g of protein is synthesized daily and a similar amount is broken down to amino acids for maintenance.

NITROGEN BALANCE

Nitrogen balance implies the balance between protein synthesis and breakdown in the body. In this state of equilibrium, nitrogen is separated out from the amino acids by the process called deamination. **Deamination** produces ammonia which is released in the bloodstream and reaches the liver where urea is formed and excreted by kidney through urine. When nitrogen intake is in equilibrium with the nitrogen excretion, it is considered that the person is in "nitrogen equilibrium" or "zero nitrogen balance". When excretion exceeds intake, the person is said to be in negative nitrogen balance and when intake exceeds excretion, it is said to be positive nitrogen balance.

- **Negative nitrogen balance** occurs in—starvation, undernutrition, fever, extensive burns, trauma, and postoperative conditions.
- **Positive nitrogen balance** occurs in growth and development. This is typically seen during pregnancy, infancy, childhood, and adolescence.

Achieving nitrogen balance: The amount and quality of dietary protein consumed determine nitrogen balance. Besides the total amount of protein being adequate as per recommendations, a suitable mix of amino acids should match demand for protein synthesis and other metabolic pathways. The demand for indispensable amino acids must be satisfied from the diet. The body also needs amino acid carbon skeletons and amino acid precursors for synthesizing a range of nonprotein products.

EVALUATION OF PROTEIN QUALITY

Protein quality is a crucial parameter that indicates the utilization of protein via digestibility and absorption of of the release of the amino acids. Two foods may contain the same amount of protein, but their quality may differ because of their amino acid composition. Protein is not considered only in terms of quantity or as complete protein but also its digestibility, i.e., the capacity of the protein to provide metabolically available nitrogen and amino acids to tissues and organs. The quality of protein is affected by the composition of the food and the absolute and relative amounts of dietary indispensable amino acids and the bioavailability of amino acids. The quality of proteins from the plant foods such as cereals, pulses and vegetables are considered poor (i) because of digestibility and (ii) because they have one or more limiting amino acid. The amino acid that has lowest amino acid score in that particular food is called 'limiting amino acid'. For example, lysine in cereals and methionine in pulses. Some of the factors are:

1. Amino acid content
2. Presence of substances that will inhibit protein digestion in small intestine, e.g. trypsin inhibitors.
3. Antinutritional factors in foods can cause digestive losses and structural changes in amino acids.
4. Interference of nonavailable carbohydrates such as dietary fiber
5. Influence of heating and processing.

Different Methods Used to Assess the Protein Quality

Biological value, NPU, and PER are older methods for evaluating protein quality, whereas PDCAAS and DIAAS are newer methods.

Assessment methods for protein quality
- Biological value
- Protein digestibility
- Net protein utilization (NPU)
- Net dietary protein energy ratio
- Protein efficiency ratio (PER)
- Net protein ratio
- Amino acid score
- Protein digestibility corrected amino acid score (PDCAAS)
- Digestible indispensable amino acid score (DIAAS)

Biological value (BV): It was developed by Mitchell in 1925. It is a measure of nitrogen retention in the body for maintenance and growth or how well the absorbed amino acids meet the metabolic demand of the body (the proportion of absorbed protein retained in the body). Two groups of experimental animals, usually albino rats are used. One group is fed the test protein (as the sole source of protein) and the other group is fed a protein-free diet. Every day the nitrogen (N) excretion in urine and feces are analyzed in both the groups and BV is calculated. If protein is of good quality, it (and nitrogen) will be better retained in the body. A protein source that has a BV of 70 or more is considered to be capable of supporting growth. However, this procedure is expensive and time-consuming.

For any food or diet, BV cannot be more than 100, since a value of 100 indicates that 100% or all of the nitrogen that has been absorbed is utilized by the body (Table 3.5).

Protein digestibility: Protein digestibility is the proportion of ingested food protein that is absorbed after the process of digestion is completed. Protein digestibility of mixed vegetarian diets is approximately 85%. This is assessed by measuring the loss of nitrogen in feces with the test protein and on a protein-

Table 3.5: Biological value (BV) of commonly consumed foods.

Foods	BV
Egg	96
Milk	90
Meat	74
Fish	80
Rice	80
Wheat	66
Bengal gram	72
Peanuts	55

Source: Gopalan, et al. and Rao BSN et.al Nutritive value of Indian Foods, 2012

Table 3.6: Protein digestibility values for some common foods.

Protein source	Digestibility
Egg	97
Indian rice diet	77
Indian rice diet + milk	87
Milk and cheese	95
Whole wheat	86
Polished rice	88
Peanuts	94
Maize	85
Soy flour	86

Source: WHO Technical Report Series 935 (2007)

free diet. Digestibility values of selected foods are given in Table 3.6.

Net protein utilization (NPU): This method was developed by Miller and Bender in 1955. Net protein utilization (NPU) calculates the N balance data in man. It is an index of quality that takes into account not only the proportion of dietary protein retained but also the amount digested. NPU of average Indian diet is approximately 65. NPU reflects both digestibility and biological value.

Net dietary protein energy (NDPE) ratio: Utilization of protein and deposition of protein in the body depends on the energy intake. If energy intake is inadequate, the body utilizes protein for obtaining the energy and consequently utilization for deposition in the body is reduced. This implies inefficient utilization of protein. Net dietary protein energy ratio takes into account the amount of protein (relative to total energy intake) and the protein quality. It is calculated by multiplying the energy obtained from protein by NPU divided by the total energy obtained from that food or diet.

$$\text{NDPE ratio} = \frac{\text{Protein energy}}{\text{Net dietary intake of kcals}} \times \text{NPU}$$

(Utilization of N under actually eaten food)

If energy intake is expressed in kcal, the result is expressed as net dietary protein calories percent or NDP kcal%.

Protein efficiency ratio (PER): Protein efficiency ratio is the simplest measure of protein quality which measures the ability of a protein to support growth. It is based on the assumption that weight gain per gram of protein intake in a growing animal (usually rats) is proportional to gain in body protein. The method was developed by Osborne, Mendel, and

Ferry in 1919. It is a good method to compare a new protein against reference protein of known PER which is casein (PER 2.5). It is to be noted that PER is not done on humans.

If PER >2.5, 45 g protein can meet RDA.

If PER <2.5, Approximately 65 g protein can meet RDA.

It assesses only weight gain which may not represent the body protein under all conditions. A limitation of PER is that using amino acid needs of rats results in overestimation of protein quality of animal protein and underestimation in case of plant protein. Also, there are differences in amino acid requirements of rats and humans. Rats apparently require more amount of sulfur-containing amino acids than do humans.

Net protein ratio (NPR): Net protein ratio is a modification of PER and was introduced by Bender and Doell (1957). It includes the allowance for protein needed for maintenance.

$$\text{NPR} = \frac{\text{Gain in weight of test group} + \text{Loss in weight of nonprotein group}}{\text{Protein intake of test group}}$$

Amino acid score (Chemical score): All the above methods involve animal experiments. Amino acid score is a chemical method, which involves comparing the amino acid content with the reference protein or reference human amino acid requirement pattern. It determines the effectiveness with which the nitrogen absorbed from a food protein is able to meet the requirement for indispensable amino acids at the safe level of protein intake.

$$\text{Amino acid score (AAC) m} = \frac{\text{mg of amino acid in 1 g of test protein}}{\text{mg of amino acid in 1 g of reference protein}}$$

This helps to identify the limiting amino acid in a protein. If the protein's limiting amino acid is 70% of the amount found in the reference protein, the amino acid score is 70. However, this method cannot estimate the digestibility of the protein.

Protein digestibility corrected amino acid score (PDCAAS): The protein digestibility corrected amino acid score was introduced by the Food and Agricultural Organization in 1991. It is internationally approved and widely used routinely to evaluate protein quality and has replaced the older traditional biological methods like PER which was performed on rats. PDCAAS is estimated by comparing the essential amino acid content of the protein with the essential amino acid pattern of a reference protein. Correction is made for differences in protein digestibility which is determined by measurement on rats. It is rapid and useful.

The following three factors are considered in PDCAAS:
- Essential amino acid content of the food protein
- Digestibility of the protein
- Ability of the protein to supply indispensable amino acids in amounts that can meet human needs.

PDCAAS is based on the amino acid requirements of 2–5-year-old children because at this age (except for infancy),

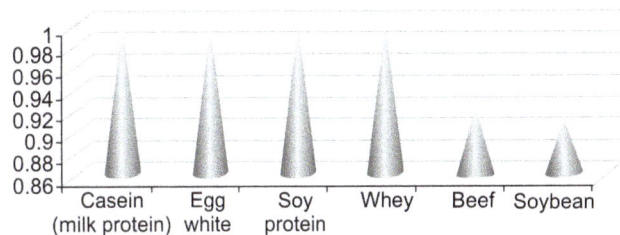

Fig. 3.6: Protein digestibility corrected amino acid score (PDCAAS) values of selected food proteins.

demand for amino acids is highest compared with other stages in the life cycle.

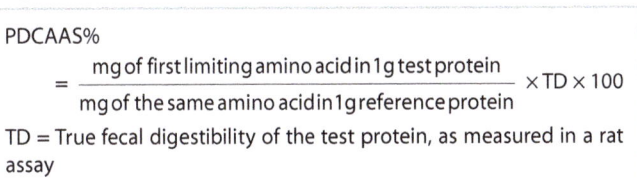

A PDCAAS value of 1 is the highest and 0 the lowest. Figure 3.6 shows the PDCAAS of selected proteins. Foods having low PDCAAS can be combined effectively with high PDCAAS food to improve the value.

Food	PDCAAS	Limiting amino acid
Grain protein	0.4–0.5	Lysine
White bean protein	0.6–0.7	Methionine
Grain + White bean protein	~1.0	Mutual complementation

DIAAS (Digestible Indispensable Amino Acid Score)

In 2011, the FAO Expert Consultation on "Protein Quality Evaluation in Human Nutrition" indicated that there is a need for accurate information on the amounts of digestible or preferably bioavailable amino acids in foods and proteins. It also recommended that dietary amino acids be treated as individual nutrients and that wherever possible data for digestible or bioavailable amino acids be given in food tables on an individual amino acid basis. Based on both these considerations, a new protein quality measure (DIAAS) has been recommended to replace PDCAAS.

DIAAS% = 100 × [(mg of digestible dietary indispensable amino acid in 1 g of the dietary protein)/(mg of the same dietary indispensable amino acid in 1g of the reference protein)].

Unlike PDCAAS, DIAAS can have values above 100.

PEPTIDES

Peptides are short chains of different amino acids linked together in a definite order using amide linkage or peptide bond. There are dipeptides, tripeptides, oligopeptides, and polypeptides. A dipeptide contains two amino acids linked by one peptide bond, e.g., an artificial sweetener consists of two amino acids namely aspartic acid and phenylalanine. Tripeptides consist of three amino acids having two peptide bonds, e.g., glutathione; and polypeptides consist of more than 20 amino acids, e.g., insulin. Oligopeptides and polypeptides are also joined by linkages like disulfide linkages besides peptide bonds. Typically, peptides can be distinguished from proteins by their relatively shorter chain length, proteins generally contain multiple peptide subunits, and proteins can be digested using enzymes to give shorter peptide fragments. Unlike proteins, because they are short in length, peptides do not fold into complex structures within the cell. Peptides are found in every cell and tissue and perform a wide range of essential functions. The function of a peptide is determined by its size and shape as well as its amino acid sequence. Some peptides act as transporters, enzymes, hormones, and structural components. Some peptides are gene-related.

Maintenance of appropriate concentration of peptides and their activity is essential for homeostasis and health. Some peptides like keratin, collagen, actin, and myosin participate in the structural part of the body, while some are used in clinical diagnosis.

Although many bioactive peptides that have important functions such as hormones or act as signaling molecules in regulatory processes, are synthesized by the human body, a variety of peptides are derived from foods during digestion. These are referred to as food-derived biologically active peptides. They act as growth factors, hormones, antimicrobial agents, and antioxidants.

Peptides Synthesized by the Body

Several peptides synthesized in the body have important biological functions. There are neuropeptides that act as critical messengers in neurosecretory cells, e.g. oxytocin or vasopressin and the parvocellular neurons synthesize corticotropin-releasing factor (CRF), thyrotropin-releasing hormone, gonadotropin-releasing hormone (GnRH), and somatostatin. Peptides are synthesized in the gastrointestinal tract like ghrelin and vasoactive intestinal peptide. Some important peptides and their functions are listed in Table 3.7.

Food-derived biologically active peptides: Bioactive peptides are food-derived components can be obtained from different plants, animals, and marine sources. Numerous bioactive peptides are derived from plants such as soy, pulses (lentil, chickpea, pea, and beans), oats, wheat, rice, maize, sunflower, hemp seed, pumpkin, canola, flaxseed, and many others including mushrooms. Milk and milk-based products are animal sources that have been intensively studied and a large number of peptides are derived from them. Peptides have also been isolated from eggs, meat, bovine blood, collagen, gelatin, various fish species including tuna, sardine, herring, salmon, and bonito, and from marine organisms.

These biologically active peptides are defined as fragments that remain inactive in precursor protein sequences, but when released by the action of proteolytic enzymes, they may interact with selected receptors and regulate the body's physiological functions. The effect exerted by such peptides may be positive or negative. Many types of bacteria applied in the production of fermented food products and occurring naturally in the gastrointestinal tract are capable of producing biologically active peptides. These bioactive peptides that are encrypted within the food protein can be released by hydrolysis by proteases in the intestinal tract (hydrolysis *in vivo*) or when food is processed (hydrolysis *in vitro*). Generally, enzymes are used such as trypsin, subtilisin, chymotrypsin, thermolysin, pepsin, papain alcalase, pronase, papain, carboxypeptidase A, and pancreatin.

Food protein-derived bioactive peptides (BAPs) have been extensively studied in relation to their potential health promoting effects in humans. Biologically active peptides can exhibit opiate-like, mineral binding, immunomodulatory, antimicrobial, antioxidant, antithrombotic, hypocholesterolemic, antidiabetic, antiobesity, and antihypertensive actions. They can modulate and improve the physiological functions and are thus considered useful in prevention or treatment of chronic diseases. These can also be commercially used as components of functional foods or nutraceuticals.

Table 3.7: Biological significance of peptides.

Peptides	Number of amino acids	Biological functions
Thyrotropin-releasing hormone (TRH)	3	Released from hypothalamus and regulates the secretion of thyroid-stimulating hormone (TSH)
Glutathione	3	Acts as an antioxidant, scavenges the free radicals via glutathione peroxidase (GSH). Plays important roles in nutrient metabolism, and regulation of cellular events such as gene expression, DNA and protein synthesis, cell proliferation and apoptosis, signal transduction, cytokine production, and immune response
Oxytocin	9	Stimulates uterine contraction before delivery
Vasopressin	9	Secreted from pituitary gland and helps kidney to retain water from urine
Gastrin	10	Helps in secretion of hydrochloric acid in the stomach
Glucagon	10	Pancreatic hormone involved in glucose metabolism. Its effects are opposite to that of insulin (antagonistic)
Vascular endothelial growth factors	Its isoforms contain 121, 145, 165, 183, 189 and 206 amino acids	Have important roles in regulation of blood vessel formation in health and disease—formation of new blood vessels (vasculogenesis) and formation of new capillaries from preexisting blood vessels (angiogenesis)

Hypotensive effects: Hypertension increases the risk of cardiovascular diseases. The renin-angiotensin system (RAS) is a major regulator of blood pressure and fluid homeostasis and dysregulation of the RAS can lead to blood pressure elevation with ensuing cardiovascular disease, chronic kidney disease, and diabetes. The regulatory mechanism takes place in the kidneys, where the hydrolytic enzyme renin is secreted. Renin cleaves plasma angiotensinogen to release a decapeptide called angiotensin I, which is subsequently hydrolyzed by angiotensin-converting enzyme (ACE) to form angiotensin II, which is a prohypertensive vasoconstrictor. Therefore, ACE and renin are two key enzymes that regulate RAS operation and ACE inhibitors have been widely used as antihypertensive agents. Various natural peptides can be obtained from a range of food proteins and have an antihypertensive effect. These peptides can be derived from milk, e.g., hydrolysates of whole milk protein, casein, whey proteins, and fermented dairy products. The antihypertensive effects have been attributed to "casokinins". Similar peptides that influence blood pressure have been found in fermented soybean products, in certain fish, meat proteins, egg yolk, and buckwheat, an edible species of mushroom (*Tricholoma giganteum*), wheat, and rapeseed.

> **Research glimpse:** Bovine milk is a source of bioactive compounds. Milk-derived bioactive peptides are usually encrypted and kept inactive within the primary structure of milk protein and they are generated by proteolysis of casein (α-, β-, γ-, and κ-casein) and whey proteins (β-lactoglobulin, α-lactalbumin, serum albumin, immunoglobulins, lactoferrin, and protease-peptone fractions). Peptides can be generated by enzymatic hydrolysis or microbial fermentation, either *in vivo* during digestion by digestive enzymes like trypsin and by gut microbial enzymes, or during food processing or ripening or by *in vitro* hydrolysis using isolated enzymes. The bioactive peptides can be absorbed from the intestine to the bloodstream and exert either local effects in the gastrointestinal system or systemic effects. These bioactive peptides have antithrombotic, antihypertensive, anti-inflammatory, antioxidative, antimicrobial, and antiobesity properties, reduce arterial stiffness and improve endothelial activity. Milk peptides have been shown to have antihypertensive effects, to influence insulin secretion and glucose control, and to have antioxidant and antithrombotic properties. They also influence lipid concentrations, immune response, inflammation, and oxidative stress. Milk proteins contain a number of ACE inhibitory peptides and potent ACE inhibitors from milk casein (casokinins) and whey proteins (lactokinins). Antihypertensive peptides may also influence blood pressure through mechanisms that are independent of ACE inhibition. Many peptides derived from lactoferrin and κ-casein have been shown to inhibit platelet aggregation and to have antithrombotic activity.
>
> *Marcone S, Belton O, Fitzgerald. Milk-derived bioactive peptides and their health-promoting effects: a potential role in atherosclerosis. British Journal of Clinical Pharmacology. 2017;83(1):152-62.*

Antioxidant effect: Peptides generated from the digestion of milk proteins have demonstrated antioxidative activities. Peptides with antioxidant effect may function by scavenging or preventing the formation of radicals, particularly free radicals released from casein peptides that may influence scavenging activity and inhibit enzymatic and nonenzymatic lipid peroxidation. Antioxidant activity of bioactive peptides has been attributed to the content of specific amino acids such as proline, histidine, tyrosine or tryptophan in the sequence. High amounts of histidine display peroxy radical trapping and chelating abilities thus increasing the accessibility of peptides to hydrophobic targets. Several milk peptides also play a regulatory role in oxidative metabolism which is essential for the survival of cells and cause oxidative changes by producing free radicals.

Antithrombotic effect: Casoplatelins derived from milk proteins have been found to inhibit the aggregation of blood platelets which may help in the prevention of thrombosis which often occurs in patients with coronary heart disease or other blood system diseases.

Antilipemic effect: Lactostatin derived from bovine milk β-lactoglobulin has been shown to have strong cholesterol-lowering effects. On the contrary, casein proteins induce elevation of cholesterol concentrations that may be due to the high ratios of methionine-glycine and lysine-arginine present. Numerous studies have shown milk bioactive peptides derived from whey may reduce serum cholesterol concentrations similar to soy proteins.

Anti-inflammatory effect: Inflammation is an essential component of the innate immune response to tissue injury. However, failure to control the magnitude and duration of inflammatory response can damage host tissues and contribute to pathology and to the development of chronic diseases such as rheumatoid arthritis, atherosclerosis. Chronic inflammation is believed to underlie autoimmune diseases, neurological diseases, cancer, metabolic disorders, diabetic complications, and pulmonary disease. Lactoferrin derived from whey exhibits anti-inflammatory effects. It regulates the LPS-induced cytokine production in monocytic cells which is thought to be involved in NF-κB activation. Also, a peptide from beta-lactoglobulin in milk has been found to have anti-inflammatory effect.

Immunoenhancing effects: These effects can be due to their influence either on some component of the immune system or due to their role as an effective antimicrobial agent. Substances derived from casein have been found to inhibit the growth of several pathogenic organisms. Immunomodulating peptides have been detected in cow's milk proteins, peptides from rice, and soybean protein. Whey protein also contains a number of immunomodulatory peptides and exhibit specific and non-specific immune responses.

Anticariogenic effects: Peptides from dairy products have anticariogenic effects. Lactoferrin has antibacterial activity toward gram-negative bacteria including the dental cariogen *Streptococcus mutans*. Acid casein (insoluble) as an active ingredient in toothpaste was effective at reducing dental caries, but was required at very high levels for activity. Sodium caseinate as an ingredient in a chocolate confectionery reduced cariogenicity, but high levels of caseinate (17%) were required to elicit an effect and the product was unpalatable. Caseinophosphopeptides (CPP) and glycomacropeptide (GMP) have been patented for use in common personal hygiene products to prevent dental caries. CPP and GMP have shown inhibitory activity to enamel demineralization and promote tooth enamel remineralization.

Antibacterial effects: Antibacterial peptides have been isolated from many sources. Several peptides have been found to possess a wide spectrum range of activity against bacteria and fungi. Lactoferrin in milk is well known for its antibacterial property. Peptides from egg white have been found to have bacteriostatic activity against gram-positive bacteria like *Escherichia coli*. Other organisms that peptides may be effective against are *Helicobacter, Listeria, Salmonella* and *Staphylococcus*, yeasts and some fungi. Antimicrobial peptides have been found to be generated through digestion of milk proteins. Thus, food proteins can be regarded as a possible resource to increase the natural defense of the person against invading pathogens. They can also enhance the shelf-life of the food product.

> Atherosclerosis is the underlying cause of heart attack and strokes. It is a progressive dyslipidemic and inflammatory disease where accumulation of oxidized lipids and inflammatory cells leads to the formation of an atherosclerotic plaque in the vessel wall. Milk-derived bioactive peptides can be released during gastrointestinal digestion, food processing or by enzymatic and bacterial fermentation and are considered to promote diverse beneficial effects such as lipid lowering, antihypertensive, immunomodulating, anti-inflammatory, and antithrombotic effects. Milk-derived peptides were already produced on an industrial scale and as a consequence, these peptides have been considered for application both as dietary supplements in "functional foods" and as drugs.

Opioid effects: Opioids are chemical substances that have analgesic effects leading to reduced perception of pain and also play a role in appetite control. The body synthesizes opioids that are called endogenous opioids or endorphins. Food-derived peptides are known as exorphins. One example is casomorphins from milk protein casein which may be involved in regulating gut functions and enhancing water and electrolyte absorption.

Opioid peptides can modulate absorption processes in the intestinal tract, mineral-binding peptides may function as carriers for different minerals, especially calcium and antithrombotic peptides inhibit fibrinogen binding to a specific receptor region on the platelet surface and inhibit aggregation of platelets. Research studies suggest that casomorphin, as opioid ligands, exert antisecretory action and stimulate endocrine responses such as secretion of insulin and somatostatin.

Decreasing risk of atherosclerosis: Peptides from egg white showed antioxidant function. When soy protein was given instead of animal protein, blood cholesterol levels were lowered. A peptide from buckwheat protein has also been shown to have a beneficial effect on serum lipids. Peptides from millet (proso millet) increased HDL level and lowered plasma total cholesterol in a rat model.

Other functions: Peptides derived from gluten the wheat protein, called "gluten exorphins" have been found to stimulate the release of insulin postprandially in experimental rats. Some food-derived peptides have been found to influence cell proliferation, differentiation, and apoptosis (programmed cell death) and have antioxidant activity. Some peptides with anticancer effect have been found in soy and amaranth. Also, some peptides have been found to stimulate bone growth.

Further research will clearly indicate the role of these peptides and how human beings can derive maximum benefits from these.

ROLES OF INDIVIDUAL AMINO ACIDS OR FUNCTIONS OF AMINO ACIDS

Amino acids are an important class of nutrients because they serve as building blocks of all peptides, polypeptides, and proteins. The amino acid sequence determines the type of protein which ultimately influences the function of protein. All amino acids serve as sources of energy when carbohydrate and fat intakes are inadequate. All amino acids are not present in all foods, but all are needed by the body to perform body functions optimally. In the human body, amino acids have important roles in different physiological processes that include skeletal muscle function, in atrophic conditions, cancer and sarcopenia. Some amino acids also have antioxidant activity. Amino acids have diverse metabolic roles which can be grouped into four categories:

1. They are substrates for messenger RNA (mRNA) translation and so are important for gene expression.
2. They act as initiators of signal transduction and neurotransmission.
3. They are essential for the biosynthesis of other nitrogen-containing compounds such as glutathione, polyamines, creatine, taurine, carnitine, nitric oxide, serotonin, and hormones like thyroxin.
4. They are important for the formation of nonnitrogenous compounds for gluconeogenesis, one-carbon methyl reactions, and anaplerotic balance of the tricarboxylic acid cycle (TCA cycle) as well as phosphorylation of proteins.

> **Functions of Amino Acids**
> Amino acids are important not only because they are part of proteins but also are sources of nitrogen. Many amino acids perform specific important functions:
> - Regulation of protein turnover by leucine
> - Transport of fatty acids in the cell by carnitine
> - Regulation of enzyme activity by arginine and phenylalanine
> - Function as neuronal agent, e.g., Gamma-aminobutyric acid (GABA)
> - Function as antioxidant, e.g. taurine
> - Methylation reactions—methionine
> - Function as precursors for neurotransmitters, e.g., tryptophan is converted to serotonin, glutamine is converted to gamma-aminobutyric acid, and phenylalanine and tyrosine are precursors of dopamine, adrenalin, and noradrenaline.
> - Regulation of gene expression.
> - Regulation of messenger RNA translation.
> - Glutamine has been found to perform several functions such as being a trophic factor for muscle and intestines, as a fuel for intestinal cells, stimulating glycogen synthesis, etc.
> - Formation of glutathione which has antioxidant function—cysteine
> - Important for synthesis of purines and pyrimidines—aspartate and glutamate
> - Important for hemoglobin (part of hemoglobin) and bile synthesis, e.g., glycine.

Essential Amino Acids

Phenylalanine

Phenylalanine and tyrosine are aromatic amino acids. Phenylalanine is required for protein synthesis. It is a precursor of tyrosine (conversion of tyrosine to phenylalanine is not possible in the human body) and thus helps in the production of catecholamines like norepinephrine, epinephrine, and dopamine which are important in transmitting nerve signals. It is also needed for production of thyroxin by thyroid gland and melanin, a pigment present in skin and eyes. An inborn error in metabolism, phenylketonuria (PKU) may occur due to lack of the enzyme required for metabolism of phenylalanine. PKU is characterized by mental retardation and neurological symptoms like hyperreflexes and seizures. Several psychotropic drugs have phenylalanine as a constituent. Phenylalanine can act as a pain reliever and has been used in treatment of premenstrual syndrome.

Tryptophan

It is a precursor of niacin and essential for the production of the neurotransmitter serotonin (5-hydroxytryptamine) which is a precursor for synthesis of melatonin in brain and retina of eye. Serotonin, a biogenic amine, regulates, in the human CNS, adaptive reactions and responses to environmental changes, e.g., mood-anxiety, cognition, nociception (perception of pain), impulsivity, aggressiveness, libido, feeding behavior, and body temperature. 5-hydroxytryptamine is also involved in gut function, immune and inflammatory responses, differentiation of blood stem cells, and hemodynamic function. Melatonin promotes immune function, may play a role in protection against oxidative stress, and also influences growth hormone and thyroid hormone status.

Methionine

This sulfur-containing amino acid is a constituent of almost all proteins and peptides in the body and is a precursor of the amino acid cysteine. It is a donor of methyl groups, required for synthesis of succinyl CoA, homocysteine, epinephrine, creatine, melatonin, phosphatidylcholine, carnitine, and many other important biological compounds. It is a constituent of hemoglobin. It works with folic acid and vitamin B_{12} and plays a significant role in DNA synthesis. It also promotes collagen synthesis and is necessary for the metabolism of polyamines. Through its metabolites, it plays an important role in the immune system and for synthesis of glutathione. Methionine has been shown to chelate lead and decrease oxidative stress.

Lysine

It is a component of numerous proteins and several peptides. It is important for synthesis of carnitine, plays a role in collagen formation and therefore is important for growth and tissue repair. It plays an important role in calcium absorption. It helps in recovery from surgery, sports injuries as well as the body's production of hormones, enzymes, and antibodies. Lysine has also been shown to have antibacterial activity. L-lysine has been explored as drug therapy for problems such as Alzheimer's dementia, hair loss, cancer, cardiovascular disease, and aging. Lysine plays an essential role in carnitine production. It is important for synthesis of muscle tissue, and it is used by athletes to support lean mass building and the overall health of muscle and bone. Cereals typically do not contain adequate amount of lysine. Lysine content of some common foods and the lysine score given by the FAO/WHO/UNU Expert Group is given in Table 3.8.

Branched Chain Amino Acids (BCAA)

The three branched chain amino acids are leucine, isoleucine, and valine. They are described as branched chain because they have side chain in their structure unlike the other amino acids. These are important for synthesis of body proteins. They regulate protein synthesis and maintain the glutamine-glutamate levels in the body. When there is a high demand for energy and during stress, BCAA are oxidized. They stimulate synthesis of muscle, lower the degradation of muscle proteins. BCAAs are primarily broken down in the extrahepatic tissues, i.e., muscle, adipose, kidney, and brain). BCAAs account for about one-third of the amino acids in muscle. They play a role in lipogenesis, glucose metabolism, glucose transportation, intestinal barrier function and absorption, milk quality,

Table 3.8: Lysine content of selected protein sources.

Protein sources	Lysine content (mg/g protein)	*Lysine score (45 mg/g protein)
Wheat	27	60
Rice	35	78
Sorghum	24	53
Millets	22	50
Nuts and seeds	35	77
Vegetables	43	96
Legumes	73	>100
Animal protein	82	>100

Source: Indian Council of Medical Research. Nutrient requirement and recommended dietary allowances for Indians. A report of the Expert Group of the Indian Council of Medical Research. 2010; p. 60.
*FAO/WHO/UNU (2007)

mammary health, embryonic development, and immunity. They are also likely to have a role in the central nervous system control of food intake and energy balance.

Their potential in management of hepatic encephalopathy is being explored. Although leucine, isoleucine and valine are structurally similar, their side chains are different in terms of structural conformation and hydrophobicity. Due to this, there are differences in their metabolism and function. Valine is a glucogenic amino acid whereas leucine is ketogenic. Deficiency symptoms of these three amino acids are different. In valine deficiency, neurological deficits have been reported; whereas in isoleucine deficiency, muscle tremors have been observed.

Due to their role in muscle protein synthesis, use of BCAA supplements has become popular. However, research studies show that high levels of circulating BCAAs and related metabolites are associated with insulin resistance and coronary heart disease. Results of epidemiological studies suggest that elevated levels of branched chain amino acids are associated with insulin resistance.

Leucine

It is a branched chain amino acid that has been studied extensively. It is an important source of energy, especially for muscle cells and to some extent for liver and intestines (hence this amino acid as well as isoleucine and valine are important during exercise). Almost all proteins contain this amino acid. It may play a role in synthesis of the neurotransmitter formed from glutamic acid. Being a ketogenic amino acid, it plays a role in synthesis of ketones, steroids, and fatty acids. It may be involved in regulating initiation of translation during cell mitogenesis and may be particularly important for promoting proliferation of beta cells of pancreas, and augmenting the growth-stimulating effects of insulin and insulin-like growth factor. Leucine plays an important role in the mTOR signaling pathway, acting as a trigger/signaling molecule for initiating protein synthesis. It enhances energy homeostasis through augmenting mitochondrial biogenesis and fatty acid oxidation.

Isoleucine

This BCAA is a source of energy for skeletal muscle and to a small extent for liver and intestines. Isoleucine has been found to prevent tumor growth in a mouse model of colon cancer. Like leucine, isoleucine also stimulates muscle protein synthesis, but it is less effective than leucine. It also acts as a regulator of glucose metabolism. In a rat model, it has been observed that isoleucine prevents a rise in plasma glucose concentration, with its effect being greater than that of leucine or valine.

Valine

This BCAA is required for protein synthesis (however, it is not as effective as leucine in stimulating muscle protein synthesis) and is a source of energy. It may play a role in synthesis of neurotransmitter from glutamic acid. It has anabolic effects on skeletal muscle. It improves the absorption of other amino acids. Valine is a glycogenic amino acid and so causes an increase in plasma glucose levels as seen in rat model studies.

Threonine

It is present in almost all proteins, is a principal part of structural proteins like collagen, elastin, which are important components of skin as well as tooth enamel and connective tissue. It is a precursor of glycine and plays a role in mucin production. It plays a role in fat metabolism and immune function. It also plays a role in mucin production and prevents buildup of fat in the liver. It functions as an immunostimulant and promotes growth of the thymus gland. In high doses, it is used for treatment of genetic spasticity disorders and multiple sclerosis.

Histidine

Histidine is required for globin synthesis. It is an essential amino acid for infants and children and is important for growth and repair of tissues. It plays a role in scavenging free radicals and protects against oxidative stress. It plays a role in the immune system. Histamine is a potent neurotransmitter produced from histidine. It may also play a role in enhancing iron absorption. It has antioxidant ability as it can scavenge free radicals and chelate divalent metal ions. Therefore, it has cytoprotective role in chronic kidney disease. Dietary histidine has been shown to improve intestinal zinc absorption. Prolonged deficiency of this amino acid results in growth failure as do deficiencies of other amino acids or protein; there is loss of muscle mass and organ damage.

Nonessential Amino Acids

Glycine

This nonessential amino acid is the simplest amino acid in nature. It is synthesized by the liver from other amino acids. It represents about one-tenth of total amino acids in the body. It is a component of glutathione. Glycine is glucogenic and plays a role in glycogen storage. It is required for synthesis of proteins, peptides, purines, heme, creatine, and glutathione. It supports wound healing. In the collagen polypeptide chain, glycine is present at every third position. The presence of glycine in enzymes provides flexibility. Glycine is needed for conjugation of bile acids. It modulates intracellular Ca^{2+} levels, and thus is involved in regulating the production of cytokines, generation of superoxide, and in immune function. It may also be involved in regulating behavior and food intake. It may be conditionally essential for LBW infants due to their limited capacity to synthesize it.

> **Research glimpse:** Plasma glycine level is low in patients with obesity or diabetes and the improvement of insulin resistance increases plasma glycine concentration. In prospective studies, hypoglycinemia at baseline predicts the risk of developing type 2 diabetes and higher serum glycine level is associated with decreased risk of incident type II diabetes. Consistently, plasma glycine concentration is lower in the lean offspring of parents with type 2 diabetes compared with healthy subjects. Among patients with type 2 diabetes, hypoglycinemia occurs before clinical manifestations of the disease, but the pathophysiological mechanisms underlying glycine deficit and its potential clinical repercussions are unclear. Glycine participates in several metabolic pathways, being required for relevant human physiological processes. Humans synthesize glycine from glyoxylate, glucose (via serine), betaine and likely from threonine and during the endogenous synthesis of L-carnitine. Glycine conjugates bile acids and other acyl moieties producing acyl-glycine derivatives. The glycine cleavage system catalyzes glycine degradation to carbon dioxide and ammonium while tetrahydrofolate is converted into 5,10-methylenetetrahydrofolate. Glycine is utilized to synthesize serine, sarcosine, purines, creatine, heme group, glutathione, and collagen. Glycine is a major quantitative component of collagen. The role of glycine maintaining collagen structure is critical, as glycine residues are required to stabilize the triple helix of the collagen molecule. This quality of glycine likely contributes to explain the occurrence of medial arterial calcification and the elevated cardiovascular risk associated with diabetes and chronic kidney disease, as emerging evidence links normal collagen content with the initiation and progression of vascular calcification in humans.
>
> *Adeva-Andany M, Souto-Adeva G, Ameneiros-Rodríguez E, Fernández-Fernández C, Donapetry-García C, Domínguez-Montero A. Insulin resistance and glycine metabolism in humans. Amino Acids. 2018;50(1):11-27.*

Alanine

It is involved in transfer of nitrogen from peripheral tissues to liver and plays an important role in cellular nitrogen homeostasis. It is the principal amino acid released from muscle. It is a major substrate for hepatic glucose synthesis (gluconeogenesis) and so aids in glucose metabolism. It is an intermediary between protein catabolism and glucose (carbohydrate) synthesis. Besides gluconeogenesis, it is closely linked to important metabolic pathways like glycolysis and citric acid cycle. It also helps in production of antibodies and thus strengthens the immune system. It is needed for protein synthesis. β-alanine is involved in synthesis of pantothenic acid.

Serine

Although it is classified as a dispensable/nonessential amino acid, it is important for many cellular processes. With glycine, this amino acid forms what is known as the serine, glycine and one-carbon network. This plays an important role in integration of cellular metabolism that is required for the cells' various biological functions. Thus, this amino acid is needed for one-carbon metabolism and sulfur metabolism, nucleotide, lipid, polyamine, and protein synthesis, as well as maintaining epigenetic status. It is also involved in glycolysis and gluconeogenesis, folate metabolism, and fat metabolism. It plays an important role in one-carbon metabolism and is required for the formation of glycine, cysteine, taurine, alanine, and phospholipids as well as D-serine. D-serine is a neuromodulator in the brain. It is also involved in the synthesis of proteins present in nervous system and antibodies.

Cysteine

It is a sulfur-containing amino acid that provides the sulfur for sulfur-containing proteins, tRNA, pantothenic acid, and many other compounds. This amino acid promotes protein structure by sulfhydryl bonding. It is a precursor of glutathione (for this it is a rate-limiting precursor), coenzyme A, taurine (necessary for bile formation and nerve function), sulfate which is needed for connective tissue, and reduced sulfur. H_2S produced from cysteine functions as a neuromodulator and smooth muscle relaxant. It is also a source of pyruvate and is important for energy production. It helps in utilization of fat. Since it is necessary for glutathione formation, it has a role in antioxidant functions and detoxification. It is conditionally essential for LBW infants. In premature infants, tyrosine, and in preterm and term infants, cysteine are considered essential amino acids. In liver disease, cysteine requirement cannot be met due to diminished transsulfuration capacity. Thus, cysteine is considered a conditionally essential amino acid. Cysteine can be oxidized to form cystine. Cysteine deficiency has been shown to be associated with impaired antioxidant defense, decreased drug-metabolizing ability (also applies to metabolism of toxic compounds), reduced immunity, and higher levels of homocysteine.

Tyrosine

This dispensable amino acid can be formed by hydroxylation of phenylalanine in the liver. It readily passes the blood-brain barrier. It is needed for synthesis of the catecholamines (epinephrine and norepinephrine) and dopamine. These neurotransmitters play an important role in the body's sympathetic nervous system. It aids in boosting memory and is also needed for the production of thyroxin, which regulates BMR and melanin. It is a part of several proteins, peptides, and enkephalins that are natural pain relievers in the body. The body regulates tyrosine content of cells. Tyrosine supplementation has no effect on anxiety symptoms or improvement of mood states but may have some effect on depression.

Aspartic Acid

It is required for synthesis of asparagine, arginine, and is needed for synthesis of proteins, pyrimidine, and purine nucleotides. It plays a role in the urea cycle and citric acid cycle. It serves as an energy fuel and as a neurotransmitter may provide resistance to fatigue. This amino acid has important roles in the urea cycle and DNA metabolism. Aspartic acid with phenylalanine is a part of the artificial sweetener, aspartame. It may be an immunostimulant of the thymus and can protect against some of the damaging effects of radiation.

Glutamic Acid or Glutamate

It is one of the most abundant amino acids and plays a highly significant role in amino acid metabolism as it takes part in deamination (removal of nitrogen). Eventually, it is also involved in urea cycle. It can also be synthesized from alpha-ketoglutarate (an intermediary compound in TCA cycle). It is also needed during conversion of pyruvate to alanine. It serves as a fuel source for enterocytes, i.e., intestinal cells. It is a substrate for synthesis of glucose in kidney, lymphocytes, and monocytes. It is used for synthesis of several amino acids such as glutamine, proline, arginine, and folate (a vitamin). Glutamate and glutamine, both are important for fetal and placental metabolism. It is also essential for brain function. It has a role in regulating energy and protein metabolism, serves as a source of fuel/energy, especially as a nutrient in muscle protein metabolic response to conditions like infections, inflammation, and muscle trauma. It is also important for maintaining immunocompetence. In foods, presence of glutamic acid is associated with typical meat flavor known as "Umami". It is part of monosodium glutamate which is used as a flavor enhancer. It helps to maintain mucosal integrity of the gastrointestinal tract when it is administered to patients with major bowel surgery. It has a protective role and is used as a supplement in total parenteral nutrition, especially for patients under intensive care.

Glutamine

Glutamine plays a central role in human nitrogen, protein, and energy metabolism. It is involved in a wide variety of metabolic and biochemical reactions and plays a pivotal role in nitrogen homeostasis. It transports nitrogen between cells and/or organs and serves as a metabolic fuel, in addition to glucose or it is used as an alternative source of fuel in rapidly proliferating cells. It is unique in that it serves as a respiratory fuel for rapidly proliferating cells such as lymphocytes and enterocytes. It is a precursor of nucleic acids, nucleotides, amino sugars, neurotransmitters, and glycoproteins since it serves as a nitrogen donor. It is used in the synthesis of purine and pyrimidines (nucleic acid) and is a substrate for synthesis of many proteins.

It is also an integral component of gamma-aminobutyric acid (GABA), a neurotransmitter and glutathione. Through removal of ammonia, it regulates acid–base balance. Glutamine is converted to ornithine and citrulline which are converted to arginine in the urea cycle. It also stimulates glycogen synthesis and enhances neutrophil phagocytosis. It plays an important role in regulating cellular pathways and related functions. Among the free amino acids, it is the most abundant amino acid in extracellular and intracellular compartments. Its concentration in blood reflects the short-term balance between dietary supply, endogenous synthesis, and its utilization by organs and cells such as enterocytes and immune cells. Muscle tissue contains more than half of the intracellular body pool. Glutamine is used for critically ill patients who are on parenteral nutrition.

Arginine

This is a conditionally essential amino acid. It can be obtained from the diet as well as by de novo synthesis from citrulline. The latter accounts for about 60% of the de novo whole-body synthesis of arginine. It plays a key role in several metabolic pathways. It plays a role in nitrogen metabolism and homeostasis, being an important metabolite of the urea cycle which converts ammonia that is toxic (an end product of amino acid degradation) into urea which is then excreted by kidneys. It aids in release of hormones such as growth hormone, insulin, glucagon, and prolactin. It plays a role in immune system. It also increases fat metabolism thereby is involved in maintenance of weight. It is a precursor of glutamine, proline, and synthesis of polyamines. This amino acid plays a significant role during growing years, hypermetabolic situations such as burns and recovery period. It is a biological precursor of nitric oxide which plays an integral role in regulating immune system by decreasing proinflammatory substances, regulating macrophages as well as activating T-lymphocyte. Nitric oxide also protects against initiation and progression of atherosclerosis.

Proline

Proline is a unique amino acid. It plays an important role in protein synthesis, structure and metabolism, particularly metabolism of arginine, polyamines, and glutamate. It is involved in collagen synthesis particularly of skin, and thus helps in wound healing. It may act as an osmolyte. It functions as a regulator in many cellular biochemical and physiological processes. It serves as a signaling molecule, as a sensor of cellular energy status, and is important for cell differentiation. It is also required for synthesis of polyamines and proteins in the intestines. Thus, it is of importance for growth and development, particularly of the fetus and neonate. It may play an important role in neurodegenerative disorders like Alzheimer's and Parkinson's diseases. It is a precursor of glutamate and for the neurotransmitter GABA. Proline-rich peptides in colostrum have unique antiviral characteristics. It may serve as a synaptic regulatory molecule. It is a part of proteins that are important for oxygen sensing in the body.

Asparagine

It is a dispensable amino acid synthesized from aspartate and glutamine. It is a constituent of most of the proteins and peptides synthesized in the body. It is utilized for synthesizing aspartic acid/aspartate and is synthesized from aspartate. It provides amino groups for synthesis of other dispensable amino acids. It plays a role in collagen assembly, enzymes and cell-to-cell recognition. It contributes its carbon skeleton in the citric acid cycle and hence contributes to cellular energy production. It is a component of the urea cycle.

Aspartate

It is used for synthesis of asparagine, purines, pyrimidines, and some nucleotides. It is a constituent of a large number of proteins and peptides synthesized in the body. It also plays a role in the synthesis of other amino acids as well as in the urea cycle and citric acid cycle. It plays an important role in urea cycle and vitamin B_6 metabolism. It is an excitatory neurotransmitter.

The requirements for different amino acids have been given by the FAO/WHO/UNU Expert Committee in 2007 (Table 3.9).

Food sources of selected amino acids are listed in Table 3.10.

Nonproteinogenic Amino Acids

Taurine

It is a sulfur-containing amino acid and is the most abundant intracellular free amino acid. Human liver cells synthesize taurine from cysteine and methionine. It plays an important role in stabilizing the pH inside the cell and prevents loss of fluid from the cells to the extracellular compartment. This is of special significance in the kidney. It is involved in formation of bile acid conjugates, i.e., taurocholic acid and is important for prevention of cholestasis. In adults, taurine concentrations in plasma decrease in starvation, surgical injury, cancer, trauma, and sepsis. It has antioxidant activity (in the form of hypotaurine). Taurine is used for therapeutic applications such as in AIDS, diabetes, congestive heart failure, athletic wounds, interstitial cystitis, fibromyalgia, and joint pain.

Table 3.9: Amino acid requirements (mg/g protein) for adults (FAO/WHO/UNU, 2007).

Amino acid	mg/kg body weight/day	mg/g protein
Histidine	10	15
Isoleucine	20	30
Leucine	39	59
Lysine	30	45
Methionine	10	16
Cysteine	4	6
Methionine + Cysteine	15	22
Threonine	15	23
Phenylalanine + Tyrosine	25	38
Tryptophan	4	6
Valine	26	39
Total essential amino acid	184	277
Total protein (high quality)	0.66 g/kg/day	
Safe level of protein (mean + 1.96 × SD)	0.83 g/kg/day	

Joint Food and Agriculture Organization of the United Nations, World Health Organization, United Nations University Expert Consultation (2007). Protein and Amino acid Requirements in Human Nutrition. WHO Technical Report Series No 935.

Table 3.10: Food sources of different amino acids.

Amino acid	Major food sources
Valine	Milk, eggs, rice, cheese, beans, mushrooms
Isoleucine	Milk, soy, meat, egg, piyal seeds, cashew nuts, and cereals
Leucine	Pulses, grains, milk and dairy products, egg, soybean, sorghum or jowar
Lysine	Pork, beef, chicken, cow's milk, eggs, and pulses including soy
Tryptophan	All protein sources, especially milk and curds/yoghurt and cheese
Methionine	Animal proteins such as fish, meat, eggs, dairy product, beans, beef, cereals, although plant proteins contain less amounts than animal sources
Phenylalanine	Legumes, eggs, and rice have higher content than milk, beef, pork and chicken, and the sweetener, aspartame
Threonine	All dietary proteins, including dairy products, beef, poultry, eggs, beans, wheat germ, cottage cheese (paneer) and sesame seeds
Cysteine	Eggs, wheat, rice, and human milk
Tyrosine	All protein-containing foods, especially soybean, cow's milk, eggs, fish, beef, pork, and chicken
Aspartic acid	All legumes/pulses including soybean, eggs, chicken, fish, rice, and meat
Glutamine	All food proteins—plant and animal sources
Arginine	Rice, oats, soy, meat, eggs, fish, and beans
Proline	All dietary sources of protein
Histidine	Pork, beef, legumes, buckwheat
Glycine	Legumes, fish, dairy products, and meat

Citrulline

Citrulline can be considered as an intermediate amino acid and is an important component of the urea cycle and hence is important for detoxification of ammonia. It accelerates clearance of plasma ammonia and lactate. Proteins containing citrulline called citrullinated proteins may have a role in diseases like multiple sclerosis (an autoimmune disease) and rheumatoid arthritis. Low citrulline levels (hypocitrullinemia) have been observed in persons with celiac disease, short bowel syndrome, and radiation-induced small bowel damage. Renal failure is associated with impaired citrulline metabolism because approximately 80% of citrulline is converted into arginine. Citrulline is synthesized exclusively in the intestines and plasma citrulline levels could be used as a biomarker for gut function. Thus, the gastrointestinal tract and the kidney play major roles in citrulline metabolism. In some cells, arginine can be produced from citrulline as part of the nitric oxide cycle (nitric oxide is an integral part of the inflammatory process involved in the regulation of angiogenesis, vasodilation, and collagen deposition at the site of wounds). In animal models, citrulline supplementation to elderly rats increased the muscle protein content and muscle synthesis. Also, it is being studied for its potential to lower blood pressure in persons with hypertension.

Ornithine

Ornithine is an non-essential and naturally occurring amino acid found in dairy, meat, and legumes. It is not involved in protein synthesis but plays an important role overall in amino acid metabolism. This is a precursor (intermediate in synthesis) of proline, citrulline, and glutamine as well as polyamines (polyamines are small polycationic molecules present in all cells. They interact with negatively charged molecules, like DNA, RNA or proteins. They are involved in several functions connected with gene expression, cell growth, survival, and proliferation as well as in cellular response to stress such as starvation and oxidative stress. Common polyamines include putrescine, spermidine and spermine, cadaverine, and diaminopropane). It promotes the release of growth hormone which helps to metabolize excess fat. It may promote cell proliferation and collagen production and in rats, it has been found to stimulate hepatic regeneration. It plays a significant role in urea cycle and helps in removing the excessive ammonia build up from the body thus supports waste removal from the body, liver detoxification, and rejuvenation. Ornithine is produced by separating arginine from urea cycle within the body.

Low doses of ornithine are used as food supplement and high doses are used therapeutically (as a medicine) to lower ammonia levels in blood to overcome the symptoms associated with hepatic encephalopathy that occurs in liver cirrhosis. Ornithine is used as a nutraceutical for enhancing muscle strength and cardiovascular activity. In some studies, it has been found that when healthy individuals were given ornithine before exercise, they were able to overcome fatigue and there was efficient excretion of cellular ammonia.

> **Laboratory laurel:** It is reported that ingestion of glutamine, arginine or ornithine before resistance exercise enhances postexercise growth hormone secretion in healthy male adults and growth hormone has lipolytic activity, facilitating the release of free fatty acids (FFAs) and glycerol from triglycerides in adipose tissue. In this study, the effect of oral L-ornithine hydrochloride (0.1 g/kg BW) on energy expenditure during a rest period from 120 minutes to 180 minutes after resistance exercise was evaluated by indirect calorimetry. Healthy male subjects instead no habit of resistance training underwent resistance exercise (chest press, lat pulldown, leg press, shoulder press, leg extension, and leg curl), with three sets of each exercise and 10 repetitions in each set at 90-second intervals, 30 minutes after ingestion of ornithine or placebo. Conclusively ornithine ingestion before resistance exercise may enhance postexercise carbohydrate oxidation without changing total energy expenditure.
>
> *Morishita K, Yamada T, Yamaji S, Aoki M, Kitabayashi T, Uchiyama M. The effect of ornithine ingestion on carbohydrate metabolism during rest after acute resistance exercise in healthy young males. Advances in Bioscience and Biotechnology. 2011;2(4):287-92.*

DIGESTION OF PROTEINS

Proteins from two sources are present in the gastrointestinal tract. The major part is of exogenous origin, i.e., diet. However, a considerable amount, about 20-30 g is of endogenous origin. This includes mostly protein of desquamated cells, a very small amount of plasma proteins (1-2 g), mostly albumin, enzymes, and mucoproteins that are secreted into the intestine. Digestion of endogenous proteins occurs slowly as compared with those of exogenous origin. Generally, about 95% of protein is digested and absorbed, since in the feces, the amount of nitrogen derived from proteins is only approximately ≤10 g per day.

Different proteins are preferentially digested in different parts of the gastrointestinal tract. Casein, the major protein in bovine milk, is precipitated and then hydrolyzed in the stomach. Whey protein or soy protein are soluble proteins. They pass rapidly through the stomach and are digested by the pancreatic enzymes. Protein digestion is also influenced by whether it is in solid or liquid form, i.e., its physical state, as well as other factors such as meal size, its composition, and osmolality, and the other nutrients that are present. The rate of gastric emptying can also influence digestion. Fate of protein intake has been explained in Figures 3.7, 3.8 and Table 3.11.

Digestion: Digestion of proteins begins in the stomach. When a person eats, gastric cells in the stomach come into contact with the food and release a hormone called gastrin. This gastrin enters the blood and stimulates the release of hydrochloric acid (HCl). Hydrochloric acid in the stomach denatures or unfolds the compact structure of the thus disrupting the protein structure. Stomach contains pepsinogen (inactive form of enzyme or proenzyme) which is turned into pepsin (active form of enzyme) in presence of hydrochloric acid. Pepsin is a protease which breaks down/hydrolyzes proteins into shorter polypeptides and some free amino acids. However, only partial digestion of protein occurs in stomach. At this stage, about 10–20% of the dietary protein

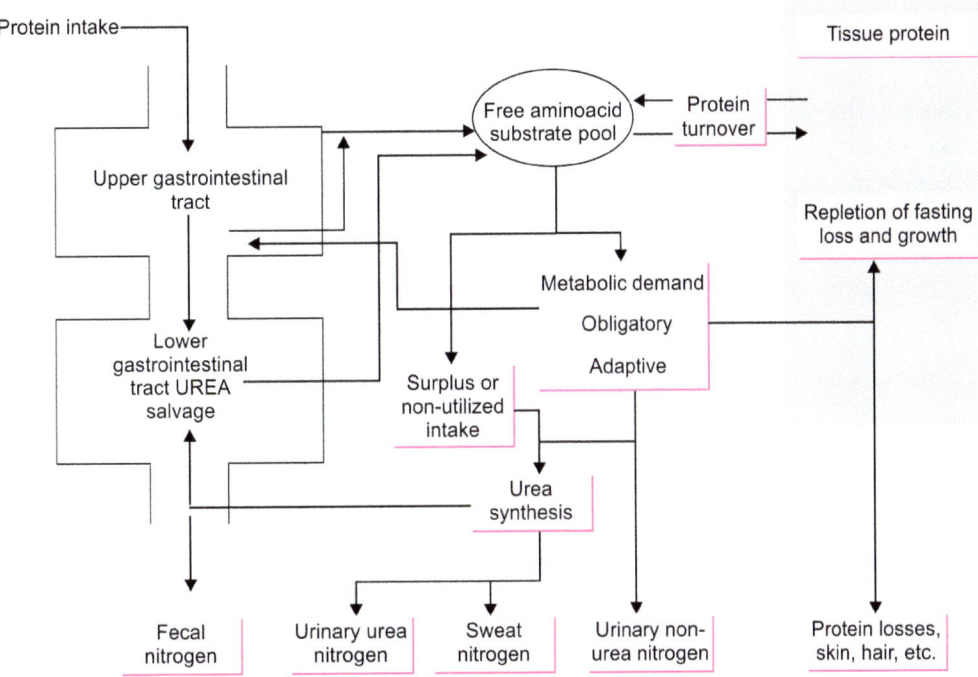

Fig. 3.7: Model of protein metabolism in humans from WHO/FAO/UNU (2007).

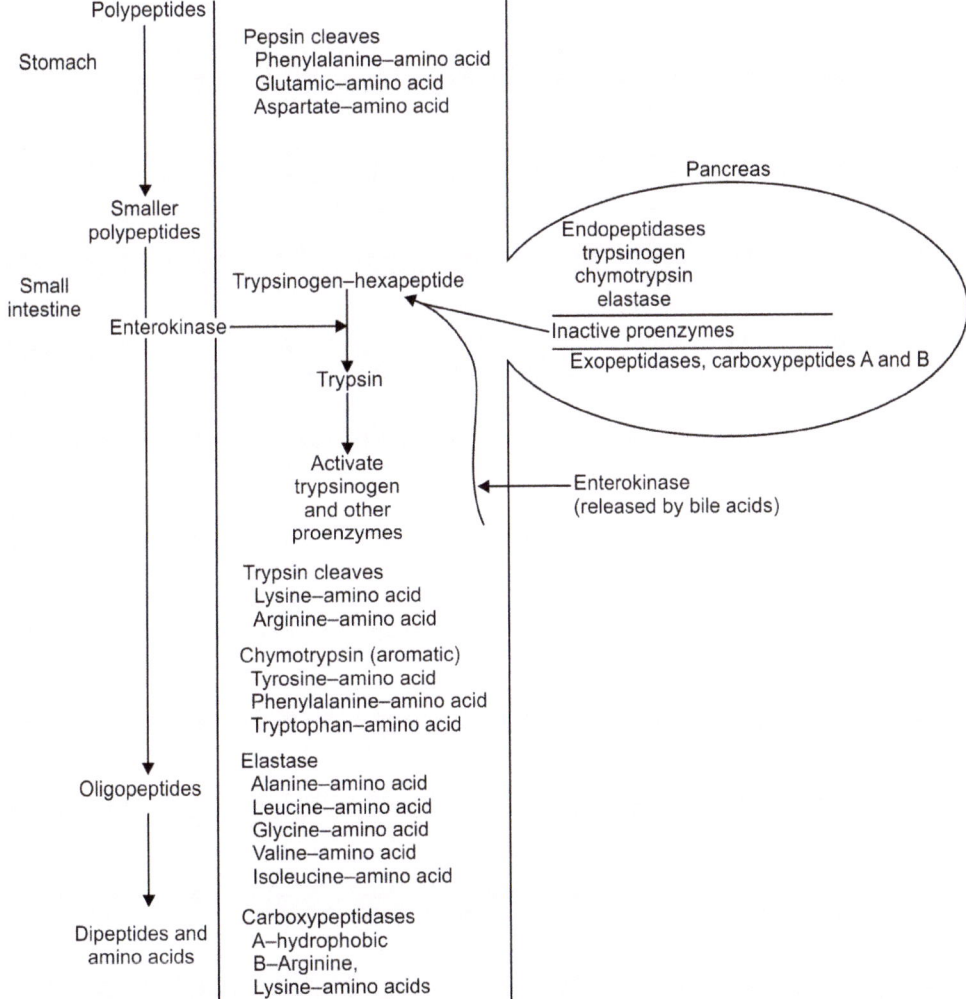

Fig. 3.8: Proteins are sequentially reduced in molecular size during passage through the stomach and the upper gastrointestinal tract. Pepsin initiates the enzymatic process. The pancreas excretes inactive proenzymes which are activated by enterokinase, a mucosal enzyme. This activates trypsinogen which, in turn, activates chymotrypsin, elastase, and carboxypeptidases A and B. Enzyme activity with a specified amino acid–amino acid peptide linkage.

Table 3.11: Proteins involved in digestion.

Inactive enzymes	Source of secretion	Hormone/juice involved	Active enzyme	Final product of protein after enzymatic action
Pepsinogen	Stomach (gastric gland)	Gastrin	Pepsin	Polypeptides
Trypsinogen	Duodenum	Pancreatic juice	Trypsin	Polypeptide and simpler peptides
Chymotrypsinogen	Duodenum	Pancreatic juice	Chymotrypsin	Polypeptide, simpler peptides, and amino acids
Endopeptidases	Present in the enteric mucosa			Cleaves peptides at the nonamino terminal
Amino peptidases	Small intestine			Amino acids and dipeptides. Amino acids Have different specificities for amino acids depending on their charge, i.e. acidic, neutral or proline or tryptophan. Activity is increased by high protein intake but decreased in starvation
Carboxypeptidases	Small intestine			Hydrolyze peptides at the C-terminal end
Dipeptidase	-	-	-	Hydrolyzes a wide range of amino acid residues

has been digested by pepsin. When the partially digested food enters the small intestine, it stimulates secretion of a hormone called secretin. Secretin signals the pancreas to release bicarbonate which neutralizes the hydrochloric acid that has come from the stomach with the partially digested food. Another hormone called cholecystokinin is also secreted in response to the presence of amino acids in the small intestines. Cholecystokinin stimulates pancreas to release pancreatic juice. Pancreatic juice contains proenzymes such as trypsinogen, chymotrypsinogen and procarboxypeptidase, and proelastase. These are activated by trypsin in the intestinal lumen. Enteropeptidase located in the brush border of the jejunal mucosa converts trypsinogen to trypsin.

Those polypeptides that are the products of digestion by pepsin are further broken down by trypsin and chymotrypsin. These two proteolytic enzymes convert protein into proteoses, polypeptides, di- and tripeptides, and free amino acids. The cells of the surface of the small intestines contain peptidases (dipeptidases and tripeptidases) which break down the di- and tripeptides into amino acids. All proteins are not digested to the same extent, because some resist hydrolysis and they or their constituent amino acids will not be absorbed to the same extent as are proteins that are digested to a greater extent.

Generally, animal proteins are better digested than plant proteins.

Gastric pepsin and pancreatic trypsin have different affinity for bonds between amino acids. Pepsin attacks peptic bonds next to aromatic amino acids such as phenylalanine, tryptophan, and tyrosine, whereas trypsin cleaves bond next to the basic amino acids, arginine and lysine. Hence, the site of digestion determines the type of peptides produced by enzymatic hydrolysis and consequently their further physiological properties. Thus, the unique physicochemical properties as well as amino acid sequence of each dietary protein predetermine the course of proteolysis and composition of peptides released.

Absorption: Approximately 80% of the products of protein digestion are absorbed. The gastrointestinal tract can absorb amino acids at the rate of about 1.3–10 g/hour. Most of the absorption occurs in the small intestines. Active transport is used for absorption of amino acids across a gradient. Also, this transport mechanism is sodium dependent. Some amino acids like glycine, proline, and hydroxyproline are transported by more than one mechanism. Also, the absorption rate of different amino acids differs. Glucose stimulates amino acid absorption. There are likely to be five different transport systems—separate ones for basic amino acids, for neutral amino acids, for imino acids. Small peptides and amino acids are water soluble and are absorbed through the villi present in the brush border of the small intestine into the bloodstream, reach portal blood, and are then taken to the liver. Generally, about 99% of the ingested protein is absorbed as amino acids. However, some small proteins may also be absorbed intact and within the cell where they have been absorbed, they are hydrolyzed to amino acids. Absorption of whole protein may provoke immune response and result in allergy. There are specific carriers which will transport amino acids with the small amount of dipeptides/tripeptides to enter intestinal cells. However, some amino acids share the same transport system. Hence, with excessive intake of one amino acid (especially if amino acid supplements are taken), there can be competition between amino acids and absorption of some amino acids can be inhibited. Within the intestinal cells, some amount of amino acids may be used or energy for synthesis of substances required by the intestinal cells. Considerable amounts of amino acids like glutamic acid, aspartic acid, glutamine, valine, lysine, leucine, and isoleucine are catabolized. Several nonessential amino acids including glutamine, glutamate, and aspartate are extensively oxidized in enterocytes such that very little comes into the portal vein. The remainder which is not utilized is transported out of the cell through the cell membrane to the surrounding fluid from where they are carried to the liver through portal blood. Generally, about 300 g of protein is synthesized by the body on daily basis. Out of this, 300 g, two-thirds, i.e., 200 g is synthesized from recycled amino acids. Nitrogen is also lost through hair, skin, GI cells, mucus, nails, and body fluids like sweat.

In conditions like starvation, absorption of both amino acids and peptides is enhanced. Absorption may also be influenced by season and time of day. It has been reported that there are diurnal and seasonal alterations in the absorptive abilities of the gut. Absorption of amino acids that are products of intestinal digestion is more (almost twice as fast) as compared with free amino acids that are ingested as a mixture.

At various stages of the digestive process, proteins and the peptides that are already present or produced through protein hydrolysis have different effects on the gastrointestinal tract. These include:

- Regulating the enzymes of the gastrointestinal tract
- Modulating nutrient absorption
- Modulating postabsorptive metabolic signals.

In case of unhealthy intestinal mucosa or during protein deficiency, absorption of amino acids is decreased further aggravating the problem of protein energy malnutrition (PEM).

While protein is essential for your body, poorly digested protein foods can putrefy. Putrefaction is the process by which undigested proteins are broken down in the lower intestine by bacteria. Byproducts of intestinal putrefaction include hydrogen sulfide (the so-called rotten egg gas), mercaptans (more of a decaying cabbage smell), inflammatory leukotrienes, ammonia, amines like cadaverine and putrescine, and a whole host of other toxic, allergenic, and potentially carcinogenic gases and compounds. This also reduces the number or population of the colonic bacteria that are good for health, while the number of gut microflora that are undesirable increase. The undigested proteins can also be absorbed into the bloodstream.

Role of liver: The liver is the master organ or the powerhouse. It is responsible for ensuring that all the 50 trillion cells in the human body have optimal nutrition. The liver is the body's largest organ. The liver routinely performs over 500 known functions to regulate the body's metabolism and plays a very important role in metabolism of amino acids. It is the only organ capable of catabolizing (breakdown) all amino acids. It removes approximately two-thirds of the amino acids that are absorbed. A major fraction is metabolized and about one-third is used for protein synthesis. Some amino acids like isoleucine, leucine, and valine are sent into circulation to be supplied to other tissues. The liver plays a key role in converting NH_3, the end product of protein and amino acid metabolism to urea. Ammonia is harmful, thus by converting ammonia into urea, liver protects the entire body. This urea is then excreted by kidneys through urine. Some of the most important activities related to protein metabolism performed by the liver are:

- Deamination and transamination of amino acids. Deamination is the process of separating out ammonia from amino acids. The non-nitrogenous part of the deaminated amino acids is converted into glucose or lipids, depending on whether they are glucogenic or ketogenic amino acids. Some of the enzymes used in these pathways such as glutamate, alanine and aspartate aminotransferases (also known as SGOT and SGPT) are commonly measured in serum to assess liver function and to determine whether there is any liver disease/damage.
- Removal of ammonia from the body by synthesis of urea: A ammonia is very toxic. It needs to be rapidly and efficiently removed from the circulation. The ammonia released through deamination of amino acids is converted to urea by the liver via the urea cycle and the urea is then sent to the kidneys for excretion via urine.
- Synthesis of nonessential amino acids.
- Liver is responsible for synthesis of most of the plasma proteins. Albumin, the major plasma protein, is synthesized almost exclusively by the liver. Also, the liver synthesizes many of the clotting factors necessary for blood coagulation.
- The liver manufactures carnitine from lysine and other nutrients. Carnitine is needed to transport fatty acids from the cytoplasm into the mitochondria for energy production. The heart muscle utilizes considerable amount of fats for its energy needs and is sensitive to deficiency or lack of cellular carnitine. Also, endurance athletes' muscles obtain considerable amount of their energy needs from fats. Carnitine is also necessary to transport the branched-chain amino acids (BCAAs) into the mitochondria. BCAAs are also used as a source of energy by muscle during prolonged, intense athletic training or performance.

RAPID FIRE

1. Name five important functions of protein.
2. Which amino acid is limiting in cereals and which one in pulses?
3. What is the difference between vegetable and animal proteins?
4. Name two proteins which increase the immunity.
5. What is a peptide and name any one with its biological function?
6. What is glutathione and its function?
7. Name essential amino acids and explain the role of lysine.
8. Under what conditions, nonessential amino acids become conditionally essential?
9. What do you mean by DIAAS, PDCAAS, and biological value?
10. Where protein is digested first in the body and what is its role in liver?

EXERCISE

1. Identify the food sources of protein in your diet (one day) and calculate the approximate amount in them.
2. Suggest five combinations of food that will help achieve protein complementation.
3. Select five cereals, five pulses and five nuts and five non-vegetarian food items, calculate the amount of protein in one serving of each food stuff.

SUGGESTED READING

1. Belitz HD, Grosch W. Food chemistry, 2nd edition. Berlin: Springer-Verlag; 1999.
2. Benyon R. Metabolism and Nutrition. Mosby: Edinburgh; 2003.
3. Food and Nutrition Board, Institute of Medicine. Dietary reference intakes for energy, carbohydrates, fiber, fat, fatty acids, cholesterol, protein and

amino acids (Macronutrients). Washington DC: National Academies Press: 2002.
4. Gary N. The Complete Guide to Health and Nutrition. London: Arlington Books; 1984.
5. Gosnell BA, Levine AS. Reward systems and food intake: Role of opioids. International Journal of Obesity. 2009;33 (Suppl 2):S54-8.
6. Grosch W, Schieberle P. Amino acids, peptides and proteins. Food Chemistry. Heidelberg: Springer; 2009. pp. 8-28.
7. Hartman R, Meisel H. Food-derived peptides with biological activity: from research to food applications. Current Opinion in Biotechnology. 2007;18:163-9.
8. Hunt RJ, Johnson LK, Roughead ZKF. Dietary protein and calcium interact to influence calcium retention: a controlled study feeding trial. American Journal of Clinical Nutrition. 2009;89(5):1357-65.
9. Jahan-Mihan A, Luhovyy BL, Khoury DL, Anderson GH. Dietary Proteins as Determinants of Metabolic and Physiologic Functions of the Gastrointestinal Tract. Nutrients. 2011;3:574-602.
10. Khan A, Khan S, Jan AA, Khan M. Health complications caused by Protein deficiency. Journal of Food Science and Nutrition. 2017;1(1):1-2.
11. Kohlmeier M. Nutrient Metabolism. Food Science and Technology International Series. Cambridge: Academic Press; 2003.
12. Kurpad A. The requirements of protein & amino acid during acute & chronic infections. Indian Journal of Medical Research. 2006;124:129-48.
13. Li P, Yin YL, Li D, Kim SW, Wu G. Amino acids and immune function. British Journal of Nutrition. 2007;98:237-52.
14. Millward DJ, Layman DK, Tomé D, Schaafsma G. Protein quality assessment: impact of expanding understanding of protein and amino acid needs for optimal health. American Journal of Clinical Nutrition. 2008;87(5):1576S-81S.
15. Nutrient Requirements and Recommended Dietary Allowances for Indians. Indian Council of Medical Research, Hyderabad (2010).
16. O'Neale Roach J. Metabolism and Nutrition, 2nd edition. Edinburgh: Mosby; 2003.
17. Pencharz PB, Young VR. Protein and Amino Acids. In: Bowman BA, Russell RM (Eds). Present Knowledge in Nutrition, 9th edition, Vol. 1. Washington DC: International Life Science Institute; 2006. pp. 59-77.
18. Puri D. Textbook of Medical Biochemistry. New Delhi: Elsevier; 2002.
19. Reeds PJ. Dispensable and indispensable amino acids for humans. Journal of Nutrition. 2000;130:1835S-40S.
20. Schaafsma G. The protein digestibility-corrected amino acid score. Journal of Nutrition. 2000;130(7):1865S-7S.
21. Woods SC, May-Zhang AA, Begg DP. How and why do gastrointestinal peptides influence food intake? Physiol Behav. 2018;193(Pt B):218-22.
22. World Health Organization. (2007). Protein and Amino Acid Requirements in Human Nutrition. Report of a Joint WHO/FAO/UNU Expert Consultation WHO Technical Report, Series 935.
23. Wu G. Dietary protein intake and human health. Food Function. 2016;7:1251.
24. Wu G. Functional Amino Acids in Growth, Reproduction, and Health. Advances in Nutrition. 2010;1:31-7.
25. Yalcin A, Hotamisligil GS. Impact of ER protein homeostasis on metabolism. Diabetes. 2013;62(3):691-3.
26. Young VR, Reeds PJ. Nutrition and Metabolism of Proteins and Amino Acids. In: Gibney MJ, Vorster HH, Kok FJ (Eds). Introduction to human nutrition. Oxford: Blackwell Publishing, The Nutrition Society; 2002. pp. 46-68.
27. Lean M, Combet E. Barasi's Human Nutrition: A Health Perspective, 3rd edn. CRC, Press, Taylor and Francis group. 2017;31-36.

4

CHAPTER

Fats, Oils, and Lipids

KEY CONCERNS
- What are lipid, fat, and fatty acid?
- What are the different types of lipids and fatty acids, and their functions?
- What can happen if we eat more or less amount of fat?
- Do different fatty acids have different impact on health?
- What is the role of cholesterol and phytosterols?
- How much fat should we consume and how much is present in various foods?

KEY CONCEPTS
- Classification of lipids and fatty acids
- Functions of different types of lipids and fatty acids
- Vegetable and animal sources of fat and their impact on health
- Cholesterol and plant sterols
- Essential fatty acids, ratio of n-6 to n-3 fatty acids and eicosanoids
- Trans-fatty acids (TFAs) and conjugated linoleic acid (CLA)
- Causes and consequences of deficiency and excess.

INTRODUCTION

Fats, oils or lipids are large, diverse or heterogeneous group of organic compounds found in food and living organisms in varied forms. They are insoluble in water and soluble in organic solvents. All fats are lipids but all lipids are not fats. Fats and lipids are predominately composed of carbon, hydrogen, and oxygen and sometimes, they also contain phosphorus, nitrogen, and sulfur.

Lipid includes different categories or fractions of fat-soluble components such as (i) fats and oils, (ii) free fatty acids, monoacylglycerols or monoglycerides, diacylglycerols/diglycerides, and triacylglycerols/triglycerides (TG), (iii) phospholipids (PL), (iv) sphingolipids, (v) glycolipids, (vi) lipoproteins, (vii) sterols such as cholesterol and cholesterol esters, and (viii) waxes. Other important lipids are eicosanoids, carotenoids, and the fat-soluble vitamins A and E as well as fatty alcohols, and hydrocarbons. Dietary fats and oils are one of the subclasses of lipids. Fats, steroids, and phospholipids are very important for the functioning of membranes in cells. Fats and oils are triglycerides composed of fatty acids and glycerol. Acylglycerol means a fatty acid is esterified to glycerol.

Lipids are insoluble in water, i.e., they are hydrophobic but are soluble in organic solvents like hexane, ether, etc., because they are mostly hydrocarbons and do not contain many polar functional groups. Most triacylglycerols consist of fatty acids that are long-chain compounds, containing 16–18 carbons. For digestion, they need the help of bile acids to emulsify them before they are absorbed in the small intestine, from where they are transported by transport proteins. This is necessary to enable the water-insoluble lipids to travel in the aqueous phase of blood and reach the target tissues.

Lipids are the form in which the mammalian body stores energy for a long period of time. They are needed for a wide range of metabolic and physiological processes, and are very important constituents of cell membranes. They are primarily obtained from dietary sources. Many forms of lipid compounds are synthesized *de novo* in the body using the substrates from the diet. Various types of lipids are present in blood, adipose tissues, cell membranes of body cells, and myelin sheath of nerve cells in varying concentrations. Triglycerides or triacylglycerols are the major lipids in the diet and the storage form of fat in adipose tissue. They are primarily made up of fatty acids that are the major building blocks of triacylglycerols or dietary fats and oils.

Fats and oils are edible substances found in certain plant, animal, and marine food sources. They are considered rich sources of energy and are necessary for growth, development, and myriad of vital functions in the body and brain. Fatty acid composition of dietary fats influences the lipid composition of the blood (lipid profile) and body tissues as well as that of the cell membranes. They are also reflected in the fat deposited in adipose tissue and other tissues which are crucial in health and disease. Deviation from the normal range influences the risk for obesity, cardiac or neurological diseases.

The term fats is used for those that are solid at room temperature and those of liquid consistency are referred to as oils. Animal fats are usually solid until melted. Fats obtained from plants are usually liquid at room temperature, although there are some exceptions. Vegetable oils obtained from various oil seeds like soybean, groundnut, sunflower, olive, etc. are oils, and coconut oil and palm kernel oil are solid at low temperatures. Fats have a high melting point whereas the melting point of oils is low. Butter, ghee, lard, and tallow are animal fats and solid in nature, however fish oil is liquid.

Other oils do not solidify under normal or low temperature unless they undergo some processing like hydrogenation.

> **Lipids**—this is a generic name, which includes the various compounds listed about and may include lipoproteins, phospholipids, etc.
>
> **Fats**—this is also a generic name, but applied mostly to fats that are solid at room temperature.
>
> **Oils**—these are liquid at room temperature.
>
> **Fatty acids**—they are the basic building blocks for fats.
>
> **Triglycerides**—these are esters of fatty acids with glycerol. Monoglycerides and diglycerides are also esters of fatty acids.

FUNCTIONS OF FATS AND LIPIDS

Functions of fats and lipids can be viewed from two perspectives: 1. Role in food and 2. Role in health and nutrition.

Role in Food

Fats and oils are important ingredients in almost every food that we eat. Many of the characteristics that we consider desirable and important in different foods such as tenderness of cakes, flavor of foods, having a lubricating effect, and producing a sensation of moistness in the mouth, are imparted by fats in foods.

Improve taste, flavor, and color: Fats and oils improve the palatability of foods. Foods containing fats have a typical mouthfeel. The typical taste of butter and ghee is well known to Indians. During cooking, particularly frying, fat undergoes oxidation resulting in formation of many volatile compounds such as aldehydes, ketones, and aromatic compounds, etc. which impart flavor to the food products. Browning usually occurs in fried or baked products.

Fatty foods or fried foods are tasty and irresistible to many people, but often such foods are consumed in more amounts than is desirable/wise, which eventually leads to overweight and obesity. If fats/oils are not stored properly, they may undergo oxidation because of exposure to heat and air. As a result, fats and oils become rancid. Rancidity is associated with a typical odor and off-flavor in the oil or foods. Consumption of rancid oil is harmful to health.

Give texture to foods: Fats and oils are used to enhance creaminess, crispiness, palatability, and mouthfeel of the food products. Creamy texture is obtained by incorporating butter and cream. Use of solid fat not oil as shortening gives light and desirable texture to biscuits and other savories. Shortening is the process of weakening/shortening the gluten strands during dough making. Crispness is obtained in fried products due to loss of moisture from the food or replacing the moisture by oil. However, frying at low temperature allows more oil to be absorbed, thus making the food oily, soggy, and undesirable. Milk foam is due to the fat and whipped cream is just an aerated fat.

Medium of heat transfer: Fat is a medium for heat transfer. Oils have lower "specific heat capacity than water", thus they get heated much quicker than water. Oils/fats tend to raise the temperature of food higher and faster because they have high heat capacity and food cooks faster in fat compared with water. Oil envelops the food during frying and heat reaches to surface of the oil and the food gets cooked. Heat is transferred by convection. Liquid convection is faster than gas or air, thus the food cooks faster by frying than baking.

Increases shelf-life: Fats/oils provide a shield to the food and prevent entry of microorganisms and spoilage of the food. Oils form a layer over the food, e.g., pickles, and thus prevent entry of microorganisms. During frying or baking, moisture content of food is reduced, limiting the growth of microorganisms. Thus fried foods like mathris, sev, and gathia, and baked foods like biscuits can be stored for longer duration in air-tight containers.

> **Research glimpse:** Fats and oils are important raw materials, and serve as functional ingredients in a wide variety of food products including confectionery and bakery items, ice creams, emulsions, and sauces, shortenings, margarines, and other specially tailored products. However, since fats are energy-dense, with the increasing prevalence of overweight and obesity, the need for developing these foods with low fat content is in focus. In addition, lowering of trans-fats due to their adverse health implications, and reducing the saturated fat content are also issues that need to be addressed. These pose considerable challenges given the varied functions that fats play in foods in terms of imparting texture, flavor, physicochemical, and sensory attributes. Products that are low in fat, need to still retain some important sensory attributes like creaminess, crispiness, rich texture, and milky and creamy appearance as well as the taste of the original food. In different food systems, the micro- or nanostructure plays a critical role in their function in which fat is a critical ingredient in products such as chocolates, biscuits, and ice creams. Fat replacers including carbohydrates, proteins, and lipids are available today and need to be studied for their incorporation into these highly popular foods.
>
> *Rios RV, Pessanha MDF, de Almeida PF, et al. Application of fats in some food products. Food Sci. Technol (Campinas). 2014;34(1):3–15.*

Role in Health and Nutrition

Lipids play a very important role in nutrition and in the human body. These include providing energy and serving as storage form of energy. They are important substrates for synthesis of several important compounds such as hormones, prostaglandins, bile acids, and cytokines. They are critical components of the cell membrane structure, for myelination, and are important for cell differentiation and growth. They also play an important role in signal transmission.

Concentrated source of energy: One gram of oil/fat provides 9 kcal. This is more than double the amount of calories provided by carbohydrates or protein (4 kcal/g). Regardless of which oil or fat it is, the calorific value is the same, except for butter. Butter gives comparatively less calories per gram (7–8 kcal) due to the presence of moisture. Energy from fat is used by the body for its energy (ATP) needs, but the excess is stored in the body in the adipose tissues (fat tissues). Thus consumption of more energy through high-calorie foods is stored as fat, leading to overweight and obesity, and its associated disorders. It can be utilized during aerobic exercise or physical activities. Energy from fat is an important fuel source not only during intensive physical activities, in sports or manual labor, but also in case of starvation.

Structural component: Cell membranes of all body cells are predominantly comprised of phospholipids, glycolipids, and cholesterol. Cell membranes are bilayers having lipids which have one polar end (soluble in water) and one nonpolar end (soluble in fat). Fat within the cell membranes helps in cell to cell communication. Some tissues also contain polyunsaturated fatty acids (PUFAs), which help to regulate transport of numerous compounds and ions across the membrane. Adipose tissue is basically made up of triglyceride and it provides a cushion, structure, and shape/contour to the body.

Thermal insulation of the body: Fat is a poor conductor of heat and thus prevents heat loss from the body. The layer of fat underneath the skin provides insulation that helps to maintain body temperature.

Shock absorber: There is a layer of lipid under the skin and surrounding the vital organs. This padding absorbs external mechanical shock and thus prevents injury. Also, it serves as a structural support to the organs.

Insulation to nerve fibers: Nerve fibers are surrounded by lipid called myelin sheath which provides insulation. Fat aids in transmission of nerve impulses via myelinated nerve fibers.

Improves absorption of fat-soluble vitamins: Many foods that are good sources of lipids contain sterols and vitamins like vitamin E. Vitamins A, D, E, and K are fat soluble, hence they require some amount of fat to be absorbed. It is advisable to add some amount of oil/fat in food preparations using vitamin A-rich foods like green leafy vegetables, carrot, etc.

Source of essential fatty acids: Essential fatty acids (EFAs) are essential for numerous vital functions in the body. Those fatty acids which are not synthesized by the body and need to be obtained from dietary sources are called essential fatty acids. Omega-3 (n-3) and omega-6 are essential fatty acids. Omega-3 fatty acids are found in seafoods, fish, flaxseeds, etc. Deficiency of EFAs can have adverse effects on health, as they are required for many vital functions in the body and they can be supplied to the body only through dietary means.

Precursor of hormones: Cholesterol is a sterol that is part of the cell membrane. It is the precursor of some steroid hormones like sex hormones and some adrenal hormones. These hormones can pass through the cell membranes and bring about changes at cellular level. Polyunsaturated fats from plant sources support hormone production released from hypothalamus and pineal gland.

Components of lipoproteins in the blood: Lipids are hydrophobic; therefore when they are transported in blood, they are combined with protein and circulate in the form of lipoproteins in blood. There are various types of lipoproteins such as low-density lipoprotein (LDL) and high-density lipoprotein (HDL), which have significance in health and disease.

Source of eicosanoids: Eicosanoids are signaling molecules that are synthesized from lipid precursors such as arachidonic acid (AA) and related polyunsaturated fatty acids (PUFA). They act like local hormones and perform important functions including regulation of body temperature, aggregation of blood platelets, and have a role in tissue inflammation.

Role in immune system: Dietary fats affect the immune system by influencing the substrate availability in the formation of cyclooxygenase and lipoxygenase products. These enzymes are important for metabolism of the dietary essential fatty acids, i.e., linoleic and linolenic acids, or arachidonic acid (n-6) and n-3 fatty acids. Their action produces eicosanoids which, in turn, act as lipid mediators in the control of the immune system. Since functioning of the cells of the immune system is associated with the components secreted by the cell membrane such as antibodies, antigens, etc.

> **Research glimpse**: Lipids are basic constituents of the human diet and contribute greatly to the acceptability, flavor, and perception of food. Lipids have many beneficial roles in the human body and are important for health. However, lipids are linked to many pathologies and diseases. Considerable research has been carried out on the diversity of molecular and supramolecular structures of dietary lipids, and related to the metabolic and nutritional effects of the multiscale structures of lipids in foods. Perception of lipids in the mouth during oral processing has been shown to modulate the production of digestive fluids and food intake. During the gastric and intestinal phases of lipid digestion, the multiscale structures of lipids play a role in the kinetics of release of the fatty acids by influencing fatty acid bioaccessibility and rate of absorption of fatty acids ingested. The structure of the lipids may influence digestion, absorption as well as metabolic and nutritional effects of lipids.
>
> *Meynier A, Genot C. Molecular and structural organization of lipids in foods: their fate during digestion and impact in nutrition. Oilseeds & Fats, Crops and Lipids. 2017;24(2):D202.*

CLASSIFICATION OF FATS, OILS, AND LIPIDS

Dietary fats are classified on the basis of food source, viz. animal fats and plant fats. Fats and oils are either visible or invisible. Visible fats are topically added to the food, e.g., butter, ghee, and vegetable oils. Invisible fats are inherently present in the food, e.g., nuts and seeds are rich in fats. Dietary fats are composed of different types of fatty acids and depending on the structure, fatty acids can be either saturated or unsaturated fatty acids. The types of fatty acids not only determine the physicochemical properties of the food but also greatly influence the body composition.

In 2008, FAO (Food and Agriculture Organization) gave a new and comprehensive system of classification of lipids. Lipids are defined as small hydrophobic or amphipathic (or amphiphilic) molecules that may originate entirely or in part through condensations of thioesters and/or isoprene units.

> Polar group has affinity with water or attract water. It is also referred as hydrophilic group.
>
> **Hydrophilic = Polar = soluble in water**
> Non-polar has affinity with oil or organic solvents but repel water. It is called hydrophobic because it repels water. It is also called lipophilic because it attracts oil.
>
> **Hydrophobic = Non-polar = insoluble in water**

In the new system, lipids from biological tissues are divided into eight categories so that lipids and their properties can be catalogued in a way that is compatible with databases for other macromolecules are presented in Table 4.1.

Earlier lipids were classified mainly in three categories as shown in Figure 4.1.

Simple Lipids

Simple lipids are abundantly available in nature. Simple lipids include fatty acyls or fatty acids, and glycerolipids such as triacylglycerol or triglycerides. They include edible fats, oils,

Table 4.1: Classes of lipids.

Classes	Example	Characteristics and significance
Fatty acyls	Oleic acid	Fatty acyls or fatty acids are a diverse group of molecules. The fatty acyl structure represents the major lipid-building block of complex lipids. The fatty acyl group is characterized by a repeating series of methylene groups which makes these compounds hydrophobic.
Glycerolipids	Triacylglycerols	It includes all glycerol-containing lipids or fatty acid esters of glycerol (acylglycerols), e.g., triacylglycerols, which is most common and nutritionally important in health and disease. They are found in seed oils and storage fat in animal tissues. It consists of glycerol to which either one or two or three fatty acids are attached. The most common is three fatty acids attached to glycerol, i.e., triacylglycerol.
Glycerophos-pholipids	Phosphatidylcholine	It is also referred to as phospholipids. They have a backbone of glycerol, two fatty acids that form the nonpolar tail, and a phosphate group that forms the polar head. Hence they are called amphipathic molecules. They are constituents of cell membranes, which occur in foods and extracted oils. Examples are phosphatidylcholine (lecithin) found in biological membranes.
Sphingolipids	Sphingosine	All sphingolipids share a common structural feature having sphingoid base backbone that is synthesized de novo and then converted into ceramides, phosphosphingolipids, and glycosphingolipids. These are found in abundance in myelin sheath.
Sterol lipids	Cholesterol	Sterol lipids/steroids have a common steroid nucleus of a fused 4-ring structure with a hydrocarbon side chain and an alcohol group. Dietary sterols are found in both animal fats and most vegetable oils (oryzanol). Cholesterol is the primary animal fat sterol and is found in vegetable oils in trace amounts. Cholesterol plays an important role in the body as it is widely distributed in almost all tissues, especially in brain, other nervous tissues, adrenals, and liver. Plant-derived sterols are collectively known as plant sterols or phytosterols. The steroid hormones also contain the same fused 4-ring core structure. The C18 steroids include the estrogen family, the C19 steroids include androgens (testosterone and androsterone) and the C21 subclass includes progestogens and glucocorticoids. Bile acids and their conjugates are also sterols, which are synthesized from cholesterol in the liver. Vitamin D is also a steroid.
Prenol lipids	Farnesol	Prenol lipids are synthesized from 5-carbon precursors, isopentenyl diphosphate and dimethylallyldiphosphate. Successive additions of these 5-carbon units (terpenes) give rise to various compounds. Those containing more than 40 carbons are known as polyterpenes. Examples are carotenoids, vitamins E and K.
Saccharolipids	N-acetylglucosamine	These are compounds in which fatty acids are linked to a sugar instead of being linked to glycerol.
Polyketides	Aflatoxin, which is a fungal metabolite. Some act as cholesterol-lowering agents, e.g., lovastatin and pravastatin	They are a diverse group of compounds that are often formed by a series of enzymes, which first condense and then modify chains of acetate or propionate units largely through reactions such as reduction, dehydration, cyclization, and aromatization. They are secondary metabolites and natural products from animal, plant, bacterial, fungal, and marine sources. Many commonly used antimicrobial, antiparasitic, and anticancer agents are polyketides or their derivatives, e.g., erythromycins and tetracyclines.

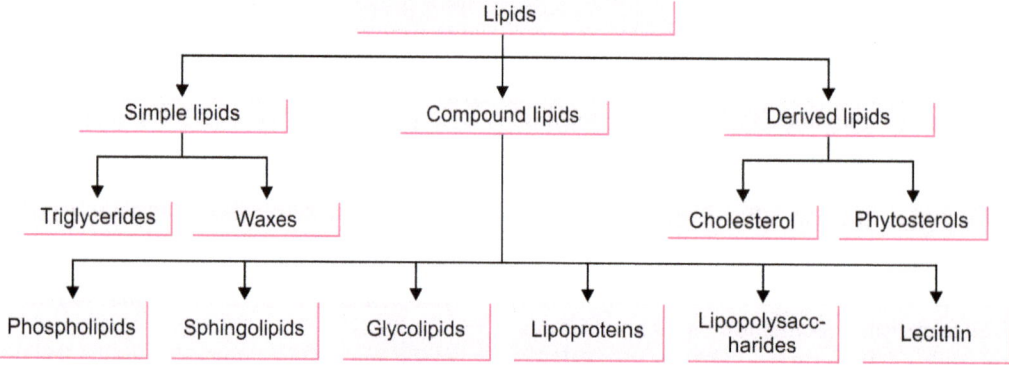

Fig. 4.1: Classification of lipids.

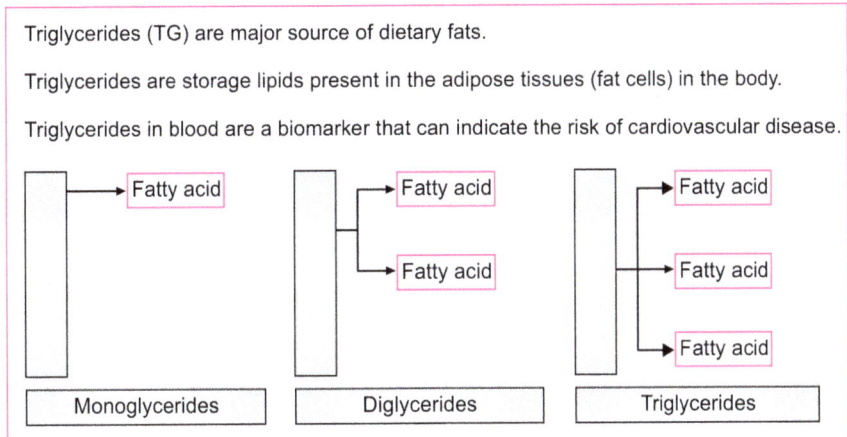

and inedible waxes. Fats are used for eating and cooking, and waxes are present naturally as a coat on the surface of some foods, thereby protecting the food from harsh environmental conditions. Fats and oils provide energy but waxes do not, because they are not digested and absorbed by the human body.

Triglycerides: This group is also known as fats/oils. Edible form of fat is primarily composed of triglycerides (TG) or triacylglycerols. They are abundantly available in natural vegetable oils, butter, and ghee as well as in animal food sources (lard and tallow). Triglycerides are composed of one molecule of glycerol that is joined by ester bonds with three molecules of fatty acids. The behavior of TG is dependent on the kind of fatty acid attached to glycerol. More than 30 kinds of fatty acids are found in nature, and are present in numerous permutations and combinations in different triglycerides. Triglycerides (TG) are major source of dietary fats.

Fatty acid composition of triglycerides varies from one food to another. Therefore, two fats/oils will not have the same effect on cell metabolism, although all fats/oils provide the same amount of energy (kcals). Hence, the nutritional and health significance of different fats/oils differs.

Triglycerides can easily be metabolized, synthesized, and stored in the body. They are broken down into glycerol and fatty acids that are metabolized in the mitochondria of the cell via β-oxidation. They can be synthesized in the liver and circulate in the blood. Triglycerides are storage lipids present in the adipose tissues (fat cells) in the body. Triglycerides in blood are a biomarker that can indicate the risk of cardiovascular disease.

Waxes: Waxes are nonedible substances but they are naturally present on the outer surface of skin and protect the food from environmental hazards and prevent loss of moisture and other valuable components in the outer layer or just underneath the skin. For example, apple skin is a good source of antioxidant compounds and many vital nutrients are present just underneath skin. Thus, the waxy coat on the skin has a protective role.

Compound Lipids

Compound lipids contain one simple lipid molecule and an organic and/or inorganic molecule. **Lipoproteins** (protein and lipid), **glycolipids** (carbohydrate and lipid), and **phospholipids** (phosphate and lipid) are all examples of compound lipids. They are components of body cells, body fluids, and are synthesized in the body. Some of them like lecithin, which is a type of phospholipid, are found in foods, e.g., egg yolk and soybean. They play a significant role in regulation of many biological functions.

Phospholipids

Phospholipids (PL) are structural lipids found in every cell membrane. Phospholipids are abundantly available in nervous tissues. Phospholipids contain a diglyceride and the third carbon in the glycerol molecule is bound to a phosphate group. Most phospholipids are composed of glycerol, fatty acids, and phosphoric acid bound in ester linkage to a nitrogenous base or one simple organic molecule as functional groups like choline, ethanolamine or inositol. Depending upon the functional group as well as the type of fatty acid, phospholipids behave differently. They can be synthesized in the body and also obtained from dietary sources like egg and soy.

The phosphate group along with the glycerol group makes the head of the phospholipid hydrophilic, whereas the fatty acid tail is hydrophobic. Thus phospholipids are amphipathic—a molecule with a polar end and a hydrophobic end. In an aqueous solution, phospholipids assemble into bilayers (also called micelles) and these structures exclude water molecules from the hydrophobic tails while keeping the hydrophilic head in contact with the aqueous solution. Similarly, phospholipids form a stable bilayer in cell membranes due to this amphipathic property. Phospholipids are arranged spherically or in a rod-like manner with the hydrophilic/polar portion on the outer side of the cell membrane while the lipophilic portion faces the inner side of the cell. This arrangement enables lipid-soluble and hydrophobic substances to cross the cell membrane from the surrounding fluid and enter the cell. Phosphatidylcholine and sphingomyelin are concentrated on the surface toward ECF (extracellular fluids), and phosphatidylethanolamine and phosphatidylinositol are present in cytosol. When present in myelin sheath along with cholesterol, it performs a structural role. Phosphatidylserine is important for apoptosis; phosphatidyl inositol is a precursor of second messengers and cardiolipin is present in mitochondrial membranes.

In the body, phospholipids play critical roles in many important biological and cellular processes, which are as follows:
- Being a structural component of cell membranes, phospholipids influence the integrity and permeability, thereby functioning of cells.
- They are components of membranes surrounding intracellular organelles such as mitochondria.
- The phospholipid membrane allows some small uncharged molecules like oxygen and carbon dioxide to freely diffuse/cross the cell membrane. However, charged ions, polar molecules or other larger molecules like glucose and amino acids are not allowed to pass. This makes the membrane semipermeable which in turn is important for the cell to maintain the composition of the cytoplasm independent of the external environment.
- They are important for keeping lipids suspended in blood and body fluids. In plasma, they are part of lipoproteins, which facilitate transport of fat and cholesterol in the body. Thus, they are important for the formation of lipoproteins like LDL and HDL.
- They help in cellular processes such as organelle division or apoptosis (programmed cell death).
- They regulate activities of membrane proteins.
- They are involved in absorption of fat from the intestine and its disposal into the lymphatics and transport as chylomicrons.
- Phosphatidylcholine (lecithin) is a major component of bile; thereby phospholipids play a major role in fat absorption.
- They play an important role in processes such as blood coagulation (by cephalin), recognition and removal of apoptotic cells.
- They aid in cell signaling via presence of specific receptor proteins on the outer surface of cell membrane. Phosphoinositol helps in anchoring these receptors.
- They are important for blood clotting.
- Phospholipid containing choline is also capable of synthesizing a neurotransmitter called acetylcholine, which is responsible for cognition and memory.
- Phospholipids are very good emulsifiers due to the typical chemical configuration. In the body, it emulsifies fat for its transport their target tissues.
- In food, it also acts like an emulsifier that facilitates the mixing of watery substances into oil phase to make the food in stable form, e.g., egg yolk contains phospholipid in lecithin that is used in making mayonnaise.
- They also maintain the integrity of mitochondrial membrane.

Different Phospholipids

- **Lecithin**: Lecithin is phosphatidylcholine, which contains choline as a functional group. It is involved in the synthesis of a neurotransmitter, acetylcholine. It is a part of every cell membrane and is important for cell membrane fluidity. It is a very good emulsifier, thus facilitates absorption of fat in the body, and transport of fat and cholesterol in the blood stream. It is also present in myelin sheath and prevents damage of the neuronal tissues. It is naturally available in foods like egg yolk, soybean, and wheat germ.
- **Cephalin**: Cephalin is phosphatidylethanolamine owing to the presence of ethanolamine or serine as the functional group. It is present in cell membranes, especially in brain, neural tissues, and spinal cord. Cephalins are present in blood platelets and, therefore, are important for blood clotting.

Sphingolipids

Sphingolipids are another type of naturally occurring lipids found in all cell membranes, and in abundance, in the nervous system (nerve cells and brain tissue). They contain **sphingosine**, an amino alcohol, choline, and a long-unsaturated hydrocarbon chain attached to glycerol. They constitute about one-fourth of the lipids in the myelin sheath that surrounds and insulates cells of the central nervous system. It constitutes about 10% of brain tissue and almost 50% of other tissues. Ceramides and sphingomyelin (SM) are common sphingolipids. **Sphingomyelin** is the most abundant sphingolipid present in animal cell membranes. It is also a precursor of ceramides that function as part of membranes and as intracellular messenger. Being amphiphilic in nature, sphingolipids play many important roles in physiological functions and in the development and progression of diseases. Interaction of lipids and proteins can reorganize the cell membrane and affects cellular functions.

> **Laboratory laurel**: Milk and dairy products, particularly cream, are important sources of sphingolipids. Sphingolipids are not "ordinary fats" but also categorized as "functional ingredients". They have structural and regulatory functions in the body. Dietary sphingolipids exhibit important role in inactivation of toxins and bacteria, cognitive function, skin homeostasis, inflammation, high cholesterol, and cancer.
>
> *Potočki S. Potential health benefits of sphingolipids in milk and dairy products. Mljekarstvo. 2016:66 (4):251–61.*

Glycolipids

Glycolipids are complex in structure, bonded to a carbohydrate, i.e., monosaccharides or polysaccharides. The most common among them are *glycosphingolipids (GSLs)*. These are found in the cell membrane of all cells from bacteria to man. GSLs are amphipathic in nature, present in vertebrate cells and body fluids especially in the nervous system in abundance. They are important to mediate signal transduction and cell adhesion. When the sugar moiety is a single glucose or galactose, they are called **cerebrosides**.

> **Research glimpse:** Sphingolipids are a diverse group of essential cellular lipids. They play an important role as structural membrane components and as signaling molecules. Source of sphingolipids in cells are de novo biosynthesis and recycling of exogenous sphingolipids; de novo sphingolipid biosynthesis in adipocytes was studied. Adipocytes were selected as the cell type for study because their lipid metabolism is highly regulated. The researchers studied the mice with an adipocyte-specific deletion of Sptlc1 that is a subunit of serine palmitoyl transferase, the enzyme responsible for the first and rate-limiting step of de novo sphingolipid biosynthesis. In these mice, first adipose tissue was developed but, there was a notable age-dependent loss of adipose tissue due to adipocyte death accompanied

Contd...

Contd...

by evidence of increased macrophage infiltration and tissue fibrosis. Sptlc1 deletion did not have any effect on adipocyte differentiation. Other observations in these mice included, raised fasting blood glucose, fatty liver, and insulin resistance. Altogether, these data indicate that adipocyte cell viability and normal metabolic function require de novo sphingolipid biosynthesis, and that reduced de novo sphingolipid biosynthesis in adipocytes is associated with adipocyte death, adipose tissue remodeling, and metabolic dysfunction.

Alexaki A, Clarke BA, Gavrilova O, et al. De novo sphingolipid biosynthesis is required for Adipocyte survival and metabolic homeostasis. J Biol Chem. 2017;292(9):3929–39.

In human red blood cells, glycolipids play a role in determining the blood group of the individual, i.e., the A, B, and O blood type antigens. Glycolipids often act as antigens and as receptors for hormones and other signaling molecules. Thus, they play significant role in signal transmission and cell recognition. They help in maintaining stability of the cell and are crucial in immune response. Many pathogenic bacteria bind to glycolipids of host cell surface for colonization and infection. Symbolic structure of different types of sphingolipids are shown in Figure 4.2.

Gangliosides are glycolipids, so named because they were first isolated from ganglion cells in the brain. A **ganglioside** is a molecule composed of a glycosphingolipid (ceramide and oligosaccharide) with one or more sialic acids (e.g., N-acetylneuraminic acid, NANA) linked on the sugar chain. They are found in tissues and fluids particularly in nervous tissues. Brain contains 20–500 times more gangliosides than most non-neuronal tissues, with their content in gray matter being more than in white matter. They recognize specific molecules at the cell surface and regulate activities of proteins in plasma membrane. They may have specialized functions in cell adhesion, cell-to-cell interaction, growth, and motility through interactions with specific proteins and signal transduction pathways, activity of insulin receptors. They play a role in formation of synapses and maintaining the integrity of axons and myelin, thus play a role in transmission of nervous impulses. Gangliosides may also play a role in memory and learning. They play crucial role in neurological disorders and psychological responses to a stimuli. Gangliosides are particularly high in breast milk. Intake of long-chain fatty acids during retinal development increases the concentration of gangliosides, which helps to stabilize retinal membrane and enhances visual function.

Research glimpse: Gangliosides are acidic glycosphingolipids, essential compounds, located on the outer leaflet of the plasma membrane. They contain at least one sialic acid residue. They interact with phospholipids, cholesterol, and transmembrane proteins, forming lipid rafts. They are involved in cell adhesion, proliferation, recognition processes, and modulate signal transduction pathways. The sugar/glycan moiety governs the functions of the ganglioside. In pathological conditions such as neuroectoderm-derived cancers, changes in ganglioside structures have been reported. Researchers are focusing on development of cancer immunotherapy targeting gangliosides.

Sphingomyelin, glycosphingolipids, and gangliosides are important polar lipids in the milk fat globule membrane. When sphingomyelin and glycosphingolipids are digested and absorbed, the bioactive metabolites ceramide, sphingosine, and sphingosine-1-phosphate (S1P) are obtained. Intact gangliosides may have beneficial effects in the gut, and could be important for gut integrity and immune maturation in the neonate. The enzymes alkaline sphingomyelinase (nucleotide phosphodiesterase pyrophosphatase 7), and neutral ceramidase are expressed in the brush border expressed at birth in both term and preterm infants. Released sphingosine is absorbed, phosphorylated to S1P, and converted to palmitic acid via S1P-lyase in the gut mucosa. It has been hypothesized that S1P also may be released from absorptive cells and exert important paracrine actions favoring epithelial integrity and renewal, as well as immune function, production of secretory IgA, and migration of T lymphocyte subpopulations. Lactase-phlorizin hydrolase is the enzyme that hydrolyzes lactose, hydrolyzes gluco-, galacto-, and lactosylceramide to ceramide. Gangliosides may adhere to the brush border. They are probably internalized, modified, and it is likely that they transported into blood. They may interact with bacteria, bacterial toxins, and the brush border, and thus have a protective role.

Groux-Degroote S, Guérardel Y, Delannoy P. Gangliosides: Structures, Biosynthesis, Analysis, and Roles in Cancer. Chembiochem 2017;18(13):1146–54.

Nilsson A. Role of sphingolipids in infant gut health and immunity. J Pediatr. 2016;173Suppl:S53–9.

Lipids in Blood

Lipoproteins

Lipids are transported in the circulation through the molecules called lipoproteins. Since lipids (cholesterol and triglycerides) are nonpolar, for circulation in blood, a polar medium is required. Hence, some special proteins (amphipathic) are required. Lipoproteins are complex particles composed of lipids and proteins. Many enzymes, transporters, structural proteins, antigens, adhesins, and toxins are lipoproteins. Lipoproteins can be differentiated on the basis of their density, size, lipid composition, and by the types of apolipoproteins they contain. Each lipoprotein carries a specific protein called "Apoprotein", which is also termed as "Apolipoproteins" (Apo), as an identity tag. There are different types of apolipoproteins, which vary according to the size, distribution in lipoproteins, and other characteristics. The lipoprotein particles have hydrophilic groups of phospholipids, free cholesterol, and apoproteins directed outward. These form the outer layer of the lipoprotein particle (called surface layer) inside which there is the hydrophobic core, i.e., triglycerides, cholesterol, and cholesterol esters, fat-soluble vitamins, and antioxidants are carried, shielded by the phospholipid monolayer and

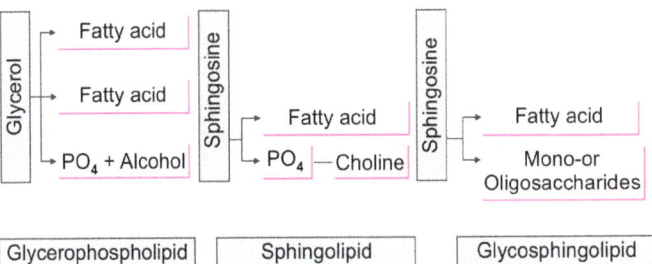

Fig. 4.2: Structure of glycerophospholipid, sphingolipid, and glycosphingolipid.

Table 4.2: Composition of lipoproteins.

Lipoprotein	Density	Protein (%)	Lipid present (%)			Apoproteins
			Triglyceride	Cholesterol	Phospholipids	
Chylomicrons	<0.95	1–2	80–95	2–7	3–9	Apo B-48, Apo C, Apo E, Apo A-I, A-II, A-IV
VLDL	0.95–1.006	5–10	55–80	5–15	10–20	Apo B-100, Apo E, Apo C
LDL	1.019–1.063	25	5–15	40–50	20–25	Apo B-100
HDL	1.063–1.21	45–50	5–10	15–25	20–30	Apo A-I, Apo A-II, Apo C, Apo E

Source: Lichtenstein AH, Jones PJH. Lipids: Absorption and Transport. In: Bowman BA, Russell RL (Eds). Present Knowledge in Nutrition, 9th edition, Volume 1. Washington, DC: ILSI Press, International Life Sciences Institute; 2006. p 119.

the apoproteins. This makes it possible for lipids to be transported in the aqueous fluids in the body. Based on their size, lipid composition, and apoprotein content, there are five classes of lipoproteins namely chylomicrons, VLDL, IDL, HDL, and LDL. In addition, in blood, chylomicron remnants and lipoprotein A (Lpa) are present. Table 4.2 and Figure 4.3 give the composition of the major lipoproteins.

Each lipoprotein performs specific roles as do each of the apoproteins present in them, such as activating/inhibiting enzymes involved in lipid metabolism, enhancing uptake of triacylglycerol. The roles of the lipoproteins are summarized in Table 4.3.

Chylomicrons: Dietary fats/TG are hydrolyzed, and long-chain fatty acids are absorbed into the walls of villi of intestines (enterocytes), where chylomicrons are synthesized. Chylomicrons (CM) are rich in triglycerides (TG) and sterols. The protein component in CM is Apo-B. CM is light in weight but large in size. Their quantity in plasma is increased following a fatty meal. Plasma becomes opaque when they are present. Their size depends on the amount of fat consumed. If a person consumes a high-fat meal, large chylomicron particles are formed, whereas in the fasting state, chylomicron size is smaller as less amount of TG is to be transported. They are rapidly taken up from the blood by the peripheral tissues, skeletal muscle, and adipose tissues.

The capillaries of these tissues contain an enzyme called "lipoprotein lipase" (LPL). This enzyme hydrolyzes (lipolysis) the TG in the chylomicrons to fatty acids and monoglycerides, which then go into the cells and circulation for oxidation. In adipose tissues, TG is resynthesized and stored. The chylomicron with the remaining lipid material is now called a chylomicron remnant (these are smaller in size than chylomicrons). Compared with chylomicrons, they contain more cholesterol and are considered proatherogenic. These particles reach the liver, where they are internalized by hepatic receptors and metabolized. Chylomicrons are rapidly cleared from circulation, and their half-life is less than an hour. If chylomicrons are not rapidly cleared, the person will have postprandial and fasting lipemia (hypertriglyceridemia).

Very low-density lipoprotein (VLDL): VLDL is similar to chylomicrons because it also contains high amount of triglycerides and cholesterol esters. The difference is that it is synthesized in the liver from fatty acids that are produced by the liver and free fatty acids that are formed by catabolism of the chylomicrons. Like chylomicrons, their size varies according to the amount of triglyceride present, but their size is smaller than that of chylomicrons. Under normal physiologic conditions, the ratio of triglycerides to cholesterol esters is 5:1. In hypertriglyceridemia, the liver produces more amount of VLDL particles and they are generally larger in size. Large VLDL particles are a marker of insulin resistance. VLDL circulates in the blood where the capillary LPL enzyme breaks down triglycerides and provides fatty acids to adipose tissue and muscles. The remaining portion is denser than VLDL and smaller in size. It is called intermediate-density lipoprotein or IDL (IDL is a VLDL particle that has lost most of its TG and some surface phospholipids). They are finally converted to LDL.

The activity of LPL is enhanced by heparin and also by apo C and apo C-II. Glucose and insulin also enhances its activity. It is under hormonal control [epinephrine, adrenocorticotropic hormone (ACTH), and growth hormone], which helps to remove the excess CM lipid taken up by the liver.

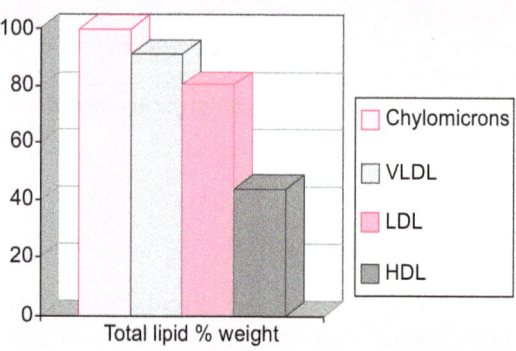

Fig. 4.3: Lipid content of lipoproteins.

Table 4.3: Roles of lipoproteins.

Lipoproteins	Major role
Chylomicrons	Carry triglycerides from intestine (where they are synthesized) to peripheral tissues and liver. Provide energy in the form of fatty acids to skeletal muscle and to adipocytes for storage
Very low-density lipoproteins (VLDLs)	Carry newly synthesized triglycerides from liver to adipose tissues. Provide energy in the form of fatty acids to skeletal muscle and to adipocytes for storage
Intermediate-density lipoproteins (IDLs)	Intermediate between VLDL and LDL; rich in cholesterol
Low-density lipoproteins (LDLs)	Carry cholesterol from liver to the body cells
High-density lipoproteins (HDLs)	Collect cholesterol from body tissues and bring back to liver.

Low-density lipoproteins (LDL): LDL contains majority of the cholesterol and delivers it to cells including liver cells where cholesterol fraction is metabolized. LDL is obtained from IDL or small VLDL after most of the TG is removed. LDL-binding domain receptors bind to apo-100. LDL contains about 20% TG and ratio of TG to cholesterol esters is 1:4. Synthesis of LDL receptors by the cells is regulated by the cholesterol content of the cells. LDL has a long half-life of about 3 days. There are LDL receptors on all cells, which bind LDL and the cholesterol is utilized by peripheral cells for cell membranes and for hormone production.

Absence of receptors can be a genetic disorder leading to familial hypercholesterolemia in which coronary heart disease can occur at very early stage. Lack of these receptors or blockage of these receptors reduces the uptake of cholesterol from blood. Thus, more amount of cholesterol remains in circulation raising the cholesterol level in the blood and increases the risk of being deposited in plaques and the risk of cardiovascular disease. LDL is therefore said to be an atherogenic lipoprotein. LDL particles are small as well as large in size. All LDL particles are atherogenic. Thus, high level of LDL increases the risk of heart disease (atherosclerosis). Therefore, LDL has gained the reputation of "bad cholesterol". Small-dense LDL and oxidized LDL are said to increase risk of coronary heart disease.

The medication given to control high cholesterol is an inhibitor of 3-hydroxy-3-methyl-glutaryl-coenzyme A reductase, the key enzyme in synthesis of cholesterol. It actually stimulates LDL receptor production and helps in clearing LDL from plasma.

High-density lipoproteins (HDL): LPL primarily carries and clears cholesterol from circulation. Increase in LPL activity increases the HDL content in plasma. High HDL is an indicator of decreased risk of coronary atherosclerosis. Hence, HDL is considered "good cholesterol". HDL particles are synthesized and secreted in the liver and intestines. Intestinal HDL contains only apo A and liver HDL apo A, apo C and apo E as the protein content. Intestinal HDL also contain phospholipid bilayer where lecithin-cholesterol acyl transferase (LCAT), a hepatic enzyme converts cholesterol to cholesterol esters. HDL enters the circulation from where esterified cholesterol returns to the liver for catabolism and excretion.

"HDL content of plasma decreases when plasma triglyceride levels increase."

There are different HDL particles with different metabolic roles. HDL particles also differ in size. HDL1 is the largest, and the size progressively decreases as follows: HDL2b>HDL2a>HDL3a>HDL3b>HDL3c. HDL contains more amount of protein (45–50%) and less amount of cholesterol. Because of its higher protein content, its density is higher than that of the other lipoproteins. Increased HDL levels are associated with decreased risk of coronary heart disease and low HDL levels are associated with increased risk. HDL particles are synthesized in the liver and intestines. Nascent (newly formed) HDL picks up free cholesterol from peripheral tissues thus reducing its accumulation. The purpose of HDL is to enable secretion of cholesterol from cells, esterify cholesterol in plasma, transfer cholesterol to other proteins, and return cholesterol to the liver for catabolism and excretion. Because of the latter, this process has been also called "reverse cholesterol transport". Thus, HDL is considered to be antiatherogenic.

They also play a role in triacylglycerol transport. They facilitate activation of lipoprotein lipase, transfer of triacylglycerols between lipoprotein classes and in removal of chylomicron remnants and VLDL that contain high amounts of triglycerides. HDL also contains antioxidant enzymes. Thus, HDL prevents oxidation of LDL and reduces risk of heart disease. High-HDL level is associated with lower risk of heart disease; hence, it is called "good cholesterol".

Lipoproteins are used as biomarkers to indicate the risk of heart disease. Standard fasting blood tests for cholesterol and lipid profiles include values for total cholesterol, HDL cholesterol, and LDL cholesterol, as well as triglycerides. Family history and life style, including factors such as blood pressure, and whether or not one smokes, affect what would be considered ideal versus non-ideal values for fasting blood lipid profiles. The National Cholesterol Education Program (NCEP) Expert Panel on Adult Treatment III (2017) has recommended blood lipid profile, which is presented in Table 4.4.

Lipids in Liver

Liver plays a very important/central role in regulating lipid metabolism (which occurs mainly in the liver) through various pathways, including synthesis of new fatty acids, and transport and removal of fats (export) through lipoprotein and cholesterol synthesis, and utilizing fat for energy. Though mechanism of lipid transport is tightly regulated under hormonal and neuronal control, alteration in anyone of these pathways can eventually lead to fatty liver diseases. High-carbohydrate foods (rich in sucrose and fructose), high FFA levels in plasma, ethanol, and insulin hormone tend to increase the production of TG and VLDL. When fat continues to accumulate in the liver beyond 5%, the condition is called

Table 4.4: Blood lipids profile (mg/100 mL plasma).

Particulars	Low	Desirable/ optimal	Above optimal	Borderline high	High	Very high
Total cholesterol	–	<200	–	200–239	>=240	–
LDL cholesterol	–	<100	100–129	130–159	160–189	>=190
HDL cholesterol	<40	–	–	–	>=60	–
Triglycerides	–	<150	–	150–199	200–499	>=500

Source: National Cholesterol Education Program (NCEP) Expert Panel on Adult Treatment [Panel ATP III (2017)]

fatty liver; it is also called hepatic steatosis. It can be due to multiple dysfunctions.

These processes are closely regulated by:
- Mobilization of fat from fat depots into the liver (increased circulating pool of nonesterified fatty acids)
- Alteration in β-oxidation of fats
- Impaired utilization of fat and poor transport from the liver including altered VLDL secretion
- Hormonal causes
- Altered hepatic synthesis of fatty acids
- Toxic overload.

Mobilization of fat from fat depot into the liver: It occurs in case of carbohydrate deprivation and fat becomes the major source of calories. Nonesterified fatty acids are released by adipose tissue into plasma. This condition occurs in case of diabetes and starvation.

Alteration in β-oxidation of fatty acids: It is possible that there may be dysfunction of the mitochondria (normal mitochondrial function is needed for oxidation of fatty acids). Lipid oxidation and oxidative damage to mitochondrial DNA could further diminish mitochondrial function. Decreased activity of the mitochondrial respiratory chain has been reported in overweight/obese patients who have hepatic steatosis.

> **Research glimpse:** Prevalence of nonalcoholic fatty liver disease (NAFLD) is rising in parallel with the rising prevalence of obesity. Earlier, pathogenesis of NAFLD was attributed to faulty lifestyle choices involving diet and exercise. Calorie restriction and low macronutrient intakes (carbohydrate and fat) were found to be helpful in controlling both obesity and NAFLD. However, in recent years, micronutrients have been found to play significant roles in disease progression. Use of vitamin A (retinoic acid), niacin, vitamin B_{12}, vitamins D and E have been demonstrated to hold promise as therapeutic supports in the treatment of NAFLD. These vitamins were found to alter the lipid metabolism, e.g., retinoic acid-enhanced hepatic fat catabolism.
>
> *Jiawei L, Cordero P, Nguyen V et al. The role of vitamins in the pathogenesis of non-alcoholic fatty liver disease. Integr Med Insights. 2016;11:19–25.*

Impaired fat utilization and poor transport from liver, decreased plasma lipoprotein production: In choline deficiency, production of VLDL is compromised. Similarly, if insulin levels are high in the postprandial state, VLDL production is less. Choline can be synthesized in the body only when certain amino acids like serine, methionine, and threonine are available for synthesis of hepatic enzymes, and vitamins such as folic acid and vitamin B_{12} are involved in choline synthesis. Essential fatty acids (EFA), pyridoxine (vitamin B_6), inositol, vitamin E, and selenium are also needed and deficiencies of these nutrients can result in fatty liver. Hence, choline, methionine, and others are called lipotropic substances and prevent fatty liver. Dietary intake of large amount of cholesterol can also induce fatty liver as it competes with essential fatty acids and causes deficiency of EFA.

Hormonal causes: In diabetes mellitus, there is risk of mobilization of lipid from tissues to liver and may cause fatty liver.

Increased de novo lipogenesis can cause hypertriglyceridemia and/or hepatic steatosis.

Toxic overload: Liver produces bile (though it is stored in gallbladder). Bile not only helps to digest fats and but also aids in elimination of excess cholesterol, heavy metals, and toxins from the body through feces. Intake of heavy metals like mercury and cadmium has shown to increase the risk of developing fatty liver disease (nonalcoholic fatty liver disease or NAFLD). Alcohol intake is toxic.

LIPIDS AND ADIPOSE TISSUE

Adipose tissue is the main storage site of lipids. It takes up lipids from the plasma and also synthesizes triglycerides from carbohydrates. It continuously releases free fatty acids into the circulation by hydrolyzing triglycerides. Adipose tissue contains adipocytes that constitute about half of the cells in adipose tissue. Adipocytes have an important role in not only lipid storage but also in energy balance and overall body homeostasis. Hormones like epinephrine, glucagon, and adrenocorticotropic hormone stimulate lipolysis while insulin promotes lipogenesis (synthesis of lipids). Increased availability of glucose to tissues lowers FFA in plasma and suppresses lipolysis. Decreased availability of glucose encourages lipolysis.

Triacylglycerol or triglycerides are the principle form of stored energy in adipocytes (fat cells) of adipose tissues. This form of stored energy is far more than the energy available from protein, glycogen, and glucose. It accounts for approximately 83% of available energy. Fatty acids are completely oxidized to ATP and therefore yield 9 kcal/g because they are much more reduced compared to glycogen. Also they are much less anhydrous than are proteins and carbohydrates. Thus can be packed more closely in storage tissues.

Excessive deposition of fat (triglycerides) in the fat cells results in obesity. Obesity is due to several endocrine disorders as well as non-endocrine reasons such as overconsumption of food and positive energy balance (intake is in excess of expenditure). Endocrine disorders that are associated with obesity include hypothyroidism, hyperinsulinemia, diabetes, insulinoma, growth hormone deficiency, Cushing's syndrome, and polycystic ovarian syndrome (PCOS). The mechanisms for development of obesity depend on the actions of these hormones on energy balance, adipose tissue, and other tissues. Dysregulation of neuronal networks in the hypothalamus that are involved in homeostatic control of energy metabolism and feeding (appetite regulation, calorie intake, as well as regulation of glucose homeostasis, and energy expenditure) is also likely to be involved in obesity development.

DERIVED LIPIDS

Sterols

Sterols are derived lipids and are structurally very different from triglycerides or triacylglycerol. The only common property is that they are hydrophobic. They are derived from a precursor squalene and are made up of four fused carbon

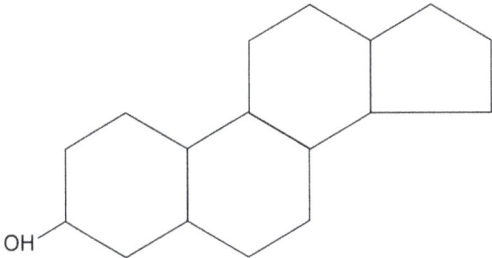

Fig. 4.4: Basic structure of sterols.

rings (Fig. 4.4). Sterols are an important group among steroids and there are different steroids.

Each steroid contains different chemical groups attached to these rings. Sterols are found in both plant and animal tissues. Two sterols, namely cholesterol and phytosterols, have received considerable attention because of their role in the body and significance to health and disease. Sterols have a number of roles; some are hormones and some are signaling molecules. Many biologically important substances are steroids derived from cholesterol in animals which include five families of hormones such as androgens, estrogens, progestins/progestogen, glucocorticoids (anti-stress hormones), and mineralocorticoids (ion uptake regulators). This is based on the receptor that the steroid binds to, and its physiological outcome. Steroids coordinate physiological and behavioral responses that are important for several biological functions that range from having anti-inflammatory effect to regulating events during pregnancy.

Table 4.5 gives the role of these steroid hormones in brief. Steroid hormones act both on peripheral target tissues and the central nervous system. The central nervous system also forms some biologically active steroids from cholesterol and these are called neurosteroids.

Squalene is a 30-carbon straight-chain hydrocarbon steroid precursor that is produced by both plant and animal cells. It is converted into phytosterols in plant cells and cholesterol in animal cells. Squalene possesses antioxidant property, which is effective in quenching singlet oxygen ROS.

Cholesterol

The term "Cholesterol" was derived from the ancient Greek word, "**Chole**"—meaning **bile** and "**Stereos**" stands for **solid**, and "**ol**" the suffix indicates **alcohol**. It is an organic waxy substance. It contains 27 carbons arranged in four fused rings and a hydrocarbon tail (Fig. 4.5), and each carbon molecule comes from acetyl-CoA. It is synthesized primarily in the liver and adrenal glands. It is an extremely hydrophobic molecule.

Cholesterol in the body is derived either from cholesterol synthesized within the body or obtained from dietary sources. It is synthesized from acetyl-CoA in most tissues (except RBC) but primarily in the liver and adrenal glands. It is an essential component of cell membranes. Therefore, it is transported from liver to peripheral tissues or it is converted to bile salts. Being amphipathic in nature, it finds its place in the bilayer of phospholipid within the cell membrane, which supports the role of cholesterol in regulating the permeability and fluidity of the cell membrane. Cholesterol is also the precursor molecule for the synthesis of steroid hormones

Table 4.5: Steroid hormones and their functions.

Steroid hormone	Functions
Gonadal steroids, e.g., androgens and estrogens, and progesterone	Influence sexual differentiation of the genitalia and of the brain, determine secondary sexual characteristics during development and sexual maturation, contribute to the maintenance of their functional state in adulthood and control or modulate sexual behavior.
Progesterone (progestogen)	Progestogens play a role in menstrual cycle Prepares uterus lining for implantation of ovum Essential for maintenance of pregnancy.
Androgens (male sex hormones), e.g., androstenedione and testosterone	Development and maintenance of secondary sexual characteristics in males Contribute to anabolic status of somatic tissues May play role in increasing bone thickness and periosteal bone formation Has a role in erythropoiesis Androstenedione and testosterone can serve as estrogen precursors.
Estrogens (female sex hormones) include estradiol and estrone	Development of female secondary sexual characteristics Regulation of menstrual cycle Important hormone in pregnancy Have a role in energy metabolism and homeostasis Help in maturation of sperm in males Increase bone formation and reduce bone resorption Help in protein synthesis (production of several proteins by liver, e.g., binding proteins, factors II, VII, IX, and X, and plasminogen that are involved in coagulation Increase platelet adhesiveness Increase HDL as well as TG Decrease LDL and promote fat deposition Cause retention of salt and water Reduce bowel motility Improve lung function and content of collagen and its quality in skin, increase skin thickness, and improve blood supply to skin Considered to play a significant role in women's mental health Protective against atherosclerosis.
Mineralocorticoids, especially aldosterone	Act on the distal tubules of the kidney to increase the reabsorption of Na^+ and the excretion of K^+ and H^+ (regulate excretion of salt and water by kidneys), which leads to an increase in blood volume and blood pressure.
Glucocorticoids, e.g., cortisol	Affect carbohydrate, protein, and lipid metabolism. Promote gluconeogenesis and the formation of glycogen, enhance the degradation of fat and protein, and inhibit the inflammatory response and response to stress.

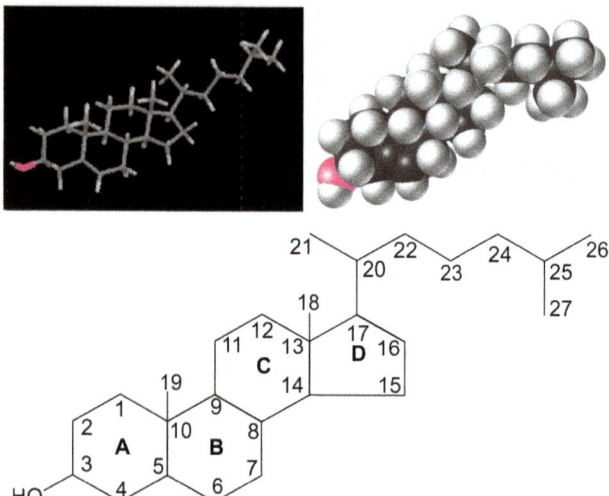

Fig. 4.5: Chemical structure of cholesterol.

such as testosterone, estrogen, progesterone, cortisol and aldosterone, bile acids, and vitamin D. About one-tenth of the cholesterol produced is used for synthesis of steroid hormones. It is also produced in central nervous system particularly during sleep. which supports learning and memory. If bile salts are not reabsorbed in the gastrointestinal tract, it is excreted in feces.

Liver can produce all the cholesterol needed by the body. Since it is naturally found in some animal foods, dietary intake of it is inevitable part of regular diet, liver adjusts its production in the body. Hence, there is no guideline for dietary intake of cholesterol.

Cholesterol is found in animal tissues only. Thus, animal foods contain varying amounts of cholesterol and organs like liver, egg yolk, and milk. Plant foods naturally do not contain cholesterol, rather they contain phytosterols (discussed separately). Thus, plant-foods or vegetable oils that are advertised as "no cholesterol" or "zero cholesterol" is just a marketing strategy and consumers should not get misled. It is important to note that the manufacturer has not done much but this is the gift of nature.

It aids in maintaining the correct fluidity of the cell membrane. However, it adjusts the amount synthesized according to the amount of cholesterol ingested through food. Despite having earned a bad name, it is important to remember that cholesterol is essential to life. Cholesterol is required by the body for a variety of functions:

Structural component of cell membrane: Cholesterol is a nonpolar molecule present in all cell membranes. In some cells, cholesterol may constitute as much as 25% of the plasma membrane. Cholesterol has a unique structure. Hence it is important not only for the maintenance of cell membrane structure, but also influences its thickness, fluidity, permeability (it reduces cell membrane permeability and increases the packing of phospholipids), and functions. It plays a role in membrane lipid composition, organization, and function. Thus, it is essential for determining which molecules can pass through the cell membrane into the cell. It prevents leakage of ions through membranes and diffusion of water-soluble molecules across the membrane. It stabilizes some proteins such as rhodopsin.

Component of bile acids: The liver synthesizes bile acids from cholesterol. Bile acids are transported to the gallbladder. Bile acids play an important role in digestion of fats. Hence, indirectly cholesterol is necessary for fat digestion. About one third to half of the cholesterol in bile (both free cholesterol and in bile acids) is reabsorbed in the large intestines. The remaining is excreted in the feces.

Component of brain lipids: Brain lipids include glycerophospholipids, sphingolipids, and cholesterol. Brain lipids contain significant amount of cholesterol (about 20% of the total body cholesterol). In fact, brain is the most cholesterol-rich organ. Brain cholesterol is mostly obtained through *de novo* synthesis, as the blood-brain barrier (BBB) does not prevent cholesterol uptake from circulation. Cholesterol is required for normal brain development, which includes synapse and dendrite formation, axonal guidance, and formation of the myelin sheath. Myelin layers wind around nerve cell axons. Myelin insulates the nerve cells and enhances the electric signal or increases the speed of signal through nerve axons. Most of the cholesterol in brain accumulates between the perinatal period and adolescence, when the neurons are surrounded by myelin.

Defects in cholesterol metabolism result in structural and functional central nervous system like Smith-Lemli-Opitz syndrome, Niemann–Pick type C (NPC) disease, Huntington's disease, and Alzheimer's disease. These metabolic defects affect different metabolic pathways such as cholesterol biosynthesis, lipid transport, and lipoprotein assembly, or receptors that mediate the cellular uptake of lipids, and signaling molecules. Lack of cholesterol may unfavorably affect the functioning of nervous system particularly memory and focus. Degradation of myelin sheath may result in blurred vision, difficulty in walking, etc.

Synthesis of hormones: It is the base material from which several important substances are synthesized in the body like sex hormones such as progesterone, testosterone, estrogen, progesterone, and some adrenal hormones like cortisol and aldosterone secreted by the adrenal glands. Hence, cholesterol is important for sexual development and metabolic control. It is the precursor of vitamin D.

Liver is capable of synthesizing enough cholesterol to fulfill the body's requirement (about 1 g of cholesterol in a 70 kg male). However, cholesterol is also consumed from dietary sources and the liver adjusts synthesis of cholesterol. Maximum 200 mg cholesterol per day from dietary sources is recommended for a healthy individual. The food sources of cholesterol and their content is shown in Table 4.6.

Phytosterols

Phytosterols are steroid compounds that occur naturally in plants and are structurally similar to cholesterol, except that they have an extra ethyl or methyl group or a double bond. Hence, they are considered as plant cholesterols or plant-derived lipid compounds. In plants, they contribute to the

Table 4.6: Cholesterol content of foods (mg/100 g).

Food item	Cholesterol	Food item	Cholesterol	Food item	Cholesterol
Butter	250	Ghee	300	Cow's milk	14
Cream	40	Cheese	100	Buffalo's milk	16
Egg whole	400	Chicken without skin	60	Skimmed milk	2
Egg yolk	1020	Chicken with skin	100	Condensed milk	40
Mutton	13	Prawns and shrimp	150	Brain	2000
Beef	70	Lean fish	45	Liver	300
Pork	90	Fatty fish	45	Kidney	370

Source: Ghafoorunissa, Krishnaswamy K. Diet and Heart Disease. Hyderabad: National Institute of Nutrition, Indian Council of Medical Research; 1995.

permeability and fluidity of cell membranes. The human body cannot synthesize phytosterols. Hence, phytosterols are obtained from plant foods only. The most common phytosterols in human diet are β-sitosterol, campesterol, and stigmasterol as shown in Figure 4.6.

Crude vegetable oils and their products are richest in phytosterols. Refining of vegetable oils strips away the phytosterol content. Seeds and nuts being rich in phytosterols contribute significantly to phytosterol intake in spite of their low consumption. Though cereal, legumes, fruits, vegetables, and berries are not rich sources, they contribute to phytosterol intake owing to the high amounts consumed in the diet. Phytosterol content in different foods is shown in Table 4.7.

Unrefined oils from plant sources are better sources than are refined oils. Nuts, seeds, and grains are also good sources. Commercially phytosterols are isolated from plant oils such as soybean, rapeseed, corn, and sunflower. When these oils are hydrogenated, the phytosterols are converted into phytostanols.

Thus, phytosterols are classified into two:
1. **Sterols:** Contain double bond in the sterol ring, so are unsaturated compounds.
2. **Stanols:** Lack a double bond in the sterol ring, so are saturated molecules.

Though both sterols and stanols are ubiquitously found in the plant world, they can effectively be used when taken with food. They are available commercially and are added/supplemented to processed foods like margarine and salad dressing. The phytosterols have been incorporated into mayonnaise, margarine, milk, vegetable oils, yoghurt, bread spreads, chocolate, cereals, snack bars, bread, hamburgers, orange juice, soups, green tea, and meat. In milk products and in nonspread vehicles, the method used for dispersion of fat, processing, use of emulsifiers, surfactants, and crystal habit modifiers will affect the extent to which plant sterols will be effective. These are also sold packaged with other functional ingredients such as fiber, with a spice mixture.

More than 40 plant sterols have been identified in the plant kingdom but campesterol, β-sitosterol, and stigmasterol are commonly found in human diet. The metabolism of both is different. Stanols may be present as free alcohols or they may be present as fatty acid esters, or bound to phenolic compounds or sugar moieties. Plant stanols are less abundant than are plant sterols. They are completely

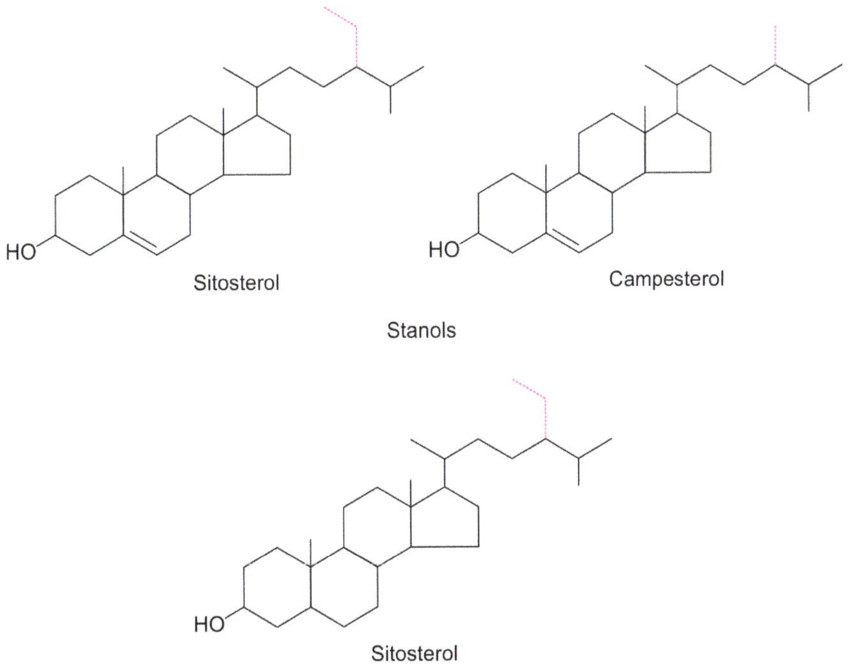

Sitosterol   Campesterol

Stanols

Sitosterol

Fig. 4.6: Chemical structures of different phytosterols.

Table 4.7: Phytosterol content in different food items.

Foods	Total phytosterols mg/100g	Foods	Total sterol mg/100g	Foods	Total sterol mg/100g
Wheat	60–78	Almond	142–208	Peanut	234
Rice	25	Cashew nuts	150–160	Coconut	112
Oats	58	Coconut	45–133	Cottonseed	355
Corn	178	Pistachios	110–297	Corn	1156
Sorghum	178	Sesame	711–714	Palm	88
Rice bran	1325	Walnuts	108–128	Palm kernel	109
Wheat germ	1970	Peanuts	116–221	Rapeseed	741
Wheat bran	200	Mustard	246	Soybean	288
Chickpea	35	Clove	256	Sunflower	366
Soybean	161	Coriander	46	Rice bran	1108
Beans	76	Cardamom	46	Sesame	686
Broad beans	124	Fenugreek	150	Safflower	348
Vegetables	2–20	Turmeric	100	Olive	210
Fruits	10–32				

Source: Ghafoorunissa. Impact of quality of dietary fat on serum cholesterol and coronary heart disease: focus on plant sterols and other non-glyceride components. Natl Med J India. 2009;22(3):126–32.

saturated, whereas phytosterols are not. Plant sterols are one kind of non-glyceride component (NGC).

Absorption: Efficiency of absorption is much lower than that of cholesterol but because they are structurally similar; phytosterols competitively inhibit intestinal absorption of cholesterol. While 60% of dietary cholesterol is absorbed, not more than 2–5% of plant sterols are absorbed. It is estimated that about 0.4–0.5% of plant sterols are absorbed, whereas 0.02–0.3% of stanols are absorbed. Therefore, blood levels of plant sterols are only a fraction of the level of cholesterol 0.1–0.14%, and in serum concentration of stanols is much lower than that of sterols. Phytosterols tend to displace cholesterol during micelle formation in the intestine thus reduce absorption of cholesterol. For absorption to occur as in the case of cholesterol, phytosterols have to be first incorporated into micelles. These sterol-containing micelles interact with the intestinal brush layer and the sterols are absorbed by enterocytes. Hence, metabolism of both is different. Phytosterols competitively inhibit intestinal absorption of cholesterol. Most of the assimilated phytosterols are directly eliminated via the liver and the biliary system and in healthy persons, and less than 1% of the ingested amount is retained in the body.

Health benefits: In 1951, sitosterol was first described as a therapeutic agent for hypercholesterolemia, because plant sterols inhibited (by competition) the absorption of dietary cholesterol and research focused a lot on the possibility of lowering serum cholesterol by using plant sterols. However, studies in the literature indicate that there are other health benefits such as anticancer, antiatherosclerosis, antioxidant, and anti-inflammatory activities. Phytosterols inhibit absorption of both dietary and biliary cholesterol. With doses of up to 2–3 g/day, clinical studies show that LDL cholesterol is lowered by about 15%. In order to achieve optimal effect, phytosterols should be consumed with a meal that contains cholesterol. Use of phytosterols is not recommended for pregnant or lactating women or for normocholesterolemic children under 5 years of age, as there is concern that consumption of plant sterols can affect adversely the absorption of fat-soluble vitamins. In infants, it has been shown that consumption upregulated cholesterol synthesis. Hence, exposure in utero or in early life may affect gene expression and physiology in later life.

Antiatherogenic effects: Phytosterols may be helpful in preventing atherosclerosis. However, there are some individuals, who are genetically prone to overabsorb sterols and stanols. In such persons, stanols accumulate and they are prone to develop atherosclerosis prematurely.

Anticancer activity: Plant sterols can suppress cancer cell growth in various types of cancers. Phytosterols may also have anti-inflammatory activity as well as decrease lipid peroxidation. Other possible benefits that are being researched are antifungal activity and reduction in body mass accumulation specifically accumulation of body fat.

> **Laboratory laurel:** This study was carried out with 409 men and 503 women aged 18–60 years to evaluate the association between dietary phytosterols and prevalence of obesity. Data was collected using validated food frequency questionnaire and measurement of body mass index (BMI), waist circumference (WC), blood glucose, serum lipid profiles. Results showed that high intake of dietary phytosterols is linked with lower prevalence of overweight/obesity and abdominal obesity in Chinese adults, as reflected in lower BMI, WC, blood pressure, serum TC and low density lipoprotein cholesterol (LDLc).
>
> *Li YC, Li CL, Li R, et al. Associations of dietary phytosterols with blood lipid profiles and prevalence of obesity in Chinese adults, a cross-sectional study. Lipids Health Dis. 2018;17(1):54.*

Besides phytosterols, plants also contain many other non-glyceride components (NGCs) like tocopherols, tocotrienols, carotenes, oryzanol, sesamin, and phenolic acids. These also show cholesterol-lowering effect and other health benefits. Hence, phytosterols have become one of popular ingredient for use in food supplement and food formulations such as snack bars, bakery products, dairy products, salad dressing, etc.

FATTY ACIDS

Fatty acids are the basic building blocks of most lipids. They are primarily composed of carbon, hydrogen, and oxygen. They naturally occur in plants and animal foods. They are also found in the body mainly as free fatty acids in plasma and in the form of triglycerides after esterification with glycerol. Most naturally occurring fatty acids contain even number of carbon atoms, although some are cyclic. Fatty acids play important roles in signal transduction, as energy stores in adipose tissue, as cellular sources of energy/fuel, as a part of important lipids, in modification of proteins, and as gene regulators.

Fatty acids are found both in foods and in the body. Chemically, they are carboxylic acids with hydrocarbon chains or aliphatic tail (the chain consists of carbon and hydrogen atoms). These hydrocarbon chains vary in length, i.e., in the number of carbon atoms, which range from 2 to 26. The hydrocarbon chain has carboxyl group (COOH) at one end (right) and methyl group (CH_3) on the other (left). The carboxyl group is a polar group having a high affinity to water (soluble in water) and the methyl group is a nonpolar group which is insoluble in water. The carboxyl group (COOH) of the fatty acid is bonded to the hydroxyl group (OH) of glycerol ester linkage (esterification). When fatty acids are esterified to the glycerol, they are referred as "glycerides or acylglycerols". The length and degree of saturation determine the physical properties of fatty acids such as melting point and fluidity. Fatty acids are also responsible for the hydrophobicity of lipids including triacylglycerols.

> In some triglycerides (TG), three molecules of the same fatty acid may be attached to glycerol, in others there may be two molecules of the same fatty acid and the third may be different or all three fatty acids may be different. When different fatty acids are present, it is known as a **"mixed triglyceride"**. The behavior of a TG is dependent on the kind of fatty acid attached to glycerol. The nutritional and health significance of triglycerides is primarily due to the fatty acids present. Most of fatty acids present in foods are generally straight-chain compounds, although branched-chain fatty acids are also found in nature.

Different fatty acids differ structurally and chemically. There are numerous permutations and combinations of fatty acids in the triglycerides present in foods. The fatty acid composition of foods, fats, and oils influences their food properties. It also has tremendous significance in nutrition, health, and disease. Fatty acids differ from each other in various ways:
1. Chain length
2. Degree of saturation
3. Position of double bond in the chain length
4. Configuration of double bond
5. Physical properties.

Chain Length

Each fatty acid differs in hydrocarbon chain length. Usually two hydrogen atoms are attached to a carbon atom. In plants and animals, usually the fatty acids have even number of carbon atoms. However, in nature fatty acids with odd number of carbon atoms occur. Depending upon the chain length, fatty acids can be divided into four categories:
1. Short-chain fatty acids (SCFAs)
2. Medium-chain fatty acids (MCFAs)
3. Long-chain fatty acids (LCFAs)
4. Very long-chain fatty acids (VLCFAs).

> H–H–H–H–H–H–H–H–H–H–H–H–H–H
> | | | | | | | | | | | | | |
> H–C–C–C–C–C–C–C–C–C–C–C–C–C–C
> | | | | | | | | | | | | | |
> H–H–H–H–H–H–H–H–H–H–H–H–H–OH
>
> The fatty acid shown above is saturated. An unsaturated fatty acid will have a double bond as shown below:
>
> H–H   H H–H–H–H–H
> | | | | | | | |
> H–C–C–C=C–C–C–C–C–C–C–C–OH
> | | | | | | | | | | |
> H–H–H–H   H–H–H–H–H–H–H

Degree of Saturation

Besides chain length, fatty acids are distinguished by other structural features, i.e., degree of saturation, viz presence of double bond, which determines the degree of saturation. They also differ in the location of the double bond and its conformation. The carbon in the carboxyl group is numbered as 1 (see box, the carboxyl group is on the extreme right) and all the carbon atoms following are numbered in increasing order.

In a hydrocarbon chain, when all the carbon atoms are saturated with hydrogen atoms, it is called "saturated", i.e., such fatty acids do not have any double bond. On the basis of degree of saturation, fatty acids can broadly be divided into two categories:
1. Saturated fatty acids
2. Unsaturated fatty acids.

Saturated fatty acids (SFA) signify that every carbon atom is attached to two hydrogen atoms with a single bond (C-C-C). Butyric, myristic, lauric, palmitic, and stearic acids are examples of SFAs.

Unsaturated fatty acids are the one in which hydrogen atoms are missing and the carbon atom is connected with adjacent carbon atom with a double bond (C=C). When a fatty acid has only one double bond, it is called monounsaturated fatty acid (MUFA), and when the hydrocarbon chain carries more than one double bond, the fatty acid is referred as polyunsaturated fatty acid (PUFA). The human body cannot produce some of the polyunsaturated fatty acids. Therefore, they have to be obtained from the diet and are called "essential fatty acids".

Position of Double Bond in the Chain Length

Double bonds occur at various positions in the hydrocarbon chain of the unsaturated fatty acid. The position of the double bond is counted from the left end [methyl group (CH_3)] of the chain which is generally denoted by the suffix omega (ω), or also noted as "**n**". Omega is the last letter of Greek alphabet. **Omega** is the last carbon of the hydrocarbon chain. The numerical position is given as per the placement of first double bond.

While writing or reading the fatty acid formula like oleic acid (18:1) (n-9), it denotes that the oleic acid contains 18 carbon atoms and one double bond which are placed on the 9th carbon atom from the methyl group on left side of the chain. By convention, a specific bond in the fatty acid chain is identified by the lower number of the 2 carbons that it joins. For example, in oleic acid, the double bond is present between carbons 9 and 10; hence it is called n-9.

First double bond	= Occurs at 9th position from methyl group - oleic acid - 18:1(n-9)
Second double bond	= Occurs at 6th position from methyl group - linoleic acid - C18:2 (n-6)
Third double bond	= Occurs at 3rd position from methyl group - linolenic acid - C18:3 (n-3)

Configuration of Double Bonds

Unsaturated fatty acids also differ in geometric placement of double bonds arranged between carbon-carbon atoms. It implies the arrangement of hydrogen across the carbon atom, which is referred to as configuration. On the basis of configuration, fatty acids are categorized as:
1. *Cis* form
2. *Trans*-fatty acid.

In the *cis* arrangement, the hydrogen atoms at the two carbons linked by the double bond are on the same side. In the *trans* arrangement, the hydrogen atoms in the chains are on opposite sides of the double bond. In a fatty acid with *cis* form, the acyl chain is bent at an angle. This gives some freedom of movement to the fatty acid. In *trans*-fatty acids, the acyl chain is more or less straight and is rigid. Fatty acids in vegetable oils are naturally in *cis* form, which can be converted into *trans* form during processing of fats and oils.

Trans and cis configuration
In *cis*-fatty acids, the hydrogen groups are on the same side of the double bond

$$\begin{array}{cc} H \quad H & H \\ | \quad\; | & | \\ C=C & C=C \\ & \quad\; | \\ & \quad H \\ (Cis) & (Trans) \end{array}$$

In *trans*, they are on opposite sides of the carbon chain

Physical Properties

Saturation level or the number of double bonds is crucial in fats. Presence or absence of double bonds in fat influences the physical properties of fat. Fatty acids differ in their physical properties such as odor, taste, consistency, and the melting point. These physical properties influence the choice of fat in different food preparations. For example, butter is chosen for its taste but it is not a good choice for cooking due to its low melting point. Some fats are solid and hard but provide good texture and are thus chosen for shortening in baked products. The fats having high melting point are selected for frying.

Each vegetable oil differs in its fatty acid composition. Mainly oils contain monounsaturated fatty acids (MUFAs), polyunsaturated fatty acids (PUFAs) and some saturated fatty acids (SFAs). Saturated fatty acids (SFAs) are present in high proportion in coconut oil, but the type of fatty acid is different from SFA in animal fats, i.e., lauric acid. In addition to different types of fatty acids, vegetable oils contain phytosterols, tocotrienols including tocopherol (vitamin E). Presence of these compounds and more of unsaturated fatty acids makes consumption of vegetable oils a good choice for protecting health and preventing chronic diseases, like coronary heart diseases (CHD).

Fats containing double bonds are usually liquid in nature, thus vegetable oils in general contain unsaturated fatty acids. Double bonds are vulnerable to oxidation in presence of heat, light, and oxygen. This makes unsaturated fatty acids more chemically reactive. In contrast, saturated fatty acids are least reactive chemically and have a longer shelf-life than unsaturated fatty acids. Therefore, more the number of double bonds, more is the risk of oxidation. On heating, double bonds easily come in contact with air (oxidation begins) and release some volatile flavor compounds, therefore fried foods are often tasty and flavorful. On prolonged exposure to heat and air, there is formation of peroxides and hydroperoxides, which cause off-odor and off-flavor in visible fats and oils, and is termed as **"rancidity"**. When fats and oils are oxidized, they are said to be rancid. The more unsaturated the fatty acids, the more susceptible the oil will be to oxidation. Therefore, linolenic acid is oxidized the fastest followed by linoleic and oleic acids. When lipid in cell membranes of the body cells is exposed to excess of free radicals, they can be oxidized and the process is termed as **lipid peroxidation** that occur in both food as well as in the body.

Lipid Peroxidation and Rancidity in Edible Fat

Rancidity of food fat can be viewed as a form of oxidative degradation in the dietary fat. In order to prevent rancidity, antioxidants like butylated hydroxyanisole quinine (BHA), butylated hydroxytoluene (BHT), and tertiary butyl hydroquinone (TBHQ) are added particularly in refined vegetable oils at industrial level. However, protective effect of these antioxidants is lost on too much heating of oils. Crude oils are relatively less susceptible to autoxidation due to presence of plant sterols. Therefore, oils and food containing refined oils should be stored in airtight containers and in a cool place. Oxidative stability is one of the most important quality parameters of edible vegetable oils as it determines their usefulness in technological processes besides determining the shelf-life/stability of the oil.

Effect of Lipid Peroxidation in the Body

Lipid peroxidation: It is the process of oxidative damage of lipids present in the cell membrane. Free radicals are generated during some metabolic processes and these oxidize lipids and other compounds upon coming into contact with lipid. Peroxidation causes cell damage and adversely affects cellular functions. It has been suggested that in due course of time, it can lead to aging, several inflammatory conditions, autoimmune diseases, and many other chronic degenerative diseases.

The human body has natural defense mechanisms to counteract lipid peroxidation and its aftereffects, in the form of vitamins, minerals, and enzymes. These act as antioxidants, which prevent oxidative damage and thus protect cells and their functions. Vitamins E and C, selenium, glutathione, and enzymes like superoxide dismutase (SOD), peroxidases, and catalases tend to inhibit the excessive generation of free radicals and thus lipid peroxidation. Vitamins are obtained from the diet and the enzymes are synthesized in the body. Antioxidants other than these vitamins also support in preventing the lipid peroxidation and cellular damage.

Nomenclature of Fatty Acids

Generally, the chemical name (nomenclature) recommended by the International Union of Pure and Applied Chemistry (IUPAC-IUB Commission on Nomenclature) is used for fatty acids. In the IUPAC system, fatty acids are named based on:
a. The number of carbon atoms
b. The number of double bonds
c. Position of unsaturated fatty acids relative to the carboxyl group.

The configuration of double bonds, the location of branched chains, and other structural features are also identified. The carbon atom of the carboxyl group is considered to be first and the subsequent carbons in the fatty acid chain are numbered from the carboxylic carbon.

Conventionally, a specific bond in the fatty acid chain is identified by the lower number of the two carbons that it joins. The double bonds are labeled with Z or E where appropriate, but are very often replaced by the terms *cis* and *trans*, respectively. For example, the systematic name of linoleic acid (LA) is "*cis*-9, *cis*-12-octadecadienoic acid", because the first double bond is between carbons 9 and 10, and the second double bond is between carbons 12 and 13.

The **IUPAC** (International Union of Pure and Applied Chemistry) nomenclature is precise and technically clear but the names are long. Therefore, in scientific articles, scientists use "trivial" names and shorthand notations. All the notations use the form **C:D,** where C stands for the number of carbon atoms and D represents the number of double bonds in the carbon chain.

Besides this, biochemists and nutritionists use the "n minus" system of notation for naturally occurring cis unsaturated fatty acids, wherein "n minus" indicates the position of the double bond of the fatty acid closest to the methyl end of the molecule, e.g., n-9, n-6, and n-3, etc. The "n minus" system is also referred to as the omega system. Omega may be signified by the symbol "ω"**or small letter w.** For example, oleic acid has one double bond located at the 6th carbon from the methyl end; hence it is abbreviated as 18:1 n-9. Linoleic acid has two double bonds, the first located at carbon 6 (6 carbons away from the methyl end), therefore it is abbreviated as 18:2 n-6.

Another widely used system is the **delta (Δ) system**. In this system, the classification is based on the number

Table 4.8: Nomenclature systems of fatty acids.

System used for nomenclature	Description with example
IUPAC (International Union of Pure and Applied Chemistry)	Use trivial names-—lauric acid Systematic name—dodecanoic acid C: D (Number of carbon atoms: Double bonds)—**C12:0**
"n minus" system or omega system	Oleic acid has one double bond located at the 6th carbon from the methyl end written as **18:1 n-9.** Linoleic acid has two double bonds, the first located at carbon 6 away from the methyl end as **18:2n-6**
Delta (Δ) system	Specifies the position of all the double bonds as well as their *cis/trans* configuration. Linoleic acid is *cis*-Δ 9, *cis*-Δ 12-18: 2. For convenience—*cis*, *cis*-Δ 9, and Δ 12-18: 2

of carbon atoms interposed between the carboxyl carbon and the nearest double bonds to the carboxylic group. This system specifies the position of all the double bonds as well as their *cis/trans* configuration. It is applicable to a large number of fatty acids, except fatty acids with branched chains and unusual structural features. According to the delta system, the shorthand notation for linoleic acid is *cis*-Δ 9, *cis*-Δ 12-18: 2. For convenience, it could be expressed as *cis*, *cis* Δ 9, and Δ 12-18:2 different systems has been explained in Table 4.8.

Classification of Fatty Acids

Fatty acids are categorized into three broad groups based on chemical classification as shown in Figure 4.7.

Saturated Fatty Acids (SFAs)

Saturated fatty acids (SFAs) are largely present in dietary fats. They are chemically less reactive and hence they are more stable. Fats containing SFAs have a long shelf-life and shorter chain length. However, butter is an exception having shorter shelf-life due to its high moisture content. Different dietary sources of SFA have varying chain lengths of fatty acids (number of carbons). Increase in chain length increases the melting point. Long-chain fatty acids are solid at normal room temperature and also high melting points. Hence fats and oils having long-chain fatty acids (>16-carbon length) and high melting points are used in cooking at high temperature and shorter-chain length SFA like butter (having 4-carbon length) has low melting point and are not used regular cooking.

Saturated fatty acids (SFAs) are present in saturated fats. They do not contain any double bond since the hydrocarbon chain is fully saturated with hydrogen atoms. They are usually derived from animal fats. Sources such as milk, meat, and poultry contain invisible form of saturated fats and curd, cream, cheese, butter, and ghee, lard, tallow, and margarines are visible form of saturated fats. Some of the vegetable oils like palm kernel oil, coconut oil also contain SFAs. Palm oil and palm kernel oil are both saturated but the percentage of SFAs in palm oil is about 49% most of it being palmitic acid, whereas palm kernel oil contains 82% saturated fat, most of

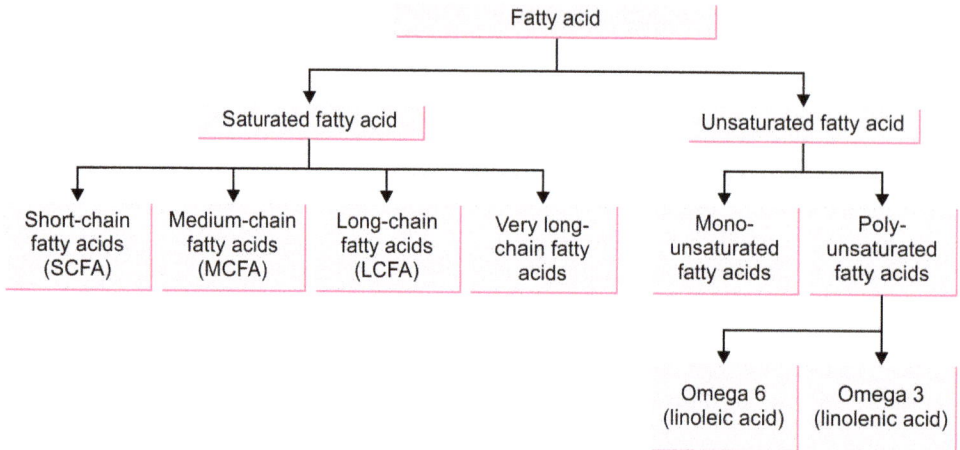

Fig. 4.7: Classification of fatty acids.

it being the SFAs with 12–14 carbons. In animals, plants and microorganisms, the most common saturated fatty acid is palmitic acid containing 16 carbons. Stearic acid containing 18 carbons is a major fatty acid present in animal tissues but is found in only minor amounts in plant food sources. Another saturated fatty acid is myristic acid with 4 carbons. It is present in a wide variety of foods. Short-chain saturated fatty acids with 8–10 carbons, e.g., caprylic acid with 8 carbons and capric acid with 10 are less common in food supply but are present in milk and coconut triglycerides. Most vegetable oils do not contain saturated fatty acids and hence they are liquid in nature. However, there are exceptions as some plant sources like palm kernel oil, coconut oil and cocoa also contain some SFAs and they are solid or semisolid at room temperature. Saturated fats are responsible for synthesis of hormones, brain compounds and cholesterol in the body. They are found in various chain lengths. Different types of saturated fatty acids along with their systematic names, food sources, and melting points are shown in Table 4.9.

Length of the fatty acid chain determines the biological functions of the fatty acids. Butter contains butyric acid that has a short chain length containing 4 carbons but it is a desirable saturated fat. Similarly, coconut oil contains lauric acid, which is made up of 12 carbon atoms and have medium chain length. On the contrary, fats containing myristic acid and palmitic acid have medium-chain and long-chain fatty acids but these are harmful for cardiac health and disturb the LDL/HDL ratio in the blood. It was a notion that all saturated fats must not be consumed, to protect the heart. However, not all saturated fatty acids are harmful to health. It is the myristic and palmitic acids that increase the risk for high levels in blood cholesterol, LDL, triglycerides, and also threat for low HDL, thrombosis, and CVDs. Saturated fatty acids have also been linked to insulin resistance.

Few saturated fatty acids such as behenic acid (C 22) and lignoceric acid (C 24), are not found suitable for human consumption as these are poorly absorbed in the body. Behenic acid is used in skin and hair care products.

Table 4.9: Saturated fatty acids—chain length, melting points and food sources.

Fatty acid	Carbon atom/ chain length	Systemic names	Melting point °C	Food sources
Short chain fatty acids (SCFA)				
Butyric acid	C-4:0	Butanoic acid	-7.9	Dairy fat
Caproic acid	C-6:0	Hexanoic acid	-3.9	Dairy fat
Caprylic acid	C-8:0	Octanoic acid	16.3	Butter, coconut oil, and palm kernel oil
Medium chain fatty acids (MUFA)				
Capric acid	C-10:0	Decanoic acid	31.3	Butter, coconut and palm kernel oils
Lauric acid	C-12:0	Dodecanoic acid	44.0	Coconut oil and palm kernel oil
Myristic acid	C-14:0	Tetradecanoic acid	54.4	Butter, dairy fat, coconut oil, and palm kernel oil
Long chain fatty acids (LCFA)				
Palmitic acid	C16:0	Hexadecanoic acid	62.9	Vegetable oils and animal fats
Stearic acid	C18:0	Octadecanoic acid	69.6	Vegetable oils and animal fats
Arachidic acid	C20:0	Eicosanoic acid	75.4	Peanut oil
Very long chain fatty acids (VLCFA)				
Behenic	C 22:0	Docosanoic acid	80.0	Egg and animal organs
Lignoceric	C 24:0	Tetracosanoic acid	84.2	Minor constituent in some plant fats including peanut oil

"In Ayurveda, consumption of butter and *desi ghee* (clarified ghee) though saturated has been given high place as it improves the vigor and vitality of the body, enhances brain power, and promotes longevity. It does so by increasing the digestive fire, i.e., *Agni* and improving the digestion and utilization of nutrients. It lubricates the connective tissues and making the body more supple and flexible. It makes the skin smooth and shiny. It also pacifies *Vata* and *Pitta, two among the tridoshas* (organizing principles that govern the physiology)." Desi ghee contains different types of fatty acids including saturated and unsaturated fatty acids and other nutrients in some amounts.

> **Reaserch glimpse:** Ghee (clarified butter) has been used as a therapeutic agent in *Ayurveda* for thousands of years. In India, it is a preferred cooking medium in some areas. Though has been implicated in increasing risk of cardiac diseases due to its content of saturated fatty acids and cholesterol, but research showed the pathogenesis of CAD is not only due to ghee intake but is also linked with the genetic predisposition to diseases. Present study revealed that 10% dietary ghee fed for 4 weeks did not have any significant effect on levels of serum total cholesterol, but did increase triglyceride levels in Fischer inbred rats. Similar results were seen with heated (oxidized) ghee, which contains cholesterol oxidation products. A preliminary clinical study showed that high doses of medicated ghee decreased serum cholesterol, triglycerides, phospholipids, and cholesterol esters in psoriasis patients. A study on a rural population in India revealed a significantly lower prevalence of coronary heart disease in men who consumed higher amounts of ghee. Research on Maharishi Amrit Kalash-4 (MAK-4), an Ayurvedic herbal mixture containing ghee, showed no effect on levels of serum cholesterol, high-density lipoprotein (HDL), LDL, or triglycerides in hyperlipidemic patients who ingested MAK-4 for 18 weeks. MAK-4 inhibited the oxidation of LDL in these patients. The article indicated that rise of CAD in Asian Indians may be attributed to the increased consumption of vanaspati (hydrogenated fat containing 40% *trans*-fatty acids), psychosocial stress, insulin resistance, and altered dietary patterns.
>
> Sharma H, Zhang X, Diwedi C. **The effect of ghee (clarified butter) on serum lipid levels and microsomal lipid peroxidation.** Ayu. 2010;31(2):134–40.

Fatty acids like caproic, caprylic, and capric acids decrease LDL secretion; C8 and C10 have hypocholesterolemic effect. C12 may have an antiviral effect, and C14 is needed for acylation of some proteins and the very long-chain fatty acids are involved in myelination in the nervous system. Saturated fatty acids are less susceptible to lipid peroxidation. Since many fats and fat-containing foods also contain many other bioactive substances, which may provide protection from the heart diseases; it is not always advisable to completely omit or cut down all kinds of saturated fats in the diet. Foods like milk, egg, and meat contain SFA but are also rich in other nutrients and bioactive compounds. SFA from butter and coconut oil provide health benefits and are useful in case of fat malabsorption. It is important to choose foods wisely. It is suggested that 7–10% of the total calories should come from the saturated fats.

Hydrogenation is an industrial food process that can make the vegetable oils into solid fat with a consistency similar to saturated fats. Hydrogenated fats such as vanaspati, mayonnaise contain significant amount of *trans*-fat, which is harmful to health. However, all governments including Government of India have restricted the amount of *trans*-fatty acids that should be present in edible fats and oils. It is advisable to restrict use of vanaspati and saturated fat-containing foods and a variety of processed foods owing to the presence of *trans*-fats. Saturated fats are used in food processing because they impart desired texture to the final food product and prolong shelf-life. The taste, flavor, and color of these foods are also attractive. These characteristics often tend to make the food attractive and energy dense resulting in overconsumption of such foods increasing the risk of obesity. Saturated fats are of different nature depending upon the chain length. Each has different physiological function.

Physiological Functions of Different Chain Length Fatty Acids

Short-chain Fatty Acids (SCFAs)

SCFAs consist of only 3–6 carbon atoms. They are formic acid (C1), acetic acid (C2), propionic acid (C3), butyric acid (C4), isobutyric acid (C4), valeric acid (C5), isovaleric acid (C5) and caproic acid (C6). Acetate, propionate, and butyrate are the common SCFAs (represent 90–95% of the SCFAs) that are produced in the gastrointestinal tract by the fermentation of mostly nondigestible carbohydrate or fiber (gut bacteria species) and proteins (to a very small extent) by the colonic microflora in large intestine. Inulin fructo-oligosaccharides (FOS), resistant starch, pectin, arabinoxylan and guar gum are good sources which tend to produce SCFA in the colon. The amount of SCFA produced depends on the diet and microorganisms present in the gut. There is inter-individual variation in the amount of SCFAs produced. The main SCFA produced by bacterial fermentation are acetate, propionate and butyrate in approximate molar ratio of 60:20:20. Alteration in this ratio determines the effect of SCFA on health. Butyric acid is present in butter and some types of cheeses. Generally, the butyric acid is bound to glycerol in the butter, however, when the butter becomes rancid, the butyric acid is in the free form. These fatty acids do not require bile for their digestion since fatty acids with chain length of 12 carbons or less are transferred directly into portal blood and taken to the liver. They are useful for persons with fat malabsorption, infants, and children. SCFAs have several effects on human health:

- Source of energy for colonocytes (epithelial cells in the colon)
- Modulate or reduce pH in the colon. Thus SCFA influence the type of microorganisms (inhibit some pathogenic organisms) that are present in the colon, and decrease solubility of bile acids. Due to the lower pH, solubility of minerals increases and absorption of ammonia decreases.
- May be important in controlling intestinal inflammation
- May have a role in appetite regulation and energy homeostasis
- Regulate cell proliferation through growth factors or gastrointestinal peptides or modulating intestinal blood flow
- Influence genes involved in regulation of cell proliferation and cell cycle

- May influence gastrointestinal motility
- Inhibits synthesis of cholesterol, thus have a lipid lowering affect.

Butyric acid is a 4-carbon fatty acid, soluble in water, a source of energy for colonic epithelial cells. It is involved in the processes that regulate cellular proliferation and differentiation as well as apoptosis and affects gene expression. Butyrate has anti-inflammatory effects in the gut. Some studies indicate that it may have a preventive role in colon cancer. It has been shown to regulate apoptosis, production of cytokines, cell proliferation, cell differentiation, and cell maturation, and control the intestinal barrier effect. Butyric acid is also responsible for the typical odor in cheese and the disagreeable odor of rancid butter, which results from hydrolysis of the triglyceride.

Medium-chain Fatty Acids (MCFAs)

Medium-chain fatty acids contain 6–13 carbon atoms, e.g., caproic (C6), caprylic (C8), capric (C10), and lauric (C12) acids. Capric acid is present in milk fat and lauric acid is a constituent of coconut and palm kernel oils. MCFAs are absorbed more efficiently than are long-chain fatty acids. They are absorbed directly into portal vein and transported directly to the liver, where they are readily oxidized and used to produce energy.

Triglycerides containing primarily medium-chain fatty acids are also known as medium-chain triglycerides or MCT. They are used in infant formulas, clinical and parenteral nutrition. Studies also indicate that MCT can increase energy expenditure, give faster satiety when they replace fats containing long-chain fatty acids and therefore, may be useful for weight management and other health conditions then connect with such as obstructive jaundice, biliary cirrhosis, pancreatitis, cystic fibrosis, celiac disease, Crohn's disease, *Candida* colonization (growth of yeast) and malabsorption in neonates. MCTs may also improve absorption of calcium, magnesium, and amino acids. MCT is also useful during convalescent period after surgery. It tends to reduce the lactate buildup in tissues and thus improves athletic performance and arrests stunted growth.

Long-chain Fatty Acids (LCFAs)

The number of carbon atoms varies between 14 and 20, e.g., palmitic and stearic acids. Palmitic acid occurs very widely and found in almost all fats such as palm oil, lard, and beef tallow. Stearic acid is a major component in tallow obtained from ruminant animals, and is also found in some vegetable fats like cocoa butter, olive oil and avocado. Animal fats and those like palm oil tend to be solid at room temperature. Fats containing LCFAs also have higher smoke point as well as high melting point as shown in Table 4.9. Food products made with these are less susceptible to rancidity and spoilage. LCFAs are components of phospholipids present in cell membrane and increase membrane rigidity. They also play a role in normal growth and development. Some long-chain fatty acids are important constituents of myelin sheath. Each fatty acid has specific functions, e.g., myristic acid may be important for protein acylation and gene regulation. Myristic acid is converted to palmitic acid; hence, it does not accumulate in the body whereas palmitic acid does. Myristic acid also plays an essential role in activation of cellular functions. It is also important for elongation of C18:3 n-3 and C18:2 n-6 into longer chain compounds and activation of sphingolipid synthesis.

Some of these individual fatty acids have been reported to increase risk for cardiovascular diseases (CVD). Stearic acid does not influence cholesterol levels much, whereas lauric, myristic and palmitic acid are atherogenic when they are in excess because they increase LDL cholesterol and the risk of CVD. Therefore, consumption of saturated fat, especially myristic and palmitic acids should be minimized. Long-chain fatty acids are digested and absorbed by a process different from medium chain fatty acids. These fatty acids are digested with the aid of bile salts and after absorption they are incorporated into chylomicrons and reach circulation via lymph.

Very Long-chain Fatty Acids (VLCFA)

These contain 21 or more carbon atoms such as behenic (22: 0) and lignoceric (24:0) acids. These fatty acids are present in very small amounts (<0.1%) in most dietary fat, although peanut oil contains a higher amount. Some of these individual fatty acids have been reported to increase risk for cardiovascular diseases (CVD).

Unsaturated Fatty Acids

Unsaturated fatty acids are divided into two subclasses: (1) Monounsaturated fatty acid (MUFA) and (2) Polyunsaturated fatty acids (PUFA).

They are usually present in a wide variety of vegetable oils and some marine sources like fish. Unsaturated fatty acids have beneficial effects on health. At the same time, they are highly susceptible to oxidation (lipid oxidation) as the double bonds can easily react with oxygen. This reaction produces free radicals that cause damage when produced in excess. Different types of MUFA and PUFA with their chain length are listed in Table 4.10.

Monounsaturated fatty acids (MUFAs): MUFAs have only one unsaturated bond. The presence of a double bond lowers the melting point of the oil and hence oils rich in MUFA are liquid at room temperature. The most commonly occurring MUFA is oleic acid (C18:1 n-9) and palmitoleic acid (C16:1, n-7). There are other MUFAs that are much less abundant. Oleic acid is present in large amount in olive oil (70–76%), mustard oil (60–65 %), canola oil (60%), and groundnut oil (40–55%). Another important MUFA is erucic acid present in mustard oil and rapeseed oil. However erucic acid is considered harmful in high doses. Some foods like avocado, nuts, seeds, and grains are also rich in MUFA. Besides obtaining MUFA from the diet, MUFA can also be synthesized by elongase and desaturase enzymes from SFAs by de novo lipogenesis.

Table 4.10: Unsaturated fatty acids—chain length, double bonds, melting points, and food sources.

Fatty acid	Carbon atom/ chain length	Melting point °C	Food sources
Monounsaturated (MUFA)			
Palmitoleic acid	C16:1	0.5	Olive oil, fish oil, and beef fat
Oleic acid	C18:1	13.4	Olive oil and canola oil
Erucic acid	C22:1	34.7	Mustard and rapeseed oil
Polyunsaturated (PUFA)			
Linoleic acid	C18:2(n-6)	-5.0	Vegetable oils
Alpha-linolenic acid	C18:3(n-3)	-11.0	Soybean oil
Arachidonic acid	C20:4(n-6)	-49.5	Lard, meat, and liver
Eicosapentaenoic acid (EPA)	C20:5 (n-3)	-54	Fish oil and shell fish
Docosahexaenoic acid (DHA)	C22:6(n-3)	-78	Fish oil and shell fish

When MUFA is substituted for SFA, it results in reduction of LDL cholesterol levels and triglycerides with slight increase in HDL cholesterol. Also replacing carbohydrates with MUFA increases HDL cholesterol concentrations and may possibly increase insulin sensitivity. Since MUFAs have a double bond, they are susceptible to oxidation but to a lesser extent than PUFAs. Substitution of a high-carbohydrate diet with a high-MUFA diet has been shown to have a beneficial effect on glycemic control, glycosylated hemoglobin levels, serum lipids, and systolic blood pressure in type 2 diabetics. Also when high MUFA was compared with high PUFA, there was a beneficial effect on fasting plasma glucose levels.

Polyunsaturated fatty acids (PUFAs): PUFAs are a heterogeneous group, divided into two subclasses: (1) Long-chain polyunsaturated fatty acids and (2) Very long-chain polyunsaturated fatty acids.

Among these, the n-3 and n-6 families have the most nutritional and health significance. They serve as precursors for important metabolic products that have structural and functional roles in biological systems. PUFAs are integral part of cell membranes and in myelin sheath of the brain cells. They participate in several important biological functions like cell signaling, gene expression, cell differentiation, and cell survival.

In all n-6/omega 6 fatty acids, the double bond is present between the 6th and 7th carbon atom from the methyl end, whereas in n-3/omega-3 fatty acids, the double bond is present between the 3rd and 4th carbon atoms. Different types of PUFA are important in health and disease. Some of them cannot be synthesized by the body and must be supplied by the diet; hence they are designated as **Essential Fatty Acids.**

> **Research glimpse:** The effect of major dietary macronutrients on glucose-insulin homeostasis is controversial. The authors assessed the influence of saturated fat (SFA), monounsaturated fat (MUFA),
>
> *Contd...*
>
> polyunsaturated fat (PUFA), on key metrics of glucose-insulin homeostasis. They searched several databases and identified published randomized clinical trials related to the effects of macronutrient intake on blood glucose, insulin, HbA1c, insulin sensitivity, and insulin secretion in adults above 18 years of age. Their analysis indicated that replacement of carbohydrate with PUFA, can significantly lower glycosylated hemoglobin (HbA1c), and fasting insulin. Replacing SFA with PUFA significantly lowered glucose, HbA1c, C-peptide, and homeostatic model assessment (HOMA). Acute insulin response in ten trials showed that PUFA significantly improved insulin secretion capacity when the PUFA replaced either carbohydrate, SFA, or MUFA. However, there was no effect of any macronutrient replacements when the 2-hour post-challenge glucose or insulin sensitivity was done. The authors concluded from this meta-analysis of randomized controlled feeding trials that dietary macronutrients have diverse effects on glucose-insulin homeostasis, and when compared with carbohydrate, SFA, or MUFA, PUFA showed favorable effects more consistently in terms of improved glycemia, insulin resistance, and insulin secretion capacity.
>
> *Imamura F, Micha R, Wu JHY, et al. Effects of saturated fat, polyunsaturated fat, monounsaturated fat, and carbohydrate on glucose-insulin homeostasis: A Systematic Review and Meta-analysis of Randomised Controlled Feeding Trials. PLoS Med. 2016;13(7):e1002087.*

The two parent fatty acids, alpha-linolenic acid (ALA) (18.3) and linoleic acid (LA) (18.2), are different, although both are acted upon by the same enzymes that are involved in the two processes of desaturation for inserting more double bonds and elongation for increasing the chain length. The desaturation and elongation process consists of a series of steps carried out by desaturases and elongases. From these two fatty acids (LA and ALA), other EFA having 20–22 carbon atoms are formed. LA is converted into gamma-linolenic acid (GLA) and AA, whereas ALA is converted into EPA and DHA. Since the same set of enzymes metabolize the n-6 and n-3 series of fatty acids, there is competition for these enzymes. The compounds obtained from n-6 are considered proinflammatory compounds and those obtained from n-3 are considered anti-inflammatory. Since many of the non-communicable and degenerative diseases are linked to inflammation, it is considered advisable to have an appropriate ratio of the n-6 to n-3 fatty acids, as both sets of fatty acids are essential for the body. In healthy young men, about 8% of dietary ALA is converted into EPA and up to a maximum of approximately 4% is converted into DHA. Women have higher capacity to generate DHA than men as it has been shown that about one-fifth of dietary ALA is converted to EPA and 9% to DHA. The difference between women and men may be due to the estrogen in women. There is also genetic variability in ability to synthesize the long-chain polyunsaturated fatty acids, making some individuals more efficient converters of the fatty acid precursors/parent molecules, namely linoleic acid and alpha-linoleic acid.

> Desaturation is carried out by two key enzymes—delta-6 desaturase (FADS2) and delta-5 desaturase (FADS1). Polymorphisms have been observed in the *FADS* genes and single nucleotide polymorphisms (SNPs) in these genes that encode these two key enzymes and influence the levels of omega-6 and omega-3 fatty acids in blood.

Contd...

Contd...

> Increased activity of both FADS1 and FADS2 is associated with haplotype D and more efficient conversion of linoleic acid and alpha-linolenic acid to the long-chain PUFAs, i.e., eicosapentaenoic acid, docosahexaenoic acid, arachidonic acid and gamma-linolenic acid. In some individuals therefore, desaturation of the parent molecules/precursors is likely to be slower and their blood lipid patterns will have higher amounts of 18:2 n-6 and 18:3 n-3 but lower levels of arachidonic acid, eicosapentaenoic acid and docosahexaenoic acid. Such polymorphisms may explain about 30% of the variability among the levels of n-6 and n-3 fatty acids in blood of different persons.

Factors that can inhibit desaturase enzyme activity, limiting the conversion of LA and ALA to the long-chain PUFA, include age, metabolic syndrome, diabetes, and deficiency of protein and minerals such as iron, zinc, copper, magnesium, and vitamins B3, B12, and B6. Dietary cholesterol and high-fat diets decrease the activity of the desaturating enzymes. Hence, it is necessary to not exceed recommended dietary intakes of both cholesterol and total fat.

ESSENTIAL FATTY ACIDS

Burr and Burr (1929) found that a fat-free diet cannot support optimal health. Cell membranes, myelin sheath, and adipose tissues are predominantly composed of different types of fatty acids. Those fatty acids that cannot be synthesized in the body and necessarily need to be obtained from the diet are called essential fatty acids (EFAs). These fatty acids have to be obtained from the diet because the human body does not have the necessary enzymes to insert a *cis* double bond either at the n-6 or n-3 position in the fatty acids. However, human body has the ability to synthesize saturated fatty acids and some monounsaturated fatty acids from carbon groups from carbohydrates or proteins.

Some of the important EFAs, which are crucial in health and disease are:
1. Alpha-linolenic acid (ALA) (18:2 n-3)
2. Gamma-linolenic acid (GLA) (18:3 n-6)
3. Arachidonic acid (AA) (20:4 n-6)
4. Eicosapentaenoic acid (EPA) (20:5 n-3)
5. Docosahexaenoic acid (DHA) (22:6 n-3).

EFAs are essential for normal growth and development of the body. They play structural, regulatory, and many other biological roles in physiological as well as pathological conditions. Important functions of EFAs are as follows:
- Structural component of cell membranes and myelin sheath. They are incorporated into the phospholipids of cell membranes and influence membrane properties such as fluidity, flexibility, permeability, as well as the activity of membrane-bound enzymes.
- Help in conversion of food energy to metabolic energy.
- Essential for visual development, especially the retina during pregnancy and infancy.
- Essential for brain development during pregnancy and infancy and other mental functions throughout life.
- Accelerate many enzymatic reactions.
- Play a role in immunity, having bactericidal effect on certain pathogens, and being part of the T cells and B cells of the immune system.
- Reduce premenstrual syndrome, aging process, and infections.
- Modulate inflammation, blood coagulation, and blood vessel constriction.
- Prevent pathogenesis of degenerative diseases.
- Provide protection to skin by regulating sebum production.
- Regulate gene expression.
- They are precursors for bioactive lipids called specialized pro-resolving mediators (SPMs) which mediate the resolution phase of inflammation. These compounds are S-resolvins, S-protectins, and S-maresins, with those derived from n-3 PUFA having a protective role. Similarly is oprostanes that are involved inflammation are also produced from PUFA.

> **Role of PUFA in regulating gene expression**
> n-3 and n-6 fatty acids modulate expression of several genes including those that have a role in fatty acid metabolism and inflammation. They interact with specific transcription factors, e.g., peroxisome-proliferator-activated receptors (PPARs). They can also function like hormones and bind to receptors thus, modulating gene transcription. Dietary PUFA can suppress SREBP-1 (a transcription factor that controls fatty acid synthesis), by decreasing the expression of the enzymes involved.

Omega-6 (n-6) Family

Linoleic acid (18:2): Linoleic acid or LA (18:2 n-6) is said to be the parent fatty acid of the n-6 family/series, because it can be elongated further to give rise to a series of fatty acids including gamma (γ)-linolenic acid (18:3 n-6), arachidonic acid (20:4n-6), and eicosanoids. It is a substrate from which many bioactive compounds are formed. It is a structural component in ceramides of the water barrier of the skin. Linoleic acid (n-6) accounts for 12–15% of the fatty acids in adipose tissues. Linoleic acid is a precursor of arachidonic acid, which itself is a precursor of prostaglandins and other eicosanoids, some of which are inflammatory. Hence linoleic acid is considered a proinflammatory compound which can initiate platelet aggregation and other inflammatory responses in the body.

It is available only in plant lipids. Vegetable oils such as safflower, corn, sunflower, sesame, cottonseed, soybean and rapeseed are rich sources of linoleic acid. These oils are also frequently used in manufacturing of vanaspati, margarines, shortening, and refined cooking oils. Consumption of excess amount of linoleic acid can contribute to inflammation and other related disorders in the body. Excess consumption may come from many food products like pizza, baked foods, French fries, etc. Some amount of LA is also present in sunflower seeds, pine nuts, pecans, Brazil nuts, cheese, etc. but presence of other constituents in them promote and protect health from natural sources of LA. LA deficiency may develop as a secondary condition in other disorders, such as protein energy malnutrition and fat malabsorption, as a consequence of total parenteral nutrition with inadequate LA intakes.

Gamma-linolenic acid (GLA): GLA, an n-6 fatty acid, is said to be a conditionally essential fatty acid when the activity of the delta-6-desaturase which is necessary for converting LA to GLA is reduced. It has 18 carbon atoms and three double bonds. The body can synthesize GLA from LA. GLA is converted into prostaglandin of series 1 (PGE_1), which is anti-inflammatory and is therapeutically used for reducing pain. PGE_1 also has other beneficial effects, e.g., it is antithrombotic, antiproliferative, and lowers lipids. Also, it enhances smooth muscle relaxation and vasodilation. Studies have shown that GLA has beneficial effects in reducing joint tenderness in rheumatoid arthritis, atopic eczema, asthma, cardiovascular disease and many other conditions. Evening primrose oil, and hemp seeds are rich sources of GLA and frequently prescribed for pre-menstrual syndrome (PMS), hot flushes, and night sweats in women. Other good sources are borage oil and black currant oil. These oils are generally not used as edible oils. Many long-term studies have shown that GLA up to 2.8 g per day is well tolerated.

One should be cautious about taking GLA supplements. It has been reported to aggravate a type of epilepsy and hence should not be consumed by persons who are taking medicines to prevent seizures. Also use of GLA for a prolonged period may lead to inflammation, blood clots, and lower immunity. Borage oil can adversely affect liver function and has been linked to increased risk of cancer.

Arachidonic acid: Arachidonic acid (AA 20:4) is a 20-carbon length, long-chain omega-6 fatty acid with four double bonds. It can be produced from LA but cannot be synthesized *de novo* by the human body hence need to obtained from dietary sources. It is predominantly found in animal-based foods such as poultry, egg yolks, seafood, fatty red meats, organ meats, and dairy products. AA content in food is proportional to the fat content of the food. It is a precursor of many eicosanoids and used to be considered as a culprit involved in increasing inflammation in the body. However, research studies have shown that this PUFA plays an important role in many ways. AA has the ability to contract smooth muscles. It inhibits as well as stimulates adhesion of blood platelets. It also influences the blood pressure. It plays significant role in immune system. It has been reported to be involved in apoptosis, necrosis, and cell death. Supplementation of preterm infant formulas with arachidonic acid and docosahexaenoic acid (DHA) has been found to improve visual acuity, visual attention, and cognitive development.

AA is a precursor of several proinflammatory eicosanoids, particularly prostaglandin of series 2 (PGE_2), prostacyclin, thromboxanes, and leukotrienes (LTB4, series B4 LT). These play a significant role in blood pressure, platelet aggregation and contraction of smooth muscles and production of other proinflammatory molecules like interleukin (IL-6 and IL-1) and cytokines. Therefore, excess consumption relative to the amount of n-3 fatty acids may exacerbate inflammatory symptoms like joint pain, swelling and some cardiac problems. Increased consumption of omega-6 (vegetable oils or western diet) tends to produce large quantities of arachidonic acid (AA) and contributed to the formation of thrombi and atheromas, the development of allergic and inflammatory disorders, and cell proliferation, thus increasing the risk of cardiovascular diseases and cancer. Consumption of n-3 foods like fish, nuts and flaxseeds can mitigate inflammatory problems caused by arachidonic acid.

AA-derived prostaglandins induce inflammation but also inhibit proinflammatory leukotrienes and cytokines, and induce anti-inflammatory lipoxins, thereby modulating the intensity and duration of the inflammatory response via negative feedback. Prostaglandins derived from AA—PGF_2 alpha, PGE_2, PGI_2 have been shown to play a role in muscle development and growth through the control of several functions such as proliferation, differentiation, migration, fusion, and survival of myoblasts. Lipoxin A4 which is derived from AA stimulates cessation of neutrophil infiltration, reduces bronchoconstriction in persons with asthma, decreases severity of eczema as well as reduces adipose inflammation, interleukin-6 and tumor necrosis factor-alpha that are associated with inflammation. PGE_2 and PGI_2 as well as leukotriene B4 and D4 all metabolites of AA, have been found to regulate production of angiogenic factors and thus promote wound healing as well as induce stem cell proliferation.

AA is an important component of phospholipids, especially phosphatidylinositol in the cell membrane and is important for its integrity, flexibility, and permeability. This fluidity is important because it influences the functions of specific membrane proteins that have a role in cell signaling, maintaining the integrity of the cell and its organelles, as well as vascular permeability. With DHA, AA constitutes a substantial amount of the brain, it is concentrated in the myelin sheath and outer membrane of the neurons. Some of the effects are attributable to the free arachidonic acid present in the cells and tissues. It is abundant in the gray matter of brain, where it modulates the uptake of neurotransmitters. Some studies in older animals suggest that arachidonic acid supplementation improved cognitive functions. The neural membranes in the tissues of the retina in the eyes contain both arachidonic acid and docosahexaenoic acid, which have a role in converting light to electrical signals that are translated by the human brain as vision. It is required for infant brain development.

Recent research studies show that AA and some of its metabolites like lipoxin A4 and epoxyeicosatrienoic acids (EETs) have anti-inflammatory effect, and may be important in both hypertension and diabetes mellitus. AA and these metabolites regulate smooth muscle function and proliferation, generation of free radicals, nitric oxide formation, inflammation, and immune functions that are involved in regulation of blood pressure and diabetes mellitus.

> **Research glimpse:** The authors undertook a systematic review and systematic analysis to determine whether intake of saturated fat and trans-unsaturated fat is associated with all-cause mortality, cardiovascular disease (CVD), and associated mortality, coronary heart disease (CHD) and associated mortality, ischemic stroke, and type 2 diabetes. Observational studies that were included if they had reported association between saturated fat and *trans*-unsaturated fat, total as well as industrially manufactured and that obtained from ruminant animals, with all-cause mortality, CHD/CVD mortality, total CHD,

Contd...

Contd...

> ischemic stroke, or type 2 diabetes. Their analysis showed that saturated fats do not have association with all-cause mortality, CVD, CHD, ischemic stroke or type 2 diabetes, although there are methodological limitations. *Trans*-fats were associated with all-cause mortality and CHD mortality that the authors attributed to higher intakes of industrial trans-fats rather than ruminant trans-fats.
>
> **De Souza RJ, Mente A, Maroleanu A, Cozma AI, et al.** Intake of saturated and *trans*-unsaturated fatty acids and risk of all-cause mortality, cardiovascular disease, and type 2 diabetes: systematic review and meta-analysis of observational studies. Brit Med J. 2015;351:h3978.
>
> Recommended dietary allowances for intakes of dietary fat and fatty acids are aimed at prevention of lifestyle diseases. However, fat composition of diets is greatly influenced by ethnic factors, region, and income. Indian diets are predominantly vegetarian; the main sources of fat are of plant origin with very little fat coming from animal sources. Thus, Indian diets have relatively low saturated fatty acid content, but supply high amounts of n-6 polyunsaturated fatty acids (PUFA), and are very low in n-3 PUFA. The increasing prevalence of noncommunicable diseases such as diabetes, obesity, and cardiovascular diseases in India, warrants scrutiny of fat intakes in Indian diets, in terms of the balance between the three macronutrients, rather than emphasizing the individual macronutrients.
>
> **Mani I and Kurpad A.** Fats & fatty acids in Indian diets: Time for serious introspection. Ind J Med Res. 2016;144(4):507–14.

Omega-3 Family

In the last two decades or so, omega-3 fatty acids have received considerable attention because of their critical roles in brain functions, normal growth, and development including fetal development, and later in adulthood. It is well accepted that omega-3 fatty acids can reduce inflammation in the body and so help the body to maintain homeostasis. They can be found mostly in animal sources and a few plant sources. Animal sources include fatty/oily fish namely tuna, salmon, mackerel, sardines, herring, fish oils, and spirulina. Plant sources include flaxseed, walnut, pistachio, pumpkin seeds, and sunflower seeds. It is important to note that omega-3 fatty acids are highly susceptible to oxidation on exposure to heat and air/oxygen and are easily destroyed. These need to be protected. Airtight storage for shorter period of time, purchase in relatively small amounts, and quick consumption are advisable for maximum benefits. Omega-3 fatty acids are important because LA and its metabolites cannot be converted into the eicosanoids that are formed from the n-3 fatty acids. The 3 important n-3 fatty acids are: 1. Alpha linolenic acid (ALA); 2. Eicosapentaenoic acid (EPA) and 3. Docosahexaenoic acid (DHA).

Functions of omega-3 fatty acids:
- Being constituents of phospholipids in the cell membranes, they influence permeability, fluidity, and thickness of the membrane, and thereby functioning of the cells in the brain, retina, and kidney.
- They support cell signaling.
- They influence cognitive functions and behavior.
- They play a significant role during pregnancy and infancy with regard to cognitive and mental development as well as visual functions (retinal development of fetus).
- They protect against cellular aging and age-related diseases.
- Eicosanoids (metabolites of omega-3 fatty acids) play a crucial role in inflammation and inflammatory diseases.
- Increased production of specialized lipid mediators (resolvins, protectins, maresins, and lipoxins) which act as anti-inflammtory compounds.
- Increased production of omega-3-derived eicosanoids (PGE3, TXA3, and LTB5)
- Decreased production of omega-6-derived eicosanoids (PGE2, TXA2, and LTB4) which are proinflammatory.
- Decreased production of interleukins (IL-I β) and TNF (tumor necrosis factor) production.
- They help to lower blood pressure, have antiarrhythmic action (stabilizes heart rhythm), reduce LDL cholesterol and have cytoprotective effects. Thus these fatty acids may help to lower risk of chronic diseases such as heart disease, cancer, and arthritis.

> **Interleukins** are signaling proteins (a type of cytokines), secreted by leukocytes in response to infection.
>
> **TNF-alpha** (a cytokine) is a signaling protein that causes inflammation and coordinates the process of inflammation.

Alpha-linolenic acid (ALA): Alpha-linolenic acid (ALA) is a long-chain omega-3 fatty acid (C18: n-3) and is the metabolic precursor for the formation of long-chain omega-3 fatty acids, such as eicosapentaenoic acid (EPA) and DHA. The conversion is not very efficient in humans, as only 8–20% of ALA is converted to EPA and an even lesser amount (0.5–9%) is converted to DHA. Efficiency of conversion is greater among women of reproductive age than in healthy men.

Alpha-linolenic acid is essential because it is the parent compound of long-chain fatty acids, i.e., EPA and DHA. EPA is the precursor of several anti-inflammatory eicosanoids such as prostaglandin. Consumption of EPA-rich foods may be useful in managing rheumatoid arthritis, allergic and inflammatory conditions such as psoriasis and eczema, lowering blood pressure and blood cholesterol, and is important for prevention of heart disease. Deficiency of ALA can lead to growth retardation and many neurological disorders. ALA is susceptible to oxidation; hence the use of oils like linseed oil in cooking is limited. Optimal intakes are about 2 g per day or 0.6–1% of the total dietary energy intake. Purslane, a leafy vegetable, is a good source of ALA.

Plant sources of omega-3 are flaxseeds (*alsi* in Hindi), pumpkin seeds, walnuts, whole pulses (namely rajma, soya, cowpea, black gram) and green leafy vegetables. Some cereals namely wheat and bajra, brussels sprouts and vegetable oils like soya bean oil, linseed oil, contain good amount of omega-3. The richest source of ALA is flaxseed oil (55%) and canola oil is also relatively high (15%). Very few adverse effects may occur except for mild gastrointestinal symptoms consumption of these foods in same persons. However, ALA supplements should be used with caution because they may increase the risk of prostate cancer.

Eicosapentaenoic acid (EPA): EPA is incorporated into cell membranes. EPA is also converted into several eicosanoids (prostaglandin E3 and leukotriene B5) that have antiatherogenic, antithrombotic, anti-inflammatory, and immunosuppressive effects. It is also converted into resolvins, which have anti-inflammatory effect. Thus, it has beneficial effects on blood clotting, platelet aggregation, triglyceride level, immune functions, and inflammatory responses. It competes with n-6 fatty acids and produces the more beneficial eicosanoids. Thus increasing the intake of EPA/n-3 PUFA relative to n-6 fatty acids helps to confer beneficial effects rather than using supplements. Supplementation with EPA and DHA has been shown to reduce the risk of coronary heart disease especially in persons with diabetes or those who have hyperlipidemia. Increasing n-3 PUFA levels in critically ill patients may help improve the outcome.

It is found almost exclusively in fatty fish like salmon, tuna, mackerel, sardine, shellfish and herring, although it can be formed from ALA after a series of reaction involving desaturation (addition of double bonds) and elongation (addition of carbon atoms). However, the conversion of ALA to EPA is not very efficient compared with direct consumption of the fatty acid from the diet. EPA is a precursor of DHA.

Docosahexaenoic acid (DHA): DHA is a vital component of phospholipids present in the cell membrane of the body cells, especially of the retina, myelin in brain, and other structures; and it greatly influences the membrane function in these tissues. It is present in phospholipids of the gray matter of the brain and is important for functioning of the central nervous system (influences thinking, concentration, cognition, memory, feeling, and other brain functions particularly during fetal stage, infancy, and childhood). It is present in abundant amounts in the cell membranes of the retina (retina conserves DHA) and is essential for neurological and visual development in the fetus and neonate. Research studies indicate that for retinal development, there is a critical period and if DHA supply is not adequate, permanent abnormalities in retinal function may be a consequence. DHA is important for regeneration of the protein rhodopsin that is critical in the visual cycle. However in later adulthood, it affects several brain activities because it is a messenger between brain cells. Its deficiency can cause neuronal disorders. Inadequate intake of n-3 fatty acids has been found to impair immune function and in the event of prolonged deficiency leads to development of dermatitis. High n-3 intake prolongs bleeding time.

Fish is the richest source of DHA. However, not all fish are good sources. Good sources include salmon, herring, mackerel, and trout. Vegetarians can obtain DHA by consuming adequate amounts of its precursor ALA.

Research glimpse: Omega-3 fatty acids that are mostly obtained from fish/fish oils or fish oil products are important for fetal development, cardiovascular function, and may be important for healthy aging. In fetal life, n-3 fatty acids are important for neuronal and retinal development as well as immune function. EPA and DHA are also important for cardiovascular function, they have anti-inflammatory and anticoagulative effects. EPA and DHA may play an important role in weight management and may help in cognitive function in Alzheimer's disease.
Swanson D, Block R, Mousa SA. Omega-3 fatty acids EPA and DHA: Health benefits throughout life. Adv Nutr. 2012;3(1):1-7.

Ratio of n-6 and n-3 Fatty Acids

Both omega-6 and omega-3 fatty acids are important for maintaining good health and to prevent numerous degenerative diseases. During human evolution, the dietary ratio of n-3 to n-6 is believed to have been 1:1. The ratio of both (n-3:n-6) is very critical for better health. It should be 5:1 to 10:1 (ICMR-NIN, 2020). Having the right balance in these two types of fatty acids has certain advantages:

- Important for health throughout the life cycle.
- Less inflammatory state (gene expression, prostaglandin and leukotriene metabolism) so reduce inflammation and inflammatory diseases including pain in arthritis.
- Improved glandular and endocrine functions in the body.
- Reduce water retention and improved kidney functions.
- Reduce platelet aggregation and thus risk of heart disease.
- Better immunity.
- Better fetal brain development.
- Influence preadipocyte differentiation and fat mass (adipose tissue) growth, thus influencing risk of overweight and obesity.
- May reduce weight gain in persons who are obese.
- Reduce adverse effects of high n-6 intake on leptin resistance and risk of diabetes.
- Reduce pathogenesis of neurological diseases.
- Produce less hunger and promote feeling of fullness. Decrease hyperactivity of the endocannabinoid system.
- Influence skeletal metabolism and functional response of muscle during exercise, muscle protein synthesis, and maintenance of muscle.

AA and EPA are acted upon by specific enzymes, viz cyclooxygenases and lipoxygenases. Several important different signaling molecules are formed, including eicosanoids.

Several epidemiological studies have shown that many Indians and people from other continents, who frequently consume fried or baked foods, consume more amounts of omega-6 fatty acids owing to its accessibility, palatability, and affordability. Excessive intake of omega-6 leads to adverse health consequences and also offset the desirable ratio. Modern dietary habits clearly indicate an imbalance in the ratio, i.e., 20–30:1. As such LA is present in a wide variety of foods, whereas ALA occurs in only a few foods, therefore it is necessary to pay attention. Hence it must be ensured that there is no excess of n-6 fatty acids.

Laboratory laurel: The percentage of calories obtained from total fat as well as saturated fat in Western diets has been decreasing along with an increased intake of n-6 fatty acids. Unfortunately, intake of n-3 fatty acids has decreased simultaneously resulting in a high ratio of n-6:n-3≥20:1, compared with a ratio of 1:1 during evolution. In parallel, there has been a significant increase in the prevalence of overweight and obesity. Results of research studies indicate that n-6 and n-3 fatty acids have different effects on adipogenesis, browning of adipose tissue, lipid homeostasis as well as systemic inflammation. Long-term follow-up studies indicate that higher n-6 to n-3 ratios increase the amount of n-6 in red cell membrane phospholipids, in contrast to n-3 which decrease these and are associated with decreased obesity risk. Human studies have shown that more than the absolute amounts of n-3 and n-6 fatty acids in the diet, the relative

Contd...

Contd...

> amounts or the ratios of these have an important influence in risk of becoming obese through the arachidonic acid metabolites and hyperactivity of the endocannabinoid system. Adequate intakes of n-3 fatty acids can help reverse this effect. A balanced ratio of the two classes of fatty acids in the diet is important for maintaining good health and to prevent as well as manage obesity.
>
> *Simpoulos AP. An Increase in the omega-6/omega-3 fatty acid ratio increases the risk for obesity. Nutrients. 2016;8:128.*

There are several ways through which desirable omega-2 intake and status can be ensured:
- Judicious selection of foods rich in omega-3 and omega-6 to increase omega-3 intake.
- Increase use of coconut, sesame and canola oil.
- Include pharmaceutical preparations if necessary.
- Use of flaxseed/flaxseed oil/chia seeds in salad dressing, milk/curd preparations/chutneys, etc.
- Omega-3 intake should not be less than 1% of total energy.
- Protect omega-3 rich-foods from heat and light.
- Consumption of antioxidant-rich foods will prevent oxidation of EFA.
- Ensure adequate intakes of vitamins A, C, E, B1, B2, B6, B12, pantothenic acid, and biotin, and minerals like copper, chromium, and magnesium, which will improve the effectiveness of EFA and help in reducing the risk of various disorders and diseases.
- Ensure adequate intake of protein because when there is deficiency of protein, the conversion of γ-linolenic acid to EPA and DHA would be adversely affected.
- Use groundnut and mustard oil in 3:1 or groundnut and canola oil in 1:1 proportion or sunflower and canola oil in 1:1.
- Balance can also be achieved by consuming 3–5% n-6 and 0.5–1% n-3.

Deficiency of Essential Fatty Acids (EFA)

Deficiency of EFA purely due to dietary inadequacy is rare. Sometimes rate of conversion of the parent fatty acids is diminished by age, or if a high-carbohydrate diet is consumed. Other causes include fasting, high intake of saturated fatty acids and *trans*-fatty acids, alcohol intake, and diabetes. Elders, children suffering from kwashiorkor, fat malabsorption, and vascular disease are likely to be at risk of developing EFA deficiency. In clinical situations, EFA deficiency has been observed, e.g., in diseases, where the patient is fed parenterally or in trauma or surgery or patients who have malabsorption syndrome. Deficiency of EFA often leads to demyelination or dysmyelination in the myelin sheath. In patients given total parenteral nutrition that is devoid of EFA, deficiency of EFA can develop within a week to 10 days. Symptoms of EFA deficiency can be dry, scaly skin, hair loss, fatty liver, retarded growth, and reproductive failure. Clinical signs of EFA deficiency is include:
- Dry scaly rashes (dermatitis). The dermatitis increases water loss from the skin
- Growth retardation in children and if mother's diets are deficient, fetal growth and development are adversely affected.
- Poor wound healing
- Susceptibility to infection.

Deficiency of omega-3 EFA is often created by higher consumption of omega-6. Western dietary pattern, processing of vegetable oils using modern technology as well as feeding of grains (high in omega-6) instead of grass to animals tend to increase the consumption of omega-6 and reduce the intake of omega-3. It disturbs the desirable ratio of omega-6 and omega-3 fatty acids and usually results in the deficiency of DHA and unfavorable health consequences.

Loss of n-3 PUFA, particularly DHA, occurs in neuronal tissues/brain and retina rods phospholipids, and there is compensatory replacement by AA. This compositional change (even a minor change) in the membrane lipids can lead to memory loss, learning disability, and visual impairment, i.e., loss of visual acuity.

The three groups/series of fatty acids namely, n-3, n-6, and n-9 are desaturated by the same enzymes and hence compete with each other. The preference for the substrates by the desaturase enzymes is n-3 > n-6 and lastly n-9. Thus, when intakes of n-3 and n-6 are inadequate, n-9 is desaturated, one of the desaturated fatty acids derived from n-9 is mead acid (20:3, n-9) that will be seen in increased amounts and can be considered as a possible marker of EFA deficiency. A ratio exceeding 0.2 of triene:tetraene in plasma is considered to be indicative of EFA deficiency.

Regular consumption of omega-3-rich foods and in the appropriate ratio of omega-6 and omega-3 fatty acids can combat the deficiency of EFA. Though vegetable oils are rich in both LA and ALA, but refining and processing reduce the ALA content and increase the LA. It is better to consume crude or cold pressed or filtered oils rather than refined oils. Although n-3 deficiency is not common, there are reports of isolated cases of deficiency. Visual problems and sensory neuropathy was reported in a girl who was given intravenous lipid emulsion with very little ALA. The condition was reversed when more ALA was included in the lipid emulsion.

> **Omega-3 index:** This is defined as the amount of EPA and DHA in the RBC and is expressed as a percentage of the total fatty acids in RBC membranes. The content of these two fatty acids in the red blood cells has been found to correlate with the content of cardiac muscle cells. It has been reported in some studies that the risk of death from coronary heart disease was greater, when the omega-3 index was lower. The proposed cutoff for this to be used as a biomarker is <4% = intermediate risk, 4–8% is low risk and >8% signifies low risk. However, the validity of these cutoffs needs to be established before it can be used in routine clinical practice.

Eicosanoids

Eicosanoids are derived from PUFA (omega-6 and omega-3 fatty acids) and contain 20 carbons. "Eikos" is a Greek word which means 20. The term eicosanoid includes biologically active lipid mediators (C20 fatty acids and their metabolites). Arachidonic acid not only produces prostaglandins but other related compounds and the whole group is referred as eicosanoids. Eicosanoids are lipid mediators of inflammation. Eicosanoids formed from AA and EPA are biologically important and more active than those formed from gamma-

linolenic acid. There are four types of eicosanoids, each having different functions:
1. Prostaglandins
2. Prostacyclins
3. Thromboxanes
4. Leukotrienes.

They are naturally synthesized from essential fatty acids (EFAs), namely GLA, AA, and EPA. These fatty acids are released from cell membranes when there is stimulation from hormones or cytokines or other stimuli. These fatty acids are then acted upon by cyclooxygenases, lipoxygenases, and cytochrome p450 monooxygenases. The 20 carbon derivatives of these EFA are utilized in the body to regulate inflammation, sensation of pain and immunity, and play a role in fever, blood clotting, reproductive processes, tissue growth, and regulation of blood pressure, sleep/wake cycle, cell signaling, platelet aggregation, blood clotting, uterine contractions, bone repair, and inflammatory diseases including heart diseases. The derivatives of eicosanoids are as shown in Table 4.11 and Figure 4.8.

The source of lipid has a strong influence on the eicosanoids that are produced. Some are synthesized from arachidonic acid (omega-6) and some can be produced from omega-3 fatty acids. Eicosanoids which are derived from omega-6 are generally proinflammatory (induce inflammation) and have an adverse effect on inflammatory processes and related disorders. However, eicosanoids derived from omega-3 are less inflammatory. The amount and ratio of omega-6 and omega-3 fatty acids from dietary sources influence the eicosanoid-regulated functions in the body.

Prostaglandins (PG): Prostaglandins were discovered in 1933 by a Swedish scientist who observed the synthesis of prostaglandins in prostate gland, hence the name prostaglandins. Later, it was discovered that they are synthesized in most tissues and organs. They are derived from arachidonic acid (AA). They are synthesized in response to inflammatory stimuli in presence of cyclooxygenase (COX) (Fig. 4.9) or lipoxgenase enzymes and behave like hormones. There are 2 types of cyclooxygenases, i.e., COX-1 and COX-2. COX-1 is located in blood vessels, stomach, and kidney. They are potent mediators of inflammation, pain, and fever as well as clotting. They also play a role in infections and cancer. Prostaglandins are involved in:
- Regulating salt and fluid balance
- Increasing blood flow in kidneys
- Increasing secretion of protective mucus in GI tract
- Inhibiting acid synthesis in GI tract
- Leukotrienes and related molecules promote constriction of bronchi associated with asthma.

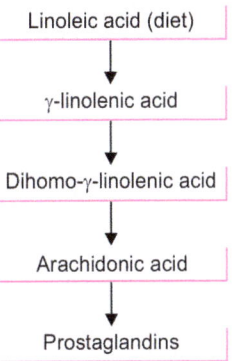

Fig. 4.9: Formation of prostaglandin.

They have a very short half-life (10 seconds to 5 minutes), so their effects are limited to cells in the nearby vicinity. Anti-inflammatory compounds inhibit the synthesis of prostaglandins at COX-1 and COX-2 and reduce the sensation of pain. There is a series of 3 prostaglandins, i.e., PGE_1, PGE_2 and PGE_3. Prostaglandin in series 1 and 3 are good, because they act as anti-inflammatory agents. PGE_2 series act opposite or induce inflammation.

PGE_1 is derived from gamma-linolenic acid (GLA) and is naturally found in evening primrose oil and borage oil. PGE_1 helps to relax smooth muscles in blood vessels and ovaries, and decrease inflammation. It brings improvement in circulation, nerve functions, and immunity.

PGE_3 is derived from EPA and DHA and prevents inflammation, blood clotting, and dilates blood vessels. It reduces pain and inflammatory response.

PGE_2 tends to produce inflammation, pain, fever, and swelling, and thereby promote progression of heart disease, arthritis, and inflammation. PGE_2 is favorably crucial in uterus contraction during pregnancy. It is derived from omega-3 fatty acids, usually found in meat and vegetable oils. It is a vasodilator, and is involved gastric cytoprotection and bone resorption.

Prostacyclin: Prostacyclins are formed in the arterial walls and inhibit platelet aggregation, but they relax the arterial wall and help in lowering the blood pressure. It prevents the formation of blood clots to certain extent. Thus, it acts as antithrombotic and anti-inflammatory substance. It is released from healthy endothelial cells.

Thromboxanes: Thromboxanes are produced by platelets, hence they participate in blood clotting and constriction of blood vessels. They are important in wound healing. There are two types of thromboxanes—Thromboxanes A2 (TXA2) and Thromboxanes B2 (TXB2). TXA2 is active and a potent

Table 4.11: Derivatives of eicosanoids.

Enzymes and the major classes of prostaglandins/products of their action on 20 carbon derivatives of EFA		
Cyclooxygenases	Lipoxygenases	Cytochrome P450 monooxidase products
Prostanoids, i.e., prostaglandins (PG), prostacyclins, and thromboxanes (Tx)	Leukotrienes and hydroxyl fatty acids	Hydroxyeicosatetraenoic acids (HETEs) Epoxides

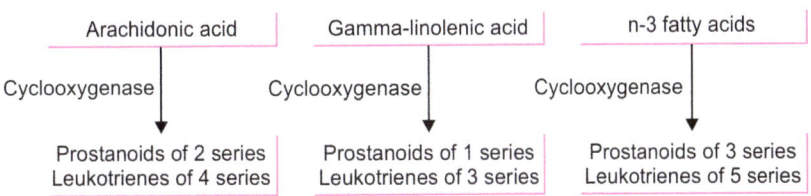

Fig. 4.8: Formation of eicosanoids.

constrictor of smooth muscle. They also reduce platelet aggregation.

Leukotrienes: Leukotrienes are produced in leukocytes by oxidation of arachidonic acid and eicosapentaenoic acid by a specific enzyme. Hence they regulate immune response and are usually accompanied by release of histamines and prostaglandins, which are part of the inflammatory response. They can also trigger smooth muscle lining of lungs and cause asthma and allergies. There are three types of leukotrienes, namely LTB4, LGT5, and LGB5. LTB4 helps in recruiting neutrophils in damaged tissue and promotes production of cytokines by immune cells. LGB5 is derived from EPA and possesses mild anti-inflammatory effect.

Each compound has a characteristic biological activity. Prostaglandins, thromboxanes, and prostacyclins together are also called prostanoids. They act on vascular cells, leukocytes and platelets. They are called local hormones because they act only locally in the area, where they are produced.

Prostaglandins and thromboxane A_2 (TXA2) are collectively termed as prostanoids. Besides prostaglandins and leukotrienes, compounds such as resolvins, protectins, and maresin 1 are derived from n-3 fatty acids, whereas lipoxins are derived from n-6 fatty acids. These enhance host immunity, reduce inflammation, prevent platelet aggregation, lower blood pressure, reduce LDL cholesterol, and have cytoprotective effects. Overall, the group of compounds formed from n-3 PUFA has anti-inflammatory effects and protect against atherosclerosis through a variety of ways. They also modulate gene expression and production of specific eicosanoid compounds.

Consumption of more omega-3 fatty acids (as previously stated) is beneficial as compared with omega-6 fatty acid-rich foods. Consumption of turmeric, pomegranate juice, flaxseed, evening primrose oil, borage and canola oils from plant sources and marine food or cod liver oil tend to suppress the production of PGE_2 and thus have been proposed in painful and rheumatic conditions to ameliorate the pain.

Conjugated Linoleic Acid (CLA)

Conjugated linoleic acid (CLA) is actually a group of positional isomers (position of double bonds) and geometric isomers (*trans*) of linoleic acid (linoleic acid is in the *cis* form). There are about 28 isomers that are collectively referred to as CLA. CLA is formed when reactions occur during which one or both the double bonds present in linoleic acid shift in location. In linoleic acid, the two double bonds are separated by two single bonds. When the shift in location of the double bond occurs, this arrangement of the two single bonds between the double bonds ceases to exist. Formation of several isomers is possible depending on where the double bond shifts and there is change from the *cis* to the *trans* form. The predominant naturally occurring CLA isomer in the human diet is c-9(*cis* -9), t-11(*trans*-11) CLA.

Most of the CLA in human diets is formed enzymatically in the rumen of ruminant animals such as cattle, goats, sheep, and buffalo, wherein LA is converted into CLA by fermentative bacteria microorganisms. Thus CLA is present in milk and meat of cattle. Cow's milk, butter, cream and cheese are good sources of CLA. Grass-fed animal foods contains more CLA as compared with grain-fed animals. Milk fat from cows fed marine algae has also been found to contain more amount of CLA. Seasonal variations significantly affect the CLA content. Skimmed milk is not a good source of CLA because the fat has been removed. Breast milk of mothers who drink whole milk contains CLA. CLA is gaining attention because of the following possible benefits:

- Animal studies show that CLA reduces body fat and changes body composition. Thus, it has been proposed to play a role in weight management. But it cannot be considered as sole remedy for obesity because this is still being investigated.
- It is being studied for its anticancer potential (inhibition of carcinogenesis). In animal studies, it was found to hinder the growth and proliferation of tumors in mammary glands, skin, liver, lungs, and colon.
- It may also have potential to reduce the risk for cardiovascular disease by reducing LDL and total cholesterol. However, it also reduces HDL cholesterol. Adverse effects such as gastrointestinal complaints and fatigue have been reported after CLA administration in humans.
- It has a role in enhancing immune response.
- It has been shown to have a role in promoting growth, improving bone metabolism, and diabetes and insulin resistance.

In 2008, CLA received the GRAS (Generally Recognized as Safe) status from the USFDA. On this basis food industry can incorporate it in fluid milk, yogurt, meal replacement shakes, nutritional bars, fruit juices, and soy milk. It must be noted that CLA may have adverse effects on insulin sensitivity and glucose levels. Therefore persons consuming CLA for a prolonged period, may be advised to monitor the HDL and glucose levels.

> **Laboratory laurel:** There is considerable interest in CLA because it has been found to have beneficial effects on health. Studies with in vitro human cell lines and animal models have demonstrated that this has protective effect against cancer, obesity, diabetes, and atherosclerosis. The biological effects are conferred largely by the following isomers: c9, t11-CLA and t10, c12-CLA.
>
> *Yang B, Chen H, Stanton C, et al. Review of the roles of conjugated linoleic acid in health and disease. J Functional Foods. 2015;15:314–25.*
>
> Conjugated linoleic acid (CLA) has been studied in animal models to favorably modify the body composition and cardiometabolic risk factors such as glycemic profile, atherosclerosis, and cancer. Now in human studies also, it has been proved to reduce adiposity through modulating properties in the lipid metabolism.
>
> *Lehnen TE, Da Silva MR, Camacho A, et al. A review on effects of conjugated linoleic fatty acid (CLA) upon body composition and energetic metabolism .J Int Soc Sports Nutr. 2015;12:36.*

Trans Fats

Most unsaturated fatty acids found in nature contain double bonds in *cis* configuration and the other configuration is *trans*, that is also found in nature but in less amount, e.g., in some seed oils, which are not used as dietary source. *Trans*-fatty acids are fatty acids with at least one double bond in the trans configuration. *Trans*-fatty acids are also produced by microbial biohydrogenation of PUFA in the rumen of ruminant animals. Industrially they are produced by partial chemical hydrogenation of PUFA. *Trans*-fatty acids usually found in the body tissues are relatively proportionate to the dietary consumption. These are deposited more in adipose tissues. It is found in phospholipids and behave as saturated fats and found in heart, liver, and brain. These fatty acids are also metabolized in the body and do not remain in tissues permanently but tend to alter the metabolism of other fatty acids. Particularly, it competes with linoleic acid (EFA) for the same enzyme. Thus, favorable effects of EFA in formation of prostaglandins are diminished. Hence use of TFA can cause deficiency of essential fatty acid and cause unfavorable metabolic effects. Addition of EFA tends to reduce the accumulation of TFA in the tissue lipids.

Trans-fats are "manufactured" fats formed by subjecting oils to a type of processing called hydrogenation (addition of hydrogen atoms to the fatty acids). The hydrogenation process is conducted at a high temperature, typically at 260ºC and pressure, during which the unsaturated oil is subjected to structural transformation wherein hydrogen is added to the double bonds. During this process, in the fatty acids that have double bonds, the naturally occurring *cis* configuration can flip to a *trans* configuration, thus creating *trans* "isomers". However, partial hydrogenation occurs and the degree of saturation increases but 100% hydrogenation need not occur. This is done to prevent the unsaturated fatty acids becoming rancid, to ensure a longer shelf-life and also to obtain a solid consistency at room temperature. The degree of hydrogenation determines the final consistency of the product. *Trans*-fatty acids are also formed during normal cooking and frying. Some *trans*-fatty acids may be fully saturated whereas some may still have double bonds. However, these fats are classified as saturated fats. TFA is found in partially hydrogenated vegetable oils (PHVO) commercially used in food processing. It should not be considered low in SFA. They are often used as hidden fat (the fats used in processed food, e.g., ready to eat mixes, fats foods, bakery and confectionery items) and also as visible fat (in cooking). However, red palm oil can replace PHVO and it will also improve the consumption of vitamin A.

> **Note:** *Trans*-fats may occur naturally in foods such as beef, pork, lamb, butter, and milk, except in CLA (conjugated linoleic acid) which is found in meat and dairy products. Thus only CLA is beneficial and all other *trans*-fats are harmful to health.

Hydrogenated fat is commercially produced in India. It is popularly known as "vanaspati" and also commonly used at household as well as industrial levels as a cheaper substitute for ghee or butter. This fat has high heat stability, high smoking point, and better shelf-life as it does not go rancid as quickly as vegetable oils. It is used extensively in bakery products such as biscuits, cakes, etc. for its plasticity and firmness. Other products that hydrogenated fats have been used in are—ready meals, snack foods, breakfast cereals, chips, soup powders, and readymade sauces. However, it has adverse effects on health. In experimental studies, *trans*-fatty acids were found to compete with other dietary long-chain fatty acids and impair their metabolism.

Trans-fats raise triglyceride levels and LDL cholesterol levels, and decrease HDL cholesterol, thus contributing to thickening of the artery walls. Besides this, they increase inflammation. TFA may be linked to endothelial dysfunction. Thus *trans*-fats may increase the risk of coronary heart disease more than saturated fats. *Trans*-fatty acids may adversely affect insulin sensitivity, especially in persons who have insulin resistance, may possibly increase risk of weight gain and development of diabetes.

Erucic acid is a long-chain monounsaturated fatty acid [*trans*-22:1(n–9)] found in high amounts in some types of rapeseed oil. Zero erucic acid rapeseed oil is being sold as "canola oil". Absorbed erucic acid is oxidized slowly and accumulates in myocardium, causing myocardial lipidosis and functional abnormalities in myocardial mitochondria. These side effects are observed at high but not at low (<1% of dietary fatty acids) levels of intake.

In 2003, the Joint Expert Committee of the World Health Organization and Food and Agriculture Organization recommended that *trans*-fatty acid (TFA) intake should be below 1% of energy intakes or less than 2.2 g/day in a 2000 kcal diet. In India, also the government is regulating the amount of *trans*-fats that can be present in a food. It has been proposed that the amount of *trans*-fatty acids should not exceed 5% in partially hydrogenated vegetable oils and should be brought down to 2% by 2022. The Food Safety and Standards Authority of India (FSSAI) has recommended that there should be mandatory labeling of TFA and SFA content on vanaspati packs, edible oils or any other product containing TFA from vanaspati sources. This is necessary to enable consumers to make informed choices.

Substitutes for *trans*-fat include oils that have been produced by modified hydrogenation so that the amount of *trans*-fats is reduced, use of selective breeding or genetic engineering to modify oils such as soybean, sunflower or cotton seeds that will have a lower unsaturated fat content. Other alternatives are to use butter and animal fat, or natural saturated oils such as palm and coconut oil, or even non-fatty texture-building substances, e.g., plant fiber or whole oats. Saturated fatty acids, especially palm oil, are being used in reformulating bakery foods, and unsaturated oils are being used in the reformulation of fried foods.

RECOMMENDED DIETARY ALLOWANCE OF FATS AND OILS

The Expert Committee of the Indian Council of Medical Research and National Institute of Nutrition (ICMR-NIN, 2020) has given recommendations for dietary fat intakes based on FAO/WHO (2008) that are shown in Table 4.12.

Requirements of fats and oils for adults were set between 15-30% E (35% E for active individuals who are in energy

Table 4.12: Requirement for total fat as percentage of total energy.

Category	RDA (2020)	Remarks
Minimum total fat intake by adults	15% E (of energy requirement) 20-40g/day	E to ensure adequate consumption of total energy, essential fatty acids and fat-soluble vitamins for most individuals.
Minimum total fat intake by women of reproductive age and adults with BMI <18.5	20 % E (of energy requirement)	To achieve adequate energy intake in malnourished populations.
Desirable/ optimal fat intake	15-30 % E	For consistent good health
Maximum total fat intake	30-35% E (of energy requirement) and above 35% will increase risk of NCDs	To fulfill recommended fat requirement
Maximum total fat intake for children up to 2 years.	30-40% E	To fulfill recommended fat requirement including of growth
Saturated fatty acids (SFAs) (C12:0 – C16:0)	An upper limit of 10% E SFAs. SFA intake should not exceed 10% of total energy intake	To prevent elevated serum LDL cholesterol which is a risk factor for CHD
Total PUFA	6-11% of total energy intake with a minimum intake of 2.5 – 3.5% of total energy	For optimal health and to prevent EFA deficiency
n-6 PUFA	5-8% of energy with minimum intake of 2.5%	For optimal health and to prevent EFA deficiency
n-3 PUFA	1-2% of energy with minimum of 0.5% of energy	For optimal health and to prevent EFA deficiency
MUFA	To be estimated by difference MUFA = Total fat intake (%E) – energy from SFA + PUFA + TFA	For optimal health and to prevent EFA deficiency
Trans Fats	Less than 1% of energy	
Cholesterol	300 mg	Optimal body functions
Desirable intakes of LA	4-10% E	To prevent risk of CHD
Desirable ratio of LA: ALA	5:1 to 10:1	To attain good health and reduce risks of EFA deficiency and other health problems

Sources:
1. Interim Summary of Conclusions and Dietary Recommendations on Total Fat and Fatty Acids From the Joint FAO/WHO Expert Consultation on Fats and Fatty Acids in Human Nutrition, 2008, WHO, Geneva.
2. Nutrient Requirements of Indians, Recommended Dietary Allowances, Estimated Average Requirements, A Reports of the Expert Group, 2020, Indian Council of Medical research, National Institute of Nutrition, Department of Health Research, Ministry of Health and Family Welfare, Government of India. pp 122.

balance), at least 20% E for women in reproductive age and 30-40% E for children up to 2 years.

Recommendations for fatty acids considered elevated serum LDL cholesterol as a major risk factor for CHD. An upper limit of 10% E SFAs and <300 mg/day of dietary cholesterol, desirable intakes of LA between 4-10% E and ratio of LA: ALA between 5:1 to 10:1 were recommended.

Intake of leafy vegetables, legumes, fish and sea foods was to be encouraged to achieve a ratio of LA: ALA between 5:1 to 10:1.

ICMR-NIN (2020) have made recommendations for dietary fats based on FAO and WHO recommendations (2008) considering the sources of dietary fats available in the country and their fatty acid composition and also to meet the requirements of the fetus, infants, mothers and combat the chronic energy deficiency (children and adults) and diet related non-communicable diseases (DR-NCD) in adults. These recommendations are given in Table 4.12 and Table 9.1A in Chapter 9.1.

Recommendations for dietary fats in Indians have been revised taking into account recent FAO and WHO recommendations for: i) total fat, individual fatty acids and health promoting non-glyceride components ii) sources of dietary fats in Indians and iii) availability of fat. The recommendations are directed towards meeting the requirements for optimal fetal and infant growth and development, maternal health and for combating chronic energy deficiency (children and adults) and DR-NCD in adults.

- **Total fat** should contribute between 15% and 30% (20-40 g per person per day) for adults of total energy intake and should not be less than 15%; in order to ensure distribution of energy supply from macronutrients and intake of fat-soluble vitamins and for consistent good health and prevent NCDs. Minimum intake of fat should be 20 % of energy for women of reproductive age and the population with BMI less than 18.5. Further minimum requirement of fat for children and adolescents has been shown to be 25 % of energy for growth and physical activity and visible fat for them can be 25-30g and 35-40g per day respectively. The upper limit for children is 35% of total energy intake. The requirement for total fat (as percentage of total energy) during pregnancy and lactation is the same as that for other adults. More than 35 % of energy may increase the risk of NCDs.

- **Ratio of LA: ALA** is important and the recommended ratio is between 5:1 and 10:1. This can be achieved with generous intake of dark green leafy vegetables, legumes (that contain this fatty acid), flaxseeds, fish, and sea

foods. It is highly crucial for pregnant women to meet the requirements, to ensure fetal and infant development.
- **Foods high in PUFA** should also contain at least 0.6 mg tocopherol, as it helps to stabilize unsaturated fatty acids. Thus consumption of foods rich in antioxidants, carotenoids, and nonglyceride components is recommended.

These recommendations include energy obtained from both visible and invisible fats. Fats are integral components of foods which is called invisible fat. Different foods contain varying amounts of fat and also differ in fatty acid composition. Fat from animal foods like butter, cream, cheese, ghee, usually contains SFA, and cholesterol. Fats from nuts and oilseeds are fairly good source of MUFA and PUFA. Fenugreek is a good source of both LA and ALA. However, LA is a major fatty acid in legumes and leafy vegetables and ALA is found in nuts like walnuts and almonds and mustard/rapeseed.

Dietary Guidelines for Fat Intake

Dietary guidelines are based on the function of fat in food and other safety concerns in health and disease.

- Dietary intake of fats and oils has been set between 15% and 30% of energy for most adults. Hence the source of fat becomes very crucial.
- Judicious selection would help to get desirable ratio of n-6 and n-3 PUFA fatty acid.
- Consume foods having high content of ALA and long-chain n-3 PUFA. Addition of whole grains, nuts, seeds, legumes, and seafoods (for fish eaters) would be advisable. These foods also contain other beneficial nutrients which support utilization of fat in the body.
- Selection of crude oil or cold-pressed vegetable oil will be better than the refined oil; as these oils will also supply phytosterols.
- Use blend of 2 or more vegetable oils (1:1).
- Use oils containing LA + oil containing both LA and ALA, e.g., groundnut, sesame, rice bran, cotton seed + mustard. Consider all vegetable oils that contain tocopherols and plant sterols, e.g., sesame lignans, oryzanols + tocotrienols, tocotrienols, and vitamins A and D. These nonglyceride components have many health benefits.
- Include MUFA-rich foods in the diet. Oils like olive oil, rice bran oil, and groundnut oil contain MUFA. Nuts like walnut also contain MUFA.
- Combinations with rapeseed and mustard reduce erucic acid content.
- While butter/ghee are important, judicious use of these in the diet is necessary as they contain SFA.
- Use frying oils having high thermal stability instead of hydrogenated fat, e.g., palmolein/palm oil/ sesame/ rice bran, and cotton seed (single or blend).
- Use coconut oil/palm kernel oil/palm oil, palmolein, palm stearin (solid fractions) or blends in bakery fat (shortening), and Indian sweets (solid fats).
- Intake of energy-dense processed foods, fried foods, and sugar-sweetened beverages should be low. It will also reduce the intake of TFA.
- It is advisable to pay attention to portion size and to avoid consuming large portions of food.
- Moderate amount of dairy products, lean meat, and poultry can be included in the diet. It will increase the intake of CLA.
- Along with this, it is important to have adequate physical activity to prevent weight gain and maintain desirable body weight in order to ensure optimal health especially for individuals who are predisposed to insulin resistance.

FOOD SOURCES OF FATS AND OILS

Dietary fats are obtained from animal and vegetable sources. Fat content (in grams) can be seen in Appendix 1.

Vegetable sources: Vegetable oils and fats are usually obtained from nuts and oilseeds by extraction and expression or cold-pressing. When fat is subjected to first extraction, it is crude and also contains phospholipids (lecithin), waxes, sterols, pigments, hormones, and some volatile oils. Further extraction reduces the amount of these compounds. Oilseeds like soybean, groundnut, sesame, sunflower, safflower, and mustard are commonly used vegetable oils. Oils from the olive fruit, coconut, and rice bran are also extracted. Refining is done to obtain colorless and odor-free vegetable oils. Refined oils contain little or no phytosterols.

Oils can be obtained from nuts like almond and walnut, but are not regularly consumed in the daily diet as they are not commercially viable. Vegetable oils are converted into solid fats such as vanaspati or margarine by the process of hydrogenation. Fat can also be obtained by churning as butter from churning of fermented milk culture.

Cold-press oils: Olive oil and few other oils are expressed by cold press method. It releases less amount of oil as compared with other methods of extraction. However, the oils contain many health-beneficial naturally occurring substances, which confer extra health benefits which are otherwise lost in refining process. However, energy value is not diminished.

Almost all foods including cereals, millets, pulses, Green leafy vegetables (GLV), and fruits, contain some fat which is invisible. However, nuts and oilseeds, fruits like olive, avocado, coconut, and palm contain considerable amount of invisible fat.

Vegetable oils have been found to protect from several chronic diseases like coronary heart diseases (CHD) on account of their fatty acid composition. Each vegetable oil differs in its fatty acid composition, i.e., saturated fatty acids (SFA), monounsaturated fatty acids (MUFA) and polyunsaturated fatty acids (PUFA) (Table 4.13). In addition, some vegetable oils also contain essential fatty acids (EFA), phytosterols, tocotrienols including tocopherol (vitamin E), and nonglycerides components which exhibit many health benefits. All the vegetable oils are rich in PUFA with varying amounts of n-6 and n-3 fatty acids.

Animal sources: Edible animal fats are usually obtained from cattle, sheep, goats, and fish. The quantity and quality of animal fats vary from species to species. Fat composition may vary in different parts of the body in the same species.

Table 4.13: Fatty acid composition of edible oils/fats (%).

Fats/ Oils	SFA	MUFA	PUFA	Linoleic acid (n-6)	α-linolenic acid (n-3)
Coconut	90.86	7.24	1.90	1.90	–
Corn oil	16.60	33.67	49.74	48.97	0.76
Cotton seed	28.17	19.66	52.16	51.81	0.35
Gingelly (sesame) oil	16.25	41.41	42.34	41.96	0.39
Groundnut	18.94	53.89	27.17	27.17	–
Mustard	5.72	67.09	27.19	15.65	11.64
Palm oil	44.98	43.53	11.49	11.18	0.30
Rice bran	23.76	44.12	32.12	31.56	0.56
Safflower (Kardi)	9.19	14.04	76.78	76.58	0.13
Safflower (Blended)	19.53	37.61	42.86	42.09	0.78
Soybean	15.96	24.06	59.98	54.78	5.20
Sunflower	11.39	25.96	62.65	62.65	–
Ghee	71.02	26.44	2.54	2.00	0.55
Vanaspati	61.44	33.87	4.69	4.69	–

(- below detectable limits)

Source: Longvah T, Ananthan R, Bhaskarachary K, et al. Indian Food Composition Tables. Hyderabad: National Institute of Nutrition, Indian Council of Medical Research; 2017.

Fat which cushions the vital organs of the animal is generally not used in cooking because it melts slowly. However, fat present underneath the layer of skin from some species like hogs, beef, and sheep is used as edible fat, e.g., lard and tallow. This fat tends to contain more MUFA and melts easily. However, it is more easily oxidized than the fat stored in fatty tissues. Fat is inherently present in egg, poultry, and fish but it is invisible fat, which cannot be separated out. This fat generally melts while cooking. Animal fats are generally solid in nature and most fats are heat-stable compared with vegetable fats.

The fat in milk can be separated and consumed independently in the form of visible fats. Examples are butter, cream, ghee (desi ghee). In general, animal fats contain more saturated fatty acids, cholesterol and some fat-soluble vitamins such as vitamin A. Butter and cream are comparatively easily digested, as they contain short-chain fatty acids, which do not require bile salts for digestion in the small intestine. Therefore for people with fat malabsorption these are better options. However, consumption of excess amount of animal fats may be harmful for health and increase one's risk for many degenerative diseases.

CONSEQUENCES OF INSUFFICIENT INTAKE OF FATS AND OILS

In India and several other low- and middle-income countries, there are segments of the population whose fat intakes are very low for several reasons such as unaffordability, weight loss and fad diets and medical prescription. Since fat is an important source of fuel (energy), insufficient fat intake leads to chronic energy deficiency (CED) syndrome which is common in underfed children and in adults. They also face deficiency of EFA and its consequences.

Zero-fat or low-fat diets (giving less than 5% of the total calories) are often consumed for weight loss by persons of different age groups. A very low-fat diet is defined as one in which ≤15% of total calories are derived from fat.

In a very large study conducted in the United States, it was observed that a low-fat diet does not offer protection against breast or colorectal cancer and cardiovascular disease. Consuming low-fat diets that supply less than 15% of total energy intakes may be too low to maintain desirable body weight. Also use of the fat-soluble vitamins A, D, E, and K may be compromised. Generally foods that contain invisible fats, may be restricted on such diets, leading to lower intakes of other important nutrients such as iron, zinc, vitamin B_{12}, and calcium. A low-fat and high-carbohydrate diet may also lead to unfavorable changes in serum triglycerides, cholesterol, and HDL.

In children, low-fat diets could result in EFA deficiency. Children with LA deficiency exhibited desquamation, thickening of skin, and faltering of growth. Consequences of omega-3 deficiency, i.e., abnormal visual function and peripheral neuropathy did not respond to LA supplementation.

Inclusion of plenty of vegetables, pulses, and fruits is advisable rather than consuming high amount of starchy foods. This can be a preventive measure to avoid risk of cardiovascular diseases. However, weight loss with such diets has been found to be short-lived, and persons often regain weight after they stop the diet, because continuing on such a diet may be difficult. Some persons switch over to their regular dietary habits and tend to indulge in the food products, which have hidden fats like bakery products and high amount of simple carbohydrates.

CONSEQUENCES OF EXCESSIVE CONSUMPTION OF FATS AND OILS

Fat is an integral part of the diet and most people relish fat-laden food preparations owing to their irresistible taste and flavor. Fat is used for various purposes in food—ranging from improving texture and color, mouthfeel, food appeal, as a gesture of happiness, prosperity or celebration and for prolonging shelf-life. Some people think fried food is microbiologically safe rather than boiled or raw food, particularly during travelling. With a high-fat intake (more than 35% of dietary calories). There can be adverse consequences, especially when:

- Intake of total amount of fat is high
- Intake of saturated fats sources is high
- Fat source contains more lauric, myristic and palmitic acids.

It is not only the quantity of fat but the fatty acid composition also plays an important role in causing adverse effects which are:

- More adipose tissue (fat deposition) in the body
- Affecting or deshaping the body contour leading to psycho-social problems.
- Overweight and obesity
- Elevated levels of serum cholesterol and low-density lipoprotein (LDL)
- High risk of coronary heart disease, certain cancers, inflammatory diseases and autoimmune diseases.

More fat in the diet results in more fat cells and amount of fat per cell in the body. It leads to weight gain thus overweight, obesity, coronary heart disease, inflammatory diseases, and certain types of cancer. Type and level of fatty acid intakes, percentage of energy from total fat, dietary cholesterol, lipoprotein levels, intakes of antioxidants and dietary fiber, and activity levels have effects on health. Excessive consumption of dietary n-6 tends to suppress the production of eicosanoids and cause many chronic diseases, inflammatory and autoimmune diseases. Dietary cholesterol elevates serum cholesterol and LDL levels, but the extent of the increase is highly variable. The saturated fatty acids—lauric, myristic, and palmitic, elevate serum cholesterol and low-density lipoprotein (LDL) levels.

WAYS TO REDUCE FAT INTAKE

- Use as little oil as possible for seasoning when making vegetable preparations, curries, dal, etc.
- Limit or avoid use of oil/ghee for chapatis, phulkas, and parathas.
- Avoid consumption of deep-fried foods like samosa, kachori, sev, puris, mathris, wadas, burgers, vegetable or non-vegetarian puffs, fried chicken or sweets containing a lot of fat.
- Avoid consuming too much of nuts like peanuts, almonds, coconut particularly dry coconut, etc.
- Keep absorption of fat during frying to a minimum. Foods which are soaked in fat tend to be less palatable and give more calories.
- Absorption of fat during frying can be minimized by heating the oil to the right temperature, keeping contact time of the food with the oil to a minimum, not overloading the frying pan (this will prolong cooking time and hence increase oil absorption), water content and fat content of the dough should not be too much (more water and fat increase fat absorption)
- Minimize use of foods like biscuits, cookies, wafers, chocolates, ice-creams, kulfis, Indian sweets, pastries, instant noodles, cakes, frankies, etc.; they contain relatively high amounts of hidden/invisible fat. Icing on pastries and cakes is visible and fat content is quite high.
- Trim all fat from nonvegetarian foods.
- Read label information very carefully when purchasing processed foods.
- Include more of fiber-containing foods in the diet.
- Use low-fat dairy products.
- Use flavorful and fragrant herbs and spices in dishes.

ADVERSE EFFECTS OF USING RANCID OR REHEATED OILS

Unsaturated fats like vegetable oils contain unsaturated fatty acids which are unstable. The PUFAs in the oils tend to be easily oxidized under the influence of heat, air and light. These conditions inevitably occur during food processing. When oil is heated repeatedly, oxidative degradation is accelerated. During deep frying the high temperatures used, the moisture in the food and air result in a series of chemical reactions such as oxidation, polymerization, hydrolysis, isomerization, and lipid peroxidation. At the same time, the natural antioxidants that are present in the oil are depleted.

Repeated heating results in both chemical and physical degradation. Characteristically, the viscosity of the oil is increased and it becomes darker in color, because of the formation of volatile and nonvolatile compounds such as free fatty acids, trans isomers, ketones, aldehydes, alcohols, hydrocarbons, and cyclic as well as epoxy compounds.

Oxidation of PUFA results in formation of hydroxides and lipid peroxides such as 4-hydroxynonenal and 4-hydroxyhexenal followed by aldehydes that are potentially toxic. Animal studies have shown that when these compounds are ingested, they cause significant damage to the gut and the liver. The polycyclic hydrocarbons that are formed have been linked to development of gastric cancers. These compounds are quite readily absorbed and have been shown to damage liver, thymus, and kidney as well as increasing risk of atherosclerosis in animal studies. Repeatedly heated oils have been shown to impair endothelium-dependent vasodilatation and have harmful effects on endothelial function as well as reduce nitric oxide levels, thus increasing the contractility of vascular smooth muscle.

Oxidized PUFA increases susceptibility to atherosclerosis by altering the cholesterol metabolism. Like PUFA, cholesterol in foods can also be oxidized and consumption of oxidized cholesterol increases risk of atherosclerosis. Chronic feeding of rats with whole oxidized oils and fats has been found to result in growth retardation, intestinal irritation, hemolytic anemia, enlarged liver and kidney, increased amount of lipid peroxides in liver as well as lower amounts of the antioxidant vitamin E in both serum and liver.

There are certain precautionary measures to prevent fats/oils from being oxidized:

- Store fats and oils in air tight containers.
- Avoid using the same oil repeatedly for deep frying (not more than 2–3 times for short durations, if it must be used)
- Avoid heating for long duration.
- Remove food particles before using oil again for frying
- Do not use if oil has thickened or darkened
- Do not mix fresh oil in used heated oil.

FAT REPLACERS

Fat is a valuable food component because it performs a wide variety of functions in foods ranging from contributing to the flavor of foods, taste, aroma, creamy texture, appearance, palatability, besides providing lubrication. They are carriers/vehicles for lipophilic flavor compounds. However, because excess consumption of fat is harmful; it becomes necessary to replace/remove fat. Fat replacement may be the need of the hour to reduce the overconsumption of fats and oils to reduce the global prevalence of obesity and associated health problems. This is especially so as consumers are becoming increasingly aware about the adverse effects of excessive fat intakes. One way to reduce fat content of the diet is to use ingredients with less fat, e.g., low fat or skimmed milk instead of whole milk. However, removing fat brings about changes in the properties of fat. Hence, when a replacement for fat is sought in order to reduce the energy (kcals) supplied by fat, all of the physical properties of the food need to be kept in mind. Fat can be replaced by reformulating the foods with lipid or protein or carbohydrate-based ingredients singly or in combination. The appearance, texture, etc. can be retained by use of fat replacers. Fat replacers are ingredients that imitate one or more of the functions of fat and hence are used to replace the fat in food products. They provide fewer calories than fat.

By definition, fat replacers are "carbohydrate-, protein-, or fat-based compounds that replace one or more of the functions of fat to reduce the calories in the food". Fat replacers can be synthetic fat substitutes, emulsifiers, starch derivatives, maltodextrins, hemicelluloses, β-glucans, bulking agents, microparticulates, composites, and functional blends. They can be categorized as follows:

Fat substitutes	Fat mimetics	Fat analogs	Fat extenders
These are synthetic compounds and and can be used to replace the fat on weight by weight basis. Structurally they are similar to fat but are not digested by the lipolytic enzymes in the human intestines.	These can imitate the physical or organoleptic properties of fat (hence their name). They are also called texturizing agents For them to be functional, a considerable amount of water needs to be used in the preparation.	These compounds have many of the characteristics of fat but are not digested in the same way in the human gastrointestinal tract.	These substances allow reduction in the amount of fat used in a food preparation by optimizing the functionality of the fat.

Fat Substitutes

Fat substitutes are compounds that resemble dietary fat in chemical structure of the dietary fat that is triglycerides but are not same. They are either chemically synthesized or the chemical structure itself is so modified enzymatically, that while the substance may retain the physicochemical properties of fat but provide fewer calories on per gram basis. During digestion, these compounds may resist lipase action on fat and are not completely absorbed in the body and eventually provide zero to low calories. They are stable at frying temperatures and high cooking temperature and thus can be used in 1:1 proportion with other fats and oils.

Fat Mimetics

Fat mimetics that mimic or imitate the physical or organoleptic properties of fat but cannot be used to replace the fat in a recipe on a gram to gram basis or one-to-one. They are generally made from carbohydrate, lipid or protein bases that have been either chemically or physically modified so that they can perform like fats functionally. Some of them are digested and they can give anything from zero calories to 4 kcal per gram of the substance. They are not suitable for frying operations because they absorb considerable amount of water and there is likelihood of either denaturation (in case of protein) or caramelization (of carbohydrates) at the typically high temperatures used for frying. However, the product can be subjected to baking or retorting. They are not able to completely give the same flavor that fat can give as they are water soluble. Therefore for incorporating lipophilic flavors, emulsifiers may need to be used.

Wide range of fat replacers is available such as modified starch, maltodextrin, polydextrose, pectin, microcrystalline cellulose, resistant starch, carrageenan gels, xanthan gum, ethoxylated glucoside tetraoleate, guar gum, gelatin, sucrose fatty acid polyester. Many of them are being used by food industries which manufacture baked goods, chocolates, salad dressings, confectionary, and frozen desserts, margarine, shortening spreads, butter, processed meat products, dairy products, soups, mayonnaise, sauces, gravies and snack products, peanut butter, yogurt, cottage cheese, fruit spreads, icing mixes, cake mixes, etc. Each type of replacer performs specific functions. Thus they can definitely impact the diet quality, e.g., if a person judiciously chooses to consume a snack containing fat replacer, it will reduce the energy intake of the person. However, portion control and physical activity are better options rather than being solely dependent on fat replacers in weight loss management.

Fat replacers can be grouped/classified into four categories:
1. Carbohydrates-based fat replacers
2. Protein-based fat replacers
3. Lipid-based fat replacers
4. Structured lipids.

Carbohydrate-based Fat Replacers

Carbohydrate-based fat replacers are fat mimetics, which partially or totally replace fat. They provide 4 kcal/g. They include modified food starches, resistant starch, dextrins, polyols or sugar alcohols, fructooligosaccharides, pectin, xanthan gum, hydrocolloids, maltodextrin, and carrageenan. These are obtained from starches of corn, waxy maize, wheat, potato, tapioca, rice, and waxy rice. Carbohydrate polymers need more liquid for obtaining creamy texture and mouthfeel. Hydrocolloids include gums, gels, and fibers, which provide thickness and used as stabilizers and emulsifiers. Corn syrups, syrup solids, and high-fructose corn syrups are used as fat replacers in some fat-free and reduced-fat cookies. These are used successfully in many baked products and frozen desserts, candies, salad dressings, soups, chewing gums, etc. Carbohydrate-based fat mimetics are not suitable for frying, but can be used as fat barriers for fried foods and in baked goods. Gums like guar gum, xanthan gum, locust bean gum, carrageenan, gum arabic, and pectins are used in combination with other systems as fat replacers or bulking agents. Their function is to retain moisture/increase water holding capacity and retard staling, texturize and provide mouthfeel, increase viscosity/thicken, gelling properties, and to stabilize gels. They are used in salad dressings, icings, glazes, desserts, ice-cream, baked products, dairy products, soups, and sauces.

Sometimes bran and pectin are used in food product development to add bulk and flavor, e.g., apple sauce and prune puree are cellulose-based fat replacers which are used in salad dressings. Powdered cellulose has the ability to retain three to ten times its weight and exploited in the manufacture of low-fat sauces. They are also used in fried batter coatings, fried cake doughnuts, to increase the volume of baked goods, because it can stabilize air bubbles and minimize shrinkage of the product after baking. Inulin and oat bran in combination with corn flour are used to impart desirable mouthfeel. They can sustain high temperatures for small duration but are not suitable for frying operations.

Inulin is nondigestible natural oligosaccharides that have similar texture factories without adversely affecting flavor. It is a good stabilizer in aqueous phase.

Protein-based Fat Replacers

Protein-based fat replacers are also fat mimetics. They are manufactured from egg white, milk, whey protein, soy, gelatin, and wheat gluten. Some of which are microparticulate and form microscopic particles. Microparticulate protein is created by heating and blending proteins at high temperature to develop microscopic particles which give creamy mouthfeel and texture of fat. They are being used for emulsification in making dairy products, salad dressings, frozen desserts, and margarines. Protein-based fat replacers have some limitations like they cannot be used for frying and baking because the protein will coagulate at high temperature and loose its creaminess. Protein-based replacers are used for texturization, providing mouthfeel, and to improve the water-holding capacity. They can be used to emulsify as well as stabilize. Protein fat substitutes are micro egg white, milk protein, whey protein, zein (maize protein) are commonly used in butter, spreads, cheese, mayonnaise, etc.

Fat-based Fat Replacers

Fat-based substitutes are developed by chemical altering of fatty acids to provide lesser calories, e.g., three fatty acids of triglycerides (form of dietary fat) from vegetable oils replaced with one or two fatty acids or mono or diglycerides using polysorbate. It provides 5 kcal /g. They may behave like emulsifiers. SALATRIM (short- and long-chain acyl triglycerides) is a good example of fat-based fat replacer. Fat- or lipid-based replacers are used as emulsifiers, carry flavor, tenderizers, dough conditioners, as well as to prevent retrogradation of starch and prevent staling, to conduct heat, help to make the product crispy, provide plasticity and spreadability, increase overrun (aeration and increase volume), provide mouthfeel. Various lipid-based fat replacers are available such as sucrose polyester, alkyl glycoside polyesters, polyesters made with raffinose, trehalose, or stachyose, medium-chain triglycerides, fatty alcohol esters of malonic and alkyl malonic acids, or polycarboxylic acids esterified with fatty alcohols.

Olestra is the first fat-based fat replacer. It is composed of hexa, hepta and octa ester of sucrose esterified with long-chain fatty acids derived from vegetable oils. It can be liquid or solid depending upon the raw material. It has similar organoleptic and thermal properties but not digested by gastric and pancreatic enzymes like normal fat, hence does not provide calories. It may cause side effect such as abdominal cramps or loose stools if the amount consumed at one time is more than 20 g, because it is neither digested nor absorbed. Also it binds with fat-soluble vitamins and reduces their absorption although absorption of other vitamins and minerals and the macronutrients is not affected. Other fat replacers similar to olestra type fat substitutes are sorbitol polyester, sorbestrin, trehalose polyester, raffinose, polyester and stachyose polyester. Sucrose fatty acid esters (SFE) are also fat substitutes, but are different from SPE because they are easily digested and absorbed. Hence unlike SPE, they provide calories. They are used to retard ripening of fruits and are used as lubricants or as anticaking, anti-thinning or antimicrobial agents.

Salatrim is the generic name for a family of structured triglycerides-containing short-chain fatty acid and one long-chain fatty acid like stearic acid randomly attached to glycerol. It provides fewer calories (5 kcal/g) than fat because short chain fatty acids have lower calorific value and because stearic acid is not completely absorbed. By varying the amounts of short chain and long chain fatty acids, salatrim compositions have different physical and functional properties such as differing melting points, hardness, etc. It is useful in making reduced fat bakery products and confectionery, particularly for lowering the *trans*-fat. It is used in products such as chocolate flavored coatings, caramels and toffees, frozen desserts, and cheese but cannot be used for frying.

Structured Lipids

Structured lipids (SLs) are triacylglycerols that are modified by chemically and/or enzymatically catalyzed reactions and/or genetic engineering. New fatty acids are incorporated or the position of the fatty acid is changed. Alternatively, novel triglycerides may be made for specific desired properties. These are generally produced with desired physical characteristics, chemical properties, and/or nutritional benefits, depending on the metabolic effect desired, such as providing simultaneous delivery of beneficial long-chain fatty acids (LCFAs) at a slower rate and medium-chain fatty acids (MCFAs) at a quicker rate. They offer a means of delivering target fatty acids for even therapeutic purposes or to alleviate a disease or metabolic condition. Applications for human health include use in enteral and parenteral nutrition, enhancing immune function, improving nitrogen balance, reducing cholesterol and triglycerides, preventing thrombosis, reducing cancer risk, and reducing caloric intake.

Besides this, they are used for their functional properties such as melting point, iodine and saponification values. The approaches used for modifications that are carried out can be: (i) the glycerol moiety in the triglyceride is replaced by another alcohol, e.g., carbohydrate or sugar alcohol or polyols; (ii) the long-chain fatty acids in the triglyceride molecule may be replaced by either a short- or medium-chain or another long-chain fatty acid by esterifying them to glycerol.

When SL is modified in the solid fats are also referred as plastic fats, e.g., margarine, modified butters and shortenings. SL composed of MCFAs and linoleic acid may be helpful in pancreatic disease or malabsorption. Several commercial products are available that have different applications such as margarine fats, cocoa butter equivalents, frying oils, fats for confectionery and candies, dairy products, and breast milk fat substitute.

Protein-based Fat Mimetics

These are manufactured from egg, milk, whey, soy, gelatin, and wheat gluten. Some of which are microparticulate and form microscopic particles mimic the mouthfeel and texture of fat. Some proteins are processed to mimic other functional properties of fat such as emulsification. They are generally used in dairy products, salad dressings, frozen desserts, and margarines. Most of the protein-based fat mimetics cannot be used for frying but can be used as ingredients in foods that will be cooked.

Carbohydrate-based Fat Mimetics

These are used to partially or totally replace fat. They are digestible carbohydrates such as modified starches, dextrins providing approximately less than half the calories given by fat, as their calorific value is 4 kcal/g. Other nondigestible carbohydrates that are used will provide fewer calories. Different types of carbohydrate-based fat mimetics are used for different purposes in varied foods. Corn syrups, syrup solids, and high-fructose corn syrups are used as fat replacers in some fat-free and reduced-fat cookies. Sugar alcohols like sorbitol, maltitol and fructooligosaccharides are used to control water activity. Xanthan gum and carageenan are used as stabilizers in fat-free salad dressings. Carbohydrate-based fat mimetics are not suitable for frying but can be used as fat barriers for fried foods and in baked goods. Gums are used as thickeners to increase viscosity, as stabilizers and gelling agents. Gums like guar gum, xanthan gum, locust bean gum, carrageenan, gum arabic, and pectin are used in combination with other systems as fat replacers or bulking agents. They are used in salad dressings, icings, glazes, desserts, ice-cream, baked products, dairy products, soups, and sauces.

Different types of starches obtained from different sources possess different functional properties and are used to provide sensory properties of oil, e.g., slippery mouthfeel. Examples are corn, waxy maize, wheat, potato, tapioca, rice, and waxy rice.

Cellulose-based Fat Replacers

These are used in salad dressings, frozen desserts, sauces, and dairy products. Powdered cellulose has the ability to retain three to ten times its weight. This property is exploited in manufacture of reduced fat sauces. It is also used in fried batter coatings, fried cake donuts, to increase the volume of baked goods, because it can stabilize air bubbles and minimize shrinkage of the product after baking.

Maltodextrins

These are used to increase viscosity, bind/control water. They give a smooth mouthfeel in foods such as table spreads, margarine, imitation sour cream, salad dressings, baked goods, frostings, fillings, sauces, processed meat, and frozen desserts.

Polydextrose

It is a polymer of glucose, sorbitol, and citric or phosphoric acid, used in either liquid or powdered and acidic or neutralized forms. Polydextrose provides 1 kcal/g. It is used as a bulking and texturizer in a wide variety of products including baked foods, salad dressings, peanut spreads, and fruit spreads, soft and hard candies, as well as chewing gum. It imparts smoothness in product with high moisture content. However, it can act as a laxative, especially if a single serving of the product contains more than 15 g.

The hull or bran of oats is enzymatically hydrolyzed and used. It can be combined with corn flour to impart desirable mouthfeel. It can be used in products that are processed at high temperatures for short periods of time but is not suitable for frying operations.

Researchers are studying use of whole foods as fat replacers. Many of them contain a range of carbohydrates, lipids, and proteins that may be advantageous in ensuring the rheological properties of the food product especially baked goods. Another important benefit is that they contain micronutrients and phytoactives that are beneficial for health. They have been found to have the least effects on the physical and sensory properties of baked goods. Some of the foods that have been tested include apricot kernel flour, chia seed mucilage, high-oleic sunflower oil, avocado puree, apple puree or pomace, bean and pea purees, oat bran or β-glucan powder, and tapioca starch.

In view to reduce the fat consumption and still make the food product tasty with cream-like mouthfeel, fat replacers mentioned above are used in wide variety of food products. The fat replacers reformulate the foods and also maintain the appearance, taste, aroma, creamy texture, appearance, palatability, lubrication, which otherwise is provided by fats and oils. Fat can be replaced by lipid- or protein- or carbohydrate-based ingredients singly or in combination. Fat replacers are ingredients that imitate one or more of the functions of fat and hence are used to replace the fat in food products. They provide fewer calories than fat.

DIGESTION AND ABSORPTION OF FAT

Most of the fats present in foodstuffs and the diet is in the form of triglycerides, with small quantities of cholesterol esters and phospholipids. The challenges in digestion are that the triglyceride molecule is rather large and most lipids are insoluble in water whereas in the gastrointestinal tract, fat has to be digested in aqueous surroundings.

Mouth: Not much digestion occurs in the mouth. At the base of the tongue, the salivary gland produces a lipase "lingual lipase". In adults, this does not have a significant role because it digests the short-chain fatty acids and medium-chain fatty acids present in milk. However, in infants, this lingual lipase is important for digestion of milk lipids.

Digestion of dietary fat occurs in three phases:
1. Gastric phase
2. Duodenal phase
3. Ileal phase.

Stomach: In the gastric phase, crude emulsification of the fats occurs, as chyme is formed as a result of the mechanical churning of the stomach contents. When food enters the stomach, it stimulates release of the hormone gastrin, which circulates in blood and stimulates release of a lipase called human gastric lipase (HGL). HGL is a component of gastric juices and it hydrolyzes approximately 10% of the ingested fat. HGL acts primarily on short-chain fatty acids. Thus most of the fat digestion actually takes place in the small intestines. The emulsified fat in chime is separated from the rest because it is less dense and the contents of the stomach are aqueous.

Small intestine: The small amount of breakdown products stimulates secretion of the following 3 vital "actors" into the intestines:
1. Cholecystokinin
2. Bile containing bile salts from the gallbladder
3. Pancreatic juice containing lipases.

Cholecystokinin is important because it inhibits gut motility. It is also important because it triggers release of bile into the duodenum by the gallbladder. Before the fat can be acted upon by the lipases, it has to be solubilized in the fluid present in the intestine. Because fat is insoluble and the enzymes are present in water, as such digestion is difficult. Bile salts therefore perform a very important role of emulsifying the fat. Bile salts are amphipathic molecules, i.e., one part of the molecule is not soluble in water (hydrophobic) and the other is soluble in water. The bile salts associate with small amounts of the fat with the hydrophobic part inward, the water-soluble part outward. This enables the fat to remain in solution. Formation of micelles helps to solubilize dietary fat anywhere from 10–1,000 times, once the fat is in solution; it becomes accessible to the pancreatic lipase. Pancreatic lipase acts on TG and the products of breakdown are—a monoglyceride and 2 fatty acids.

- Pancreatic lipase does most of the work of digestion. Pancreatic lipase for its activity requires colipase which is also secreted by the pancreas. For digestion of dietary phopsholipids and cholesterol esters different enzymes are required. Dietary phospholipids are hydrolyzed by pancreatic phospholipase A_2 and cholesterol esters by pancreatic cholesterol ester hydrolase. About 40% of dietary cholesterol is absorbed directly.

> Bile is a mixture of bile acids, free cholesterol, and phospholipids. Bile acids and phospholipids are amphipathic, i.e., they possess both hydrophilic and hydrophobic groups. The hydrophilic groups associate with water and the hydrophobic groups with the lipid. This helps the large droplets of fat to be emulsified into micelles and prevents them from coalescing together. This also stabilizes the lipid particles and increases the surface area exposing more ester bonds to the lipases (action is like that of detergents).

Hence in cases/conditions where fat digestion poses a problem, consumption of fats containing short-chain fatty acids or medium-chain fatty acids, i.e., medium-chain triglyceride is advised.

ABSORPTION

Absorption of fat/ileal phase: This is basically the process by which dietary fats from the mixed micelles enter the enterocyte. The process is known as "translocation". This translocation of the long-chain fatty acids and the monoglyceride takes place with the help of a fatty acid-binding protein (FABP), which is present within the cell membrane and the cell also. Different FABPs have preference (specificity) for different LCFA. As the LCFA and 2-monoglyceride exit the mixed micelle, within the enterocyte itself, the LCFA is again combined with (re-esterification) the monoglyceride. This reaction is carried out (catalyzed) by the enzyme acyl-CoA cholesterol acyl transferase or called ACAT in brief.

Similarly, phospholipids are also reassembled in the enterocyte. Almost 90% of the fatty acids and monoglyceride that have been produced as a result of digestion are incorporated back into TG/phospholipids. Most of the free cholesterol that was absorbed is also reesterified by the enzyme.

The products of digestion, i.e., the monoglycerides and the fatty acids are now transported into the enterocyte, where triacylglycerols are reassembled. The triacylglycerols are then assembled together with cholesterol, phospholipid, and apoproteins into chylomicrons. However, there is a difference among fatty acids, determined by their chain length.

- Fatty acids containing <12 carbon atoms, i.e., SCFA and MCFA are directly absorbed into portal circulation may be transported as unesterified fatty acids bound to albumin. They are transported to the liver, which oxidizes these fatty acids.

- Long-chain fatty acids having more than 12 carbon atoms are unable to pass into the enterocyte directly. Hence they associate with bile salts and micelles are again formed. This complex may also contain fat-soluble vitamins and cholesterol. Such a micelle is called a "mixed" micelle. The micelle is absorbed (by diffusion) into the enterocyte where it is acted upon further.

The next stage is transport of the lipids out of the enterocyte. This essentially consists of formation of lipoproteins and their secretion, i.e., the resynthesized lipid is combined with a protein molecule which is known as lipoprotein. In the intestinal cells, the newly formed triglyceride and cholesterol esters as well as phospholipids are assembled with proteins to form the lipoprotein "chylomicrons" (lipids are covered by a protein layer and thus stabilizes the lipid for transport in lymph and blood, i.e., in an aqueous environment). These chylomicrons via lymph enter circulation through the thoracic duct and the lipids reach to different parts of the body. In the blood vessels, there is an enzyme "lipoprotein lipase", which is located on the surface of capillaries and acts on the lipid in the chylomicrons. It hydrolyzes the fatty acids from the TG. These fatty acids, then, are utilized by muscle cells and oxidized for energy or are released into the systemic circulation and returned to the liver. In adipose tissue, they will be re-esterified again to form TG which is stored. The chylomicron without the fatty acids still contains other lipids in its core. It is now renamed "chylomicron remnant", which is then transferred to the liver.

Within the intestines, bile is reabsorbed in the ileum. It then reaches blood and then to liver to be reutilized. Bile is stored in the gallbladder. In case of gallstones, bile does not reach the gut and hence fat digestion may be affected. Absorption of vitamins A, D, E, and K is also impaired. Liver is the key organ for fat metabolism. Level of lipids including cholesterol in blood is controlled by the liver. If triglyceride level is low, the liver can synthesize the triglyceride (called de novo synthesis).

In summary digestion and absorption of LCFA consists of five different phases are described in Figure 4.10.

Digestion and absorption of fat is influenced by the following factors:
- **Amount of fat consumed**: When fat-rich foods are taken in one meal, it takes longer for the fat to be digested and absorbed. All of the fat may not be digested and absorbed.

- **Kind of fatty acid in the fat**: Long-chain fatty acid takes longer time than SCFA and MCT. Degree of saturation of fatty acids also affects digestion. Saturated fatty acids are less well digested.
- **High calcium** intakes may hinder, since calcium can bind with the fatty acids and form soaps.
- **Presence of emulsifying agent**: Bile works as emulsifying agent due to the presence of lecithin. However, if there is a problem with either the liver or the gallbladder, digestion can be affected.

RAPID FIRE

1. What is the basic difference in fats and oils and their fatty acid composition?
2. What are the different lipids?
3. How fat is important in cellular function?
4. List the functions of phospholipids.
5. What is the major role of different types of fatty acids?
6. Why excess of omega-6 is harmful and omega-3 is beneficial?
7. What is the percent contribution of fat to total calories?
8. What is role of invisible fat in health?
9. Which fats are healthy and which ones are unhealthy and why?
10. What are the functions of cholesterol and phytosterols?
11. What are fat replacers?
12. Why is MUFA important?

EXERCISE

1. Find out the amount of visible and invisible fat in your one-day diet. Are your intakes within the recommended levels? Pinpoint the unhealthy fat or food preparation in the diet.
2. Prepare a plan to guidelines for few obese persons or heart patients with regard to fat intake.
3. Find out the fatty acid composition in different brands of fats and oils available in the market and give comments with regard to their use to control high serum cholesterol and high LDL.

SUGGESTED READING

1. Akoh CC, Min DB. Food lipids: chemistry, nutrition, and biotechnology, 3rd edition. New York: Marcel Dekker; 2008.
2. Akoh CC. Fat Replacers: A Scientific Status Summary. IFT. 1998;52(3):47–53.
3. American Dietetic Association (ADA). Position of the American Dietetic Association: Fat Replacers. J Am Diet Assoc. 2005;105:266–75.
4. AOCS Lipid Library. Lipids: Definitions, Classification and Nomenclature.
5. Belitz HD, Grosch W. Food chemistry, 2nd edition. Berlin: Springer-Verlag; 1999.
6. Benatti P, Peluso G, Nicolai R, et al. Polyunsaturated fatty acids: biochemical, nutritional and epigenetic properties. J Am Coll Nutr. 2004;23(4):281–302.
7. Beresford SA, Johnson KC, Ritenbaugh C, et al. Low-fat dietary pattern and risk of colorectal cancer: the Women's Health Initiative Randomized Controlled Dietary Modification Trial. JAMA. 2006; 95:643–54.
8. Chow CK. Fatty acids in foods and their health implication, 3rd edition. New York: Marcel Dekker; 2008.
9. Eritsland J. Safety considerations of polyunsaturated fatty acids. Am J Clin Nutr. 2000;71(1Suppl):197S–201.
10. Esterbauer H. Cytotoxicity and genotoxicity of lipid oxidation products. Am J Clin Nutr 57(5Suppl) 779S–86.

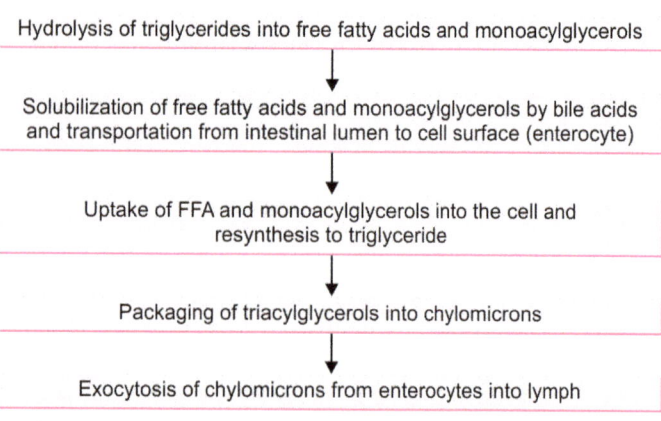

Fig. 4.10: Digestion and absorption of long-chain fatty acids (LCFA).

11. Fahy E, Subramaniam S, Brown HA, et al. A Comprehensive Classification System for Lipids. J Lipid Res. 2005;46(5):839–61.
12. Feingold KR, Grunfeld C. Introduction to Lipids and Lipoproteins. Endotext (Internet). South Dartmouth (MA): MD Text. Com, Inc; 2018.
13. Ghafoorunissa, Krishnaswamy K. Diet and Heart Disease. Hyderabad: National Institute of Nutrition, Indian Council of Medical Research; 2004.
14. Ghafoorunissa. Impact of quality of dietary fat on serum cholesterol and coronary heart disease: focus on plant sterols and other non-glyceride components. Natl Med J India. 2009;22(3):126–32.
15. Gopalan C, Shatri BVR, Balasubrahmanium. Nutritive value of Indian foods. Hyderabad: National Institute of Nutrition Indian Council of Medical Research Hyderabad; 2004.
16. Howard BV, Manson JE, Stefanick ML, et al. Low-fat dietary pattern and weight change over 7 years: the Women's Health Initiative Dietary Modification Trial. JAMA. 2006;295:39–49.
17. Howard BV, Van Horn L, Hsia J, et al. Low-fat dietary pattern and risk of cardiovascular disease: the Women's Health Initiative Randomized Controlled Dietary Modification Trial. JAMA. 2006;295:655–66.
18. HT Osborn HT, Akoh CC. Structured Lipids–Novel Fats with Medical, Nutraceutical, and Food Applications. Comprehensive reviews in food science and food safety. 2002;1(3):110–20.
19. http://www.chem.qmul.ac.uk/iupac/misc/glylp.html
20. Interim Summary of Conclusions and Dietary Recommendations on Total Fat and Fatty Acids from the Joint FAO/WHO Expert Consultation on Fats and Fatty Acids in Human Nutrition, 10-14 November, 2008, WHO, Geneva https://www.who.int/nutrition/topics/FFA_summary_rec_conclusion.pdf?ua=1
21. Interim Summary of Conclusions and Dietary Recommendations on Total Fat and Fatty Acids From the Joint FAO/WHO Expert Consultation on Fats and Fatty Acids in Human Nutrition, 2008, WHO, Geneva.
22. Kaur N, Chugh V, Gupta AK. Essential fatty acids as functional components of foods-a review. J Food Sci Technol. 2014;51(10): 2289–303.
23. Kelly GS. Conjugated Linoleic acid: A Review. Altern Med Rev. 2001;6(4):367–82.
24. Kris-Etherton PM. Monounsaturated fatty acids and risk of cardiovascular disease. Circulation.1999;100:1253–8.
25. Linder MC. Nutritional Biochemistry and Metabolism with Clinical Applications, 2nd edition. London: Prentice-Hall International Limited; 1999.
26. lipidlibrary.aocs.org/lipids/sph/index.htm
27. Mahan LK, Arlin M. Krause's Food nutrition & diet therapy, 8th edition. Philadelphia: WB Saunders Company; 2007.
28. Manchanda SC, Passi SJ. Selecting healthy edible oil in the Indian context. Indian Heart J. 2016;68(4):447–9.
29. Mani I, Kurpad AV. Fats and fatty acids in Indian diets: Time for serious introspection. Indian J Med Res. 2016; 144(4): 507–14.
30. Molendi-Coste O, Legry V, Leclerq IA. Why and How Meet n-3 PUFA Dietary Recommendations? Gastroenterol Res and Pract. 2011;2011:364040. Mozaffarian D, Aro A, Willett WC. Health effects of trans-fatty acids: experimental and observational evidence. Eur J Clin Nutr. 2009;63Suppl2:S5–21.
31. Mudambi SR, Rajagopal MV. Fundamentals of Food Nutrition and Diet Theory. New Delhi: New Age International Publisher; 2007.
32. Narsinga Rao BS, Sivakumar B. Nutrient Requirements and Recommended Dietary Allowances for Indians, 2nd edition. Hyderabad: Indian Council of Medical Research; 2010.
33. Narsinga Rao BS, Sivakumar B. Nutrient requirements and recommended dietary allowances for Indians, 2nd edition. Hyderabad: Indian Council of Medical Research; 2010. p. 103.
34. National Institute of Nutrition. (2010). Dietary Guidelines for Indians—a manual. [online]. Available from http://ninindia.org/DietaryGuidelinesforNINwebsite.pdf. [last accessed July 2019].
35. Nietzel JJ. Fatty acid molecules: A role in cell signaling. Nature Education. 2010;3(9):57.
36. O'Neale Roach J. Metabolism and Nutrition, 2nd edition. Edinburgh: Mosley, an imprint of Elsevier Ltd.; 2003.
37. Prentice RL, Caan B, Chlebowski RT, et al. Low-fat dietary pattern and risk of invasive breast cancer: the Women's Health Initiative Randomized Controlled Dietary Modification Trial. JAMA. 2006; 295(6): 629–42.
38. Puri D. Textbook of Medical Biochemistry. New Delhi: Elsevier; 2002.
39. Ratnayake WM, Galli C. Fat and fatty acid terminology, methods of analysis and fat digestion and metabolism: background review paper. Ann Nutr Metab. 2009;55:8–43.
40. St-Onge MP, Jones PJ. Physiological effects of medium-chain triglycerides: Potential agents in the prevention of obesity. J Nutr. 2002;132(3): 329–32.
41. Whitney EN, Sizer WF. Nutrition: Concepts & Controversies. Australia: Wadsworth Thomson Learning; 2002.
42. Wijendran V, Hayes KC. Dietary n-6 and n-3 fatty acid balance and cardiovascular health. Annu Rev Nutr. 2004;24:597–615.
43. World Health Organization (WHO). Population Nutrient Intake Goals for Preventing Diet-related Chronic Diseases. [online]. Available from http://www.who.int/nutrition/topics/5_population_nutrient/en/index.html (Last accessed on July 2019).
44. Yehuda S. Omega-6/Omega -3 ratio and brain related functions. World Review of Nutrition and Dietetics. 2002;92:37–56.
45. Youdim KA, Martin A, Joseph JA. Essential fatty acids and the brain: possible health implications. Int J Dev Neurosci. 2000;18(4-5): 383–99.
46. Yu RK, Nakatani Y, Yanagisawa M. The role of glycosphingolipid metabolism in the developing brain. J. Lipid Res. 2009;50Suppl:S440–5.

5
CHAPTER

Energy Metabolism, Energy Balance and Body Weight

KEY CONCERNS
- How is energy generated in the body?
- What are the components of energy expenditure?
- How is energy expenditure estimated?
- How is food intake regulated?
- What are the factors influencing body weight?
- What is energy balance and what are the consequences of energy imbalance?
- What are the energy requirements of different persons?
- What is body composition and how is it estimated?

KEY CONCEPTS
- Energy metabolism and energy generating pathways
- Energy balance
- Energy expenditure
- Body composition and methods of assessment
- Basal metabolic rate (BMR)
- Calculation of energy requirements
- Regulation of food intake and eating disorders
- Body weight regulation

The human body requires energy to perform millions of vital functions such as respiration, digestion, blood circulation, body temperature regulation, muscle contraction and movement, nerve transmission, synthesis and transport of various important biomolecules. Unlike plants, the human body cannot synthesize energy from sunlight. Therefore, energy has to be provided by food, specifically the energy yielding components/macronutrients—carbohydrate, fat, and protein. Another source of energy is alcohol.

WHAT IS ENERGY?

Energy can be explained simply as "the ability or capacity to do work". Energy can be broadly grouped into potential energy and kinetic energy.

There are different forms of energy, the four most common forms being chemical, mechanical, electrical, and thermal. The first law of thermodynamics (the law of conservation of energy) states "**Energy can neither be created nor it is destroyed, however, energy can be converted from one form to any other form of energy**". This implies that energy is conserved. Steam is thermal energy that is used to run an engine (mechanical energy). Electrical energy is converted into thermal energy when we use it for heating water. In a torch or flashlight, chemical energy is converted into electrical energy.

Kinetic energy is the motion of waves, electrons, atoms, molecules, substances, and objects.

Potential energy is stored energy—the energy of position, e.g., gravitational energy.

Mechanical energy is energy possessed by an object because of its motion or its position.

Nuclear energy is the energy stored in the nucleus of an atom and that holds the atom together.

Chemical energy is a form of potential energy in the bonds between atoms within a molecule. This energy holds molecules together and is released when chemicals react. Petroleum and natural gas are examples of stored chemical energy. Chemical energy of a substance can be transformed into other forms of energy. Example—when kerosene is burnt, chemical energy is converted to heat. When food is metabolized, it is converted into another form of energy. Green plants transform solar energy to chemical energy via photosynthesis. In electrochemical reactions, electrical energy can be converted to chemical energy.

Thermal energy is the internal energy of substances because of vibration of the atoms and molecules present in that substance or it is the energy given off by heat.

Radiant energy is electromagnetic energy that travels in transverse waves. Solar energy and light are examples of radiant energy. Other examples are X-rays, gamma rays, and radio waves.

Sound energy is released by vibrating objects that produce sound when a force causes an object to vibrate. This energy is transferred through the substance in a wave.

Potential Energy (Stored energy or energy of position)	Kinetic energy (Energy of motion)
- Gravitational - Stored mechanical - Chemical - Nuclear	- Motion - Sound - Radiant - Thermal - Electrical

There are other examples of energy being converted into other forms of energy. For example, solar panels convert light energy into electricity. Coal goes through different phases from the chemical energy that is stored in coal. When it is burned, heat and light energies are released. Coal is used to produce steam and coal will change into mechanical energy when it is used in a generator.

In food also, energy is stored in the three macronutrients viz. carbohydrates, protein, and fat. When food is consumed, the metabolic processes of the body convert these macronutrients into chemical and thermal energy that helps to maintain body temperature (heat), pH, and move the body, i.e., mechanical energy for muscle contraction and movement. Chemical energy is also converted into electrical energy in brain and nerve activities.

In the human body, energy is required to build, repair and maintain and mainly involve mechanical, chemical and electrical forms of energy.

> One calorie = 4.184 joules
> 1,000 calories = 1 kilocalorie (kcal)
> 1,000 joules = 1 kilojoule (kJ)
> To calculate the energy content in kJ, multiply 4.2 × kcal = kJ
> To calculate the energy content in kcal, multiply 0.239 × kJ = kcal
> Internationally, energy is measured in kilojoules or mega joules. Because the human body utilizes considerable amount of energy and humans consume large amount of energy, generally kilojoules or mega joules is used. However, both measurements—kcal and kJ are used.
> Unit of nutritional energy is the amount of energy in a food or drink and measured in calories. This calorie is too small to measure as energy value of food. Hence, **calorie value of food is written as "kcal", i.e., kilocalories. Similarly, kJ is for kilojoules.**

When a substance is burnt in the presence of oxygen, it generates heat and that can be measured as energy and the unit of that energy is calorie or joules. Energy is measured in joules, i.e., the unit of energy in the International System of Units. It can be defined as "the energy expended/used when 1 kg is moved through a distance of 1 m by the force of one Newton". Joule is the accepted and recommended standard unit of energy used in human energetics, both in terms of energy intake and expenditure. Previously, energy was measured in calories. Calorie is the amount of heat required to raise the temperature of 1 g of water by 1°C from 14.5°C to 15.5°C.

ENERGY METABOLISM

Metabolism refers to all the chemical reactions that take place within the body in order to maintain the living state of cells and the organism as a whole. Complex molecules are broken down to produce energy that is then used to build complex molecules by the body. For example, when a person eats some food, the carbohydrates, proteins, and fats are broken down into molecules that release energy that is used by the body for various functions.

The body requires energy even to move a molecule from one side of a cell membrane to another, such as occurs in active transport (the Na^+-K^+ pump, for example) or in vesicular transport (exocytosis and endocytosis).

All metabolic reactions can be categorized as: (a) catabolic or (b) anabolic reactions. Catabolism is the process by which large molecules are broken down into smaller ones. Anabolism is the process of synthesis of complex compounds. Anabolic processes require energy. The three energy yielding macronutrients in food—after digestion and absorption are oxidized by a complex series of chemical reactions in cells to obtain chemical/metabolic energy from food energy. Metabolic energy is converted into different forms of energy for various purposes in the body (Table 5.1).

Table 5.1: Different forms of energy used for different body functions.

Forms of energy	Body functions
Chemical	Needed for all metabolic reactions including synthesis of new compounds; for growth during pregnancy and childhood and synthesis of milk during lactation. Used to form bonds during chemical reactions, such as the bond formation that occurs when small molecules are used to synthesize large molecules.
Mechanical	Needed for muscle contraction, movement, and physical activity. Uses intracellular protein filaments to generate movement, such as occurs in muscle contraction or the beating of cilia lining the respiratory tract.
Electro-mechanical	Osmosis, active transport for exchange of fluid across cell membrane.
Thermal	Required to maintain body temperature and keep the body warm in cold environment.
Electrical	Involved in the flow of charged particles, needed for brain and nerve activities.

Energy released by oxidation of the macronutrients always takes two forms- heat and work. About 60% of the energy derived from the three macronutrients is used for heat production, which is necessary to maintain body temperature. Most of the remaining 40% of energy is used to synthesize adenosine triphosphate (ATP), which is used to perform cellular work (a process that releases still more heat).

Adenosine Triphosphate: The Currency for Energy

Metabolic energy is also known as chemical energy and its currency is termed ATP (adenosine triphosphate). ATP is an energy-bearing molecule present in all cells and is almost universally used as a molecule for energy transfer.

> **High Energy Compound and High Energy Bonds**
> - ATP (adenosine triphosphate) is a high energy compound due to the presence of two high energy phosphate bonds denoted by the symbol ~.
> - It is produced through biochemical reactions occurring in metabolic cycles, such as tricarboxylic acid (TCA) cycle and oxidation of fatty acids.
> - ATP is broken down into adenosine diphosphate (ADP) and one (Mono) phosphate; free energy is released that is used for various purposes or transformed into other forms of energy (Fig. 5.1).

Cells require constant supply of energy for their metabolic activities. ATP is also required to synthesize the myriad number of molecules that each cell requires to function and exist; ATP is used for many cell functions, such as transporting substances across cell membranes, muscle contraction for body movements as well contraction of heart muscle that is vital for blood circulation. It is also

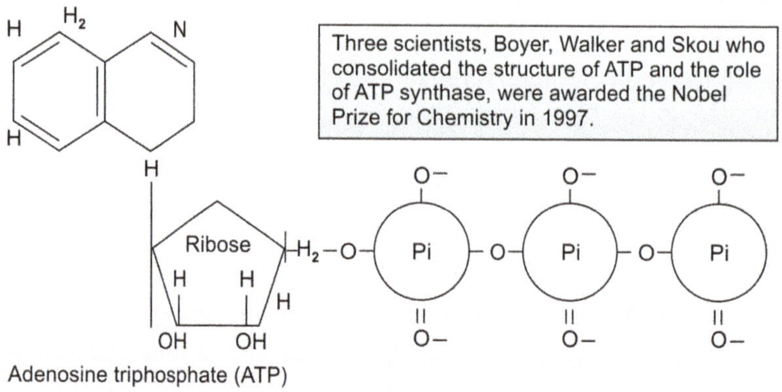

Fig. 5.1: Adenosine triphosphate (ATP) structure.

Three scientists, Boyer, Walker and Skou who consolidated the structure of ATP and the role of ATP synthase, were awarded the Nobel Prize for Chemistry in 1997.

used to control chemical reactions through bonding to protein molecules thus determining their activity. When cells are damaged, their release of ATP is involved in eliciting pain. It can also be released from carotid body to signal the shortage of oxygen in blood. It is released by taste receptor cells that trigger action potentials in sensory nerves, which carry the signal to the brain. Also, it is released to signal a need to empty the bladder when it is full and the bladder wall is stretched.

Energy-consuming activities of cells
- Anabolic reactions, such as protein synthesis
- Synthesis of DNA and RNA
- Synthesis of polysaccharides and lipids
- For active transport of molecules and ions
- Nerve impulses
- Maintenance of cell volume by osmosis

All activities that require energy obtain it from ATP. The human body is made up of approximately one hundred trillion cells, each containing about one billion ATP molecules. This amount of ATP can meet the cells' need for energy for only a few minutes. Hence, ATP needs to be continuously formed.

The covalent bonds that unite the phosphate units in ATP are high-energy bonds (Fig. 5.1). When an ATP molecule is broken down by an enzyme, the third (terminal) phosphate unit is released as a phosphate group that is an ion and an enormous amount of energy is released as shown in Figure 5.2.

Cells obtain ATP not only by oxidation of the three macronutrients but also by regenerating ATP from ADP, for which energy is required, as shown in the equation. With adequate supply of oxygen, ADP$^+$, Pi, and H$^+$ are again converted back into ATP by the enzyme ATP synthase, within the mitochondria (an organelle within the cell that is known as a power house of energy). When oxygen supply is limited, less ATP is formed.

This conversion of ATP to ADP is crucial because by breaking one high energy bond and their arrangement of the molecule, it liberates about 7.5 kcals per mole. This process is efficient. Synthesis of ATP occurs in all organisms. In mammalian cells, it is synthesized during glycolysis in the cytoplasm/cytosol and in the mitochondria by cellular respiration.

Energy Generating Pathways

Various energy generating pathways are involved in the process of ATP formation that essentially occurs in three stages:
1. Glycolysis
2. TCA Cycle
3. Electron Transport Chain.

Glycolysis

It is the primary step in the energy generation process that occurs in the cell cytosol. One molecule of glucose (glucose is a six carbon molecule) is broken down into two molecules of an intermediate compound called glyceraldehyde 3-phosphate, which is then converted into pyruvate (pyruvate is a three carbon molecule). For this reaction, two ATP molecules are required/utilized. The glyceraldehyde 3-phosphate is further broken down, during which two NADH molecules are formed and energy is released, whereby the phosphate group combines with ADP and thus forms two molecules of ATP. Further breakdown to pyruvate will give two more molecules of ATP. However, since two ATP have been utilized until this step, net gain is two molecules of ATP. Pyruvate can also be generated from glycerol and some glucogenic amino acids like alanine, glycine, glutamine, and arginine. Pyruvate is further converted into Acetyl CoA (a two carbon molecule) by decarboxylation. Acetyl CoA enters into the mitochondria where a series of reactions occur in the TCA cycle.

TCA Cycle

Tricarboxylic acid (TCA) cycle is also known as citric acid cycle or Krebs cycle that completes the oxidation of glucose,

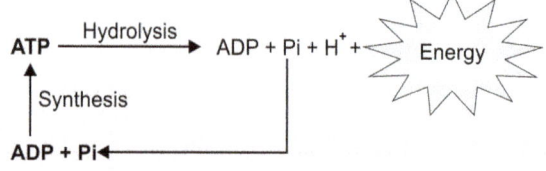

Fig. 5.2: Release of energy from ATP.

amino acids, and fatty acids. It occurs in the mitochondria where all the enzymes and coenzymes needed to produce high energy compounds are present. During the TCA cycle, acetyl CoA that was formed from all three macronutrients is metabolized by a series of reactions ultimately generating carbon dioxide, hydrogen, and electrons. NADH and $FADH_2$ are formed. The hydrogen and electrons are then passed through a series of intermediate compounds (transferred to specific substrates) and ultimately to molecular oxygen in the electron transport chain.

> **Oxidation:** It is a stepwise process that breaks down fat into glycerol and fatty acids. During β-oxidation, at a time, two carbons are taken off from a long chain of fatty acids, thus shortening it until all fatty acids are broken down into acetyl CoA. Glycerol can be converted into pyruvate.

The TCA cycle is important because it is the ultimate stage for oxidation of all three macronutrients. The citric acid cycle starts with acetyl coenzyme A (acetyl CoA). All three macronutrients, i.e., glucose, amino acids, and fatty acids are first converted to acetyl CoA. Fatty acids are converted to acetyl CoA (through the β-oxidation pathway). Among the amino acids, some, which are glucogenic, such as alanine, glycine, glutamine, and arginine are converted into pyruvate. Some others are ketogenic, e.g., leucine and lysine and are converted into acetyl CoA that is a common intermediate. This has been summarized in Figure 5.3.

Electron Transport Chain

Most of the ATP produced by our body is formed by a process called oxidative phosphorylation. Electron transport chain occurs in the mitochondrial membrane. It is a sequence of reduction-oxidation reactions through which energy is released by converting ADP and phosphate into ATP. This is the stage of electron transfer in which NADH and $FADH_2$ give up the electrons they gained from glycolysis and the TCA cycle. This process requires molecular oxygen that comes from regular respiration. Oxidative phosphorylation gives 34 molecules of ATP for every molecule of glucose.

> **Oxidative phosphorylation:** This is a metabolic pathway wherein energy is obtained by oxidation of nutrients to produce ATP. This pathway is used by almost all aerobic organisms and is a highly efficient way of releasing energy.

Generally, the body ensures that ATP is made available for all biochemical and mechanical activities of cells, tissues, and organs, for which the body makes available substrates for ATP production. These processes are regulated by various hormones, such as insulin, glucagon, glucocorticoids, growth hormone, and adrenaline (epinephrine) so that the circulating level of the energy nutrients are maintained at relatively constant level, although the amount of macronutrients obtained from the diet may vary substantially.

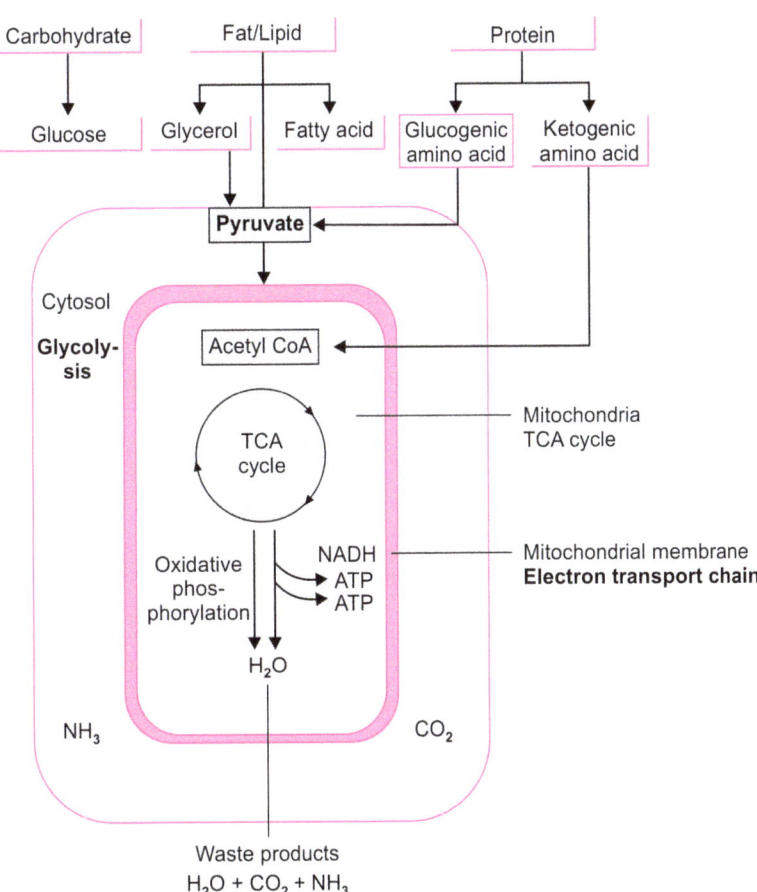

Fig. 5.3: Generation of energy (ATP) from carbohydrates, proteins and lipids.

Energy metabolism is a continuous process and the rate of metabolism influences health. It has an impact on energy balance that is influenced by the supply of energy yielding nutrients. Thus, weight gain and loss in weight is governed by energy metabolism. Energy balance is needed for maintaining body weight, keeping good health and preventing disease.

ENERGY BALANCE

Energy balance is a state of equilibrium (homeostasis) between energy intake and total energy expenditure of the body. Energy intake comes from food intake. Energy expenditure is energy spent on vital functions of the body and physical activities. Energy intake and energy expenditure must be balanced. Deviation in energy balance can result either in positive or negative energy balance (Fig. 5.4).

Energy balance	Energy intake	=	Energy expenditure
Positive energy balance	Energy intake	>	Energy expenditure
Negative energy balance	Energy intake	<	Energy expenditure

When energy balance is maintained over a prolonged period, an individual is considered to be in a steady state resulting in a stable and healthy body weight. An optimal steady state is achieved when energy intake compensates for total energy expenditure and allows for adequate growth in children, meets the energy requirements during pregnancy and lactation in women, without imposing metabolic, physiological or behavioral restrictions that limit the full expression of a person's biological, social, and economic potential. Mammals including humans have evolved a finely tuned system for controlling energy balance. This involves processes in adipose organs such as lipid storage when there is excess or mobilization of lipid stores under circumstances of inadequate intake. Also, there are endocrine signals given by hormones and other signaling molecules. Energy intakes in healthy individuals are generally regulated by the brain. There are mechanisms that integrate food intake regulation, energy expenditure, and environmental cues with the endocrine signals in order to achieve metabolic balance.

Positive Energy Balance

When consumption of energy from food exceeds the energy expenditure, the body is in a state of positive energy balance. If positive energy balance is prolonged, it can lead to overweight, obesity and related disorders. Major energy fuels are carbohydrates and fat. Both can be stored in the body. Carbohydrates are stored in the form of glycogen and if there is still an excess, it is converted into fat that is stored in fat cells of adipose tissues.

Negative Energy Balance

When energy expenditure exceeds the energy consumption, the body is in negative energy balance. There is depletion of body reserves and could result in loss of body weight. If this state continues for a considerable period of time, the person becomes underweight and is said to be undernourished.

Both underweight and overweight/obesity have health implications. Appropriate food selection is important to ensure adequate energy intake so that energy needs are met. But food should not be consumed in excess. Physical activity is necessary to ensure that energy expenditure matches or is in balance with intake. Energy balance varies on a day-to-day basis depending upon the environmental factors that affect the food intake and energy expenditure.

ENERGY EXPENDITURE

Energy expenditure is the amount of energy (calories) needed for "Total energy expenditure (TEE)" that is total energy spent in 24 hours by an individual. It may not be the same each and every day, because activity pattern may vary on different days. Based on energy expenditure, requirements are estimated, however, they are influenced by many biological and environmental factors.

Predominantly, there are three components of total energy expenditure, namely basal metabolism, diet-induced thermogenesis (DIT) or thermic effect of food and physical activity. At some stages in life, energy is required for growth, for example, in intrauterine life or pregnancy, during lactation for milk synthesis and from birth throughout infancy, childhood, and adolescence. Energy expenditure is usually maximum for basal metabolism (50–60% of total energy) followed by physical activity that can be 20–30% but is highly variable and very less energy is expended on diet-induced thermogenesis (10%).

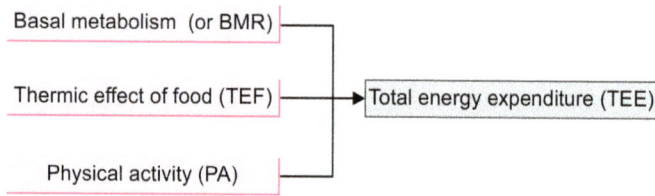

Basal Metabolism

Basal metabolism involves the vital metabolic activities necessary to sustain life. It includes cellular functions, turnover or replacement of cells, synthesis, secretion, and transport of many molecules. Including synthesis, secretion and metabolism of enzymes and hormones, and transport proteins. Energy is also required for maintenance of body temperature, uninterrupted work of cardiac and respiratory muscles, and brain function. These functions occur even during rest/sleep and in the fasting state. These are involuntary activities performed by all cells, especially metabolically

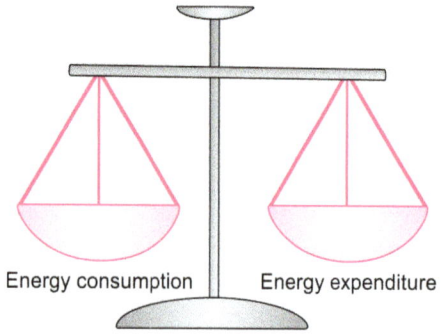

Fig. 5.4: Energy balance.

active tissues, such as brain, liver, gastrointestinal tract, heart, and kidney. The energy required for these activities must be met before energy can be used for anything else. Hence, energy expenditure for these activities is high and usually comprises about half of the body's total energy requirement.

> **Basal metabolic rate (BMR)** is the minimal energy requirement of the body to sustain life. It is estimated in supine position, standard conditions of fasting, and resting stage. It is usually expressed as kcal per minute/per hour or per 24 hours. This accounts for more than 50–60% of total energy requirement. It varies widely among individuals for variety of reasons.

The total amount of energy used in basal metabolism in a given period of time is called Basal Metabolic Rate (BMR). It can also be stated as the rate at which the body invests energy in these maintenance activities. It is usually constant for an individual but varies from one individual to another. BMR also varies with physical condition, gender, body size, body composition, body surface area, and age. Thus, depending on a person's age and lifestyle, BMR represents 45–70% of daily total energy expenditure. It remains relatively constant. BMR is higher during periods of growth/anabolic states, if there is hormonal imbalance, fever, in cold climate whereas it decreases when there is less physical activity and more amount of adipose tissue in the body. BMR represents energy requirement of performing such necessary tasks as pumping blood and transporting ions. Therefore, this rate generally increases as body weight increases, because a larger mass of tissue requires greater energy expenditure for its upkeep. Most of this expenditure is due to activity in the nervous system and skeletal muscles, which accounts for 40% and 20–30% of the BMR, respectively. BMR varies from tissue to tissue, e.g., accumulation of adipose tissue in the body lowers the BMR, therefore the metabolic rate of the body.

It is lowest when a person is lying down (at rest) in a room with a comfortable thermoneutral environment (neither too hot nor too cold) and in a fasting state. In this situation, the oxygen consumption is lowest and the heat generated by cells through metabolic activities is also lowest. Therefore, BMR is measured under standardized conditions, when a person is in complete physical, emotional, and physiological rest, hence usually in the morning. It is measured after 10–12 hours of fasting, 8 hours of physical rest and is awake, lying in a supine position. The person should be in a state of mental relaxation in an ambient environmental temperature that will neither elicit heat-generating processes nor elicit heat-dissipating processes. BMR is usually expressed as kilocalories per 24 hours (kcal/24 h). For adults, BMR on average is 20–25 kcal per kg of body weight per day.

Measurement of BMR requires stringent conditions that are difficult to attain. Hence, resting metabolic rate (RMR) is often measured, where such stringent conditions are not required. Even if one of the conditions for measuring BMR is not met, the measurement is termed RMR. RMR is approximately 10–20% higher than the BMR because of the energy spent as a result of the additional energy accounted for the post exercise oxygen consumption. RMR also encompasses the energy needed for respiration, circulation, the synthesis of organic compounds, the pumping of ions across membranes, the energy required by the central nervous system, and the maintenance of body temperature. Practically, RMR is often used more than BMR. Liver, kidney, heart, and brain account for about 60% of the RMR, there are various factors as shown in Figure 5.5 although they represent only approximately 5%

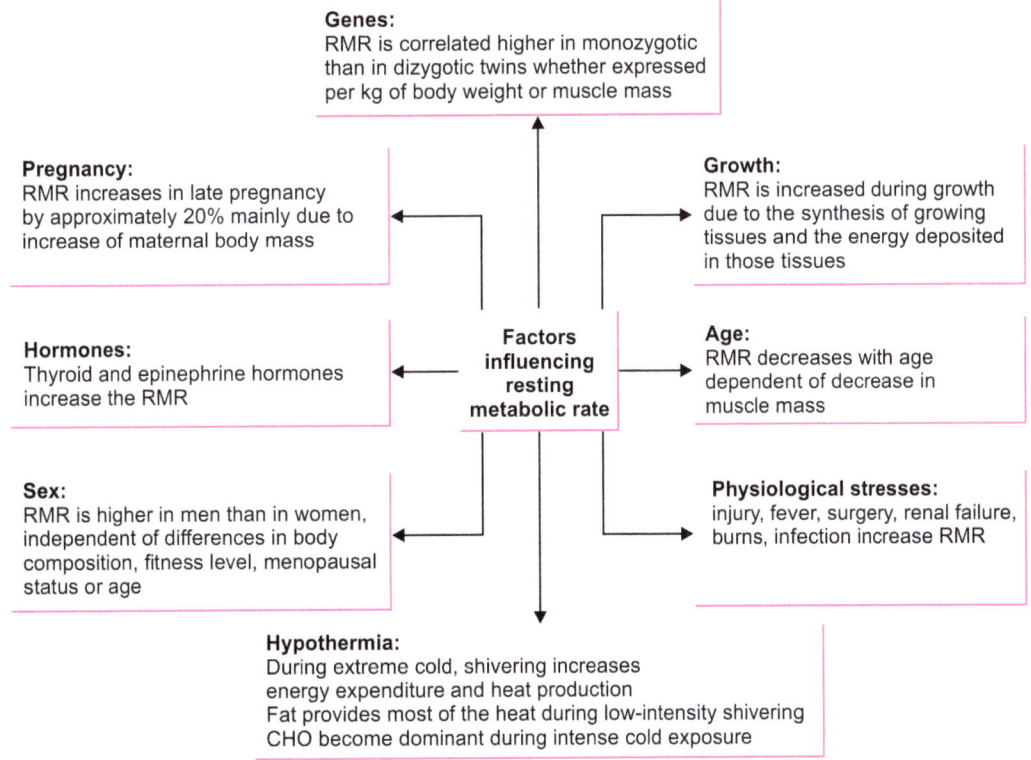

Fig. 5.5: Influence of various factors on RMR.

of body weight. This is because their metabolic rates are 15–40 times greater than that of the equivalent weight of muscle mass (~10–15 kcal/kg/day) and 50–100 times greater than that of adipose tissue (~4.5 kcal/kg/day).

Factors Affecting Basal Metabolic Rate

Many factors influence the body's metabolic rate:

Body surface area/body size: BMR is related to the body surface area as heat production is dependent on the body surface area. Larger body size means higher BMR. Body surface area can be estimated through "Dubois body surface chart" or Nomogram. Dubois' surface area in square meters is based on weight and height and can also be calculated by the following equation:

$$\text{Body surface area (m}^2\text{)} = [\text{Weight (kg)}\ 0.425 \times \text{Height (cm)}\ 0.725] \times 0.007184$$

BMR is influenced by body surface area but not weight. Two persons may have the same weight but may differ in height, one being short and stout and the other being tall and thin. The one who is taller will have a greater body surface area, i.e., more skin surface, from which heat is lost by radiation. Thus, more heat is generated by the taller and thinner person's body.

Body composition: Lean body mass (LBM) means muscle tissue that is metabolically active tissue and influences BMR. People with high LBM have higher BMR. Adipose tissue is metabolically not as active as lean or muscle tissues, thus overweight persons tend to have lower BMR. In adults, muscle mass presents the largest tissue of the whole body and accounts for about 40–50% in a lean adult man.

Gender: Women have more adipose tissue that are metabolically and relatively less active tissues than muscle tissue, thus women have about 5–10% lower BMR than men. Thus, energy requirement of women is lower than men. Men have more muscle mass, thus have higher BMR corresponding to the higher energy requirement. RMR of adolescent girls or women fluctuates during menstruation, wherein TEE may increase by approximately 150 kcal/day.

Age: Infants, children, and adolescents have high BMR because they are in the growing phase that implies multiplication of cells and a higher rate of cellular processes, i.e., higher proportion of metabolically active tissues (5 kcal per gram of tissue synthesis). This raises the BMR by 15–20%, thus raising the energy requirement. Once growth stops after the age of 20 years, there is 2% reduction in BMR per decade in women and 3% in men, due to the reduction of LBM with age. Also, activity level tends to decline with age, thus decreasing energy expenditure and thereby the requirement. Therefore, in sedentary individuals, BMR accounts for a fairly large proportion of total energy expenditure.

Pregnancy: Growth of the fetus and maternal tissues like uterus requires extra energy. The woman also needs to put in extra efforts for physical activity. BMR is also raised during pregnancy. Energy needs increase by 20–25% of the basic requirement, or 350 extra kcals are needed during pregnancy. Basal metabolism increases in pregnancy as a result of accelerated tissue synthesis, increased active tissue mass, and increased cardiovascular and respiratory work. Several studies have measured basal or resting metabolic rate at different stages of pregnancy.

Lactation: Mother requires extra energy for the process of milk secretion. Also, milk provides energy (65 kcal/100 mL of mother's milk) that enhances the calorie requirement of lactating mother.

Physical activity: Physical activities are either obligatory (those than cannot be avoided and must be performed) and discretionary (done voluntarily or by choice). Human beings perform both on regular basis. Obligatory activities are those which the individual cannot avoid within his/her given setting, and they are imposed on the individual by economic, cultural or societal demands such as work, daily activities—going to school, office, etc. Discretionary activities include the regular practice of physical activity for fitness and health; household tasks doing and visiting outside for a purpose or for enjoyment, social interaction, and community development.

Climate: In cold climates, the body attempts to produce more heat to counteract the effect of the cold environment in order to maintain the body temperature. Thus, metabolic rate increases. However, use of protective clothing and insulation provided by body fat affects the RMR. Persons living in tropical climates have lower BMR. Exercise in temperatures above 86°F increases metabolic load by 5% due to sweating. In extremely cold climates, RMR can be even tripled.

Sleep: Rate of physiological function is reduced during sleep, the person is in a state of total relaxation (muscular and emotional) and there is no physical activity, therefore BMR is lowered by 10–15%.

Body temperature: Heat acts as a catalyst for all biochemical reactions occurring in the body. Hence, basal metabolism increases when body temperature rises.

Nutritional status: In case of fasting, BMR is lowered. This is an adaptive response to preserve the body's energy reserves. In undernutrition or starvation, there is loss of lean body mass (LBM) resulting in lower BMR. Reduction may be as much as 20% depending upon the duration of undernutrition. In overweight, there is more of adipose tissue that is less metabolically active and hence BMR is lower. Thus, in both cases, BMR is lowered. Highly calorie-restricted diet also lowers the BMR and weight loss is not maintained on such diet.

Hormonal influences: Thyroid gland regulates energy expenditure through the hormone thyroxin. When activity of thyroid gland is reduced or serum thyroxin level is low, BMR can go down by as much as 30%. This implies that a person suffering from hypothyroidism requires less energy than a person having normal thyroid activity. In case of hyperthyroidism, BMR increases, may be by 50–75%.

Stress: Physiological, neurological or behavior changes can be stressful conditions for the body resulting in the release of stress-hormones to beat the stress. This leads to increase in the BMR. In fever, BMR increases. A rise in body temperature by 1°F leads to an average 7% increase in BMR, although in some conditions, it may increase by as much as 15%.

Estimation of Basal Metabolic Rate

Basal metabolic rate (BMR) is calculated as equivalent to the heat produced by the body or oxygen consumed. It is measured by calorimetry, which measures the amount of heat emitted by the human body. It can be estimated by direct method and indirect method.

Direct method: This is based on the first law of thermodynamics and the assumptions of thermal stability and low energy storage capacity. It is assumed that energy spent in all physiological processes is ultimately dissipated as heat and thus total energy expenditure can be assessed by directly measuring heat production. The direct method requires a specially constructed equipment called calorimeter (Fig. 5.6). In direct calorimetry, a person is made to sit in a large specialized chamber and the amount of body heat produced is measured. It is more accurate but a costly and cumbersome method. Also, it is not possible to obtain measurements for large numbers of people. Thus, its use is limited to research and is hardly used nowadays. Another limitation is that the person being measured is confined to a chamber and with this method, it is not possible to measure free living energy expenditure. Also, it is technically challenging as all heat transfers including radiation, convection, and conduction as well as heat loss due to evaporation have to be measured. Hence, indirect methods are used more often.

Indirect method: Indirect calorimetry assesses energy expenditure by calculating the amount of energy released when energy substrates are oxidized. An indirect method for estimating BMR (Indirect Calorimetry) involves asking the person to lie down in a ventilated hood and measuring the oxygen consumption and/or carbon dioxide exhaled at one-minute intervals. An equation is then used to calculate the BMR. Heart rate is another method used to estimate BMR. The De Weir equation can be used to predict energy expenditure, i.e.,

Total heat output (kcal) = 3.9 × oxygen used (L) + 1.11 × carbon dioxide produced (L)

For this, it is necessary to collect urine for 24 hours and measure the nitrogen content besides measuring in milliliters per minute, the amount of oxygen consumption and volume of carbon dioxide produced.

Indirect calorimetry: This entails measuring the exchange of gases during respiration for a period varying from 10 minutes to 30 minutes and calculated as respiratory quotient (RQ). RQ usually corresponds to the volume of carbon dioxide given off by lungs and the volume of oxygen inhaled by lungs.

$$RQ = \frac{\text{Volume of } CO_2 \text{ produced or given off by tissues}}{\text{Volume of } O_2 \text{ consumed by tissues}}$$

Utilization of 1 L of oxygen generates about 5 kcals. This ratio varies with the nutrient. RQ for lipid oxidation is 0.7, for glucose or carbohydrate metabolism it is 1.0, and for protein –0.8. When carbohydrate loading occurs, RQ will be close to 1. During starvation, when fat reserves of the body are used for energy, RQ will be 0.7. If energy consumption is more than required and fat deposition (storage of energy, i.e., fat in the adipose tissues) occurs, RQ will be 1.0. There are simple equations that can be used to predict energy expenditure. Indirect calorimetry can be used to assess energy expenditure in clinical research settings. It has the advantage of continuous measurement of energy expenditure measurement. The oxygen consumption can also be measured in field settings as well, while performing defined tasks, e.g., resting, standing, walking, running, etc.

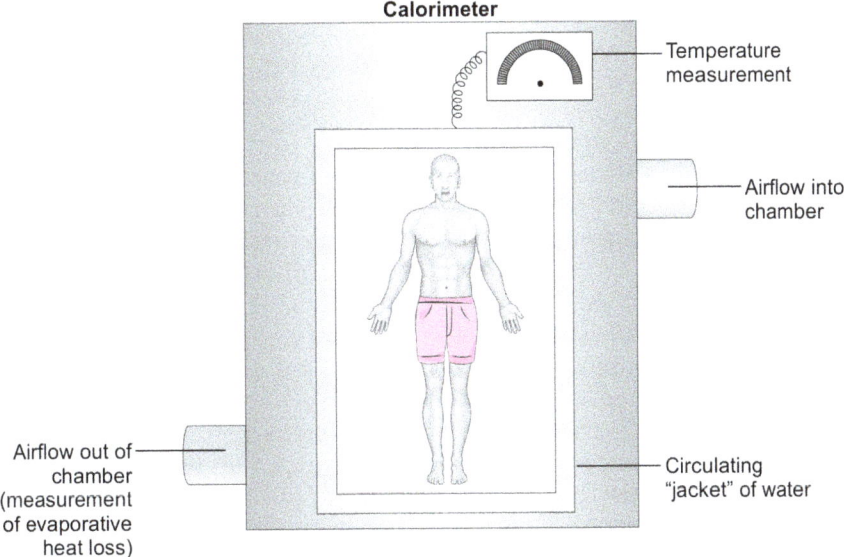

Fig. 5.6: Direct calorimeter.

However, the major limitation is the inability to measure BMR for large numbers and that laboratory conditions are required for the measurement. Hence, FAO/WHO/UNU as well as ICMR have proposed several equations for predicting BMR that use other measurements that are easier to obtain. Besides these, there are several equations used for various purposes. One of the most commonly used equations is the Harris–Benedict equation that is as follows:

BMR (Women) = 655.1 + [9.563 × weight (kg)] + [1.850 × height (cm)] – [4.676 × age (years)]

BMR (Men) = 66.5 + [13.7 × weight (kg)] + [(5.003 × height (cm)] – [6.775 × age (years)]

Nowadays, doubly labeled water is used. It is considered to be a gold standard to assess total energy expenditure. It can be used in a wide range of populations including pregnant and lactating women and infants. It is suitable for use with free-living persons. Its advantages are that it is noninvasive, burden on the participants is minimal, and it is relatively easy to perform. However, one needs to use isotopes and it requires sophisticated laboratory equipment. Turnover rates of ^2H and ^{18}O are determined by quantifying isotope concentrations in body fluids (most commonly urine) using mass spectrometry. The differential disappearance of the two isotopes provides a measure of carbon dioxide production. The method is safe as both ^{18}O and ^2H are naturally occurring isotopes, which are present in the body prior to the administration of doubly labeled water. The two stable isotopes are administered via a drink of water.

The difference between the elimination rates of ^2H and ^{18}O is equivalent to the rate of carbon dioxide production that can then be converted to average total daily energy expenditure.

AEE can be calculated—assumed that TEF constitutes 10% of TEE.

AEE (kcal/day) = 0.9 × TEE (kcal/day) – REE (kcal/day)

AEE represents all energy expended above the resting level and energy costs associated with the ingestion and assimilation of food.

Thermic Effect of Food

Energy is required to digest food, absorb, transport, and store nutrients in the body. These processes increase oxygen consumption. It is called **Thermic Effect of Food (TEF) or Thermogenesis or Diet-Induced Thermogenesis (DIT)**. Previously, this was known as Specific Dynamic Action (SDA) of food. When food is eaten, muscles move to chew it, then to move it through the digestive system, other cells synthesize the required enzymes, hormones, and other substances required for digestion, absorption, and transport of the nutrients. Thermogenesis reaches a maximum within 1 hour after a meal (postprandial). The energy used for all these processes is approximately 7–13% (average 10%) and increases total energy expenditure by about 10% of the BMR over a 24-hour period in individuals eating a mixed diet, and is proportional to the amount of food and calories consumed.

However, there are individual differences. Thermic effect varies from food to food, depending on the food composition and capacity to process the food inside the body. TEF is proportional to the size of the meal, thus larger meals are more thermogenic. Protein is more thermogenic in comparison to fat and carbohydrate. The thermic effect of carbohydrate is 5–10%, fat 0–5% and with protein the increment in energy expenditure during digestion, above baseline rates is 20–30%. Among the three macronutrients, fat is the least thermogenic. Thus, a high protein and/or carbohydrate diet induces a greater thermic response. A high fiber meal has been found to reduce TEF. Also, TEF declines with advancing age. TEF may be lower in obese persons compared to persons of normal weight.

Physical Activity

Physical activity involves use of muscles for bodily movement to contract and do work. The more physically active a person is, the more the muscular movement and contraction, hence greater the energy expenditure. Also, metabolic rate increases during physical activity. Physical activity on average accounts for approximately 30% of total energy requirement. Energy required for physical activity may also be called exercise thermogenesis. All persons perform obligatory and discretionary activities.

> ***Physical activity*** is any bodily movement produced by skeletal muscles resulting in energy expenditure and leading to elevation in energy expenditure above resting levels. Physical activity is a global term. It can be for recreation purpose or for any occupation.
> ***Obligatory activities*** are those one cannot avoid and are usually those that are linked to one's occupation and role and responsibilities in the home. These include daily activities performed by the person, depending upon the life stage and the socioeconomic and cultural environment.
> ***Discretionary activities*** are performed by choice. This can include exercise and sports, gardening, social, and community activities. These activities are undertaken voluntarily and individually for various purposes, such as personal enjoyment, social interaction, social service, and community development. Exercise, sports, and activities that result in energy expenditure and improve physical fitness contribute to good physical health. Overall engagement in discretionary activities is important for well-being and quality of life.
> ***Exercise*** is planned, structured, and repetitive movements with the intention of promoting or maintaining one or more components of physical fitness.

The physical activity component of energy expenditure is most variable because of differences in the activity pattern, intensity of the activity and its duration. Mode/type of physical activity vary, e.g., walking, running, swimming, jogging, and dancing. Energy expenditure on voluntary physical activities can vary from 15% to 40% of total energy expenditure (TEE) and in some cases, it may be even more if a person does a lot of manual work. However, in institutionalized and hospitalized persons, energy expenditure on physical activity may be less than 20% of TEE. The amount of energy utilized for physical activity or exercise/sports depends upon:

- **Duration**—the amount of time spent doing a particular activity.

- **Frequency of the activity**—how often or number of times the activity is performed per unit time.
- **Intensity**—how intensely one uses the muscles, i.e., the demand put on the muscles.
- **Mode/Type of activity**—how many muscles are being used—the more the muscles used, the more the energy expended.
- **The amount of weight being moved by the muscles**—the heavier a person, the more the energy used for the same activity as compared to a lighter person.
- **The level of fitness** also affects the energy expenditure.

Energy expended on physical activities is influenced by body weight, muscle mass, and the activity itself. It should be noted that mental activity does not require much energy, hence persons involved in intellectual activities who feel fatigued are not in essence physically fatigued, and rather, what they experience is mental fatigue. Besides this, shivering in a cold environment also involves muscular activity and increases energy expenditure.

Depending upon the intensity of activity and energy spent on them, different activities are grouped as sedentary, moderate, and heavy and very vigorous type of activities. Therefore, people occupied in different type of activities or occupations have been categorized as sedentary, moderate and heavy activities and person is refered accordingly.

> - **Sedentary workers:** Those persons who are involved in more of desk jobs and use less muscular movements are referred to as sedentary workers, e.g., executives, teachers, clerks, students, and some housewives, and the people who use energy saving devices and equipment and keep domestic help. These people often spend half of the day in very light to light activities like recreational activities like TV watching, internet surfing, and computer games.
> - **Moderate workers:** The people who use considerable amount of muscle movements and spend more time on moderate to vigorous physical activities like regular exercise, playing outdoor sports, long distance walking, using a staircase, running, cycling, dancing, floor cleaning, pottery making, gardening, etc.
> - **Heavy workers:** These persons regularly perform strenuous work for several hours such as construction and mine workers, swimmers, agricultural laborers, rickshaw pullers, coolies, etc. This category also includes sportsmen and athletes who practice or play for long hours a day.

In spite of the person's occupation, there is wide variability in the physical activities of any person on regular basis. Sometimes a person works hard or spends time in leisure.

The following factors affect physical activities and thus influence energy expenditure:
- **Biological**: Heredity, sex/gender, adiposity, nutritional status, health status, sexual maturity, proficiency in motor skills, and physical fitness.
- **Psychological**: Self-efficacy, self-concept of activity, perception of barriers to activity, perception of physical competence, attitude about activity, and belief about activity.
- **Social activity**: Attitude and behavior of the parents, peer group; socioeconomic status, time spent on computer games, and cultural values.
- **Physical environment**: Area of residence, availability of facilities, safety considerations, day of the week and holidays, season of the year, and climate.

Estimation of Energy Expenditure

Estimation of total energy expenditure is important for estimating total energy requirement. Total energy expenditure (TEE) is the energy spent by an individual in a day on all voluntary and involuntary activities.

Total Energy Expenditure (TEE)

"The energy spent, on average, in a 24-hour period by an individual or a group of individuals. By definition, it reflects the average amount of energy spent in a typical day, but it is not the exact amount of energy spent each and every day. BMR times PAL is equal to TEE or the daily energy requirement" (FAO, 2004).

Energy expenditure can be calculated from:
1. Basal metabolic rate (BMR)
2. Energy spent on physical activities.

Basal metabolic rate (BMR): BMR is calculated based on age and gender. The ICMR (2010) has given a set of equations taking into account the recommendations of the expert group of the FAO/WHO/UNU as shown in Table 5.2.

Energy spent on physical activities: Energy spent on physical activities varies considerably and can be calculated by the following ways:
1. Physical activity level (PAL)
2. Physical activity ratio (PAR)
3. Metabolic equivalent of task (MET).

Physical activity level or PAL: It is the total energy required for a 24-hour period divided by the energy needed for basal metabolism in 24 hours. PAL is calculated from physical activity ratio or PAR (Tables 5.3 and 5.4).

$$\text{PAL for the day} = \frac{\text{Total PAR} \times \text{hours}}{\text{Total time (24 hours)}}$$

The physical activity level (PAL) for Indian reference adult man and woman are: sedentary work- 1.40, moderate work- 1.80 and heavy work- 2.30. (ICMR-NIN, 2020). Differences in body composition are generally not related to differences in physical activity. According to ICMR-NIN (2020) PAL values for sedentary, moderate and heavy work is 1.4, 1.8 and 2.3 respectively.

Table 5.2: Equations for prediction of BMR (kcal/24h): FAO/WHO/UNU, 2004.

Age (years)	Prediction equation proposed by FAO/WHO/UNU Consultation (2004)		
Men		Women	
18–30	15.1 × B.W.(kg) + 692.2	18–30	14.8 × B.W.(kg) + 486.6
30–60	11.5 × B.W.(kg) + 873	30–60	8.1 × B.W.(kg) + 845.6
> 60	11.7 × B.W.(kg) + 587.7	> 60	9.1 × B.W.(kg) + 658.5

Table 5.3: PAL Values for boys and girls by level of physical activity.

PAL values for boys by level of physical activity				PAL values for Girls by level of physical activity		
		Level of activity			Level of activity	
Age (years)	Weight (kg)	Sedentary	Vigorous	Weight (kg)	Sedentary	Vigorous
5-6	18.5	1.3	1.8	18.3	1.3	1.8
6 – 7	20.5	1.3	1.8	20.2	1.4	1.8
7 – 8	22.9	1.3	1.8	22.4	1.4	1.9
8 – 9	25.4	1.4	1.9	25.0	1.4	1.9
9 – 10	28.1	1.4	1.9	28.2	1.4	1.9
10 – 11	31.2	1.5	1.9	31.9	1.5	2.0
11 – 12	34.6	1.5	2.0	36.2	1.5	2.0
12 – 13	38.9	1.5	2.0	41.2	1.5	2.0
13 – 14	44.3	1.5	2.1	46.0	1.5	2.0
14 – 15	50.6	1.5	2.1	50.1	1.5	2.0
15 – 16	56.6	1.6	2.1	52.8	1.5	2.0
16 – 17	61.3	1.6	2.1	54.7	1.5	2.1
17 – 18	64.8	1.6	2.1	55.7		

Table 5.4: PAR values for some activities.

Activities	Male	Female
Sleeping	1.0	1.0
Sitting quietly	1.2	1.2
Reading	1.3	1.5
Standing	1.4	1.5
Dressing	2.4	3.3
Walking slowly	2.8	3.0
Walking briskly	3.8	3.8
Cycling	5.6	3.6
Running—long distance	6.3	6.6
Basketball	7.0	7.7
Football	8.0	–
Swimming	9	–

Source: Nutrient Requirements and Recommended Dietary Allowances for Indians. A Report of the Expert Group of the Indian Council of Medical Research. 2010. p. 36.

Physical activity ratio (PAR): It is the energy cost of an activity per unit time (usually a minute or an hour) expressed as a multiple of BMR.

$$\text{Physical activity ratio (PAR)} = \frac{\text{Energy cost of an activity per minute}}{\text{Energy cost of basal metabolism per minute}}$$

Activity record is kept for a 24-hour period and the total number of minutes spent on each activity is calculated. PAR values for adults have been given by the Indian Expert Group for some common daily activities that have been categorized as occupational and non-occupational activity. ICMR-NIN (2020) has given PAR values as follows: mean PAR for sedentary individuals is 1.41 and for moderately active- 1.80, heavy or vigorously active- 2.33.

Metabolic equivalent of task (MET): This is a widely used physiological concept that represents a simple way of expressing energy cost of physical activities as multiples of resting metabolic rate (RMR). A MET is the ratio of the rate of energy expended during an activity to the rate of energy expended at rest. It is a numerical value that represents a multiple of the resting metabolic rate for a particular activity. One MET equates with the oxygen consumption (O_2) required at rest or sitting quietly and is assumed to be 3.5 mL/O_2/min/kg body weight. The index is used to express O_2 uptake or intensity of activities as multiples of the resting or 1 MET value. It is useful for describing and prescribing exercise of different intensities. The list of energy expenditure estimations for different physical activities has been developed, and using these values, it is possible to convert the time spent on physical activity to energy equivalents. Activities range from 0.9 MET (sleeping) to 18 METs (running at 10.9 mph).

In medical field and in sports activities, calculation of energy expenditure is simplified and new values have been developed. The exercise physiologist is required to interpret test results and estimate energy expenditure, optimize exercise protocols, prescribe exercises, and make recommendations for weight loss or maintenance of body weight. Similarly, it is used to prescribe exercise in clinical settings. Energy expenditure on different activities is calculated as metabolic equivalent of task (MET) or metabolic equivalent.

1 MET = 3.5 mL O_2 per kg of body weight per minute (can be used as a proxy for RMR).

1 MET = metabolic rate consuming 1 kcal per kg body weight per hour.

It is equal to the energy cost at rest or sitting quietly. Generally, it is assumed that the REE of any individual is equal to 1 MET. A 3 MET activity means that one expends three times the energy used by the body at rest.

This value applies to the level of energy expenditure during the performance of a specific activity at a designated intensity and provides a way of expressing the total caloric cost of the activity. MET values between 1.0 and 12.0 represent the typical range of PAL, from light to moderate to vigorous. The PAL provides information about the duration and intensity of a set of different activities performed during a 24-hour period and the relative differences in usual levels of physical activity. MET is used as a practical means of expressing the intensity and energy expenditure of physical activities in a way that allows comparison among persons of different weights. Actual energy expenditure (e.g., in kcal or Joules) during a physical activity depends on the person's body mass.

Each activity has a specific MET value. As stated previously, MET expresses energy cost of physical activity as multiples of RMR. Thus, for various physical activities as multiples of the standard resting energy value (1 MET) have been described, ranging from sleeping (0.9 MET) to running at 17.4 km/h (18 METs). All activities are assigned an intensity level in METs, and the energy cost of that physical activity is calculated as the MET level multiplied by the standard RMR value (1.0 kcal or 4.184 kJ) per kg of body weight per hour.

Some examples for METs per hour for various activities are given below. The range for activities that are light intensity, moderate intensity, and vigorous are as follows:

Light intensity activities are	1.1–2.9 MET
Moderate intensity activities are	3.0–5.9 MET
Vigorous intensity activities are	6.0 MET or more

MET can be converted in kcal consumed per minute by the formula:

MET: Body weight (kg)/60 (minutes in an hour)

For example, MET for office work is 2.0 for a man weighing 60 kg, hence energy (kcal) used is 2 × 60/60 = 2.0 kcal/minutes or 120 kcal per hour.

Other methods for estimating energy expenditure and energy requirements are:
- Heart rate monitoring
- Use of motion sensors such as pedometers, accelerometers, and use of sense wear armbands.

Heart rate monitoring: Heart rate monitoring for estimation of energy expenditure and physical activity is popular, convenient, relatively inexpensive, noninvasive, and versatile. Monitoring heart rate minute-by-minute enables detailed information on frequency, intensity, and duration of free-living physical activities. The assumption made is that there is a linear relationship between heart rate and VO_2.

Pedometers are widely used and are very popular. They were originally used to register steps taken during walking and running. Pedometers were used to popularize, motivate, and encourage sedentary/inactive individuals to become physically active. The target for physical activity is given in terms of steps per day and the commonly used benchmark is 10,000 steps per day. The rationale is that 30 minutes of brisk walking is equivalent to 3,000–4,000 steps and 1,250–1,550 steps/km. Individuals can be categorized as sedentary or active based on the number of steps taken (Table 5.5).

Table 5.5: Number of steps per day and corresponding physical activity level.

Physical activity level	Steps per day
Sedentary or inactive lifestyle	<5000
Low active	5000–7499
Somewhat active	7500–9999
Active	10,000–12,500
Highly active	>12,500

Accelerometers: These are motion sensors that detect acceleration of the body. Because acceleration is the rate of change in velocity over a given time; it allows assessment of the frequency, intensity, and duration of PA as a function of body movement. With accelerometers one can estimate the intensity and duration of movement and classify physical activity by intensity. Accelerometers are more sophisticated than pedometers and can record data over an extended period of time. However, accelerometers have low sensitivity to sedentary activity and are not really able to register static activity.

Since heart rate monitoring, pedometry and accelerometry all have limitations, combinations are used to complement the advantages of these technologies.

Sense wear armbands: Information is collected through these sensors that enable assessment type and intensity of activities. These bands are commercially available and worn on arm.

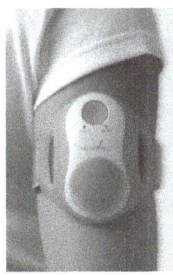

ENERGY REQUIREMENTS

The basic concept of estimating energy requirements is fundamentally different from that of protein and other nutrients. Unlike energy, protein is not stored in the body as a reserve and the daily protein intake should match the daily protein metabolism to satisfy a man's daily protein requirements.

Since energy can be stored as fat when its intake is in excess of the requirement, only the average requirement is used, called the estimated energy requirement (EER). The requirement represents the average daily requirements corresponding to daily average energy expenditure of an individual.

This is the amount of energy intake required (to be obtained) from food that balances (neither more nor less) energy expenditure when the individual has a body size and composition and level of physical activity, that is consistent with long-term good health. Also, it allows the individual to maintain economically, essential and socially desirable activities. In children and pregnant and lactating women, it includes the energy required for deposition of tissues during growth, or secretion of milk at rates consistent with good health.

Currently, it is recommended that energy requirement must be assessed in terms of energy expenditure rather than in terms of energy intake. This is because of several reasons.

Energy intakes that are derived from dietary recalls are prone to reporting errors as well as many assumptions that relate to converting cooked food portions to energy. The energy intake also is known to vary substantially from day to day; on some days, it may be above the energy expenditure and sometimes, below it. Body energy reserves (fat) help to maintain normal energy expenditure over short periods even when the daily intake is below expenditure. Over a period of time, however, adults tend to maintain energy balance and constant body weight.

The present expert committee deliberated on which reference body weight to use for the single value for the daily energy requirement and decided that for the purpose of this specific recommendation, the 95th percentile height value and a BMI of 21 kg/m² would be used. However, it also recommended that as far as possible, energy intake recommendations for a normal healthy population should be based on the actual weight and physical activity level of the target population. When this is unknown, the single value recommendation can be used. In most nutrients, requirements are set up such that the needs of almost all healthy individuals at a given life stage and a specific age group can be provided for. This is possible for nutrients that the body can dispose or get rid of in case the intake is in excess of requirements. This is not the case for energy because the body does not have the ability to get rid of excess energy that is consumed. It is converted into fat and the person gains weight. Hence, energy requirements that are set should be in balance with and be similar to the energy expenditure of individuals.

Energy requirement has been defined by experts as: "Energy requirement is the amount of food energy needed to balance energy expenditure in order to maintain body size, body composition, and a level of necessary and desirable physical activity consistent with long-term good health.

> "Human energy requirements are estimated from measures of energy expenditure plus the additional energy needs for growth, pregnancy, and lactation. Recommendations for dietary energy intake from food must satisfy these requirements for the attainment and maintenance of optimal health, physiological function, and well-being. The latter (i.e., well-being) depends not only on health, but also on the ability to satisfy the demands imposed by society and the environment, as well as all the other energy-demanding activities that fulfill individual needs" (FAO, 2004).
>
> "This includes the energy needed for the optimal growth and development of children, for the deposition of tissues during pregnancy, and for the secretion of milk during lactation consistent with the good health of mother and child".

Thus, if a person is overweight or obese, his/her energy intake should be less than the energy expended. Conversely, if a person is undernourished and underweight, the energy intake should be more than the expenditure. It is necessary to standardize desirable level of energy intake level that can easily be accessed, consumed, and within affordable resources and still balance the energy expenditure. Total energy expenditure varies with age, sex, activity, and physiological status. Thus, energy requirements vary with age, sex, and physiological state as well as the level of physical activity. The total energy expenditure (TEE) can be satisfied with dietary sources. An adequate healthy diet can fulfill the body's need for all the energy as well as all the essential nutrients and in case of adults; the bodyweight will be stable. Males have more lean body mass (that is metabolically active), hence their energy requirements are higher than females of the same age and stature.

For infants and children as well as adolescents, energy intakes should balance not only energy expenditure at the level of physical activity consistent with normal development and maturation as deposition of tissues (growth) at a rate that is consistent with health and yet not result in overweight and obesity. Thus, as children grow energy requirements increase and are generally higher for boys. Similarly, energy requirements during pregnancy and lactation are higher than requirements for nonpregnant, nonlactating females. Energy requirements are prescribed by national and international organizations for a population/group based on age, gender, bodyweight (desirable weight), physical activity, and physiological condition like pregnancy and lactation. The expert group of the Indian Council of Medical Research (2010) has recommended the use of the following equation:

Total energy requirement = Basal metabolic rate × Physical activity level (PAL)

> For example: Calculate energy requirement of a housewife weighing 52 kg and age 32 years.
>
> BMR equation selected: 8.3 × body weight (kg) + 788
> = 8.3 × 52 + 788
> = 431.6 + 788
> Hence BMR is = 1,220 kcal
> Assume PAL is = 1.8
> Total energy requirement (TER) = BMR × PAL = 1,220 × 1.8
> = 2,196 kcal

The recommended levels of dietary energy intakes are intended for healthy, well-nourished and active population. Energy requirements for male and female adults are given in terms of Reference man and Reference woman. Body weight of a normal healthy Indian adult male is taken as 60 kg and for a woman as 55 kg. No allowance is to be made for any safety margin, in contrast to other nutrients (such as protein). This is because excess intake of energy can lead to weight gain that may be undesirable.

During pregnancy, additional allowance is given to ensure growth of the fetus and maternal tissues, to meet energy needs of increased BMR, and woman also needs to put in extra efforts for physical activity. During lactation, women require extra energy for milk synthesis and secretion. During infancy and childhood, energy requirements for growth are considered. Energy requirements then level off during adulthood (when growth stops) and declines in later years. By 75 years of age, there is approximately 30% decrease in energy requirement due to loss of functioning capacity of cells, loss of muscle mass, and lower BMR. ICMR-NIN (2020) has given recommendations for energy allowances for Indian population in Appendix 3 in different age groups.

ENERGY INTAKE

Energy intake comes from dietary sources. Food energy can be measured by the bomb calorimeter and the unit of measurement for energy is "Calorie" or "Joule" that is referred as kilocalorie (kcal). (1 kcal = 4.184 kilojoules). Energy is obtained from the three energy yielding nutrients namely, carbohydrates, proteins, and fats as well as dietary fiber.

Carbohydrate	–	4 kcal/g or 17 kJ/g
Protein	–	4 kcal/g or 17 kJ/g
Fat	–	9 kcal/g or 37 kJ/g
Dietary fiber	–	2 kcals/g or 8.5 kJ/g

Other sources of energy are sugar alcohols — (7 kcal/g).

Though dietary fiber, short chain fatty acids (SCFA), sugar alcohols (~2 kcal/g) and alcohol also provide some amount of calories (7 kcal/g), these (except dietary fiber) are not regular/daily sources of energy in general. Energy intake can be calculated by the calorific value of food consumed.

Each food varies in its calorie (energy) contents depending upon its composition and the content of the three energy yielding nutrients. For example, 100 g of potato contains 0.23 g fat and 70 kcal whereas 100 g whole Bengal gram contains 5.1 g fat and 287 kcal. Energy values (in kcal and kj) of commonly consumed raw foods are given in Appendix 1 along with other nutrients.

Individuals consume a wide variety of food preparations supplying varying amounts of energy and nutrients. How much food and what food a person consumes, are determined by his/her food choice and accessibility that are physiologically and psychologically governed by hunger, appetite, and satiety. The hypothalamic and brainstem centers act as the control centers for controlling food intake and energy expenditure in animals and humans. In most individuals who maintain stable body weight, there is spontaneous adaptation of energy intake to their energy expenditure through accurate mechanisms controlling food intake. Hunger, appetite, and satiety play a significant role in regulation of food intake, body weight, and endocrine function.

Hunger

Hunger is a biological drive that impels individuals to search for food and describes the sensations that promote food consumption. Hunger sensation is elicited after absorption of nutrients contained in the previous meal. It is the stimulus or signal that drives a person's need to eat. The feeling of hunger is important in determining what, how much, and when to eat. It is a sensation that compels the individual to eat something (food). It is a mechanical feeling that is felt through the contraction of abdominal muscles (hunger pangs). Hunger is a crucial factor in determining energy balance. When the body needs energy, signals are sent from an empty stomach and intestines that trigger the feeling of hunger. These signals are processed by the brain. However, human beings possess the ability to override these signals and delay eating even when they are hungry. People who fast or starve have diminished hunger responses. On the other hand, some people adapt by eating more. In such persons, the signal of fullness may be ignored and the person becomes used to "overeating".

> *Hunger* is a physiological drive for food intake. It is defined as a sensation felt by the person that makes him/her search for and consume/ingest food.
>
> *Appetite* is psychological drive for food intake. It is a natural desire for a specific food that is stimulated by the sight, smell, and thought of food. It is strongly influenced by memory and other associations.
>
> *Satiety* is a hypothalamic signal to stop food intake. It refers to the complete absence of hunger that occurs very rapidly.

The feeling of hunger is important in determining what, how much, and when to eat, however, it is influenced by the several factors:

> **Factors affecting hunger and embed in hunger**
> Nutrients present in the bloodstream, Size and composition of previous meal, Customary eating patterns, Prevailing weather conditions (hot weather reduces food intake), The quantum of exercise/physical activities Hormones, Physical and mental states, Disease, Stomach: Adaptable to the size of the meal. It does not shrink except in the case of starvation.

Thus, hunger signals are upregulated whenever there is an increased demand or need for more energy, e.g., after fasting, during lactation, and after physical activity. Hunger peptides also have an awakening effect and stimulate the seeking and collection of food.

Appetite

Appetite is another signal to eat and is a complex phenomenon that arises from a sequence of interactions between the brain and peripheral mechanisms. Appetite is psychological drive for food intake. "It is a natural and strong urge or desire or craving for a specific food. However, unlike hunger, it can occur with or without hunger since it is often stimulated by the sight, smell, and thought of food. It is strongly influenced by memory and other associations. Appetite can be stimulated in some persons and repressed in others by stress. Many environmental, psychological, and physiological factors influence appetite such as:

> **Smell and sight of the food**
> Thought or talks of food, availability of food, hormonal triggers and disruption in hypothalamic region, physiological status and disease condition, mood and depression, stress and emotional disturbances, previous experience, exhaustion and exercise.

The gastrointestinal tract contains mechanoreceptors and chemoreceptors. These give information about the nutrient content via the vagus nerve to the brain.

Satiety and Satiation

Satiety is a feeling of fullness or satisfaction after food intake that leads a person to stop eating. Satiety delays onset of the next meal and can reduce food consumption. Termination of the period of satiety coincides with the resurgence of feeling hungry. The satiety center of the hypothalamus creates the distension in the stomach that suppresses the desire to eat food further.

Satiation is the sensation of fullness during an eating episode that contributes to the cessation of eating. It reduces termination of desire to eat further. It is governed by the hormones and receptors in the brain and abdomen respectively. Satiation is a hypothalamic signal to stop eating. Satiation and the period of satiety are influenced by different factors. Overall food intake is governed by physiological and environmental factors:

- **Physical state of food:** Volume and weight of the food also influence satiety. Solid and dense food provides better satiety.
- **Particle size:** Larger particles take more time and effort to chew, thus slows down food intake and gastric emptying.
- **Macronutrient composition of foods:** Protein rich food gives more satiety than food rich in fat or carbohydrate or both. Fiber content also produces more fullness as fiber increases volume or bulk of the food.
- **Energy density of foods:** Energy value of food is associated with water and fat content. It also modifies the physical state of food and affects satiety. Energy value influences food volume, palatability, and satiety.
- **Mastication:** Food that requires more chewing leads to fatigue and so quicker feeling of fullness.
- **Taste and palatability:** Decrease in good taste often reduces the food intake. Highly palatable food delays the satiety.
- Temperature and texture of food also affects the satiety.
- **State of health:** Many a times during illness, persons have lack of appetite.
- **Mood:** Some persons eat less when they are anxious and stressed, whereas some over eat.
- Habits, experiences, and culture influence food intake.
- Knowledge and attitudes are also important influencing factors.

Since overeating and excess energy consumption are important, and many factors are involved in development of obesity, there is considerable research on satiety. A Satiety index has been developed. It is calculated on the same lines as is the Glycemic index. Equicaloric/isocaloric (same calorific values) portions of food are fed to the subject and white bread is used as a standard and the feeling of fullness is registered. Researchers also call it a fullness factor evidence show that foods containing large amount of water, protein, dietary fiber have higher fullness factor.

Advances in research on the physiological basis for food intake and satiety have revealed there is a physiological basis governed by a network of hormonal and neural signals. There are two types of hormones in circulation—those which initiate and terminate a meal (secreted mainly during meals) and the second type that reflect body adipose tissue and energy balance. Physiological regulation of food intake is a complex homeostatic process regulated by many endocrine and metabolic factors in combination with visual, olfactory and taste sensations, emotions, memory, and health status.

Hormonal Regulation of Food Intake

Food intake is largely regulated by brain through certain hormones and neuropeptides, such as ghrelin, leptin, insulin, cholecystokinin (CCK), and neuropeptide Y (NPY). Understanding the role of each can be of help in regulating energy balance. Food intake can be modulated by short-term mechanisms and there is also long-term regulation of food intake as shown in Figure 5.7.

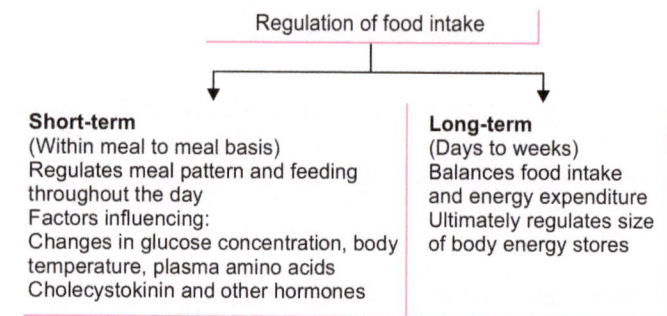

Fig. 5.7: Short-term and long-term regulation of food intake.

The central nervous system plays an important role in the physiology of neuroendocrine regulation of food intake. Central regulation of food intake is mainly done by the hypothalamus and some neurohormones. Short- and long-term peripheral regulation of satiety and energy balance is done by hormones secreted by the gastrointestinal tract, adipose tissue hormones, and pancreatic hormones. The hypothalamus is the key region involved in appetite regulation. Peptides from the gut and adiposity signals give feedback (send signals) to the hypothalamus that ultimately influences the drive to eat and energy expenditure is adjusted so that over time, body weight of the person remains stable.

Ghrelin: It is a peptide hormone consisting of 28 amino acids. It is produced in the epithelial lining of the stomach in response to hunger. Ghrelin stimulates appetite by acting on a region in the hypothalamus that controls food intake. It is one of the most powerful orexigenic agents (substance that stimulates appetite). It circulates in the bloodstream under fasting conditions or voluntary energy deprivation during weight loss. Hence, it may serve as a peripheral signal of hunger and the need to consume food to the central nervous system. Plasma ghrelin levels are higher before a meal and drop soon after eating. Ghrelin secretion is influenced by the nutrient composition of meal. Ghrelin functions in association with another orexigenic hormone called orexin, are also involved in regulating food intake.

Hormones involved in food intake and satiety
Orexigenic (stimulate appetite): Ghrelin
Anorexigenic (decrease appetite) cholecystokinin (CCK), leptin, insulin, and neuropeptide Y (NPY)

Ghrelin stimulates orexin neurons whereas glucose and leptin inhibit them. Ghrelin also suppresses fat utilization in adipose tissue and so can slow down the metabolism and reduce ability to burn fat. Ghrelin has also been found to be involved in other body functions as well, such as cardiovascular functions and stimulating release of growth hormone.

Leptin: It is a hormone, produced by the fat cells (adipocytes) in response to feeling of fullness. It is involved in long-term regulation of body weight and is thus involved in suppression of food intake. It influences the amount of food consumed relative to the energy intake. Leptin levels do not increase after a meal and by itself; this hormone does not lead to termination of a meal/food intake. Leptin with the other components of the long-term system interact with the components of the short-term system and modulate the amount of food consumed. Low leptin levels are generally indicative of low fat stores.

Circulating leptin levels in blood influence the appetite and satiety centers (that control feeding behavior and hunger) in the hypothalamus to reduce appetite and stop food intake. Leptin has also been associated with regulating onset of puberty. Leptin's effects are opposite to those of Ghrelin. When there is weight gain, more leptin is produced and it results in decreased food and energy intake and greater energy expenditure and vice versa. Since leptin is produced by the fat cells, obese people have more fat cells so more leptin is produced. It has been suggested that in obese persons there may be leptin resistance. Leptin resistance leads to food cravings, sweet tooth, overeating or eating when the person is under stress and results in weight gain. This in turn increases the risk of elevated blood sugar, increased level of visceral fat, insulin resistance, diabetes, high blood pressure, heart disease, sleep disorders, and accelerated aging. Persons with leptin resistance also suffer weight rebounds even after weight loss. Circulating leptin levels are proportional to fat mass. Leptin also increases sympathetic activity, thyroid-stimulating hormone, growth hormone, luteinizing hormone, and follicle-stimulating hormone and hence is linked to puberty and reproduction. It enhances hematopoiesis. A decrease in leptin levels is an indicator of energy imbalance.

Insulin: It is produced by the beta cells in the pancreas primarily in response to a rise in blood sugar level. Like leptin, insulin circulates in blood in proportion to the fat mass. Short-term underfeeding decreases leptin and insulin concentrations whereas short-term overfeeding increases the concentrations of both hormones. During fasting conditions, insulin levels are low and increase during and immediately after a meal or glucose ingestion/administration. Insulin enters the brain from circulation and food intake is then reduced. Like leptin, it is an important adiposity signal and both increase sensitivity of the brain to meal-generated satiety signals. The postprandial rise in insulin is an important factor that influences and determines meal termination.

Insulin acts in synergistically with leptin. Insulin inhibits food intake by acting through central receptors.

> **Research Glimpses:** Eating behavior is regulated by energy homeostasis and appetite control which includes homeostatic and hedonic control. Gut-derived hormones play an important role as signals in appetite regulation. They are produced by enteroendocrine cells in response to nutrient and energy intake, and evoke their effects through their influence on brain structures involved in food intake
>
> *Contd...*
>
> regulation, the key role played by the hypothalamus. Gut hormones reach the hypothalamus from circulation or by the vagal nerve via the nucleus of the solitary tract. Different gut peptides are synthesized among which the only orexigenic hormone is ghrelin, i.e., it increases food intake and body weight. All the other gut peptides namely cholecystokinin, glucagon like peptide-1, oxyntomodulin, peptide tyrosine-tyrosine or pancreatic polypeptide, are anorexigenic, and therefore they generally reduce in food intake. Besides gut peptides, there are gut-derived endocannabinoids that have an orexigenic effect on appetite. Understanding the mechanisms of action of these substances is highly relevant to the management of obesity which is increasing in prevalence. These gut-derived peptides or their analogues have the potential to be used as therapeutic agents.
>
> *Marić G, Gazibara T, Zaletel I, Borović ML, Tomanović N, Ćirić M, Puškaš N. The role of gut hormones in appetite regulation (Review). Acta Physiologica Hungarica. 2014;101(4):395–407*
>
> Combating obesity requires a good understanding of body weight regulation, energy homeostasis, food intake behaviors, the role of hormones, peptides, and neurotransmitters in the periphery and central nervous system. Understanding the mechanism of action of both centrally and peripherally secreted peptides/hormones will be useful in development of therapeutic substances that either suppress the orexigenic response and/or have anorexigenic function. Dysfunction in feeding signals by the brain play a role in obesity. "The hypothalamic (arcuate nucleus) and brainstem (nucleus tractus solitarius) areas integrate behavioral, endocrine, and autonomic responses via afferent and efferent pathways from and to the brainstem and peripheral organs. Neurons present in the arcuate nucleus express proopiomelanocortin, neuropeptide Y, and agouti-related peptide. Among these, proopiomelanocortin lowers food intake, whereas neuropeptide Y and agouti-related peptide acutely increase eating. Hormones are secreted peripherally but the gut, pancreas, adipose, and liver play important roles in regulating energy homeostasis, as do the vagal afferent neurons. Peripheral signals respond to the level of stored and currently available fuel. Ongoing research is focused on development of therapeutics that could be used in treatment of obesity.
>
> *Miller GD. Appetite Regulation: Hormones, Peptides, and Neurotransmitters and Their Role in Obesity. American Journal of Lifestyle Medicine. 2017. https://doi.org/10.1177/1559827617716376*

Other hormones that decrease meal size are the bombesin family, glucagon, glucagon-like peptides 1 and 2, amylin, somatostatin, enterostatin, peptide YY, and adiponectin. Endorphins, cortisol, and insulin lead to decreased satiety or increased hunger. Another hormone is amylin that is secreted by the pancreatic beta cells with insulin in a ratio of ten and one hundred. Amylin functions as a signal for satiety as well as of adiposity. Plasma amylin levels are low during fasting and increase after food intake or glucose administration.

Gastrointestinal hormones: The gastrointestinal tract has numerous sensory receptors. More than 40 gastrointestinal hormones have been discovered so far. Satiety signals arise from different parts of the gastrointestinal system including the stomach, proximal and distal small intestine, colon, and pancreas. When food is eaten, two main effects are seen: (i) gastric distention and (ii) peptides are released from the enteroendocrine cells. The gut hormones are believed to have an important role in meal initiation and termination. Table 5.6 in lists some hormones that play a role in regulating food intake.

Contd...

Table 5.6: Hormones affecting food intake.

Hormone	Site of synthesis	Effect on food intake
Cholecystokinin	Intestinal cells	Decrease
Ghrelin	Stomach	Increase
Pancreatic polypeptide	Pancreas	Decrease
Peptide YY	Intestinal cells	Decrease
Glucagon-like peptide -1	Intestinal cells	Decrease
Leptin	Adipocytes in adipose tissues	Decrease
Serotonin	Specific neurons of central nervous system	Decrease
Norepinephrine	Noradrenergic neurons of CNS and adrenal medulla	Decrease
Corticotropin-releasing hormone	Hypothalamus	Decrease
Alpha melanocyte-stimulating hormone	Anterior lobe of the pituitary gland	Decrease
Agouti-related protein	AgRP/NPY neuron in the brain	Increase
Melanin-concentrating hormone	Magnocellular neurons of the lateral hypothalamus	Increase
Endorphins	Anterior pituitary gland	Increase
Glutamate and gamma-aminobutyric acid (GABA)	Nervous system	Increase
Cortisol	Adrenal cortex	Increase
Galanin	Amygdala in the brain	Increase

The vagal afferent nerves are sensitive to signals such as gastrointestinal distention, presence of macronutrients in the intestinal lumen and carry the message to the brain, and the peptides that are produced by endocrine cells in the gut.

Cholecystokinin (CCK): CCK is found within the brain (in the hypothalamus) and the gastrointestinal tract. It is a short-term satiety signal produced in specialized cells in the epithelium of the small intestines (duodenum and upper jejunum) and functions as a satiety hormone and is a neurotransmitter. CCK is rapidly released locally in response to the presence of protein and fat (or products of the digestion). Carbohydrates are weak stimulants for CCK release. CCK stimulates the pancreas to release digestive enzymes into the duodenum and also stimulates release of bile from gallbladder to facilitate the digestion. It is a major regulator of gallbladder contraction. Cholecystokinin slows down gastric emptying and suppresses energy intake. Its level increases gradually over 10–30 minutes after a person starts eating and then gradually falls and the person senses satiety. There appears to be a dose-dependent decrease in food intake. CCK has been shown to reduce both meal size and meal duration. However, CCK levels may remain elevated for even 3–5 hours after a meal. CCK is an important regulator of meal size. CCK works in synergy with leptin to produce sensory consequences that may be associated with satiety. Chronic ingestion of large size meal or fatty meal may disrupt the functioning of hormonal signals to brain that control appetite. Though CCK tends to decrease the meal size, it does not much influence body weight. Low level of CCK in the bloodstream has been found to result in binge eating. It mediates satiation and early phase satiety.

Neuropeptide Y (NPY): It is a neurotransmitter that is secreted by the hypothalamus. It has been found to be associated with a drive for food intake or feeding (a potent stimulator of feeding behavior) and hence may play a role in energy balance. It is an important mediator of central leptin signaling. Its function has been found to be linked also with insulin. In case of leptin resistance and insulin resistance, it may increase food intake and decrease physical activity. Thus, NPY plays a role in obesity as well.

Pancreatic polypeptide (PP): This is an anorexigenic peptide containing 36 amino acids. It is largely synthesized in the pancreas and to some extent in the colon and rectum. In fasting condition, the levels of this peptide are low and it rises in proportion to the caloric intake. The hypothalamus is believed to have an important role in pancreatic polypeptide-mediated reduction in food intake. Its secretion is under vagal control and is stimulated postprandially in proportion to the calories ingested. It influences exocrine pancreatic function, gastrointestinal motility, and gastric acid secretion.

Peptide YY: It is synthesized and released from the cells of the gastrointestinal tract. Circulating levels of this peptide are influenced by meal composition and calorie content, and become elevated within 1 hour after intake of food. Levels are often lower in obese persons. It has been shown to have anorexigenic effects in normal weight and obese individuals. It slows gastric emptying as well as gastrointestinal motility and inhibits gastric acid secretion. It is secreted in proportion to the caloric load.

Glucagon-like peptide 1 (GLP-1): It is released from the small intestinal and colonic cells in proportion to the energy (calories) intake. It has been shown to exert anorexigenic effect in both lean and obese persons. It may also be linked to reducing gastric emptying and suppression of gastric acid secretion. Besides enhancing satiety and reducing food intake, it has been shown to promote weight loss.

Oxyntomodulin: It shares the same precursor as GLP-1, and following food intake it is generally cosecreted with GLP-1, in proportion to the calories ingested. It increases satiation and decreases food intake. Repeated injections

Table 5.7: Factors regulating satiety and hunger.

Factors influencing Satiety	Factors influencing Hunger
Distention of stomach and duodenum	Hunger contractions
Heat	Cold
Increase in blood levels of glucose, amino acids, and lipids	Decrease in blood levels of glucose, amino acids, and lipids
Catecholamines	Orexins
Serotonin	Endorphins
Insulin (postprandial state)	Glutamic acid
Leptin	Cortisol
Glucagon	Ghrelin
Peptide YY	Gamma amino butyric acid (GABA) and AMP-activated protein kinase (AMPK)

have been found to result in weight loss. It also promotes energy expenditure.

Amylin: This is also known as islet amyloid polypeptide (IAPP), and is cosecreted postprandially along with insulin by the beta cells of the pancreas. It is a short-term satiety peptide that inhibits gastric emptying, as well as secretion of gastric acid and glucagon. It also decreases meal size and food intake. An analog of amylin is used in treatment of diabetes for improving insulin sensitivity and causes weight loss.

Certain neurotransmitters, such as serotonin, dopamine, and endorphin are also found to be involved in appetite and satiety. Serotonin may play a role in consumption of carbohydrate-rich foods and conferring satiety. Dopamine is associated with food cravings. Endorphins also known as opiate peptides may play a role in response to sugar and fat.

Table 5.7 summarizes the factors regulating food intake.

EATING DISORDERS

Eating is often an illusionary distraction of the mind. Eating behavior of humans (when, what, and how much) is influenced by the following factors that sometimes due to unfavorable conditions lead to eating disorders (ED). Eating disorder is a disturbed pattern of eating particularly among adolescents and women. Eating behavior and disorders are influenced by various factors:

Sociocultural factors: In some cultures, food is in abundance but slimness has high value and there is pressure to be thin. Individuals tend to develop dissatisfaction with body weight and shape and indulge in unusual ways of diet even resorting to use of pharmacological agents. Media also plays a significant role in development of eating disorders because it portrays an often unrealistic picture of the human body in a glamorous way. Young teenage girls may be driven by these advertisements to try and achieve unrealistic ideal body shape. Sometimes fear of weight gain may begin in school age itself. Also, there are negative images and perceptions in society about persons who are overweight or obese.

Family dynamics: Eating disorders are common in members of the family where communication is poor and expectations from each other are high. Children often feel pressure to please their parents and avoid conflict. In some cases, parent(s) may be alcoholic, depressed or emotionally upset. Some children may develop eating disorders to gain attention.

Personality traits: Some persons are always preoccupied with the thought of food and thus indulge in binging. Persons having low self-esteem, lack of confidence, anxiety, and feeling of helplessness may also have ED. Some persons react to stress by finding comfort in eating whereas in others, anxiety and stress results in lack of appetite. Chronic stress may result in eating disorders.

Biological: Sometimes, there is a disturbance in the nervous or endocrine signals or hormonal secretion, which may lead to ED. ED occurs when the eating pattern of the individual is disordered or disturbed by self choice in order to satisfy any psychological need rather than fulfilling physiological requirement. There is consistently undereating or overeating, with food being used as the mechanism, by which the person tries to feel better about self. Such irregularities in eating have adverse effects on physical and psychological health of the person.

There are largely three types of eating disorders:
1. Anorexia nervosa
2. Bulimia
3. Binge eating.

Anorexia Nervosa

The term anorexia means loss of appetite. Anorexia nervosa refers to an abnormal lack of appetite or lack of desire to consume food even when there is a physiological need for food and it is expected that the individual should have a desire to consume food.

Anorexia nervosa involves self-denial of appetite and eating even if the person feels hungry due to psychological reasons. In essence, it is self-induced starvation. It is often seen in adolescent girls who desire an imaginary or glamorous kind of self-image and think they are fat. They avoid eating or shun food to have low body weight. Over a period of time, this may have adverse effects on health—the person may become severely underweight (85% or less of normal weight for height and age) and undernourished. Girls having anorexia nervosa may also suffer from amenorrhea, lack of concentration, vertigo, and fainting. It can affect electrolyte levels leading to changes in muscle and nerve function. In some cases, anorexia nervosa has been fatal.

Bulimia Nervosa

Bulimia means great irresistible hunger. Bulimia nervosa is again a nervous disorder when the person is afraid to gain weight and eats large amounts of food (could be a particular kind of food) followed by a feeling of regret about eating. Such a person indulges in episodes of rapid eating (within 2 hours) followed by vomiting, strict dieting, taking diuretics or laxatives. This act is also called "binge eating and purging". This disorder is more common among girls than boys. If this is not treated, it may become chronic.

Binge Eating

Bingeing is episodes of uncontrolled eating large quantity of food, two or three times in a week. There is irresistible desire to eat and the person eats rapidly till he/she is uncomfortably full, even when he/she is not hungry. It is similar to bulimia but in this case, there is no purging or other compensatory behavior. The person indulges in such kind of eating when he/she is alone or has no one to share feelings with, is depressed or disgusted with oneself. Often the person eats alone. Binge eaters usually are in positive energy balance and are at high risk of diabetes, atherosclerosis, gallstones, and hyperlipidemia. Binge eating occurs in both males and females. In many persons, childhood obesity, negative self-image, repeatedly being told negative things about body weight and shape and a desire for perfectionism, have been found to be causes of binge eating.

Eating behavior and the type of food composition influences body weight and body composition, which in turn influence the nutritional status and health of the individual. It is not just the body weight and body frame but body composition, i.e., the proportion of lean tissue, bone, fat, and water also makes the difference in terms of health and risk of disease; stamina and fatigue. Body composition can be studied at different levels: (i) atomic, (ii) molecular, (iii) cellular, and (iv) tissue level. Information on body composition is widely used in various fields. Various techniques are used to assess body composition.

BODY COMPOSITION

Concept of body composition existed in ancient times. Ayurveda which dates back thousands of years states that the human body is made of the same five basic elements or "Panch Mahabhootas", namely Aakash (Ether), Vayu (Air), Agni (Fire), Aapa (Water), and Prithvi (Earth) which make up the Universe as well. The human body is made of three Doshas viz Vata, Pitta, and Kapha, which are physiological entities of the body that are responsible for carrying out all the functions of the body. The body is also made of seven Dhatus/the structural entities of the body and include Rasa/Plasma, Rakta/ Blood cells, Mamsa/Muscle tissue, Meda/Fatty tissue, Asthi/Bone tissue, Majja/Bone marrow, and Shukra, i.e., Hormonal and other secretions.

These doshas are derived from the five elements of nature and their properties: Vata is composed of space and air, Kapha of fire and water, and Pitta of earth and water. Based on these, each person has a particular Prakriti and body type. In Ayurveda, the characteristics of each body type are described in detail.

Greek records dated much later than Ayurveda, around 400 BC, show that the Greeks also believed that human body is made up of the same elements as in the universe, i.e., fire, earth, water, and air, and the qualities of these elements could be dry or moist and hot or cold. Ingested food has the same qualities and digestion of food helps to convert it into blood, phlegm, yellow bile, and black bile.

Modern technologies have identified various components of the body which can be assessed by various field and laboratory methods with varying degrees of precision. Body composition of an individual implies that the human body has different components such as water, protein, minerals, and fat mass; fat free mass including skeletal and lean body mass which when added together constitutes body weight.

Primarily, the body is composed of innumerable atoms of carbon, oxygen, hydrogen, and nitrogen. These atoms join together and form various organic and inorganic molecules, such as carbohydrates, lipid, protein, minerals, and water. These molecules constitute the cell mass and body fluids. Eventually, different tissues and organs in the body are formed and each of these consists of different types of cells. It is possible to assess body composition at different levels, such as atomic, molecular, and cellular and tissue levels (Fig. 5.8).

Body composition of humans varies widely. Within the same individual, changes occur with age and with health status/disease state. Thus, body composition varies considerably with age, gender, physiological states like pregnancy, type, and level of physical activity including

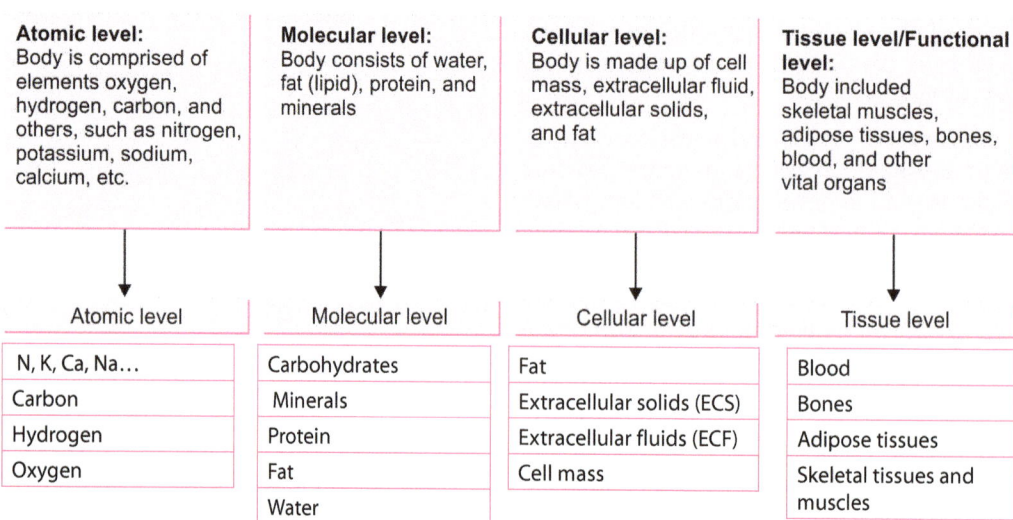

Fig. 5.8: Body composition at various levels.

Table 5.8: Body composition of adults.

Parameters	Women	Men
Age (years)	20–24	20–24
Height (cm)	163.8	174.0
Total body mass (kg)	56.7	70.0
Total fat (%)	27.0 (15.3 kg)	15.0 (10.5 kg)
Storage fat (%)	15.0 (8.5 kg)	12.0 (8.4 kg)
Essential fat (%)	12.0 (6.8 kg)	3.0 (2.1 kg)
Lean body mass (kg)	48.2	61.7
Muscles (%)	36.0 (20.4 kg)	44.7 (31.3 kg)
Bones (%)	12.0 (6.8 kg)	14.9 (10.4 kg)

Source: McArdle WD, Katch FI, Katch BM. Essentials of Exercise Physiology. Baltimore: Williams and Wilkins; 1994. p. 453.

sports. Several environmental factors like food composition, certain clinical conditions such as malnutrition, edema, ascites, massive tumor growth, cellular atrophy, etc. bring about significant changes in body composition and also in body weight. Table 5.8 gives body composition for women and men in the age group of 20–24 years. However, body composition is influenced by race, climate, physical activity, age, and gender.

Fat generally constitutes 12–20% of an adult male body and 20–30% of an adult female body. The remaining is lean body mass comprising water, muscle, bone, and connective tissue. These two components largely affect metabolism and are altered in various physiological and pathological conditions. Generally, body composition is assessed by measuring lean body mass and fat mass. Body composition is depicted in Figure 5.9.

Lean Body Mass

Lean body mass (LBM) includes weight of muscles, bones, and of the vital organs, such as liver, heart, kidney, brain, and skin. It indicates the amount of muscle mass present in the body and includes the muscle present in all tissues and organs. Since, it does not include the fat mass at all, therefore it is also called fat free mass (FFM).

Fat free mass = ECS + ECF + protein + carbohydrates + minerals (soft tissue minerals) + bone minerals

Lean soft tissue = ECS + ECF + protein + carbohydrates + minerals (soft tissue minerals) except bone minerals

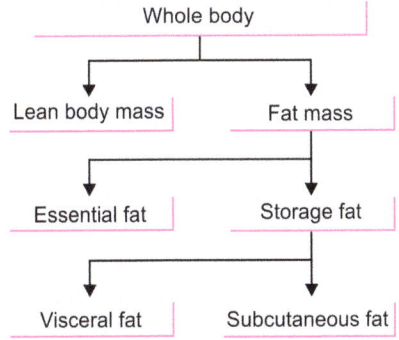

Fig. 5.9: Body composition.

LBM determines strength, stamina, and work capacity of the person. Since, it is the metabolically active component, its proportion influences the energy and protein requirement of the individual. Increment in LBM is favorable whereas a decline in LBM is not, since it affects body functioning. LBM is important for survival and is regulated by metabolic pathways so that the amount of protein that the body requires for optimal function is maintained to the extent possible. Greater muscle mass is associated with better strength and power, better metabolic health, and decreased risk of chronic diseases. Therefore, loss of lean body mass is associated with morbidity, impaired immunity and increased infections, weakness, and decreased wound healing. When there is loss of 30% or more of lean body mass, the patient may be too weak; there is risk of pressure sores and increased risk of mortality. The percentage of muscle mass is also critical for specific sports. LBM is influenced by several factors.

Growth: LBM increases during periods of growth as there is growth and development of tissues and organs (multiplication of cells and accretion of protein). Thus, the requirement for energy and protein is high during growth. Between the ages of 10 years and 20 years, LBM increases on an average by 33 kg in boys, but is much less (16 kg) in girls. This difference is also observed in relation to velocity of height gain. The sex difference in LBM, weight, and height is due to the production of testosterone that is six times higher in males than females. Adult women have approximately 70% less LBM than adult men. Therefore, energy and protein requirements of women are comparatively less than men.

Age: Age also affects LBM. With increasing age, there is loss of muscle mass and decrease in LBM. Between 70 years and 79 years, skeletal muscle declines by about 1% per year. This loss of muscle mass is called sarcopenia. It may be due to lower production of hormones, lower level of physical activities involving muscles and altered fat metabolism. It can easily be seen in people who find difficulty in getting out of a chair, standing or walking long distances, and climbing a staircase. However, similar symptoms are also observed in undernourished, obese or sick people that are due to poor dietary habits, inadequate physical exercise or prolonged illness. In addition, there may be reduced physical activity that predispose to accumulation and redistribution of fat in the body that in turn may increase the risk of obesity.

Exercise: Exercise tends to build more muscles and thus increases LBM. Development of muscles is also governed by the sex hormones particularly testosterone. Males produce more testosterone, thus they have more muscle mass and are able to perform more intense physical work. LBM has also been found to increase with resistance training and aerobic physical exercise. This is because when a person exercises, some amount of damage occurs to the muscle cells. This stimulates proliferation of muscle cells as well as hypertrophy (increase in cell size) at the site. A single bout of exercise stimulates protein synthesis within 2–4 hours after the workout and protein synthesis may occur at a higher level for up to 24 hours. High LBM indicates low body fat and vice versa. Low LBM thus implies that there is accumulation and redistribution of fat in the body and signifies higher percentage of body fat that is not desirable. It implies low stamina, poor performance, and the risks of many diseases, such as obesity, insulin resistance, and osteoporosis because it alters the metabolic functions and body homeostasis.

Nutrient intake: Consumption of high quality protein, adequate amount of potassium, carbohydrate, and fat to provide adequate energy (with emphasis on complex carbohydrates and adequate fiber intake) can help to improve LBM. Thus, dietary intake of food sources of protein in moderation can help to increase LBM provided enough exercises are done regularly. It is not necessary to increase total protein intake drastically. Studies show that when consumption of protein is more than 10 g, there is diminishing increase in muscle anabolism following exercise and the excess protein is oxidized to obtain energy rather than being used for muscle building.

Body Fat

Body fat is generally the fat accumulated in adipose tissues that shapes the body and is also involved in numerous vital functions. Total body fat is comprised of two types of fat, i.e., essential fat and storage fat that behave differently and are present at different sites of the body. Type of body fat varies with age, heredity, gender, and physiological status. It alters during pregnancy and lactation.

Essential fat: Essential fat plays a vital role to sustain life and is present in the cell membranes, fat in bone marrow, heart, lungs, liver, spleen, kidneys, intestines, muscles, and lipid-rich tissues throughout the central nervous system. It is not used as a source of energy and cannot be separated out from the body. There is a gender difference with regard to the amount of essential fat. Men have only 3% essential fat, whereas women carry more amounts (12%) to provide support in childbearing activities. It is present in breast, thighs, and pelvic regions that are required during pregnancy and lactation. Low levels of essential fat may pose health risks.

Storage fat: Storage fat is predominantly present in fat cells (adipocytes) of adipose tissues. Adipocytes contain fat in the form of triglycerides. Both men and women accumulate fat at different sites that design their anatomy. Men have more fat around waist and abdomen whereas women carry fat around hips and thighs. Storage fat is a concentrated source of energy used for various life processes. Storage fat is again of two types depending upon the site of distribution, i.e., subcutaneous fat and visceral fat located around internal organs (internal storage fat).

Subcutaneous fat: The fat present underneath the skin is known as subcutaneous fat. It is responsible for shape and size of the body; texture of the skin and transport of fat-soluble substances, such as fat-soluble vitamins, cosmetics, pharmaceutical products, and even toxic substances. It provides protection to the body from physical and environmental traumas. Subcutaneous fat is the major source of energy used for fuel. Excessive intake of energy may result in excessive subcutaneous fat that can deshape, desize the body, and make the person bulky, lumpy, and lethargic. Excessive subcutaneous fat does not increase the risk of degenerative diseases possibly because it does not participate in metabolic activities. Reduction of subcutaneous fat is possible by adoption of appropriate diet and exercise. The body of a Sumo wrestler is large and bulky and his body weight is also extraordinarily high that is attributed to their body density. Persons with excess storage fat are also at the risk of chronic diseases.

Visceral fat: Visceral fat is the fat present underneath the abdominal muscles and around the vital organs. It provides protection to the vital organs and facilitates their functions. There is no gender difference with regard to the amount of visceral fat; both men and women carry approximately 3% of it. Under normal conditions, it does not increase or decrease, but poor dietary intake and imbalanced lifestyle for a prolonged period may increase it. High visceral fat impairs functionality of vital organs and tends to initiate high-risk diseases, such as abdominal obesity, insulin resistance, type II diabetes, and atherosclerosis. Some body fat is needed for health but too much (>25%) and too little (<5% for males and <10% for females) have adverse effects on health.

> Adipose tissue can be divided into truncal region or peripheral region. Truncal adipose tissue includes subcutaneous fat in thoracic and abdominal region and also fat in intrathoracic and intra-abdominal regions.
> Peripheral adipose tissue includes subcutaneous depots in upper and lower extremities.
> In intra-abdominal adipose tissue, metabolic activity in terms of lipogenesis and lipolysis is more. There is a portal vein hypothesis that free fatty acids that are produced by lipolysis of this adipose tissue are directly transported via the portal vein to the liver. In the liver, they are substrates for lipid synthesis, gluconeogenesis, and give rise to insulin resistance. The consequences of this are hyperlipidemia, glucose intolerance, hypertension, and ultimately atherosclerosis. Excess free fatty acids are able to inhibit the glucose uptake by skeletal muscle resulting in peripheral insulin resistance.

Scientific evidence indicates that not just a high body mass index (BMI) but where the adipose tissue is stored in various body locations can have differ impact on metabolic health. Adverse risk for metabolic disorders is associated with greater trunk adiposity. Some studies are now focusing on leg fat mass and that larger leg fat mass is associated with lower fasting and post glucose load in oral glucose tolerance tests. Besides this, sarcopenia in which there is characteristically less amount of muscle mass is associated with insulin resistance.

Adipose tissue is an endocrine organ that produces numerous biologically active substances called "adipocytokines/adipokines". Some important adipokines include adiponectin, leptin, plasminogen activator inhibitor (PAI-1), tumor necrosis factor (TNF-α), interleukin 6 (IL-6), and resistin. These adipokines play an important role in regulating energy metabolism, in appetite, insulin sensitivity, inflammation, atherosclerosis, cell proliferation, among others. In obesity, there is dysregulation of adipokine production. Particularly, adiponectin plays an important role in energy metabolism, inflammation, and cell proliferation. It is important because it is insulin sensitizing, antiatherogenic, and anti-inflammatory.

According to the American Diabetic Association (2007), visceral fat causes impairment in blood sugar control and adipocytes produce some inflammatory substances (adipokines), such as interleukin (IL)-6, resistin, etc. that induce insulin resistance. Visceral fat is broken down by the liver and creates more low-density lipoprotein (LDL), thereby increasing the risk of atherosclerosis. Reduction of visceral fat is rather difficult but low glycemic food; aerobic exercise can reduce visceral fat. Liposuction does not remove visceral fat.

With aging, initially fat mass increases and then levels off. Intramuscular and visceral fat tend to increase whereas subcutaneous fat decreases. Increased infiltration of fat occurs in muscle. This decreases lower muscle strength and results in reduced lower extremity performance.

Why Measure Body Composition?

Maintaining body health and level of body fatness is key to healthier and longer life. Body composition analysis is necessary to yield data about normal growth, maturity, and longer life.

Appropriate body composition is important for physical fitness. Having information about body composition:
- Can help predict the status/the risk of onset of disease/the progression or repression of diseases like cardiovascular disease, diabetes, cancers, osteoporosis, and osteoarthritis.
- Decisions to be made about whether weight loss or weight gain is needed and whether the body composition is conducive to good metabolic health and fitness.
- Helps the team of health practitioners including the dietitian, trainer, physical therapist, and physician to set realistic goals about achieving desirable or favorable body composition in terms of body fat and nonfat compartments, especially lean body mass.
- Helps to make decisions about the type of exercise regimen and its duration.
- Monitors whether the diet and exercise regimens that are undertaken are helping the individual to achieve a favorable body composition.
- It is easy to find out the reason for symptoms like inability to use muscle(s) properly, the state of sarcopenia (due to loss of muscle mass), commonly seen in elder population, and even in obese people. Treatment can be planned to increase the muscle mass. Similarly, rapid loss of body weight leading to cachexia in cancer patients and in people with metabolic disorders, assessment of body composition is very helpful.

It is an objective method. Further, its measurement is extremely useful in assessment of malnutrition, physical fitness, for sports persons, and in various clinical settings to monitor: (i) changes in weight and in which body compartment loss is more and (ii) effects of therapy. It determines the LBM and body fat percentage and fat distribution. It reflects physical fitness, endurance, and cardiorespiratory levels. It helps to predict suitability of the individual sportsperson for specific sport event(s). It also helps to know the risk of chronic disease in advance so treatment becomes easy and economical. Further the assessment data support the diet plan as well as drug dose, if required.

Techniques of Measuring Body Composition

Various methods have been developed for assessment of body composition. These include anthropometric measurements isotopic determination of total body water, whole body potassium ^{40}K counting, radiography, electrical conductance, and bioelectric impedance.

Based on the knowledge of chemical composition, three models of body composition have been developed and measurements are based on the two compartments, three compartments, and four compartments models (Fig. 5.10):

In the two-compartment model, the body is assumed to have fat and lean body mass. Fat is assumed to have a stable density of 0.900 g/cm^3 and the density of lean body mass is 1.095 g/cm^3.

According to the three-compartment model, the human body has four main components, namely water, proteins, minerals, and glycogen. Generally, the proportion of each of these components is stable, but they could vary. The three-compartment model was developed by Siri who assigned a density of 1.565 g/cm^3 to a "combined residual mass component". This density reflects the density of protein (1.34 g/cm^3) and minerals (3.00 g/cm^3).

The four-compartment model was developed because it was recognized that the contribution of bone should be taken into account. Later, other models have been developed such as dividing body composition into five levels, i.e., atomic, molecular, cellular, tissue-system, and whole body. Figure 5.10 depicts the different compartmental models of body composition.

Body composition can be measured using many highly sensitive instruments and techniques.

Skinfold measurement: Skinfold measurement is a popular method that can measure body fat percentage, muscle mass, and bone mass. **Skinfold caliper** is used that holds the double skin and fat layer at various sites in the body (Fig. 5.11).

The underlying principle is that a large proportion of body fat is stored underneath the skin. Therefore, thickness of the subcutaneous fat at various sites in the body, such as upper arm, forearm biceps, triceps, mid-thigh, calf, subscapula, suprailiac (iliac crest), and abdominal fat are measured. Generally, three or seven sites are measured using a skinfold caliper. If the measurement is done properly, the error is less than 3%. It is inexpensive and easy to do once the skill is mastered. It is difficult to measure obese and very lean persons. Also, distribution of body fat varies with age, sex, race, and athletic activity. Body fat can be calculated using equations. Several such equations are available.

Bioelectrical impedance analysis (BIA): Bioelectrical impedance is based on the principle of Ohm's law. Different biological tissues can act as good conductors and insulators (bad conductor). Bone and fat contain less water thus they

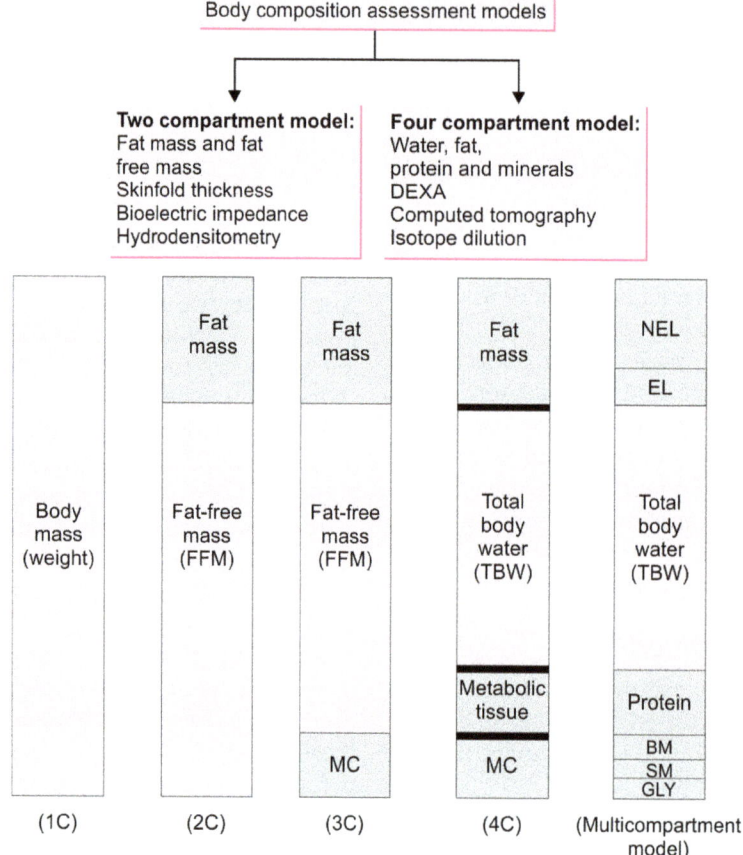

Fig. 5.10: Assessment models of Body composition.
Source: Kuriyan R. Body composition techniques. Indian Journal of Medical Research. 2018;148:648–58.

Seven sites for measuring body fat
Chest or Pectoral
Triceps
Subscapular
Axilla (Midaxilliary)
Suprailiac
Abdomen
Thigh

Three sites for measuring body fat

Men	Women
Chest	Triceps
Abdomen	Suprailiac
Thigh	Thigh

Fig. 5.11: Different sites of measuring body fat.

are poor conductors, hence the resistance (impedance), whereas blood, visceral organs, and muscles are good conductors, as they contain fluid and electrolytes. Fat is a very poor conductor of electricity, hence, the more the fat, the more it will impede the current as compared to lean tissue. Among the different body components, water and electrolytes are able to conduct a small alternating current that is applied to the body. The small alternating current flows between two electrodes and passes more rapidly through fat-free body tissues and extracellular water that it will through fat or bone, because the fat-free component has greater electrolyte content. Hence, BIA measures the fat content by the impedance or opposition of the body tissue to flow of electric current (<1 mA or less than 1 milliampere) alternating electric current to the body at the frequency of 50 kHz or kilohertz. It helps in prediction of fat free mass and body fat percentage. Impedance is proportional to the total body water volume (TBW), e.g., a muscular person will have lower resistance or impedance than an obese person. Body water is assumed to be approximately 73% of the fat free mass. Advantage of BIA is that it can be used in field and clinical settings to measure the body fat or body composition. It is quick, precise, safe, portable, and noninvasive. It is easy to perform and testing takes only about a minute.

Once the procedure is performed, body density, etc. can be estimated. However, the impedance analysis should be performed under standardized conditions in terms of hydration status, recent food and beverage consumption, skin temperature, and recent physical activity. This is because hydration status affects the accuracy of the measurement. When there is considerable loss of body water, for example, due to exercise or if there is fluid restriction or, impedance is lower giving lower body fat percentage readings. The reverse will be seen under conditions of over hydration. With reference to skin temperature, impedance to electric flow is less in a warm environment and therefore percent body fat will appear to be lower.

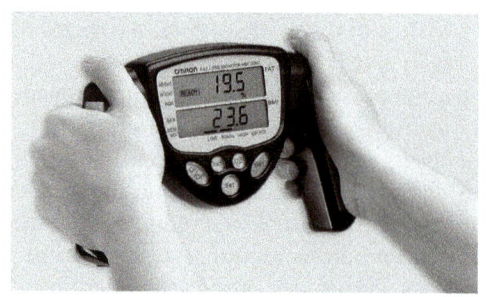

Table 5.9: General multicomponents of the body composition.

Compartments	Amount (grams)	% body
Water	42	60
Extracellular	-18	-26
Intracellular	-24	-34
Fat	12	17
Protein	10.6	15
Bone minerals (osseous)	3.7	5.3

Source: Benjamin J (Ed). Assessment of nutritional status in clinical practice. Joshi YK Basics of Clinical Nutrition. New Delhi: 2008. p. 54.

Body weight = Fat Mass + Total Body Water + Minerals + Protein (Table 5.9).

Compared to underwater weighing, it has generally been seen that BIA tends to overestimate body fat in lean and athletic persons, whereas it underestimates body fat in obese persons. It also allows the monitoring of hydration and body cell mass. Some precautions need to be taken when doing BIA measurements. These are:

- At least 2 hours should elapse after ingesting a meal before doing BIA measurements
- If the person has consumed any alcoholic beverage, BIA measurement should be done after a gap of 24 hours
- If the person has exercised, a gap of 3-4 hours should be kept between the exercise and measurement
- The persons should not have used any hand cream or lotions at least 2 hours before the measurement
- BIA measurements should preferably not be taken during a woman's menstrual cycle.

Underwater weighing or Hydrostatic weighing: Underwater weighing is considered the **Gold Standard** and is based on Archimedes principle. It gives highest level of accuracy, but it is not a very viable method owing to its costly instrument and water tank. It is an indirect method. It considers that the body volume is equal to reduction in body weight in water. It is based on the two compartment/component model. Since, fat is lighter than water but bone and muscle are more dense, it considers that the density of lean tissue is denser than water and the density of fat tissue is less dense than water. The fat free or lean mass is assumed to have a density of 1.10 kg/L and the fat component has a density of 0.90 kg/L. Thus, the density of the whole body is influenced by the relative size of the two compartments. A person having more body fat will weigh less underwater. This technique requires highly sophisticated equipment, considerable amount of space, and consumes lot of time in execution and computation. The equation given by Siri (1961) is used to calculate percent body fat:

    Percent body fat = (495/body density) – 450.
    Body density = Body weight in air/body volume
    Body volume = (Body weight in air – body weight underwater)/water temperature) – residual lung volume
    Percent lean body mass = 100 – percent body fat
    Absolute mass of body fat = (Percent body fat × body weight)/100

Absolute lean body mass = Body weight – absolute mass of body fat

The person is submerged in water and the volume of the human body is measured. Weight is measured and the decrease in body weight when the person is submerged is equal to the weight of the water that is displaced. Since we know the density of water, the volume of water displaced is calculated and the volume of the person's body is determined. However, air in the lungs and in the gastrointestinal tract need to be accounted for. This is done by instructing the person to exhale as much air from the lungs as possible and measuring the amount of air that is exhaled, i.e., residual volume. For air in the gastrointestinal tract, it is assumed that when a person is in fasting state, the volume is about 0.1 L.

Dual energy X-ray absorptiometry (DXA, previously DEXA): DXA is widely used to assess the bone mineral density (BMD) of the whole body and of different parts of the body, such as legs, trunk, spine, femur and arms, i.e., regional body composition and also fat content of the body. Typically, bone weight constitutes approximately 4–6% of total body weight. DXA is a valid and precise method for measuring body composition and is the method of choice when it comes to measuring bone mineral density. For DXA, the body is divided into three components—bone, lean body mass + bone – free tissue and fat.

It can be used to measure whole body composition even in severely obese persons whose body weight is 150 kg or more, except that very large body size can be a limitation in terms of fitting inside the scanning area of the equipment. It also enables estimation of android and gynoid fat distribution. Although it is quick and noninvasive, DXA is expensive. It is considered to be safe for repeated measurements for clinical purposes even if there is a very small amount of exposure to radiation. Accuracy may be affected by hydration status.

Magnetic resonance imaging (MRI) or Magnetic resonance tomography (MRT): It is a technique to visualize the internal structure and function of the body, when the body is placed in a strong magnetic field. It gives precise information about body composition. MRI has also been developed to measure adipose tissues and the distribution of fat in the body as well as help in characterizing a disease due to the association between different patterns of adiposity. MRI is used to image every part of the body, and is particularly useful for neurological conditions, for disorders of the muscles and joints, for evaluating tumors, and for showing abnormalities in the heart and blood vessels. It is a valid and precise as well as noninvasive method.

Computed tomography (CT): CT scan involves visualization of the body tissues in cross sectional slices by use of X-rays. It helps to assess body fat in specific parts of the body. It can accurately give quantitative measures of body composition. Axial CT uses cross-sectional images that are taken around a single axis of rotation. It permits measuring body components at the tissue level and can give measurement of total body fat area as well as visceral and subcutaneous adipose fat area. Visceral fat volume and skeletal muscle index can also be measured. Besides this, in research studies, pericardial fat, intrathoracic fat, and epicardial fat has also been measured. However, one concern is that it exposes the person to radiation.

Near infrared interactance (NIR): This method is based on the principles of light absorption, reflection, and near infrared spectroscopy, in which a computerized spectrophotometer equipped with a scan and probe is used. Measurement is done on the biceps of the dominant arm and a light beam at specific wavelengths is sent into the arm. The degree of infrared light that is absorbed and reflected are related to the body composition of the tissues through which the light passes and the specific wavelength that is emitted by the light. When the probe is placed on the site where fat mass is to be measured, it emits infrared light that passes through both fat and muscle (light absorption is different in the fat mass and the lean mass) and is reflected back to the probe and the percent body fat and lean tissue are estimated and displayed. Unlike BIA, this method directly measures fat. It is a simple and rapid as well as non-invasive method and does not have many limitations. One important limitation is for persons who have very dark or black tattoos because the NIR light is low energy that could be totally absorbed by a black tattoo.

Bod Pod (Air displacement plethysmography): The principle underlying this method is similar to that of measuring body volume with water. However, instead of water, air displacement is used to measure the body volume. It is noninvasive and does not require much technical expertise for use of the equipment. The equipment consists of two chambers. One is a test chamber in which the person being measured sits and the other is a reference chamber containing the instrumentation that is used to measure changes in pressure between the two chambers. The method is based on determining pressure changes that occur between the test and the reference chambers respectively and is based on Boyle's law, i.e., $P1/P2 = V2/V1$

V1 and P1 are the volume and pressure in the test chamber before the person enters it and V2 and P2 are the volume and pressure while the person is in the test chamber.

The volume of the person's body is equal to the difference in volume pre- and post entry of the person into the chamber. Some precautions are advised such as the person should be dry, the test should be conducted prior to exercise and the environment temperature should remain stable.

Ultrasound: This is an older method compared to others. It is based on reflection of echoes and represents two-dimension gray scale images between white that are strong reflections and black that are no echoes. With this, the borders of subcutaneous fat, fat-muscle, and muscle-bone interfaces are seen. The method is fairly simple, not expensive, and noninvasive, but it is not a standardized procedure. It may be useful to predictor visceral adipose tissue through measurement of intra-abdominal thickness.

Use of anthropometry: The above techniques are useful for assessing body composition. However, when large numbers of persons are to be measured, cost and time are constraints.

When nutritional status is to be assessed, nutritionists use anthropometric measurements to determine—whether the person is having normal weight or otherwise. Anthropometry is the measurement of size, weight, and proportions of the human body. Various measurements are used but whichever the measurement, what is critical is to have precise measurements. Many factors affect anthropometric variations such as age, gender, race and ethnic factors, occupation, socioeconomic status, lifestyle and diet, and circadian and secular trends.

There are two types of anthropometric data: (a) physical or static anthropometry which is concerned with measuring the basic physical dimensions of the body and (b) functional anthropometry in which physical dimensions are measured in relation to particular activities or tasks. Newtonian data is also used. Newtonian data is concerned with body segment data and data about forces that can be exerted in different postures or different tasks.

Body Mass Index (BMI): It is the ratio of body weight to height [Wt (kg)/Ht (m^2)]. It is also known as Quetelet's index. It is highly correlated with body fat. The WHO has given cut off points for determining whether individuals are underweight, normal or overweight/obese Based on WHO (2004), Asian cut offs are shown in Figure 5.12. High BMI (>30) is associated with increased risk of chronic diseases. It should be noted that the cut off points for Asians are lower than for persons in other parts of the world, since Asians have a higher risk for type II diabetes. BMI is age-independent and the cut-offs are the same for both males and females. However, this does not always reflect fatness. For example, an athlete or weight lifter may have a high BMI that is largely attributable to muscle mass. Therefore, it is advisable to use BMI along with a circumference measurement, such as waist circumference or the ratio of waist to hip circumferences. More recently waist to height ratio is recommended to assess abdominal adiposity.

Circumference measurements: Typically, waist and hip circumference measurements are taken. They should be taken in the morning, before eating, and after emptying the bladder. Measurements are taken when the person is standing upright and for the same person, two or three measurements should be taken and the average is calculated, if the two measurements differ by less than 1 cm. But, if the difference between the two measurements is more than 1 cm, the two measurements should be repeated. The following are important considerations:
- Where exactly the tape is placed, i.e., the anatomical site
- The type of tape used
- How tight is the tape
- The posture of the person being measured
- What is the phase of respiration (measurements should be taken at the end of a normal respiration)
- What is the abdominal tension
- Type of clothing worn by the person who is being measured
- The stomach contents, i.e., the amount of water and food that the person has consumed.

The World Health Organization has given the protocol for these measurements.

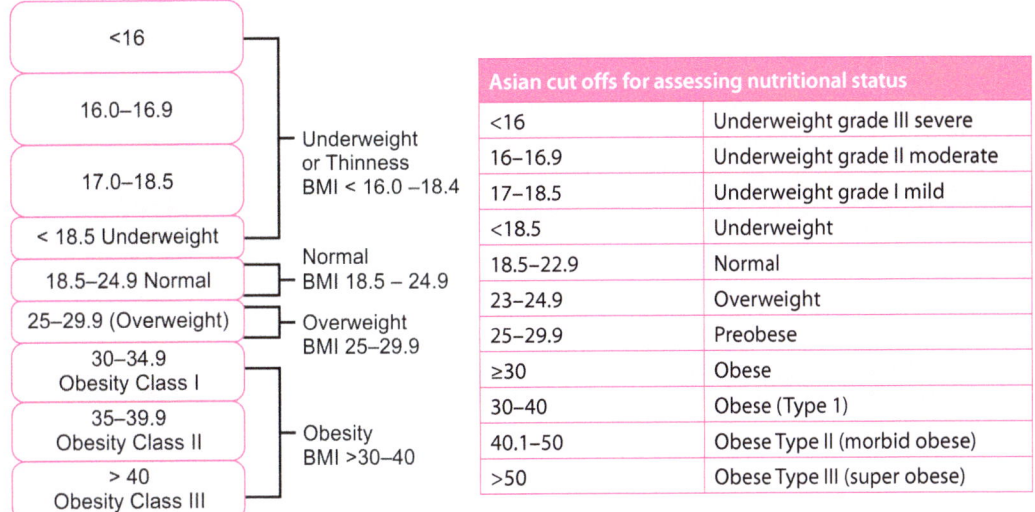

Fig. 5.12: Body mass index (BMI).

Waist circumference (WC): It indicates upper body fat storage. Both WC and WHR are surrogate measures for abdominal adiposity. A waist circumference exceeding 94 cm is indicative of higher BMI and adiposity. Persons having a waist circumference >94 cm should take appropriate action. However, for Asians the cutoff points are lower—for males the cutoff is 90 cm and for women the cutoff is 80 cm. This measurement measures the amount of abdominal fat with more precision than does WHR. Waist circumference measurement should be made at the approximate midpoint between the lower margin of the last palpable rib and the top of the iliac crest. Hip circumference should be taken around the widest portion of the buttocks. WC is likely to be a better indicator of abdominal adiposity.

Waist-to-Hip ratio (WHR): The waist circumference measurement is divided by the hip circumference measurement. It is not just the amount of body fat that is important. Where the fat is deposited is of concern. WHR is better predictor of the fat distribution. It is an easy method for field studies and patients in bed, but it is not a good measurement for elder population because it is difficult to interpret, as waist circumference may be higher and hip circumference may be lower due to loss of lean body mass. WHR above 0.90 for men and 0.80 for women is indicative of health risk since more fat is distributed in upper part of the body. It can also predict the progression of disease such as diabetes.

Waist-to-Height ratio (WHtR): WC has been used as an indicator for abdominal adiposity. However, different expert groups recommend different sites for measurement and there are differences in the cutoff values as well. Hsieh and Yoshinaga (1999) demonstrated that metabolic risks were different for people whose waist circumferences were similar, but they had different heights. Simultaneously, Ashwell and other scientists in the UK proposed that waist-to-height ratio is a good indicator for monitoring risk. A WHtR value of 0.5 has been suggested as the cutoff and values exceeding 0.6 indicate that the person is at a substantially increased risk.

Studies undertaken later have shown that WHtR is a better predictor of risk for cardiovascular disease and diabetes than WC. With this indicator, a simple message that can be given to people has been proposed that one's WC should be less than half of one's height.

BODY WEIGHT

Body weight is the sum total weight of body fat, bones, muscle, organ tissues, skin, and total body water. On an average, 60–70% of the body weight comes from total body water (TBW). Total water includes ECF and ICF and other fluids, whereas solid mass is composed of adipose tissues, muscles, vital organs, bones, and skin. Body weight influences one's personality, physical appearance, psychological response, and physiological reactions.

Whole body weight is influenced by age, sex, height, lean body mass, body fat, and body water and is largely governed by several biological and environmental factors. Body weight measurement is one of the most popular, practical, useful, and economic measurements. It is frequently used to assess nutritional and health status at home, in physical fitness and sports activities, in clinical practice as well as in field studies.

> Body weight = Total body water + muscle + bones + body fat + organ + tissues (Brain + liver + kidney + GI tract + skin)

Body weight fluctuates because of alterations in food intake, body composition, physical and metabolic activities, and environmental stressors. Frequent and drastic fluctuations indicate energy imbalance, nutritional imbalance or deficiencies, disorders, and diseases. Increase in body weight during growth period and pregnancy is desirable, but weight gain in mature adults is undesirable. Even during periods of growth and pregnancy, excess weight gain is not desirable. Both overweight and underweight may predispose the individual to some imbalances or diseases. A person whose weight is 10% below the desired weight range is said to be underweight. The human body has mechanisms for energy homeostasis and body weight regulation. These comprise control of food intake, regulation of energy expenditure by autonomic nervous system, and endocrine hormones. Body weight can be regulated by short-term and long-term controls. Short-term controls generally include initiation and termination of feeding in which gastrointestinal signals play a role. Long-term control is connected with alterations in energy balance and stores in the body, and the relationship between the two.

Theories for Body Weight Regulation

Theories for body weight regulation are based on epidemiological observations that body composition and body weight remain relatively the same/stable over a long period of time, although energy intake and expenditure varies, considerably long-term benefits of weight loss therapies are not very long-lasting (most people including children regain most of the weight they had lost). There are many theories in relation to regulation of the body weight:

Fat Cell Theory

According to fat cell theory, size or number of fat cells determines body size. There are two types of obesity.

Hyperplastic obesity: It is because of the increase in the number of fat cells and usually occurs in infancy, childhood or adolescence. One cause of obesity may be the development of excess fat cells during childhood. During the period of growth, the number of fat cells increases and then level off. It may be because of overfeeding. This type of obesity is rather difficult to manage because the number of fat cells once formed may not reduce.

Hypertrophic obesity: Fat cells have the capacity of expanding several times their original size. It usually occurs in adults and largely due to overconsumption of energy dense foods. In certain cases, it may be due to the increase in the rate of fat synthesis. During adulthood, the numbers of fat cells are rather fixed after growth ceases, but the size of fat cell can vary. A fat cell can expand 8- to 10-fold in size by storing excess energy in the form of triglycerides. Once they reach a certain size, adipose cells may also divide. Fat cells of obese people also contain more LPL so they are likely to reach a large size more quickly. This type of obesity can be controlled by dietary management and intense exercise.

Set Point Theory

According to the set point theory, a person's body will maintain body weight in a given range over a long period of time (years together) even if there are changes in food intake or exercise. When the adipose tissue increases beyond the "set point", a signal causes food intake to be reduced (there is a feedback mechanism that is designed to regulate the body weight to a predetermined weight) while energy expenditure may or may not increase, so that weight is lost. On the other hand, when there is decrease in the fat stores, food intake increases with possible reduction in energy expenditure, such that the body weight increases. Every individual's body has an inbuilt system that regulates and monitor for specific amount of fat stores and body weight, i.e., the individual's metabolism adjusts itself to maintain a given weight and a defect in this homeostatic mechanism may be responsible for obesity. Some people may have high set point whereas others have a low set point. It is considered that at set point or constant body weight the person will work efficiently and remain stable. It is not clear yet but assumed that certain centers in brain may resist the change. Hence, however much a person tries, he/she is not able to lose weight beyond a certain point. However, recent research provides evidence that challenges this set point theory.

In this, it is assumed that the body does not have an active mechanism for predefined regulation of body weight, and that body weight is largely influenced by "settles" by environmental and socioeconomic factors, such as diet and lifestyle, in interaction with genetic predisposition, or, to phrase this more generally, in interaction with the individual's constitution. Thus, there is no fixed set point and many factors contribute to regulation of body weight. An example given to illustrate the settling point model for body weight regulation is the level of water in a lake. Water in a lake or a reservoir equilibrates naturally, i.e., when there is inflow of water due to rain, the extra water flows out and the amount that flows out is equal to the amount of inflow. In the settling point theory, the increasing prevalence of obesity is explained to be a result of the greater availability of food or being more exposed to food cues, leading to higher food intake. Alternatively there may be decrease in physical activity and energy expenditure.

Enzymatic Theory

This theory links fat storage with elevated concentrations of the enzyme that enables fat cells to store triglycerides. Lipoprotein lipase (LPL) is the key enzyme in lipid metabolism. It is present in endothelial cell lining of the capillaries of heart, muscles, and adipose tissues. In a lean, healthy individual, LPL is evenly distributed in equal amounts between muscle cells and fat tissues. Insulin tends to increase synthesis of LPL. LPL is increased by meals but decreased by fasting. In addition, leptin also accelerates LPL activity, since it is synthesized in adipose tissue. LPL level varies with gender and site of fat deposition in the body. High LPL activity accelerates storage of fat in adipocytes. Obesity is associated with increased LPL activity in adipose tissue.

The LPL activity is inversely regulated in fat cells and muscle tissues in response to eating cycles. Eating a meal increases LPL activity in fat cells whereas activity in muscle cells is decreased. Thus, it allows the body to store as much energy (as fat) as possible when food is available. Between meals, or when food is not available, LPL activity decreases in fat cells whereas it is increased in muscle cells in order to increase energy output during periods of food-seeking behavior.

Research has shown that diets rich in refined carbohydrates require more insulin. High level of insulin (hyperinsulinemia) stimulates transport of glucose into adipocytes; induces LPL synthesis, thereby promotes fat storage. At the same time, it inhibits breakdown of fat and limits weight loss. Further, it may lead to insulin resistance followed by type II diabetes.

Therefore, consuming complex carbohydrate instead of refined carbohydrates and low glycemic foods may be helpful.

Theory of Thermogenesis

Adipose tissue contains white adipose tissue cells and brown fat cells. White adipose tissue (WAT) contains relatively few mitochondria and thus the white adipose tissue has a slower metabolic rate. Its main function is to serve as a reservoir for energy. However, it is also involved in immune function and production of adipocytokines (leptin) as well as growth factors. White adipose tissue has receptors for hormones such as insulin, growth hormones, norepinephrine, and glucocorticoids.

In comparison, the metabolic rate of the brown adipose tissue (BAT) is higher because it has numerous mitochondria. It is abundant in newborn babies and hibernating mammals. Brown adipose tissue dissipates a lot of heat and the stored energy that is released as heat through nonshivering and diet-induced thermogenesis. It has been suggested that those who are lean may have more brown adipose tissue and that in obese persons; both the brown and white adipose tissue cells may burn off less energy compared to those who are of normal weight or lean persons. There is also a beige adipose tissue or beige fat that is a mixture of brown and white adipose tissue. Beige fat is induced in white fat in response to several factors that stimulate the transformation, e.g., cold stress, norepinephrine, and surgical denervation. The activity of brown or beige adipose tissue has been reported to be inversely associated with body mass index and visceral fat mass and is low in obese persons. Induction of beige fat is being studied for its potential as therapy for diseases such as obesity, diabetes, and fatty liver.

> **Research Glimpse:** Excess visceral adiposity, especially the adipose tissue located adjacent to the heart and coronary arteries is associated with increased cardiovascular risk. Dysfunctional adipose tissue secretes many factors that have an effect on vascular function and increases the risk of atherogenesis. However, brown and beige adipose tissues are beneficial for cardiometabolic health because these tissues utilize glucose and lipids for generating heat. Cardiac and thoracic perivascular adipose tissues reportedly contain brown adipose tissue in the healthy state, but in obesity, the brown adipose tissue probably is converted into white adipose tissue. This may increase the propensity for development of cardiovascular disease. There are mechanisms by which white adipose tissue can be converted into brown adipose tissue (browning). Some of these include specific components of the diet such as dietary nitrates, conjugated linoleic acid, and omega-3 fatty acids.
>
> *Aldiss P, Davies G, Woods R, Budge H, Sacks HS, Symonds ME. 'Browning' the cardiac and peri-vascular adipose tissues to modulate cardiovascular risk. International Journal of Cardiology. 2017;228:265–74.*

> **Research Glimpse:** There is a unique uncoupling protein (UCP1) in brown adipose tissue (BAT). When UCP1 is activated, heat is rapidly generated and lipids and/or glucose are oxidized. UCP1 is present in relatively small amounts in adult humans, but it is rapidly activated at birth and plays an important role in preventing hypothermia in newborns. Newborns are able to rapidly generate large amounts of heat through nonshivering thermogenesis. BAT was found to be
>
> *Contd...*
>
> *Contd...*
>
> present in adult humans about a decade ago. Along with this research has shown that we have beige fat. This type of fat consists of white adipocytes and has discrete areas of UCP1-containing cells. Beige fat depots contain about 10% of the UCP1 that is present in BAT. In obese persons, the abundance of brown and/or beige fat is reduced, as also in ageing. There is interest in strategies to either preventing age-related loss and/or to reactivate the depots. However, there are difficulties because BAT function is assessed in humans by measurement of radio-labeled glucose uptake when the person is fasting, and depends on exposure to cold environment. Repeat scans have shown that in the same person positive and negative scans are obtained. In rodents, multiple pathways that are involved in modulating brown fat and beige fat function have been identified but the relevance of these findings to humans is to be considered because the studies have been typically done in cool-adapted conditions. Also, BAT can adapt rapidly to changes in the environmental temperature so that glucose oxidation occurs and there is heat production.
>
> *Symonds ME, Aldiss P, Pope M, Budge H. Recent advances in our understanding of brown and beige adipose tissue: the good fat that keeps you healthy. F1000 Research. 2018;7:F1000 Faculty Rev-1129.*

BODY TYPES

Body types are also known as phenotypes. Phenotype is defined as "the physical appearance or biochemical characteristic of an organism as a result of the interaction of its genotype and the environment. The expression of a particular trait, for example, skin color, height, behavior, etc. according to the individual's genetic makeup and environment".

Since ages, various efforts have been made to categorize human body on the basis of physical structure. In 1940, William Sheldon proposed a theory that there are three body types or somatotypes (Soma means body) that are inherited through genetic makeup. Some persons look lean or thin, others look fat and some we think are normal. According to this theory, the type of body mainly determines one's body size and shape that are based on skeletal frame and body composition. The three body somatotypes are as follows:

Endomorph (round and fat type): Soft, round and broad size and extremities are tapering from trunk, underdeveloped muscles. Considered to have more body fat and can gain weight easily.

Mesomorph (muscular type): Medium and muscular built, hard muscular body. Can gain or lose weight relatively equally.

Ectomorph (slim or linear type): Thin, slender with long bones and narrow upper body and fingers, delicately built and lightly muscled. Have less fat and may find it difficult to gain weight.

Endomorph

These are on average heavier, taller, and have relatively more fat. The body shape looks wide, round, soft, and curvy. They usually have a round face and heavier fat accumulation around their waist. Buttocks and thighs also tend to be larger. Extreme endomorphs have pear-shaped bodies with wide shoulders and wide hips. Endomorphs usually have higher number of fat cells and low BMR (requires less energy for their metabolism). Being broad and heavy, they are not very active and quick to move, therefore, they are always at high risk to gain weight and find it difficult to lose weight and they also tend to regain weight easily. They require more energy in physical activity to maintain energy balance otherwise they may undergo positive energy balance or overweight. Endomorphs may feel quickly fatigued after doing some work.

Mesomorph

Mesomorphs have more muscle and bone mass, less body fat, broad shoulders, and narrow hips. They have less risk of obesity; however, they can become overweight or obese through lack of exercise and/or poor nutrition. They are usually more involved in physical activities and sport without much effort.

Ectomorph

They are tall, lean, and slim. They have less muscle and find it difficult to gain weight. A rating for degree of type was developed by Sheldon in 1940, using a seven point scale for the three main components, i.e., fat, muscle, and bone. Based on this an extreme endomorph's rating is 7:1:1, the scale rating for an extreme mesomorph is 1:7:1, and for an extreme ectomorph it is 1:1:7.

> **Laboratory Laurel:** In this study, 176 male and 110 female students were categorized as per their somatotypes and the contribution of the somatotype to their coordinate abilities was determined. Among males, the mesomorphic endomorph somatotype was more prevalent and among females, the balanced endomorph somatotype was seen. The endomorph somatotype was seen to contribute to constant balance and agility among males, and the mesomorph and ectomorph somatotypes contributed to dynamic balance and agility among females. The researcher recommended that it is necessary to improve the mesomorphic traits/characteristics through appropriate training programs.
>
> Khasawneh A. Prevailing Somatotypes and Their Contribution Rate to the Coordination Abilities among the Students of the Physical Education College. Advances in Physical Education. 2015;5:176–87.

The above is a typical classification. In reality, most persons will show characteristics of more than one phenotype, i.e., have some tendencies for one phenotype while having the main characteristics of another phenotype. Thus, most persons are said to have a mixed type of physique. For example, a mesomorph may show endomorphic characteristics around the waist and abdominal area. These phenotypic differences are visible, but it is possible that such somatotypes may differ metabolically.

There are broadly two body types namely android and gynoid and they are characterized by the body shapes.

Android (Apple-shape)

The upper part of the body or trunk (around shoulder, neck, and face) has more fat deposition. Apple-shaped bodies tend to have increased risk for high cholesterol, higher triglycerides, higher blood glucose levels, and hypertension indicating risk of diabetes, CVD, i.e., metabolic and cardiovascular disease and cancer. Android obesity is also known as truncal obesity.

Gynoid (Pear-shape)

Fat deposition is more in lower parts of the body (around waist and abdomen) and such individuals may have abdominal obesity and are at high risk of its associated disorders. Studies have shown that there is association in between the android/gynoid ratio and metabolic and cardiovascular disease. It is related to insulin resistance and is a measure of obesity.

Assessment of Body Weight

Individuals vary considerably in their body weights even when their heights are the same; it becomes difficult to spell out "ideal" body weight. The terms "healthy weight and desirable body weight" are generally used. Experts recommend reference values compared to which, it is possible to assess whether the person's weight is appropriate for his/her height.

Healthy weight: It is the body weight at which there is no harm or risk to health. It implies absence of any medical conditions that would improve with weight loss. And fat distribution is not associated with any risk of disease. Healthy weight is that weight which is appropriate for a person's height.

Desirable body weight: Longevity and health of the person is proportional to weight. Traditionally, desirable weight was previously considered in relation to the height. Now desirable weight is considered in relation to gender, body frame size, and body composition. "Frame size is an estimate of the proportion of body weight that is due to bones". Devine's formula helps to assess one's desirable formula as shown in Table 5.10. The other methods are:

1. **Broca's index:** Measure the height in centimeters and subtract 100 from the height. The figure obtained gives the approximate desirable weight in kilograms, e.g., if height is 165 cm the weight can be
   165 – 100 = 65 kg
2. **Hamwi's equation:** For males weight = 106 lbs for first 5' of height + 6 lbs for each additional inch over 5', for females weight = 100 lbs for first 5' in height + 5 lbs for each additional inch over 5'.

Table 5.10: Calculation of desirable body weight based on frame size.

Body build	Women	Men
Medium frame	For 5 feet height—45.5 kg weight For additional inch, add 2.3 kg, e.g., for 5'3" height, weight can be 52.4 kg	For 5 feet height—48.0 kg For additional inch, add 2.7 kg, e.g., for 5'8" height, weight can be 69.6 kg
Small frame	Subtract to base line by 10%, e.g., 5' height, weight can be 40.9 kg	Subtract to base line by 10%, e.g., 5' height, weight can be 44.8 kg
Large frame	Add to base line by 10%, e.g., 5' height, weight can be 50.1 kg	Add to base line by 10%, e.g., 5' height, weight can be 52.8 kg

Adapted from Committees of American Dietetic Association 1974.

3. **Based on body fat mass:** Normally desirable body fat in woman is 25% and man 15%. Desirable body weight (DBW) = Lean body weight/1 – % body fat.

   For example: A woman weighs 70 kg with 30% fat in the body. Normally, desirable body fat in woman is 25% and man 15%. Therefore, her DBW will be

70 × 0.30	= 21.0 kg body fat
70 – 21	= 49 kg is lean body weight
Desirable body weight	= 49/ (1 – 0.25) = 49/0.75
	= 65 kg

   Use of LIC Tables: Life Insurance Corporation (LIC) has given standard height and weight table depending upon the life expectancy.

Deviations in Body Weight

Body weight is an approximate measure of energy stores and nutrient build up. Although the human body has mechanisms to maintain body weight, the latter is not static. The human body is constantly exposed to various biological and environmental factors (Table 5.11) that often lead to alterations in food and energy intake and/or in energy expenditure. These results in deviations in body weight and efforts have to be made to achieve and maintain homeostasis or balance. Body weight is affected by a person's genetic background, developmental history, physiology, age, physical activity level, diet, environment, and social background. Some factors like physiology, genetics, and age are biologically programmed, whereas other factors are in the individual's control such as diet and level of physical activity. Some factors are occupational and environmental such as the type of work and worksite design and the facilities available.

Biological Factors

By and large body weight is not different in boys and girls, till the age of 7–9 years or prepubertal stage but thereafter it differs. Body constitution is genetic, for example, endomorphs are plump and are short-statured whereas ectomorphs are slender and tall. Such conditions are natural, difficult to reverse, and must be accepted.

Table 5.11: Biological and environmental factors responsible for deviation in body weight.

Biological factors	Environmental factors
Gender	Food intake
Genetics	Exercise
Parental body makeup	Cultural influence
Body type	Childhood food habits
Body constitution	Psychological reactions to food
Cell size and cell number	Fad diets
Metabolic rate	Social group
Hormones	Advertisement and media
Thermogenesis	Urbanization
Physiological condition	Industrialization
Sickness and infection	Transport
Chronic diseases	Pollution and pollutants

Children of fat parents are usually fat or vice versa. One view is that children inherit the genes from either or both the parents. Another view is that the children grow and develop in the same environment, in which their parents had developed the obesity. This environment can be the food habits, lifestyle, lack of knowledge, etc.

Prenatal Factors

During fetal stage, maternal nutrition plays a role in determining body weight. Low birth weight and its after effects in adulthood is an issue of concern in our country. Studies on animals and humans show that if the mother was nutritionally deprived during the first and/or second trimester of pregnancy, prevalence of obesity and its consequences in adult life are higher. Lower birth weight has been associated with obesity in adulthood and increased risk of cardiovascular disease.

Infancy and Childhood

In extrauterine life, body weight is influenced more by environmental and nutritional factors. If the baby is well-nourished and cared for in a hygienic environment, the child will grow and develop into a healthy well-nourished child. However, episodes of illness and infection can affect body weight. Frequent infections and prolonged persistence of infectious diseases, such as measles, typhoid, etc. may adversely affect the body and body weight and as seen in this country, and put young children at risk of being underweight and undernourished.

From birth until 1 year of age, adipose tissue increases and then declines to a minimum by 6 years of age. Although plump chubby young children are considered to be charming; this may not be necessarily healthy. Some children between 5 years and 7 years of age show increased adiposity. This is known as "adiposity rebound" and such children are at increased risk (3- to 6-fold) of increased BMI as adults. Such children are often observed to have wrong eating habits with insufficient exercise and may soon become obese. This may make them targets for teasing in schooling, putting them in psychological distress as well as being at high risk for pathological conditions.

Adolescence

In some countries, it has been estimated that for about one-third of the persons who are obese, obesity may have been initiated in childhood. For others, adolescence is a critical period. This is the age when children want to establish their independence, follow their peers, and may have aberrant food patterns. Some may want to be very thin whereas others may indulge in energy dense and "junk" foods, putting them at risk of deviations in body weight, sometimes to extremes and adversely influencing nutritional status.

Hormonal Factors

Besides diet, age, and physical activity, several hormones influence body weight. Thyroid gland and the hormone secreted by it, i.e., thyroxin, influences the metabolic rate of the body that directly influences body weight and the level of physical activity. Underactive thyroid reduces the BMR, makes the person lethargic. There is a tendency to accumulate body fat and for the body weight to increase. Excess of thyroid hormone results in higher BMR and the person may lose weight.

Several hormones, such as leptin, ghrelin and insulin and neurotransmitters, such as neuropeptide Y, influence appetite, hunger and satiety and in turn influence body weight. When there is leptin resistance or insulin resistance, body weight is found to increase and the person may find it difficult to reduce and maintain the reduced body weight. Sex hormones and growth hormone also influence appetite, metabolism, and body fat distribution.

Estrogen hormone in females also affects body weight, therefore, women tend to gain and retain weight to some extent during and after menopause. Women in their reproductive years tend to store fat in the lower body whereas postmenopausal women and older men tend to have more fat stores in the upper part of the body. Weight gain before menstruation is also related to female hormones that normally subside after menopause. Lack of estrogen may also lead to weight gain.

Growth hormone influences stature and height. It influences metabolism and there are studies that show that growth hormone levels are lower in obese persons than individuals with normal body weight.

Cortisol is another hormone that affects weight. It is a steroid hormone produced by the adrenal cortex under stress conditions, such as fasting, food intake, exercising, awakening, and psychosocial stressors. It performs two important functions: Energy regulation and mobilization. It influences mobilization of fat stores. In order to counteract the effect of stress, individuals often resort to eating foods that are rich in carbohydrate and fat (called stress or emotional eating). Some persons may crave salty food as well. Consumption of such foods might make the person feel less stressed and relax but if this occurs persistently, it can adversely influence body weight. Some studies have shown that stress and elevated cortisol tend to cause fat deposition in the abdominal area rather than in the hips.

Obese people have hormone levels that encourage the accumulation of body fat. It seems that behaviors, such as overeating and lack of regular exercise, over time, "reset" the processes that regulate appetite and body fat distribution to make the person physiologically more inclined to gain weight. Since hormones are regulators of body weight and influence obesity. Hence endocrine disruptors and obesogens will also affect appetite, satiety, adipose tissues, insulin sensitivity metabolic rate, etc. thereby body weight.

Environmental Factors

Body weight changes with changes in food intake, stress, exercise, and other environmental factors. These changes are reflected not only in fat depots but also in body fluids, bone minerals, muscles, etc. These changes can result in short-term or long-term deviations in body weight. Short-term fluctuations can be due to changes in water balance, changes in glycogen stores, infection, trauma, enforced bed rest, and malignancy. These can be relatively managed by diet and medical treatments. Long-term changes can result in overweight or underweight and generally involve appetite control (physiological mechanism) and the metabolic rate (hormonal control). Lifetime adjustments in lifestyle may be required to handle such deviations.

> The chemical environmental which have the capacity to disrupt the action of hormones are called endocrine-disrupting chemicals (EDCs) or Endocrine disruptors. The EDC which may bring imbalance in body weight or which can lead to obesity are called "obesogens"). These can be present in house hold products, pesticides, herbicides. Plastics bags, containers and personal care products.

Food intake considerably influences body weight. Both the amounts of food intake as well as the composition of food are important. Energy intake is of paramount importance. Inadequate energy, i.e., food intake may lead to chronic fatigue and undernutrition in adults and underweight or undernutrition in children whereas an excess of energy intake results in overweight progressing toward obesity and its related disorders. Starvation, intended restriction, and deficient food intake over a period of time lead to weight loss. Many people adopt very restricted diets for weight loss; but these may not be appropriate. Many a times, people follow fad diets. Fad diet is a term that refers to some popular diets that are intended to promote quick weight loss. These diets often lack scientific evidences and may cause some health problems or deficiency diseases.

It is necessary to assess body composition and pay attention to the nutrient composition of the foods included in weight loss program for better health outcome. Very low calorie diets that are highly restricted in energy and other nutrients lead to underweight due to loss of body reserves of fat but with fat loss there is loss of lean body mass and body fluids.

Planning a healthy balanced diet in accordance to dietary guidelines can help maintain appropriate body weight. Food intake is influenced by sociocultural circumstances. There are many occasions where the person tends to consume food whatever is available. Such situations are common in highly stressful and job-oriented situations. High energy foods are often easily available and accessible. In social gatherings also, generally energy dense foods are part of the menu.

Eating patterns and eating habits play a major role in food intake. Eating pattern includes portion size, variety, frequency, regularity, snacking, skipping meals, consumption of energy rich beverages and snacks, eating fast foods, junk foods and eating out, eating more on festivals, holidays, social gatherings, parties, etc. Eating habits are linked with taste preferences of the individual, interest, mood/emotional factors, time of eating, skipping breakfast, dietary restraint, and cultural and societal norms.

Food intake is influenced by mental and emotional state. Some people eat less when they are under stress whereas others tend to eat when they are stressed or depressed as a compensation for being bored. Industrialization and urbanization have limited the time available to eat proper balanced meals in spite of availability and affordability. Advertisements and availability of ready-to-eat foods and food outlets in urban areas have greatly influenced eating patterns and food intake. Digitalization and social media have also triggered the rising trend of obesity, largely due to reduced physical activity and consumption of high energy beverages and snacks.

In the urban working scenario, people are busy but they lead sedentary lives. There are facilities, such as public transport or personal vehicles; hence people do not like to walk much. Many face constraints of time to undertake separate exercise sessions. They do not have much physical activity and hence weight gain is visible over a period of time. Housewives do household chores using easy to do appliances but most do not have enough physical activity and exercise.

Regular exercise, not necessarily gym or sports, can help in reducing and maintaining the body weight. Exercise and appropriate physical activity not only influence weight but also brings favorable changes in body composition, flexibility, agility, speed, muscular strength and endurance, balance, and cardiorespiratory fitness.

Urbanization and industrialization have not improved the circumstances of children and adults belonging to physically and economically challenged groups. People residing in villages and hamlets far away from urban areas, those who face drought or other natural calamities or live in disaster-struck areas are forced to limit their food intake for variable periods of time. Among these communities, the risk of undernutrition and underweight is high.

Biological factors, such as age, gender, genes and certain physiological conditions are unavoidable but food intake and exercise are within a person's control and should be used wisely to maintain appropriate body weight. Sharp fluctuation and deviation in body weight needs to be attended to and body weight should be checked regularly.

Further evidence are available that air quality in cities have decline. Population exposed to high levels of air pollutants is at higher risk of gaining unhealthy body weight through alteration in metabolism and disruption in regular physical activities.

RAPID FIRE

1. Which pathways and cycles are involved in energy metabolism?
2. What is chemical energy?
3. How is ATP important in energy metabolism?
4. What is the significance of BMR in energy expenditure?
5. What is the advantage of assessing PAL?
6. What is BMI and give the classification for BMI?
7. Why is assessment of body composition important?
8. What is importance of LBM and different types of fat in the body?
9. Which hormones affect the food intake?
10. What are the theories linked with body weight?
11. Which factors will increase risk of weight gain?
12. What is the difference in appetite and hunger and what factors affect them?
13. What is the difference in hyperplastic and hypertrophic obesity?
14. What is set point theory?
15. Why does body weight deviate so much and why is it important to maintain?

EXERCISES

1. Prepare a questionnaire and survey five people each from sedentary, moderate, and heavy workers regarding their weight management practices/energy expenditure.
2. Assess the body composition based on BMI and waist-hip ratio of 10 people and comment on their weight status.
3. Meet five obese people and find out their knowledge, attitude, and practice with regard to food intake and energy expenditure.

SUGGESTED READING

1. Ainsworth BE, Haskell WL, Herrmann SD, Meckes N, Bassett DR Jr, Tudor-Locke C, et al. 2011 Compendium of Physical Activities: a second update of codes and MET values. Med Sci Sports Exerc. 2011;43(8):1575-81.
2. Alberts B, Johnson A, Lewis J, et al. Molecular Biology of the Cell. 4th edition. New York: Garland Science; 2002.
3. Bandini L, Flynn A. Overnutrition. In: Gibney MJ, MacDonald IA, Roche HM (Eds). Nutrition and Metabolism. Chichester: Blackwell Publishing, The Nutrition Society; 2003. pp. 324-33.
4. Bergman J. ATP: The perfect energy currency for the cell. Creation. 1999.
5. Bergman RN, Kim SP, Catalano KJ, et al. Why visceral fat is bad: Mechanisms of the metabolic syndrome. Obesity. 2006;14:16S–9S.
6. Darbe PD. Endocrine disruptors and obesity. Curr obes rep. 2017;62(1):18-27.
7. Das SK, Roberts SB. Energy metabolism. In: Bowman BA, Russell RM (Eds). Present Knowledge in Nutrition. 9th edition, Vol I. Washington: International Life Sciences Institute; 2006. pp. 45-58.
8. Deurenberg P, Roubenoff R. Body composition. In: Gibney MJ, Vorster HH, Kok FJ (Eds). Introduction to Human Nutrition. Chichester: Blackwell Publishing, The Nutrition Society; 2002. pp. 12-30.
9. Drewnowski A, Monsivais P. Taste and food selection. In: Bowman BA, Russell RM (Eds). Present Knowledge in Nutrition. 9th edition, Vol I. Washington: International Life Sciences Institute; 2006. pp. 807-15.
10. DuBois D, DuBois EF. A formula to estimate the approximate surface area if height and weight be known. Archives of Internal Medicine. 1916;17:863-71.
11. FAO. Human Energy Requirements. Food and Agricultural Organization, 2004.
12. Food and Nutrition Board. Dietary Reference Intakes for Energy, Carbohydrate, Fiber, Fat, Fatty acids, Cholesterol, Protein and Amino Acids (Macronutrients). Washington: Institute of Medicine, The National Academies Press; 2005.
13. Friedman JM. The function of leptin in nutrition, weight, and physiology. Nutrition Reviews. 2002;60(10):S1-14.
14. Goran MI, Astrup A. Energy metabolism. In: Gibney MJ, Vorster HH, Kok FJ (Eds). Introduction to Human Nutrition. Chichester: Blackwell Publishing, The Nutrition Society; 2002. pp. 31-46.
15. Guthrie HA. Introductory Nutrition. Toronto: Times Mirror Mosby College Publishing; 1986. pp. 131-54, 157-79, 465-86.
16. Harris J, Benedict F. A biometric study of basal metabolism in man. Washington DC: Carnegie Institute of Washington; 1919.
17. Hoeger WWK, Hoeger SA. Body composition in life time physical fitness and wellness: a personalized program. Cenage Learning. 2008;110.
18. https://www.biology-online.org/dictionary/Phenotype
19. Jéquier E, Tappy L. Regulation of body weight in humans. Physiological Reviews. 1999;7(2):451-80.
20. Kang J. Bioenergetics Primer for Exercise Science. Primers in Exercise Science Series. USA: Human Kinetics; 2008.
21. Keijer J, Hoevenaars FPM, Nieuwenhuizen A, Schothorst EMV. Nutrigenomics and body weight regulation: A rationale for careful dissection of individual contributors. Nutrients. 2014;6(10):4531–551.

22. Kojima M, Kangawa K. Ghrelin: Structure and function. Physiological Reviews. 2005;85:495–522.
23. Kurpad AV. Assessment of physical activity. In: Gibney MJ, Margetts BM, Kearney JM, Arab L (Eds). Public Health Nutrition. Chichester: Blackwell Publishing, The Nutrition Society; 2004. pp. 83-104.
24. Mcrory MA. Energy intake, obesity and eating behaviors. In: Bowman BA, Russell RM, (Eds). Present Knowledge in Nutrition. 9th edition, Vol I. Washington: International Life Sciences Institute; 2006. pp. 816-21.
25. Moran TH, Kinzig KP. Gastrointestinal satiety signals II. Cholecystokinin. American Journal of Physiology Gastrointestinal and Liver Physiology. 2004;286:G183-8.
26. Recommended Dietary Allowances, Estimated Average Requirements-Nutrient Requirements of Indians A report of the Expert Group, Indian Council of Medical Research, National Institute of Nutrition, Department of Health Research, Ministry of Health and Family Welfare, Government of India, 2020.
27. Nutrient Requirements and Recommended Dietary Allowances for Indians-A Report of the Export Group of the ICMR. Indian Council of Medical Research Hyderabad. 2010.
28. Raj KR, Krupad AV. Nutrition in Obesity and Diabetes. New Delhi: Jaypee Brothers Medical Publishers; 2015.
29. Rao BNS. Energy requirements of Indians. In: Towards National Nutrition Security. Silver Jubilee Symposium 29th Nov–1st Dec. Nutrition Foundation of India; 2004. pp. 101-9.
30. Schneiter BCP, Tappy L. Energy expenditure, physical activity and body weight control. Proceedings of the Nutrition Society. 2003;62:663-6.
31. Shetty P. Assessing human energy requirements. In: Towards National Nutrition Security. Silver Jubilee Symposium 29th Nov–1st Dec. Nutrition Foundation of India; 2004. pp. 93–100.
32. Wang Y, Moss J, Thisted R. Predictors of body surface area. Journal of Clinical Anesthesia. 1992;4(1):4-10.
33. Whitney EN, Sizer FS. Nutrition: Concepts and Controversies. Australia: Wadsworth Thompson Learning; 2002.
34. Woods C. Gastrointestinal satiety signals: An overview of gastrointestinal signals that influence food intake. American Journal of Physiology–Gastrointestinal and Liver Physiology. 2004;286:G7-13.
35. Woods SC, Lutz TA, Geary N, Langhans W. Pancreatic signals controlling food intake; insulin, glucagon and amylin. Philosophical Transactions of the Royal Society. 2006;361:1219-35.

6

CHAPTER

Vitamins

> **KEY CONCERNS**
> - What are the roles of different vitamins in the human body?
> - What are their food sources?
> - How much of each vitamin is required at different ages?
> - What are the effects of their deficiencies and excess?
>
> **KEY CONCEPTS**
> - Classification of fat-soluble and water-soluble vitamins
> - Functions, food sources, and recommended dietary allowances
> - Causes and consequences of deficiency and excess of each vitamin

Vitamins are diverse organic compounds which are essential for optimal functioning of the body, maintenance of health, and protection from diseases. They themselves do not provide energy, but some vitamins facilitate energy release from the macronutrients. They need to be obtained from the diet on a daily basis because the body cannot synthesize almost all of them. The body requires them in very minute amounts, i.e., milligrams or micrograms. Their deficiency can impair normal body functions and affect health. Deficiency can be prevented by a regular and adequate supply of vitamins (which is applicable to all nutrients). Deficiency can be due to insufficient intake as well as losses during food handling and processing at different stages. With advancement in science, isolation and synthesis of chemical compounds behaving like vitamins followed. Now many vitamin preparations are available for commercial and therapeutic purposes at a relatively low cost. However, it must be emphasized that synthetic vitamins are not good substitutes for a healthy balanced diet.

CLASSIFICATION OF VITAMINS

There are 13 vitamins which are critical for numerous biological purposes from playing a role in important metabolic processes, energy production to being important for growth, serving as antioxidants, and possibly preventing development of some diseases. FG Hopkins an English biochemist was awarded the Nobel Prize in Physiology or Medicine in 1929, with Christiaan Eijkman, for the discovery of essential nutrient factors i.e., vitamins. Casimir Funk, a Polish biochemist, is also credited with discovering vitamins. Vitamins are classified according to their solubility in water. There are two major categories: (1) fat-soluble vitamins and (2) water-soluble vitamins (Fig. 6.1).

Fat-soluble Vitamins

Vitamins A, D, E, and K are soluble in fat and organic solvents but are insoluble in water. They are absorbed in the small

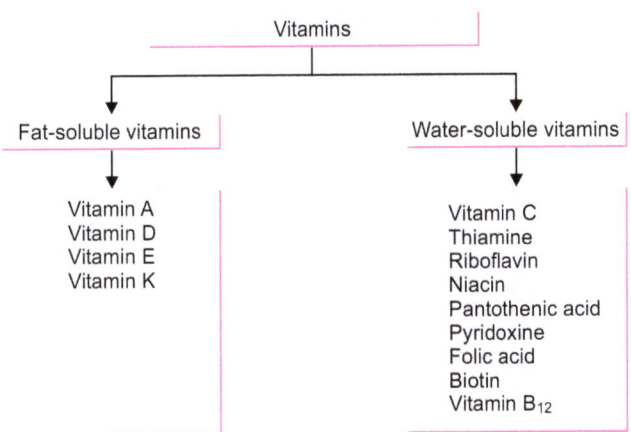

Fig. 6.1: Classification of vitamins.

intestines with the help of fat and travel through lymphatic system. They are then incorporated into chylomicrons that transport fat-soluble vitamins through blood and reach them to other organs and tissues.

Vitamin A

In 1912, an English biochemist HG Hopkins found a compound in milk which could support growth of rats. In 1929, he received the Nobel prize for his discovery. In 1913, they coined the term "fat-soluble A" and thereby attributed for the first time, the growth stimulating property of these extracts to a single compound. Though β carotene was isolated from plants 100 years ago, its vitamin activity was recognized in 1919 by Steenbock. The role of vitamin A in vision was established much later in 1935.

Vitamin A is a group of unsaturated organic compounds which play different roles in visual system, growth and development, and maintenance of epithelial cells and strengthen immunity and reproduction.

There are two forms of vitamin A: (1) Preformed vitamin A or retinol, and (2) carotenoids or provitamin A. Retinol,

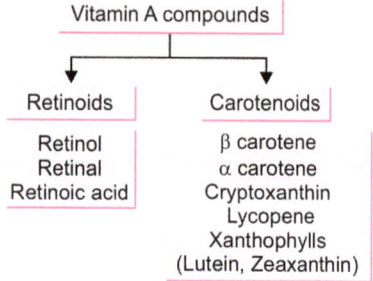

Fig. 6.2: Different compounds of vitamin A.

retinaldehyde, and retinoic acid (RA) comprise the group "preformed vitamin A." These pigments are found in plants and are converted (by enzymatic cleavage) into vitamin A in the body. Hence, vitamin A is a generic term for two groups of fat-soluble substances (Fig. 6.2):

1. Retinoids — preformed vitamin A — obtained mainly from animal sources
2. Carotenoids — provitamin A — obtained mainly from plant sources

Retinoids: The term "Retinoid" is used for both natural and synthetic forms of vitamin A that may or may not show vitamin activity but they are biologically active. They are found to regulate epithelial cell growth. It is being used in pharmaceutical and cosmetic industries. Retinoids include retinol, retinal (retinaldehyde) and retinoic acid (RA).

Retinol: Retinol is the alcohol form of vitamin A and performs many biological functions such as visual cycle, skin, growth and immunity. It is obtained from animal foods like fish liver oils, egg yolk, liver, meat, and dairy products like butter, cheese, milk fat, etc. It is stored in the liver in the form of retinyl esters. Excess intake can cause hypervitaminosis. It can be converted into 11-cis retinal and retinoic acid (RA).

Retinaldehyde (Retinal): Retinaldehyde is the aldehyde form of vitamin A and is crucial for normal vision. It also plays a role in intercellular communication and can be converted into RA. Retinol and retinal are also interconvertible.

Retinoic acid (RA): Retinoic acid does not participate in the visual cycle because it cannot be converted back into retinol. However, it is significant in embryonic development and epithelial functions due to its participation in cell signaling, gene transcription, and cell differentiation. Retinoic acid plays a significant role in skin and skin diseases like acne.

Carotenoids: Carotenoids are a group of more than 600 pigment compounds synthesized by plants, algae, and photosynthetic bacteria. Among these, a few carotenoids have been observed to have tremendous potential for health promotion and disease prevention. β carotene, α carotene, and β cryptoxanthin display vitamin A activity. The carotenoids showing vitamin A activity can be converted into the retinoids. Hence, these are also referred as provitamin A carotenoids. Among all, β carotene is the most potent carotenoid, its chemical structure is shown in Figure 6.3.

Other carotenoids like xanthophylls (lutein and zeaxanthin) and lycopene do not show vitamin A activity. These six major carotenoids are found in human plasma. Carotenoids are found in human plasma and tissues. Lutein and zeaxanthin are present in macula of the eyes and protect them. Lycopene is associated with decreased risk for many chronic diseases including cancer. Xanthophylls determine the hue or color of the fruits and vegetables as well as flesh and feathers in animals. Carotenoids are abundantly found in yellow, orange, and red colored fruits and vegetables. Apricot, carrot, mango, papaya, tomato, watermelon, dark green leafy vegetables, and sweet potatoes are good sources of β carotene. Though color of the dark green leafy vegetables looks green but underneath it is the yellow pigment containing carotenoids which is visible after photo-oxidation of chlorophyll.

> **Laboratory Laurel:** Beta-cryptoxanthin is found in fruits, and also in human blood and tissues. Rich sources of this carotenoid are tangerines, persimmons, and oranges. It plays important roles in antioxidant defense and cell-to-cell communication in addition to its role in eye sight, growth, development, and immune response. In animal model and in human studies, it has been observed that beta-cryptoxanthin has greater bioavailability from common food sources than alpha- and beta-carotene present in foods. Hence, it is advocated that beta-cryptoxanthin-rich foods are also good sources of vitamin A.
>
> *Schweiggert RM, Kopec RE, Villalobos-Gutierrez MG, et al. Carotenoids are more bioavailable from papaya than from tomato and carrot in humans: a randomised cross-over study. Br J Nutr. 2014;111(3):490-8.*

Relationship of β carotene and retinol/conversion of β carotene into retinol

Conversion of β carotene into retinol occurs in the intestinal cells (enterocytes) by cleavage, for which the enzyme carotene dioxygenase is required. At this point, both retinol and β carotene are indistinguishable and follow the same pathway. After the triglycerides have been removed from chylomicrons, the remnants go to the liver which takes up the chylomicron remnants. The liver also converts β carotene into retinol. Most of the dietary retinoids, i.e., 70–90% of the preformed vitamin A esters in the diet, are absorbed and utilized by the body and any excess is stored.

Conversion process of β carotene to vitamin A and absorption of vitamin A from plant (in the form of carotenoids) as well as animal sources is shown in Figure 6.4.

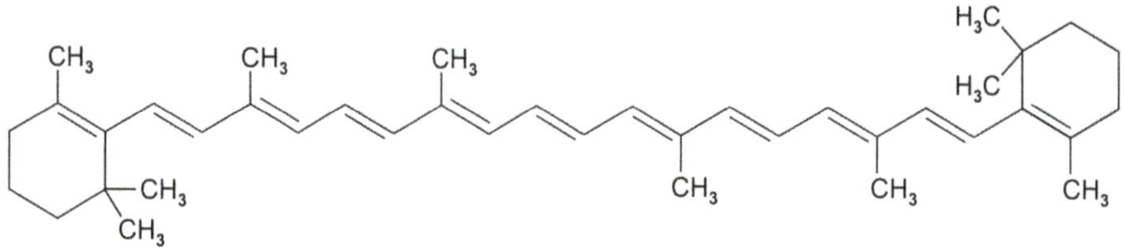

Fig. 6.3: Chemical structure of β carotene.

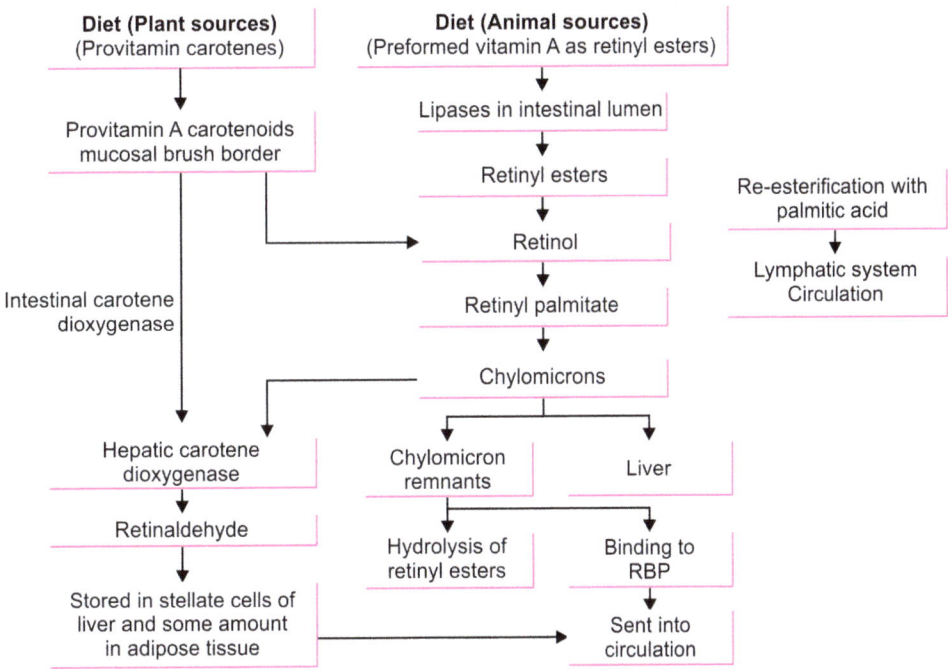

Fig. 6.4: Absorption of vitamin A and carotenoids.

In contrast to preformed vitamin A, absorption and assimilation of β carotene is much less. The efficiency of absorption of carotenoids varies from as little as 5% to 60%, being influenced by several factors. Among the carotenoids, efficiency of conversion of β carotene is higher compared to the other carotenoids. Studies on bioavailability (the amount of carotenoids absorbed in the GI tract) and bioconversion show that this is lower with leafy vegetables as compared to oranges. Therefore, a larger amount of β carotene must be consumed to obtain the amount of vitamin A required by the body. Absorption of vitamin A is also governed by the level in the diet as well as serum retinol concentration in the individual. Two aspects are relevant to carotenoids as a source of vitamin A:
1. Bioconversion (how much is converted into vitamin A).
2. Bioavailability (how much is absorbed).

Bioavailability: Bioavailability indicates how much of a consumed nutrient or dietary constituent (i.e., the proportion of the ingested nutrient) is accessible for utilization/absorbed by intestinal cells and transported in bloodstream under normal physiological conditions, metabolism, or storage.

Bioconversion: Bioconversion deals with the amount of carotenoids that are converted into retinoids. This is influenced by the following factors:
- Nutritional status of the person with reference to the specific nutrient under consideration
- Presence or absence of other nutrients (like energy, fat, iron, and zinc in case of provitamin A)
- Physiological state, e.g., aging and health status
- Injury or malfunction of intestinal cells
- Pathological condition of the individual.

Factors affecting absorption of carotenoids
Many factors influence the absorption of carotenoids:
- Type of carotenoid
- Amount of carotenoid
- Presence of other carotenoids that inhibit activity of carotene dioxygenase
- Food matrix
- Amount of fat present in food containing carotenes
- Presence of inhibitory factors, e.g., pectin, cellulose, plant sterol
- Food processing techniques
- Quantity of fat in the food preparation
- Body stores of vitamin A
- Malabsorption syndrome
- Parasitic infection.

For example, absorption of β carotene from green leafy vegetables is much higher than from carrot and papaya. β carotene in cooked carrot is more bioavailable than from raw or mashed. Absorption of both retinol and carotene requires lipid/fat in the food. Carotene from spinach soup with cream is better absorbed because it is cooked, pureed, and there is some fat. Similarly, salad with oil dressing enhances the vitamin uptake. However, if fat intake is very low (less than 10% of the total energy intake), absorption is impaired. This can increase the risk of vitamin A deficiency.

The ICMR-NIN (2020) has given the minimum acceptable liver stores, i.e., liver retinol concentration should be 0.07 μmol/g or 20 μg/g of liver in healthy persons. It is assumed that this amount will be sufficient to meet physiological needs and maintain reserves for about three months for adults as well as children.

Liver stores most of the vitamin A in the body (50–80%) in the form of retinyl esters/palmitate. When the vitamin A stores are low, conversion of β carotene to retinol is enhanced. Retinol is released from the liver (hepatic stores) and transported in blood, after it is bound to a protein, i.e., retinol-binding protein (RBP). This ensures that this lipophilic vitamin remains in solution in blood; it delivers

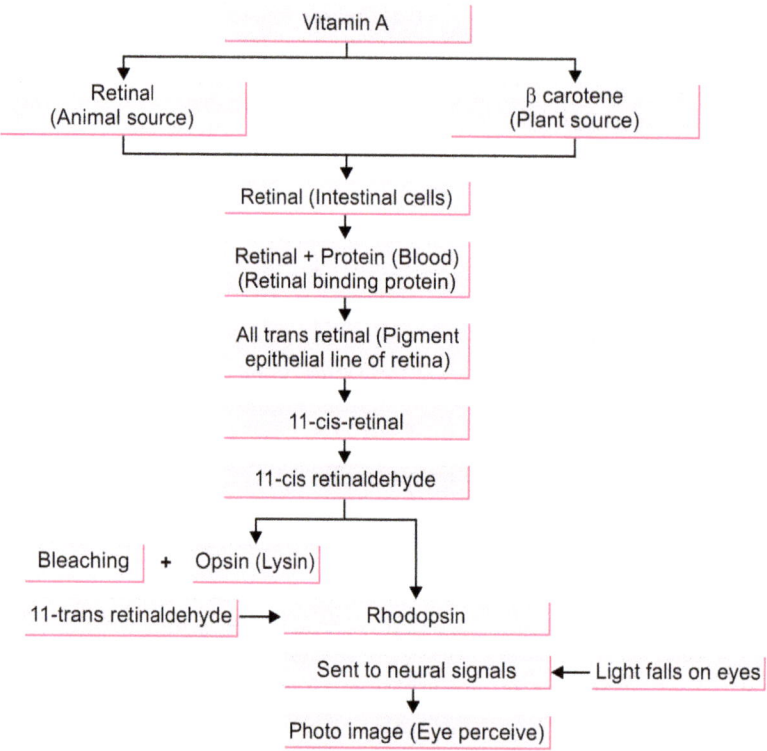

Fig. 6.5: Visual cycle.

the vitamin to the target tissues and protects it from being oxidized. Liver secretes RBP as a complex with thyroxine-binding prealbumin and transthyretin. This is done to ensure that RBP which is a relatively small molecule will not be filtered out by the kidney. Thus, urinary loss of vitamin A is prevented.

There are cell surface receptors on target tissues. The RBP-transthyretin complex binds to these and transfers the complex to an intracellular RBP. Here the RBP molecule is modified so that its affinity for retinol is reduced.

FUNCTIONS OF VITAMIN A

Vitamin A is an essential vitamin for all vertebrate animals. It participates in several biological processes that include vision, maintenance of epithelial tissue surface, immunity, reproduction, and growth and development.

Role in vision: Vitamin A is indispensable for normal vision. It is involved in the generation of rhodopsin, the visual pigment in rod photoreceptors, which allows the retina to detect light in dark-adapted conditions. 11-cis-retinaldehyde is a critical component present in the photoreceptor cells of the eyes. In the retina of the eye, 11-cis-retinal binds with a protein called opsin and forms rhodopsin which plays a key role in the visual cycle. Opsin proteins are sensitive to light. There are two proteins that have a role—(1) rhodopsin in the rods and (2) iodopsin in the cones. When light falls on the eye, it passes through the cornea and reaches the retina, 11-cis-retinaldehyde is converted from the 11-cis form to the all-trans form and is released from the opsin. The release of retinaldehyde initiates a cascade of events ultimately initiating a nerve impulse. A signal is sent to the brain through the optic nerve which results in the person being able to see the object.

Also, after some chemical reaction, all trans-retinol is formed again, converted to 11-cis retinol which is then converted to retinaldehyde followed by the recombination of opsin and 11-cis-retinaldehyde, and this cycle goes on as shown in Figure 6.5.

> **Black and white vision is due to Rhodopsin.**
>
> **Color vision** is due to three pigments present in the cones—(1) the blue cone is activated by blue, violet, magenta colors and to some extent green color, (2) green cone is activated by green and yellow colors and (3) the red cone is activated by red, orange, magenta and partially by violet, yellow. White activates all three cones.

Maintains integrity of epithelial tissues: Vitamin A is necessary for lubricatory compound, mucus production by the epithelial cells lining the different tissues like cornea, respiratory tract, digestive tract, urinary tract, and vagina. It is necessary for the production and maturation of columnar epithelial cells in various tissues which support various secretions like mucus, juices, hormones, and enzymes for proper functioning of these tissues. They enhance the absorption of nutrients from digested food.

Role in infection and immunity: The skin and mucosal cells that line the airways, digestive tract, and urinary tract act as a barrier and are the body's first line of defense against infection. It has a critical role in the morphological formation of the epithelium, epithelial keratinization, stratification, differentiation, and functional maturation of epithelial cells. Thus, vitamin A helps in maintenance of integrity of the epithelial lining of different tissues, thereby prevents colonization by bacteria and infection. It promotes mucin secretion and so improves the nonspecific immune function of epithelial tissues. Vitamin A is also important for differentiation of the cells of the immune system. The various differentiated cells/lymphocytes (B-cells, T-cells, natural killer cells, neutrophils, and macrophages) confer different types of immunity, i.e., humoral and cell-mediated. This vitamin has a role in both innate and adaptive immunity.

Two forms of vitamin A, namely all-trans RA and 9-cis-retinoic acid play an important role in regulating cell differentiation and turnover. In vitamin A deficiency, immune response is depressed because the number of lymphocytes and immunity is lowered. Also synthesis of retinol binding protein is reduced, thus there is decrease in circulating vitamin A. This in turn impairs the immune response and further lowers resistance to infection.

> **Research glimpse:** Vitamin A is important for maintaining vision, promoting growth and development and protecting integrity of epithelial cells and mucus layers in the body. It enhances immune function and is involved in the development of the immune system. It is the "front line" of the body's defense against pathogens due to its critical role in maintaining epithelial tissues, especially for mucus formation in the respiratory tract and the intestines. It has a role in regulating cellular and humoral immune responses. It affects cell differentiation, maturity, and immune functioning of cells in the innate immune system. Its role in pneumonia, measles, and infantile diarrhea is well demonstrated. The role of vitamin A in TB needs to be studied further.
>
> *Huang Z, Liu Y, Qi G, et al. Role of Vitamin A in the Immune System. J Clin Med. 2018;7:258-73.*

Gene expression: Since vitamin A is needed for growth and development, role of vitamin in gene expression is inevitable. Retinol, all-*trans* and 9-*cis* RA are the bioactive components which activate the nuclear receptors and regulate target genes. The two, forms trans retinoic acid and 9-cis RA are both transported to cell nucleus where all-*trans* RA is bound to RA receptor (RAR) in the nucleus and 9-*cis* is bound to retinoid X receptor (RXR). This binding results in formation of a complex which regulates the rate of gene transcription and thereby influences the synthesis of some specific proteins. A large number of genes in different tissues are sensitive to RA. In the cytosol, RA binds to cellular retinoic acid-binding protein (CRABPII). RA regulates the expression of several target genes through several families of nuclear receptors—RARs, RXRs, and peroxisome-proliferator-activated receptor β (PPARβ), PPARδ, polymorphic RA response elements, and multiple coregulators. For example, retinoic acid may be involved in upregulating mRNA expression of mucin proteins in conjunctiva and respiratory system and development of fetal lungs. Nuclear RA receptors appear in cells of different tissues at different stages during development. Vitamin A itself, in the cytosol, has been found to regulate translation and cell plasticity.

Cell differentiation: Cell differentiation involves transformation of one type of cells into highly specialized cells for very specific function(s) in the body. Immature cells are also converted into mature cells. During this process, cells change dramatically in their specific sizes, shapes, membranes, activity, and responsiveness to signals and physiological roles. RA directs differentiation of immature skin cells (keratinocytes) into mature epidermal cells. Secretory epithelia and inhibit the formation of highly keratinized, cornified epithelial cells. Red blood cells (RBC) are derived from precursor stem cells. Normal differentiation of these stem cells into red blood cells is dependent on retinoids. Vitamin A has an important role during embryonic development as well as tissue regeneration in adults.

In rat models, it has been demonstrated that retinoids are involved in control of endometrial growth and differentiation, probably by modulating the hormonal regulation of cellular differentiation. RA may also play a role in adipocyte differentiation and has been found to exert highly specific effects on neuronal differentiation of precursor and embryonic stem cells. It is well known that retinoids are involved in regulation of epithelial cell differentiation, wherein they are important for formation of secretory epithelia whereas highly keratinized, cornified epithelia are inhibited.

Cell signalling: Cell communication can be self-self, i.e., intracrine or autocrine, between nearby cells, i.e., juxtacrine, and indirect communication that is local, over a short distance known as paracrine and synaptic signaling or over a longer distance as in case of hormones and their effects (endocrine). Adjacent cells normally communicate with each other which are important for the integrity and functioning of tissues. Communication between cells is critically important for morphogenesis, cell differentiation, cell growth, homeostasis, and cell to cell interaction. Cells contain various receptors for these signals which are connected to intracellular networks of interacting proteins, nucleic acids, and small molecules. These networks integrate and process the inputs from various signals and based on this, multiple effects occur in terms of functioning of cells. Cell-to-cell communication is generally achieved by signaling mechanisms at "gap junctions" (i.e., junctions between cells) involving the "connexin 36 mechanism." RA affects cell membranes by increasing the number of gap junctions. All-*trans* retinol and RA have been found to inhibit the connexin mechanism. Within the nucleus, RA induces adhesion proteins and membrane complexes that are important for cell adhesion and communication. Cell signaling is important for cell differentiation that occurs during different developmental stages. During embryonic development, RA is an essential signaling molecule and its level and distribution are tightly regulated in the developing embryo, as either deficiency or excess as well as abnormal distribution can disrupt embryonic development.

Role in growth and development: Retinol and RA both are needed for embryonic development. Signaling by retinoids begins in the early phase of embryonic life itself, i.e., during gastrulation. Vitamin A may be involved in fetal lung maturation. Retinoid signaling plays a role in expression of several proteins such as collagen, proteoglycans, etc. Vitamin A is required for synthesis of hemoglobin through its role in mobilizing iron from stores. Thus, vitamin A plays a role in formation of RBC. Retinoic acid has a role in limb development, in formation of heart, ears, and eyes, lungs, limbs, visceral organs, and in bone formation. It regulates expression of the gene for growth hormone and other hormones. Retinoic acid controls myelin formation during development of peripheral nervous system through its binding to retinoic acid receptor (RAR). Both deficiency and excess can cause birth defects.

Other functions: Retinoic acid is important for normal responses to vitamin D, thyroid hormone, and derivatives of long-chain polyunsaturated fatty acid (PUFA). Besides this, vitamin A plays a role in inhibiting cell proliferation and promoting apoptosis. Hence, retinoids may play an important role in preventing cancer. Besides these, recent research shows that vitamin A may play an important role in lipid metabolism, insulin response, energy balance, and in the nervous system, wherein it is likely that active metabolites of retinol especially 11-cis-retinaldehyde may be involved. It may also have a beneficial effect on bone health. However, supplements may not be advocated as some studies suggest that increased vitamin A intake along with low vitamin D concentrations in blood may increase bone fragility. The carotenes also act as antioxidants, also as they help in scavenging free radicals or ROS.

Recommended dietary allowance of vitamin A

Recommended dietary allowance (RDA) for vitamin A are given by ICMR NIN (2020) and given in Table 9.1B in Chapter 9.

> Traditionally, vitamin A activity was expressed in IU (International Unit). However, the FAO/WHO Expert Committee recommended that vitamin A activity to be expressed as RE (retinol equivalent). In 2001, the US Institute of Medicine used retinol activity equivalents (RAE). RE or RAE includes vitamin A plus the retinol obtained from β carotene using the conversion factor recommended by experts.
> 1 RE or RAE = 1 μg retinol 2-4 μg of β-carotene in supplements, 12 μg of beta-carotene found in the diet, or 24 μg of the provitamin-A carotenoids α-carotene, γ-carotene and β-cryptoxanthin. The conversion factors are 1:21 for a fruit/vegetable mix and 1:26 for vegetables

Food sources of vitamin A

Retinol is obtained from animal foods—liver, cow's milk, butter, egg yolk, and fish in the form of retinyl esters. Provitamin A or β carotene is available in plant foods like yellow-orange bright colored fruits and vegetables like carrot, papaya, mango, pumpkin, etc. Dark green leafy vegetables contain much higher concentration of β carotene. Though the efficiency of β carotene conversion into retinol is variable and poor, in India, carotene-containing foods are the major sources of vitamin A. β carotene content of some commonly consumed foods is given in Figure 6.6. α carotene is also a source but the efficiency of conversion is less than that of β carotene. The ICMR-NIN (2020) have recommended the use of conversion ratio of 6:1 for beta carotene and 12:1 for alpha-carotene and beta-cryptoxanthine into vitamin A.

There are several other carotenoids that are nutritionally important in health and disease. Some of them are found in foods like dried apricot, plum, tomato, peas, sweet corn, watermelon, and red palm oil. Table 6.1 lists the different carotenoids and their sources.

Table 6.1: Food sources of different types of carotenoids.

Name of the carotenoids	Food sources
β carotene	Broccoli, carrot, pumpkin, mango, papaya, green leafy vegetables like colocasia, mint, fenugreek, spinach, etc.
Alpha carotene	Carrot, pumpkin, tomato, cantaloupe, winter squash
Cryptoxanthin	Yellow pepper, melon, grape fruit, raw yellow pumpkin, peas, yellow corn, carrot, sweet potato, pineapple, watermelon, etc.
Xanthophylls—lutein and zeaxanthin	Corn and corn products, pumpkin, peas, lettuce, egg and egg products, pistachio, celery, broccoli, spinach
Lycopene	Tomato paste, tomato juice, watermelon, grape fruit

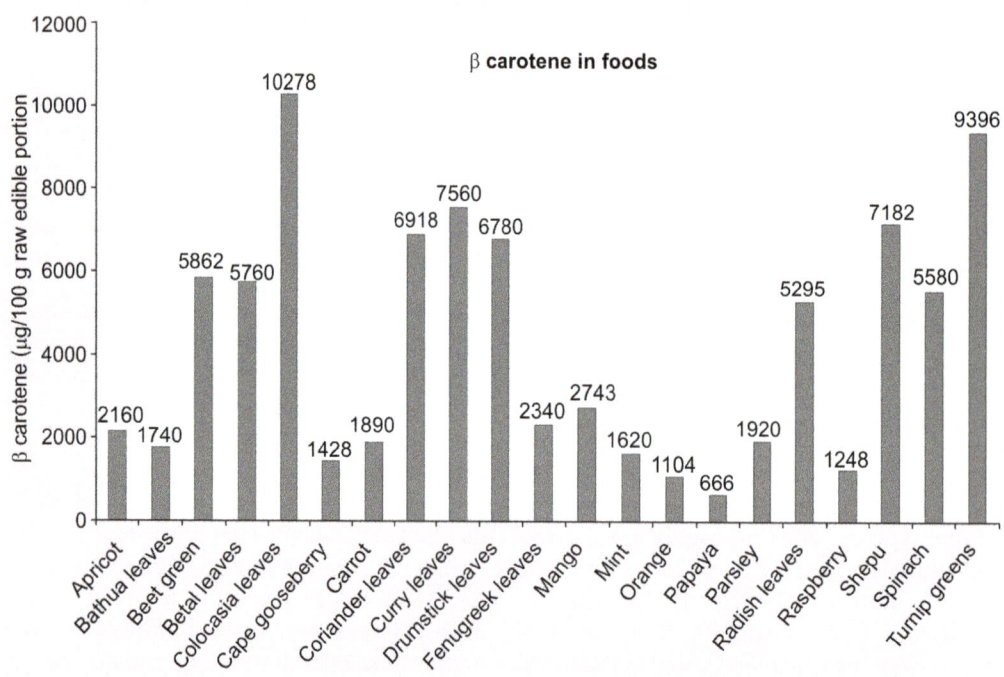

Fig. 6.6: β carotene content in commonly consumed foods.

The provitamin A content is also influenced by many agro-climatic factors like season, growing conditions, stage of maturity at the time of harvest, plant variety, and many steps in post-harvest handling, during marketing and storage, as well as processing techniques. Fortified foods are important sources of vitamin A. Several countries are working on vitamin A for fortification of foods. Oil, butter, margarine and hydrogenated fats are suitable vehicles. Red palm oil is also very rich source of vitamin A precursors but its use is limited because of its intense color. Mustard oil has also been selected for fortification trial but its use is narrowed down by regional preferences. Some countries are using fortified breakfast cereals, flours, and sugar. Retinyl palmitate is the fortificant used for fortification. Scientists are making efforts to increase intake of provitamin A through biofortification, e.g., sweet potatoes and genetically modified foods, e.g., golden rice (Biofortification is discussed in Chapter 12).

Deficiency of vitamin A—causes and consequences
Inadequate consumption of vitamin A rich foods over a long period of time (months or years) is one of the major causes of vitamin A deficiency. Inadequate consumption can be due to poverty, poor accessibility and perishability, and high costs of such foods. Some people also dislike some food sources of provitamin A such as leafy vegetables. It is also related to some religious concerns with regard to animal foods that are rich source of vitamin A. Other causes can be:
- Poor handling of food sources during post-harvest and especially processing and cooking
- Ignorance about the essentiality of vitamin A for protection of health and prevention of diseases
- Protein energy malnutrition
- Zinc deficiency limits the transport of vitamin A stores from the liver to other body tissues
- Fat malabsorption
- Diarrheal diseases and intestinal parasites also interfere with absorption of vitamin A
- Liver disease like hepatitis reduces the capacity of the liver to store and release vitamin A
- Insufficient bile production
- Inflammatory conditions and illness
- Acute phase of illness increases the utilization of the vitamin by peripheral tissues and subsequently urinary losses.

Vitamin A Deficiency is briefly referred to as VAD, and is a public health problem. It is a preventable cause of blindness, growth retardation, morbidity, as well as maternal and child mortality. It can affect people of all age groups but the most afflicted are preschool children and pregnant women. Night blindness is the primary symptom of VAD.

Strategies for prevention of VAD
- Food-based strategies—dietary diversification
- Home gardening of vitamin A rich foods
- Poultry keeping
- Medication
- Vitamin A supplementation in drops and syrups
- Fortification and biofortification
- Health and nutrition education.

Insufficient intakes result in depletion of liver store of retinyl esters. Many children who have VAD also suffer from PEM. Vitamin A deficiency has clinical and functional manifestations that affect eyes and immune system. VAD may cause intrauterine growth retardation (IUGR), fetal malformation, and congenital abnormalities. In young children, growth retardation occurs. Besides this, VAD can exacerbate iron deficiency anemia.

In vitamin A deficiency, the secreting cells are replaced by squamous epithelial non-mucus producing cells, making the skin dry and scaly. The process is called keratinization.

Causes and consequences of excessive intake of vitamin A
Excess vitamin A that is ingested is stored in the liver. The condition caused by excessive intake of vitamin A greater than 10 times the RDA is known as hypervitaminosis A. It is indicated by elevated plasma retinol level. This may result from exposure to very high doses over a short time period or high intakes over a prolonged period. However, some subgroups may be susceptible with lower intakes, e.g., elderly persons, individuals who consume alcohol regularly for long periods, and some persons who have genetic predisposition to hypercholesterolemia. In children, toxicity occurs at lower doses. In the elderly, high intakes may be associated with risk of fractures. Bone mineral density was found to be highest in the elderly when intakes were close to the RDA. Excess vitamin A can also impair responsiveness to vitamin D and hormones.

Use of synthetic retinoids for acne therapy for prolonged periods can also cause hypervitaminosis A. Excessive consumption of β carotene, i.e., 10 times of RDA, can also be the cause of hypervitaminosis but it is relatively less harmful in comparison to retinoid consumption except showing of yellow pigmentation in the hands and other parts of the body. Recovery is also rapid when the supplementation is withdrawn. The Institute of Medicine (2001) has given 3,000 μg/day as the tolerable upper limit of intake (UL) for preformed vitamin A for adults (Table 6.2).

Both lack and excess of vitamin A during embryonic development can lead to congenital malformations. During pregnancy, vitamin A supplements should be used with caution and should not exceed 3,000 μg/day or 10,000 IU/day. Excess intake of preformed vitamin A has resulted in birth defects. Even preparations containing synthetic retinoids that are used for topical applications should be avoided during pregnancy since there is potential for systemic absorption.

Table 6.2: Upper tolerable limit of intake for preformed vitamin A.

Age groups	Age	Upper limit (μg)
Infants and toddlers	Up to 3 years of age	600
Children	4–8 yrs 9–13 yrs	900 1,700
Adolescents	14–18 yrs	2,800
Adults (include men, women, pregnant and lactating women)	≥ 19 yrs	3,000

Vitamin D

In the 17th century, Whistler and Glisson gave scientific descriptions of rickets which was common among children of the upper class who avoided sunlight and those who lived in slums in big industrialized cities and did not have the opportunity to be exposed to sunlight. In the 20th century, Mellanby in the UK and McCollum in the US discovered the nutritional importance of vitamin D. Mellanby and his coworkers named this anti-rachitic agent as Vitamin D. Steenbock demonstrated that exposing vegetable oil to UV radiation produced vitamin D2. In 1938, Windaus earned the Nobel Prize for the chemical identification and synthesis of vitamin D. In 1969, a biologically active form of vitamin D was identified.

Vitamin D has long been known for its role in regulating blood levels of calcium and phosphorus, and bone mineralization. Research has shown that receptors for vitamin D are present in almost all cells, and that this vitamin acts as a hormone. Its biologic effects extend far beyond control of mineral metabolism. Vitamin D itself is biologically inactive, and it must be metabolized to its biologically active forms, 25-hydroxycholecalciferol and 1,25-dihydroxycholecalciferol.

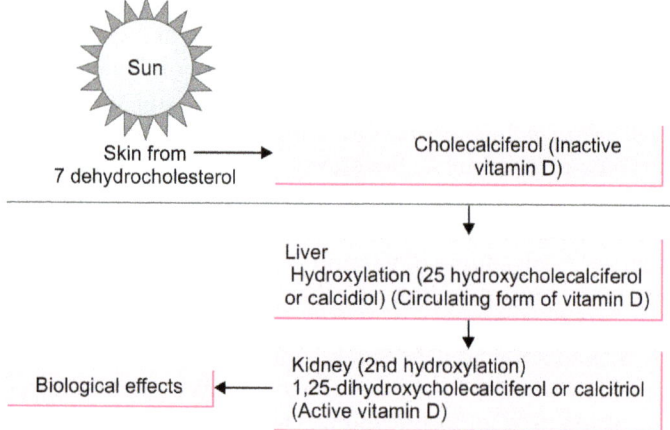

Fig. 6.7: Synthesis of vitamin D.

Forms of Vitamin D

Cholecalciferol is synthesized in the skin of the body when exposed to sun. It is an inactive form of vitamin D also referred as precursor or provitamin D.

Calcidiol or 25-hydroxycholecalciferol (25 OH D) is synthesized in liver by hydroxylation of cholecalciferol. It is a good indicator of the body vitamin D status. Greater exposure to sunlight or increased intake of vitamin D from diet raises the 25-hydroxyvitamin D serum levels. Thus, serum 25-hydroxyvitamin D concentration is a useful indicator of vitamin D status of a person.

Calcitriol or 1,25-dihydroxycholecalciferol is synthesized in the kidney by second hydroxylation. It is the most biologically active form and functions like steroid hormone. This form is also used in nutritional supplements in the treatment of bone disease and chronic kidney failure.

Cholecalciferol is synthesized in the epidermis of skin from 7 dehydrocholesterol on exposure to ultraviolet rays of the sun (wavelength 290–315 nm). Its synthesis is greatly influenced by season, clouds, latitude (zenith angle of the sun), altitude, age, air quality, and amount of skin exposed to sun as well as the color of skin/pigmentation (melanin).

Cholecalciferol from diet is absorbed in the small intestine (nearly all the ingested vitamin D is absorbed) with the help of bile salts and is then incorporated into:

Chylomicrons ⟶ Circulation ⟶ Transported to the liver.

In the liver, it is hydroxylated (first hydroxylation) to form calcidiol, the major circulating form of vitamin D in the presence of an enzyme (hepatic D3-5–hydroxylase) and is then bound to a vitamin D-binding protein (globulin). The activity of the enzyme is stimulated by parathyroid hormone (PTH) which is important in maintaining calcium homeostasis.

Calcidiol is then transported to kidney for next hydroxylation at C-1 and the compound formed is calcitriol. Calcitriol is produced in the cells of the proximal tubule of nephron in the kidney. This step is catalyzed by the enzyme 25-hydroxyvitamin D3-1-hydroxylase. Besides renal synthesis, hydroxylation can also occur in "ectopic sites" muscles, colon, prostrate, immune system, and pancreas. In extra renal sites, this is probably to meet the needs of the local organ/tissue. Final stage of hydroxylation is promoted by PTH. Vitamin D is transported in plasma bound to a vitamin D-binding protein. In this form, vitamin D3 and all its metabolites are transported to the various target organs (Fig. 6.7).

After vitamin D is absorbed, it is incorporated into chylomicrons and transported to blood. In blood, it binds to the D-binding protein (DBP) and is transported to the liver where one of four enzymes (CYP2R1, CYP2J2 and CYP3A4, CYP27A1, the most active one being CYP2R1) hydroxylate the molecule at the 25 position. Serum vitamin D levels reflect both dietary intake by an individual and the synthesis in the skin.

Sun plays a significant role in our health. It not only initiates the synthesis of vitamin D but also biorhythmic cycle of the body that refers to the patterns of energy and exhaustion, functioning and resting, and wakefulness and sleep that characterize everyday life. The circadian rhythm affects core body temperature, brain wave activity, hormone production, cell regeneration, and other biological activities.

Laboratory Laurel: The active form of vitamin D, $1\alpha,25\text{-}(OH)_2D_3$, has been found to play a role in numerous functions such as metabolism control, cell growth, differentiation, anti-proliferation, apoptosis, and adaptive/innate immune responses, in addition to its well-known role in bone and calcium homeostasis. Many of the functions of $1\alpha,25\text{-}(OH)_2D_3$ may be regulated by circadian rhythm. In this study, the authors studied the role of this vitamin in the expression of circadian genes, namely, *BMAL1* and *PER2*, in adipose-derived stem cells (ADSCs), using different conditions over a 60-h period. Measurements were done at 4 hour intervals, in serum shocked ADSCs, serum shocked ADSCs supplemented with $1\alpha,25\text{-}(OH)_2D_3$, and ADSCs under the presence of only $1\alpha,25\text{-}(OH)_2D_3$. They found that $1\alpha,25\text{-}(OH)_2D_3$ was able to synchronize circadian clock gene expression in ADSCs. The expression profile of circadian genes *BMAL1* and *PER2* in ADSCs containing only $1\alpha,25\text{-}(OH)_2D_3$ was similar to that found in the ADSCs synchronized by a serum shock. The authors concluded that $1\alpha,25\text{-}(OH)_2D_3$ may play an important role in regulating the molecular clock.

Gutierrez-Monreal MA, Cuevas-Diaz Duran R, Moreno-Cuevas JE, et al. A role for 1α,25-dihydroxyvitamin d3 in the expression of circadian genes. J Biol Rhythms. 2014;29(5);384-8.

Functions of vitamin D

Primarily vitamin D plays a significant role in calcium absorption in the intestine and maintains the calcium level in the blood. Hence, it influences the mineralization of bones and plays an important role in prevention of bone diseases like rickets, osteomalacia, and osteoporosis. Calcium levels in serum/blood are maintained in a narrow range.

Calcitriol
↓
Increases synthesis of calcium binding protein (calbindin)
↓
Increase absorption of calcium in intestines
↓
Increase blood calcium level

Enhances calcium absorption: Calcitriol stimulates the absorption of calcium in small intestines through its nuclear vitamin D receptors (VDR). It also stimulates the synthesis of calbindin, a protein that transports calcium across the intestines and thereby increases blood calcium level. It also stimulates phosphorus absorption to some extent.

Calcium balance/homeostasis and maintenance of normal serum calcium level is vital for normal functioning of nervous system as well as for development and maintenance of bone. Essentially, $1\alpha,25$-dihydroxyvitamin D binds to and activates VDR in the target cells. This leads to alterations in gene expression in order to maintain normal serum calcium level. Calcitriol acts on three target tissues, namely, the intestines, the kidney, and bone. The process involves two hormones, calcitonin secreted by thyroid gland and parathormone (PTH) secreted by parathyroid gland. Parathyroid gland senses serum calcium concentration and when blood calcium level is low, it secretes PTH. Calcitonin regulates serum calcium and phosphorus by opposing the action of PTH tends to increase PTH. PTH further stimulates the hydroxylase enzyme in the kidney and increases synthesis of calcitriol (active form of vitamin D) which in turn increases intestinal absorption of calcium by increased synthesis of the protein calbindin and stimulates reabsorption of calcium in renal tubules. Simultaneously, it also acts on osteoclasts on the bone surface, stimulating them to release calcium from bone (especially when dietary calcium intake is inadequate). All three together contribute to normalization of serum calcium. When serum calcium levels rise, PTH levels drop as a result of which calcium mobilization decreases. Thus, vitamin D plays a very important role in regulation of calcium homeostasis. Similarly, it is important for phosphate homeostasis.

Formation of bones: Vitamin D is believed to control bone metabolism largely by regulating calcium homeostasis. In adults, bone is continuously remodeled wherein bone mass is maintained by a balance between bone resorption by osteoclasts and bone formation by osteoblasts. In children and adolescents, bone growth, i.e., increase in length, depends on the coordinated growth and differentiation of the chondrocytes. Calcitriol is important for bone mineralization. Calcitriol stimulates rapid influx of calcium into osteoblasts and increases expression of bone matrix proteins such as osteocalcin, osteopontin, alkaline phosphatase, bone Gla protein, matrix Gla protein (MGP), and type I collagen. VDR plays a significant role in the formation of bones in more mature osteoblasts, VDR activity has been found to exert anabolic and anticatabolic activity and thus increases bone mass. Growth plate chondrocytes have also been found to express the VDR. Vitamin D receptor influences bone resorption and negatively regulates bone mass through its signaling in osteoprogenitors and has a positive effect on osteoclast formation.

Vitamin D as a hormone: Vitamin D is structurally a steroid and closely allied to estradiol, cortisol, and aldosterone. Calcitriol acts as a steroid hormone that enhances the absorption of calcium in the intestine. Essentially every tissue and cell in the body has a VDR and the biological actions of vitamin D are mediated by the VDR. VDR belongs to the family of steroid receptors. This family includes receptors for RA, thyroid hormone, sex hormones, and adrenal steroids. This subfamily of nuclear receptors acts as transcription factors. VDR forms a complex with RXR which then binds to the VDR element in the promoter region of target genes or at distant sites and regulates their expression either positively or negatively. VDR is present in and interacts with intranuclear receptors of all cell types including gut, bone, breast, prostate, brain, skeletal muscle, and the immune system. Besides influencing transcription, VDR also interacts with basal transcription factors. VDR signaling has been found to be initiated by low affinity ligands such as curcumin (present in turmeric), PUFAs, and anthocyanidins (present in many fruits and vegetables). Resveratrol and sirtuin A (molecules involved in influencing longevity) have been found to potentiate VDR signaling.

Vitamin D receptor binding sites have been found to change during cell differentiation and maturation as well as disease activation and thus affect gene expression. Mutations in VDR affect the functionality resulting in vitamin D-resistant rickets or type II rickets. In this, due to the mutation binding to VDR, nuclear location of the vitamin D and receptor complex and VDR binding get modified.

> **Research glimpse:** The Vitamin D system consists of hormone precursors, active metabolites, carriers, enzymes, and receptors involved in genomic and non-genomic effects, that activate numerous mediators and have several physiological functions. In vitro and in vivo studies vitamin D has shown many "non-calcemic" actions such as maintenance of glucose homeostasis, cardiovascular morbidity, autoimmunity, inflammation and cancer. In multiple ways, it is found associated with brain development, functions and diseases. Hence optimal blood levels of vitamin D supports neurological development and protects the adult brain. Since prevalence of vitamin D deficiency is high, the authors have reviewed the relationship between vitamin D and neurological diseases.
>
> Di Somma C, Scarano E, Barrea L, Zhukouskaya VV, Savastano S, Mele C, Scacchi M, Aimaretti G, Colao A, Marzullo P (2017) Vitamin D and Neurological Diseases: An Endocrine View. Int J Mol Sci. 18(11): 2482.

Gene expression: VDR affects numerous genes in humans and mediates gene regulation in a great variety of target cells generating extra-skeletal biological responses and regulates numerous cellular processes in normal tissues like breast, colon, prostrate (inhibits cancer cell progression in these tissues), influences the cardiovascular system, differentiation of keratinocytes, innate and adaptive immunity, and with other hormones. Some genes are responsible for antimicrobial peptides and some prompt the release of cytokines linked with autoimmune diseases such as inflammatory bowel disease, multiple sclerosis, etc. Many are involved in bone forming cells (osteoblasts) and cell division. VDR tends to modulate the expression of 3,000 genes in various tissues. These regulate reproductive tissues such as the ovaries, uterus, and vagina and also the serum levels of luteinizing hormone, sex hormone-binding globulin, testosterone, and insulin.

Cell differentiation: Vitamin D has been found to inhibit proliferation and stimulate differentiation of cells. Studies have demonstrated that $1,25(OH)_2D_3$ and its analogs retard the growth of cancer cells by arresting cells in the G0/G1 phase of the cell. They also induce their differentiation and/or induce apoptotic cell death. Vitamin D3 also has a role in angiogenesis, cell adhesion, and migration, and has been found to reduce the invasiveness of cancer cells. Thus, it may have a role to play in cancer by promoting apoptosis and retarding metastasis, influencing quiescence, and modulating growth factors. This is an important area for development of vitamin D analogs which may be useful in cancer but will not raise serum calcium levels and cause hypercalcemia.

Vitamin D receptor (VDR) belongs to the family of nuclear receptors involved in gene expression.

Nuclear receptors are a class of proteins found within the cell that are capable of sensing the presence of foreign as well as innate molecules like steroid hormones. These can directly bind with deoxyribo nucleic acid (DNA) and regulate gene expression.

Vitamin D3 binds to intracellular receptors that then function as transcription factors to modulate gene expression. Like the receptors for other steroid hormones and thyroid hormones, VDR has domains for binding hormones and DNA.

After vitamin D binds to VDR, it forms a complex with another intracellular receptor, the RXR. This complex binds to vitamin D responsive elements (VDRE) in the nucleus.

VDRE initiates a cascade of molecular interactions that modulate expression/transcription of more than 50 genes (of proteins such as osteocalcin, osteopontin, alkaline phosphatase, calcium transporting ATPase) that are involved in development, homeostasis, and metabolism such as:
- Formation of bone matrix proteins
- Bone remodeling through osteoblast and osteoclast activities
- Calcium homeostasis
- Anti-proliferative—cancer
- Anti-inflammatory markers
- Most cell types of immune system
- Keratinocytes

Role in immune system: Most cells of the immune system such as antigen-presenting-cells, T cells, B cells, and monocytes contain vitamin D metabolizing enzymes and VDR. This includes most cells, i.e., T lymphocytes, neutrophils, antigen-presenting cells, like macrophages and dendritic cells that support conversion of 25-hydroxyvitamin D to calcitriol. Vitamin D regulates innate immunity. Thus, it is important for immunity toward bacteria, fungi, and viruses and it has been shown that if vitamin D status is good, it provides broad protection against a range of bacteria and viruses besides inhibiting development of autoimmunity. Vitamin D is also involved in inflammatory response. It can downregulate the production of pro-inflammatory cytokines.

Evidence from human studies shows that vitamin D may be associated with inflammatory and autoimmune diseases such as rheumatoid arthritis, inflammatory bowel disease, multiple sclerosis, Crohn's disease, periodontal disease, hypertension, cardiovascular disease (CDC), and impaired glucose tolerance.

Other roles: Vitamin D may be involved in regulation of the renin-angiotensin system, influence muscle strength, muscle size, and neuromuscular performance.

Laboratory Laurel: Vitamin D has long been known to be important for its "classical role" enhancing intestinal calcium absorption, maintaining serum calcium and phosphate, its action on bone development, and its effects on osteoclasts and osteoblasts. In the last two decades, numerous other functions have been discovered such as cell proliferation and differentiation, and that it has an important role in the nervous system and in immune responses/immune regulation and resistance to a broad range of bacteria and viruses. Other pleiotropic effects are detoxification of xenobiotics, reducing oxidative stress, neuroprotection, anti-cancer effect, anti-inflammatory, and cardiovascular health.

Gil Á, Plaza-Diaz J, Mesa MD. Vitamin D: Classic and Novel actions. Ann Nutr Metab. 2018;72:87-95.

Research glimpse: Vitamin D improves intestinal absorption of calcium and phosphate, thereby stimulates osteoclast differentiation and calcium reabsorption from bone and promotes mineralization of the bone matrix. The vitamin D receptor (VDR) and the vitamin D activating enzyme 1-α-hydroxylase (CYP27B1) are also expressed in T and B cell types which are not involved in bone and mineral metabolism, such as intestine, pancreas, prostate, and cells of the immune system. Vitamin D status of the individual is low in winters. Circulating levels of calcitriol are mainly determined by renal CYP27B1 activity. Low calcitriol concentrations have also been linked to elevated mortality caused by severe infections in end-stage renal disease patients, and low serum 25(OH)D levels have been associated with upper respiratory tract infections (URTIs), including influenza, chronic obstructive pulmonary disease, and allergic asthma. Vitamin D supplementation studies have shown beneficial effects on immune function and on the regulation of inflammatory responses, as well as regulatory mechanisms connected to autoimmune diseases particularly in type 1 diabetes mellitus (T1D). Vitamin D deficiency is commonly found in autoimmune diseases, such as T1D, MS, systemic lupus erythematosus, rheumatoid arthritis, and inflammatory bowel disease.

Prietl B, Treiber G, Pieber TR, et al. Vitamin D and immune function. Nutrients. 2013;5(7):2502-21.

Recommended dietary allowance of vitamin D

Based on IOM recommendations, ICMR-NIN (2020) has extended the recommendations for vitamin D provided calcium intake is adequate. RDA for infants i is 400 IU (10 µg) AI and thereafter for all age groups it is 600 IU (15 µg).

Research glimpse: The IOM committee concluded based on the scientific evidence that supports the role of calcium and vitamin D in skeletal health as well as extra-skeletal outcomes, including cancer, CDC, diabetes, and autoimmune disorders. For bone health, RDAs for calcium are from 700 mg/day to 1,300 mg/day for infant to adults. For RDAs, vitamin D is for 600 IU/day for ages 1–70 years and 800 IU/day for ages 71 years and older. RDAs for vitamin D were derived based on conditions of minimal sun exposure due to wide variability in vitamin D synthesis from ultraviolet light and the risks of skin cancer.

Contd...

Contd...

> *Ross AC, Manson JE, Abrams SA, et al. The 2011 report on dietary reference intakes for calcium and vitamin D from the institute of Medicine: what clinicians need to know. J Clin Endocrinol Metab. 2011;96(1):53-8.*

Sources of vitamin D

Sunlight is a major and important source because about 50 to 90% of vitamin D is produced cutaneously upon exposure of skin to sunlight, i.e., ultraviolet B (UVB) radiation with wavelength of 290-320 nm. <Maximal synthesis of vitamin from UV-B rays is said to occur between 11 am–3 pm. Further it is governed by many factors such as geographical location where latitude is 35 degrees and season of year. Studies suggest that 20 minutes of direct sun exposure (with 10 % body surface area exposure) at solar noon in summer may be sufficient for vitamin D synthesis in different parts of the country, However, this may not apply to places like Srinagar. Similar wavelengths can also be obtained from mercury vapor sunlamps. Skin color influences cutaneous synthesis and more amount of melanin is associated with reduced production. Clothing also affects synthesis. Lightweight, non-synthetic fabrics like linen and cotton block UV radiation less as compared to wool, silk, nylon, and polyester. Cutaneous synthesis of vitamin D declines as age advances due to change in skin morphology and low levels of 7-dehydrocholesterol levels in the skin. Furthermore, skin temperature, body surface area and portion of the body exposed to the sun influence the cutaneous synthesis. Being a fat soluble vitamin, evidence indicates that it is sequestered in the fat tissue and higher body fat may be associated with lower levels of circulating vitamin D. In addition ozone layer, aerosols, optical thickness, surface reflectance, and cloud constellations also influence synthesis of vitamin D in the skin.

Black carbon particulates that are generated by burning fossil fuels and biomass reduce surface radiation by up to 5% to 81% depending upon how extensive the biomass burning is.

Recent studies suggest that magnesium deficiency may influence vitamin D status because this mineral regulates activity of many enzymes that are involved in vitamin D metabolism.

> **Laboratory laurel:** Proportions of VDI varied from 57% to 100% depending on gender and age. Overall, the prevalence of vitamin D insufficiency (VDI) was 67.5%. Awareness or proper knowledge is prerequisite for favorable practice. Proper information, education, and communication materials regarding various aspects of sun exposure and vitamin D should be prepared with due consultation of field experts and disseminated to increase awareness among the community. Exposure of face (3.5%), forearm (6%), hand (6%), and neck (2%) for "1" hour may give sufficient vitamin D levels. Participants of all age groups, in both genders, in urban and rural areas and different parts of the country with a larger sample should be studied in the future.
>
> *Garg S, Dasgupta A, Maharana SP, et al. Sun exposure and Vitamin D in rural India: A cross-sectional study. Indian J Public Health. 2018;62:175-81.*

Dietary sources of cholecalciferol are very few and include mushrooms, egg (if the hens have been fed vitamin D), liver oil, milk and butter, ocean fish specifically fatty fish like salmon, sardines, and mackerel. Yogurt and cheese are not good sources of vitamin D. Plants sources do not contain sufficient amounts of it. Ergosterol is a form of vitamin D found in plants, however, they do not contain sufficient amounts. Fortification of packaged milk and vanaspati with vitamin D is used in India. Vitamin D is stable and is not destroyed on heating or during storage. Estimating the contribution of vitamin D from diet is difficult in Indian context.

Deficiency of vitamin D—its causes and consequences

Vitamin D deficiency is widely prevalent worldwide including India although sunshine is in abundance in most parts of this country. It is caused by lack of exposure to sunrays, dark skin pigmentation, clothing, and latitude, chronic use of anticoagulant, and chronic steroid therapies. In vitamin D deficiency, calcium absorption is adversely affected. Decreased absorption results in a small reduction in serum calcium that is sufficient for increased PTH secretion. As a result, calcium is mobilized from bone in order to maintain serum calcium levels. Vitamin D deficiency has adverse consequences on bone health. Deficiency can be due to lack of exposure to UV rays from sunlight or some medical/physical conditions.

Lack of/inadequate exposure to sun: The time spent in the sun in day time is crucial. However, there are important factors which influence the role of sun in synthesis of vitamin D. Sunrays are more effective between 10 am and 2 pm. UV rays cannot penetrate through the window glass and sunrays are more intense in areas near equator. In some communities, "Parda" system where women and infants are covered and stay inside the house for months and years together for social and cultural reasons are not or less exposed to sunlight. In winters or in temperate climate, people usually remain inside and thus exposure to sun is limited. Besides season, latitude, zenith angle, and time of day are crucial. Layers of clothing can also limit the sun exposure of skin. Pollution can also interfere with the penetration of the atmosphere by UV rays of the sun.

> **Laboratory laurel:** A cross-sectional population-based study was conducted on 325 middle- and high-school adolescents (both sexes) to evaluate the association between ambient air pollution and bone turnover in and to compare the prevalence of vitamin D deficiency between polluted and non-polluted areas of Tehran. Data for serum levels of calcium, phosphorus, PTH, bone-specific alkaline phosphatase, 25(OH) vitamin D, osteocalcin, cross-linked C-telopeptide, total protein, albumin, and creatinine were obtained. Vitamin D deficiency was more prevalent in polluted areas than in non-polluted areas. Subjects from polluted area showed a statistically significant positive association with vitamin D deficiency and a statistically significant negative association with bone turnover. High calcium intake (>5,000 mg/week) protects against the effects of air pollution on bone turnover. Air pollution limits the amount of solar UVB that reaches the earth's surface and thus contributes to vitamin D deficiency.
>
> *Feizabad E, Hossein-Nezhad A, Maghbooli Z, et al. Impact of air pollution on vitamin D deficiency and bone health in adolescents. Arch Osteoporos. 2017;12(1):34.*

> **Laboratory laurel:** It is believed that vitamin D deficiency is common among pregnant women and has been linked to increased risk of pre-eclampsia, gestational diabetes mellitus, preterm birth, and other tissue-specific conditions. Sufficient evidence is not available in terms of assessing either benefits or ill effects and risks of vitamin D supplementation to pregnant women, on maternal and infant health outcomes. "Vitamin D supplementation is not recommended during pregnancy to prevent the development of pre-eclampsia and its complications." "The use of this intervention during pregnancy as part of routine antenatal care is also not recommended." The remarks in this guideline are as follows:
>
> - "In cases of documented deficiency, vitamin D supplements may be given at the current recommended nutrient intake (RNI) [5 µg (200 IU) per day as recommended by WHO/FAO or according to national guidelines].
> - Vitamin D may be given alone or as part of a multiple micronutrient supplement, to improve maternal serum vitamin D concentrations. The benefit of this intervention for other maternal or birth outcomes remains unclear.
> - Pregnant women should be encouraged to receive adequate nutrition, which is best achieved through consumption of a healthy balanced diet during pregnancy.
> - There is limited evidence on the safety of vitamin D supplementation during pregnancy."
>
> *World Health Organization (2012). Guideline: Vitamin D supplementation in pregnant women.*

> **Laboratory laurel:** This study was done to observe the link between serum vitamin D levels and the menstrual cycle in young women with different body weights. The subjects were divided into two groups. One group had one group had low Vitamin D levels (<30 ng/mL) and the other had normal levels (>30 negative <=80 ng/ml). In LD group, 40% of participants had long cycles, 27% oligomenorrhea, and 13% amenorrhea. In the ND group, only 12% reported menstrual cycle disorders, 6% had oligomenorrhea, and 6% had amenorrhea. This study indicates close relationship between the frequency of menstrual disorders and low levels of vitamin D. Supplementation is necessary in women with low levels of vitamin D in order to compensate for this deficiency and to assess its effect in order to menstrual disorders. Low vitamin D levels can also lead to insulin resistance, hirsutism, and infertility and polycystic ovary syndrome (PCOS). In addition, it has been postulated that increased serum vitamin D and calcium levels may improve reproductive function in women with PCOS.
>
> *Lagowska K. The Relationship between Vitamin D Status and the Menstrual Cycle in Young Women: A Preliminary Study. Nutrients. 2018;10(11):1729.*

Skin type: People with fair skin can synthesize vitamin D faster than dark color skin type because of the presence of a pigment, "melanin" which provides color to the skin and is opaque. More melanin delays synthesis of vitamin D in the skin.

Age: The capacity of synthesizing cholecalciferol in the skin is diminished with advancing age and therefore calcium metabolism is also altered. However, older persons who are regularly exposed to sun and participate in outdoor activities may possess the same capability of synthesizing vitamin D as young ones. Reduced mobility and institutionalization puts them at risk.

Window glass prevents penetration of UV rays.

Digestion and absorption of dietary vitamin D: Vitamin D is fat soluble and is incorporated into micelles during digestion. Most of the dietary vitamin D is absorbed. After absorption, with fat, vitamin D is incorporated into chylomicrons and is taken to lymph vessels and finally to blood. Liver takes up approximately half of the vitamin D from chylomicrons, bone marrow, and bone takes up about 20% and other tissues take up the remaining 30%. Liver secretes vitamin D into circulation bound to vitamin D binding protein.

Storage: Vitamin D is stored in the liver. This helps people who may not be exposed to sun throughout the year, especially in winter season. Small amounts may also be stored in other tissues besides the liver.

Dietary deficiencies of other nutrients: Vitamin D is a fat-soluble vitamin; hence low fat diet reduces its absorption in the body. Low cholesterol limits its synthesis in the skin from 7-dehydrocholesterol and magnesium deficiency can restrict its conversion from inactive to active form. In obese persons, although vitamin D is synthesized, it is deposited in adipose tissue and is less bioavailable.

Some medical/physical conditions can increase risk such as fat malabsorption, cystic fibrosis, inflammatory bowel disease, Crohn's disease, and sprue. Persons who have epilepsy and are on anticonvulsant drugs are also at risk because these drugs probably induce catabolism of calcitriol. Liver and kidney both are involved in synthesis of active form of vitamin D, hence hepatic and renal disorders will impair hydroxylation or activation, thus the vitamin D status. Vitamin D has been linked to several chronic, non-communicable diseases like non-alcoholic fatty liver disease (NAFLD), obesity, diabetes, cancer, asthma, CDC, autoimmune diseases, skin diseases, hypertension, arthritis, sleep disorders, and some psychiatric illness like obsessive compulsive disorder (OCD). However, further scientific evidence from clinical studies is required in order to determine whether vitamin D has a preventive role in many of these diseases and whether it can be used in medical management. Vitamin D deficiency has been associated with infectious diseases like tuberculosis since it has a role in immunity. There is lot of evidence that people having obstructive sleep apnea (OSA) and sleep disturbance are vitamin D deficient. Some of them also suffer excessive daytime sleepiness (EDS) which is characterized by general debility, gastrointestinal disturbances, cognitive impairment, emotional impairment, pain, physical discomfort as well as depression.

Low blood calcidiol can affect bone mineralization leading to softening of bones and its associated disorders like rickets in children and osteomalacia in adults. Severe vitamin D deficiency causes rickets and osteomalacia where osteoid tissue cannot be mineralized whereas in less severe deficiency, there is increase in serum PTH level which causes bone resorption resulting in porous bones or osteopenia, osteoporosis, and fractures. Vitamin D deficiency also causes muscle pain.

> **Research glimpse:** The meta-analysis was done to clarify the association between vitamin D and sleep disorders risks using PubMed, EMBASE, and Web of Science. It indicated that persons with
>
> *Contd...*

Contd...

> vitamin D deficiency have very high risk of sleep disorders. More high-quality cohort studies and randomized controlled trials (RCTs) are needed to verify this association. National Sleep Foundation recommends that adults should get 7-8 hours sleep every day, albeit sleep demands may vary in age and gender. The daily sleep–wake cycle is controlled by circadian clock, different neurons, and hormones produced by the hypothalamus and environmental signal (dark/light). Several studies reported that VDR are expressed in brain areas that regulate the sleep–wake cycle, such as the hypothalamus. Many mechanisms have been discussed in this article.
>
> *Gao Q, Kou T, Zhuang B, et al. The Association between Vitamin D Deficiency and Sleep Disorders: A Systematic Review and Meta-Analysis. Nutrients. 2018;10(10):1395.*

Rickets: Rickets occurs in young children. It commonly occur in cases of codeficiency of calcium and vitamin D. There is defective mineralization of bone matrix and growth plate cartilage (before epiphyseal closure). It results in misshaped deformed or weak bones. Rickets is characterized by improper mineralization during developmental stages of the bones. Rapidly growing bones are most affected. The growth plate of the bones enlarges but mineralization does not occur adequately resulting in the weight bearing limbs like legs and arms becoming bowed. Bowed legs or knocked knees in young children are typical signs of rickets. Pigeon breast due to deformities of the rib cage, and delayed closure of fontanels in the skull are other clinical features of rickets. New bone cell osteoid is not mineralized. Subtle symptoms may be regarded as a warning for medical examination. These include bone pain in legs, problem in standing or walking for long, falling frequently, and delayed growth. Vitamin D deficiency in infants may lead to tetany and convulsions as a result of hypocalcemia. This may be the first sign of rickets.

Osteomalacia: Osteomalacia occurs in adults. It a disease characterized by softening of bones due to vitamin D deficiency. Although bone growth has stopped in adults, remodeling or turnover of bone occurs. In severe deficiency, the collagenous matrix is not affected but there is progressive loss of bone mineral resulting in softening of bones. Fractures occur with very little injury. Common symptoms are pain in bones, muscle weakness, and bone tenderness and pain in the thorax, shoulder, hips, thighs, forearms, and feet. Metabolic acidosis and liver or kidney diseases may also cause osteomalacia. There is negative calcium balance. Elevated level of alkaline phosphatase and low plasma level of calcium and phosphorus are biomarkers of negative calcium balance and indicator of vitamin D deficiency and onset of osteomalacia.

Osteoporosis: Osteoporosis occurs when vitamin D deficiency is not corrected and calcium is continuously resorbed from the bones which make the bones thin, porous, and weak that is a typical characteristic of osteoporosis. Bone mass density (BMD) is low due to resorption of bone minerals. It usually occurs in postmenopausal women and affects bones of wrist, rib, hip, and spine. Fracture risk is high in osteoporosis and many daily activities like bending, climbing stairs, even sitting, and getting up from bed or chair are hampered that deteriorates with age. Regular intake of calcium and vitamin D is advocated for the osteoporotic patients. Maintaining serum vitamin D level up to 50-70 nmol/L in old age may be beneficial to prevent falls. Various suggestions are being given in different clinical and residential settings with regard to vitamin D supplementation that may range from 400-800 IU per day. However, any supplementation should be taken after testing and medical consultation. It is equally important to maintain adequate intake of calcium while taking vitamin D supplementation.

Regular exposure to sunshine for at least 10-15 minutes for two to three times a day is advisable. Under certain cases, use of ultraviolet irradiation is prescribed. Use of cod liver oil and large quantity of homemade fresh butter has been found to be useful for rickets. Vitamin D supplements are prescribed in clinical practice in the form of powder or intramuscular injections as a weekly dose. Use of fortified vanaspati and milk may promote vitamin D intake. Fortification with vitamin D is being practiced in US and Canada and now it is practiced in certain parts of India.

Effect of excessive intake of vitamin D

Prolonged exposure to sun does not cause vitamin D toxicity. However, excessive intake of vitamin D through supplements or fortified products (above 155 units per day) can cause hypervitaminosis D or vitamin D toxicity. Symptoms of toxicity can be constipation, polyuria, backache, and hyperlipidemia. If any reference can be given of vitamin D intake is 25 µg/day for infants, 62.5 µg for children aged 1-3 years, 75 µg for children 4-8 years of age, and 100 µg for children above 9 years of age and adults. In this case, blood level of calcidiol, calcium, and phosphorus may be elevated. Infants are at high risk if they are given 100 times of adult dose.

If circulating 25(OH)D is <150 ng/mL, there may be no clinical symptoms and if >150 ng/mL, there may be calcium hyperabsorption, hypercalcemia, and calcification of soft tissues. Symptoms of hypercalcemia are bone pain, head ache, anorexia, and irritability. Hypercalcemia is a common feature of vitamin D toxicity and has been observed when daily doses of 50,000-60,000 IU were ingested in the form D_3 supplement. If untreated, it can cause calcification of soft tissues like kidney, lung, and heart. Pregnant and lactating women are at high risk of vitamin D toxicity if given high doses of supplements. They should consult the doctor before taking vitamin D supplement.

Vitamin E

Vitamin E was discovered in 1922 by Evans and Bishop who observed that laboratory rats failed to reproduce when lard was their only source of food fat. They reported that there was a compound in both wheat germ and lettuce that corrected the problem. For a time, the unknown component was termed the "anti-sterility factor". In 1925, Evans decided that the component should be renamed vitamin E since this discovered after the discovery of vitamin D. Evans and his co-worker Gladys A Emerson isolated vitamin E from wheat germ oil, corn oil, and cotton seed oil in 1936. In 1938, it was synthesized by Paul Karrer (1889–1971) et al. Later its biochemical function as an antioxidant was elucidated. In 1968, vitamin E was finally recognized as an essential nutrient for humans.

Forms of vitamin E

Vitamin E is a collective name for eight lipid-soluble molecules: four tocopherols [alpha (α), beta (β), gamma (γ), and delta (Δ)] and four tocotrienols compounds (alpha, beta, gamma, and delta). They are structurally related but differ slightly in their chemical structures which make the difference in their vitamin E activities. Alpha (α) tocopherol is the most potent biologically active form of vitamin E and is the only form that meets the human body's requirement for vitamin E. Among the eight compounds, it is also present in largest amounts in blood and tissues. Both tocopherols and tocotrienols possess antioxidant property and are available in nature for human consumption.

Naturally occurring forms of vitamin E	
α-Tocopherol	α-Tocotrienol
β-Tocopherol	β-Tocotrienol
γ-Tocopherol	γ-Tocotrienol
δ-Tocopherol	δ-Tocotrienol

Functions of vitamin E

Antioxidant Activity: The major biological function of vitamin E is that of a lipid-soluble antioxidant preventing the propagation of free-radical reactions. It is an integral part of cell and organelle membranes. Free radicals are formed during normal metabolic processes and upon exposure to exogenous toxic agents like cigarette smoke, pollutants, etc. Vitamin E is an important chain-breaking antioxidant. It protects PUFAs and other components like phospholipids of cellular membranes from oxidative damage (lipid peroxidation) by free radicals, as the first line of defense. Apart from maintaining the integrity of the cell membranes in the human body, it also protects the lipids in low density lipoprotein (LDL) from oxidation. This is especially relevant to risk of CVD because oxidized LDL has been linked to development of CVD. When a molecule of alpha-tocopherol neutralizes a free radical, it gets oxidized (tocopheroxyl radical is formed) and loses its antioxidant capacity.

The tocopheroxyl radicals that are formed are capable of further reactions such as oxidizing other lipids. They can also be further oxidized to form tocopheryl quinones. A third possibility is that tocopheroxyl radicals can interact with each other and form tocopherol dimers that are nonreactive. The fourth is that the radicals can be reduced by antioxidants and tocopherol can be regenerated. Generally, other antioxidants such as vitamin C are present in the cell cytosol and regenerate the antioxidant capacity of alpha-tocopherol. However, oxidative stress and deficiency of antioxidants like vitamin E, C, or others can increase the rate of production of free radicals and degradation of lipids (PUFA) in the cell membrane.

Oxidative stress (OS) is the physiological condition, an imbalance between the production of reactive oxygen species (ROS) (the kind of free radicals), and antioxidant defenses. ROS are very unstable and highly reactive. They attack lipids, nucleic acids, proteins, carbohydrates, and other biomolecules located nearby and cause a cascade of reactions. It may be the result of nutritional imbalance/inadequacy, exposure to chemical and physical agents in the environment, strenuous physical activities, injury, and hereditary disorders. OS is cytotoxic. However, it plays an important role in modulating messengers involved in regulating cell membrane functions needed for survival. When intracellular redox status is altered, protein kinases within the cell are activated, e.g., protein kinase C and mitogen activated protein (MAP) protein kinase cascade. The protein kinases are important for cell activation, proliferation, differentiation, and other functions. OS influences biological processes including apoptosis, inflammation, and viral proliferation. It is recognized as a key element involved in the pathogenesis of diseases like cancer, CVD, atherosclerosis, diabetes, arthritis, neurodegenerative disorders, skin diseases, autoimmune diseases and pulmonary, renal, and hepatic diseases. Increasing the consumption of vitamin E, A, C, and variety of antioxidant compounds found in food can prevent occurrence of oxidative stress. Lifestyle and environmental factors including diet, smoking, etc. also contribute to generation of active oxygen species and DNA damage.

It is likely that α-tocopherol inhibits generation of new free radicals whereas gamma tocopherol reacts with and neutralizes those that are existing/already formed.

Non-Oxidant Functions: Non-antioxidant functions of α-tocopherol have been identified. α-tocopherol inhibits protein kinase C activity, which is involved in cell signaling. Vitamin E inhibits platelet aggregation and enhances vasodilation, by increasing the release of prostacyclins which is a vasodilator and inhibitor of platelet aggregation through inhibition of protein kinase C activity and the activity of nitric oxide synthase. For inhibition of protein kinase C, α-tocopherol is much more effective than the other forms of vitamin E. Vitamin E plays a role in adhesion of blood cell components to the endothelium of the blood vessels. Also, gamma tocopherol has been found to possess anti-inflammatory activity. Vitamin E may have a role in prevention of chronic diseases such as atherosclerosis and age-related macular degeneration of eyes, cataract, and lower risk of contracting upper respiratory tract infection in the elderly. Vitamin E promotes better packaging of the cell membrane. In muscle tissue, vitamin E has been found to play a role in muscle homeostasis by promoting repair of injured muscle tissue.

The other isomers of α-tocopherol also have biological action. Tocotrienols have been shown to have potential in preclinical trials to be helpful in preventing chronic disease. δ-tocotrienol particularly as the other tocotrienols, in cancer cell lines, has been shown to be more effective in their anti-proliferative effects and apoptosis than α-tocopherol. However, further studies are required to provide confirmed evidence about efficacy and effectiveness of these isomers.

Digestion and absorption of vitamin E are similar to that of fats/lipids. Almost all forms of vitamin E are well absorbed from the intestines after they are incorporated into mixed micelles (formation of which requires biliary and pancreatic secretions). Fat is required for absorption. Vitamin E is then incorporated into chylomicrons which pass into the lymphatic system and then enter circulation. A small amount of vitamin E is transferred to peripheral tissues but the majority of the vitamin E is carried by the chylomicron remnants that carry the vitamin E to liver where it is taken up by hepatic cells which have receptors. α-tocopherol is specifically selected by alpha-tocopherol transfer protein (α-TTP), a small cytoplasmic hepatic protein which has affinity for α-tocopherol and differentiates this isomer from the others. Besides liver, α-TTP is also expressed in brain and placenta. Excess α-tocopherol is excreted into bile and metabolized and degraded to form carboxyethyl hydroxychroman that is mostly excreted in urine, when the plasma threshold for the vitamin is exceeded.

Plasma lipid status influences the uptake of this vitamin. Intestinal absorption is lowered by the presence of vitamin C, polyphenols, and carotenoids. Other factors influencing absorption are genetic regulation, intracellular trafficking, and lipoprotein secretion of vitamin E.

Recommended Dietary Allowance of Vitamin E

Alpha-tocopherol requirement is related to its antioxidant property and the essential fatty acids (EFA) content in the diet. ICMR-NIN-2020 has suggested an intake of 0.8 mg of vitamin E per gram of dietary essential fatty acids which is approximately 8–10 mg tocopherol/day, depending on the oil used. In Indian diets, unrefined vegetable oils and invisible fat from cereals, nuts, and vegetables are good sources of α-tocopherol.

Increased consumption of PUFA through vegetable oils and its use in frying increases the requirement of vitamin E, because it is lost during frying. Further use of refined foods, smoking, certain drugs, coloring agents, preservatives, and other additives may also raise the requirement for vitamin E. Requirement of vitamin E may be higher when there is malabsorption of fat or greater oxidative stress, e.g., in endurance exercise. In addition, pregnancy, lactation, infancy, and old age have comparatively high demand of vitamin E.

Food Sources of Vitamin E

Unrefined vegetable oils (olive, soya beans, palm, corn, safflower, sunflower, etc.), nuts, whole grains, and wheat germ are the most important sources of vitamin E. Other sources are seeds and green leafy vegetables. The vitamin E content of vegetables, fruits, dairy products, fish, and meat is relatively low. The vitamin E content in foods is often reported as α-tocopherol equivalents (α-TE). This term was established to account for the differences in biological activity of the various forms of vitamin E; 1 mg of α-tocopherol is equivalent to 1 TE. Other tocopherols and tocotrienols in the diet are assigned the following values: 1 mg β-tocopherol = 0.5 TE; 1 mg γ-tocopherol = 0.1 TE; 1 mg δ-tocopherol = 0.03 TE; 1 mg α-tocotrienol = 0.3 TE; 1 mg β-tocotrienol = 0.05 TE.

During cooking, heat treatment and exposure to air (oxygen) lead to loss of vitamin E. There is significant loss of tocopherol at high heat. During refining of vegetable oils, considerable loss of the vitamin occurs. Extent of loss varies from 30% to 70% depending on how severe the processing parameters are, i.e., temperature, pressure, and steam flow as well as the length of processing. In both chemical and physical refining processes, the steam deodorization and distillation lead to losses.

Deficiency of vitamin E—causes and consequences

Severe vitamin E deficiency may occur in malnourished persons or in individuals who suffer from fat malabsorption syndromes or cholestatic liver disease and persons having specific genetic defects affecting the transport of α-tocopherol by α-tocopherol transfer protein (α-TTP) and lipoproteins. Vitamin E status can be affected by high production of free radicals in the body due to several various reasons including smoking, and low amount of vitamin E/insufficient consumption. Low intake of vitamin E rich foods tend to cause poor vitamin E status. Vitamin E deficiency may occur when the diet mainly consists of refined foods, fried foods, and the foods containing coloring agents, preservatives, and other additives. Use of certain medications in some diseases like heart disease, some pathological conditions, chronic liver disease or neurodegenerative diseases, pancreatic disease, and malabsorption of fat may tend to reduce the utilization of vitamin E in the body and cause deficiency. Low intake of vitamin E for longer duration can result in the following symptoms:

- Leg cramps and muscle weakness
- Progressive peripheral neuropathy due to injury to sensory nerves
- Impaired balance and coordination (due to spinocerebellar ataxia)
- Lack of energy
- Poor immunity
- Aging
- Pigmentation of skin
- Myopathy/muscle weakness
- Retinopathy and in persons with inherited defect in α-TTP, there can be visual impairment and early-onset macular degeneration.

During embryonic and fetal life, the developing nervous system is vulnerable to deficiency. In children with severe deficiency at birth, if the problem is left untreated, they can have irreversible neurological symptoms. Marginal intakes of vitamin E are very likely. Research reports indicate that inadequate vitamin E status in pregnant women may be linked with risk of miscarriage. There may be the damage of cell membrane and leakage of cell content into the external fluids.

Consequences of Excessive Intake of Vitamin E

At high concentrations, vitamin E has been shown to have a pro-oxidant action. Hence, it is necessary to assess the presence of vitamin C and other antioxidants also. High amounts of vitamin E may interfere with apoptosis, cell adherence, and immune response. High oral doses of vitamin E could increase the risk of prostate cancer. Upper limit of vitamin E has been set (>100 mg alpha tocopherol for prolonged periods) for vitamin E supplements but not for dietary sources. People on anticoagulants need to be monitored when on vitamin E supplements.

Vitamin E excess in doses exceeding 1,000 mg (in any form) interferes with blood clotting, increases tendency to bleed, and increases the risk of hemorrhagic stroke. Patients who are prescribed anticoagulants need to be extremely careful with vitamin E supplementation and should ensure that intakes of vitamin E are adequate. People with diabetes and autoimmune diseases need to consult a physician before taking vitamin E supplements. However, supplementation with both vitamin E and C may slow down the progression of atherosclerosis and Alzheimer's disease (AD). Vitamin E supplementation should always be taken under medical supervision rather than taking as over the counter (OTC) medicine.

VITAMIN K

The existence of the vitamin K group was discovered by a Danish scientist Henrik Dam in 1929 while studying cholesterol metabolism in chicks. He noted a new deficiency syndrome in the young birds fed a fat-deficient diet. The characteristic features were lengthened blood clotting time, anemia, and hemorrhage. In 1939, he named this vitamin "vitamin K," choosing the letter "K" from a German word "Koagulation" meaning coagulation. Ten years later, EA Doisy isolated the vitamin from hexane extracts. Although at this time the structure had not been established, chemical and physical properties were correctly attributed to a substituted 1,4-naphthoquinone. Dam was awarded the Nobel Prize for medicine in 1943 for his discovery of vitamin K and Doisy for his discovery of the chemical nature of vitamin K.

Vitamin K is known as the clotting vitamin, because without it, blood would not clot. It also helps maintain strong bones. Vitamin K is a family of various compounds, namely, phylloquinone (K1) and menaquinones (K2), menadione (K3), and hydroquinone. Phylloquinone is the major dietary source primarily obtained from plant foods whereas menaquinones are obtained from animal sources and are synthesized by bacteria (in gut as well as in fermented foods) and other compounds that are synthetic in form and are less active than the previous ones.

Vitamin K is absorbed along with the dietary fat from small intestine and transported to blood via chylomicrons. The efficiency of absorption of free phylloquinone is about 80% but vitamin K from leafy vegetables is not well absorbed as it is embedded in the chloroplasts and not easily released. Chylomicrons with vitamin K are transported to the lymph ducts and then to blood. Bioavailability of vitamin K1 may be reduced by high intakes of vitamin A, E, and lutein. Chylomicron remnants are taken up by liver, bone, and other tissues. Liver contains the largest amount of vitamin K. It contains approximately 90% menaquinones and 10% phylloquinone. Bones also contain significant amount and some amount is present in adipose tissue.

Functions of Vitamin K

The fat-soluble vitamin K plays two crucial roles, one in the mechanism of blood clotting and its unique function in post-translational chemical modification of a group of calcium-binding proteins, known as vitamin K-dependent proteins or Gla-proteins. However, in the last few years, evidence has accumulated about the role of vitamin K2 in osteoporosis, vascular calcification, osteoarthritis, cancer, and cognition.

Formation of blood clot: Vitamin K is critically involved in many reactions occurring during the process of blood clotting (blood coagulation). This is achieved by a cascade that involves seven proteins/coagulation factors that are vitamin K dependent. There are four proteins—prothrombin (Factor II), Factors VII, IX, and X, that participate in the cascade resulting in the formation of a fibrin clot. Three proteins counteract (i.e., inhibit blood clotting) these four factors and are vitamin K-dependent. The three proteins are Factors C, S, and Z.

Vitamin K acts as a cofactor in a specific carboxylation reaction that converts specific glutamic acid residues in the protein to gamma glutamic acid. Due to this, the proteins (inactive clotting factors) are able to bind calcium. Binding to calcium converts these four vitamin K-dependent clotting factors into active clotting factors. Thus, vitamin K stimulates the conversion from preprothrombin to prothrombin then to thrombin and further thrombin catalyzes the conversion of fibrinogen into fibrin clot (blood clot). Thrombin is involved in promotion of platelet aggregation, inflammation, and atherosclerosis.

Role in bone formation: Vitamin K1 and K2 are predominantly involved in the γ-glutamyl carboxylation of Gla proteins, produced in bone cells. Some of these proteins are osteocalcin, Matrix Gla-Protein (MGP), and protein S. These proteins are calcium-binding proteins and become active only in the presence of vitamin K-dependent enzyme (carboxylase). Children with inherited protein S deficiency have been reported to have decreased bone density and complications related to increased blood clotting. The role of osteocalcin is not clear, although in vitamin K deficiency, osteocalcin is only partially carboxylated. Osteocalcin synthesis is stimulated by vitamin D. It is possible that osteocalcin has a negative regulatory role in bone formation. MGP inhibits mineralization in bones.

Other functions: Vitamin K-dependent MGP is found in soft tissues including the smooth muscle cells in blood vessels. It prevents calcification of vascular tissues especially in the arterial walls of the heart. Recent research shows that adequate vitamin K intakes in the form of menaquinone (MK 7) and phylloquinone (vitamin K1) may be important for maintaining elastic properties of arteries, and lower the risk of heart disease.

> **Laboratory Laurel:** Multi-Ethnic Study of Atherosclerosis was carried out to determine the association between vitamin K status and coronary artery calcium (CAC) progression in 296 participants with extreme CAC progression and 561 randomly selected participants without extreme CAC progression. Serum phylloquinone (vitamin K1) was measured. A significant interaction between low vitamin K1 and anti-hypertension medication use was detected. Hypertension medication users with low serum vitamin K1 were more likely to have extreme CAC progression than were medication users without

Contd...

Contd...

> extreme CAC progression. In replication, baseline antihypertensive medication users in the supplementation group had less CAC progression than did those in the control group. It is suggested that the low serum vitamin K1 is associated with greater CAC progression particularly in anti-hypertension medication users. Intervention trials are needed to determine whether improving serum vitamin K1 reduces CAC progression, especially in hypertensive individuals. This trial was registered at clinicaltrials.gov as NCT00183001.
>
> *Shea MK, Booth SL, Miller ME, et al. Association between circulating vitamin K1 and coronary calcium progression in community-dwelling adults: the Multi-Ethnic Study of Atherosclerosis. Am J Clin Nutr. 2013;98(1):197-208.*

Proteins C and S are two vitamin K-dependent plasma proteins which regulate the blood clotting, and are vital in wound healing and prevent organ damage. Deficiency of protein C, that is often genetic, can be serious due to abnormal blood clotting. Activated Protein C (APC) has anti-inflammatory, antithrombotic, and neuroprotective properties particularly in stroke. Protein S is synthesized in several tissues including walls of blood vessels. It appears to be involved in apoptosis, vision, and promotion of phagocytosis. Like protein C, it has been found to be neuroprotective in ischemic and hypoxic mice.

Another vitamin K-dependent protein is Gas-6 or (Growth-Arrest-Specific Gene 6). Structurally, it is similar to protein S associated with anticoagulating system and inflammation. It is found in nervous system and several other tissues. It is involved in a wide number of functions related to cell physiology such as cell adhesion, cell proliferation, chemotaxis, phagocytosis and apoptosis, and promoting growth and survival of different cells and neurons. It is involved in nervous system, vision, platelet metabolism, bone metabolism, and renal system. Overall Gas-6 is important for cell physiology.

MK-4 is a form of vitamin K which is produced from phylloquinone (vitamin K1) in the body. Besides its role in gamma carboxylation, it may be involved in expression of some genes and may be inversely related to the risk of heart disease. It may protect neurons against oxidative stress.

Gas-6, a K-dependent protein is associated with central nervous system rather than liver or bone. It has been shown to have a role in cell survival, chemotaxis, mitogenesis, myelination, and cell growth of neurons and glial cells in the brain. Vitamin K occurs mostly as MK-4 in the brain.

Role of Vitamin K2: It has been shown to improve bone quality and thereby reduce risk of fractures although bone density may not be necessarily affected. This is possibly by inhibiting osteoclasts and stimulating osteoblasts resulting in net bone anabolism. It helps to incorporate calcium into bones and bone matrix. It has shown benefits in a trial where low dose supplements of K1 did not. Along with vitamin D and calcium supplementation, K2 was effective in reducing under carboxylated osteocalcin. It also inhibits vascular calcification and may have a role in preventing osteoarthritis as well as reducing inflammation since c-reactive protein (CRP) levels are reduced. Thus, it may help in decreasing the inflammation in rheumatoid arthritis. In the kidneys, urinary GLa protein inhibits calcium salt precipitation, thus vitamin K may be important for reducing renal stone formation. It may also be involved in insulin sensitivity. In this case, K1 and K2 may both play a role. It may also have a protective role in cancer. Vitamin K2 activated MGP (Matrix GLa protein) may prevent tissue calcification and risk of coronary heart disease.

Recommended dietary allowance of vitamin K

ICMR-NIN (2020) has recommended that an intake of 55 µg per day would be sufficient for adults (both men and women) as well as during pregnancy and lactation. The FAO/WHO joint report (2004) has given recommendations for vitamin K intake for adult males including elders, adult females including pregnancy, lactation and menopausal period to be 65 and 55 µg/day; whereas infants, children and adolescents need 5-10 µg, 15-25 µg and 35-55 µg per day respectively.

Food sources of vitamin K

Most of the commonly consumed food items contain ample amounts of vitamin K1. Dark green leafy vegetables especially spinach, lettuce, turnip greens, mustard greens, peas and beans, cabbage, broccoli, and Brussels sprouts are rich sources of phylloquinone, although there are varietal differences. Outer layer of leaves (cabbage) contain relatively more amount of vitamin K than inner leaves. Certain vegetable oils like olive, canola, cotton seed, and soybean are also good sources; however, hydrogenation destroys the vitamin. Exposure of these foods to light and alkali tends to reduce their vitamin content. K1 is also present in asparagus, plums, and kidney beans. Intestinal microflora synthesizes large amounts of menaquinones that may be a source for humans. However, the bioavailability of menaquinones of bacterial origin is poor. Sources of K2 are natto (fermented soy like Natto is the richest source), hard cheese (Gouda), and soft cheese (Blue cheese), egg yolk, chicken, liver, salami, sauerkraut, and kefir (a type of fermented milk). In natto, the organism responsible for K2 synthesis is *Bacillus subtilis natto* which produces mostly MK-7. Lactic acid bacteria produce MK-8 and MK-9 and propionic acid bacteria produce MK-10. Butter, animal fats, olive oil, avocado oil support absorption of vitamin.

Deficiency of vitamin K—causes and consequences

Deficiency of vitamin K is considered to be not common in India due to the dietary pattern. However, its deficiency has been reported in persons with problems associated with food digestion and/or absorption particularly fat malabsorption and/or obstruction in the bile duct. These conditions are inflammatory bowel disease, celiac disease, or liver disease. Medications which interfere with the gut flora can also exacerbate the vitamin K deficiency. However there is possibility of vitamin K_2 deficiency. It may increase the risk of hip fracture.

Consequences of vitamin K deficiency result in increased blood clotting time because clotting is impaired. This is used as a laboratory test. It can lead to hemorrhage which can be fatal in certain conditions. Problems like heavy menstrual bleeding, bleeding gums, nose bleeds, and fecal blood loss (seen as tarry and black stools) are also causes. Infants are at risk since intracranial hemorrhage is life-threatening. The American Academy of Pediatrics and other similar international organizations recommend that a prophylactic injection of phylloquinone (vitamin K1) be administered to all newborns to prevent hemorrhagic disease in them. This deficiency syndrome is now known as Vitamin K deficiency bleeding (VKDB). Earlier it was believed that VKDB occurs only in newborns. However, it is now seen that VKDB can occur in the first few months of life. Premature babies are at higher risk of vitamin K deficiency, hence smaller amount of supplements is recommended. Persons with high doses of vitamin E and low intake of potassium have shown symptoms of vitamin K deficiency. Some cholesterol lowering drugs, antacids, salicylic acid (aspirin), and sulfonamides can reduce the absorption of vitamin K and cause deficiency. Consumption of transfats and high intake of PUFA also retard the absorption of vitamin K_2 in the digestive system.

Causes and consequences of excessive intake of vitamin K
Usually, toxic effects of excess of natural vitamin K are not observed because excess is excreted from urine more rapidly than any other fat-soluble vitamin. Intakes of 10–20 mg of phylloquinone have not resulted in any toxic effects. However, synthetic preparations of menadione and its salt should not be used for infants, since it can be toxic to newborns. This can result in neonatal hemolysis and liver damage. It can also be toxic to patients on anticoagulants like warfarin. Menadione interferes with glutathione functions and oxidative damage to cell membranes can occur.

WATER-SOLUBLE VITAMINS

As the name suggests water-soluble vitamins are soluble in water and are widely distributed in nature. Water-soluble vitamins include the B-complex vitamins and vitamin C. Vitamin B-complex includes eight vitamins, namely, vitamin B_1 (thiamine), vitamin B_2 (riboflavin), vitamin B_3 (niacin), vitamin B_5 (pantothenic acid), vitamin B_6 (pyridoxine), vitamin B_9 (folate), vitamin B12 and biotin. Few water-soluble compounds behave like vitamins in the body which are para amino benzoic acid (PABA), inositol, choline, and lipoic acid.

Each vitamin has one or more pivotal role(s) in energy metabolic pathways, cell division, and utilization of other nutrients and formation of other biological compounds in the body. They are involved in myriad cellular functions and are required in miniscule amounts. Deficiency of each adversely affects biochemical/physiological functions of the body. The body neither can synthesize nor store the water-soluble vitamins; hence, they have to be obtained from dietary sources on a regular basis. If excess amount is ingested, it is gets excreted. Thus, there are less chances of toxicity with water-soluble vitamins unlike fat-soluble vitamins. However, in certain cases, when large doses of supplements were consumed, some adverse effects have been observed.

Most of them are sensitive to heat, air, light, radiation, and many food processing techniques. Thiamine, folic acid, and vitamin C are most sensitive, hence they are lost maximum during food processing steps such as washing, soaking, cooking, and milling. Careful handling and some innovative food processing methods can reduce the loss of vitamins and traditional cooking methods like germination can enhance the content of vitamin C. The functions, recommendations, and food sources of individual vitamins along with deficiency symptoms are described herein.

Vitamin C

During ancient times, sailors had to sustain on poor diets while travelling on long voyages by sea. Many suffered from a disease called scurvy, characterized by poor wound healing, bleeding gums, and severe joint pains. In 1747, James Lind, an officer and naval surgeon in the British Royal Navy discovered that citrus foods could prevent scurvy among sailors. It took Lind decades to convince the British Royal Navy to implement his recommendation to include fruits in sailors' diets. Thereafter, the incidence of scurvy declined sharply.

Vitamin C is also referred to as ascorbic acid (AA)/ascorbate. It appears to be important for plants and animals in order to combat oxidative stress and modulate gene expression. Highly evolved mammalian species seem to have lost the ability to synthesize vitamin C. Hence, it must be supplied by the diet in some vertebrates including man, primates, and guinea pigs. Vitamin C is water-soluble and tends to get easily destroyed on exposure to air (oxygen), light, alkali, and heat, particularly in the presence of iron or copper. There are two interchangeable forms of the vitamin—(1) the reduced form called AA and (2) oxidized form called dehydroascorbic acid (DHA). It acts as a reducing agent and is used wherever electron or hydrogen needs to be donated. The reduced form is very important in biological functions. It reduces the ferric iron (Fe^3) to the ferrous state (Fe^2) of iron, which facilitates iron absorption. It also plays a significant role in collagen synthesis and helps combat stress and infection.

Small amounts consumed in the diet are almost completely absorbed. However, when intakes are >200 mg, only 1/5th of the vitamin is absorbed. The body does not store much AA (approximately 1–2 g). If the stores are <300 mg, it may increase the risk of deficiency symptoms. Some tissues have higher concentrations of AA, e.g., leukocytes, adrenal gland, pituitary gland, and brain.

When AA is oxidized, it is converted to DHA, which is rapidly taken up by several types of cells and is reduced back to AA. This mechanism ensures intracellular antioxidant capacity. However, in certain conditions like diabetes mellitus and smoking, this uptake and recycling of DHA to AA is compromised. In blood, DHA is very rapidly and irreversibly hydrolyzed to 2,3-diketogulonic acid, that is then excreted.

Functions of Vitamin C

Ascorbic acid is a cofactor for several enzymes such as monooxygenases and hydroxylases and has many physiological roles. Its role is to maintain the metal ions, specifically copper and iron, in reduced form and thus maintain optimal activity of the enzymes. Table 6.3 indicates biochemical and physiological functions.

Collagen synthesis: Collagen is a fibrous protein (one of the most abundant) that binds cells like glue. It is present

Table 6.3: Functions of vitamin C.

Biochemical functions	Physiological functions
• Synthesis of macromolecules like collagen, carnitine, norepinephrine • Possibly involved in regulating several genes for apolipoprotein E, transferrin, and tyrosine hydroxylase • Antioxidant activity and thus helps in reducing oxidative stress	• Immunity • Role in reducing risk of atherosclerosis • Anticancer agent • Reducing progression of diseases linked to oxidative stress, e.g., cataract, Alzheimer's disease, rheumatoid arthritis • Aids in iron absorption

in connective tissue of our skin, teeth, bones, tendon, cartilages. About 33 percent of body protein is collagen. This protein is necessary for formation of scar tissue. Therefore patients, with burns, injuries or who have undergone surgery i.e., wherever wound healing is required, require adequate vitamin C intakes. Collagen formation is a lifelong process. Vitamin C is required for synthesis of collagen and procollagen as it is needed for hydroxylation of two amino acids—proline and lysine and their conversion to hydroxyproline and hydroxylysine, respectively. These amino acids are important components of collagen. Ascorbic acid maintains the metal ions iron and copper that are present in certain metalloenzymes in a reduced state.

Skin health: The role of vitamin C in collagen synthesis extends to its role in firmness and resiliency in skin which prevent aging and wrinkling. Vitamin C supports the formation of muscle fibers in connective tissues and speeds up the healing process. Therefore, vitamin C is important in wound healing and formation of scar tissue. Vitamin C is important for skin health as it reduces the damage caused by ultraviolet light, by functioning as an antioxidant.

Ascorbic acid maintains the metal ions, iron, and copper, present in certain metalloenzymes in a reduced state. These enzymes are involved in modification, i.e., hydroxylation of two amino acids, proline and lysine to hydroxyproline and hydroxylysine, which are important components of collagen. Collagen is a fibrous protein (one of the most abundant proteins) present in skin, bone, tendon, cartilages, and teeth. Vitamin C supports the formation of muscle fibers in connective tissues and speeds up the healing process. Therefore, vitamin C is important in wound healing, formation of scar tissue, and formation of matrix of bones, cartilages, and connective tissues. Therefore patients with burns, injuries, or who have undergone surgery need adequate vitamin C intakes. It is also a cofactor for enzymes required for osteocalcin synthesis.

Acts as an antioxidant: End product of oxidation is free radical which is a highly reactive and rapid process. Vitamin C is one of the most potent antioxidants. It works in association with vitamin E. Vitamin C helps to regenerate vitamin E by donating electrons to oxidized vitamin E. Thus, it tends to reduce lipid peroxidation, oxidation of DNA, and LDL. It has been suggested to be helpful in reducing the risk of many chronic diseases.

However, it should be noted that under certain conditions, vitamin C can act like a pro-oxidant, especially in the presence of free transition metal ions like iron and copper. Its pro-oxidant activity leads to the formation of reactive oxygen species or glycated proteins, both of which are linked to development of non-communicable diseases.

Iron absorption: Vitamin C converts ferric form (Fe^{+++}) of iron into the ferrous form (Fe^{++}) of iron and thereby improves the iron absorption. Vitamin C is required to facilitate absorption of ferric iron or non-heme iron from plant foods.

Promotes immune function: It helps to prevent infections and to control inflammation. It enhances T-cell proliferation in response to infection. T-cells play an important role by killing the organisms and help B cells to produce immunoglobulins. Vitamin C may have anti-viral activity and may help in reducing the severity of symptoms of cold. Linus Pauling a Nobel Laureate strongly recommended that vitamin C can help combat common cold. It enhances the activity of natural killer cells that are part of the body's surveillance against tumor cells in the early stages of tumor development. Vitamin C may also provide protection against cancer by neutralizing free radicals which otherwise can damage DNA and thereby initiate tumor growth. Also, it can function as a pro-oxidant to produce more free radicals which will destroy tumor cells in early stages of tumor development.

Synthesis of carnitine: Carnitine is a molecule needed to transport fatty acids into the mitochondria. Vitamin C is required for carnitine synthesis. Carnitine plays a role in fatty acid metabolism and energy production because it helps to move fatty acids from cytosol to mitochondria for beta oxidation.

Amino acid metabolism: Ascorbic acid is also involved in metabolism of phenylalanine and tyrosine.

Stress management: Cortisol is a stress hormone which is raised during "fight and flight" mechanism in stressful situations. Synthesis of adrenalin, a stress hormone, requires vitamin C. Ascorbate is also involved in conversion of tryptophan to serotonin, a relaxing neurotransmitter. The enzyme involved in synthesis of norepinephrine from dopamine is vitamin C dependent. Vitamin C also plays a role in enzymatic reactions necessary for maximum activity of hormones such as oxytocin, vasopressin, and cholecystokinin.

Detoxification: Helps in neutralizing toxins and heavy metals like lead and cadmium. (Present in polluted environment, cigarette smoke, water pipe lines, and certain utensils). It suppresses formation of nitrosamines (which are carcinogenic) from nitrites present in food.

Other physiological functions: Ascorbic acid stimulates synthesis of nitric oxide in endothelium of blood vessels. Nitric oxide plays an important role in vasodilation and protects LDL against oxidation. Reduced nitric oxide synthesis is associated with elevated blood cholesterol (hypercholesterolemia), hypertension, and diabetes. Thus, vitamin C may help in reducing blood pressure and provide

Table 6.4: Food sources of vitamin C.

Food source	Vitamin C content (mg/100 g)	Food source	Vitamin C content (mg/100 g)	Food source	Vitamin C content (mg/100 g)
Amla (gooseberry)	252	Green chillies	94.0	Coriander leaves	23
Guava (pink flesh)	222	Drumstick leaves	71.9	Papaya (ripe)	43.1
Guava (white flesh)	214	Mango (harsingar)	49.1	Pineapple	36.4
Yellow capsicum	127	Lemon juice	48.1	Strawberry	50.2
Grapes (green)	16.5	Lime pulp	47.0	Cauliflower	47.0
Grapes (black)	22.8	Orange pulp	42.7	Potato big	23.2

Source: IFCT, 2017.

protection against cardiovascular disease. It is also involved in prostaglandin synthesis. Vitamin C is also needed for modification of a protein that activates Factor V that is involved in blood clotting. Ascorbate has been shown to play a role in the hydroxylation of hypoxia-inducible factor 1 (HIF-1), which is effected by prolyl and lysyl hydroxylases. HIF-1 is a transcription factor that is responsible for the cellular response when there is less oxygen. HIF-1 activates the genes involved in the cellular transduction pathways by regulating growth and apoptosis, cell migration, energy metabolism, angiogenesis, vasomotor regulation, extracellular matrix and barrier functions, and transport of metal ions and glucose.

Vitamin C has been found to improve the responsiveness of arteries to vasoconstrictors like vasopressin, angiotensin, and norepinephrine. This may be helpful in preventing hypotension and perhaps edema. It may be useful with other antioxidant vitamins in reducing the rate of development of cataract, age-related macular degeneration, and thus the loss of visual acuity. However, its role in diabetic retinopathy needs to be well studied. Ascorbic acid is also a cofactor for osteocalcin synthesis.

Recommended Dietary Allowance of Vitamin C

FAO/WHO recommended intake of 40-45 mg/day ascorbic acid. Globally four criteria are used to establish the recommendations for vitamin C (ascorbic acid). These are to (i) prevent scurvy (ii) improve saturation of immune cells (neutrophils) with ascorbic acid while limiting its excretion (iii) replace daily turnover to maintain adequate plasma levels (iv) optimize health by optimal intake of vitamin C.

ICMR-NIN (2020) has recommended RDA for vitamin C for different age groups that can seen in Table 9.1B in Chapter 9. Also ICMR-NIN (2020) has given the EAR for vitamin C. (Appendix 4)

The minimum requirement for preventing scurvy is 10 mg/day and for wound healing is 20 mg/day. The Institute of Medicine (IOM, 2000) in the US has pointed out that persons who smoke need more vitamin C since they face more oxidative stress as compared to non-smokers. The IOM and ICMR-NIN have set the Upper Tolerable Intake Level for oral vitamin C ingestion at 2 g daily for adults based on gastrointestinal disturbances.

Food Sources of Vitamin C

Many fruits and vegetables are sources of vitamin C. However, the vitamin is highly labile since it is easily destroyed by prolonged storage, heating, and exposure to air/light. Hence, it is advisable to obtain vitamin C from raw fruits and vegetables. Some rich sources of vitamin C are listed in Table 6.4.

Causes and consequences of deficient intake of vitamin C

Inadequate intake of vitamin C rich foods is the main cause of the deficiency symptoms. Scurvy is caused by the deficiency of vitamin C. It is characterized by depleted body stores of vitamin C, fragile blood vessels, and poor linkage of collagen fibers. Primary symptoms are listlessness, fatigue, weakness, muscle cramps, loss of appetite, and aching bones. Clinical symptoms include gingivitis (bleeding gums) and petechiae (small hemorrhagic spots on skin). Depression, pain in joints, hypotension, poor performance, and delayed wound healing are other common features of vitamin C deficiency. Secondary bacterial infection in gums, loss of dental cement, and loosening of teeth can occur in scurvy. Older persons, smokers, diabetics, and people suffering from depression or trauma are at increased risk of poor vitamin C status.

Insufficiency and deficiency will decline the collagen synthesis making skin to wrinkles, the sign of aging. Depleted collagen makes the skin more susceptible for bruising, bleeding, and delayed wound healing. Lack of vitamin C will alter the configuration and weaken the collagen making the cells susceptible to damage.

Consequences of excessive intake of vitamin C

Adverse effect of excessive consumption is rare because vitamin C is water soluble and excess is removed through urine. If it is consumed in doses exceeding 1,000 mg daily for a prolonged period, it may cause imbalance in other nutrients. Massive doses can interfere with anticoagulant therapy in ischemic heart disease or people with sickle cell anemia. Some individuals who consumed more than 3 g per day suffered from gastrointestinal problems like nausea, diarrhea, and abdominal cramps. Saturable intestinal absorption and renal tubular reabsorption data suggest that overload of ascorbic acid is unlikely in humans. High doses of vitamin C for prolonged periods should be taken with caution, as ascorbic acid is converted to oxalate and may increase the risk of kidney stones.

UL is not meant to apply to individuals who are receiving vitamin C under medical supervision.

> **Interactions with other nutrients**
>
> **Vitamin C and Bioflavonoids:** Both are water-soluble compounds that act as antioxidants and often occur together in foods that are also rich in vitamin C. Bioflavonoids such as citrin, hesperidin, rutin, flavones, flavonols, catechin, and quercetin are found in citrus fruits like lemons, grapefruits, oranges, apricots, cherries, grapes, black currants, plums, blackberries, green pepper, broccoli, and tomatoes. Bioflavonoids perform a wide variety of functions in promoting and protecting the health. They may act synergistically with vitamin C in strengthening capillary walls, preventing oxidative stress, cell membranes, and maintaining collagen.
>
> **Vitamin C and Iron:** It reduces ferric iron into ferrous and facilitates absorption of non-heme iron from plant sources. ICMR has recommended that at least 20 mg of ascorbic acid (AA) should be consumed in a day (through meals) with the AA to iron in a molar ratio of 2:1 in order to improve iron absorption.
>
> **Vitamin C and Vitamin E:** Vitamin E is present in the cell membrane and quenches free radicals. When vitamin E is oxidized, vitamin C which is present in the cytosol helps in its regeneration. Eventually damage caused by oxidation and free radical generation is minimized.
>
> **Vitamin C and copper:** Copper helps in synthesis of hemoglobin. Absence or excess of vitamin C can disturb normal status of copper in the blood.

Thiamine

Thiamine which is also referred as vitamin B1 plays a significant role in carbohydrate metabolism and neural functions. This is the first water-soluble vitamin that was discovered by Christiaan Eijkman in 1897 while treating neurological disorder called beriberi. Thiamine works as a coenzyme for different enzymes involved in the production of adenosine triphosphate (ATP), acetylcholine, gamma aminobutyric acid (GABA), nicotinamide adenine dinucleotide phosphate (NADPH), myelin sheath, DNA, and many other compounds. Hence, vitamin B1 is important for healthy functioning of the body and prevents many neurological disorders including neuropathy and Alzheimer's and Parkinson's diseases. Christiaan Eijkman a Dutch medical officer had established that deficiency of vitamin B1 causes beriberi which is characterized by weakness, abdominal discomforts, confusion, irritability, and sleep disturbances.

In Asian countries where polished white rice is a staple food, **beriberi**, a neurological disorder was endemic. This was confirmed by Christiaan Eijkman in 1897, when he fed unpolished rice instead of the polished variety to chickens and demonstrated that unpolished rice could cure and prevent beriberi. In 1885, Dr Takaki, a Surgeon-General of the Japanese navy, improved the quality of naval diets and reduced prevalence of beriberi. Later, Christiaan Eijkman fed polished rice to chickens to induce a polyneuritic disease resembling beriberi in humans. He observed that feeding them rice polishings or rice bran prevented the problem. He gave it the name "anti-beriberi factor." Later the anti-beriberi factor was called vitamin B1, being the first water-soluble vitamin and was named thiamine. In 1929, Christiaan Eijkman and Sir Fredrick G Hopkins shared the Nobel Prize in Physiology or Medicine for their discovery of the antineuritic vitamin and growth-stimulating vitamins, respectively.

Dietary thiamine is absorbed in the small intestine, most of it in the duodenum, and transferred to portal circulation. Almost all of dietary thiamine is absorbed. In deficiency states, absorption increases. However, absorption decreases as age advances and in folate deficiency or with alcohol intake. Alcohol may reduce absorption of a single dose of thiamine by almost one-third. Some drugs may also reduce availability of thiamine.

Once thiamine is absorbed, it is taken up by various organs and tissues including liver, heart, etc. In case of neuronal tissues, thiamine is transported from blood via the blood–brain barrier into the cerebrospinal fluid. Within the cell, it is then transported through the mitochondrial and nuclear membranes. Thiamine is transported with the help of a transporter. In the cell, thiamine is converted to thiamine pyrophosphate, the biologically active form by the enzyme thiamine diphosphokinase.

Deficiency or lack of this transporter has been reported to lead to thiamine-responsive megaloblastic anemia. Persons who had this thiamine-responsive megaloblastic anemia were found to have a mutation in the gene that encodes a transporter protein for thiamine. Such patients respond to megadoses or pharmacological doses.

Functions of thiamine

The main function of thiamine is to act as a coenzyme that with thiamine pyrophosphate (TPP). Enzyme activity is not complete without the presence of coenzyme and it is an important cofactor in tricarboxylic acid (TCA) cycle and pentose phosphate pathway. These pathways are important in generation of ATP and are associated with oxidation of glucose, decarboxylation of pyruvic acid in carbohydrate metabolism, and energy metabolism.

There are mainly three enzymes for which TPP is crucial and they are transketolase, pyruvate dehydrogenase, and α ketoglutarate dehydrogenase. These enzymes support conversion of glucose-6-phosphate into two products, namely, ribose-5 phosphates and NADPH via pentose phosphate pathway. Ribose is involved in biosynthesis of nucleic acids, complex sugars, and NADPH. Hence, it plays a role in formation of coenzymes, steroids, fatty acids, amino acids, neurotransmitters, and glutathione. The major role of thiamine is as a coenzyme—TPP. TPP is important for decarboxylation reactions associated with energy metabolism and for the nervous system. Important functions of thiamine are:

Alpha (α) ketoglutarate dehydrogenase also participates in metabolism of branched chain amino acids, namely, leucine, isoleucine, and valine.

Carbohydrate, protein, and fat metabolism: TPP is required during glycolysis for conversion of glucose into pyruvate. TPP is also involved in the decarboxylation of branched chain amino acids. TPP is a coenzyme for another group of enzymes in the pentose phosphate pathway that generates ribose and supplies NADPH which is used in a variety of biosynthetic reactions, especially fatty acid synthesis.

Table 6.5: Food sources of thiamine.

Food sources	Thiamine mg/100 g	Food sources	Thiamine mg/100 g	Food sources	Thiamine mg/100 g
Wheat flour atta	0.42	Soyabean	0.61	Cashew nut	0.61
Jowar	0.35	Peas dry	0.56	Groundnut	0.57
Barley	0.36	Bengal gram dhal (Chana dal)	0.35	Pistachio nut	0.98
Ragi	0.37	Green gram dhal	0.35	Sesame seeds white	0.36
Puffed rice	0.11	Lentil brown	0.40	Walnut	0.40
Rawa (semolina)	0.29	Moth bean	0.45	Sunflower seed	0.85

Source: IFCT, 2017.

Nervous system: Thiamine is required for smooth functioning of nervous system. Glucose is completely oxidized in the brain through TCA cycle for which TPP is required. Pyruvate dehydrogenase for which TPP is a cofactor is necessary for the synthesis of acetylcholine. It facilitates neurotransmission. Thiamine is also necessary for the synthesis of acetylcholine and GABA that facilitate neurotransmission. Acetyl coenzyme A (CoA) is also a precursor for acetylcholine and for myelin synthesis. It has been found to be involved in transmission of nerve signals to peripheral nerves. In genetic defects where thiamine deficiency occurs during fetal development or infancy, degeneration of the cerebral cortex has been observed.

Pyruvate dehydrogenase and α ketoglutarate dehydrogenase are important for numerous cellular processes including in the brain. Pyruvate dehydrogenase is essential for production of acetylcholine and formation of myelin sheath around neurons. Alpha-ketoglutarate dehydrogenase supports the maintenance of the level of GABA, glutamate, and aspartate. All these compounds in the brain play a role in neuronal signaling.

Formation of genetic material: Glucose is metabolized into 5-carbon compounds, i.e., ribose and deoxyribose, that are integral components of ribonucleic acid (RNA) and DNA and contain genetic information.

Recommended dietary allowance for thiamine
Thiamine requirement is influenced by energy intake. Thiamine intake below 0.12 mg/1,000 kcal can cause deficiency symptoms like beriberi. Requirement is higher during chronic illness, fever, alcoholism, and strenuous exercise and for sports persons. During periods of growth, i.e., adolescence, pregnancy, lactation, and infancy, extra thiamine is needed because of high requirements of energy in these physiological states. In old age, there is high metabolic demand, high risk of cardiac diseases, and dementia where thiamine plays an important role, hence thiamine requirements are high. In old age or persons suffering from neurodegenerative diseases like Alzheimer's and Parkinson's, the level of thiamine-dependent enzymes is depleted, hence requirements are raised. Requirements are increased with high intake of carbohydrate.

Food sources of thiamine
Thiamine is found in most food items but in relatively small amounts. Good food sources are those which provide more than 0.3 mg thiamine per 1,000 kcal. Most animal foods are not good sources of vitamin B_1 but yeast and pork are exceptions. In plant foods, groundnuts, sesame seeds, pistachio, cashew nuts, and sunflower seeds are excellent sources. Whole wheat and pulses are also considered good sources of vitamin B_1. Some of the good food sources are shown in Table 6.5.

Processing has significant effect on vitamin content. Being water soluble, it leaches out into cooking water and being heat labile, significant amounts are destroyed during heat treatment like pasteurization. On average, processing and cooking lead to 40-50% losses, baking leads to approx 30% loss whereas losses with pasteurization are much lower 10-20%. Significant loss of thiamine also occurs in alkaline medium, e.g., addition of soda to soften whole pulse or/and to preserve green color in green leafy vegetables; sulfite in fruit juices; and use of preservatives like potassium metabisulfite for preserving wine and dried fruits. Milling of grains also causes significant loss of thiamine due to removal of the aleurone layer of the grain which is where thiamine is mostly present.

There are certain foods which naturally contain antithiaminase enzyme which destroys or inhibits the use of thiamine in the body. These foods include sea foods, raw fish, fermented fish, or uncooked fish. Some compounds such as polyphenols (chlorogenic acid, tannin, and caffeic acid) and some flavonoids (quercetin and rutin) tend to interfere with the digestion of thiamine. Such compounds are widely distributed in numerous plant foods including betel leaf and tea. In some countries, processed food products like bread and cornflakes are fortified with thiamine.

Deficiency of thiamine—causes and consequences
Deficiency of thiamine can be tested by **erythrocyte transketolase activity (ETK)**. Normal range is 1.00–1.15; mild deficient cases may have 1.16–1.24; and in deficiency, the value is >1.24. Increased pyruvic levels are also indicative of thiamine deficiency.

Besides low dietary intake, many other factors are found responsible for thiamine deficiency. Poor quality diet, poor absorption in the body, food processing methods, and many other health states can cause thiamine deficiency. Consumption of high amount of carbohydrates or simple sugars, refined flour, and polished rice can increase the metabolic demand of vitamin B_1 to release the energy. Foods containing high amount of polyphenols (tea, coffee, betel nut) and foods with thiaminase enzyme (raw sea foods) also inhibit absorption. People practice extra washing and long soaking of rice, pulses, and other foods and discarding water after cooking; adding cooking soda for quick cooking; overcooking and cooking on high heat; and use of irradiation and high extraction milling. These practices lead to loss of thiamine and increase the risk of deficiency. Hypomagnesemia, conditions in which metabolic demands are high, e.g., hyperthyroidism, fever, pregnancy, lactation, strenuous work, adolescence, and trauma after surgery often make individuals susceptible to thiamine deficiency. Others who are at risk and likely to have thiamine deficiency are alcoholics, chronic dialysis patients, persons with autism, or neuropathy conditions, malnourished persons and those suffering from HIV/AIDS, diabetes, Alzheimer disease, peptic ulcer, and/or who have undergone duodenal or bariatric surgery, and people on restrictive diets.

> **Research glimpse:** Malnutrition is found that 15.5–29% obese patients seeking bariatric surgery and they have shown thiamine deficiency. The vague signs and symptoms are often overlooked in them. It is attributed that the current RDA of thiamine is often not sufficient to meet the metabolic needs of overweight or obese adults. Thiamine is essential for the metabolism of glucose and is thus critical for normal tissue and organ function and its deficiency can lead to severe (or even fatal) cardiovascular and neurologic complications, including heart failure, neuropathy leading to ataxia and paralysis, confusion, or delirium.
>
> *Kerns JC, Arundel C, Chawla LS. Thiamin deficiency in people with obesity. Adv Nutr. 2015;6(2):147-53.*

Thiamine is not stored in the body. Therefore, deficiency can be observed using biochemical indicators within a few days of subsisting on a thiamine-free diet. Even in the late 1990s, endemic thiamine deficiency has been reported in some countries.

Mild thiamine deficiency is characterized by muscle weakness, fatigue, apathy, loss of appetite, mental confusion, irritability, and peripheral neuropathy. It can leads to cell damage including of the brain resulting in neuropathy, neuralgia, cognitive deficit, and memory loss. Since thiamine is a cofactor for enzymes responsible for releasing cellular energy, glucose metabolism, and biosynthesis of crucial compounds like glutathione, acetylcholine, and GABA, etc. deficiency of thiamine impairs the energy metabolism and diminishes the functioning of the body at cellular level.

Beriberi is the name of the disease caused by thiamine deficiency. It adversely affects the functioning of cardiovascular, gastrointestinal, and nervous systems. Primary deficiency symptoms are like constipation. Beriberi is classified into four types based on the different symptoms present: These are (1) dry beriberi where there is no edema, (2) wet beriberi in which edema is present, (3) Wernicke-Korsakoff syndrome and (4) infantile beriberi.

Dry beriberi: Dry beriberi is generally associated with prolonged but possibly less severe deficiency and poor food intake whereas wet beriberi is associated with high carbohydrate intake and physical inactivity. Symptoms of dry beriberi are bilateral (two sides) and symmetric. Symptoms of dry beriberi generally begin with abnormal sensation in toes (paresthesia), pins and needles (tingling), or/and loss of sensation in feet and hands, burning or pain (more intense at night), stiffness, cramps or/and pain in calves, lower legs; difficulty in rising from squatting position, inability to walk long distances, difficulty in speaking, mental confusion, poor coordination of motor activities (like involuntary eye movements), and peripheral neuropathy. **Paresthesia** is an abnormal sensation due to peripheral nerve damage. Neuromuscular disorders are predominant with no edema. There is degeneration and demyelination of sensory and motor nerves.

Wet beriberi: It usually affects the cardiovascular system. Common symptoms are high cardiac output, palpitation, restlessness, sweating, warm skin, acidosis, and edema. It can also be fatal due to heart failure. Edema is a notable feature, being present in legs, face, trunk, and serous cavities. In the absence of TPP, glucose is not metabolized completely and there is accumulation of pyruvic acid or lactic acid in tissues. Signs of peripheral neuritis as seen in dry beriberi may not be present.

Wernicke-Korsakoff syndrome: Wernicke-Korsakoff syndrome or Wernicke-Korsakoff encephalopathy is characterized by decreased reflexes, confusion, impaired memory, poor recall especially of recent events or impairment of short-term memory, although memory for past events may not be affected there may be confabulation; changes in response and reactions of eyes and vision and deterioration in the functions of the central nervous system (CNS) leading to coma. It is commonly found in alcoholics whose food intake is poor. However, it may also occur in some patients who are seriously ill and are put on parenteral nutritional support. If thiamine is administered intravenously to such patients, in doses of 100 to 500 mg/day, it can relieve life-threatening deficiency conditions. Gastrectomy patients may also at risk in the long term, if their diets are deficient in thiamine.

Infantile beriberi: It usually occurs in infants in 2–4 months of age and is characterized by excessive crying without sound and face may turn bluish. It can be fatal too if left unnoticed. Immediate medical attention is needed. It is common in developing countries and a cause for high infant mortality. It occurs in breast fed babies whose mothers' diets are thiamine deficient or when they are not fed due to some infection. Intake of thiamine rich diet by lactating mothers may help to reduce such episodes in the child.

> **Laboratory Laurel:** Brain glucose hypometabolism is correlated with cognitive impairment and disease progression of Alzheimer's disease. In this study, patients with AD and control subjects were studied to evaluate brain glucose metabolism using positron emission tomography with 2-(18F) fluoro-2-deoxy-D-glucose (FDG-PET). AD patients with clinically diagnosed AD, brain amyloid-β (Aβ) deposition was quantified. Study was also carried out on mice to examine the effect of thiamine deprivation. In both the human subjects and the mice, levels of blood thiamine metabolites were measured and in mice, brain samples were also analyzed. In the patients with AD, it was observed that in different parts of the brain, the FDG values were correlated with the blood thiamine diphosphate (TDP) levels and their cognitive abilities but there was no correlation with the brain Aβ deposition. In the thiamine-deprived mice, there was significant decline in brain glucose metabolism in several brain regions that

Contd...

Contd...

> was strongly correlated with TDP levels in blood and brain but not with the amyloid precursor protein (presenilin-1). The investigators concluded that TDP reduction is strongly related to brain glucose hypometabolism and that is one mechanism that needs to be studied for pathogenesis and the therapy for AD.
>
> *Sang S, Pan X, Chen Z, et al. Thiamine diphosphate reduction strongly correlates with brain glucose hypometabolism in Alzheimer's disease, whereas amyloid deposition does not. Alzheimer's Res Ther. 2018;10:26.*

Consequences of excessive intake of thiamine

Being water soluble, it is excreted through urine. No adverse effects have been observed with oral intakes as high as 10 g/day. However, reactions have been reported with high doses administered parenterally.

For treatment of mild thiamine deficiency, The World Health Organization recommends daily oral doses of 10 mg thiamine for a week, followed by 3–5 mg/daily for at least 6 weeks, followed by 3–5 mg/day orally. In severe cases, 25–30 mg intravenously for infants and 50–100 mg in adults, then 10 mg can be given under medical supervision.

Riboflavin (Vitamin B$_2$)

In 1879, a water-soluble pigment with yellow-green fluorescence was discovered in milk. It was named lactoflavin—*lacto* for milk and *flavin*, for the yellow color. In the 1930s, Otto Warburg, a chemist, isolated a yellowish substance from yeast and observed that it consisted of a protein as well a non-protein factor that appeared to be important for cell repair. Later, Warburg and his team then observed this substance, important for cell repair. Richard Kuhn in Germany, and Paul Karrer (1889-1971) in Switzerland, isolated and crystallized vitamin B$_2$, which they observed was identical to lactoflavin. In 1935, Kuhn and Karrer synthesized the vitamin. Karrer was awarded the Nobel Prize for his work on riboflavin in 1937 and Kuhn in 1938.

Riboflavin is a water-soluble vitamin present in a variety of foods and critical in maintaining health. Biologically active forms of riboflavin are flavin mononucleotide or 5' riboflavin-phosphate (FMN) and flavin adenine dinucleotide (FAD). These two compounds act as coenzymes and are also known flavoenzymes. They participate in a range of redox reactions which are essential for aerobic cell functions.

Most of the riboflavin in foods is present in the form of FMN, FAD, and their covalently bound forms. Thus, in almost all foods, riboflavin is in bound form except for dairy foods which contain a small amount of free riboflavin. Therefore, the phosphorylated riboflavin needs to be released by digestive enzymes before it is transported into enterocytes. There are specific saturable transporters. Riboflavin is absorbed in the jejunum. Bile salts increase absorption. Longer rate of gastric emptying is favorable because it increases absorption of riboflavin by facilitating longer contact of the vitamin with the intestinal mucosal cells. Diets that contain large amounts of psyllium gum decrease the rate of absorption. Alcohol interferes with both digestion and absorption.

Functions of riboflavin

Flavoproteins are involved in a wide array of biological functions which include energy metabolism, reducing oxidative stress, DNA repair, and formation of hemoglobin. The coenzymes of riboflavin play an important role as electron carriers and participate in numerous key reactions such as the citric acid cycle, the electron transport chain for formation of ATP, and in oxidation of fatty acids and amino acids as well as cell signaling, protein folding as well as metabolism of lipids, drugs, and xenobiotics. Since flavin nucleotides undergo redox reactions, they are important in a wide array of cellular processes and are necessary for enzymes such as electron transferases, dehydrogenases, oxidoreductases, monooxygenases, hydroxylases, and oxidases. It is important for growth and development.

Energy release from energy nutrients: Two coenzymes FMN and FAD of riboflavin act as electron carriers and participate in numerous key reactions in the citric acid cycle (TCA cycle) and electron transport chain (ETC) for formation of ATP via oxidation–reduction reactions. Riboflavin plays a critical role in controlling the 2-electron acceptor/donor and 1-electron acceptor/donor complexes in the electron transport chain. There are four complexes in the inner mitochondrial membrane, among which Complexes I and II contain flavoprotein reductases or dehydrogenases and electron transferring flavoproteins. Thus, FMN and FAD play a very important role in the respiratory chain/the electron transport chain.

Riboflavin is also involved in various metabolic pathways involved in fatty acid metabolism. This vitamin is also helpful in releasing energy under anaerobic conditions. Thus, riboflavin is essential for metabolism of carbohydrates, fats, and proteins. Riboflavin is necessary for fatty acid desaturation, cholesterol metabolism, 1-carbon metabolism, and sphingosine formation. FMN is associated with enzymes such as cytochrome C reductase and L-amino acid dehydrogenase and FAD is associated with xanthine oxidase, liver aldehyde oxidase, and acyl S-CoA dehydrogenase. Adrenal hormone facilitates conversion of riboflavin into FMN coenzymes that increases the absorption of the vitamin. Adrenal hormone is also associated with carbohydrate metabolism that involves riboflavin. Thyroid hormone stimulates absorption of riboflavin and synthesis of FMN/FAD.

Antioxidant: Flavoproteins in the form of FAD are required for the action of glutathione reductase enzyme that has antioxidant activity and prevents lipid peroxidation. FAD is required to regenerate reduced glutathione from oxidized glutathione. This is known as the glutathione/glutathione disulfide (GSH/GSSG) redox cycle. In riboflavin deficiency, antioxidant defense is compromised. Another enzyme involved in combating oxidative stress is xanthine oxidase. This FAD-dependent enzyme is important for oxidation of hypoxanthine and xanthine to uric acid which is an important water-soluble antioxidant in blood.

Formation of myelin sheath: Riboflavin participates in the formation of myelin and thus supports normal functioning of the CNS.

Supports vitamin metabolism: Flavoproteins are involved in metabolism of folate, vitamin B_{12}, and vitamin B_6. It also supports conversion from retinal (retinaldehyde) to RA and tryptophan into niacin.

Cell signaling: Many flavoproteins have a role in signal transduction pathways, programmed cell death, including nitric oxide synthetase, apoptosis-inducing factor, proline dehydrogenase, and NADPH oxidase.

Tissue building, growth and development: It helps in metabolism of amino acids, conversion of glycogen into glucose, and in synthesis of tissues and vital organs.

Formation of red blood cells: FAD is important for the formation of hemoglobin.

Protective role to skin: Riboflavin protects some dermal tissues and prevents lesions in the skin, eye, and epithelial cells.

Other functions: Pre-eclampsia during pregnancy may be linked to riboflavin deficiency. Risk of pre-eclampsia has been found to be associated with the presence of a genetic variant in the methylenetetrahydrofolate reductase gene. In adults suffering from migraine, riboflavin has been shown to reduce the severity of headaches.

Recommended dietary allowance of riboflavin
Like thiamine, riboflavin requirement is based on energy requirement.

Food sources of riboflavin
Skimmed milk powder, whey water, walnuts, almonds, niger seeds, radish leaves, beet greens, and eggs are all rich sources of riboflavin. On average, cooking losses are about 20%. Milk contains the vitamin, but riboflavin is light sensitive, thus exposing milk in the sunlight may damage it. Hence, it is advisable to avoid exposing milk to light. When milk is coagulated to make paneer, the riboflavin is in the whey water rather than paneer. Therefore, it is advisable to use whey water while making curries or dough rather than discarding it. Vegetable vendors often keep green vegetables exposed under the sun; this results in loss of the vitamin. Table 6.6 lists the sources and their riboflavin content.

Deficiency of Riboflavin—Causes and Consequences
Riboflavin deficiency is also known as ariboflavinosis. According to a survey conducted by National Nutrition Monitoring Bureau (NNMB), 2006, riboflavin intake among Indian population is less than 42% of the RDA particularly among children and women of low income group. Its deficiency is fairly widespread; however, it is not fatal, because the body is capable of efficiently reutilizing the riboflavin from the flavoproteins when they are metabolized. Riboflavin deficiency generally does not occur in isolation and most often it occurs along with deficiencies of other B-complex vitamins.

Poor intake of riboflavin rich foods like milk or milk products and green leafy vegetables for several months leads to riboflavin deficiency. Loss of the vitamin due to exposure to light (UV rays), cooking in open pan, and refining of cereals is also responsible for poor intakes. Diet low in riboflavin contributes to anemia particularly when iron intake is also low. Deficiency of vitamin B_2 alters the metabolism of other B vitamins notably folate and vitamin B_6. It is because it interferes with utilization of riboflavin. Adrenal or thyroid insufficiency (hypothyroidism) may be associated since conversion of the vitamin to its coenzyme forms is inhibited. Deficiency of riboflavin adversely affects the structure and functioning of the hormones particularly, adrenal and thyroid glands. Since this vitamin is associated with FAD, it affects all biological processes including energy production and hormonal regulation. Excretion is higher in heat, stress, and during strenuous physical exercise. Riboflavin utilization is increased during respiratory infection which increases the urinary loss of the vitamin and causes its deficiency.

Symptoms of riboflavin deficiency in early stages are generally weakness, sore throat, fatigue, swelling of the lining of the mouth, mouth pain, and tenderness, and burning and itching of eyes. In later stages, typical riboflavin deficiency signs are angular stomatitis (cracks or fissures at corners of mouth), outside of the lips (cheilosis), and glossitis (red, dry atrophic, magenta tongue with flattening of papillae). Sometimes moist, scaly skin inflammation (seborrheic dermatitis), greasiness, and fissures in the folds of ears and nose are also observed. Photophobia occurs in which eyes become sensitive to light leading to their itching, watering, and burning in the eyes that may lead to cataract and reduces the visual acuity. Also, blood vessels may form in the clear covering of the eye (known as vascularization of the cornea). RBC count decreases although the hemoglobin level is

Table 6.6: Food Sources of riboflavin.

Food source	Riboflavin mg /100 g	Food source	Riboflavin mg /100 g	Food source	Riboflavin mg /100 g
Bajra	0.20	Red amaranth leaves	0.27	Almond	0.26
Barley	0.18	Drumstick leaves	0.45	Niger seeds gray	0.35
Whole wheat	0.15	Beet green	0.17	Mustard seeds	0.33
Bengal gram whole	0.24	Radish leaves	0.13	Coriander seeds	0.23
Horse gram	0.24	Fenugreek leaves	0.22	Omum	0.23
Lentil whole	0.22	Mint leaves	0.19	Red chillies dry	0.83
Green gram whole	0.27	Garlic big	0.25	Cloves	0.22

Source: IFCT, 2017.

normal and the size of the RBCs is normal. This anemia is called normochromic, normocytic anemia.

> **Research glimpse:** Recently, riboflavin has been recognized as an essential component of cellular biochemistry. The mechanisms and regulation of its intestinal absorption have been shown to be involved in various diseases and metabolic disorders such as migraine, anemia, cancer, hyperglycemia, hypertension, diabetes mellitus, and oxidative stress directly or indirectly. Deficiency of vitamin B_2 has profound effect on iron absorption, metabolism of tryptophan, mitochondrial dysfunction, gastrointestinal tract, brain dysfunction, and metabolism of other vitamins as well as is associated with skin disorders. The vitamin is also used in many treatments as an adjunct therapy.
>
> *Thakur K, Tomar SK, Singh AK, et al. Riboflavin and health: A review of recent human research. Crit Rev Food Sci Nutr. 2017;57(17):3650-60.*

> **Research Glimpse:** Multiple sclerosis (MS) is an inflammatory demyelinating disease of the central nervous system (CNS). Since riboflavin is important in myelin formation, its deficiency is a risk factor for MS and can also trigger peripheral neuropathies. Some RCTs and case-control studies report that riboflavin supplementation or higher dietary riboflavin intake showed improvements in neurological motor disability in MS patients. Riboflavin is a cofactor of xanthine oxidase and its deficiency exacerbates low uric acid caused by high copper levels, leading to myelin degeneration. The vitamin also plays a role in the normal functioning of glutathione reductase (GR) and its deficiency leads to oxidative damage. Riboflavin promotes the gene and protein levels of brain-derived neurotrophic factor (BDNF) in the CNS which showed beneficial effect of riboflavin on neurological motor disability. Further observational and interventional studies on human populations are warranted to validate the effects of riboflavin.
>
> *Naghashpour M, Jafarirad S, Amani R, et.al Update on riboflavin and multiple sclerosis: a systematic review, Iran J Basic Med Sci. 2017;20(9):958–66.*

Riboflavin deficiency tends to impair psychomotor development, reduces iron absorption leading to anemia due to poor conversion of ferric iron to ferrous iron, and reduces wound healing due to the poor cross-linking in collagen. Persons with low energy, reduced hand grip strength, depression, or hysteria have been found to have low riboflavin level, when assessed by glutathione reductase activity in red blood cells. Poor riboflavin status has been linked to oxidative stress. Low glutathione levels are observed along with low levels of riboflavin. Low glutathione levels tend to increase the synthesis of proinflammatory cytokines and oxidative stress which may further lead to the onset of autoimmune diseases, migraine, and neurological dysfunctioning such as Parkinson disease, high blood pressure, cataract, cancer, etc.

Consequences of excessive intake

Being water soluble, excess intake of riboflavin is removed through urine. Toxicity of riboflavin has not been reported yet, even when intakes are several times more than the RDA (as high as 10 g/day). This is because absorption of riboflavin is limited to approximately 25 mg. However, effects have been reported with high doses administered parenterally. Excess may reduce the capacity of gastrointestinal tract to absorb the vitamin when it is consumed at the rate of 400 mg/day for 3 months. In such cases, toxicity can occur. However, such doses are given in clinical practice in the treatment of cancer, severe skin disorder, and migraine under medical supervision.

Niacin (Vitamin B_3)

In the early 20th century (1915-26), Dr Joseph Goldberger, a public health physician who was nominated five times for the Nobel Prize struggled and with his studies conducted in orphanages and patients in mental asylums. He was able to successfully prove the close link between onset of a deadly and painful skin disease known as pellagra, which was caused by a corn diet which was also deficient in meat, milk, and vegetables. Until Goldberger's discovery, pellagra was believed to be caused by a germ. In 1937, a renowned biochemist Conrad A Elvehjem successfully recognized the compound called niacin as anti-pellagra vitamin. Nicotinic acid and nicotinamide is a collective name for Niacin which has the capacity of preventing and treating the deadly skin disease called pellagra.

It functions as a vitamin through formation of two coenzymes, namely, nicotinamide adenine dinucleotide (NAD) and nicotinamide adenine dinucleotide phosphate (NADP) that are involved in cell metabolism to convert food into fuel/energy. Niacin can be obtained by dietary sources. The body can also synthesize nicotinic acid from tryptophan, i.e., 60 mg of dietary tryptophan is converted into 1 mg niacin and which is also reported as 1 niacin equivalent/NE (mg) = 1 mg niacin or 1 mg derived from conversion of 60 mg of dietary tryptophan.

Both nicotinamide and nicotinic acid are absorbed to a small extent in the stomach. In animal sources, the vitamin is present as NAD and NADP. Although niacin is not stored in large amounts, however in some organs, i.e., liver, kidney, and heart as well as skeletal muscle, the concentration of NAD is high. In the face of inadequate dietary intakes, this NAD is utilized and can last for a few weeks.

Functions of niacin

Supports energy generation: NAD and NADP participate in several oxidation and reduction reactions in energy metabolism, where nicotinamide acts as an electron acceptor or donor. Niacin is first incorporated into NAD which can then undergo phosphorylation resulting in the formation of NADP. NAD accepts hydrogen and electrons and is converted into NADH (reduced form). These, under aerobic conditions, are involved in cellular respiration and electron transport chain to produce ATP. These coenzymes are usually associated with dehydrogenase enzymes involved in oxidation of molecules such as pyruvic acid, lactic acid, alcohol, and glyceraldehyde-3-phosphate, which ultimately yield energy from fats and carbohydrates. More than 400 enzymes require NAD or NADP as electron acceptors or donors in the oxidation–reduction reactions that these enzymes catalyze. NAD is generally involved in catabolism of carbohydrates, fats, proteins, and alcohol, whereas NADP is involved in anabolic reactions. Therefore, within the cell, NAD is maintained in an oxidized state (largely by the action of the electron transport chain) so that it can be involved as an oxidizing agent in catabolic reactions. At the same time, NADP (in the form of NADPH) is kept in the reduced state so as to donate electrons that are required in reduction reactions. These two coenzymes play important roles in glycolysis, the Krebs cycle, alcohol metabolism among others.

Formation of important biological compounds: NADP is a hydrogen donor for synthesis of fatty acids and steroids including cholesterol, bile acids, and steroid hormones. NADP participates in the pentose phosphate pathway which is important for synthesis of ribose, an important constituent of RNA and DNA. NAD is also involved in the actions of enzymes that catalyze the transfer of ADP-ribosyl groups, in sirtuins [silent information regulator-2 (Sir2)-like proteins] that are involved in removal of acetyl groups from acetylated proteins and enzymes involved in intracellular calcium signaling.

> **Sirtuins** are regulatory proteins involved in signaling pathways. They are energy sensing and are believed to play a role in gene silencing, repair of damaged DNA, cell cycle regulation, cell differentiation, and delaying the onset of age-related diseases such as dementia, cancer, and cardiovascular disease.
>
> **Calcium signaling** plays a very important role in many biological processes including muscle contraction, neurotransmission, release of insulin from the beta cells of the pancreas, and activation of T lymphocytes.

Helps in formation of serotonin: Serotonin is a relaxing neurotransmitter which is formed from an amino acid, tryptophan, which can be obtained from niacin.

Other functions: It is involved in the DNA repair mechanism. It acts as a regulator of cellular calcium transport. NAD and NADP may also be involved in the anti-inflammatory and anti-oxidant mechanism. NAD is also required for activity of enzymes involved in regulation of transcription, protection of neurons, and cell signaling. Thus, it may be important for modulating or regulating critical cellular processes as well as immune responses. NADP is required for the regeneration of components of detoxification and antioxidant systems. Nicotinic acid is well known to reduce serum cholesterol and may help improve abnormal lipid profiles (in doses of 1–4 g). *In vitro* studies indicate that this vitamin may modulate inflammation, oxidative stress, and may be involved in the regulation of cell adhesion, cell migration, and cell differentiation.

Studies suggest that this vitamin may be beneficial in reducing risk of neurodegenerative diseases, and may sensitize tumors to drugs that are used for cancer treatment.

Recommended dietary allowance of niacin

Niacin requirement is related to energy intake. Since niacin can be obtained from tryptophan but its conversion is dependent upon intakes of protein and energy, hormonal status, and vitamin B_6 and riboflavin status. ICMR-NIN (2020) has given EAR for niacin in Appendix 4 and RDA in Table 9.1b, Chapter 9 for different life stages. The EAR for niacin is recommended per 1000 kcal. The diet should provide extra niacin during pregnancy and lactation to take care of the growing fetus and infant.

Food Sources of Niacin

Some foods are rich in niacin and some contain tryptophan. Both can fulfill the need of niacin. Some foods are good sources of both niacin and tryptophan. Foods that are good sources of protein are also good sources of niacin. Eggs, fish, poultry, meat, liver, cheese, groundnuts, peanut butter, legumes, and green leafy vegetables are rich sources of niacin. Milk contains enough tryptophan that can be easily converted into niacin and helps to fulfill the requirement. Gelatin is completely devoid of tryptophan.

In cereal grains, the outer bran layer (aleurone layer) is rich in niacin where it may be complexed with either carbohydrate or peptides. The bioavailability from these complexes is believed to be low. Treatment with alkali such as soaking overnight in lime (calcium hydroxide) or baking with sodium bicarbonate which are alkaline helps to release a large proportion of the bound niacin. Coffee beans are a good source of a compound trigonelline, some of which is converted to nicotinic acid when coffee beans are roasted. It has been suggested that cooking losses can reach to 25%.

Deficiency of niacin—causes and consequences

Diet low in niacin and its precursor or corn-based diet contributes to niacin deficiency. PEM and pellagra often coexist. Diet rich in leucine or sorghum alters the tryptophan metabolism resulting in niacin deficiency. The disease caused by niacin deficiency is referred as "Pellagra." Pellagra is a 3"Ds" disease which stands for diarrhea, dermatitis, dementia or depression. In extreme cases, pellagra is 4D and fourth D implies death. Pellagra affects the gastrointestinal system, skin, and nervous system.

- **Diarrhea**: Diarrhea due to niacin deficiency occurs due to intestinal inflammation. The patient feels nausea and has poor appetite and abdominal pain. Anorexia and malabsorption exacerbate the malnutrition.
- **Dermatitis:** Dermatitis is a specific feature of pellagra. Skin becomes thicker and hyperpigmented. It occurs on dorsal sides of hands, legs, feet, and cheeks in symmetrical fashion and also forehead and neck. There is pigmented rash on the skin especially parts of the body that are exposed to sunlight and those that are subject to pressure like elbows, knees, wrists, and ankles. In chronic case, darker pigmentation may occur.
- **Dementia:** It starts with muscle weakness, frequent mental problems, progressing toward lethargy, apathy, depression, anxiety, and visual and auditory hallucination followed by paranoid and aggressive behavior.
- Niacin deficiency weakens the brain signaling rather than altering the brain structure.
- Death may occur when there is deficiency of other vitamins also due to depletion of NAD.
- **Neurological problems** are depression, headache, apathy, and loss of memory. The dementia is probably because of the lack of the neurotransmitter, serotonin which is formed from tryptophan. Symptoms of pellagra coincide with deficiency symptoms of other B vitamins also such as weakness, lack of appetite, lethargy irritability, confusion, and impaired memory. In later stages, hallucination,

delusion, and severe depression can also occur followed by death.

> *Tryptophan is the precursor of serotonin. Serotonin is a neurotransmitter which facilitates the communication between neuronal cells in the brain. It is a regulatory neurotransmitter which helps to manage stress, overexcitement, negative thoughts, libido, sleep cycle, and appetite.*
>
> *Tryptophan can cross the blood–brain barrier but not niacin. Hence, foods rich in tryptophan support synthesis of serotonin. Vitamins B_1, B_3, B_6, and B_9 help to convert tryptophan to serotonin.*
>
> *Serotonin is formed in two steps: use of L-tryptophan from food that we eat and converting it into another intermediary chemical called 5 HTP that is finally converted to serotonin. This conversion needs decarboxylase enzyme and that requires vitamin B_6 as cofactor. Hence deficiency of vitamin B_6 can also lower serotonin level.*

Consequences of excessive intake of niacin

Toxicity of niacin is not common in healthy persons. Being water-soluble, the excess is excreted. However, mega dose is given to treat certain medical conditions that may cause side effects like reddening of skin, burning, tingling, and itching and increased incidence of gouty arthritis as nicotinic acid aggravates hyperuricemia (elevated levels of uric acid in blood). Doses of 3 to 9 g have been found to increase utilization of muscle glycogen stores, as well as a lowering of serum lipids, and during exercise result in mobilizing the fatty acids in adipose tissue. These problems are not encountered with nicotinamide. High doses of nicotinic acid may also cause gastrointestinal problems, headache, and liver or muscle damage. Intakes above 36 mg/day result in flushing, burning, and itching of face, arms, and chest. Intakes exceeding 500 mg/day can cause liver damage, especially if the dose is >3,000 mg/day and prolonged use can culminate in hepatic failure. However, mega dose (may be 1,500–3,000 mg/day) may be given to treat certain medical conditions like depression.

Recent studies have focused on problems associated with pharmacological doses of the vitamin taken to improve lipid profiles. There are reports of niacin therapy increase fasting glycemia and development of new-onset diabetes. It has been linked to insulin resistance in muscles. In experimental models, it has been observed that dietary precursors of NAD could counteract age-related diseases such as neurodegenerative diseases. However, the role of this vitamin in anti-aging processes is still a subject of research and supplements should not be taken without medical advice.

> **Research glimpse**: The gut microbiome plays role in energy homeostasis and in obesity. In rodent models, niacin showed beneficial effect on host–microbiome interaction. Researchers characterized >500 persons with different metabolic phenotypes with reference to their nicotinic acid (NA) and nicotinamide (NAM) status and the gut microbiome. They prepared NA and NAM delayed-release capsules to target the ileocolonic regions so that increased amounts of NA and NAM are delivered to the microbiome, while simultaneously preventing systemic resorption and preventing side effects like flushing of the face. They conducted *in vitro* studies and two intervention trials, on bioavailability and proof-of concept/safety. They observed that obese subjects whose dietary niacin intakes were low had reduced diversity and there was abundance of Bacteroidetes in the microbiome.
>
> *Contd...*
>
> Results of the *in vitro* studies showed that the compounds were released at pH 7.4 being stable at pH 1.4, 4.5, and 6.8. NA administration led to a favorably significant increase in Bacteroidetes whereas NAM did not. Along with this, there was improvement in biomarkers for systemic insulin sensitivity and metabolic inflammation. The authors concluded that intervention using delayed-release NA can be a therapeutic option for prediabetes and type 2 diabetes.
>
> *Fangmann D, Theismann EM, Türk K. et al. Targeted Microbiome Intervention by Microencapsulated Delayed-Release Niacin Beneficially Affects Insulin Sensitivity in Humans. Diabetes Care. 2018;41:398-405.*

Pantothenic Acid

Pantothenic acid, generally referred to as vitamin B_5, is named from a Greek word *Pantos* which means "everywhere" as it is widely distributed in all living cells in the form of CoA, which is a vital coenzyme in many chemical reactions. Pantothenic acid was discovered by Williams et al. 1933. By 1939, pantothenic acid was determined to be chemically identical to the anti-dermatitis factor found in chicks. Beta-alanine played an important role in pantothenic acid production, and in 1940, a method to synthesize and crystallize pantothenic acid was established. In 1950, acetyl CoA, a derivative of pantothenic acid which is a key compound in the start of the Krebs cycle or citric acid cycle, was discovered.

Pantothenic acid is easily converted to CoA and acyl carrier protein. They are its functional forms and act as the carriers of acyl group. Being a part of acetyl CoA, pantothenic acid participates in many energy generating pathways like glycolysis, TCA, and β oxidation. Only the D-isomer of pantothenic acid has biological activity.

In foods, most (85%) of the pantothenic acid is combined with CoA or in the form of 4 phosphopantetheine. These substances have to be hydrolyzed in the intestines by the hydrolases, alkaline phosphatase, and pantetheine hydrolase. Small amounts of crystalline pantothenic acid are almost fully absorbed. Some amount of the vitamin may be obtained from synthesis by the gut bacteria. After absorption, it enters the circulation. Limited amount of the vitamin is stored mainly in RBC and adipose tissue in the form of pantetheine.

About 40 to 63% of the ingested pantothenic acid is absorbed. Absorption is fairly rapid; within about 6 hours, tissue levels are increased. Within 6 to 24 hours, levels of pantothenic acid and CoA are increased in leukocytes and in urine. After it is absorbed and taken up by cells, it is either converted into CoA or acyl carrier protein.

Functions of pantothenic acid

Pantothenic acid is the main component of CoA which is essential for all living cells. Coenzyme A functions in more than 70 enzymatic pathways. Acetyl CoA is formed from metabolism of fatty acids, glucose, and amino acids. It is involved in acetylation for the formation of acetylcholine, mucopolysaccharides, and in detoxification. It is involved in synthesis of cholesterol and some steroid hormones.

Involved in energy generation: Coenzyme A is composed of pantothenic acid, phosphate group, and adenine molecule.

CoA is a major component of acetyl CoA which plays a critical role in metabolism of carbohydrate, protein, or fat and further participates in Kreb's cycle to release energy.

Synthesis of fat and cholesterol: Acyl carrier protein and CoA are involved in synthesis of fatty acids and sphingolipids. CoA is involved in synthesis of cholesterol and other steroid hormones produced by adrenal glands.

Role in nerve transmission: Acetyl CoA helps in the formation of acetylcholine which is implicated for memory and better functioning of the autonomic nervous system. It is also needed in transmission of nerve impulses. Pantothenic acid is required for the synthesis of sphingomyelin that enhances the nerve transmission.

Detoxification of drugs: Acetylcholine helps to detoxify certain drugs.

Formation of hemoglobin and antibodies: CoA is essential for antibody formation as well as the formation of the hemoglobin.

Other functions: It is needed for acetylation of proteins. Acetylation affects the three-dimensional structure of proteins and their function such as altering the activity of peptide hormones, influencing cell division, gene expression, and cell signaling.

Recommended dietary allowance of pantothenic acid
It is widely distributed in all edible foods. Normal diet can fulfill the pantothenic acid requirement. Since no deficiency has been found, it was difficult to establish the minimum requirement. During physical exercise and physiological needs like pregnancy and lactation, pantothenic acid requirement is increased and can be fulfilled through a balanced diet. Requirements for this vitamin are increased by smoking (as much as 50%), strenuous physical exercise, heat, infections, and injuries.

Food sources of pantothenic acid
Most foods including peanut butter, peanuts, almonds, whole grains, vegetables, avocado, shiitake mushroom, sunflower seeds, sweet potato, tomato products and cheese, skimmed milk powder, egg yolk, fish, chicken, beef, lobster, and organ meats like liver and kidney are rich sources of pantothenic acid. It is comparatively stable; however, it is readily lost when exposed to heat or in acid or alkali medium and is easily oxidized. Also refining and freezing foods lead to losses. Hence, processing and cooking lead to losses of the vitamin. Losses range from 20% to as much as 78% with canning and freezing resulting in higher losses.

Causes and consequences of deficient intake of pantothenic acid
Because of widespread availability in food, deficiency is rare. However, low intake of normal diet for prolonged duration or malnutrition can slow down the metabolic processes, which can further cause certain subclinical symptoms like restlessness, irritability, easy fatigue, muscle cramps, burning feet syndrome, and many respiratory and gastrointestinal disturbances. Signs and symptoms of other vitamin deficiencies are seen before signs or pantothenic acid deficiency are seen. Deficiency caused by medication was associated with mild, reversible symptoms such as tingling of toes and feet, fatigue, vomiting, sleeplessness, and more susceptibility to infections. Severe deficiency can cause demyelination (destruction or loss of myelin sheath) and peripheral nerve damage.

Consequences of excessive intake of pantothenic acid
No side effects have been observed under normal conditions. Mega doses up to 10 to 20 g/day appear to be well tolerated but along with some medical treatment can cause gastrointestinal disturbances like accumulation of gas, abdominal pain, and mild diarrhea. Limited studies have been carried out on the potential of pantothenic acid as a therapeutic agent for *acne vulgaris,* alopecia, and rheumatoid arthritis, improving adrenal function, healing wounds. However, there is limited information and supplements and should not be taken.

> Biological effects of pantothenic acid are believed to be the result of incorporation of acyl and acetyl groups that pantothenic acid carries and transfers, as this vitamin is used in CoA and acyl carrier proteins. CoA serves as a cofactor in fatty acid oxidation, lipid elongation, and fatty acid synthesis. It plays a part in the synthesis of many secondary metabolites such as polyisoprenoid-containing compounds such as dolichol, ubiquinone (CoQ10), squalene, and cholesterol, steroid molecules (e.g., steroid hormones, vitamin D, and bile acids). It is also required for synthesis of acetylated derivatives of amino sugars like N-acetylglucosamine, acetylated neurotransmitters such as N-acetylserotonin, acetylcholine, and prostaglandins. It is required for degradation of pyrimidines, as well as synthesis of phospholipids.

Pyridoxine (Vitamin B_6)

In 1930s, Rudolf Peters observed "rat acrodynia," a condition characterized by severe cutaneous lesions on young rats. In 1934, Paul György cured it with a compound, first isolated and crystallized in 1938 by Samuel Lepovsky of the University of California, Berkeley. György proposed the term pyridoxine (PN) for this derivative, and in 1939, Folkers and his colleague Stanton Harris determined the structure of PN. Further studies showed that there are various forms, i.e., pyridoxal (PL), pyridoxamine, and pyridoxine. Vitamin activity is high in the form of pyridoxal-5-phosphate which plays significant roles in a wide variety of enzyme systems, especially in the metabolic utilization and transformation of amino acids.

Vitamin B_6 is a group of six compounds—pyridoxine, pyridoxal, and pyridoxamine (PM) and their phosphorylated forms called pyridoxine phosphate (PNP), pyridoxal phosphate (PLP), and pyridoxamine phosphate (PMP). All six forms called vitamers are inter-convertible, contain a pyridine core, and can be metabolically converted into the biologically active form that is PLP. They differ in the group at the 4' position in the pyridine ring. Thus, pyridoxamine has an amino methyl group, in PN, there is a hydroxyl methyl group PN, and in PL, there is an aldehyde group. All vitamers have equal biological activity. Vitamers are chemically related compounds of the same vitamin having similar biological activities. Vitamin B_6 is a central molecule for cellular metabolism. It is said to be a cofactor in more than 140 cellular biochemical reactions.

Pyridoxal phosphate is the active form of vitamin B_6. PLP is a coenzyme for more than 100 enzymes that are involved in protein metabolism, synthesis of blood cells, formation of neurotransmitters, and carbohydrate metabolism. Approximately 80 to 90% of the body's vitamin B_6 is present as PLP in muscle although this does not serve as a store. In young men, the total amount stored is approximately 110 mg and in women, 60 mg is stored. In the 1950s, infant formulas which contained inadequate amount of B_6 led to an outbreak of B_6 deficiency. These infants suffered from convulsions which stopped after being treated with vitamin B_6.

During digestion, the vitamin is released from the glycosides and peptides, to which it is bound in various foods. Vitamin B_6 is absorbed in the upper jejunum. In the intestinal mucosa, the phosphorylated vitamers are first dephosphorylated by enzymes, namely, alkaline phosphatase or other phosphatases. The nonphosphorylated form enters the mucosal cell based on the luminal concentration. When the concentration is low, the vitamers are absorbed by an active process depending on the requirements. When cell concentrations are high, the vitamers are absorbed via nonsaturable passive diffusion. In the cell, a process called metabolic trapping occurs, that is, the vitamers are phosphorylated by the action of ATP-dependent PN kinase. However, the phosphorylated form cannot cross the cell membrane and therefore in order to cross the basolateral membrane of the mucosal cell, it needs to be dephosphorylated again.

When the vitamers enter circulation, most of the vitamers are first taken to the liver which again phosphorylates them to either PN phosphate, PLP, or PMP, respectively after which these vitamers are released into the plasma. More than 70% of the vitamin is absorbed from a mixed meal. However, availability of B_6 which is present as glycosides is approximately 50%. High fiber intake decreases availability as it slows down the process of dephosphorylation. Most of the absorbed vitamin is taken up by the liver which puts it out into circulation in the form of PLP and PL. In fact, almost 60% of plasma B_6 is in the form of PLP, about 15% is PN and 4% is PL. All of these are bound to albumin. In circulation, PLP can enter the red blood cells where it is bound to hemoglobin, and PLP increases hemoglobin's affinity to oxygen.

Functions of vitamin B_6

Pyridoxine in the form of PLP participates in protein metabolism. It is important in maintaining brain functions and formation of RBCs. It helps in the synthesis of antibodies. The catalytic action is attributable to the carbonyl group in PLP reacting with the α-amine group of lysine and formation of a Schiff's base.

Protein metabolism: PLP is directly involved in transfer of amino group (NH_2), carboxyl group (COOH), and water (as H or OH). The process of transfer of amino group from an amino acid to another substance (new amino acid or keto acid) is called transamination whereas the process of removal of amino group from an amino acid is known as deamination. Thus, PLP is involved in the synthesis of many nonessential amino acids including taurine, glutamic acid, glycine, aspartic acid, methionine, and proline. Vitamin B_6 is important for protein synthesis and cell metabolism. In amino acid metabolism, the binding of PLP is important for further reactions to occur/proceed. B_6 is also involved in decarboxylation of L-amino acids leading to the formation of important biological molecules such as amines which function as neurotransmitters, hormones, or biogenic amines.

Carbohydrate metabolism: Several tissues contain enzymes (glycogen phosphorylases) that require PLP as a cofactor for the breakdown of glycogen into glucose. Thus, vitamin B_6 is needed for the conversion of glycogen present in liver and muscle into glucose. PLP is also a coenzyme required for gluconeogenesis, i.e., conversion of glucogenic amino acids to glucose.

Lipid metabolism: Vitamin B_6 is involved in fatty acid metabolism. It also participates in the synthesis of sphingosine from serine (as a coenzyme in serine palmitoyltransferase), for synthesis of phospholipids, with enzymes which extend the chain length of some fatty acids, such as production of eicosapentaenoic acid (EPA) and docosahexaenoic acid (DHA) from γ-linolenic acid. These essential fatty acids are required in cellular functions, hence vitamin B_6 is also required.

Growth: Since B_6 is necessary for protein metabolism and protein turn over, it is inevitably required for growth and development.

Role in blood cell synthesis: Vitamin B_6 participates in synthesis of white blood cells (WBCs) as well as in synthesis of heme that is a part of hemoglobin. It is involved in the formation of delta amino levulinic acid, a precursor of heme.

Formation of neurotransmitters: In the nervous system, its role in transaminases and L-amino acid decarboxylases is crucial because there are PLP-dependent steps in the synthesis of neurotransmitters. It functions as a coenzyme in nonoxidative decarboxylation of some amino acids or their derivatives, e.g., 3, 4 dihydroxyphenylalanine to dopamine + CO_2; glutamic acid to GABA + CO_2; and tyrosine to tyramine + CO_2. Removal COOH from amino acid is essential for the formation of certain neurotransmitters, e.g., serotonin from tryptophan or conversion of tryptophan to nitric acid, norepinephrine from tyrosine, and histamine from histidine. B_6 is necessary for production of several other neurotransmitters—dopamine, tryptamine, GABA from glutamic acid, epinephrine, and norepinephrine.

Role in hormones: PLP has been found to affect the activity of steroid receptors and decrease the effects of steroid hormones on gene expression. This may be relevant to steroid receptors for reproductive hormones such as for estrogen, progesterone, testosterone, as well as other steroid hormones.

Formation of niacin: Conversion of tryptophan to niacin requires B_6.

Other functions: This vitamin is also involved in selenium metabolism. It is a coenzyme for the enzymes involved in catabolism of thyroid hormone. It also facilitates the transport of amino acids and some cations across the cell membrane. Vitamin B_6 also plays an important role in one-carbon metabolism wherein one-carbon or methyl units are transferred from serine to tetrahydrofolate (THF) to form 5,10 methylene THF. This reaction is catalyzed by a PLP-dependent enzyme serine hydroxymethyltransferase. This compound ultimately serves as a methyl donor for synthesis of thymidylated purines, i.e., for nucleic acid synthesis or for biological methylations as well as methionine synthesis.

Methionine is converted to form S-adenosylmethionine (SAM) that is a universal methyl donor in a variety of reactions. In the brain, SAM is required for synthesis of several neurotransmitters, e.g., catecholamines and indoleamines, phospholipids.

Elevated levels of homocysteine are recognized as a cardiovascular risk factor. Homocysteine is generally methylated to methionine and one of the pathways is PLP dependent.

Recent research studies indicate that systemic inflammation that is associated with most chronic diseases/non-communicable diseases may impair vitamin B_6 metabolism. Vitamin B_6 may be involved in immune system impairment.

Recommended dietary allowance of pyridoxine
ICMR-NIN (2020) has recommended RDA and EAR for B6 on the basis of energy intakes. The requirement for all age groups is shown in Table 9.1B in Chapter 9 and Appendix 4.

Food sources of vitamin B_6
Vitamin B_6 is widely distributed in foods. The PN form occurs predominately in plant foods whereas PL and PLP are found in animal foods. PL and PLP is usually lost during cooking while PN is relatively heat stable. Among rich sources of vitamin B_6, banana, potato, sweet potato, avocado, organ meats, muscle, fish, milk, and eggs are worth mentioning. Citrus fruits are poor sources. Crude rice bran is also a good source. Cooking leads to loss of the vitamin. Since it is water soluble, it can leach out into the water used for cooking and would not be available, if this water is discarded.

Causes and consequences of deficiency of vitamin B_6
It can be due to:
- Inadequate intake of vitamin B_6 rich foods along with protein-rich foods
- Impaired activity of active form, i.e., PLP to be used as coenzyme
- Defective intestinal absorption
- Metabolic defect in its utilization
- Excessive loss of the vitamin through kidney
- Use of oral contraceptives can also cause the deficiency.

In alcoholics, metabolism of the vitamin is impaired which along with low intakes place them at risk of deficiency. The elderly also may be at risk of deficiency. Some drugs/medications that are prescribed such as isoniazid for treatment of tuberculosis are antagonistic; also treatment for Parkinson's disease, nonsteroidal anti-inflammatory drugs could lead to B_6 deficiency, if dietary intakes are inadequate. Severe deficiency is not encountered much, but moderate deficiency may occur. Generally, B_6 deficiency has been found to occur with deficiencies of other B-complex vitamins.

Deficiency of vitamin B_6 can cause many neurological symptoms like irritability, depression, confusion headaches, and convulsions. Normocytic, microcytic anemia, or sideroblastic anemia may also occur and there is decrease in circulating lymphocytes, platelet, and clotting dysfunction.

> **Microcytic hypochromic anemia:** It is caused primarily due to deficiency of vitamin B_6, but iron deficiency can also cause this. This type of anemia is characterized by smaller size of RBC and lack of sufficient hemoglobin to carry oxygen.

Other effects are inflammation of the tongue, sores in the mouth, and ulcers at the corner of the mouth. Due to its participation in energy release, it can result in physical weakness and pain in legs.

Homocystinuria and cystathioninuria may also be due to the deficiency of vitamin B_6 because of its involvement in metabolism of methionine.

Consequences of excessive intake of vitamin B_6
Adverse effects have been observed only with vitamin B_6 supplements and never from food sources. Sometimes people self-prescribe supplemental vitamin B_6. Prolonged used of massive dose of PN (2–6 g/day) can result in neurological symptoms, i.e., neuropathy (when doses exceed 1,000 mg/day) which can be reversed by withdrawal of the vitamin. However, some persons have developed neuropathy with smaller doses <500 mg/day. Severe toxicity has been observed in adults who ingested 500 mg/day. In certain cases, it can cause irreversible nerve damage. High dose has been taken to treat premenstrual syndrome (PMS) but its effect/benefit has not been proven scientifically. The Food and Nutrition Board of the Institute of Medicine, USA, has stated that the tolerable upper intake level for B_6 is 100 mg/day for adults.

Folic Acid

Folic acid was discovered in Bombay hospital by Lucy Wills in 1934. Wills and Mehta observed the effect of liver and yeast extracts on tropical macrocytic anemia and concluded that this disorder must be due to a dietary deficiency. She recognized that yeast contains a curative agent equal in potency to that of liver. The substance was found in spinach leaves and hence named "folic acid" after the Latin word "folium" meaning foliage.

Folic acid is also referred to as folate, folacin, or vitamin B_9 with the chemical structure of pteroylglutamic acid (PGA). Folate is a generic term that includes naturally occurring compounds—several biologically active vitamers and folic acid—the synthetic form. Folic acid contains glutamic acid, pteridine group, and para amino benzoic acid (PABA). Most naturally occurring folates contain a number of glutamic acid residues, from 1 to 7. These glutamic acid residues are linked together by peptide bonds. The active form of folate is tetrahydrofolic acid in the body and circulates as 5-methyl tetrahydrofolate (5 Met-THF) in the blood. Folic acid is the more stable synthetic form, but is rarely found in foods or the human body. It is the form generally used in vitamin supplements and fortified foods.

About 80% of the folates present in the diet are polyglutamates. These need to be first converted to the monoglutamate form, by the enzyme folate conjugase, in the jejunum. Folate conjugates are zinc—dependent pancreatic and intestinal mucopeptidases; hence, in zinc deficiency, folate absorption can be impaired. Free folate is absorbed mostly in the ileum and then enters portal blood and it carried to the liver. Not all dietary folate is absorbed and bioavailability from different foods varies. However, bioavailability of the synthetic form, i.e., folic acid is very high, its bioavailability is 85%. Availability of the vitamin from liver and egg yolk is fairly good (75% and 56%, respectively) whereas from orange juice, it is estimated to be comparatively lower (21%) and very low from vegetables (3–6%). Considerable amount of folate is present in the liver in the polyglutamate form.

Functions of folic acid

Folic acid mediates one-carbon transfer in numerous biosynthetic and catabolic reactions. It is closely involved in some reactions with vitamin B_{12}. Thus, it is involved in the synthesis of purines, pyrimidines, amino acids, carnitine, creatine, lipids, and hormones, and serves as a cofactor for some proteins. It is also critical for cell replication.

Formation of mature red blood cells: Folate plays a major role in formation of heme in the red blood cells (erythrocytes) multiplication, and maturation of red blood cells. Folic acid closely works with vitamin B_{12} in production RBC.

Synthesis of DNA/RNA: Folic acid mediates one carbon transfer reaction. This is important for formation of purines and pyrimidines. Folic acid is essential for the synthesis of purines (adenine and guanine) and pyrimidines (cytosine and thymine), which are nucleic acids and are the basic building blocks of RNA/DNA.

Growth and development: Folic acid is utilized in synthesis of nucleic acids which are important for cell division. Thus, it is extremely essential for growth, particularly growth of the embryo and fetus. Its supply is critical for neurological development of the fetus. In the first weeks, i.e., in the first trimester of pregnancy, inadequate supply of folic acid to the developing fetus increases the risk of neural tube defects, cleft palate, congenital heart disease, as well as malformations of other organs.

Methylation: Folate is important for conversion of homocysteine to methionine. SAM is a one-carbon donor, i.e., methyl group donor for most biological methylation reactions such as within DNA and RNA. These reactions include methylation of sites within DNA, RNA, proteins, and phospholipids. DNA methylation plays an important role in controlling gene expression and in cell differentiation. Folate functions in inter-conversion of glycine to serine and serine to glycine, and conversion of histidine to glutamate. It acts as a coenzyme for transferring single carbon unit during trans-methylation and trans-sulfuration pathways.

Amino acid metabolism: Metabolism of many important amino acids like methionine, cysteine, serine, glycine, and histidine requires folate coenzymes. Deficiency of folate can lead to decreased methionine synthesis and results in accumulation of homocysteine. High homocysteine levels an indicator not the pathogenesis of cardiovascular diseases.

Other functions: Folate is also essential for synthesis of catecholamines, carnitine, creatine, melatonin, and choline. It interacts with vitamin B_{12} and vitamin B_6. Folate interacts with vitamin B_{12} for synthesis of SAM. For synthesis of methionine from homocysteine, both B_{12} and folate are required. Homocysteine, an intermediate in the metabolism of sulfur-containing amino acids, is converted to cysteine for which vitamin B_6 is required. The homocysteine levels in blood are regulated by folate, vitamin B_{12}, and vitamin B_6.

Recommended dietary allowance of folate

RDA for folate is given in Table 9.1B in Chapter 9 and EAR in Appendix 4 for different age groups and in physiological states. Its requirement is increased during pregnancy as it plays significant role in cell division and maturation of RBC. ICMR-NIN (2020) has estimated EAR and RDA based on the dietary intake required to maintain normal plasma folate and homocystein level.

There may be genetic variations in folate requirements. This is due to a common polymorphism in the gene for the enzyme, 10-methylenetetrahydrofolate reductase known as the *MTHFR* c.677C>T polymorphism. MTHFR catalyzes the reduction of 5,10-methylenetetrahydrofolate (5,10-methylene THF) into 5-methyl tetrahydrofolate (5-MeTHF). Persons with genetic mutations may have lower folate concentrations in red blood cells and higher concentrations of homocysteine in blood and such persons are likely to have a higher folate requirement.

Dietary folate equivalents

The Food and Nutrition Board of the Institute of Medicine, USA, has introduced the dietary folate equivalent (DFE) as a new unit. This has been done in order to reflect the higher bioavailability of synthetic folic acid that is present in supplements and fortified food than that of naturally occurring food folates. According to this,

- 1 microgram (µg) of food folate provides 1 µg of DFEs
- 1 µg of folic acid taken with meals or as fortified food provides 1.7 µg of DFEs
- 1 µg of folic acid (supplement) taken on an empty stomach provides 2 µg of DFEs.

DFEs were determined in studies with adults. Hence, this may not be applicable to human milk and therefore it is not advisable to use DFEs for determining folate requirements for infants.

Food sources

Folate is found in plant and animal food sources. Among plant foods, green leafy vegetables, ladies finger, cowpea (lobia/chaouli), Bengal gram (chana), and among animal sources, liver is an excellent source of folic acid. Milk is not a good source of folate. Other foods that also contain folate are shown in Table 6.7. In some countries, many foods especially cereal products like bread and pasta are fortified with folate.

Causes and consequences of deficient intake of folate

Folic acid deficiency is commonly caused by inadequate intake of folate rich foods and frequent consumption of refined foods. Folate is rapidly lost during processing, cooking, and storage. There is about 33% cooking loss of the vitamin with the Indian style of cooking due to high sensitivity

Table 6.7: Food sources of total folic acid.

Food sources	Total folic acid µg/100 g	Food sources	Total folic acid µg/100 g	Food sources	Total folic acid µg/100 g
Maize tender	63.0	Colocasia green leaves	159.0	Fresh peas	55.0
Bajra	36.1	Mint Leaves	106.0	Capsicum	51.8
Jowar	39.4	Spinach	142.0	French bean	45.5
Wheat flour atta	29.2	Nigar seed black	140.0	Lady finger	63.7
Ragi	34.6	Sesame seeds white	131.0	Mango	82-90
Rajmah black	332.0	Groundnut	90.9	Khoa	94.3
Bengal gram whole	233.0	Sunflower seeds	81.8	Paneer	93.3

Source: IFCT, 2017.

of folic acid to heat. Low intake may also be because of inability to afford such foods. Other causes are poor intestinal absorption, increased demand of folic acid during pregnancy and lactation as well as in parasitic infestation, infection, and use of certain medications. These include methotrexate used for the treatment of cancer, as well as for rheumatoid arthritis, psoriasis, asthma, and inflammatory bowel disease. Other drugs are anticonvulsants, anti-inflammatory drugs, and biguanides (used for controlling blood sugar levels in diabetes). Chronic alcohol consumption also increases risk of folate deficiency especially if the dietary intake is inadequate. Alcoholics are at risk because absorption is low and so are dietary intakes.

Folate deficiency has serious implication on fetal development resulting in preterm delivery, low birth weight, fetal growth retardation, spontaneous abortions, and pre-eclampsia. Deficiency adversely affects the development of spinal cord and brain during fetal development and leads to congenital anomalies such as neural tube defects, cleft palate, and spina bifida in infants.

In the early stages, symptoms may not be obvious, although blood levels of homocysteine are increased. High level of homocysteine increases the risk of heart disease. Folate deficiency often underlines the deficiency of vitamin B_{12}. It has also been observed in persons with coronary heart disease, depression, neurotic disorders, and cancer. Personality changes, paranoid behavior, and apathy and lack of interest are common in women with folic acid deficiency.

Since folate is required for DNA synthesis, in folate deficiency, those cells that divide rapidly are affected. Those affected include the cells in bone marrow which eventually form red blood cells. Thus, immature precursors of RBC called megaloblasts (enlarged red blood cells with hypersegmented nuclei) are released into circulation. Hence, the anemia caused by folate deficiency is called megaloblastic or macrocytic anemia. Macrocytic anemia is characterized by big size of RBC but reduced capacity to carry oxygen. The oxygen carrying capacity is lowered resulting in shortness of breath, fatigue, and weakness. The level of white blood cells and platelets decreases due to impairment of cell division. Similarly, epithelial cells of the intestinal mucosa are continually regenerated and replaced every 3 days. In severe folate deficiency, gastrointestinal symptoms may occur due to impairment of gastrointestinal function.

Consequences of excessive intake of folate

Apparently there is no toxicity with excessive doses. However, larger amounts (>100 times of RDA) can interfere with the action of drugs like anticoagulants and may promote certain cancers. Also, consuming/ingesting too much folate especially if B_{12} intakes are inadequate may mask the vitamin B_{12} deficiency and there is risk of nerve damage. The elderly may be especially at risk. The main concern of excess intake is with synthetic folic acid, largely because of masking of vitamin B_{12} deficiencies which often go unnoticed and undiagnosed.

Vitamin B_{12}

In 1926, Castle observed an abnormal gastric secretion in persons with pernicious anemia which was considered to be fatal at that time. He postulated that there is an intrinsic factor (IF) in normal gastric secretion and extrinsic factor in animal food like liver; both together could have encouraging effect in the treatment of this disease. Whipple, Minot, and Murphy showed that feeding large amounts of liver stimulated production of red blood cells in persons with pernicious anemia. They were awarded the Nobel Prize in 1934. Later the discovery of the microorganism *Lactobacillus lactis* as an anti-pernicious factor further led to the discovery of vitamin B_{12} which is now known as cobalamin as it contains cobalt in its structure.

The term "vitamin B_{12}" is a generic descriptor for cobalamins which are cobalt-containing compounds and have the biological activity of the vitamin. There are various forms of cobalamin with vitamin B_{12} activity, e.g., cyanocobalamin, hydroxocobalamin, or methylcobalamin. Cyanocobalamin is a vitamer and can be metabolized in the body; however, this form does not occur in nature. Methylcobalamin, another vitamer, is required in the synthesis of methionine. Among all vitamins, B_{12} has the largest and most complex structure. Hydroxocobalamin is man made form and used in clinical practice only.

Vitamin B_{12} in food is generally bound to protein from which it has to be released before it is absorbed. In the acidic pH of the stomach, the action of pepsin releases B_{12} from the proteins. (Hence, use of antacids can hamper B_{12} absorption.) Similarly, decreased gastric acid secretion such as in the elderly is a problem. After B_{12} is released from the food proteins, it binds to a protein cobalophilin. In the intestines, cobalophilin is hydrolyzed by pancreatic enzymes, B_{12} is freed and then binds to IF. Without binding to IF, free B_{12} is not absorbed. In the absence of IF, only 1% is absorbed. In the intestines, the alkaline pH favors absorption of the vitamin. B_{12} is taken up by the enterocyte, primarily in the ileum. B_{12} undergoes enterohepatic circulation, providing a means of conserving the vitamin in the body. In a well-nourished person, approximately 2–5 mg of B_{12} is stored in the liver. However, in older population, maintenance of vitamin B_{12} depends upon normal functioning of the gastrointestinal tract, secretion of gastric acid, and amount of IF.

Functions of Vitamin B_{12}

Vitamin B_{12} is essential for formation of red blood cells and nerve cells. It is essential for the regeneration of THF in folate metabolism and formation of DNA. Methylcobalamin is required for the function of the enzyme methionine synthase that is required for the synthesis of the amino acid, methionine, from homocysteine. B_{12} plays a critical role in metabolism of amino acids, fatty acids, phospholipids, hormones, and other compounds. Vitamin B_{12} plays an important role in DNA synthesis and neurological function. It is important for conversion of homocysteine to SAM, the methyl donor which is important for DNA methylation. In B_{12} deficiency, DNA is impaired. SAM is important for methylation reactions that are essential for synthesis of proteins, lipids, and neurotransmitters in the CNS. If there is abnormal methylation of DNA and protein, it results in altered chromatin structure as well as gene expression.

Growth and maintenance: Vitamin B_{12} along with folate is required for synthesis of DNA and cell division. Thus, it plays a role in growth and maintenance of nervous tissues and normal blood formation.

Role in red blood cell formation: Vitamin B_{12} is required for the synthesis of all cells but its role is more pronounced in RBC or erythrocytes as it provides methyl group to the erythroblasts in the bone marrow. If there is B_{12} deficiency, erythropoiesis is ineffective.

Role in nervous system: Vitamin B_{12} plays a significant role in formation of myelin that surrounds nerve fibers. Deficiency of the vitamin affects neural function in general and neurological development in infancy. B_{12} may also be important for cognitive function.

Protects heart: In B_{12} deficiency, homocysteine levels are elevated because it cannot be converted into SAM and high levels of homocysteine in blood are associated with the risk of heart disease.

Recommended dietary allowance of vitamin B_{12}

The ICMR-NIN (2020) recommendations for vitamin B_{12} for adult men and women are 2.5 µg/day (RDA; EAR 2 micrograms/day). which is increased during pregnancy and during lactation. Infants and preschool children 5 months to 5 years need 1.2 mg/day (RDA; EAR 1.0 micrograms/day) and children and adolescents from 5 year to 17 years of age require need 2.5 mg/day (RDA; EAR 2.0 micrograms/day).

Food sources

It is found mainly in animal foods such as liver, meat, sea food, egg, milk, and cheese. Those who avoid non-vegetarian foods including milk are likely to have low intakes of B_{12}. Adequate consumption of milk and milk products protects vegetarians from its deficiency. A high concentration of AA can degrade B_{12} in foods.

Causes and consequences of deficiency of vitamin B_{12}

Poor intake of foods containing vitamin B_{12} is one of the major reasons, particularly among vegetarians. Achlorhydria (low secretion of gastric acid), lack of IF, and dysfunction of the cubam receptor (special receptors at ileum site for absorption of vitamin B_{12}) predispose vitamin B_{12} deficiency. Lack of IF is usually due to atrophic gastritis which reduces the number of IF secreting parietal cells. Endocrine disorder (hypothyroidism), celiac disease, sprue, infection with *Helicobacter pylori*, and inadequate absorption are other causes. The deficiency may occur in late adulthood. Atrophic gastritis is estimated to affect anywhere from 10% to 30% of people who are above 60 years of age. In persons whose gastric function is compromised/diminished gastric function and in individuals with atrophic gastritis, there can be bacterial overgrowth in the small intestine which can result in food-bound vitamin B_{12} malabsorption. In people who have *H. pylori* infection, serum/plasma vitamin B_{12} levels are low, besides their having significantly less amount of gastric fluids. Generally, treatment that eradicates the *H. pylori* leads to significant improvement in vitamin B_{12} status as assessed by their serum levels. Food cobalamin malabsorption is mainly caused by gastric atrophy which is very common in elder patients. Any surgery to gastrointestinal tract may also reduce the ability to produce IF.

Causes of dietary deficiency of vitamin B_{12}	
Dietary deficiency	Vegans (strict vegetarians), low intake of animal foods
Malabsorption	Pernicious anemia, gastrectomy/gastric bypass
	Protein bound B_{12} absorption
	Ileal disease/resection—Crohn's disease
	Pancreatic insufficiency
	Drug-induced malabsorption
	Congenital absence or dysfunction of IF
	Chronic alcoholism
Biological completion	Bacterial overgrowth syndrome
	Fish, tape worm infestation
Impaired utilization	Congenial deficiency

Although rare, there are cases of inborn errors of B_{12} metabolism. One example is the Imerslund-Gräsbeck syndrome. It is an inherited syndrome characterized by B_{12} malabsorption that results in megaloblastic anemia, neurologic disorders, and the severity of which vary among the persons with this inherited problem. Also, there are mutations that affect B_{12} transport.

Deficiency of vitamin B_{12} leads to megaloblastic anemia which reflects morphological and functional changes in RBC, WBC, platelets, and their precursors in blood and bone marrow due to the disturbances in the synthesis of DNA. It usually occurs in case of dual deficiency of vitamin B_{12} and folic acid. The effect of folic acid is observed much before the symptoms of B_{12} deficiency. Pernicious anemia is the major disease caused by inadequate amount of vitamin B_{12} for the formation of RBC in bone marrow. Food and Nutrition Board of the Institute of Medicine, USA, recommends that for adults who consume foods fortified with folic acid, their intake of folic acid should not exceed 1 mg per day.

Vitamin B_{12} deficiency also leads to neurological abnormalities. It includes myelopathy, neuropathy, dementia, neuropsychiatric abnormalities, and sometimes optic nerve atrophy. While the hematologic abnormality can be cured with folic acid therapy, the neurological problems worsen, particularly when large doses of folic acid are given. Neurological abnormalities include demyelination of CNS, swelling of myelin sheath, degeneration of spinal cord, and lesions in the brain and optic nerves. The most common symptom is painful paresthesia of extremities. Patients also have sense of vibration in toes and ankles. There is numbness and tingling of the hands, numbness and feet. The person has difficulty in walking, experiences loss of memory, and may be disoriented. Person may also have dementia and sometimes there can be mood changes. If the neurological changes are of long standing duration, B_{12} supplements may not fully reverse these problems. Neurological problems may not be accompanied by megaloblastic anemia and about one-fourth of patients with B_{12} deficiency may exhibit only neurological symptoms. Methylcobalamin is used in the treatment of peripheral neuropathy and diabetic neuropathy. It is also common in patients with OCD (obsessive compulsive disorder).

Megaloblastic anemia which is a consequence of B_{12} deficiency cannot be distinguished easily from the anemia associated with folate deficiency. During vitamin B_{12} deficiency, carbohydrate metabolism is affected depriving the nervous tissues of energy as a result they are damaged leading to peripheral neuropathy. Symptoms can be soreness and inflammation of tongue, numbness, and tingling in fingers and toes. There is increase in the level of pyruvic acid and lactic acid.

Patients may also have gastrointestinal problems such as soreness of the tongue, loss of appetite, and constipation. Although the origin of these symptoms is not clear, it has been linked to inflammation of the stomach and progressive destruction of the stomach lining. However, approximately three-fourths of patients who have pernicious anemia develop neurological abnormalities. In some cases, hematologic parameters are normal but may have spinal cord symptoms without anemia. Other symptoms include glossitis, weight loss, mental changes, and infertility.

Drug and B_{12} interactions

Several therapeutic drugs decrease absorption of the vitamin. Table 6.8 lists the drugs and the disease and mechanisms through which this occurs. Diabetics may not even know that they are at risk of B12 deficiency if they are taking Metformin, the most commonly used drug.

Consequences of excessive intake of vitamin B_{12}

There are no reports in the literature to indicate that high intakes are harmful, even when patients with pernicious anemia have been treated with very high doses either orally 2 mg (2,000 μg) daily or 1 mg monthly by intramuscular injection. Also, no adverse effects have been seen in intervention trials on diabetics or patients with acute myocardial infarction on intakes of 400 μg to 1mg for prolonged periods. Clinically high serum level of vitamin B_{12} is called hypercobalaminemia that may be indicative of liver or bone disorders.

Table 6.8: Drugs and B_{12} interactions.

Drug	Condition	Mechanism through which absorption is reduced
Proton-pump inhibitors like omeprazole and lansoprazole	Zollinger-Ellison syndrome, gastroesophageal reflux disease	Decrease acid secretion in stomach Note: However, B_{12} absorption from supplements is not adversely affected
Gastric acid inhibitors, i.e., histamine$_2$ (H_2)-receptor antagonists (e.g., cimetidine, famotidine, and ranitidine)	Peptic ulcer	Decrease absorption due to inhibition of gastric acid secretion
Cholestyramine	Treatment for hypercholesterolemia	Inhibit B_{12} absorption
Antibiotics like chloramphenicol and neomycin	For infections	Inhibit B_{12} absorption
Colchicine	For gout	Inhibit B_{12} absorption
Metformin	Type 2 diabetes mellitus	Inhibit B_{12} absorption
Nitrous oxide	Anesthetic	Oxidizes and inactivates the vitamin

> **Megaloblastic anemia:** In case of cellular deficiency of folate or B_{12} or both, DNA synthesis is impaired and cell division is restricted but RNA continues to synthesize the protein which increases the size of cells and this is called megaloblast. When new DNA is not formed in the bone marrow, RBC continues to form but is large and bizarre in shape, fragile, and has short life. This is characteristic of megaloblastic anemia. Megaloblast soon matures into macrocytes (abnormally large cells). Megaloblasts and macrocytes replace normal RBC and thus RBC cannot perform their normal function particularly oxygen carrying capacity and they die before their normal lifespan (120 days). It results in weakness and fatigue. Folate deficiency anemia is characterized by depression, irritability, forgetfulness, and disturbed sleep as it adversely affects the neurological behavior and myelin damage.
>
> **Macrocytic anemia:** Mean corpuscular volume (MCV) indicates the volume of RBC, and high value indicate deficiency of folic acid and MCV is more, it is referred as macrocytic anemia.
>
> **Pernicious anemia:** This is mainly due to an autoimmune disease which destroys the parietal cells in the stomach which secrete IF and hydrochloric acid. In the absence of IF, absorption of vitamin B_{12} is also impaired. It is characterized by nerve damage and reduced oxygen supply to cells resulting in shortness of breath.

> **Homocysteine:** Homocysteine is a non-protein amino acid and it is biosynthesized from methionine by the removal of its terminal Cε methyl group. It can be recycled into methionine or converted into

Contd...

Contd...

> cysteine in the presence of some B-vitamins. The recycling process uses N5 methyl tetrahydrofolate as the methyl donor and cobalamin (vitamin B_{12}). It is not obtained from dietary sources. Deficiencies of folic acid, pyridoxine, or vitamin B_{12} can lead to high homocysteine level. Supplementation with these or betaine (trimethylglycine) reduces the concentration of homocysteine level in the blood. Some evidence suggests that long duration exercise raises plasma homocysteine. Homocysteine normally does not affect the bone density but interferes with cross linking between collagen fiber and the tissues.
>
> **Causes of elevated homocysteine level:**
> - Deficiency of folate, pyridoxine, or vitamin B_{12}
> - Chronic alcohol consumption
> - Prolonged exercise
> - Oxidative stress.
>
> **Consequences of elevated homocysteine level:**
> - Risk of thrombosis and cardiovascular disease
> - Risk of preeclampsia and premature delivery
> - Risk of osteoporosis.

Biotin

Biotin was referred as vitamin H or vitamin B_7 and was discovered in 1927. Biotin is known by its name rather than its number. The word biotin might have come from a Greek word *bios* meaning life. Biotin is essential for many enzymes which participate in the Krebs' cycle, production of fatty acids, and metabolism of fat and amino acids. It is widely distributed in foods and can also be synthesized by microorganisms. It inhabits the intestinal tract of humans and animals. Biotin is one among vitamin B complex.

Biotin is present in foods mostly in the form of biocytin where it is complexed with protein. The biotin-containing proteins in food are first acted upon by proteases (proteolytic enzymes) and converted to biocytin/lysyl biotin or lysyl biotin-containing peptides. These are hydrolyzed further by the enzyme biotinidase which is present in pancreatic juice. The products of digestion then cross into intestinal enterocytes. Small amounts of biotin-containing peptides may be absorbed without hydrolysis. The rate of absorption is faster in the jejunum than the ileum and is almost completely absorbed.

Functions of biotin

Biotin acts as a coenzyme in carboxylation reactions for certain enzymes involved in Krebs' cycle, fatty acid synthesis, and amino acid metabolism. It functions as a covalently bound cofactor, serving as a prosthetic group for five carboxylases which have important roles in:

> Biotinylation is a term that refers to covalent addition of biotin to molecules including the apo carboxylases for which it serves as a prosthetic group as well as histones. Biotinylation converts the inactive apo carboxylase into an active holocarboxylase. Biotin can be released from the biotinylated histones and the holocarboxylases by the enzyme biotinidase.

Lipid metabolism: It is involved in the elongation of fatty acids in tissues such as adipose tissue, placenta, kidney, and pancreas. It also participates during catabolism of fatty acids with odd number of carbon atoms.

Carbohydrate metabolism: It helps in formation of oxaloacetate, the precursor of glucose production through gluconeogenesis. Oxaloacetate also participates in the TCA cycle which is important for ATP production.

Amino acid metabolism: Catabolism of valine, leucine, isoleucine, methionine, and threonine.

Gene expression: Biotin appears to affect gene expression. Recent studies show that there are more than 2,000 biotin-dependent genes in human lymphoid and liver cells. This vitamin may also play a role in control of gene expression and genomic stability, gene silencing, cell proliferation, and cellular response to DNA damage.

Food sources of biotin

Biotin is available in a wide variety of foods like cereals, legumes especially sprouts, nuts, egg yolk, soybean, and liver. Most vegetables and fruits are poor sources except cauliflower and mushrooms. Milk and meat are also not good sources.

Causes and consequences of deficient intake of biotin

People consuming raw egg in large amount are more susceptible to the deficiency because avidin, present in raw egg, binds biotin tightly, however it gets denatured when egg is cooked; hence biotin is available in cooked egg. Absorption of biotin is also impaired in conditions like inflammatory bowel disease, achlorhydria, and excessive alcohol ingestion. People on sulfur drugs may also be at risk of biotin deficiency. The deficiency symptoms are conjunctivitis, skin infections, scaly red rash near eyes, nose, and mouth, dermatitis, ataxia, seizures, and developmental delays in children. Immune response is also impaired.

Biotin deficiency may be aggravated by pantothenic acid deficiency. Deficiency of biotin causes abnormalities in fatty acid composition, as a result of impaired lipogenesis. Impairment of gluconeogenesis occurs and there may be fasting hyperglycemia. In some cases, hypoglycemia may occur. Requirements may be increased for persons who are on anticonvulsant therapy. Persons who have been maintained on total parenteral nutrition without biotin supplementation have been found to suffer from biotin deficiency.

Consequence of excessive intake of biotin

Toxicity of biotin has not been reported even with consumption of 60 mg/day.

VITAMIN-LIKE COMPOUNDS

There are some compounds which are considered to be essential nutrients because they play many physiological roles in the body and at the same time they can be synthesized in the body. Many of them are also available in commonly consumed foods. Recommended intake for vitamin-like compounds has not been established and their content in food is also not usually reported in food composition tables. Since they have structural or metabolic role(s) in the body, they are often added in infant formula or given as supplement. These vitamin-like essential nutrients are choline, inositol, carnitine, and lipoic acid.

Choline

Previously, choline was not considered an essential nutrient since the body synthesizes some amount, although it was discovered by Adolph Strecker in 1864 and chemically synthesized in 1866. Almost 130 years later, in 1998, the Food and Nutrition Board of Institute of Medicine (USA) has classified choline as an essential nutrient. Choline is a quaternary amine (trimethyl-beta-hydroxyethyl ammonium) that is present in free or esterified forms in all mammalian tissues. The esterified forms are phosphocholine, phospatidylcholine, sphingomyelin, and glycerophosphorylcholine. The three methyl groups that are present play an important role in metabolic reactions, making choline an important methyl group donor in numerous physiological processes.

Choline is said to be "lipotropic" meaning the ability to breakdown the fat in the body. It is water soluble and is synthesized by the liver (liver is probably the major site where it is in the form of phosphatidylcholine), to some extent by the brain and the mammary glands. The quantity synthesized in the liver is enough to meet the requirement of the body. Its physiological role is associated as a methyl donor; the methyl group is essential for methylation in many metabolic pathways. For persons who are nourished intravenously with solutions that have low amounts of choline, some metabolic abnormalities were observed which were treated successfully with choline. Choline is used for the synthesis of several biologically important molecules such as the neurotransmitter acetylcholine.

Choline is available in both water-soluble and fat-soluble forms. Water-soluble compounds are phosphocholine, glycerophosphocholine, and free choline. Fat-soluble forms which the body synthesizes are phosphatidylcholine and sphingomyelin which are vital components of cell membranes. Both forms are found in foods.

In food, choline is present in the free form or is bound with phospholipids. These phospholipids are acted upon by the pancreatic enzyme phospholipase A2. The product is phosphatidylcholine which is incorporated into micelles and then taken up into the enterocytes of the small intestines. A considerable amount of the choline that is absorbed is incorporated into phospholipids in the chylomicrons and secreted into lymph. Free choline is also absorbed in the small intestines. This unesterified/free choline enters portal circulation and is rapidly removed by the liver.

Pancreatic and mucosal enzymes convert some choline compounds into free choline. Water-soluble compounds are absorbed in the small intestine and directly enter the portal circulation and are stored in the liver where they are subsequently phosphorylated and distributed throughout the body to make cell membrane. The remaining fat-soluble compounds are absorbed and incorporated into chylomicrons, and secreted into the lymphatic circulation where they are distributed to tissues and organs including brain and placenta.

Functions of Choline

Choline is the precursor of many biologically important molecules such as acetylcholine, lecithin, and sphingomyelin. Phosphatidylcholine comprises approximately 95% the choline in tissues.

Important source of methyl groups: Choline is one of the major sources of methyl group. It supplies the methyl group for the conversion of homocysteine to methionine. Thus, its metabolism is linked with that of other nutrients, viz., folate, vitamin B_{12}, methionine, and homocysteine as well as being involved in one-carbon metabolism. It is also important for fat metabolism. Choline can be oxidized both in the liver (in mitochondria) and the kidneys and converted to betaine. This molecule is the source of about 60% of the methyl groups that are required for methylation of homocysteine. Thus, betaine is involved in one-carbon metabolism.

Structural integrity of cells/cell membranes: Some of the water-soluble and fat-soluble compounds, i.e., phospholipids particularly phosphatidylcholine (also known as lecithin) and sphingomyelin, are integral part of the cell membrane and support its functioning. It is also a part of sphingomyelin that is present in the fatty sheath that surrounds the myelinated nerve fiber and therefore is important for nerve conductivity.

Cell signaling: Phosphatidylcholine and sphingomyelin, both of which contain choline, are precursors of diacylglycerol and ceramide which function as intracellular messenger molecules. Phosphatidylcholine and sphingomyelin are degraded to phosphocholine and ceramide, respectively, by the phospholipases (sphingomyelin phosphodiesterases). There are other choline-derived metabolites that are involved in cell signaling such as platelet activating factor and sphingophosphocholine.

Brain development: Phosphatidylcholine and sphingomyelin both aid in brain development. Breakdown products of these phospholipids are involved in cell signaling process.

Formation of acetylcholine: Choline is used for the synthesis of acetylcholine, an important neurotransmitter. Acetylcholine is synthesized by cholinergic neurons and plays an important role in memory and mood, muscle control, circadian rhythm, modulates the brain development and other functions of the nervous system. Acetylcholine is formed by the acetylation of choline and the reaction is catalyzed by the enzyme choline acetyl transferase. It is also involved in regulating the heart rate, breathing, sweating, salivation, and contraction of skeletal muscles. Non-neuronal cells of different tissues and organs also synthesize acetyl choline which when released by the cells binds and stimulates the cholinergic receptors present on the target cells.

Component of complex lipids: It is a part of many lipids—lipoproteins, lipids involved in intracellular signaling, and platelet-activating factor. Thus, choline plays an important role in the transport and metabolism of lipids.

Phosphatidylcholine is necessary for assembly of very low density lipoproteins (VLDL) and its secretion from hepatic tissues. If there is insufficient amount of phosphatidyl choline, then fat and cholesterol accumulate in the liver. Phosphatidylcholine increases the activity of some enzymes.

Functions as an osmolyte: Betaine, a metabolite of choline, plays an important role in the epithelial cells in the kidney medulla for reabsorption of water and concentration of urine. Thus, as an osmolyte, betaine regulates the cell volume and contributes to maintenance of cell integrity by protecting against osmotic stress. Choline is irreversibly metabolized to betaine.

Prevents fatty liver: Choline is a component of lecithin. Thus, it helps in the transport of fat (triglycerides) from the liver; prevents accumulation of fat and cholesterol in liver and helps in removal of fat from adipose tissues. The relation between choline deficiency and accumulation of lipids in the liver has been recognized more than 5 decades ago. However, not much is known about the role of choline in prevention and treatment of non-alcoholic fatty liver disease in which there is accumulation of fat in hepatic tissues.

Other possible roles: Increasing research evidence suggests that choline is involved in several other functions such as gene expression, prevention of cancer, cell cycle regulation and apoptosis (programmed cell death), synthesis of lung surfactant, as well as brain development in early life. The gut microbiome has also been found to play a role in choline metabolism. The gut microflora may metabolize choline and thus alter its bioavailability and possibly alter the risk of choline deficiency. At least eight different organisms have been identified as being avid choline metabolizers. Conversely, it is likely that dietary choline can also influence the gut microflora. It is also likely that genetic factors may influence the type of microflora in an individual's gut.

Food Sources of Choline

In normal diets, choline is consumed in the form of choline phosphates such as lecithin and sphingomyelin. The richest food sources of lecithin are egg yolk, liver, and other organ meats, soybean, wheat germ, and peanuts. Human milk is a good source of choline. Choline is found in grains, legumes, spices like coriander seeds, and herbs of daily use. Cauliflower and cabbages are good sources but in general fruits and vegetables are poor sources of choline.

> **Laboratory Laurel:** Choline and its derivative betaine play a very important role in the donation of methyl groups to homocysteine to form methionine. Choline is present in the body and food in various forms like choline, glycerophosphocholine, phosphocholine, phosphatidylcholine, and sphingomyelin in varying concentrations. It plays a role in normal membrane function and acetylcholine synthesis. The researchers have assayed the choline content in about 145 common foods using liquid chromatography-mass spectrometry and measured in mg/100 g. It was found to be highest in beef liver (418 mg), eggs (251 mg), wheat germ (152 mg), bacon (125 mg),
>
> *Contd...*
>
> *Contd...*
>
> dried soybeans (116 mg), and pork (103 mg). The foods with the highest betaine concentration (mg/100 g) were: wheat bran (1,339 mg), wheat germ (1,241 mg), spinach (645 mg), shrimp (218 mg), and wheat bread (201 mg). Both folate and choline are methyl donors and their roles may be interchangeable in reducing homocysteine level. Thus, choline may be helpful in cancer and heart disease.
>
> *Zeisel SH, Mar MH, Howe JC, et al. Concentrations of choline-containing compounds and betaine in common foods. J Nutr. 2013;133(5):1302-7.*

Causes and Consequences of Deficient Intake of Choline

Poor dietary intake of choline may cause fatty liver. Choline supplement was found to be effective in reducing accumulation of fat in liver. Choline deficiency may decrease the amount of acetylcholine and result in impaired brain functions and impaired memory. Since choline and folate metabolism are linked, choline deficiency may be involved in risk of neural tube defects. In infants, it may impair cognitive development and retard growth. Deficiency of choline has been observed in case of kwashiorkor as well as among alcoholics. Deficiency of niacin, folate, or methionine can also cause choline deficiency because these three are involved in its synthesis.

Consequences of Excessive Intake of Choline

Dietary sources of choline have not been found to cause toxicity in healthy individuals. However, patients with neurological disorder on pharmacological doses >3.5 g/day show some symptoms like nausea or diarrhea, salivation, and fishy body odor. Toxicity can cause liver damage.

Inositol

Inositol or myo-inositol (or hexahydroxy cyclohexane, or cis-1,2,3,5-trans-4,6-cyclohexanehexol) is a six-carbon polyol. It is found in plasma and cell membrane. Inositol is a term that refers to nine possible stereoisomers, the most common among them being myo-inositol. Inositol is considered to be a pseudovitamin, i.e., it is neither an essential vitamin nor a mineral but it has physiological importance. It is a precursor for phosphoinositides. These compounds are involved in cell signal transduction and other second messengers like diacyl glycerol that regulates some of the protein kinase C family. Inositol is involved in glucose metabolism. Inositol polyphosphates and pyrophosphates are ubiquitous eukaryotic messengers that are involved in numerous cellular processes, including insulin signaling and cell migration. Inositol is a precursor of inositol phosphoglycans (IPG) that consist of two groups: the P-type, P-inositol phosphoglycans (P-IPG), and the A-type, A-inositol phosphoglycans (A-IPG). P-IPG and A-IPG are antagonistic to each other. P-IPG that activates pyruvate dehydrogenase phosphatases activate the pyruvate dehydrogenase complex which is an important/key process in glycolysis. In contrast, A-IPG is known to inhibit these phosphatase enzymes. When there is insulin resistance, urinary inositol metabolites, mainly P-IPG class/group metabolites are increased. Consequently, the ratio shifts in favor of A-IPGs and there is suppression of activity of pyruvate dehydrogenase. It has been observed that inositol supplementation corrects/normalizes the ratio of P-IPG to A-IPG. Inositol-1,4,5-triphosphate modifies intracellular calcium levels, and phosphatidylinositol-3,4,5-biphosphate is involved in signal transduction.

Phosphatidylinositol is a phospholipid that is found in the cell membranes of kidney, eyes, heart, brain, and other organs and body fluids in varying concentrations. Inositol is present in blood mostly in the free form and a small amount is present in lipoproteins in the form of phosphatidyl inositol. Inositol is present as free inositol and is also bound to lipids. In animal tissues, it occurs as myo-inositol in free form.

The inositol bound to phospholipids (phosphatidyl inositol is the main dietary source) needs to be hydrolyzed first by pancreatic phospholipase A2 after which it is absorbed. Efficiency of absorption of both the free and bound forms is very good and occurs in the small intestines. However, in plant foods, inositol is also combined with polyphosphates particularly inositol hexaphosphate, i.e., phytate. The human gastrointestinal tract does not contain the enzyme phytase which is required to release inositol from inositol polyphosphates. However, many foods contain the phytase enzyme, which can hydrolyze the phytate in plant foods. Processing techniques typically used in Indian cooking like soaking, germination, and fermentation as well as malting help to increase phytase activity and release the inositol.

As such inositol needs not be supplied by the diet since adequate amounts are synthesized by the body. However, infants may need more inositol than the amount that can be synthesized by their bodies. Blood concentrations are influenced by dietary intakes. Inositol is metabolized in the kidney, being broken down to D-glucuronic acid and D-xylulose-5-phosphate. Therefore, when kidney function is compromised, blood inositol concentrations increase.

Functions of Inositol

Inositol acts as the second messenger and is concentrated in brain. It is important for relaying messages by nerves to cells. In the body, inositol is synthesized from glucose. It has been found to improve liver functions. Its importance has been much studied in case of diabetes, multiple sclerosis, and kidney failure.

Since inositol is a part of phospholipids, it is a precursor for compounds that are required for cell membrane synthesis. Thus, it has a structural role in cell membranes. It is important for intracellular signaling and intracellular responses to peptide hormones and neurotransmitters.

Phosphatidylinositol is a source of arachidonic acid and other long-chain PUFA. These fatty acids are metabolized into prostaglandins, thromboxanes, and leukotrienes. Inositol is one of the compounds that protect cells from damage caused by high osmotic pressure. Inositol may also play a role in nerve conduction velocity, mental health, and prevention of lung cancer, although further research is required to confirm these roles of inositol.

Inositol is considered to be an insulin sensitizing agent. It is also being used as a therapeutic agent for polycystic ovarian syndrome.

> **Laboratory Laurel:** Myo-inositol is used in correcting insulin resistance (IR) that has been found to play role in onset of polycystic ovarian syndrome (PCOS). In this study, 50 anovulatory (no periods and no pregnancy) PCOS patients with insulin resistance were selected who were given myo-inositol for three spontaneous cycles. Anovulatory patients were further given combination of myo-inositol and clomiphene citrate in the next three cycles. They were assessed for ovulation and pregnancy rate, changes in body mass index (BMI) and homeostatic model assessment (HOMA) index, and any adverse event. Out of 50, 29 women (61.7%) showed ovulation after myo-inositol treatment and 18 (38.3%) remained IR. Of the ovulatory women, 11 became pregnant (37.9%). In the next three cycles with combination treatment, 13 (72.2%) ovulated and among them 6 (42.6%) became pregnant. During follow-up, a reduction of body mass index and HOMA index was also observed. It can be concluded that myo-inositol treatment can treat insulin resistance and lower body weight, and improves ovarian activity in PCOS patients.
>
> *Kamenov Z, Kolarov G, Gateva A, et al. Ovulation induction with myo-inositol alone and in combination with clomiphene citrate in polycystic ovarian syndrome patients with insulin resistance. Gynecol Endocrinol. 2015;31(2):131-5.*

Food Sources of Inositol

Meat, poultry, fish, milk, and milk products are good sources. Grains, nuts, and seeds are good sources especially cashew nut, poppy seeds, groundnuts, and sunflower seeds. Vegetables, fruits, and tubers also contribute some amount to the total intake. Tea is also a good source of inositol. Myo-inositol can also be synthesized from glucose. The immediate precursor is fructose 6-phosphate, which is converted to myo-inositol.

Causes and Consequences of Deficient or Excessive Intake of Inositol

To date, there are no reports of clinical symptoms due to deficiency of inositol. However, excessive intakes of inositol in the form of supplements may increase risk of diabetic neuropathy. Also inositol polyphosphates, i.e., phytate can inhibit absorption of iron and zinc. It has been reported that 12 g of myo-inositol intake daily was accompanied by mild gastrointestinal side effects including nausea, flatus and diarrhea, although the severity of these problems did not increase when the dose was increased above 12 g/day.

Para Amino Benzoic Acid (PABA)

Para amino benzoic acid is a cyclic amino acid that belongs to the B vitamin group. PABA is an intermediate compound in folate synthesis. It is present in both plant and animal tissues and is sometimes also called bacterial vitamin H_1 or B_x or B_{10}. Pteridine and PABA are components of folic acid. Thus, PABA is not considered as an independent vitamin.

It is found in many foods like grains, mushroom, eggs, milk, and meat. This vitamin-like compound has found its role in cosmetic industry to treat many skin diseases like vitiligo, dermatitis, and hair problems like gray hair and hair loss. It acts as a sunscreen. It is also used in pharmaceutical preparations used for supporting gut health.

PABA has been found to have several therapeutic benefits that include antioxidant potential, antibacterial, antimutagenic, and anticoagulant properties. It is also a fibrinolytic and immunomodulating agent. It has been found to confer protection against UV irradiation. It has been found to induce endogenous interferon. It has been found to have synergistic antiviral effect.

Carnitine

L-carnitine was discovered in 1905 but its functions were discovered in 1955. L-carnitine is obtained from two amino acids, lysine and methionine. It is synthesized in the body from ε-trimethyllysine, an amino acid derived from post-translational modification of lysine. It is a quaternary amine and its structure is somewhat similar to choline. Most of this ε-trimethyllysine is present in muscle proteins. The body can synthesize L-carnitine and the synthesis occurs largely in the liver and to some extent in the kidneys and brain (from the amino acids lysine and methionine) and is then transported to other body tissues especially those tissues like skeletal and cardiac muscle that use fatty acids as the source of energy. Only the L-isomer of carnitine is biologically active whereas the D-isomer is not. L-carnitine contains a hydroxyl group that is utilized for the synthesis of esters of organic and fatty acids. However, it is estimated that only about one-fourth of the body's needs are met by endogenous synthesis. When requirements exceed the body's capacity for synthesis, it must be supplied by the diet and it becomes a conditionally essential micronutrient. It is stored mostly (95%) in heart and skeletal muscle (muscles contain about 70 times more carnitine than the amount present in plasma) and very small amounts are stored in liver and kidney. Availability of dietary carnitine is much better than from supplements.

L-carnitine plays an important role in beta-oxidation of fatty acids in the mitochondria. It facilitates the transport of long-chain fatty acids. It is a cofactor that is required to transform long-chain fatty acids into acyl carnitines by esterification. This step is very essential because otherwise these fatty acids are unable to cross the mitochondrial membrane (from cytosol into mitochondrial matrix where beta-oxidation takes place). On the outer mitochondrial membrane is present an enzyme carnitine-palmitoyltransferase I which catalyzes the transfer of long-chain fatty acids in the cytoplasm from acetyl coenzyme A to L-carnitine. The acylcarnitine esters are then transported across the inner mitochondrial membrane with the help of a transport protein carnitine: acylcarnitinetranslocase.

The next step is the transfer of fatty acids from L-carnitine to free CoA in the mitochondrial matrix. This step is catalyzed by the enzyme carnitine-palmitoyltransferase II. In the mitochondria, the fatty acids then undergo beta-oxidation.

Carnitine may also have physiological and pharmacological roles such as synthesis and remodeling of phospholipids, repair of phospholipids that have been exposed to reactive oxygen species, minimizing the effect of oxidative stress on mitochondria, increasing stability of erythrocyte membranes as well as some therapeutic properties of glucocorticoids, and possibly reversing decline of mental (cognitive) and physical function associated with aging. However, substantial scientific evidence is required to confirm all these biological activities.

There are specific transport mechanisms in the heart, liver, kidneys, and skeletal muscle that enable these tissues to concentrate carnitine.

Although carnitine is marketed commercially as a supplement or ergogenic aid that can enhance performance, there is no scientific evidence for such claims. It is sold on the hypothesis that L carnitine supports conversion of fat into energy and thus improves the athletic performance.

> **Research glimpse:** Carnitine plays a critical role in lipid oxidation by mediating the translocation of long chained fatty acids into mitochondria. During the past 30 years, carnitine supplementation is widely being used in order to enhance lipid oxidation and increase exercise performance. However, studies on its ergogenic effect are limited. There is no evidence that muscle carnitine content can be increased by carnitine feeding in healthy men. Present study reveals that 3 months of dietary supplementation with a combination of carnitine and CHO had no effect, but after 6 months, muscle carnitine content increased by 21%. The necessity of using a very long supplementation period demonstrates the difficulties involved in many of the previous studies. Another finding in this work was that at high-intensity exercise (80% $VO_{2\,max}$) muscle lactate was reduced after carnitine supplementation.
>
> *Sahlin K. Boosting fat burning with carnitine: an old friend comes out from the shadow. J Physiol. 2011;589 (pt7):1509-10.*

Food Sources of Carnitine

Food sources include meat, red meat, poultry, fish, and dairy products, being an important source. Fruits and vegetables are poor sources of L-carnitine. Absorption is likely to be due to a combination of both passive diffusion and active transport. Bioavailability of carnitine has been reported to vary from 54% to 86%. When supplements are consumed up to even 2 g per day, only about 9–25% of the dose is absorbed. Doses above 2 g are not likely to confer any additional benefit, since there appears to be saturation at a dose of 2 g. Studies with animal models indicate that the unabsorbed carnitine is probably metabolized by the gut microflora. Thus, availability of dietary carnitine is much better than from supplements.

It is excreted through the kidneys. Most (95%) of the carnitine is reabsorbed and hence little is eliminated from the body. High fat, low carbohydrate diets increase carnitine excretion.

Causes and Consequences of Deficiency of Carnitine

Nutritional deficiency of carnitine has not been reported in healthy persons including vegans. Presently, there is no RDA or DRI recommended by any expert group for this nutrient. However, studies indicate that in certain conditions, exogenous supplementation of L-carnitine may be useful, e.g., for anorexia, chronic fatigue, cardiovascular disease, diphtheria, hypoglycemia, male infertility, muscular myopathies, and Rett syndrome. Other groups that may benefit include preterm infants, persons undergoing dialysis, and HIV-positive individuals since they seem to be prone to deficiency of L-carnitine.

There are reports of primary as well as secondary deficiencies of carnitine. Deficiency can be acquired or be caused by inborn error of metabolism. Primary carnitine deficiency is rare. In primary deficiency, carnitine levels in tissues, plasma, and red cells are low. The person will have symptoms like muscle fatigue, cramps, and myoglobinemia after performing exercise. Symptoms of chronic deficiency may include hypoglycemia, progressive myasthenia, hypotonia, or lethargy.

Preterm infants are at risk because synthesis is inadequate or impaired and renal tubular reabsorption is insufficient. Secondary deficiency is not so rare as primary deficiency and is seen in persons undergoing dialysis, in those who have undergone intestinal resection, patients with severe infection or liver disease, cancer, diabetes, cardiac failure, and Alzheimer's disease.

Pathological manifestations of chronic deficiency include accumulation of neutral lipid within skeletal muscle, cardiac muscle, and liver; a disruption of muscle fibers; and an accumulation of large aggregates of mitochondria within skeletal and smooth muscle.

Consequences of deficiency include cardiomyopathy, congestive heart failure, encephalopathy, hepatomegaly, impaired growth and development in infants, and neuromuscular disorders.

Supplementation has been found to be beneficial for some groups. For example, in children with infantile anorexia, carnitine supplementation along with adenosylcobalamin improved their appetite. Similarly in persons with anorexia nervosa, this combination was found to increase the rate of weight gain, normalize their gastrointestinal function, decrease fatigue, and improve physical performance. Athletic performance seems to have improved as assessed by running speed, decrease in oxygen consumption and heart rate, plasma lactic acid levels, and muscle recovery after exercise. However, this should be viewed with caution as many researchers have not found either acute or chronic supplementation to be a useful ergogenic aid.

Benefits have been reported for patients with ischemia and angina when 900 to 3,000 mg were administered on a daily basis as supplements. About one-fifth of patients became angina-free during the supplementation. L-carnitine is believed to reduce oxidative stress, improve endothelial function, and enhance blood flow and oxygen supply to muscle tissue. In older adults, L-carnitine could increase muscle mass and reduce physical and mental fatigue. It is suggested to consider supplementation with other health issues and taken under guidance only.

L-carnitine supplementation has been reported to result in nausea, vomiting, abdominal cramps, diarrhea, fishy body odor, muscle weakness in patients with renal disease, and increased frequency of seizures in persons who have this disorder. D-carnitine can increase the risk of L-carnitine deficiency since it is not biologically active but it competes with L-carnitine for absorption and transport.

Lipoic Acid

Lipoic acid is also called thioctic acid. Alpha lipoic acid is an eight-sulfur containing cofactor found in plant and animal tissues, that is synthesized from the intermediates obtained from mitochondrial fatty acid synthesis type II, S-adenosylmethionine, and iron-sulfur clusters. There are two isomers—R and S, with the R isomer being biologically active. In the cell, lipoic acid exists primarily as lipoamide, in an amide linkage to the ε amino group of a lysine residue on a lipoyl carrier protein (LCP).

It is a prerequisite cofactor, required in several multienzyme complexes that are involved in oxidative decarboxylation of various α-keto acids (two ketoacid dehydrogenase complexes) and glycine, e.g., in the pyruvate and α ketoglutaric acid dehydrogenase complexes, and branched-chain ketoacid dehydrogenase. It plays a very important role in stabilizing and regulating these multienzyme complexes. Several of these dehydrogenases are regulated by reactive oxygen species. The disulfide bond in lipoic acid is the source of reductive potential and thus lipoic acid helps to stabilize these enzymes. Lipoic acid is therefore important for cell growth, oxidation of carbohydrates and proteins, and for regulating mitochondrial redox balance.

Lipoic acid can be obtained from the diet and can also be synthesized in the body. It is found in both vegetable and animal foods as lipoyl-lysine. Plant-based rich sources are spinach, broccoli, and tomatoes that contain the R-isomer and animal-based sources are bovine kidney, heart, and liver. It is rapidly transported from the gastrointestinal tract into plasma and from there into tissues like heart, brain, liver, and skeletal muscle. It is excreted by the kidneys.

Alpha lipoic acid has recently gained attention in pharmacology in the treatment of many neurological disorders and chronic diseases. Lipoic acid behaved as antioxidant (it offers more protection from oxidative damage compared to glutathione) and prevented age-related effects of oxidative stress. It has also shown favorable influence on decreasing body weight, reversing insulin resistance, and attenuating high fat-induced oxidative damage in liver and in the CNS. Thus, it may be advocated for weight loss and Alzheimer and Parkinson diseases in future.

Lipoic acid has both hydrophilic and hydrophobic properties, due to which it can function both in the cytosol and in the cell membrane. Thus, it is an important mitochondrial antioxidant as well as having a role in cell redox modulation. These are critical for regulating cell proliferation, differentiation, apoptosis, and necrosis. Lipoic acid thus helps in recycling other cellular antioxidants like coenzyme Q, vitamin C, vitamin E, and glutathione. It has the ability to regulate transcription of genes that are associated with pathways involved in inflammation and oxidative stress.

Besides this, lipoic acid has been found to stimulate glucose uptake (stimulates tyrosine and serine/threonine kinases) and regulate the intrinsic activity of glucose transporters. Lipoic acid has been found to redistribute GLUT 1 and GLUT4 whereby there was stimulation of glucose uptake by adipocytes. Thus, this molecule may be important in terms of insulin signaling pathway.

Laboratory Laurel: In a randomized, double-blind, placebo-controlled clinical trial, 67 patients with stroke were divided into two groups [taking a 600 mg alpha-lipoic acid (ALA) supplement or placebo daily for 12 weeks]. The parameters measured were body weight, waist circumference, body mass index (BMI), and intakes for energy, carbohydrate, protein, and fat intake were assessed before and after intervention. The patients, taking supplementation with 600 mg ALA for 12-week, have showed significant decrease in waist circumference and food intake (energy, carbohydrate, protein, and fat).

Mohammadi V, Khorvash F, Feizi A, et al. The effect of alpha-lipoic acid supplementation on anthropometric indices and food intake in patients who experienced stroke: A randomized, double-blind, placebo-controlled clinical trial. J Res Med Sci. 2017;22:98.

Lipoic acid may play a beneficial role in diseases linked to oxidative stress such as diabetes, cataract, neurodegeneration, and age-related cognitive dysfunction. Lipoic acid supplementation are often advised under medical guidance.

RAPID FIRE

- What is common in vitamins A, E, and C and how these affect the body?
- How does vitamin A deficiency cause infection in the body?
- Define different forms of vitamin D and E.
- Explain the role of vitamin E as an antioxidant.
- How vitamin K is linked with bone health?
- How B-vitamins are linked with energy metabolism?
- Explain the role of folate and vitamin B_{12} in nutritional anemia.
- How vitamin C is associated in wound healing?
- Give one importance of each—biotin, choline, and pantothenic acid in the body.
- Which vitamins have their RDA linked with energy intake?

EXERCISE

1. Design a table for RDA and 10 food sources for vitamins A, C, Riboflavin, folic acid and pyridoxin for sedentary women and 14 year boy.
2. Discuss your weekly food intake in terms of different vitamins in relation to deficiency symptoms if present and how you can prevent them.
3. Explain the role of vitamins D and K in relation to bone health.
4. Write the interaction of the following nutrients:
   a. Vitamin C and bioflavonoid
   b. Thiamine and carbohydrates
   c. Folic acid and vitamin B_{12}.
5. Write about 200-300 words on the sale and selection criteria of any 5 vitamin supplements in your nearby area. Who buys them and why?

SUGGESTED READING

1. Agarwal R, Chhillar N, Kushwaha S, et al. Role of vitamin B(12), folate, and thyroid stimulating hormone in dementia: A hospital-based study in north Indian population. Ann Indian Acad Neurol. 2010;13(4): 257-62.
2. Almeida LF de, Coimbra TM. Vitamin D actions on cell differentiation, proliferation and inflammation. Int J Complement Alt Med. 2017;6(5):00201.
3. Antje L. Vitamin A deficiency: diverse causes, diverse solutions, A report prepared for Greenpeace International, 2005.
4. Burri BJ. Beta-cryptoxanthin as a source of vitamin A. J Sci food Agric. 2015;95(9):1786-94.
5. Cornish S, Mehl-Madrona L. The role of vitamins and minerals in psychiatry. Integr Med Insights. 2008;3:33-42.
6. Degnan PH, Taga ME, Goodman AL. Vitamin B12 as a modulator of gut microbial ecology. Cell Metab. 2014;20(5):769-78.
7. Dinicola S, Minini M, Unfer V, et al. Nutritional and acquired deficiencies in inositol bioavailability. Correlations with metabolic disorders. Int J Molsci. 2017;18(10):2187.
8. Indian Council of Medical Research. Nutrient Requirements and Recommended Dietary Allowances for Indians. A report of the Expert Group of the Indian Council of Medical Research (2010).
9. Insel P, Ross D, McMahon K, et al. Nutrition, 4th edition. Boston: Jones and Bartlett Publishers; 2012. pp. 387-502.
10. Joint FAO/WHO. Vitamin and mineral requirements in human nutrition. A report of the joint FAO/WHO expert consultation, Bangkok, Thailand, 21-30 September 1998, Second Edition, 2004.
11. Kennedy DO. B Vitamins and the Brain: Mechanisms, Dose and Efficacy—A Review. Nutrients. 2016;8(2):68.
12. Kohlmeier M, Salomon A, Saupe J, et al. Transport of vitamin K to bone in humans. J Nutr. 1996;126:1192S-6S.
13. Kulkarni ML. Vitamins in Health and Disease. New Delhi: Jaypee Brothers Medical Publishers (P) Ltd; 2012.
14. Laird E, Ward M, McSorley M, et al. Vitamin D and bone health: potential mechanisms. Nutrients. 2010;2:693-724.
15. Linder, MC. Nutritional Biochemistry and Metabolism with Clinical Applications, 2nd edition. London: Prentice-hall International Limited; 1991.
16. Longo DL, Fauci AS, Kasper DL, Hauser SL, Jameson J, Loscalzo J (Eds). Vitamin D is a hormone because it is made in one organ (skin) and transported by body fluid (blood) to act or activate other body parts. In: Harrison's Principles of Internal Medicine, 18th edition. New York, NY: McGraw-Hill; 2012.
17. Longvah T, Ananthan R, Bhaskarachary K, et al. Indian Food Composition Tables National Institute of Nutrition, (Indian Council of Medical Research) Department of Health Research, Ministry of Health and Family Welfare, Government of India, Hyderabad (2017).
18. Mahan LK, Stump SE, Raymond JL. Krause's Food nutrition & Diet Therapy, 13th edition. Philadelphia: WB Saunders Company; 2007.
19. McCann JC, Ames BN. Vitamin K, an example of triage theory: is micronutrient inadequacy linked to diseases of aging? Am J Clin Nutr. 2007;90:889-907.
20. Misra D, Booth SL, Tolstykh I, et al. Vitamin K deficiency is associated with incident knee osteoarthritis. Am J Med. 2013;126(3):243-8.
21. Morris HA. Vitamin D: A Hormone for All Seasons. Clinical Biochemist Review. 2005;26(1):21-32.
22. Mostafa WZ, Hegazy RA. Vitamin D and the skin: Focus on a complex relationship: A review. J Adv Res. 2015;6:793-804.
23. Nutrient Requirements of Indians, Recommended Dietary Allowances, Estimated Average Requirements, A reports of the Expert Group, 2020, Indian Council of Medical research, National Institute of Nutrition, Department of Health Research, Ministry of Health and Family Welfare, Government of India.
24. Oghbaei M, Prakash J, Yildiz F. Effect of primary processing of cereals and legumes on its nutritional quality: A comprehensive review. Cogent Food and Agriculture. 2016;2(1).
25. Peter RM, Singleton CK, Sturmhöfel SH. National Institute of Alcohol Abuse and Alcoholism. The role of thiamine deficiency in alcoholic brain disease. Alcohol Research & Health. 2003;27(2):134-42.
26. Prietl B, Treiber G, Pieber TR, et al. Vitamin D and immune function. Nutrients. 2013;5(7):2502-21.

27. Ravisankar P, Reddy A, Nagalakshmi B, et al. The Comprehensive Review on Fat Soluble Vitamins. IOSRPHR. 2015;5(11):2250-3013.
28. Rolfes SR, Pinna K, Whitney E. Understanding Normal and Clinical nutrition, 7th edition, International student edition; 2006.
29. Rusinka A, Pludowski P, Walczak M, et al. Vitamin D Supplementation Guidelines for General Population and Groups at Risk of Vitamin D Deficiency in Poland—Recommendations of the Polish Society of Pediatric Endocrinology and Diabetes and the Expert Panel With Participation of National Specialist Consultants and Representatives of Scientific Societies—2018 Update. Front Endocrinol (Lausanne). 2018;9:246.
30. Russell RM, Beard JL, Cousins RJ, Dunn JT, Ferland G, Hambidge KM, Lynch S, Penland JG, Ross AC, Stoecker BJ, Suttie JW. Dietary reference intakes for vitamin A, vitamin K, arsenic, boron, chromium, copper, iodine, iron, manganese, molybdenum, nickel, silicon, vanadium, and zinc. A Report of the Panel on Micronutrients, Subcommittees on Upper Reference Levels of Nutrients and of Interpretation and Uses of Dietary Reference Intakes, and the Standing Committee on the Scientific Evaluation of Dietary Reference Intakes Food and Nutrition Board Institute of Medicine. 2001.
31. Srilakshmi B. Nutrition Science (Revised Second Edition). New Delhi: New Age International Publishers; 2006.
32. Szczuko M, Ziętek M, Kulpa D, Seidler T. Riboflavin - properties, occurrence and its use in medicine Pteridines. 2019;30:33-47.
33. Thacher TD, Clarke BL. Vitamin D insufficiency. Mayo Clinic Proceedings. 2011;86(1):50-60.
34. Vieth R. Why "Vitamin D" is not a hormone, and not a synonym for 1,25-dihydroxy-vitamin D, its analogs or deltanoids. J Steroid Biochem Mol Biol. 2004;89-90:571-3.
35. Whitney EN, Sizer FS. Nutrition: Concepts and Controversies. Australia: Wadsworth Thompson Learning; 2002.
36. WHO/NHD/99.13. Thiamine deficiency and its prevention and control in major emergencies, 1999. Available from https://optimumwellness.co.za/Vitamin-C-Booklet.pdf [Last accessed August, 2019].
37. WHO Global prevalence of vitamin A deficiency in populations at risk 1995–2005 WHO Global Database on Vitamin A Deficiency.
38. WHO Regional Office for the Eastern Mediterranean, FAO Regional Office for the Near East. FAO/WHO technical consultation on national food-based dietary guidelines. (2006). Available from https://www.who.int/nutrition/publications/nutrientrequirements/dietguide_emro/en/ [Last accessed August, 2019].
39. World Health Organization and Food and Agriculture Organization of the United Nations. Vitamin and mineral requirements in human nutrition. (2004). Available from https://apps.who.int/iris/bitstream/handle/10665/42716/9241546123.pdf [Last accessed August, 2019].
40. Zhang R, Naughton DP. Vitamin D in health and disease: Current Perspectives. Nutr J. 2010;9:65-77.

7
CHAPTER

Minerals

KEY CONCERNS	KEY CONCEPTS
• What are the different minerals and trace elements? • What are the roles of different minerals and trace elements in the human body? • What are the food sources and the requirements of each mineral? • How do deficiency and excess of minerals influence health?	• Classification of minerals • Functions, food sources, and recommended dietary allowances • Causes and consequences of deficiency and excess of each minerals

INTRODUCTION

Minerals are inorganic elements widely distributed in nature—the earth's crust, sea, plants, and animals. Minerals are important for their structural, metabolic, and regulatory roles in the body. Like vitamins, they do not provide calories or energy and are required in very small amounts. Unlike vitamins, they are not destroyed by heat, light, air, and changes in pH. They can chelate (bind) with other compounds and may become unavailable to the body. However, food processing techniques like germination and fermentation may increase the bioavailability of some minerals. Most minerals are present in dietary sources but their mineral content differs greatly in different regions depending upon the mineral content of the soil and other environmental factors. Even the maturity of the plant can make a difference. Since they play many critical roles in sustaining life, their deficiency can be devastating for health, productivity, and influence national economy, e.g., anemia due to iron deficiency and iodine deficiency disorder (IDD) due to iodine deficiency.

Each mineral has diverse roles. Some minerals are integral parts of body structure or molecules, like calcium in bones, iron in hemoglobin and myoglobin and sodium, potassium, chloride, zinc and copper in nerves. Minerals are classified on the basis of quantity of the mineral needed in the body.

CLASSIFICATION OF MINERALS (FIG. 7.1)

Major Minerals

Major minerals are present in larger quantities in the body compared to the trace and ultratrace elements. Thus, their daily dietary needs are greater (more than 100 mg). Major minerals are calcium, phosphorus, magnesium, sodium, potassium, chloride, and sulfur. They have structural and functional roles in the body. They play significant roles in body movements and support brain functions and acid–base, electrolyte balance, as well as gene expression. The functions of some of the minerals are interrelated and linked with vitamins and other nutrients. Hence, besides being concerned about the adequate intake of one mineral, it is necessary to consider the minerals/nutrients whose functions are related, as lower or excessive intakes of one or both can disturb the ratio of these minerals/nutrients with adverse consequences on health. For example, a lower intake of calcium and higher intake of phosphorus can deplete the calcium from bones resulting in bone diseases. Disturbance in the ratio of sodium

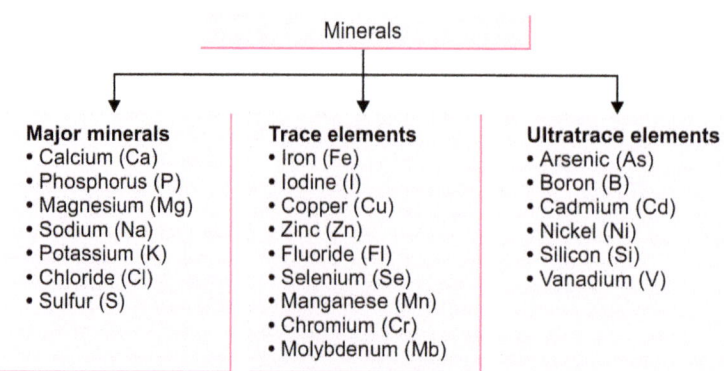

Fig. 7.1: Classification of minerals.

and potassium can affect cardiac function. Most minerals are present in the earth's crust, rocks, sea, and plants. They can be obtained from commonly consumed foods from plant, animal, and marine sources.

Calcium

Calcium was first recognized as an element in 1808 by Davy. Subsequently, the role of calcium in mammalian bones and mineralized tissues was recognized. Calcium is the most abundant mineral in the body. 99% of body calcium is present in bones; remaining 1% is found in teeth and soft tissues and out of this, only 0.1% is present in extracellular fluid (ECF). ECF and plasma contain ionized Ca^{++}. Calcium concentration in blood is tightly regulated in a narrow range by three hormones, namely calcitriol (vitamin D or 1,25-dihydroxycholecalciferol), parathyroid hormone (PTH), and calcitonin. Calcium can be mobilized from bones (resorption) to plasma and ECF when the calcium supply from dietary sources is insufficient and when serum calcium levels fall (because its physiological roles are extremely important). Normal serum calcium levels are 8–10 mg/dL.

Functions of Calcium

Calcium performs several vital functions. Calcium salts provide rigidity to bones and calcium ion participates in numerous metabolic activities in the body. Calcium in its ionic form (calcium ions—Ca^{2+}) is needed for intracellular signaling, neurotransmission, muscle contraction, regulation of cell growth, and blood clotting. Calcium ions have a central role as second messenger in intracellular signaling, in muscle contraction, secretion, glycolysis and gluconeogenesis, ion transport, cell division, and growth. Calcium along with vitamin D may has a preventive role in weight management and a protective role in polycystic ovarian syndrome (PCOS).

Formation of skeletal structure: Calcium is essential for formation and maintenance of bones and teeth. Bones are formed from a protein matrix within which calcium and other minerals or salts, i.e., phosphorus, magnesium, sodium, carbonate, citrate, chloride, fluoride, etc. are embedded.

Calcium and phosphorus ions combine with hydroxide (OH^-) ion to form a compound called hydroxyapatite [$Ca_5(PO_4)_3(OH)$], with hexagonal and crystalline structure which is propagated on collagen fibrils. It is a hard mineral and hence provides structural rigidity to bones and also prevents them from injury when exposed to mechanical pressure. This rigidity of the skeleton is critical for vertebrates including humans to move rapidly and with precise control. Hydroxyapatite constitutes up to 70% of the weight of bone. In dental enamel, the percentage of hydroxyapatite is much higher, giving teeth their mechanical resistance.

Calcium is deposited during the developmental periods and used later in life, if required. Hence, bones are a reservoir of calcium. Calcium is mobilized from bone, to maintain blood calcium level, but cannot be mobilized from teeth. Inadequate mineralization of bones in the growing years and adulthood increases the risk of fractures.

Bones are hard tissues and are made up of 40% organic and 60% inorganic compounds. Organic compounds include collagen, proteoglycans, special proteins, and other substances while inorganic compounds are calcium hydroxyapatite and ostocalcium phosphate. All these compounds have specific roles in formation and mineralization of bones, providing strength and maintaining bone turnover and bone cell differentiation. Bones provide skeletal structure, protect many organs, produce red and white blood cells in the bone marrow, store minerals, and enable mobility to the body.

Bone is a type of connective tissue that is highly dynamic. Three types of cells—osteoblasts, osteoclasts and osteocytes—are involved in bone formation. Bone is formed in layers, wherein the layers (matrix) contain collagen fibers that are arranged in almost parallel manner. Besides collagen, the matrix also contains proteoglycans and other substances. The inner surface enclosing the marrow cavity is lined with a thin connective tissue—the endosteum. The cells of the endosteum and the inner layer of the periosteum (on the outer surface of bone) differentiate into osteoblasts upon stimulation.

Osteoblasts are the bone forming cells. Osteoblasts lay down the calcifiable organic matrix which is mineralized. Ossification is formation of bone by the activity of osteoblasts and osteoclasts and the addition of minerals and salts. Calcium is essential for ossification. Osteoblasts do not make these minerals, but take them from the blood and deposit them in the bone. By the time we are born, many of the bones have been at least partly ossified.

Osteoblasts remain relatively stationary while laying down the matrix and become completely embedded in matrix, at which time, they become known as Osteocytes. Throughout life bone remodeling occurs, hence bone is a metabolically active tissue. Similar activities occur in dentine for tooth formation. With age, activity of osteoblasts decreases (after the age of 40 years) and bones are at risk of fracture. However, physical exercise or muscular activity accelerates deposition of calcium to maintain osteoblast activity. During injury, osteoblasts secrete more substances within the matrix for formation of new bone cells, provided that the essential nutrients calcium, phosphorus, and protein are available. Vitamins A and C are also needed for bone development. Vitamin D increases calcium absorption in the small intestine. Vitamin C is required for hydroxylation of proline, which is an essential step in collagen synthesis. Vitamin A stimulates the release of enzymes from lysosomes needed for bone resorption. Bone formation is also influenced by hormones such as growth hormone, parathyroid hormone, thyroxin, and estrogen.

Osteocytes are mature osteoblasts that no longer lay down the bone matrix. They are active and are in metabolic exchange with the blood that flows through the bones and are involved in regulating calcium level in the blood. They are actively involved in bone turnover through their cell to matrix contact surface, are involved in ion exchange, and are the mechanosensory cells of bone and play an important role in functional adaptation of bone.

The third type of bone cells, osteoclasts are much bigger than osteoblasts and are generally located at sites of bone resorption. Balance between activities of osteoblasts and osteoclasts are important for bone remodeling and maintaining skeletal structure. Osteoclasts remain at a site of bone resorption in small concentrated masses and remove bone mineral. Their activity is important for preventing excess bone growth during the process of bone formation. Once their activity is completed, osteoblasts appear at the site.

BONE BANK: Like a bank, calcium can easily be deposited and withdrawn from the bones throughout life. Extra demand needs to be fulfilled during pregnancy and lactation. In adulthood, bone mineralization or deposition ceases and one has to rely on diet for fulfilling calcium requirements. If the diet supplies insufficient calcium, it is withdrawn from bones. Bones may become bankrupt in case of calcium deficiency. It results in weak bones, less strength to walk, poor locomotor coordination, osteoporosis, and increases risk for bone fractures and disability.

> **PEAK BONE MASS:** Peak bone mass is the amount of bony tissue present at the end of skeletal maturation. Adolescence is the most critical period for deposition because bone accumulates rapidly and accounts for almost half of adult peak bone mass. On average, 99% of the bone mineralization is completed by 26–30 years. Adequate bone mass built up/accumulated in the critical period will help to reduce risk of osteoporosis, bone fragility, and risk of fractures in late life.

Blood clotting: Calcium is bound with the proteins particularly the amino acids which have a carboxyl group (at the terminal gamma-carboxy residues). When there is an injury, platelets and a network of fibrin together form a clot. Calcium ions participate in (i) certain steps of the blood clotting cascade by activating some of the proteins involved, (ii) platelet aggregation, and (iii) conversion of the inactive form, i.e., prothrombin is converted into active form of the enzyme called thrombin. Thrombin converts the inactive protein fibrinogen to fibrin. Fibrin is a fibrous protein. It forms strands that stick to platelets and endothelial cells at the site of injury/wound and forms a mesh/web that in turn traps other cells.

Calcium is required for two complexes to function, namely the tenase and prothrombinase complexes. These complexes bind to phospholipid surfaces and procoagulant microvesicles shed from the platelets as well as at other points in the coagulation cascade.

Blood clotting occurs through two pathways known as the intrinsic and extrinsic pathways which ultimately lead to fibrin formation. In the intrinsic pathway (known as contact activation pathway), Ca ions are required to convert/activate Factor XIA to Factor IX and in the extrinsic pathway (known as tissue factor pathway), Ca is required to convert and activate Factor X to Factor XA. These factors are vitamin K-dependent proteins involved in clotting of blood.

Muscle contraction and relaxation: Skeletal muscle cells contain an organelle called the sarcoplasmic reticulum (SR), which stores large quantities of calcium. On contraction of skeletal or heart muscles, calcium ions are released from SR and bind to actin containing thin filaments of myofibrils. This also stimulates neurotransmission.

When a muscle contracts, its constituent fibers shorten. Skeletal muscle cells contain an organelle called the sarcoplasmic reticulum (SR), which stores large quantities of calcium. When muscles are stimulated by a nerve impulse, they respond by contracting. Events in muscle contraction are as follows:

- When an electrical signal, i.e., action potential travels down a nerve cell, there is release of a neurotransmitter, acetylcholine (ACh), into the synapse.
- The ACh binds to a receptor protein on the membrane of the muscle cell and causes an action potential in the muscle cell.
- This action potential spreads rapidly along the muscle cells and travels to the sarcoplasmic reticulum (SR). The endoplasmic reticulum releases calcium into the cytoplasm.
- Calcium ions now flow into the cytoplasm, calcium floods in and around the myofibrils, and bath that are composed of repeating sections of sarcomeres.
- In the cytoplasm, filaments of two proteins, actin and myosin, are present. The actin filaments have a groove that contains troponin-tropomyosin molecules, to which the calcium ions bind.
- Once calcium has bound to troponin, its shape changes, tropomyosin slides out of the groove. Myosin interacts with actin, cross-bridges are formed and the muscle creates force and shortens, i.e., sarcomere contraction occurs. The contraction of one muscle fiber is really the net result of the shortening of all the tiny sarcomeres in each myofibril within that cell.
- Further, the contraction of the muscle itself is the net result of contraction and shortening of muscle fibers that make up that muscle.
- Once the action potential has passed, i.e., the calcium gates close and calcium pumps located on the sarcoplasmic reticulum remove calcium from the cytoplasm. As the calcium is pumped back into the sarcoplasmic reticulum, calcium ions move away from troponin, which now returns to its normal shape, tropomyosin now covers the actin-myosin binding sites. As a result, cross-bridges formation is not possible and the muscle relaxes.

Cell signaling and nerve transmission: Calcium plays an important role in release of neurotransmitters, e.g., acetylcholine from nerve terminals. Since calcium is a positively charged molecule, in its ionic form (Ca^{++}), it is useful for the conduction of a nerve impulse to a muscle fiber. In fact, calcium ions are central to numerous functions including constriction and relaxation of blood vessels, i.e., vasoconstriction and vasodilation, muscle contraction, and secretion of hormones. Skeletal muscle cells and nerve cells have voltage channels in the cell membranes. When muscle fiber is stimulated, these calcium channels open so that calcium ions can enter the muscle cell. Clay Armstrong, a neurobiologist, has stated that calcium is in charge of gated channels that release potassium and sodium to facilitate a nerve impulse. When calcium returns, the impulse stops and homeostasis is maintained.

Cell membrane permeability: Calcium has a fundamental role in controlling membrane permeability and the cell's response to stimulation. Cell membrane is semi-permeable due to which ionic concentration on both sides of the cell can be maintained. The membrane develops a membrane potential or voltage to maintain the ion concentration which is different in intracellular fluid (ICF) and extracellular fluid (ECF). Voltage change in the cell membrane brings changes in cell permeability. Calcium concentrations in ICF are lower than in the ECF but the intracellular concentrations can increase in response to stressors and hormones. There are specific calcium channels which open in response to a signaling protein. When the channels open, calcium from ECF enters the cytosol. When sufficient calcium enters the cytosol, it increases permeability of membranes or cells like endothelial cells to macromolecules. Also, permeability of human red cell membranes to sodium and potassium is regulated by internal calcium, which in turn is controlled by a calcium pump that utilizes ATP. Cell excitability and cell-to-cell communication depend on the concentration of free calcium ions in ECF.

Other functions: Calcium is involved in initiation of DNA synthesis, sorting of chromosomes, regulation of cell division, and differentiation. It also plays a role in the vestibular system in the ear which perceives balances and provides information about the position of the body. Calcium carbonate crystals are embedded in a gelatinous layer called the otolithic membrane. When there is a change in position, sensory hair cells in the vestibular system detect even the smallest amount of displacement of the layer of calcium carbonate crystals. Calcium is also required to stabilize many proteins and optimize activities of enzymes.

Absorption of Calcium from Food
Absorption of calcium in the body is equally important as is the amount of calcium present in the diet. Calcium is absorbed in the duodenum, jejunum, and ileum. Efficiency of absorption varies widely from as little as 15% to as much as 50%. Several factors which increase or decrease the calcium absorption from the intestines and influence bone health and other functions of calcium (Fig. 7.2). The amount or dose also influences the amount that is absorbed. Among the various factors, 1,25-dihydroxycholecalciferol (vitamin D/calcitriol) is one of the most important. The form in which calcium is present, i.e., whether it is soluble and whether the calcium ion can dissociate easily, influences availability. Inhibition is more when calcium intakes are low. High phosphorus intakes inhibit absorption because it forms a poorly soluble complex with calcium. In leafy vegetables with low oxalate content, calcium absorption is fairly good and may be better than absorption of calcium from dairy products.

Two pathways are probably used for calcium absorption. One is the paracellular pathway and the transcellular pathway. The paracellular pathway uses passive diffusion (that is not saturable) when the calcium concentration in the intestinal lumen is high. Movement of calcium is favored by the concentration gradient due to the lower intracellular concentration compared to the intestinal lumen concentration. It may account for half to two-thirds of the calcium absorbed. This pathway is likely to be influenced by 1,25-dihydroxyvitamin D3 because the vitamin can alter the structure of the intercellular tight junctions and make them more permeable to calcium.

Calcium moves down this concentration gradient through a calcium transporter or a calcium channel. At the apical portion of the intestinal cell, calcium is bound reversibly to the calmodulin-actin-myosin I complex. This calcium can then either diffuse to the basolateral part of the cell either by diffusion in the form of ionized calcium or it may be moved by microvesicular transport. However, binding to calmodulin is a saturable process. Here, vitamin D has a favorable influence because it causes the intestinal epithelial cells to increase calbindin synthesis. Calcium binds to calbindin and thus the calmodulin becomes available for picking up more calcium. The calcium then dissociates from the calbindin-calcium complex and is now present in free form within the cell. This free calcium is then extruded by Ca ATPase or by a sodium-calcium exchanger. Here again, vitamin D is important because it increases the synthesis of the Ca ATPase in the plasma membrane.

Calcium is excreted by the kidneys. It is filtered in the glomerulus from the plasma. Iso-osmotic reabsorption occurs with 60–70% of the filtered calcium being reabsorbed. Reabsorption is stimulated by calcitonin. Normally, the major proportion of calcium absorption is a passive process and is paracellular, being favored by the electrochemical gradient. However, some active transport does occur under the influence of vitamin D and PTH.

Recommended Dietary Allowances for Calcium
The Food and Nutrition Board, Institute of Medicine, USA (2010) suggests that infants should receive 200 mg and children (1–3 years of age) require 700 mg/day. Thereafter calcium requirements may coincide with increase in height and other developmental concerns. However, calcium requirement is increased during pregnancy and lactation of course, and during postmenopausal stage in women.

Requirements for calcium are established with the objectives of calcium accretion during growth period for attaining optimal bone mineral density (BMD) and achieving good bone health and bone integrity for the rest of lifespan. Utilization of calcium in the body is regulated by several factors such as race; geographical location; intake of animal protein; body status of sodium and vitamin D; and of course, intake of calcium. There are obligatory losses of calcium in urine, bile, sweat and stool and that cal also be considered. According to ICMR-NIN (2020) calcium requirements for adults including pregnant women is 1000 mg/day (EAR-800 mg/d). It should be noted that calcium requirements during lactation as well as post-menopausal period is the same, i.e., 1200 mg/day (EAR-1000 mg/d). For lactating women, the calcium is required for milk and in old age to preserve the bone mass. Calcium requirements are different for various age groups and are shown in Table 9.1A in Chapter 9 and EAR in Appendix 4. To achieve this level intake, minimum 200 mL of milk per day is advisable. Dietary protein and calcium are associated with BMD. Protein helps in calcium absorption, but it can also increase calcium excretion, since high protein affects the acid balance. Increasing protein intake in older population by 10–20% of energy may improve the calcium absorption and compensate the urinary loss of calcium. Studies show that protein and sodium intake influences the excretion of urinary

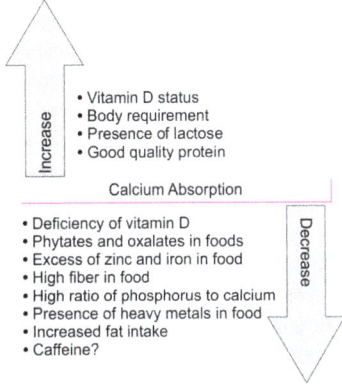

Fig. 7.2: Factors affecting calcium absorption.

calcium. If the animal protein intake is decreased from 60 g/day to 20 g/day and sodium intake from 150 to 50 mmol per day calcium requirement can be reduced by as much as 200 mg/day. For every gram of animal protein, 1 mg of calcium is lost in urine. In developed countries, intake of animal protein is higher than in less developed countries.

Food Sources of Calcium

Milk and milk products are rich sources of calcium. It is preferable to use milk or curd as a source of calcium rather than cheese because it contains high amount of sodium which increases excretion of calcium in urine. Meat also increases the urinary acidity thus calcium excretion. There are many other sources of calcium in plant foods such as sesame seeds, ragi, and green leafy vegetables but their calcium is less utilized due to the presence of phytates and oxalates in them. Enough quantities of cumin, ajwain, and coriander make good contribution for calcium intake. Several food sources of calcium are shown in Figure 7.3 as per IFCT (2017) values.

Addition of neutralizers to milk and milk products or other foods can cause increased mineral concentration in body fluids and soft organs, leading to kidney stone development. Commercial preparation of neutralizers might even be contaminated with heavy metals like arsenic, lead, etc. Continuous use of such milk and milk products may cause health hazards. Since the frequency and quantity of milk consumed by infants and children are much more compared to adults, the health risk is more for them. Hence, use of neutralizers in milk is prohibited as per food laws (FSSAI, 2012).

Deficiency of Calcium: Causes and Consequences

Poor dietary intake of calcium is one of the major causes of calcium deficiency which is further accentuated by the deficiency of vitamin D. The ratio of calcium to phosphorus should be 1:1. Excess phosphorus intake will precipitate as insoluble calcium phosphate. Reduced absorption of calcium and loss of calcium in urine contributes to calcium deficiency. Calcium deficiency adversely influences bone composition, muscle contraction, and nerve transmission. It affects growth and bone mineralization in childhood and in adolescence and in adults; it results in loss of bone mineral. Thus, in older persons, inadequate calcium intakes and low bone mineral content, increase risk of osteoporosis and fractures increase the risk of fractures. Deficiency of the mineral also affects muscle contraction (skeletal muscles and smooth muscles). Muscle cramps are common. Smooth muscles of heart are adversely affected. In children, tetany can occur. Calcium deficiency leads to rickets in children and osteomalacia and osteoporosis in adults. These diseases signify poor bone health. Adequate calcium intakes are recommended as a strategy for reduction of high blood pressure. Increasing calcium intakes may also reduce the risk of colon cancer as well as breast cancer. Adequate dietary calcium is also important for reducing risk of renal stones.

Calcium deficiency can easily be corrected by increasing dietary intake and reducing the calcium inhibitors from the diet, especially at the time of taking calcium-rich foods. At meal time, other factors like gastric acid may improve absorption. Vitamin D or exposure to sun for about 20–30 minutes improves calcium utilization in the body.

Calcium supplements: Calcium supplements are used either to prevent the deficiency or furnish the additional demand of calcium under certain conditions. These are available in tablets or powder form. Many calcium compounds are used as supplements such as calcium carbonate, calcium citrate, calcium malate, calcium phosphate, calcium gluconate, and calcium lactate. Availability of calcium from these compounds differs, for example, availability from calcium formate is better as compared to calcium carbonate and calcium citrate. The least expensive supplement is calcium carbonate. For persons with achlorhydria or if a person is on medications that blocks H^+ ion/gastric acid secretion, calcium citrate is a better choice. However, calcium supplement may also compete with zinc or iron supplements. Therefore, it is advisable to consume the calcium and zinc supplements at different times. Use of calcium supplements should be taken under the supervision of health professionals because of its side effects like formation of kidney stones and stiffening of arteries. Overall, it is advisable to obtain the calcium we need from food sources/diet, because foods will supply other important nutrients as well.

Calcium supplements are frequently prescribed and consumed in many parts of the globe to keep bone diseases

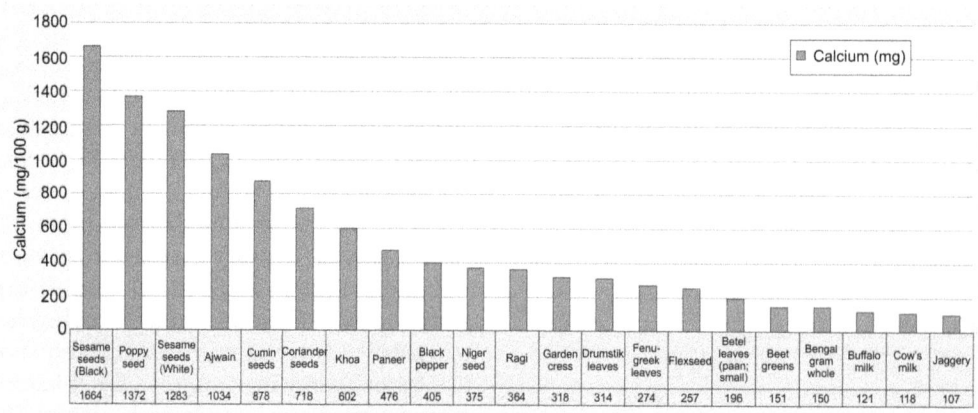

Fig. 7.3: Food sources of calcium.

at bay. Many chemical forms are available and many of them interact with several types of medications. These supplements when taken together with such medicines could decrease the absorption of some medicines or drugs. Also, there is risk of hypercalcemia or hypercalciuria.

Consequences of Excessive Intake of Calcium

Adverse effects of high calcium diets may occur at intakes exceeding the tolerable upper limit (TUL) of 2500 mg/day by adults and 3000 mg/day by children and adolescents (9-17 years) as per ICMR-NIN (2020). For children TUL for 1-3 year children is 1500 mg and for 4-9 years-2500 mg. Excess calcium level in blood is known as "hypercalcemia". It rarely occurs due to excessive intake of calcium from dietary sources but is found in people who ingest calcium and vitamin D supplements in large quantity for prolonged period without medical advice. The most common cause of hypercalcemia is overproduction of parathyroid hormone. However, it may occur in people who take calcium and vitamin D supplements for prolonged duration. Such persons may complain of constipation, large urine volume, and nausea. Hypercalcemia is characterized by elevated blood calcium level; calcification (deposition of calcium) of joints, muscles, liver, pancreas, heart, kidney or lungs, and painful arthritis and hardened arteries. High calcium intake might interfere with the absorption of other minerals like zinc and iron and exacerbate their deficiencies.

> **Research Glimpse:** Vascular calcification may increase the risk of cardiovascular mortality in chronic kidney disease (CKD) patients. It is mainly due to the dysregulation of calcium and phosphate metabolism. Elevated Ca and P adversely affect vascular smooth muscle cells (VSMCs) leading to vascular calcification. Accelerated calcification in medial and intimal arteries progresses in patients on dialysis. There is loss of inhibitor function and development of a calcifiable extracellular matrix. Dysregulated mineral metabolism is characterized by long-term elevation of serum phosphate levels as well as transient bouts of hypercalcemia. Research is ongoing for this complex mechanism involving gut and bones using calcium and phosphorus.
>
> *Shanahan CM, Crouthamel MH, Kapustin A, et al. Arterial Calcification in Chronic Kidney Disease: Key Roles for Calcium and Phosphate. Circulation Research. 2011;109:697–711.*

Phosphorus

Phosphorus is the 6th most abundant mineral in the human body, constituting about 1% of body weight. It works in close association with calcium. Most of the phosphorus in the body is present as phosphate ions (HPO_4^{-2}) in biological fluids. Most of the P is in bones (about 85%) and the remaining 15% is found in cells, cell membranes, and extracellular fluids. Phosphorus is an integral component of phospholipids, nucleic acids, and high energy compounds like ATP. It is important for various metabolic activities like phosphorylation and is required for growth. The normal serum PO_4 concentration in adults ranges from 2.5 mg/dL to 4.5 mg/dL (0.81–1.45 mmol/L). Its concentration in intracellular fluid is about 100 times more than in plasma.

Phosphate levels in serum along with calcium ions are regulated by parathyroid hormone (PTH) and calcitriol. Phosphate is released from bone, secondary to regulation of blood calcium concentration. Phosphate ions in body fluids are regulated by insulin, growth hormone, and steroid hormones, all of which act on the kidneys. Most of the phosphate is excreted through urine and kidneys are important for extracellular homeostasis of phosphate ions by either reabsorption or allowing its excretion. Excretion is also influenced by dietary intake. Low intakes of phosphorus or hypophosphatemia increase reabsorption. Excretion of phosphate by kidney is also regulated by phosphatonins.

In foods, phosphorus is present as phosphate salts (inorganic form), nucleotides, and phospholipids (organic form). Phosphorus is also a component of many food additives. Considerable amount (60–70%) of dietary P is absorbed over a wide range of intakes. When P intake is low, vitamin D may be important in enhancing intestinal absorption. Most of the phosphate is present in phospholipids of the lipoproteins and in the membranes of blood cells. Also, a small amount is present as the inorganic phosphate ion.

Phosphorus homeostasis is influenced by the absorption/secretion in the gastrointestinal tract, filtration/absorption in the kidneys, and ferry from bone.

Functions of Phosphorus

Phosphorus plays essential roles in cellular functions and bone mineralization for which the organic form is utilized. In human blood, 70% of the phosphorus is organic and the remaining 30% is inorganic. Phosphorus is essential for the growth, maintenance, and repair of all tissues and cells for the production DNA and RNA and metabolism/utilization of vitamins and other minerals like iodine, magnesium, and zinc. Phosphorus is present in many phosphorylated compounds that have important biological roles. Phosphorus plays a role as buffer and helps to maintain acid–base balance. As part of the molecule 2,3-diphosphoglycerate (2,3-DPG), phosphorus is important for delivering oxygen to cells. 2,3-DPG binds to hemoglobin in the red blood cells and thus regulates oxygen delivery.

Component of cell membrane: Phosphorus is an integral component of phospholipids which are present in all cell membranes including brain cells; hence, it provides structural stability to the cell and performs myriad functions in the body and brain. Phosphatidylcholine that is present in cell membranes is a phospholipid.

Component of biological compounds: It is a component of many organic compounds of biological importance such as phosphatides, nucleotides, DNA/RNA and many enzymes like phosphatase, kinase, etc. It is also a component of lecithin, which helps to break down and emulsify the fat.

Energy metabolism and high energy phosphate bond: Phosphorus is a component of high energy phosphate bonds (chemical energy) which are present in ADP and ATP, the predominant sources of metabolic energy used in energy metabolism. It is also present in specialized forms such as creatine phosphate, GTP, and arginine phosphate. These are essential building blocks for DNA and RNA synthesis. Cyclic

AMP is important for intracellular signaling. Phosphorus is also required for glucose utilization by muscle.

Bone mineralization: Phosphate is present in the bone as calcium phosphate and as a component of hydroxyapatite that is deposited in bone matrix.

Phosphorylation: It is a process of combining phosphate group with protein, glucose or glycerol for metabolic reactions. Oxidative phosphorylation is a metabolic pathway, where nutrients are oxidized to release ATP. Phosphorylation is necessary for intestinal absorption, glycolysis, oxidation of carbohydrates, transport of fatty acids, exchange of amino acids, and renal excretion. Activity of several proteins is regulated by phosphorylation and dephosphorylation. Phosphorylation is an important and critical step for activation of enzymes, hormones, and cell-signaling molecules.

Buffer system: Phosphate buffer (HPO_4^{-2}) has major role in acid–base balance.

Phosphoproteins: It is part of phosphoproteins like stathmin, which is involved in cell proliferation and cell differentiation and other phosphoproteins associated with highly specific functions in kidney, brain, and heart. Besides this, some types of osteoblasts contain polyphosphates which may contain up to thousands of phosphates linked together. It is speculated that these polyphosphates may have a role in inhibiting bone mineralization, apoptosis, amino acid chelation, pH regulation, and protection against osmotic stress among other roles.

Regulation of phosphorus levels: Maintaining the physiological balance for phosphate is extremely important for bone health. Body homeostasis for this mineral depends on the intake and absorption, reabsorption by the kidneys and excretion as well as between the phosphate in extracellular pool and the bone storage. Phosphate homeostasis is regulated by transporters called phosphatonins that are present in the gastrointestinal tract, bone, and kidney. Excess phosphorus is excreted by the kidneys whose functioning is regulated by vitamin D, parathyroid hormone (like calcium), and fibroblast growth factor 23 (FGF-23). Besides these, there is evidence that other factors like epidermal growth factor, glucocorticoids, estrogens, and secreted frizzled related protein 4 (sFRP-4) influence intestinal absorption.

When serum calcium levels drop even slightly, PTH is secreted by the parathyroid glands and urinary calcium excretion is decreased. However, urinary excretion of phosphorus increases and bone resorption is stimulated. These actions lead to restoration of serum calcium concentration. Vitamin D increases intestinal absorption of not only calcium but also that of phosphorus. FGF-23 is secreted by osteoblasts when the phosphorus intake increases. FGF-23 through negative feedback inhibits the production of 1,25-dihydroxyvitamin D and increases its degradation. It also promotes excretion of phosphorus in urine and this action is independent of both vitamin D and PTH.

> **FGF-23** is expressed mostly in bone but also in brain, thymus, small intestine, heart, lung, liver, kidney, thyroid, parathyroid, lymph node, skeletal muscle, spleen, skin, stomach, and testis and exerts its effects in all these tissues. It is largely secreted by osteoclasts and a small amount is secreted by osteoblasts. It downregulates sodium phosphate cotransporters in the renal proximal tubule and causes a decrease in phosphate reabsorption, thus increasing phosphorus excretion in urine and lowering the serum phosphate levels. Also, it inhibits the activity of renal 1α-hydroxylase and stimulates that of 24-hydroxylase, thus reducing the production of calcitriol and inhibits secretion of PTH. Thus, it serves to regulate phosphate homeostasis besides regulation by PTH, the main regulator.

Recommended Dietary Allowances for Phosphorus

Since calcium:phosphorus ratio of 1:1 is found to be beneficial and Indian dietary pattern has not shown the deficiency of phosphorus, ICMR-NIN (2020) has given same RDA for phosphorus as calcium for different population groups except for infants. Infants need little higher than calcium, i.e., for infants adequate intake recommended is 450 mg/day, i.e., 1.5 times the value recommended for calcium. RDA for phosphorus for Indian population is presented in Table 9.1A in Chapter 9.

Food Sources of Phosphorus

Most of the foods of daily use contain phosphorus, however, protein foods like meat, fish, egg, dairy products, legumes, nuts, and whole grains are rich sources and content in different foods as per IFCT, 2017 is shown in Figure 7.4.

Phosphorus is also high in processed foods because it is a component of several additives, such as phosphoric acid, monosodium phosphate, disodium phosphate, trisodium phosphate, monopotassium phosphate, dipotassium phosphate, tripotassium phosphate, etc. They are used for a variety of purposes, example as anticaking agent, to form ionic bridges, to interact with proteins and other charged hydrocolloids, and to prevent loss of carbonation caused by heavy metals and acidification in beverages. Cold drinks contain high amount of phosphorus in the form of phosphoric acid. Food grade phosphoric acid (additive E338) is used to provide sour and tangy taste and it is cheap in comparison to flavors obtained from lemons and limes. Excess of P disturbs the ratio of calcium:phosphorus and weakens the bones and other body systems.

Phosphorus is absorbed throughout the small intestine but the rate is higher from the jejunum. Most of the absorption is by passive diffusion. An active process is used by the body when phosphorus intakes are low. Bioavailability of phosphorus is lower from organic food, e.g., legumes (40%) while it is high from inorganic phosphorus sources like additives (nearly 100% has been observed in some studies). In plant foods, about three-fourths of the phosphorus is in the form of phytate. Therefore, not all of the phosphorus is absorbed unless the phytate has been degraded, by the phytase enzyme. Bioavailability is influenced by calcium intakes. If calcium intake is high, insoluble salts with P are formed, thus reducing absorption.

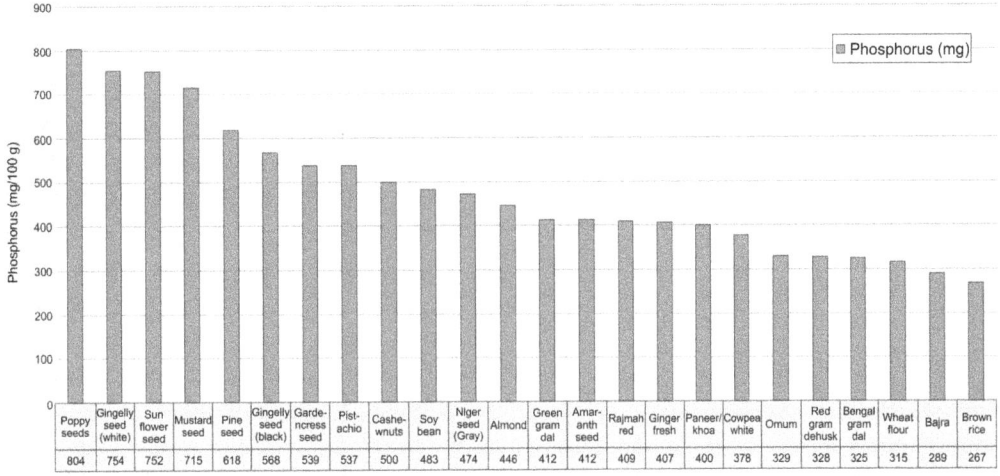

Fig. 7.4: Food sources of phosphorus.

Causes and Consequences of Deficient Intake of Phosphorus

Since phosphorus is abundantly available in dietary sources, deficiency of phosphorus alone is rare. Also, reabsorption by kidney is efficient and compensates for low intakes. However, it may occur along with calcium deficiency, since their absorption and metabolism are interlinked. Phosphate deficiency may also occur in starvation, if food intake is very poor and in the elderly.

Some underlying pathological conditions may result in low serum phosphorus level (hypophosphatemia). Phosphorus loss may occur in Crohn's disease and Celiac disease. Certain medications like antacids and diuretics may lower blood P levels. People suffering from hyperparathyroidism, diabetic ketoacidosis, liver cirrhosis, renal disease, bone disease, and sprue are found to have hypophosphatemia. Due to lack of P, there is accelerated bone loss and increased risk of fractures. Symptoms of phosphorus deficiency include loss of appetite, anemia, anxiety, bone pain, fragile bones, stiff joints, fatigue, irregular breathing, irritability, numbness, muscle weakness, and weight change. In children, decreased growth and poor bone and tooth development, and rickets may occur. Adults may suffer from osteomalacia. Patients may find difficulty in walking, numbness, and tingling of extremities, there is increased susceptibility to infection and likelihood of respiratory failure. Inherited disorders of homeostasis leading to wasting of phosphorus, can also lead to hypophosphatemia.

Causes and Consequences of Excessive Consumption of Phosphorus

Excessive phosphorus intakes are often accompanied by low calcium intake. High serum level of phosphorus is referred as hyperphosphatemia. High intake of phosphorus and low intake of calcium adversely affects the bone, disturbs calcium:phosphorus ratio in the bones, resulting in insufficient bone accretion and direct stimulation of the parathyroid gland. A high phosphorus diet has been shown to induce parathyroid hormone and FGF-23 release from bone. This has adverse effects like arterial calcification, endothelial dysfunction, and left ventricular hypertrophy. Bone loss is accelerated in certain pathological conditions like renal insufficiency. In chronic renal failure, there is less production of the biologically active form of vitamin D, calcium and P homeostasis is affected, parathyroid hyperplasia and secondary hyperparathyroidism can occur. Overuse of phosphate-containing laxatives can also lead to excessive intake of P. There is calcification of soft tissues, such as arteries, kidneys, muscles, and tendons. Some studies reveal that one of the causes of osteoporosis is also high serum level of phosphorus and that consumption of excessive amounts of cola beverages containing phosphoric acid is a risk factor.

> **Laboratory Laurel:** Though phosphorus is required for cell structure, cell signaling, energy transfer, and other important functions but excessive intakes of P can adversely affect skeletal, renal, and cardiovascular systems. Patients with chronic kidney disease (CKD) are more susceptible. Serum phosphorus is elevated with decrease in renal functions. These disturbances of bone mineral metabolism indicate increased risk of end-stage renal disease (ESRD), cardiovascular disease (CVD), and death. Authors have given the average intake in different stages of life and many other aspects of phosphorus metabolism. Animal studies are revealing but more human studies are needed.
>
> *Chang AR, Anderson C. Dietary Phosphorus Intake and the Kidney. Annu Rev Nutr. 2017;37:321-46.*

Phosphorus toxicity disrupts calcium metabolism and reduces utilization of calcium. It results in bone resorption as indicated by increased level of PTH and urinary excretion of calcium. Regular high phosphorus intakes can induce systemic complications. It induces aging process in mammals.

Magnesium

Magnesium was first used as medicine in the form of Epsom salts in 1697. Epsom salts were used to treat a wide variety of conditions. Later in 1755, Sir Joseph Black recognized it as an element and was isolated by Sir Humphry Davy from magnesia in 1808. But it is in 1926 that its essentiality for life was demonstrated by Johan Leroy. It is the 7th most abundant mineral in the earth's crust.

Magnesium (Mg) is of great importance in photosynthesis as it is centrally present in chlorophyll, as iron is present in hemoglobin. Mg is a major intracellular divalent cation, next to potassium and is a cofactor for hundreds of enzymes that are used in fundamental cellular reactions as well as phosphorylation involving ATP or GTP. The human body contains about 25 g of Mg and Mg^{++} is the second most abundant cation present in the intracellular compartment. At birth, the human body contains approximately 760 mg of magnesium which increases to about 5 g 4-5 months postnatally and then to the adult level. About 30-40% is found in muscles and soft tissues, and 1% is found in extracellular fluid in ionic form. It is present in serum, cerebrospinal fluid, sweat, and other body secretions—bile, saliva, and gastric juice. There may be several binding proteins for Mg^{++} such as calmodulin, troponin C, parvalbumin, and S100 protein.

Approximately one-third to two-thirds of the Mg that is ingested is absorbed, mainly through the jejunum and ileum, most probably through a saturable mechanism. Absorption is lower when the dose is higher and vice versa. However, the amount absorbed depends more on Mg status than on the intake. Its absorption is inhibited by phytate, phosphate, and protein. In the diet as well as in supplements, Mg is present in the form of one of the following: magnesium sulfate, magnesium hydroxide, magnesium chloride, magnesium oxide, magnesium oxalate, magnesium gluconate, and magnesium citrate. The solubility and efficiency of absorption of each of these is different, with magnesium citrate being the most soluble and magnesium oxide the least. Mg may also function as a second messenger. It is also required for metabolic activation and utilization of vitamin D, thiamine, and glutathione.

When magnesium enters the cell, it is buffered very fast by ATP, phosphonucleotides, and proteins. Magnesium is primarily found in bones (60-65%) but is not part of hydroxyapatite and the remainder is found in muscles, soft tissues, intracellular fluids, and other cells. It is largely excreted by the kidney. Hence, kidney has a major role in Mg homeostasis. Urinary loss is correlated with Mg and Ca concentrations in blood and with Mg intakes. Also, it may be influenced by hormones such as PTH, calcitonin, ADH (antidiuretic hormone), and glucagon.

Functions of Magnesium

Magnesium is required as a cofactor for more than 600 metabolic reactions and serves as an activator in about 200 reactions. Mg has an important role in physiological functions of the brain, heart, and skeletal muscles. It also has anti-inflammatory properties and is an antagonist to calcium. In essence, Mg has a role in almost every cellular process.

Energy metabolism: Mg plays a very important role in aerobic and anaerobic reactions, such as glycolysis, TCA, and oxidative phosphorylation. Most of the enzymatic reactions in carbohydrate and fat metabolism which particularly involve ATP or ADP, require magnesium (Mg^{++}) as the cofactor. ATP is generally complexed with Mg as Mg-ATP. Mg is required by the ATP synthesizing protein in mitochondria.

Structural role: Magnesium is a major constituent of bone matrix and is a part of cell membranes and chromosomes. It contributes to the synthesis of DNA and RNA and several proteins.

Ion transport: Magnesium is a cation that is essential for active transport of calcium and potassium across the cell membrane. Since it is present in ionic form in ECF, it helps to maintain balance and function of the sodium potassium pump. Mg affects conduction of nerve impulses, muscle contraction, and maintenance of normal heart rhythm. Thus, it helps to regulate blood pressure, blood sugar level, and muscle relaxation.

Synthesis of protein and other essential molecules: Mg is required in many steps for synthesis of nucleic acids and proteins. Enzymes involved in carbohydrate and lipid synthesis need Mg. Synthesis of glutathione which is an antioxidant is Mg dependent. It is also important for cell signaling and cell migration. It is necessary for the structure and activity of DNA and RNA polymerases. Other enzymes that need Mg are topoisomerases, helicases, protein kinases, exonucleases, cyclases, and ATPases. This implies that Mg is critical for amino acid and protein synthesis, DNA replication and RNA transcription, as well as maintaining genomic and genetic stability.

Muscle relaxation and muscle contraction: Magnesium present in smooth muscles facilitates the contraction as well as relaxation of muscles and helps to reduce muscle cramps. Mg influences the optimal functioning of muscles of organs, thus functioning of the heart and the kidney.

> ***Research Glimpse:*** Magnesium plays a role in several biochemical processes and its deficiency contributes to many health conditions. Evidence supports the use of magnesium in the prevention and treatment of many health problems such as migraine headache, metabolic syndrome, diabetes, hyperlipidemia, asthma, premenstrual syndrome, preeclampsia, and various cardiac arrhythmias, renal calculi, cataract formation, musculoskeletal diseases, and depression. Improving Mg intake can be a safe and useful therapy for several medical conditions. This review mentions where 300 Mg dependent enzymes are involved, e.g., in protein synthesis, muscle contraction, nerve functions, blood glucose control, hormone receptor binding, blood pressure regulation, cardiac excitability, transmembrane ion flux, gating of calcium channels, and energy metabolism. Researchers have described the causes of Mg deficiency.
>
> ***Schwalfenberg GK, Genuis SJ. The importance of magnesium in clinical healthcare. Scientifica (Cairo). 2017:4179326.***

Cell proliferation: Mg is involved in different phases of the cell cycle. The sensitivity of different cells varies in relation to availability of Mg; endothelial cells are highly sensitive, whereas tumor cells are very resistant.

Recommended Dietary Allowances for Magnesium

Wide variability in magnesium intake has been observed in different regional diets of India (540-1002 mg/day) and absorption also varies widely (13-50%). With these intakes, deficiency of magnesium has not been reported. ICMR-NIN (2020) has given the RDA and EAR for magnesium in Table 9.1A in Chapter 9 and in Appendix 4, respectively.

Food Sources of Magnesium

Magnesium is an integral part of chlorophyll, hence it is found in abundance in green leafy vegetables like spinach, etc. Nuts and seeds like pumpkin seeds, sesame seeds,

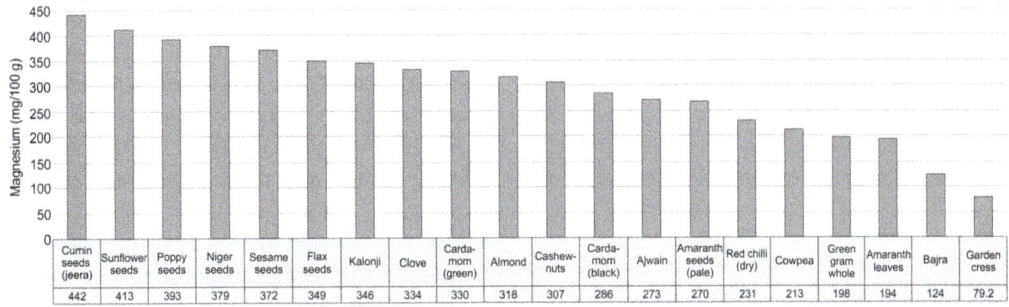

Fig. 7.5: Food sources of magnesium (mg/100 g).

hazel nuts, pine nuts, cashew nuts, and almonds are good sources. Among cereals, brown rice, buck wheat, whole grain cereals, bananas, and oat flakes contain magnesium. Peas, dried beans, and cocoa are also rich in magnesium. The Mg content according to the values given in the IFCT (2017) are depicted in Figure 7.5. Animal foods are not a good source of magnesium but seafoods like oysters and crabs are. Refining of foods reduces the magnesium content. Water is also an important source of Mg.

Deficiency of Magnesium—Causes and Consequences

Inadequate intake of magnesium impairs several biochemical processes dependent on this element. Hence, it can lead to many pathological conditions associated with these biochemical processes.

Mild and moderate stress can increase the demand for magnesium and if not met, lead to deficiency symptoms such as cramps, pain, and tingling in foot, hands, and calf muscles. Poor dietary pattern that contains more of refined foods can result in lower intakes of Mg. Since Mg is relatively soluble in water, it is readily depleted from the food. High fiber content (>40–50 g/day) and phytates bind Mg and reduce absorption and availability of Mg to the body. High intake of zinc (>140 mg/day) also reduces the Mg availability. Further, in case of PEM, there is reduced intestinal absorption and increased excretion of magnesium (diarrhea, use of laxatives), thus reducing the availability of magnesium. Vitamin D deficiency and use of certain drugs (some antibiotics, chemotherapeutic agents, diuretics) also tend to reduce absorption resulting in deficiency of this mineral. Pregnancy and stress can increase the requirement.

Treating deficiency even at subclinical level can prevent public health crisis, human suffering, and monetary loss. Its deficiency is also associated with alcoholism or use of excessive diuretics and malabsorption. Symptoms of magnesium deficiency (hypomagnesemia) include weakness and fatigue, muscle cramps, irritability, confusion, disorientation and loss of appetite, nausea, vomiting and hypertension, and personality changes. However, when the deficiency is more pronounced, there could be tremors due to increased neuromuscular excitability, muscle cramps, tetany, and generalized seizures. Mg deficiency may lead to hypocalcemia, osteoporosis, diabetes mellitus, and cardiac complications including cardiac dysrhythmia/arrhythmia, atrial and ventricular tachycardia, angina pectoris, dyslipidemia, and myocardial infarction. Mg deficiency is also associated with electrolyte abnormalities such as hypokalemia and hypocalcemia. Most of these are reversed by Mg supplementation.

In clinical settings, severe hypomagnesemia was associated with increased mortality. Low serum magnesium is commonly found in patients with type I and type II diabetes mellitus due to increased loss. Antacids, analgesics, anti-inflammatory drugs, medicines for diabetics, and BP and cholesterol lowering drugs reduce the absorption of Mg and increase its depletion. Hypomagnesemia due to loss of Mg can be caused by antibiotics, chemotherapeutic agents, diuretics, and proton pump inhibitors. Conditions that may lead to hypomagnesemia include alcoholism, poorly-controlled diabetes, and malabsorption (e.g., Crohn's disease, ulcerative colitis, celiac disease, short bowel syndrome, hyperparathyroidism and hyperthyroidism, aldosteronism, chronic kidney failure, and dialysis).

Magnesium deficiency has also been found to be linked to genetic defects such as Bartter syndrome or genetic transport disorders, autosomal dominant hypomagnesemia, Gitelman syndrome (kidney disorder having imbalance in charged ions like calcium, magnesium and potassium), maturity-onset diabetes of young, and SeSAME syndrome (genetic disorder seizures, characterized by ataxia (lack of muscle coordination intellectual disability and electrolyte imbalance).

Laboratory Laurel: A double-blind randomized clinical trial was conducted in 46 elderly subjects. Experimental group received 500 mg magnesium daily for 8 weeks and the other group received a placebo. Questionnaires of insomnia severity index (ISI), physical activity, and sleep log were completed at baseline and after the intervention period. Anthropometric confounding factors, daily intake of magnesium, calcium, potassium, caffeine, calories from carbohydrates, and total calorie intake were obtained using 24-hour recall for 3 days. Blood samples were taken at baseline and after the intervention period for analysis of serum magnesium, renin, melatonin, and cortisol. There was no significant difference in assessed variables between the two groups at the baseline. But after the intervention period, experimental group (Mg intake) showed significant improvement in sleep time, sleep efficiency concentration of serum renin, and melatonin, and simultaneously significant decrease of ISI score, sleep onset latency, and serum cortisol concentration. However, there was not much difference in the two groups with regard to sleep time in elderly people.

Abbasi B, Kimiagar M, Sadeghniiat K, et al. The effect of magnesium supplementation on primary insomnia in elderly: A double-blind placebo-controlled clinical trial. J Res Med Sci. 2012;17(12):1161-9.

Consequences of Excessive Intake of Magnesium

High intake of magnesium present in natural foods does not have any adverse effect. However, excessive use of magnesium supplements, magnesium-containing diuretics or antacids for prolonged duration can lead to toxicity. Excessive Mg intake can lead to diarrhea, nausea, loss of appetite, muscle weakness, irregular heartbeat, and impaired kidney function.

Sulfur

Sulfur is one of the most abundant elements (the 8th most abundant) in the earth's crust. Oxidation of elemental sulfur, sulfide minerals, or organic sulfur in the environment results in production of sulfate. Sulfur is an integral component of some organic compounds—the sulfur-containing amino acids, methionine and cysteine; vitamins like thiamine and biotin. It is present in glutathione, coenzyme A (CoA), lipoic acid, and sulfolipids. Sulfonic acid and chondroitin are present in cartilages and tendons. Inorganic sulfate is required for the synthesis of a compound called PAPS, i.e., 3'-phosphoadenosine-5'-phosphosulfate which is used by the body to synthesize important sulfur-containing compounds like chondroitin sulfate (cartilage around joints), keratan sulfate (cornea), heparan sulfate (extracellular matrix), and cerebroside sulfate (brain).

Sulfur is released during catabolism of protein in small intestine and is stored in all cells particularly of hair, nails, and skin. Sulfate is absorbed throughout the gastrointestinal tract. Absorption depends on sodium. More than 80% of soluble sulfate salts are absorbed but very little, almost next to nil absorption occurs when insoluble salts are ingested. Sulfate that is not absorbed in the upper gastrointestinal tract goes to large intestine and colon, from where it is reabsorbed or metabolized by anaerobic bacteria and the remaining is excreted in the feces. One of the metabolites is hydrogen sulfide.

Functions of Sulfur

The human body contains numerous sulfur-containing compounds:

1. It is present in disulfide linkages, which help to fold and shape the protein structures. These linkages further strengthen the structural part of the muscles, cartilages, and skin.
2. Being a component of many nutrients and metabolites, sulfur is directly or indirectly associated with the functions of compounds such as:
   a. Methionine, which is involved in transmethylation
   b. Cysteine, an important amino acid that is involved in disulfide linkages
   c. Thiamine, a vitamin and insulin, a hormone involved in carbohydrate metabolism
   d. Coenzyme A (CoA) needed for energy metabolism, metabolism of fatty acids, and formation of acetylcholine
   e. Sulfation and metabolism of phenolic compounds.
3. Detoxification is another advantage as liver uses sulfur to process the end products of normal metabolism or drugs.
4. It is a part of hydrogen sulfide (H_2S) that has several regulatory functions related to the central and peripheral nervous system, cellular metabolism, immunological/inflammatory responses, as well as vasodilatation, angiogenesis, inhibition of leukocyte adhesion, and cell death processes. Overproduction of H_2S has been implicated in pathogenesis of β-cell dysfunction.
5. Keratin is a sulfur-containing protein present in the outer layer of skin and is an important component of hair and nails.
6. Sulfur is needed for insulin production.
7. Sulfur is a part of glutathione, a very important antioxidant.

Research Glimpse: Sulfur is taken from amino acids methionine and cysteine, vitamins thiamine and biotin, and other valuable compounds like alliin (a precursor of allicin), glucosinolates (GSL), glutathione (GSH), and methylsulfonylmethane (MSM). Although cysteine is not an essential amino acid, its derivative—acetylcysteine or N-acetylcysteine—is used for pharmacological purposes such as mucus-dissolving therapy, acute renal failure, and psychiatric disorders. Allicin is used to prevent cardiovascular disorders. Glucosinolates from broccoli, cabbage, and turnip is reported to be useful in curing cancer. Glutathionate (GSH) reduces oxidative stresses and associated disorders like PEM, AIDS, burns, chronic digestive diseases, and alcoholism. Methylsulfonylmethane (MSM) is used for treating arthritis. Since plants obtain their sulfur from soil, adequate sulfur fertilization can play an important role in producing plant products with higher amounts of S-compounds.

Prasad R. Major sulphur compounds in plants and their role in human nutrition and health—An overview. Proc Indian Natn Sci Acad. 2014;80(5):1045-54.

Recommended Dietary Allowances for Sulfur

Sulfur requirements of the body are largely met by the degradation and turnover of methionine and cysteine. Hence, if the requirements for these two amino acids are met, sulfur requirements are met easily. Due to this, expert groups have not recommended an AI or EAR for sulfur.

Food Sources of Sulfur

Dietary intake comes from foods rich in protein, especially sulfur amino acids and other compounds. Vegetables of *Brassica* family like broccoli, cauliflower, cabbage, and turnip as well as onion and garlic are good sources. Drinking water is also a source of sulfur.

Deficiency of Sulfur

Diet high in processed foods containing cereals is usually deficient in sulfur. It is attributed to low intake of sulfur-containing amino acids. In laboratory animals, deficiency was associated with stunting. Inadequate intake of sulfur-containing amino acids is a risk. Deficiency of vitamins affects the functioning of the cell involving the sulfur-containing metabolites, leading to the production of dysfunctional cells. Cartilage remains weak due to poor formation of disulfide linkages. Since it is present in hair protein, keratin deficiency causes hair fall. Hence, increasing allicin-rich vegetable like garlic is found to be helpful in many chronic diseases.

Sulfur Toxicity

Usually, sulfur toxicity does not occur due to dietary sources. But consumption of inorganic sulfur (drugs and supplements) can be dangerous. Individuals whose intakes were high because of the high content of inorganic sulfate in drinking water have exhibited osmotic diarrhea caused by unabsorbed sulfate. The sulfate in the intestines also causes production of hydrogen sulfide, and excess of the hydrogen sulfide burdens the mucosal detoxification system in the intestines, leading to impairment in butyrate oxidation and inflammation of the epithelium in the colon. Consumption of "flowers of sulfur" has been found to cause metabolic acidosis. In rare cases, inborn error in sulfur metabolism is seen where utilization is abnormal.

In renal failure, serum sulfate levels are generally elevated. This can lead to complexation with calcium and in turn stimulate the parathyroid gland. The trans-sulfuration pathway is also affected and it contributes to elevated homocysteine levels seen in these patients. In hyperthyroidism, sulfate levels are increased possibly because of increased breakdown of protein and metabolism of amino acids including the sulfur-containing amino acids.

> **Methylsulfonylmethane (MSM)** is a naturally occurring sulfur compound and often used by body builders to reduce rigidity and inflammation in the body and eventually improve the workout.
>
> **Onion tears:** Onions contain sulfur-containing compounds. During cutting, cells are ruptured and odoriferous and volatile compound is released and irritates the eyes and tears come out. Vegetables of *Brassica* family like cabbage, cauliflower release sulfur-containing compounds on cooking, which give typical flavor.
>
> **Acid rain:** Sulfur dioxide emissions are of concern, since this gas reacts with water in the atmosphere and produces sulfuric acid, which results in acid rain. When this rain water enters the soil, it increases soil acidity and the sulfate content in ground water. Drinking water in these regions is likely to have higher sulfur content.
>
> **Sulfur spring:** It is a natural hot spring containing sulfur and believed to have curative properties.
>
> **Flower of sulfur:** It is a bright yellow powder of sulfur obtained from natural deposits of the mineral (also known as brimstone). Under a microscope, the tiny crystal resembles flower, hence the name. It is a natural and pure product.

Sodium

Sodium (Na) is an important micronutrient that has a vital role in maintaining body fluid balance. It is a major cation (Na^+) present in ECF (along with chloride) and can easily pass in and out of cells opposite to potassium. It is the principal ion in plasma, interstitial fluid, cerebrospinal fluid, and fluid between the joints. Table salt, i.e., sodium chloride, is the most common source of sodium. Dietary sodium is measured in milligrams and in milliequivalents or millimoles.

Sodium and its salts are highly soluble in the aqueous milieu in the intestines. Sodium is almost completely absorbed into the enterocytes with glucose, using the sodium/glucose co-transporter. Sodium concentration in blood is approximately 142 mmol/L. In a 70 kg adult, approximately 100 g of Na^+ is present, with half in bone and 40% in ECF. Sodium is lost mostly through urine, sweat and feces. Kidney plays an important role in regulation of sodium. Urinary excretion is the only means by which the body maintains sodium balance. Even in hot and humid environment, there is little loss through sweat and feces, since Na is lost through sweat, physical exertion and high levels of physical activity that results in more sweating, also result in Na loss. Sweating is increased by sympathetic activity whereas several hormones such as cholecystokinin and leptin decrease it. Renal excretion is modulated by glucocorticoids, insulin, PTH, epinephrine, norepinephrine, dopamine, and vasoactive intestinal peptide. Glucagon induces Na excretion. Persons who are insulin resistant have an impaired natriuretic (sodium excretion in urine) response to high-sodium intakes. Urinary losses increase with potassium administration.

Functions of Sodium

Maintains water and electrolyte balance: Sodium determines the concentration of both water and electrolytes in ECF and ICF and tightly regulates the gradients across cell membrane. All reactions, which require catalytic action of enzymes, require specific ionic strength that is provided by Na in ECF. Some reactions specifically require Na ions.

Maintains acid–base balance: Sodium works with chloride and bicarbonate ions to regulate acidity and alkalinity of the body fluids.

Helps in uptake of nutrients: Nutrients and metabolites are moved across the cell membrane by using the power of the sodium gradient. These nutrients include some amino acids, glucose as well as water. These mechanisms are also important in the kidneys for reabsorption of these nutrients. Sodium is an important determinant of membrane potential and hence active transport of substances across cell membrane.

Cell permeability and membrane potential: There are many transport systems through which biochemical substances and metabolites including the metabolic waste pass across the cell membrane. Sodium as an electrolyte (with chloride) plays an important role in cellular exchange via sodium pump and ATPase pump. Na^+ plays a role in maintaining concentration and charge differences across membranes. Generally, the concentration of potassium is approximately 30 times higher within the cell whereas that of sodium is about 10 times lower as compared to outside the cell. It is this difference that creates the electrochemical gradient or membrane potential. The control of cell membrane potential is very important for transmission of nerve impulses, muscle contraction, and cardiac function.

Muscle excitability: Sodium ions take part in transmitting nerve impulses along the nerve and muscle membrane resulting in nerve excitability and muscle contraction.

Maintenance of blood volume and blood pressure: Sodium produces osmotic pressure and has capacity to hold water in ECF, hence influences the blood pressure and the blood volume. There are baroreceptors in the circulatory system, which sense alterations in blood pressure. With any change, a signal is sent to both the nervous system and endocrine glands that in turn influence the kidneys to either retain sodium or vice versa. Under normal physiological conditions, sodium level in ECF is regulated. Kidney plays a role in retention of sodium and water to maintain blood volume. This is regulated by antidiuretic hormone and renin-angiotensin system. Sodium is excreted from the body and helps in maintaining the blood volume and blood pressure.

Provides taste: Salt is one of the basic tastes. It is used in almost all food preparations in almost every meal.

Food preservative: Since salt is hygroscopic, it draws water from the food making the surroundings such that microorganisms cannot grow. Also, due to osmotic effect, microorganisms are destroyed. Hence, salt acts like a preservative. Use of more than 12–16% salt in food preparations like pickles and sauces reduces the chances of food spoilage. Processed foods and savories contain high amount of sodium thus it is often advised to reduce their intakes.

> ***Research Glimpse:*** Sodium supports cellular homeostasis and several physiological functions. Though excess dietary intake of sodium is associated with high blood pressure (BP), its mechanisms are not yet completely understood. There is wide variability in salt sensitivity. Beyond high BP, sodium is also involved in alterations in renal function, fluid volume, fluid regulatory hormones, the vasculature, cardiac function, and the autonomic nervous system. Thus, high intake of sodium adversely affects the target organs, including the blood vessels, heart, kidneys, and brain. There are some controversies and some strategies for reducing dietary sodium and damage of vital organs.
>
> *Farquhar WB, Edwards DG, Jurkovitz CT, et al. Dietary sodium and health: More than just blood pressure. J Am Coll Cardiol. 2015;65(10):1042-50.*

Recommended Intakes for Sodium

People use salt without knowing its critical role in the body and its consequences. It provides taste to food and threshold value varies widely among people. Different food preparations need different amounts of salt. According to ICMR-NIN (2020), human body need less sodium from external sources like food. Table 7.1 gives the RDA for both sodium and potassium based on energy intake as well as maintaining the homeostasis across the cell membranes (K inside the cell and Na outside the cells) as both. The minimal amount of Na to replace losses is as little as 0.18 g or 8 mmol/day. ICMR-NIN (2020) has stated that one teaspoon of salt contains 2.3 g of sodium. In a day a healthy person can consume up to 1 teaspoon of salt per day. A person with hypertension is recommended to consume not more than 1500 mg sodium in a day. The World Health Organization in 2012 strongly recommended that adults' intake should be 5 g of salt or 2 g of sodium per day in order to reduce blood pressure and to reduce the risk of cardiovascular disease. Even for children and adolescents, parents/guardians must ensure that sodium intake should not exceed recommendations and intake of salt-containing snacks and other foods should be in controlled amounts. Persons, who are on medication and on supervised diets including those with type 1 diabetes mellitus or with cardiac failure, are not included.

> 1 g salt = 400 mg sodium (40%) and 6 g salt is 2,400 mg sodium

The World Health Organization further recommended that the guidelines for sodium should be implemented in conjunction with the guidelines for potassium and other nutrients. When it is extremely hot and a person is involved in intense physical activity that leads to profuse sweating, although sodium is lost in more amount in sweat, yet the food that is consumed is able to supply and replace the sodium that is lost and there is no need to make dietary changes or consume either supplements or specially formulated products.

It is noteworthy that there are persons who are salt sensitive because there are some individuals who will tend to retain fluid and their blood pressure could rise on the same level of salt intake compared to other persons who exhibit no change. The latter are said to be salt resistant. Alternatively, when the salt intake decreases, salt-sensitive persons will show a decrease in blood pressure. In normotensive adults, salt sensitivity is believed to predict the risk of developing hypertension in the future.

Food Sources of Sodium

Table salt or cooking salt is the major source of sodium. There are many other ingredients that are commonly used in food preparations that contain sodium such as baking soda or cooking soda (sodium bicarbonate), ajinomoto or MSG (monosodium glutamate), and sodium nitrite. In food preservation, salt is used as a preservative (12–16%) in pickles, papad, sauces, salting the fish, making brine in canned foods, etc. Salt is also present in butter, margarine, spreads, dips, cheese, some breakfast cereals, soup powders, bakery items, and several other processed and ready to eat foods, in varying quantities. Topical application of salt over salad or bland foods is a usual practice. Fried snacks usually contain more salt than non-fried ones. Sodium is inherently found in many fruits and vegetables. Meats also contain Na.

Some amount of sodium is naturally present in raw foods and the content given in the Indian Food Composition Tables (2017).

Salt replacers: Sodium intake is restricted in edema, high blood pressure, other cardiac problems, and renal disease. Such persons require other flavor enhancers to make food edible and tasty. Use of herbs, lemon, and change in cooking process can enhance the taste of the meal with minimum use of salt. Low-sodium salts generally contain potassium.

Table 7.1: Recommendations for sodium and potassium.

Life stage	Molar ratio	Sodium (mg/d)	Potassium (mg/d)
Adult men	1:1	2000	3500
Adult women	1:1	2000	3500
Infant −0−6 months	1:1	500	900
Infant − 6−12 months	1:1	650	1100
Children −1−3 years	1:1	1000	1750
Children −4−6 years	1:1	1300	2250
Children −7−9 years	1:1	1600	2825

Source: ICMR-NIN (2020). p 164.

Rock salt: It is obtained from rocks without processing. It is black in color hence referred as kala namak. It contains other minerals other than sodium and provides more salty taste. It is found useful in many digestive disorders.

Himalayan Pink salt: It has nothing to do with Himalaya. It has less sodium and also contain many other minerals in trace amounts. It is found useful in many aliments.

Sea salt: It is also known as Himalayan pink salt and there is variation in color. It also contains minerals and trace and ultratrace elements. It is also known as sendha namak that is popularly used during religious Hindu fasts.

Celtic salt: Celtic salt is also a sea salt, and gray in color. It is found in clay ponds near the seashore. Initially, it was harvested off the northwest coast of France using wooden tools and then left out in the sun and air to dry completely. It tastes less salty than table salt or other sea salts. Though Celtic sea salt is high in sodium, it also contains many other minerals and trace elements like magnesium, iron, manganese, zinc, iodine, and potassium. It is not processed mechanically or treated chemically. It is found useful in clearing mucus and lungs.

Kosher salt: It is normal kitchen salt but does not contain iodine. It is not often used as table salt. It is used in brining, flavoring herbs, spices and food. It is not a type of fine crystals but has rough edged crystals. Hence it is also used as abrasive in cleaning.

Deficiency of Sodium: Causes and Consequences

Sodium is depleted with the loss of body fluids particularly in diarrhea and vomiting. Athletes, heavy workers, or people, who often sweat more, lose sodium in sweat. Excessive use of diuretics can also decrease serum sodium level. Sodium excretion increases in Addison's disease.

> **Addison's disease:** It is a disorder where production of aldosterone hormone is reduced. This hormone is responsible for regulating the excretion of sodium and potassium from the kidney. Lack of aldosterone causes hyperkalemia.

When serum sodium level is below 125 mEq/L, the condition is called **hyponatremia.** It is characterized by weakness, giddiness, muscle cramps, lack of energy, convulsions, and cold extremities.

Consequences of Excess Sodium Intake

Many people habitually consume more salt for its taste. Excessive salt intake is injurious to health. When serum sodium level is above 150 mEq/L, the condition is called **hypernatremia.** Infants and elderly are at risk of developing hypernatremia. It is generally caused by reduced intake of water or increased loss of water or increased sodium intake. Some drugs also cause retention of salt in the body. There is decreased excretion of sodium as in case of high-lactate level during intense exercise. There is hyperactivity of adrenal cortex as in Cushing syndrome, leading to higher sodium levels.

In India, salt consumption habitually can go up to 10–20 g/day. Fluid retention and hypertension are common problems due to excessive intake of salt. This is especially so in susceptible persons (salt-sensitive) and in obese individuals. Salt sensitivity is a characteristic of an individual who responds to a high-salt intake with an increase in blood pressure. People with high blood pressure, diabetes, and renal disorder are usually salt sensitive. High-sodium intake is associated with increased calcium excretion.

Potassium

Potassium (K^+) is the most abundant cation in intracellular fluids (ICF) in the body. It works in conjunction with sodium to maintain the electrolyte balance. In blood, K level is 3.5–5.0 mEq/L; whereas in cells, K content is 155 mEq/L. K plays a significant role in cardiac muscle activity and any disturbances in potassium metabolism can have serious physiological consequences. Even small changes in the concentration of extracellular potassium affect the extracellular to intracellular potassium ratio, which in turn affects neural transmission, muscle contraction, and vascular tone. In the cell, the high concentration of K is maintained by the Na^+/K^+-ATPase pump, which is stimulated by insulin. Thus altered insulin concentrations in plasma can influence the influx of K into the cell and plasma concentration of K.

The Advisory Committee for Dietary Guidelines for Americans, in 2010, labeled potassium as a "shortfall" nutrient because many people do not make appropriate food choices and consume less amount of this mineral from their diets. It has been designated as a nutrient of concern.

Almost all (85–90%) of the dietary potassium is absorbed in healthy persons. K is excreted through urine (approximately 200 mg daily through urine). The ingested potassium does not greatly/significantly increase serum K^+. Excretion increases when intake increases. Small amounts are lost through feces and sweat and other secretions. Diarrhea causes large losses through feces. Body K is maintained by varying renal excretion. In the kidney, potassium is largely reabsorbed in the proximal tubule. Aldosterone hormone increases excretion. Catecholamines and insulin promote redistribution of K to the liver and skeletal muscles. Since kidney plays a very important role in excretion, when renal function is compromised, more K is retained in the body and its concentrations increase in blood. The body makes an attempt to regulate balance by increasing excretion (about one-third of dietary intake) through feces.

Homeostasis of K^+

Normal plasma levels for potassium in adults are 3.5–5.0 mEq/L. K^+ homeostasis is regulated by several factors. When a person consumes a K-rich meal, the pancreas is induced to secrete insulin. This hormone stimulates the Na-K pump, which in turn promotes K^+ uptake into muscle cells, thereby, minimizing the increase in plasma K^+. Aldosterone also regulates K^+ levels in plasma by increasing the activity of the Na-K ATPase pump promoting renal excretion by the kidney when K^+ levels in plasma rise. It also enhances K^+ secretion along the colon. This function becomes especially relevant in persons who have kidney disease. When K intake is low and/or there is loss of K^+ through urine, and the extracellular K^+ is reduced, K^+ is released from the intracellular compartment into plasma. When this happens, the skeletal muscle becomes insulin resistant to K^+, even prior to a decrease in the plasma level. Hypokalemia downregulates one of the isoforms of muscle Na-K ATPase resulting in entry of K^+ into plasma, there is inhibition of aldosterone release and urinary K⁺ secretion/excretion is reduced.

Other factors can also play a role. Activation of β2-adrenergic receptors by epinephrine leads to K⁺ moving into the intracellular compartment. Thus, any medications that block the β2-adrenergic receptors prevent the uptake of K⁺ into cells. Any disease or pathological state that affects the activity of Na-K pump or acid–base balance will disturb K homeostasis. Cell death or necrosis results in release of K⁺ from the intracellular compartment and disrupts homeostasis. Also, when exercise is strenuous or done for long duration, K is released by muscles. Generally, this is not a problem, but this may be of concern in special subgroups such as persons with diabetes mellitus or those who are prescribed beta blockers. Glucagon secretion can also promote renal excretion.

Functions of Potassium

Potassium is important for several cellular functions and acts as a cofactor for enzymes like Na-K-ATPase. Thus is essential for all cells, tissues, and organs for heart function, smooth muscle, and skeletal muscle contraction and thus, it is important for normal gastrointestinal and muscle function. It is important for cellular biochemical reactions, energy metabolism, protein synthesis, carbohydrate metabolism as well as for growth.

Electrolyte balance: Being the major cation (or electrolyte) inside the cell, it helps in maintaining the osmotic pressure and controls the entry of sodium into the cell. It is part of the Na/K pump. It is a major intracellular inorganic buffer (in the form of potassium bicarbonate). Potassium enters the cell and initiates sodium–potassium exchange across the cell membranes.

Acid–base balance: It is present in ionized form, aids in regulating the hydrogen concentration in the body fluid, and thus acid–base balance.

Maintenance of membrane potential: The differences in concentrations of K and Na across the cell membranes create an electrochemical gradient, i.e., membrane potential which is maintained by ion pumps especially the Na-K-ATPase pump. The pumps remove Na from the cell in exchange for Na. ATP is used for this process and about 20–40% of resting energy expenditure is used by the adult body for this activity. Control and regulation of membrane potential are vital for nerve impulse transmission, cardiac function, and muscle contraction. Both deficiency and excess result in disturbances.

Muscle activity: Along with sodium and calcium ions, K creates electrochemical impulses and tightly regulates the nerve transmission and nerve excitability. Thus, it regulates the activities of skeletal and cardiac muscles. It plays a key role in contraction of skeletal and smooth muscles. Thus, it is important for all muscular functions including digestion.

Cardiac function: Electrochemical impulses are dependent upon serum potassium concentration and the electrical gradient (potential) that is the result of the sodium–potassium flux. The electrical potential gradient helps to generate muscle contractions and also regulates the heartbeat. Slight alterations cause changes in the ECG. In hypokalemia, there is a characteristic additional U wave preceding and in the opposite direction of the normal T-wave.

Carbohydrate metabolism: When blood glucose is converted into glycogen, potassium also gets stored along with it. When glycogen is rapidly utilized, potassium is also lost, which needs replacement. The enzymes used in glycolysis and oxidative phosphorylation are potassium dependent such as pyruvate kinase and pyruvate carboxylase.

Protein synthesis: Muscle protein contains potassium. When muscle protein is broken down, potassium is lost and needs to be replaced. Potassium is also required for nitrogen retention.

Cofactor for enzymes: Some enzymes like require potassium, Na⁺/K⁺-ATPase and pyruvate kinase.

Recommended Intakes for Potassium

Desirable molar ratio of potassium:sodium (1:1 in mmol) is needed from diet to balance sodium intake. Potassium recommendations are important in pathological conditions like diarrhea, liver and kidney problems, and cardiac problems and during use of diuretics or other drugs. In certain conditions, supplements may be required other than dietary regulation of potassium intake. Adequate dietary K intake may have a preventive role in osteoporosis, hypertension, and stroke, although supplements may not have beneficial effect. About 3.5g/day potassium is recommended for adults in ICMR-NIN (2020). Recommended intakes for different age groups is given in Table 7.1.

Food Sources of Potassium

Potassium is generally found in plant and animal foods. Some of the rich sources are bananas, oats, mackerel, tuna, salmon, potato, sweet lime, orange, and coconut. Good sources are pulses, fruits, and vegetables. Nuts and oilseeds also contribute good amount of potassium. Some of the good food sources of potassium are reflected in Figure 7.6 using values from IFCT (2017). Wheat flour, rice, milk, eggs, and cheese are not good sources. Discarding water used for soaking or boiling results in loss of K due to leaching out from foods.

In unprocessed foods, potassium is mainly associated with bicarbonate-generating precursors like citrate and, to some extent, with phosphate. In processed foods and in supplements, potassium is generally present in the form of potassium chloride. Potassium metabisulfite (KMS) is commonly used food preservative. For persons with renal insufficiency, foods should be chosen very carefully.

Deficiency Symptoms of Potassium: Causes and Consequences

Most foods contain enough potassium and low-dietary intakes do not result in hypokalemia (serum K concentration < 3.5 mmol/L). Hypokalemia can result from excessive losses due to prolonged vomiting, use of diuretics, alcoholism, excessive use of laxatives, metabolic disturbances, and some forms of renal disease. However, deficiency is generally seen in anorexia and bulimia. There is redistribution of potassium

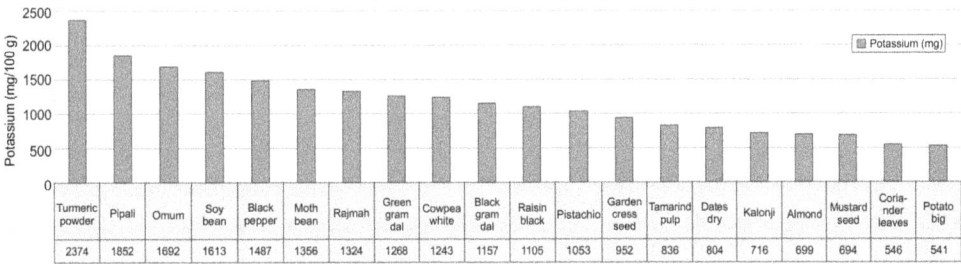

Fig. 7.6: Food sources of potassium (mg/100 g).

in case of excessive insulin, catecholamines or there is increased loss from the body. Coffee and alcohol can increase K excretion in the urine. Inadequate K intake is associated with increased risk of cardiovascular disease, in particular stroke. K deprivation has been found to increase urinary excretion of calcium.

Common deficiency symptoms are muscle cramps, weakness, lack of energy, stomach disturbances, lack of appetite, and mental apathy. Other neuromuscular symptoms are seen, e.g., paralysis, tetany. These symptoms are related to the alterations in membrane potential and cell metabolism. Intestinal function is affected resulting in constipation, bloating and abdominal pain, and vomiting. There may be polyuria. Moderate deficiency without hypokalemia is associated with elevated blood pressure, increased salt sensitivity, increased bone turnover and higher urinary calcium excretion, higher bone resorption, and higher risk of kidney stone formation. Severe hypokalemia results in cardiac arrhythmia, abnormal ECG, irregular pulse, rapid heartbeat, muscle paralysis, which may affect respiration, and decrease in blood pressure. Other cardiac effects are dysrhythmias. Acid–base imbalance and electrolyte disorders have been found to be associated with diabetes.

> **Laboratory Laurel:** Besides obesity, elevated blood pressure (BP) is also a risk factor in children and adolescents. Emerging findings indicate high dietary intake of sodium, is associated with high BP in them. Clinical studies have shown that higher potassium intake is able to lower blood pressure. Potassium deficit leads to an increase in blood pressure. However, studies on relationships of potassium intake with blood pressure in childhood are less. Some reports provide evidence that dietary intake of potassium-rich foods may lower blood pressure in adolescents with elevated blood pressure. Hence, it is advisable to encourage a diet for children that is high in potassium-rich foods.
>
> *Falkner B. Does Potassium Deficiency Contribute to Hypertension in Children and Adolescents? Curr Hypertens Rep. 2017;19(5):37.*

Consequences of Excessive Intake of Potassium

Elevated serum potassium level is referred to as hyperkalemia (blood values of potassium >5 mEq/L) that occurs when potassium intake exceeds the capacity of the kidneys to eliminate it. It is a serious matter in case of end-stage renal disease (ESRD) particularly in hemodialytic patients. Its causes are acute or chronic renal failure, hypoaldosteronism, and use of potassium—diuretics. Even in persons with normal kidney function, very high intakes, i.e., a single oral dose exceeding 18 grams may result in severe hyperkalemia. Hyperkalemia may also occur, if there is a shift of intracellular potassium into circulation, which is seen with hemolysis or tissue damage, in trauma or severe burns. Many a times, there may be no sign and there is a sudden rise in serum level of potassium leading to sudden death. To prevent and manage hyperkalemia, ESRD patients are advised to restrict potassium-rich foods such as nuts, seeds, beans, peas, lentils and tomatoes, potatoes, bananas at 2,000–3,000 mg/day or >200 mg/portion. Symptoms of hyperkalemia are irritability, nausea, decreased urine production, and cardiac arrest. Symptoms include tingling, numbness or burning of hands, feet, arms, or legs, paresthesiae, muscle weakness, and temporary paralysis. Elevated K levels (hyperkalemia) can cause cardiac arrhythmia and can result in cardiac arrest (one of the most important manifestations). Medical conditions associated with impaired urinary potassium excretion include diabetes, chronic renal insufficiency, end-stage renal disease, severe heart failure, and adrenal insufficiency. Elderly individuals are at increased risk of hyperkalemia because they often have one or more of these conditions or are treated with one of these medications.

Some persons manifest adverse reactions to potassium supplements. The most common side effects are gastrointestinal symptoms including nausea, vomiting, abdominal discomfort, and diarrhea. Ingestion of enteric-coated potassium chloride tablets has been associated with intestinal ulceration. Use of microencapsulated form may reduce gastrointestinal side effects; alternatively, the supplement should be ingested with the meal.

Chlorine

Chlorine is a halogen and is essential for life. It is an anion that usually occurs in association with sodium, is largely present in ECF (70%), and the rest in connective tissue. It is found in gastrointestinal secretions particularly HCl and cerebrospinal fluid. Chloride concentrations are maintained by the body within a narrow range. Normal plasma range of chlorine is 95–105 mEq/L. It is estimated that a 70 kg adult's body contains approximately 33 mmol per kg of body weight. In food, chloride ion (Cl^-) is commonly present. The Cl^- in both ECF and ICF, like Na^+ and K^+, is crucial. With Na^+ and K^+, chloride influences the amount of body fluid through their effects on osmolality and acid–base balance. The metabolism of sodium, chloride, and potassium are closely related. The body does not store Cl^-, hence, the body does not have the capacity to cope with either inadequate or excessive intakes for a prolonged period.

Most of the chloride in the diet comes from salt, i.e., NaCl. Some chloride is also absorbed with other nutrients, viz. cationic and neutral amino acids, carnitine, taurine, proline, and hydroxyproline. Besides this, chloride is secreted in large amounts in the stomach as part of hydrochloric acid. Some chloride is also secreted by the intestinal epithelium and pancreas. Almost all of the chloride, obtained from diet or of endogenous origin, is absorbed completely.

Functions of Chloride

Provides salty taste: Chloride ion in salt (sodium chloride) is responsible for salty taste.

Electrolyte balance: Chloride ion helps to maintain electrochemical gradient and normal osmotic pressure in ECF along with sodium and determines ECF volume.

Acid–base balance: It plays a significant role in maintaining pH in blood through bicarbonate buffer.

Acid production: Chloride is part of the hydrochloric acid secreted by the stomach. The HCl provides acid medium in the stomach, which is necessary for digestion of protein. HCl also provides an unfavorable environment for many microorganisms.

Immune response: White blood cells (WBCs) like macrophages and monocytes use chloride ion to secrete myeloperoxidase, hypochlorous acid with hydrogen peroxide in order to kill invading pathogenic bacteria.

Activation of enzymes: Some enzymes require Cl^- for their activity, which depends on ionic strength. One example is angiotensin-I converting enzyme (ACE), which plays an important role in regulating blood pressure.

Helps in transmission of nerve impulse: Chloride ion coordinates with cations like Na^+, K^+/Ca^{++} in transmission of nerve impulses. When cells are excited, there is rapid change in movement, which generates some current (–70 mV to 40 mV).

It is also important for transport of important biological compounds. During transport of some compounds, chloride is exchanged for another anion, e.g., alpha-taurine and L-glutamate.

> Chlorine is a highly reactive molecule composed of 2 atoms. It is also a poisonous/corrosive gas. However, it is used in chlorination of water for water purification but the content of residual; chlorine should not exceed 1 PPM in potable water.
>
> **Chloride** is an ion, which is essential to body functioning in humans.
>
> **Chlorine** is an element, which helps to make drinking water safe, free from germs.

Recommended Dietary Allowances for Chloride

No RDA has been recommended. Intakes need to balance with the amount lost. The Institute of Medicine, USA has set the AI at a level equivalent to that of sodium on a molar basis. The AI (Adequate intake) for younger adults is 2.3 g or 65 mmol/day.

Food Sources of Chloride

Food sources include meat, pickles, and all foods containing salt. Fruits and vegetables do not contain much chloride. Salt substitutes like potassium chloride can contribute to intake. Chloride content of processed foods from sodium contents can be calculated from sodium contents by a simple formula:

$$\text{Chloride content} = 1.5 \times \text{Na content}$$

Average consumption of salt 6 g (2,400 mg sodium)

$$\text{Chloride content} = 1.5 \times \text{Na content} = 3{,}600 \text{ mg chloride}$$

Deficiency of Chloride: Causes and Consequences

Kidney excretes excess chloride (urine is the main route) and some is lost through sweat and feces. Loss through sweat is estimated to be approximately 1 g/L. However, losses are more under conditions when sweating increases such as physical exertion or fever and in a highly humid climate. Use of diuretics can increase urinary loss. Urinary losses generally reflect dietary intake. Chloride losses generally occur along with sodium losses. Vomiting is an important cause of chlorine deficiency due to loss of chloride with gastrointestinal hydrochloric acid. Similarly, very low intakes or conditions associated with excessive loss can cause deficiency. Fasting may also lead to low intake. Due to deficiency, there is hypotension resulting in weakness and dizziness. Chloride deficiency results in hypochloremic metabolic alkalosis. In children, deficiency was found to result in growth failure, lethargy, irritability, gastrointestinal symptoms, and weakness.

Causes and Consequences of Excessive Intake of Chloride

Excessive intakes can elevate blood pressure. Some individuals have been found to be genetically susceptible. Blood pressure can rise when other risk factors like obesity are present. Hyperchloremia occurs when blood chloride level exceeds the normal range. Rise in blood pH can be dangerous (5% can be fatal). Oral/intravenous fluid administration of chlorine and other minerals needs to be replenished to restore the blood pH.

> Chloride ion in cut fruits and vegetables prevents discoloration.
>
> Sucralose, an artificial sweetener, contains chloride, which makes sucralose more stable as compared to other sweeteners.

TRACE ELEMENTS

Trace elements are nutritionally essential minerals required in trace amounts. They differ from major minerals in terms of their daily requirement and the amount present in the body. The body contains less than 5 g of the trace elements. Daily requirements of the trace elements are less than 100 mg/day. They are found in both plant and animal food sources. They play vital roles in numerous regulatory and structural roles. Trace elements include iron, iodine, zinc, selenium copper, fluoride, manganese, chromium, and molybdenum. Trace elements are also referred to as microminerals. Trace elements are difficult to measure and their roles in human nutrition and health are important areas for research. They participate in many chemical reactions having the role of cofactors. Deficiency of any one of these can halt some

cellular functions like cellular respiration, DNA synthesis, and energy metabolism. There are certain situations when the need for trace elements may be more significant. These are:
- Inborn errors of metabolism
- Malnutrition, diseases, injury, or stress
- Drug nutrient interaction
- Enhanced requirement
- Cumulative effect of the deficiency over a long period of time.

Iron

Iron is one of the most abundant elements (4th most abundant) in the earth's crust. It has a legacy as a constituent of hemoglobin and is virtually utilized by all living cells. Iron is a part of biologically important compounds like heme. Heme is part of some biologically important proteins known as hemoproteins. Hemoglobin has the unique property to pick oxygen from lungs and deliver through the capillary bed in tissues. It provides red color to the red blood cells. One of the major functions of iron is to transport oxygen to the cells. It is important for metabolism of all living organisms because it is a component of innumerable proteins including enzymes. Thus iron plays an important role in biological functions that include oxygen transport, DNA synthesis, cell growth, and replication. Iron is needed for biosynthesis of lipids and cholesterol.

Iron has been used by man since the beginning of civilization for various health ailments. Although it is ubiquitous, its deficiency is widespread in both industrialized and developing countries. In biological systems, the oxidation states are generally Fe^{2+}, i.e., ferrous, and Fe^{3+}, i.e., ferric; both forms being interchangeable. Addition of an electron to Fe^{2+} converts to the ferric (Fe^{3+}) and subtraction/removal from the ferric brings it back to the ferrous state. Thus, iron participates readily in various oxidation–reduction reactions. It can give rise to the hydroxyl radical (OH^-). This hydroxyl radical can cause oxidative stress resulting in lipid peroxidation as well as damage to proteins, carbohydrates, and nucleic acids. Perhaps due to this, in the cell, the amount of free iron is restricted to prevent the possibility of toxic damage.

Iron metabolism is unique in some aspects:
- There is no efficient physiological mechanism for getting rid of excess iron.
- It has mechanisms for maintaining balance, preventing deficiency as well as overload.
- Its absorption is regulated.
- Iron present in the RBC is reutilized.
- There is a storage protein (ferritin).

Functions of Iron

Iron plays an important role in several metabolic functions:

Oxygen transport: Iron is a constituent of hemoglobin and myoglobin. Both proteins contain heme and are oxygen-binding proteins and iron is the main acceptor of oxygen. Hemoglobin, which is present in the red blood cells continuously transports oxygen to all parts of the body. It contains about two-thirds of total body iron. Similarly, myoglobin transports oxygen to muscle cells to fulfill their demand for oxygen. Neuroglobin another protein is present in the central nervous system. It increases the availability of oxygen to the brain and provides protection even under hypoxia (lack of O_2 supply).

Energy metabolism: Iron is bound to heme and participates in electron transfer reactions when it is associated with cofactors such as Cytochrome P450 and some of the enzymes involved in the respiratory chain such as NADH dehydrogenase, Cytochrome C oxidase. Thus, iron is important for release of ATP. Cytochromes are the proteins in which heme is a cofactor. Cytochromes play an important role in the electron transport chain that occurs in the mitochondria and produces energy. Cytochromes are electron carriers and are important in ATP synthesis. Cytochrome P450 plays a role in metabolism of fatty acids, prostaglandins, steroids, sterols including the three fat-soluble vitamins—A, D, and K, besides being very important for drug/xenobiotic metabolism and detoxification. Other iron-containing enzymes (do not contain heme) play a role in the citric acid cycle and thus iron contributes to energy metabolism.

Brain functions: Iron is required for the formation of myelin sheath around nerve fibers and synthesis of neurotransmitters, which are necessary for optimal functioning of the brain. Iron, in the brain, is required for oxygen transportation. Iron homeostasis is needed to maintain normal physiological brain and neurological functions. Brain iron concentrations increase with age. In deficiency, brain iron decreases. Myelin synthesis as well as its maintenance requires high amount of iron, with oligodendrocytes requiring a constant supply. In brain, white matter contains more amount of iron than does gray matter. Iron is extremely essential for normal cognitive functions.

Component of nonheme proteins: Iron is present in many transport and storage, such as ferritin, transferrin, haptoglobin, hemopexin, and lactoferrin.

Component of many enzymes: There are many iron-containing enzymes, which play significant roles in oxidation and reduction reactions that are needed for anabolic and catabolic functions such as the synthesis of purines, RNA, DNA, and steroid hormones. It is also a part of several enzymes that are involved in metabolism of many nutrients such as enzymes involved in niacin synthesis, and those involved in degradation of serotonin and melatonin. Iron is a part of enzymes that generate peroxides and nitrous oxide, which have a role in cell signaling pathways. These include aconitase, catalase, cytochrome C, cytochrome C reductase, cytochrome oxidase, aconitase, succinic dehydrogenase, formiminotransferase, peroxidase, xanthine oxidase, and tryptophan pyrrolase, tryptophan hydroxylase. Iron is needed for ribonucleotide reductase that reduces the sugar group of nucleotides to corresponding deoxy derivatives, the precursors of DNA. If this enzyme is decreased, DNA synthesis will be impaired with resultant effects on all cell functions.

Cofactor for enzymes: Iron is required as a cofactor by enzymes like phenylalanine hydroxylase, tyrosine hydroxylase, tryptophan hydroxylase, lysine hydroxylase, prolyl hydroxylase and asparaginyl hydroxylase, as well as ribonucleotide reductase and hypoxia-inducible factor (HIF) is a transcription factor that binds to response elements in genes that code for proteins that are involved in the body's response to hypoxia. When HIF binds to these genes, there is increased synthesis of the proteins involved in the compensatory response to hypoxia.

> **Iron-containing enzymes involved in metabolism of different nutrients are:**
>
> β-carotene 15,15′-dioxygenase—converts beta carotene into vitamin A
> Retinal dehydrogenase—converts retinaldehyde to retinoic acid
> Phenylalanine hydroxylase—important for metabolism of phenylalanine
> Tyrosine 3-monooxygenase—involves in catecholamine and melanin synthesis
> Tryptophan 5-monooxygenase—involves in serotonin metabolism

Pro-oxidants, immunity, and detoxification: Fe^{2+} readily converts hydrogen peroxide into hydroxyl radicals, which are highly reactive. These are important in defense systems used by WBC but an imbalance between highly reactive free radicals and antioxidant defense systems may cause damage. Heme-containing enzymes protect the cells from the hydrogen peroxide and convert it in oxygen and water. It also helps to metabolize drugs and pollutants.

However, it is important to remember that some antioxidant enzymes like catalase and peroxidases contain heme, and these enzymes have a protective role in terms of protecting the cells against accumulation of hydrogen peroxide—a reactive oxygen species. Its role as a pro-oxidant can also be viewed as beneficial from the perspective of immunity. WBCs expose bacteria that they have engulfed to reactive oxygen species and use this as the mechanism to destroy pathogens. For synthesis of the required ROS, the cells have the enzyme myeloperoxidase, which is also a heme-containing enzyme.

Very low "free" iron concentrations are generally maintained to limit free radical generation and to prevent iron becoming available to pathogens that need iron.

Thyroid hormones: Iodide peroxidase—a heme enzyme—oxidizes iodide and is involved in generation of thyroxin and triiodothyronine.

Protein modification: Some proteins undergo post-translational modification. The enzymes involved in this process are iron-containing enzymes.

Fatty acid metabolism: The enzyme stearoyl-CoA desaturase is involved in production of oleic acid and linoleoyl-CoA desaturase is involved in production of arachidonic acid from linoleic acid. Both these enzymes add double bonds to the fatty acyl chains that contain iron.

DNA replication and repair: Repair of DNA as well as DNA replication requires deoxyribonucleotides, the synthesis of which is catalyzed by ribonucleotide reductases, which are iron-dependent enzymes. Other enzymes involved in DNA synthesis and repair are DNA polymerases and DNA helicases, which are Fe-S cluster proteins. It has been found that when intracellular iron was depleted, there was inhibition of cell cycle progression, growth, and division.

Iron Homeostasis in the Body

The human male body contains approximately 3.8 g iron (female body contains 2.3 mg). There are 3 forms of iron in the body, shown below, and each perform different functions.
1. **Functional iron:** Hemoglobin, myoglobin, and cytochromes
2. **Transport iron:** Transferrin
3. **Storage iron:** Ferritin and hemosiderin.

A large amount (80%) of functional iron is present in hemoglobin and the rest is in myoglobin and cytochromes. It is transported in the form of transferrin and stored as ferritin and hemosiderin in liver, spleen, and bone marrow.

Very little body iron is excreted but there are basal losses and menstrual losses, and iron is used for new tissue synthesis. This is compensated by absorption of about 1–2 mg of dietary iron. Body regulates it by balancing the absorption, transport, storage, and losses. Iron absorption (1–2 mg) occurs in small intestine (duodenum and jejunum). Absorption is better in the duodenum than in the rest of the small intestine.

Iron metabolism is tightly regulated, so that the amounts of the metal entering the circulation from its 2 major sources—macrophages that recycle iron from red blood cells (RBCs) and duodenal epithelial cells that absorb iron from the diet—are kept in balance with systemic requirements.

Free iron is potentially toxic because it is involved in generation of free radicals that can lead to oxidative stress and cell damage. Therefore, it is critical that there is regulation of iron homeostasis. There are several proteins, i.e., hepcidin, ferroportin (FPN) transferrin receptors and ferritin which play crucial role in iron metabolism and homeostasis.

More importantly, iron transport through different compartments in the body is tightly regulated. This includes those cells in which iron is stored, such as erythroblasts, circulating macrophages, hepatocytes, and other tissues. The intracellular stores of iron are regulated based on the body's needs. Hepcidin is an important peptide involved in regulation. It is synthesized by hepatic cells and induces the internalization and degradation of ferroportin-1. The role of ferroportin-1 is to regulate release of iron from different cells like enterocytes, hepatocytes, and macrophages into plasma. Not much hepcidin will be synthesized when there is iron deficiency anemia and the body does not have much iron. As a result, iron from the diet can be absorbed and iron can be mobilized from its storage sites. If the body iron stores are adequate or under conditions of iron overload, hepcidin will inhibit dietary iron absorption, promote sequestration of iron into cells, and overall reduce the availability of iron. Hepcidin is upregulated in inflammation; it is suggested that it has a role in innate immunity because it limits the amount of iron available to the infecting organisms.

Thus, the body has proteins that are involved in storage, transport, and utilization of iron. In the messenger RNAs of these proteins, there are iron-responsive elements known

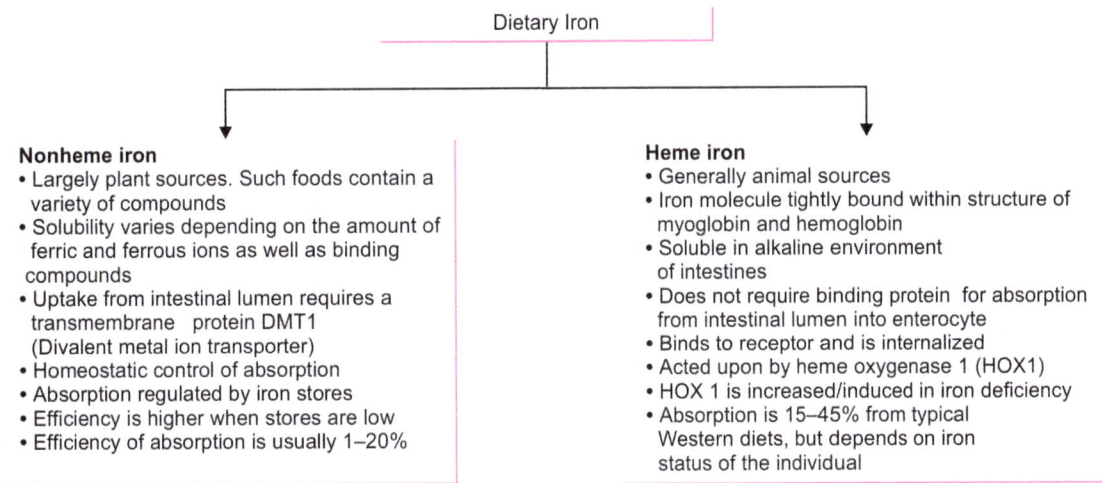

Fig. 7.7: Forms of dietary iron.

also as IREs. Iron regulatory proteins bind to IREs (on mRNA) and influence stability and translation of the mRNAs, thus they control how much of ferritin and transferrin receptor-1 are synthesized.

When body iron is low, less iron will bind to IRPs, which can then bind to IREs and vice versa. When more iron binds to IRPs, their binding to IREs on mRNA is prevented. As a result, more storage proteins but fewer amounts of the transporters are synthesized.

Most of the body iron is in the RBCs (approximately 3.5 mg per gram of hemoglobin). Aged RBCs are destroyed in the spleen and the heme is recycled (approximately 20 mg per day). This iron, which is released, is either deposited with ferritin in the spleen macrophages or exported by ferroportin-1 to transferrin the carrier protein that will deliver iron to other tissues.

To avoid iron toxicity, body regulates iron absorption through intestinal cells. In the diet, iron is present in two forms: heme and nonheme iron (Fig. 7.7).

Dietary iron is exposed to the acid in the stomach and then pancreatic and intestinal enzymes. In the stomach, inorganic iron is solubilized and ionized by the gastric acid and reduced to the ferrous form. It is kept solubilized since it is chelated to citric acid and ascorbic acid. The nonheme iron in the diet is said to enter a "pool" of iron in the upper gastrointestinal tract. Absorption from the intestines depends on whether the iron is heme or nonheme iron:

i. **Heme iron:** It is absorbed intact into the intestinal mucosal cell. Here, it is acted upon by the enzyme heme oxygenase and the iron (Fe^{3+}) is released. Absorption of heme iron is neither increased nor decreased by any factors such as citrate or any inhibitors. This mechanism is not fully understood but a heme-binding protein (HEBP-1) contributes to iron transport across the brush border membrane.

ii. **Nonheme iron**: There are separate pathways for uptake of ferrous and ferric ions (Fig. 7.8). Absorption is influenced by composition of the meal. Phytates, tannins, and polyphenols are inhibitors and hence bioavailability of iron from foods containing these and fiber is low.

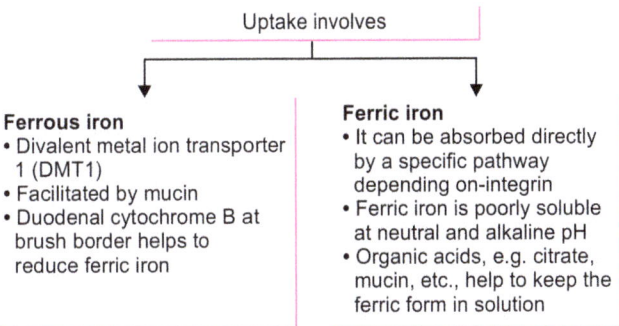

Fig. 7.8: Uptake of ferrous and ferric iron.

Within the enterocyte, the ferric form is converted to ferrous iron by a pathway involving a number of compounds such as β2-macroglobulin, integrin, mobilferrin, and GTP-binding protein. Some amount of iron is then combined with ferritin and stored within the enterocyte. When the enterocyte is shed (lifespan of enterocytes is 2–3 days), with it iron enters the intestinal lumen again. This mechanism is effective in limiting iron absorption.

The remaining iron (not bound to ferritin in the enterocyte) is bound to ferroportin 1 or metal transport protein 1 (MTP1), which moves the iron across the membrane into blood plasma where the iron may associate with ceruloplasmin or hephaestin. The ferrous iron "pool" is now oxidized into ferric ions by oxidizing enzymes ferroxidase, hephaestin, and ceruloplasmin.

Whether the iron in the enterocyte is to cross the basolateral membrane or not appears to be determined by a compound that is a "signal" to the enterocytes. This compound present in plasma is hepcidin, a plasma protein released from liver in proportion to iron stores. Hepcidin is regulated by binding receptors, which alter the release of iron. Hepcidin communicates:

- To the binding proteins within the cell to move iron to ferritin (binding would happen, if iron status is good and vice versa).
- To the luminal membrane to change the amount of iron taken into the cell, thus it prevents iron overload.

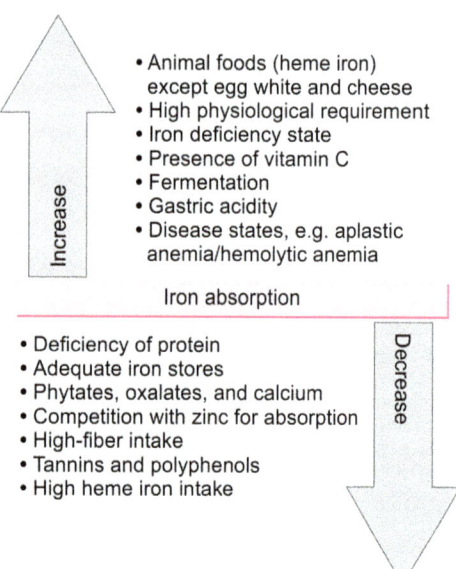

Fig. 7.9: Factors affecting iron absorption.

In blood, the iron is bound to transferrin, which ferries the iron from one organ to another. Transferrin production and saturation also depend on iron status. In an iron-replete person, transferrin saturation is high. In severe deficiency, it can be as low as 5%. When transferrin saturation is less than 15%, the person is said to be iron-deficient.

The body regulates iron absorption based on the iron status and the poorer the status, more is the amount of iron that is absorbed. Normally, about 8% of dietary iron from typical Indian mixed vegetarian diets that are cereal-pulse based. Iron absorption is increased during infancy (6–24 months), pregnancy (IIIrd trimester), blood loss, and in case of iron deficiency. In older persons, absorption is reduced due to decline in HCl secretion in the stomach. Many other factors affect iron absorption in the body as shown in Figure 7.9.

Storage: In a well-nourished adult man, about 30–40 mg iron per kilogram of body weight is present, although in women the amount is lower. Iron is stored in ferritin from which it can be mobilized, whenever there is need for iron. When there is more iron than can be bound by ferritin, the iron is bound to hemosiderin. Unlike ferritin, hemosiderin releases iron slowly.

Excretion and losses: Small amounts of iron are excreted through bile, urine, and skin. Women lose some iron through menstrual blood loss. It is estimated that approximately 30 mL blood is lost during each cycle, which is equivalent to approximately 1.5–2.0 mg iron. Women who use oral contraceptives have lower losses, whereas with use of intrauterine devices, loss may be more.

Recommended Dietary Allowances of Iron

Recommendation of iron is largely based on bioavailability of iron and basal iron losses from the body. Basal or obligatory loss is the loss from skin or exfoliated skin, desquamated gastrointestinal cells, bile, and urine and is proportional to body size or body surface area. Total basal loss of iron in an adult man weighing 65 kg can be 14 µg/kg body weight/day. For adult women, taking into consideration daily basal loss and menstrual iron loss, the RDA for iron is estimated to be 29 mg/day. During growth, expansion of blood volume and increase in lean body mass occur. These two factors are taken into consideration for computing the iron requirement during growth, i.e., for infants, children, and adolescence. It is also taken into consideration that allowances should allow for iron stores to be built up and maintained. Iron requirements vary with body weight as well as periods of growth including pregnancy. RDA and EAR for iron is given in Table 9.1A in Chapter 9 and Appendix 4.

Food Sources of Iron

Both plant and animal foods are good sources of iron but both contain two different types of iron, which significantly affect utility of iron in the body. These two types of iron are:

1. **Heme iron:** It is found in animal foods except dairy products and is better absorbed.
2. **Nonheme iron:** It is found in plant foods like green leafy vegetables, legumes, wholegrain cereals.

This type of iron is poorly absorbed but addition of vitamin C can enhance its absorption/uptake into mucosal cells and prevent the formation of insoluble and unabsorbable iron compounds. Therefore, it is advisable to consume vitamin C-rich foods like lemon, amla, guava, and orange along with major meals. Green leafy vegetables, like coriander, mint and curry leaves, dried beans (black gram, cowpeas), peaches, apricot, dates, cherries, and raisins, are rich sources of iron. Turmeric is also a good source of iron. As per ICFT (2017) values some of the food sources of iron are given in Figure 7.10.

In general, yeast and animal products like meat, liver, and egg are excellent source of bioavailable iron. However, milk and milk products are poor sources of iron.

Deficiency of Iron: Causes and Consequences

Iron deficiency is widely prevalent, affecting billons of people worldwide. Children and pregnant women are most afflicted. In India, 50–70% of women, infants and young children, and

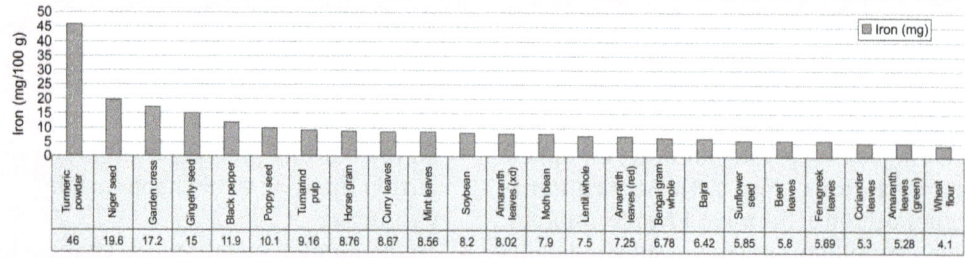

Fig. 7.10: Food sources of iron (mg/100 g).

adolescents suffer from anemia, most of which is caused by iron deficiency. Iron deficiency occurs due to several reasons:
- Low intake of iron-rich foods
- Low intake of animal foods containing heme iron
- Low intake of vitamin C-rich foods along with food containing nonheme iron
- High intake of plant foods containing phytates, oxalates, and polyphenols, which inhibit iron absorption
- High intake of tea and coffee
- Poor absorption of iron in the intestine
- Less amount of acid secretion in stomach, particularly in old age
- High body requirement and low supply of iron, e.g. pregnancy
- Worm infestation, *Helicobacter pylori* infection
- Malaria (*Plasmodium falciparum* requires and utilizes iron)
- Low immunity
- Low birth weight
- Physiological blood loss during menstruation and at the time of delivery
- Blood loss during accident, hemorrhage including gastrointestinal hemorrhage, surgery, or donation of blood
- Gross abnormalities in bone marrow particularly in the presence of vitamin E deficiency
- Use of some drugs such as aspirin, nonsteroidal anti-inflammatory drugs, and corticosteroids
- Ulcerative colitis, colon cancer
- Regular and frequent blood donation.

Iron deficiency results in symptoms which are nonspecific. Common symptoms of anemia are general weakness, apathy, tiredness/fatigue, shortness of breath upon exertion, chest pain, intolerance to cold or heat, irritability, headache, dizziness or lightheadedness, uncomfortable tingling or crawling sensation in legs and other changes such as increased susceptibility to infection due to decreased immunity. Clinical signs include glossitis, angular stomatitis, koilonychia (spoon-shaped nails). In children, there may be poor appetite. Some persons develop craving for non-nutritive substances, e.g., dirt or mud (pica including geophagia), ice (pagophagia). Examination of RBC will show microcytic hypochromic anemia. These symptoms can vary depending upon different stages of anemia. Anemia is seen in the third stage, when iron stores are depleted.

There are many types of anemias commonly referred as nutritional anemia. All anemias are not due to the deficiency of iron. They can be caused by deficiency of other nutrients like vitamin B_6, folic acid, and vitamin B_{12}.

Stages of Anemia
Anemia is a condition in which the body has less than the normal number of healthy red blood cells. A person is said to be anemic when his/her hemoglobin is less than the normal value. There are three stages before anemia, i.e., low hemoglobin level occurs. Characteristics of different stages are (Fig. 7.11):

Stage I: Iron stores are beginning to be depleted and there is reduction of ferritin but there are no symptoms of deficiency. At this stage, hemoglobin levels are normal.

Stage II: There is decrease in transferrin and increase in erythrocyte protoporphyrin resulting in symptoms like fatigue. In this stage, there is inadequate iron for sufficient hemoglobin in new RBC and for other physiological functions.

Stage III: Iron deficiency (anemia) is visible with low-hemoglobin level in blood. There is decrease in red blood cell size and hematocrit (concentration of RBC in blood).

In iron deficiency, because of less hemoglobin, the RBC is small and the anemia is called microcytic hypochromic anemia. Iron deficiency also results in other changes, which adversely affect health and well-being as well as productivity. These are the functional consequences of iron deficiency. These effects are due to reduction in hemoglobin, myoglobin, as well as the various iron-containing enzymes. They include:
- Alterations in immune function/immunity
- Alterations in endurance capacity and metabolic functions
- Changes in behavior and cognitive functions.

Alterations in immune function/immunity: In under-nourished persons, iron deficiency has been found to be associated with impaired immunity. Iron is necessary for proliferation and maturation of immune cells, particularly lymphocytes, which can generate specific response to infection. Iron deficiency alters the proportion and function of various T cell subsets and leads to immunologic dysfunction. Immune response is compromised in subclinical iron deficiency in which hemoglobin is normal, but there is reduced serum ferritin, decreased transferrin saturation, and elevated free erythrocyte protoporphyrin. The body has the capacity to reduce the iron availability to be consumed by infectious elements by proteins such as transferrin and lactoferrin.

Iron is also essential for the proliferation of bacteria, parasites, and neoplastic cells. Hence, extra iron dose may facilitate growth of bacteria, which is already in excess during infection. Certain immune cells interfere with bacterial growth and reduce availability of iron.

Muscle endurance: Due to decreased availability of oxygen (since there is less hemoglobin and myoglobin), oxygen diffusion within the muscle is decreased, in turn compromising oxidative capacity of muscle. This has direct implications for work productivity, which has been

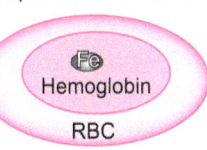

Normal RBC

Stage I
Depletion of iron store

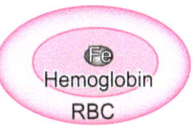

Stage II
Reduced functionality

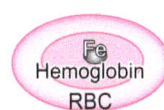

Stage III
Iron deficiency anemia

Fig. 7.11: Stages of anemia.

found to be reduced in persons working in sugar and tea plantations as well as factories. Most effects have been seen on endurance and aerobic capacity in iron-deficient persons. Iron deficiency limits the work capacity hence productivity of the person is seriously depressed. It has major impact on the national economy also.

Cognitive functions: Iron is required for myelination of white matter in brain and is a cofactor for synthesis of neurotransmitters. Therefore, deficiency of iron in early life adversely influences myelination and brain development. It could delay motor maturation hence resulting in developmental delays. In iron-deficient infants, deficits in cognitive performance persist. In older children and adults, attention and learning are adversely affected.

> **Research Glimpse:** Many iron-containing proteins are involved in oxygen transportation, oxidative phosphorylation, myelin production, and the synthesis and metabolism of neurotransmitters. Any abnormality in iron homoeostasis of CNS can lead to cellular damage resulting in oxidation and modification of lipids, proteins, carbohydrates, and DNA. Sometimes iron complexes are accumulated in certain regions of the brain resulting in motor and cognitive impairment with age and in different neurodegenerative diseases, such as Alzheimer's disease and Parkinson's disease. These changes are identified by MRI. Iron chelators are used to reduce iron accumulation, which can cross the blood–brain barrier, penetrate cells and thereby affording neuroprotection.
>
> *Ward RJ, Zuca FA, Duyn JF, et al. The role of iron in brain ageing and neurodegenerative disorders. Lancet Neurol. 2014;13(10):1045-60.*

Besides these, iron deficiency in pregnancy has been associated with low-birth weight and morbidity as well as mortality of the mother and the infant.

Consequences of Excessive Intake of Iron

ICMR-NIN (2020) has given TUL (tolerable upper limit) values for iron which are 40 mg/day for infants and children up to 13 years and 45 mg/day for adolescents (14-18 years) and adults. Overdose (20–60 mg/day) through iron supplementation is found to exhibit more toxic effects in children and pregnant women. One time high dose, e.g., 60 mg/kg may be more toxic. Excessive iron tends to reduce zinc absorption.

Excess is equally dangerous especially because the body does not have an efficient mechanism for getting rid of excess iron. When too much iron is absorbed from the gastrointestinal tract and builds up in the body, the condition is called hemochromatosis. There are two forms of hemochromatosis:

1. **Primary hemochromatosis:** The iron overload is due to a genetic defect. The excess iron is generally stored in the form of ferritin and hemosiderin in liver, spleen, and bone marrow. Excess iron, ultimately damages the pancreas, spleen, and liver leading to liver cirrhosis.
2. **Secondary hemochromatosis** is due to disease like thalassemia because the person needs to undergo blood transfusions frequently. Other conditions associated with hemochromatosis are hemolytic anemia and chronic alcoholism. Symptoms include abdominal pain, joint pains, loss of body hair, weight loss, weakness, and lassitude. Excess iron in skin gives the skin a gray bronze color.

Chelation therapy is used to eliminate excess iron from the body.

If iron supplements are consumed with certain medications, it reduces the absorption of the medicines and some other nutrients. High intakes of iron can cause necrotizing gastritis, enteritis, pallor, lassitude, and diarrhea.

> **Research Glimpse:** Oxidative stress is implicated in aging that is also attributed to excess of free iron in the body. It has been observed that patients with Alzheimer's disease or Parkinson's disease usually have high-iron content in their brain and disturbances in brain iron homeostasis. Though the exact cause of iron accumulation is unknown, the production of reactive oxygen species (ROS) lead to neurodegeneration. A role for iron is also proposed in atherosclerosis. However, further studies and evidence in this regard may be useful.
>
> *Altamura S, Muckenthaler MU. Iron toxicity in diseases of aging: Alzheimer's disease, Parkinson's disease and atherosclerosis. J Alzheimers Dis. 2009;16(4):879-95.*

> **Laboratory Laurel:** In order to see the linkage among the tissue iron stores, insulin resistance (IR), and cognition in the obese population, this study was taken up to identify the factors that contribute to increased hepatic iron concentration (HIC) and brain iron overload (BIO) by MRI, and to evaluate their impact on cognitive performance in 23 middle-aged obese subjects without diabetes (13 women; age 50.4 ± 7.7 years; BMI 43.7 ± 4.48 kg/m^2) and 20 healthy nonobese volunteers (10 women; age 48.8 ± 9.5 years; BMI 24.3 ± 3.54 kg/m^2). These subjects were recruited because they had iron load in their white and gray matter and the liver as indicated by MRI. Their IR was measured from HOMA-IR and an oral glucose tolerance test. Cognitive performance was tested by several neuropsychological tests. Obese subjects had significant increase in iron load at the caudate nucleus, lenticular nucleus hypothalamus, hippocampus, and liver. There was a positive correlation between HIC and BIO at caudate, hypothalamus, and hippocampus. The study indicates close link between obesity and IR and obesity-associated cognitive dysfunction, which may be attributed to the increased HIC and BIO.
>
> *Blasco G, Puig J, Daunis-I-Estadella J, et al. Brain Iron Overload, Insulin Resistance, and Cognitive Performance in Obese Subjects: A Preliminary MRI Case-Control Study. Diabetes Care. 2014;37(11):3076-3083.*

Iodine

Iodine is an essential (nonmetallic trace element) constituent of thyroid hormones [triiodothyronine (T_3) and thyroxin (T_4)], produced by the thyroid gland. These hormones are important for growth, development, and metabolism. It is critical in fetal stage because its deficiency can adversely affect mental functions and may lead to congenital defects in the baby. Iodine occurs in the form of iodide (I^-) or iodate (IO_3^-) in foods.

Dietary iodine is rapidly absorbed in the stomach and duodenum. The mechanism of absorption is not completely elucidated, but it is believed that transport may need a transporter. Once iodine is absorbed, it is taken into circulation and taken up by the thyroid gland and kidneys. Almost all (>90%) of iodine is excreted via the kidneys. More than 60% of iodine is stored in the thyroid gland. Absorption is increased when body requirement is high or body is in the state of iodine deficiency. Following absorption, free iodide is distributed through ECF from where it reaches to all tissues.

Selectively, it is concentrated in thyroid gland. It is also found in salivary, gastric, and mammary glands.

In healthy adults, the estimated iodine store is 15–20 mg from which the major fraction (70–80%) is in the thyroid gland. The thyroid gland takes up about 60 μg of iodine daily for maintaining synthesis of thyroid hormones. Iodine is carried into the thyroid gland by the protein thyroglobulin. Thyroglobulin is then hydrolyzed to give two thyroid hormones. In healthy adults, about three-fourths of the total body iodine is concentrated by the thyroid gland, which utilizes approximately 80 micrograms of iodine on daily basis for synthesis of thyroid hormones.

Thyroid hormones, which contain iodine, are T3 andT4. Synthesis of these hormones occurs in the colloidal space of the thyroid gland and, to a small extent, in brain and possibly other organs. Their synthesis is a three-step process catalyzed by the heme-containing enzyme iodide peroxidase. These three steps are:
i. Oxidation of iodide
ii. Iodination of the tyrosine residues in thyroglobulin, i.e., attachment of the iodide to tyrosine residues on thyroglobulin to produce monoiodothyronine and diiodothyronine, which are precursors of the thyroid hormones, and
iii. Coupling of iodothyronine to generate the hormones T3 and T4. Selenium and zinc play important roles in this stage.

The half-life of the hormones is 1.5–3 days for T3 and 5 days for T4. When these hormones are degraded, the iodine is released into plasma, from where it may be either taken up by the thyroid gland or excreted through urine.

Functions of Iodine
Thyroid hormone plays an important role in regulating reproductive function, growth, and development.

Formation of thyroid hormone: Iodine is an integral part of thyroid hormones, namely triiodothyronine (T3) and tetraiodothyronine, which is also called thyroxin (T4). T3 is converted into T4 in presence of glutathione and selenium, thus T4 is a biologically active form of thyroid hormone and is the more abundant in circulation. However, T3 is more physiologically active. Synthesis of thyroid hormones is regulated by thyroid-stimulating hormone (TSH) that is secreted by pituitary gland that is located in the brain. TSH is released in response to stimulation of the pituitary by thyrotropin-releasing hormone (TRH) secreted by the hypothalamus. When the T4 levels in circulation decrease, feedback from systemic circulation stimulates release of TRH, which in turn stimulates TSH secretion. Under the influence of TSH, the thyroid gland traps more iodine and also produces more of both T3 and T4. After synthesis, T3 and T4 are stored and when required they are released into circulation. In target tissues, T4 is converted to T3 by iodothyronine deiodinases (these enzymes contain selenium). This T3 now can bind to thyroid receptors in cell nuclei and regulate gene expression thereby involving iodine in growth, development, metabolism, and reproductive functions.

Growth and development: Iodine is important for development and maturation including myelination of nervous system, skeletal muscle, and lungs. In the developing brain, iodine influences cell growth and migration. Thyroid hormones play an important role during linear growth and skeletal maturation from childhood to adulthood. Secretion of these hormones is mediated by the hypothalamic-pituitary thyroid axis, hence is associated with the skeletal strength in early childhood and later in life. Thyroid hormone (TH) plays an important role in normal endochondral ossification and is essential for skeletal development, linear growth, maintenance of bone mass, and efficient fracture healing.

During the first 9 weeks of gestation, some thyroid hormone receptors are formed in central nervous system due to which thyroid hormones play myriad functions in the brain that include myelination, cell migration, cell differentiation, and maturation. They also modulate the gene expression (influencing mRNA transcription), which is involved in synaptic activity and memory. During pregnancy, the thyroid gland increases in size by about 10% in regions where there is sufficient iodine; however, in iodine-deficient geographic location, the increase is much more (20–40%).

Energy metabolism: Iodine influences metabolism of carbohydrates and the process of lipogenesis. It increases energy metabolism and raises the basal metabolic rate and affects oxidative phosphorylation. It also affects heart rate and respiratory rate. Thyroxin is important for cellular metabolism thereby increasing the utilization of ATP and releasing energy.

Other functions: It may be important for immune function and may modify risk for gastric cancer. Thyroid hormones influence transport of several nutrients, e.g., glucose and sodium, and affect activities of many enzymes, e.g., pyruvate kinase, and action of smooth muscles in blood vessels.

Recommended Dietary Allowance
ICMR-NIN (2020) has given RDA for iodine, based on urinary excretion and cooking losses. There is about 40% loss in cooking. Since iodized salt is the major source of iodine intake and given the proportion of salt intake, iodine intake is recommended to be 150 μg/day (RDA) for adults and children above the age of 10 years. Iodine requirement is 250 μg/day during pregnancy due to the following reasons: need for increased level of thyroid hormone in the mother; transfer of hormones from mother to fetus (since its own thyroid gland is not functional until 16–20 weeks of fetal life); and renal clearance (increased excretion) of iodine. Also, the mother's body synthesizes about 50% more iodine-containing thyroid hormones in order to maintain maternal euthyroidism. In lactation, iodine is transferred to the infant through breast milk. The RDA for lactating women is 280 μg/day of iodine. Adequate intake (AI) for infants (0–6 months and 6–12 months is 100 and 130 μg/day. RDA and EAR for children in different age groups can be seen Table 9.1A in Chapter 9 and Appendix 4, respectively.

Food Sources of Iodine
Iodine is primarily present in upper crust of earth from where it is leached out and found in soil and sea water. Hence, iodine content of food is largely dependent upon the soil

in which the foods are grown. Iodine content in fish and seafood also depends on the iodine content of sea water. In general, food and beverages of daily use contain low levels of iodine. However, high concentration of iodine is present in foods of marine origin including seaweeds. Largely, iodine content is influenced by iodine-containing compounds used in irrigation, fertilizers, and livestock. Iodine content of food cultivated in the soil of hilly regions is much less due to soil erosions and other factors. Hence, iodine content in foods varies widely around the globe. However, drinking water, particularly hard tap water, is a good source of iodine.

Besides these, iodine is ingested from other sources such as use of iodophors in many dairies to wash milk cans; use of red-color pigments (erythrosine) in foods, medicines, water purification tablets, and iodate as dough conditioner (now banned); however, these substances contribute to very low level. Some bread makers have replaced iodine with bromine that is also a halogen or chemical, which can cause toxicity in high doses.

Seeing the critical need of this nutrient, iodine is supplied to the population in different parts of the world through fortification of common salt. In India, universal iodization of the salt is indicated.

Due to the high prevalence of IDD, India and other countries are fortifying common salt with iodine. Hence, iodized salt has become the major source of iodine. However, certain communities in India still do not consume iodized salt for various reasons.

Iodine Deficiency: Causes and Consequences

Thyroid adapts to low-iodine intake (<100 mg/day) by significantly increasing the activity of TSH by pituitary gland and reduced clearance from the kidney. TSH is an indicator of iodine status in the body.

Environmental factors like formation of glaciers, soil erosions, rivers changing course, and flooding are some of the main factors causing iodine deficiency in many regions of the world particularly mountains and flood laden areas. Iodine intake varies in different parts of the world and from region to region within a country. People residing in hilly areas are often deficient in iodine and suffer iodine deficiency symptoms; it may be because iodine is leached out during soil erosion.

There is leaching of iodine from the upper crust of the soil. Deforestation and excavation aggravate the problems. Since there is low-iodine content in the food grown in those regions, people living in such areas and consuming those foods are at high risk of iodine deficiency and IDD. Further, the physiological demand of iodine is high during fetal stage, pregnancy, lactation and other growth spurts and dietary intake is low, deficiency occurs in persons in these life stages. Even in some European countries, it is said that iodine deficiency exists.

In case of iodine deficiency, production of thyroxin is inhibited and as a result, body keeps on producing thyroid-stimulating hormone (TSH). TSH causes thyroid gland to enlarge and enlargement of thyroid gland is called goiter. Hence, goiter is commonly seen in people particularly in women of hilly regions of Uttarakhand in India.

Mother is not able to transfer sufficient amount of iodine to the fetus and later to infant; hence, growth retardation occurs in children born to iodine-deficient mothers. There is also high risk of mental retardation in such children because synthesis of thyroid hormones may get limited and which further limits activities needed for brain development. It also results in stunting due to limited cell division, poor gene expression, and maturation. Children born in iodine-deficient areas are at risk of neurological disorders and mental retardation because of the combined effects of maternal, fetal, and neonatal hypothyroxinemia. Severe deficiency during this critical period may result in hypothyroidism and brain damage.

Thus, if the mother's iodine status is poor and there is fetal iodine deficiency, adverse effects are seen in the form of pregnancy complications such as fetal loss, abruptio placentae, preeclampsia, preterm delivery, and congenital hypothyroidism in the baby. The severity and type of effect depend on the timing and severity of iodine deficiency. In its severe form, there will be cretinism, i.e., severe mental retardation, physical retardation, and deafness. It has been reported in the India Iodine Survey 2018-2019 that children born in iodine deficient areas exhibit 13.5 lower IQ points, than children born in iodine -sufficient areas.

In certain parts of the globe, foods eaten contain good amount of goitrogens. Goitrogens are sulfur-containing compounds, viz. thiocyanate, isothiocyanate, glucosinolates, cyanogenic glycosides, and goitrin. These compounds prevent uptake of iodine by the thyroid gland, interfere with iodine metabolism, and aggravate iodine deficiency. Several commonly consumed foods contain goitrogens. Some of them are cassava, cruciferous vegetables like cabbage, kale, cauliflower, turnips, rapeseed, pear, peaches, bamboo shoots, broccoli, strawberry, lima beans, maize, millet, mustard, peanuts, sweet potato, millet and tea. Cabbage, kale, cauliflower, broccoli, turnips, pear, peaches, bamboo shoots, and rapeseed contain glucosinolates. Cassava, lima beans, linseed, sorghum, strawberry, maize, millet, mustard, peanuts, sweet potato, and tea contain cyanogenic glucosides. Among these, the compound in cassava called linamarin is of concern; since in many regions, cassava is used as a staple food. Linamarin can be removed by soaking cassava in water. The goitrogens present in other foods can be largely inactivated by soaking and cooking food. Cooking at high temperature in open pan tends to cause more loss of iodine from food. Hence, it is advocated to add salt after completion of cooking. Iodine loss also occurs during poor storage of food including salt. Iodine is lost with sun exposure, high humidity, and moisture. Quite often, salt and/or food containing iodine are transported through railway and open trucks in poorly packaged bags and are exposed to such conditions. Drinking large amounts of tea may affect iodine uptake and usage.

Flavonoids in plant foods, especially in pearl millet and phenolic compounds in tea, inhibit the enzyme thyroid peroxidase. This enzyme plays an important role in the formation of iodinated compounds—mono- and diiodotyrosine, which couple to form T3 and T4. Recent studies support that the cooking losses of iodine and many micro-environmental factors are also responsible for IDD.

In many regions, formation of glaciers, soil erosion, and flooding lead to loss of iodide from the surface soil. Thus, concentration in some geographic regions is very low especially in hilly regions. Hence, the drinking water and plants/crops grown in such regions have low amounts of iodine. Impurities in polluted drinking water, some industrial pollutants as well as tobacco smoke block iodine uptake and act as goitrogenic agents.

Cigarette smoking is also associated with higher serum levels of thiocyanate that may compete with iodine for uptake particularly in mammary gland; hence, smoking during lactation limits the iodine levels in breast milk and causes iodine deficiency in breastfed babies. People living in iodine-deficient areas and whose staple diets include the foods that contain goitrogens, are the main section of society suffering from iodine deficiency disorder (IDD). Thus, inadequacy in iodine intake is the primary cause of iodine deficiency.

Apart from iodine, a number of factors can affect iodine levels. Deficiencies of selenium, iron, and vitamin A exacerbate iodine deficiency. Selenium and iron deficiency adversely affect synthesis of thyroid hormone in children with goiter, it has been observed that iron supplementation improves the efficacy of iodine supplementation through iodized salt. In animals, high intakes of minerals such as calcium, fluorine and arsenic, deficient or excess intakes of cobalt, and low manganese intakes have been found to interfere with iodine metabolism.

A wide spectrum of abnormalities occurs in physiological functions, collectively known as iodine deficiency disorders (IDD). It is shown in Chapter 12. Since iodine is required at every stage of life from intrauterine to old age, IDD leaves serious marks on health and productivity of the people and it is a public health problem, which is preventable. Consequences of deficiency are more serious in women than men, with pregnant women being at greater risk for adverse effects.

Insufficient dietary iodine affects synthesis of thyroxin in the thyroid gland resulting in hyperthyroidism. Hypothyroidism is characterized by unexpected weight gain, feeling tired, feeling weak, hair loss, swollen neck, learning problem, and menstrual and pregnancy issues. Hyperthyroidism is indicated by hyperactive thyroid gland that is indicated by nervousness, anxiety, rapid heartbeat, hand tremors, excessive sweating, weight loss, and sleep problems.

The thyroid gland gets enlarged in an attempt to adapt to chronic deficiency of iodine, which is known as goiter. Goiter is a noninflammatory, nontumorous, and nontoxic condition, which is characterized by high-blood level of thyroid-stimulating hormone (TSH) followed by low thyroxin (T4) in blood level. It results in disproportionate increase in size and number of cells of the thyroid gland, which appears as enlarged thyroid or goiter. Endemic goiter is common in regions where the soil has been deprived of iodine such as hilly regions of Uttarakhand.

The effects of deficiency can range from mild goiter where the thyroid gland is enlarged to severe impact on the developing fetus/child, if there is deficiency during pregnancy or up to 3 years of age.

Infants born from iodine-deficient mothers develop cretinism (stunted growth). The consequences of iodine deficiency during pregnancy include stillbirth, spontaneous abortion, congenital anomalies such as cretinism (mild-to-severe mental retardation) and perinatal mortality. Thus, iodine deficiency has tremendous impact on productivity, quality-of-life, and socioeconomic development. Age-old identification of iodine deficiency symptom was endemic cretinism, which was characterized by brain damage, mental retardation, and where iodine deficiency was combined with deficiency of selenium. It was more prevalent in regions where cassava was the staple food. Normal thyroid carries high concentration of selenium due to which thyroid detoxifies ROS using glutathione peroxidase and superoxide dismutase.

Preventive measures: Universal salt Iodization is now widely accepted strategy to prevent and correct the iodine deficiency. Increased awareness in IDD-prone areas can be one of the actions to prevent IDD. Fortification of salt with iodine is another way for which Government of India has taken steps to fortify salt and make it available to all at reasonable price. Adding salt at end of cooking minimizes cooking losses. Some foods eg coconut oil have a protective effect on thyroid problems. One of them is coconut oil.

Unrefined coconut oil contains monounsaturated fats containing medium chain triglycerides (MCT) and is quite stable at room temperature. It does not get oxidized or rancid easily and is also processed differently in the system. It prevents cell membrane damage and also does not inhibit the conversion of T4 to T3, which other refined vegetable oils do. MCT rather helps in rebuilding the cell membranes and increases enzyme production, which assists the conversion of T4 to T3 hormones. Fortified micronutrient biscuits have also been successfully used to raise the urinary iodine concentration (UIC) of schoolgirls (aged 10–15 years) in India. Low UIC is a good biomarker for the risk of goiter and hypothyroidism, though UIC does not directly assess thyroid function and size.

Consequences of Excessive Intake of Iodine
Upper tolerable limit for iodine intake for healthy adults (but lactating or pregnant) is suggested to be 1,100 µg per day by US Institute of Medicine, WHO, United Nations Children's Fund (UNICEF) and the International Council for the Control of Iodine Deficiency Disorders (ICCIDD) as well as ICMR_NIN (2020).

Excessive intake of iodine usually comes from prolonged used of some medicines like iodine solution dressing or intravenous administration of iodine-containing substances or may be during radiological studies and supplements. In certain cases, iodine is administered in iodine-deficient population via iodized oil orally and intramuscularly; introduced into the water supply used in crop irrigation, incorporated into animal fodder, and introduced into food through salt iodization, bread iodophors, and other products. UIC is considered a good marker of iodine intake. UIC >300 µg/L is considered excessive in children and adults but > 500 µg/L during pregnancy. According to WHO, the desired adequate (median urinary iodine concentration) mUIC should be between 100-200 µg/L for children, adolescents, adult men, adult women and lactating mothers. Over consumption of iodine intake may inhibit the synthesis of thyroid hormones by the thyroid gland. This condition is called Wolff-Chaikoff effect as an autoregulatory phenomenon, whereby a large amount of ingested iodine acutely inhibits thyroid hormone synthesis within the follicular cells, irrespective of the serum level of thyroid-stimulating hormone (TSH). This condition is believed to be transient.

Overconsumption of iodine-rich foods such as kelp, dairy foods, sea foods including iodized salt or intake of iodine exceeding 350 mg from nonfood sources including supplements can also cause the symptoms such as diarrhea, nausea, anorexia and muscle weakness, difficulty in breathing and certain mental activities, irregular heartbeat and low blood pressure. Kidney function may be adversely affected. Iodine-induced hyperthyroidism has been found to occur in people who increased their iodine intake very fast, viz. if iodine content of soil may be too high or may be caused by medications containing iodine. This results in excess thyroid hormone production leading to weight loss, tachycardia, and muscle weakness. Intakes exceeding 2 g for prolonged periods are not safe. In persons with adequate iodine status, excess intakes can increase TSH although T3 and T4 levels are not low. The condition is called "subclinical hypothyroidism" resulting in goiter. This can occur even in newborns and children.

It is noteworthy that in Southeast Asian countries seaweed is relished for example in Japan. Some seaweed species can contribute substantial amounts of iodine to the diet and the problem of excess intake can be addressed by limiting or restricting the intake of such seaweeds. Prolonged intakes >18,000 µg per day can increase the risk of goiter. Persons who have undergone partial thyroidectomy or those having Graves' disease, autoimmune thyroiditis, or nodular goiter may not be able to tolerate intakes that are prescribed as safe for general population.

> **Laboratory Laurel:** This study was conducted on 298 children between 18 months and 48 months of age residing in Algerian refugee camps to explore the association of thyroid dysfunction with children's developmental status, in an area of chronic excessive iodine exposure. Early child development was measured using the Ages and Stages Questionnaires, third edition (ASQ-3), consisting of five domains: Communication, Gross Motor, Fine Motor, Problem Solving, and Personal-Social. Due to poor discriminatory ability in the Gross Motor domain, the total ASQ-3 scores were calculated both including and excluding this domain. Urinary iodine concentration (UIC), thyroid hormones (TSH, FT3, and FT4), thyroid antibodies, and serum thyroglobulin (Tg) were also measured. About 72% of the children had a UIC above 300 µg/L, while median UIC was 451.6 µg/L. 14% had thyroid disturbances and 10% of the children had TSH outside the reference range. The children with thyroid disturbances and TSH outside the reference ranges had lower ASQ scores. It was concluded that high iodine intake may cause thyroid dysfunction and hence delay developmental status. This aspect needs further exploration because optimal child development is important for a sustainable future.
>
> *Aakre I, Strand TA, Moubarek K, et al. Associations between thyroid dysfunction and developmental status in children with excessive iodine status. PLoS One. 2017;12(11):e0187241.*

Zinc

The essentiality of zinc for humans was discovered as late as 1961. Zinc is a metal present in all cells, is a cofactor for more than 300 enzymes, and is thus necessary for a wide variety of biological functions. It is also a component of more than 100 transcription factors (as zinc fingers, e.g., in DNA). Hence, zinc plays many vital roles in protein synthesis, integrity of cell membrane, DNA synthesis, normal growth, gene expression, gene regulation, cell division, and immunity. It is also crucial in recovery from infection and wound healing. About 2 grams of zinc is present in the human body, which is found in bones (30%), muscles (60%), hair and skin, and plasma. In plasma, it is bound with albumin. It interacts with a number of nutrients. In contrast to iron (which is restricted to specific cellular components and has defined physiological roles), zinc is ubiquitous in cells. The amount of zinc stored is higher in men (2.5 g) than women (1.5 g) as males have more amount of muscle. More than half of the zinc is found in muscle tissues. Rest is found in other parts of the body, which include bones, eyes, skin, kidney and prostate gland, and testes (men). Zn is excreted through feces (<1 mg/day), sweat, skin, and hair together accounting for approximately 1 mg/day and urine (0.4–0.6 mg/day).

Zinc is absorbed from the small intestines, mostly the duodenum and jejunum. As digestion progresses, Zn is bound to peptides or amino acids or nucleotides and a small amount is present in the free form. Absorption of the free form is influenced by its solubility. The zinc ions that have been released during digestion are bound to endogenously secreted ligands and then transported into the duodenum and jejunum where it is bound to metallothionein (the amount of metallothionein is correlated with zinc intakes). Here, in the cell membrane, there may be specific transporters that facilitate the transport of zinc into portal circulation. When zinc intakes are high, zinc may be absorbed passively through a paracellular route. From portal circulation, zinc is taken to the liver and then into systemic circulation (where it is bound to albumin) from where it is taken up by tissues. Absorption is influenced by zinc intake with a higher percentage being absorbed when zinc intakes are low and vice-versa.

Several factors influence its absorption, some inhibiting and others promoting absorption. Inhibitory factors include phytate, some metals like iron and high calcium intakes, and decreased secretion of gastric acid. Promoting factors include amino acids like histidine, cysteine, and organic acids. In food, zinc is bound to proteins. Efficiency of absorption is generally about 30% but can be as low as 10–15% from typical cereal- and legume-based diets. Besides the above factors, extent of digestion and transit time influence absorption. The intestines adapt zinc absorption vis-à-vis zinc status. The better the zinc status, lower the absorption. Also high-Zn intakes are associated with lower absorption and when intakes are low, absorption is higher. Zinc competes with copper, iron, and calcium during absorption because all are divalent ions. Hence, excess of one element may affect the bioavailability of the other. Excess dietary intake of Zn can impair the absorption of iron and copper. Absorption is inhibited by phytates and fiber commonly found in cereal-based diet and enhanced from meat-based diet.

Zinc Homeostasis

As you have learnt the human body contains about 2–3 g of zinc of which most is present in muscle and bone. The remaining is present in organs such as prostate, liver, gastrointestinal tract, kidney, skin, lungs, brain, heart, and pancreas. Within the cell, about one-third of the zinc is present in the nucleus; about half in the cytosol and the remaining is part of the membranes. This mechanism protects the body from accumulating excess zinc. The cellular homeostasis is due to two protein families namely the zinc importer family and the zinc transporter family. These protein families also regulate intracellular distribution of zinc in the mitochondria, golgi apparatus, and endoplasmic reticulum. In many mammals, there are zincosomes, which are zinc in the cell and release it when they are stimulated.

Zinc homeostasis also involves metallothioneins, which complex about one-fifth of the zinc within the cell. It is maintained synergistically by regulation of gastrointestinal absorption and endogenous excretion. When zinc intakes are low, the adaptation occurs at the level of the GI tract as well as changes in urinary zinc excretion. Turnover of plasma zinc also changes, although in some tissues, zinc may be retained in order to maintain function.

Most of the zinc in blood is present in red blood cells, as part of the enzyme carbonic anhydrase, and, to a smaller extent, in superoxide dismutase. WBC also contain zinc. Plasma Zn levels are influenced by Zn intakes as well as infections and other stress. A small reduction of approximately 15% occurs after consumption of a meal, possibly attributable to postprandial changes in glucose and insulin levels. Fasting increases plasma Zn, possibly because lean body mass is broken down.

Functions of Zinc

Zinc has catalytic, structural and regulatory roles. It is a component of enzymes, hormones, and has an important role in immunity.

Digestion: Zinc is a cofactor of proteases, phosphatases and carbonic anhydrases that are required for digestion of food and absorption. Other enzymes are gamma glutamyl carboxypeptidase that hydrolyses glutamate from the polyglutamate chain of folate, alkaline phosphatase that is involved in digestion of complexes containing thiamine, riboflavin, panthothenic acid as well as carbonic anhydrases that are involved in production of gastric acid.

Peptidases, carboxypeptidase	Protein digestion
Gamma glutamyl carboxypeptidase	Removal of glutamate from polyglutamate in dietary folates
Alkaline phosphatase	Digestion of complexes containing thiamine, riboflavin, and pantothenic acid
Carbonic anhydrases	Production of gastric acid

Regulation of blood pH: Carbonic anhydrase catalyzes conversion of carbon dioxide to a weak acid.

Metabolism of nutrients: Alcohol dehydrogenase is a zinc-containing enzyme required for converting retinol to retinaldehyde, which is important for vision. Similarly, a zinc-dependent enzyme is needed for folate metabolism.

Cell division, gene expression: Zinc is involved in synthesis of RNA, DNA, and, hence, is important for cell division. In these enzymes, there are zinc-complexing structures called "zinc fingers". Zinc is also necessary for editing of RNA. Through its binding to factors responsible for regulating expression of certain genes, Zn may be important for gene expression.

Brain functions: Zinc plays structural and functional roles in the brain. Zinc is also involved in neurogenesis, neuronal migration, and synaptogenesis. High concentrations of zinc are present in synaptic vesicles of hippocampal neurons (which are centrally involved in learning and memory), and has the ability to modulate some neurotransmitters and gamma-aminobutyric acid (GABA) receptors.

Growth: Since Zn is important for cell division, it is important for growth. In children, zinc supplementation reversed stunting, improved cognitive ability and activity levels. Zinc deficiency adversely affects sexual maturity in males.

Immunity: The thymus gland secretes a hormone thymulin, which is Zn-dependent. Thymulin activates T-lymphocytes and enhances activity of natural killer cells. Lack of zinc in total parenteral nutrition solutions has been found to decrease natural killer cell activity. Some studies suggest that zinc supplements may be beneficial for persons with HIV and tuberculosis.

Metallothionein (MT) is a protein that binds with zinc. Intracellular zinc is bound to MT that helps to maintain cellular zinc homeostasis. It chelates heavy metals and reduces their toxicity and oxidative stress, hence, protects the person from environmental stress.

Defense against free radicals: Zn is part of superoxide dismutases and hence protects against oxidative stress and lipid peroxidation as well as protein oxidation.

Bone mineralization: Alkaline phosphatase (ALP) is responsible for osteoblastic activity. It is synthesized in liver, bones, intestines, pancreas, and kidney and in placenta. It plays an important role in connective tissue metabolism for the enzyme collagenase, which is needed for the collagen that is essential for bone structure. Normal range of serum ALP is 20–140 IU/L. High ALP levels may indicate presence of either liver or bone disorders.

Other Functions

- Zinc appears to be important for taste acuity.
- It is a cofactor for nitric oxide synthesis. Nitric oxide is important for vascular function. Therefore, zinc indirectly influences vascular tone.
- It chelates insulin during storage and hence has a role in controlling insulin secretion. Some zinc transporters are expressed in beta cells of pancreas, where they support maturation and secretion of insulin.

- It opposes the effect of cyclic AMP on glycolysis.
- It has a role in cell apoptosis (programmed cell death).
- It protects against toxic compounds including reactive oxygen species (ROS), X-radiation, and gamma radiation.
- Carbonic anhydrases are involved in signaling, respiration, and bone resorption.
- Some Zn-finger proteins are involved in differentiation, proliferation, and adhesion.

Zinc fingers: The zinc finger contains 26 amino acids that form a structure, which binds to specific sequences in DNA. Zinc fingers are small motifs that are structurally diverse containing finger-like protrusions. Zn finger proteins are abundant in eukaryotic cells. Zinc fingers play key role in cell differentiation and development of several tissues. They have diverse functions such as DNA recognition, RNA packaging, transcriptional activation, regulation of apoptosis, protein folding and assembly, and lipid binding (Fig. 7.12).

Recommended Dietary Allowances of Zinc

Zinc requirement in humans is influenced by life stage, health state, and climatic condition, type of diet consumed, and parasitic infestation and infection. The Expert Committee of ICMR-NIN (2020) has recommended zinc requirements that can be referred from Table 9.1A in Chapter 9 and for EAR in Appendix 4. When making the recommendations, the Committee has taken into consideration that the Indian diets are primarily mixed cereal-based and high in phytates that may tend to reduce the bioavailability of zinc. Computation of zinc requirements has been done using the factorial approach, considering all the average losses of zinc through body fluids and additional requirements for growth (tissue and blood volume expansion), and during lactation and pregnancy. The RDA has been derived by multiplying the EAR with a factor of 1.2.

Food Sources of Zinc

Zinc is found in a wide variety of food sources, although its bioavailability may vary. Animal foods like shellfish, oysters, red meat, sea foods, and dairy products are rich in zinc. It is commonly seen that protein-rich foods are also rich in zinc. Plant sources of zinc include whole grains, beans, kabuli chana, cashew nuts, and pumpkin seeds. Fruits and vegetables are poor sources of zinc. Some of the important dietary sources of zinc are given in Figure 7.13 as per ICFT (2017).

Bioavailability of zinc is important. Bioavailability is reduced by phytates and oxalates. Zinc from animal sources is better absorbed and zinc from whole grain cereals or pulses is poorly absorbed. The bioavailability of zinc is increased after germination or fermentation of whole pulses and cereals. These are traditional processing techniques used for generations in India. During germination or fermentation, there is enzymatic hydrolysis of phytic acid by activating the endogenous phytase enzyme. Milling also reduces phytate since a considerable proportion of phytate is present in bran; however, with thermal processing and extrusion, the reduction in phytate is only moderate. Refining process reduces the zinc content but germination improves the bioavailability of zinc. Although absorption of the mineral is increased particularly in pregnancy, bioavailability of zinc is drastically reduced and body reserves are likely to be lower.

Zinc bioavailability is influenced by a number of dietary factors. Inhibitors are phytic acid, with molar ratios of 15:1 (phytate to zinc), as per the WHO or 18:1, as per

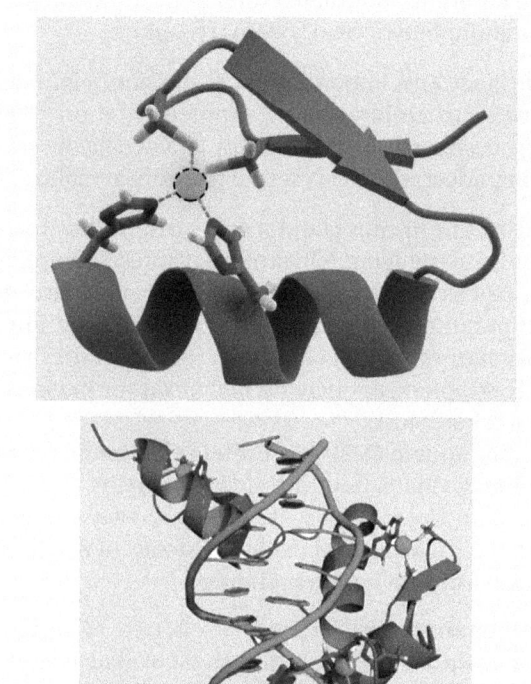

Fig. 7.12: Zinc fingers.

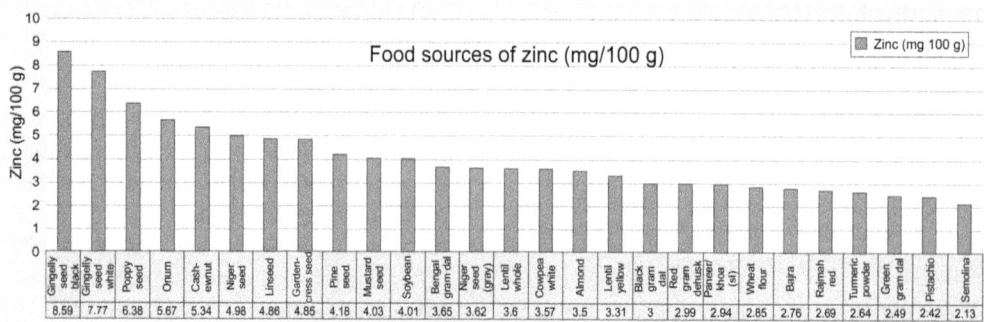

Fig. 7.13: Food sources of zinc, IFCT (2017).

the International Zinc Consultative Group. Increasing ratio of phytate:zinc progressively inhibits absorption. Zinc bioavailability can be predicted by multiplying the phytate:zinc molar ratio by the dietary calcium concentration.

High doses of inorganic iron also inhibit zinc absorption when zinc intakes are low, but the interaction between these two minerals is much less when the zinc intake is closer to physiological levels. It appears that iron exerts an inhibitory effect on zinc absorption when the ratio of iron to zinc is high in water solution. This implies that iron fortification of foods should not pose a very big problem for iron absorption. This has been demonstrated in experiments with fortified bread, weaning cereal, and infant formula.

Enhancers include protein and absorption increases with increase in protein intake. Proteins from animal sources are better enhancers than plant proteins that are likely to also contain phytate. The amino acids in animal proteins keep the zinc in solution. If zinc is bound to any soluble ligand or chelator, it will have a positive effect on zinc solubility and availability.

Deficiency of Zinc: Causes and Consequences
Zinc deficiency worldwide occurs with malnutrition and due to consuming foods with low bioavailability. Also it is associated with aging, certain diseases, or deregulated homeostasis. High consumption of cereal-based diet that is rich in phytates chelates zinc and limits its bioavailability. Another reason is low-protein intake and most zinc-rich food sources are also rich in protein. Most people do not consume enough protein for various reasons.

Its deficiency has also been observed in premature infants and undernourished children.

Zinc deficiency is also connected with diarrheal diseases. Zinc supplementation lessens the duration and frequency of diarrheal episodes in undernourished children. Deficiency also occurs due to increased requirement and excretion, low-dietary intake, and genetic causes. Alcoholism, liver disease, and renal disease potentiate it. Severe zinc deficiency results in:

- Growth retardation, there may be even cessation of growth and development
- Reduced immunity
- Lesions in skin and mucous membranes permitting entry of microorganisms
- Delayed wound healing due to lack of zinc fingers or cross-linkage in collagen formation
- Poor appetite due to hypogeusia (impaired sense of taste) and hyposmia (impaired sense of smell)
- Skeletal abnormalities
- Characteristic skin rashes
- Delayed sexual maturation, impaired reproductive ability, and sexual immaturity in males
- Poor cognitive and motor development affecting attention and motor activities because zinc deficiency could interfere with neurotransmission and subsequent neuropsychological behavior
- Chronic and severe diarrhea
- Night blindness, swelling, and clouding of corneas
- Behavioral disturbances

- It can cause defect in zinc transporters resulting in production, maturation, and secretion of insulin and subsequent glucose metabolism.

Severe zinc deficiency affects all the body systems including central nervous, gastrointestinal, epidermal, reproductive, and skeletal. However, severe zinc deficiency generally occurs in persons having acrodermatitis enteropathica, a genetic disorder in which uptake and transport of zinc are both impaired. Oral zinc therapy results in remission of symptoms. Generally, dietary zinc deficiency is not likely to be severe; however, severe deficiency could occur, if there is zinc malabsorption or a person is suffering from severe burns or prolonged diarrhea, in persons who abuse alcohol or are prescribed medications like penicillamine that interact with zinc.

In contrast to severe deficiency, marginal zinc deficiency is more common especially among children from low- and middle-income countries. It has been estimated that about 2 billion people have dietary zinc deficiency. Studies have shown that due to marginal zinc deficiency, there are impairments in physical and neuropsychological development along with increased susceptibility to life-threatening infections. Among children below 5 years of age, it is estimated that annually, deaths of almost 5% of children are attributable to zinc deficiency.

Those at risk of zinc deficiency include preterm, low birth weight infants, older breast fed infants who are fed. These include older breastfed infants and toddlers fed complementary foods that are zinc-poor, adolescents, pregnant and lactating women, patients on total parenteral nutrition or intravenous feeds, malnourished persons, individuals suffering from protein–energy malnutrition, those with anorexia nervosa, malabsorption syndrome. Inflammatory bowel disease as well as those with severe and prolonged diarrhea, those who abuse alcohol (urinary zinc excretion is more) or have alcoholic liver disease (liver zinc levels are low), persons suffering from chronic renal disease or sickle cell anemia, all increase the risk of zinc deficiency. Any therapeutic drug, which decreases zinc absorption or increases excretion or impairs it, increases risk of deficiency. Besides this, elderly persons and strict vegetarians are at risk.

Zinc supplementation alone exhibits positive effect on linear growth as compared to when zinc is supplemented along with iron supplementation. It is because the iron interferes with absorption or bioavailability of zinc supplementation can improve the condition in cases of diarrhea and pneumonia. now it is also being practiced in health clinics as per WHO guidelines.

Consequences of Excessive Intake of Zinc
High intake (150–450 mg/day) through supplements or pharmacological intakes may manifest in symptoms like nausea, vomiting, and fever. Intakes above 40 mg/day can lead to a decrease in copper stores, lower HDL levels, and impair immune function. It also leads to low serum level of copper, iron and increases risk of copper deficiency (because there is competition between copper and zinc for absorption and metallothionein has more affinity for copper as compared to zinc). Immune functions are also reduced.

Besides oral intake, zinc in the body can increase through occupational exposure such as inhalation of smoke from industries that are involved in galvanization. Workers who work at such manufacturing plants are at risk of inhaling zinc. Zinc chloride or zinc oxide smoke bombs put soldiers and others, who inhale the zinc-containing fumes from these bombs, at risk. Inhalation of zinc oxide fumes causes metal fume fever. Workers who work in welding and zinc smelting are at risk when they inhale fresh metal fumes in which the size of zinc particles is <1 μm. This syndrome is reversible and symptoms are evident within a few hours of exposure. They include fever, muscle soreness, nausea, fatigue, chest pain, cough, and dyspnea. These symptoms are temporary and the respiratory symptoms disappear within a period of 1–4 days.

Selenium

Selenium (Se) is a nonmetallic element. The role of selenium in human nutrition was recognized in 1957 by Schwarz and Foltz who observed the consequences of selenium deficiency along with that of vitamin E in rats. It is a component of glutathione peroxidase, which is associated with antioxidant functions and protects the cell membrane from oxidation. Thus, selenium acts as an antioxidant; although it performs other functions as well. The level of glutathione peroxidase is dependent on selenium intake. Selenium is present in many other proteins affecting thyroid and insulin functions, regulation of cell growth among others. It replaces sulfur in many organic compounds and forms numerous organic selenium compounds, and also combines with amino acids like methionine and cysteine to form selenomethionine and selenocysteine, respectively. Selenium is found in approximately 25 proteins called "selenoproteins" that contain cysteine. In all, about 100 selenoprotein families have been discovered. The amino acid selenocysteine (this amino acid is regarded as the 21st amino acid in the genetic code) is incorporated into proteins during translation (protein synthesis) and functional selenoproteins are formed. The selenoproteins that are formed include glutathione peroxidases, thioredoxin reductases, iodothyronine deiodinases, selenoprotein P, selenoprotein W, selenophosphate synthetase 2, methionine-R-sulfoxide reductase B1/selenoprotein R, selenoprotein S. Table 7.2 gives the functions of these proteins in brief.

The human body contains about 5–6 mg of selenium. While small amounts are essential, at high levels, it leads to toxicity. On a per unit weight basis, the highest concentration is found in kidney followed by liver, spleen, pancreas, heart, brain and lungs, bone and skeletal muscle. About one-third of the selenium in the body is present in the skeleton. Storage is in liver, kidney and to some extent in skeletal muscle in the form of selenoproteins. Se content in foods depends on the soil content. Se is absorbed from the intestinal lumen, with the amount being 60–70%.

In nature, Se is present in both the organic and inorganic form in food. The organic forms are selenocysteine (SeCys) and selenomethionine (SeMet) and inorganic forms are selenite, selenate, and selenide. Both forms can be ingested through dietary sources or dietary supplements but utilized in the body in varying capacity. In general, absorption of organic compounds is better than that from inorganic compounds. This is because a considerable proportion of Se compounds in plant foods are organic, e.g., selenomethionine (where Se replaces the sulfur in the methionine molecule). SeMet is better absorbed from foods rich in methionine. In animal foods, Se occurs in a greater variety of forms like sulfides, selenides besides being present as selenomethionine or selenocysteine. Absorption of selenium from fish is very low (<10%) due to the likelihood of Se being complexed with other substances. Presence of vitamin A, C, E and reduced glutathione enhances the absorption while presence of heavy metals, sulfur, mercury and deficiency of vitamin B_2, B_6, vitamin E and methionine reduces the bioavailability of selenium.

In blood, Se is transported as either selenoproteins or bound to glutathione. In the body, Se is bound to Se-binding proteins or is incorporated in selenoproteins during translation using the amino acid selenocysteine. Selenoproteins constitute a considerable percentage of total body selenium. It is mostly excreted through urine, which is probably important for selenium homeostasis. Selenides are excreted through breath as dimethyl selenide, which imparts garlic-like odor. A small amount (50 μg) is lost through feces.

Functions of Selenium

Selenium is a part of numerous selenoproteins and is necessary for several important functions:

- **Antioxidant function:** Many enzymes that are important for antioxidant defense contain selenocysteine. Glutathione peroxidase is a selenoprotein enzyme that participates in a wide range of biochemical reactions mainly to prevent cell damage from free radicals. Hence, selenium plays a role in prevention of cell damage. Glutathione peroxidase catalyzes the reaction that converts hydrogen peroxide into water. This enzyme uses reduced glutathione and is important for preventing DNA damage proteins by lipid peroxides. This enzyme is present even in the gastrointestinal tract where it probably protects against oxidative damage caused by agents present in the diet. It is also secreted in human milk.

- **Formation of thyroid hormones:** Thyroxin and triiodothyronine require thyroxin deiodinase, which contains selenocysteine. Similarly, enzymes involved in release of active thyroid hormone also contain selenium. Iodothyronine deiodinase is essential for the conversion of thyroxin, or tetraiodothyronine (T4), into its active form, triiodothyronine (T3).

- **Immune function:** Dietary Se is important for both innate and acquired immunity. It influence functions of neutrophils. Neutrophils produce superoxide radicals which participate in killing of microbes. It is also important in functioning of both T and B lymphocytes. Selenium as selenocysteine was found to influence the immune system and it may be because the antioxidant glutathione peroxidase may play role in protection of neutrophils from

Table 7.2: Selenoproteins and their roles.

Selenoprotein	Site of production	Role in brief
Glutathione peroxidases (GPxs): GPx1 GPx2 GPx3 GPx4 GPx6	Cytosol Intestinal lining and lungs Thyroid glands and kidneys Olfactory epithelium	Antioxidant enzymes, reduce ROS and thus minimize oxidative damage Also enable sperm motility, maturation
Thioredoxin reductases (TrxR): TrxR 1 TrxR 2 TGR	Cytosol Mitochondria Testes specific	Catalyze reduction of several substrates, including thioredoxin and protein disulfide isomerase Are electron donors and help to regenerate antioxidants like vitamin C, alpha-tocopherol, coenzyme Q, and lipoic acid Regulation of cell growth and survival
Iodothyronine deiodinases (DIOs): DIOs type 1 and 2 DIO type 3	D1 is expressed mainly in the liver, the kidneys and the thyroid. D1 also catalyzes the degradation of thyroid hormone. D2 expression changes in response to alterations in thyroid state, thus helps to maintain tissue T3 levels if plasma T4 and T3 levels vary. D3 mediates the degradation of thyroid hormone and is present in placenta and fetal tissues. High D3 activities at these sites probably prevent exposure of fetal tissues to high T3 levels, allowing the growth of these tissues.	Deiodinate T4 and increase circulating T3 DIO1 is involved in iodine homeostasis Convert T3 and T4 to inactive metabolites DIO type 2 and 3 involved in maturation of auditory and visual systems in the fetus activities like the conversion of T4 to T3 through removal of iodine
Selenoprotein P	Produced by liver	Storage of selenium, functions as an antioxidant, important for selenium homeostasis in brain and testes, may be involved in regulation of glucose metabolism and insulin sensitivity
Selenoprotein W exists in different isoforms	Expressed in many tissues, highest level in skeletal muscle and heart	Protects neuronal cells against oxidative stress and death May be involved in activation of muscle cell differentiation genes
Methionine-R-sulfoxide reductase B1/selenoprotein R		Protects against oxidative stress especially regeneration of proteins damaged by oxidative stress
15-kDa selenoprotein	Expressed in several tissues, such as prostate, kidney, testes, liver, brain and T-cells	Function not known but studies show its involvement in glycoprotein folding, early opacification of lens, anti-cancer effects
Selenoprotein S	Located in endoplasmic reticulum	Involved in response to endoplasmic reticulum stress, regulation of inflammatory and immune responses, may influence susceptibility to preeclampsia, coronary artery disease, gastrointestinal cancers

oxygen derived radicals that are produced to kill ingested foreign organisms.

- **Other functions:** It may be important for insulin metabolism, gene expression, cell proliferation, cell differentiation, and fertility. It may be important for protection against cancer.

Recommended Dietary Allowances of Selenium

Selenium requirements are based on the activity of glutathione peroxidase. Plasma Se and glutathione peroxidase activities (GSHPx) activity indicate the short-term status, whereas, red blood cell Se and GSHPX activity reflect long-term Se status. Platelet GSHPx activity is considered as a good indicator for assessing changes in selenium status. ICMR-NIN (2020) has recommended that 40 microgram per day is the acceptable intake for Indians. Recently the FAO/WHO Committee has recommended a Se intake of 26 µg/day for adult women and 36 µg/day for adult men. RDA varies with age and during pregnancy and lactation, and it is increased under stressful conditions.

Food Sources of Selenium

Main chemical form of dietary selenium is selenomethionine (SE-Met). Brazil nut is the richest vegetarian source of selenium, but it is not commonly eaten. However, taking 1–2 pieces only can raise the selenium level. Further, mixed nuts containing sunflower seeds, chia seeds, mushroom, some spices, dairy products, and tofu are good sources of selenium. Some of the important dietary sources of selenium are given in Figure 7.14 based on the values published in the IFCT (2017).

Some amount is also present in oats, rice, lentils, broccoli, green peas, berries, dates, and raisins. Among non-vegetarian sources, fish, lamb, pork, sea foods, and liver are the richest sources. Most of the cereals and pulses contain selenium ranging from 30 µg/g to 400 µg/g. Commercial Se supplements are also available but should be taken judiciously.

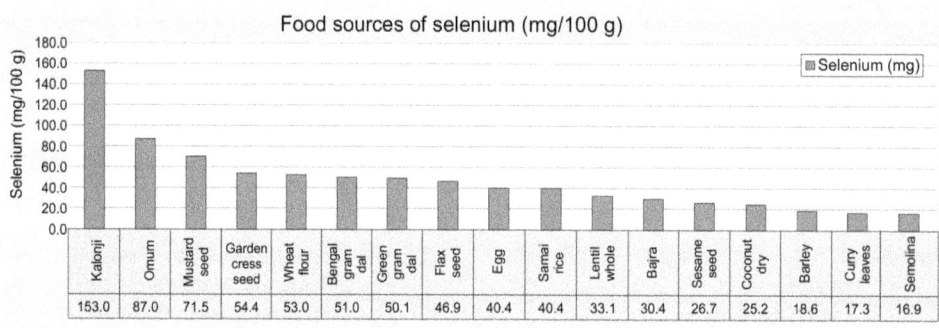

Fig. 7.14: Food sources of selenium.

Deficiency of Selenium

Low dietary intake of selenium usually does not show immediate effect on thyroid activities but gradually affects the conversion of T4 into T3 resulting in increase in T4 and decrease in T3, which is associated with hypothyroidism. Selenium deficiency exacerbates the deficiency of iodine. Deficiency of both trace elements increases the risk of myxedematous cretinism that is characterized by mental growth retardation, in young population in certain geographical regions.

Selenium deficiency is endemic in certain parts of China, Tibet, Siberia, and New Zealand owing to low-selenium content in these regions. Phenylketonuria and maple syrup urine disease in some children from New Zealand, Kashin–Beck disease (deformed arthritis) from Siberia and Asia, and *Keshan disease* (endemic cardiomyopathy) were observed there. Low selenium is observed in volcano-prone areas.

Selenium deficiency is known as Keshan's disease and is found in people residing in hilly and mountainous regions where the soil content of the mineral is low. It is associated with cardiomyopathy in children and women of childbearing age. In the acute form, there is sudden onset of cardiac insufficiency. In the chronic form, there is moderate and sometimes severe cardiac enlargement along with cardiac insufficiency, which may vary in severity. It is possible that accompanying viral infection may be associated, since seasonal and yearly variations have been observed. Some studies indicate involvement of the *Coxsackievirus B3*, either because the virus causes cardiac inflammation or selenium deficiency converts the virus from a harmless virus into a myocarditis-causing strain, due to alterations in the virus' genome. Selenium supplementation using sodium selenite has a protective role against development of the disease but does not help to reverse the damage to cardiac muscle. Genetic studies reveal that there is glutathione peroxidase 1 (GPx1) polymorphism in patients with Keshan's disease and it is likely that this polymorphism places individuals at greater risk of developing the disease when selenium intake and selenium status are poor.

Another endemic disease called Kashin–Beck disease affects millions in Northern China, Tibet, Northern Korea, and South East Siberia. This disease affects articular cartilage and occurs in preadolescent and adolescent children. The cartilage degeneration leads to osteoarthritis. Severe disease can lead to joint deformities and dwarfism. While Keshan's disease can be ameliorated by selenium supplements, Kashin–Beck disease does not respond to selenium supplementation. However, recent attempts have shown that giving sodium selenite supplements for at least 1 year increased the rate of repair of bone lesions in children suffering from the disease. It has been suggested that due to poor selenium intake, and because antioxidant status may be compromised due to polymorphisms in the *GPx* genes, the persons become susceptible to developing this disease. However, other factors that might be associated are consuming grains that contain fungal toxins, iodine deficiency, and drinking contaminated water.

Besides populations at risk these two diseases, there are subgroups who are at risk. Se deficiency also can occur clinically in patients on TPN (total parenteral nutrition) for prolonged periods. Others who have been found to have Se deficiency include patients suffering from HIV or cirrhosis, since these patients have been found to have low selenium status. It has also been observed in patients with Crohn's disease.

Supplementation of selenium was found to slow down the progression of these diseases. Se deficiency or inadequate intake is likely to affect the activity of many selenium containing/selenium-responsive enzymes like GPx1, GPx3, iodothyronine deiodinases, selenoprotein W, and methionine-R-sulfoxide reductase B1 (MsrB1). However, selenium deficiency might predispose the person to additional physiological stresses.

Selenium deficiency alters the activity of glutathione-requiring enzymes. It increases release of glutathione from liver to the periphery resulting in concentration of glutathione in the plasma. Reduced level of glutathione peroxidase tends to increase the generation of free radicals, which further increases the peroxidation and its adverse consequences. Se deficiency may encourage formation of proinflammatory compounds and predispose many diseases.

Selenium deficiency may cause fatigue, hair loss, and skin changes. Poor selenium status has also been observed in patients with cancer, atherosclerosis, and in other diseases such as rheumatoid arthritis, ulcerative colitis, pancreatitis, and asthma. It is also found associated with chronic muscle pain. Since selenium is also required during conversion of thyroid hormones; hence, it can be confused with hypothyroidism. Infection also further brings down the selenium level.

Since selenium prevents lipid, lipoprotein and DNA from oxidative damage, its deficiency can increase the risk of atherosclerosis and cancer.

In case of selenium deficiency, there is elevation of T4 and reduction of T3 level in blood, which is associated with goiter and cretinism, since selenium deficiency exacerbates iodine deficiency. Treatment with selenium alone has been found to aggravate the problem because selenium-dependent deiodinase activity is restored, which leads to increased synthesis and use of thyroxin and iodine, which is still deficient. Iodine deficiency also aggravates selenium deficiency.

Selenium supplementation has shown drastic improvements in cases of Hashimoto thyroiditis, an autoimmune disease, and Graves' disease (a condition of hyperthyroidism). Selenium also provides protection from excess of iodine exposure. Selenium supplementation significantly elevates NaK-ATPase activity and decreases formation of lipid peroxides and is thus a great support in preventing oxidative damage.

> **Research Glimpse:** Selenium (Se) has several biological functions through expression of selenoenzymes. It also has the potential as anti-tumorigenic in high doses but very high can produce adverse effects. Some Se biomarkers, such as the selenoproteins and particularly GPx3 and SEPP1, can provide indication of nutritional Se deficiency and need for Se treatment. Se deficiency is indicated humans is for humans <55 µg/day and for animals <20 µg/kg diet. Other Se biomarkers provide information indirectly through inferences based on Se levels of foods, tissues, urine, or feces. Recent analytical advances using tandem liquid chromatography–mass spectrometry suggest prospects for detecting these metabolites.
>
> *Comb GF. Biomarkers of selenium status. Nutrients. 2015;7(4):2209-36.*

Consequences of Excess Intake of Selenium

Selenium toxicity was commonly found in grazing animals that graze on selenium-rich weeds. Selenium poisoning has been observed in humans with occupational exposures or in those who reside in seleniferous areas. Daily intakes above 700 µg/day or acute consumption of 1-7 mg Se/kg/day results in toxicity in humans. Dermatitis, depression and brittle finger nails, excessive tooth decay, numbness and hemiplegia are some of the non-specific symptoms of poisoning. Animal suffer mild or acute toxicity symptoms in liver, respiratory tract, and vision. Plants grown in seleniferous soil are also rich in selenium. Chronic consumption of selenium (700 µg/day or acute consumption of 1-7 mg Se/kg/day), especially the inorganic form of Se, usually associated occupational exposure may result in peripheral neuropathy, nausea, diarrhea, hair loss, brittle nails, garlic odor on breath, dermatitis, secondary infection, and mottling of teeth.

Hydrogen selenide is a gas and is the most toxic form of selenium. Selenium toxicity was found in people working in various industries like mining, paper, printing, plastic, and infrastructure raw material like cement. Inhalation of selenium through environment may irritate the eyes, produce garlicky odor, and cause headache, fatigue, and indigestion. Selenium intoxication has been found in people consuming supplements. Care should be taken since Se can become a potential environmental and health hazard, as it is used in several industries including electronics, glass, pharmaceuticals, rubber, feed supplements, and fertilizers in agriculture.

Copper

Copper is widely distributed in biological tissues (almost in every cell), particularly in saliva and gastric juice. It is present mostly in the form of metalloprotein. Copper is utilized in reactions involving oxygen where single electron is transferred. It is essential for energy metabolism, synthesis of neurotransmitters, metabolism of nutrients, for collagen synthesis, and antioxidant defense. It is required at every stage from fetal life to old age.

Copper is absorbed largely in the stomach and small intestines, with half to three-fourths of dietary copper being absorbed. Pepsin and HCl in the stomach facilitate the release of copper, which is absorbed through the enterocytes in the brush border of the intestines. In the stomach, ionic copper is released from partially digested food. This ionic copper combines with amino acids, organic acids, and other compounds. If these complexes are soluble, they are absorbed. Copper absorption is regulated by a protein metallothionein, which is present in a numberof tissues including the mucosal cells of the intestines. As the amount of copper in the dietincreases, the percentage absorbed decreases. Absorption is enhanced when low dietaryavailability of copper is low and in presence of organic acids other than ascorbic acid and citrate inthe food. Copper absorption is adversely influenced, if one has high intakes of nutrients like iron,zinc, molybdenum, ascorbic acid, and certain amino acids like sulfur-containing aminoacids as well as sucrose and fructose. Some medications like excessive ingestion of antacidsinhibit absorption. Phytate may also decrease absorption. On the other hand, high-protein diets enhance its absorption. In human milk, ceruloplasmin promotes copper absorption in breastfed infants. After copper is absorbed, ionic copper (Cu^{++}) is bound to albumin and transcuprein in portalblood and transported to the liver. Some amount of Cu^{++} also reaches the kidney and other tissues.

Copper-transporting enzymes assist copperto enter into the main circulation and to the liver (hepatocytes). Liver utilizes copper for itsmetabolic needs like respiration and defense mechanism. In circulation, the copper forms acomplex with protein that is called ceruloplasmin. The ceruloplasmin prevents overload ofcopper in the body and excretes into the bile.

Approximately, 100 mg of copper is present in the body. About one-fourth is present in muscle. It is important that the newborn infant have adequate stores of copper, since human milk contains small amounts of copper. Copper

> **Copper-dependent enzymes:**
> - Amine oxidase
> - Ceruloplasmin
> - Cytochrome-c oxidase
> - Dopamine
> - β-monooxygenase
> - Superoxide dismutase
> - Lysyl oxidase
> - Hephaestin
> - Tyrosinase

concentration in blood is 75–130 µg/L. Metallothioneins (MTs) regulate homeostasis of zinc (Zn) and copper (Cu), mitigate heavy metal poisoning, and alleviate superoxide stress.

Copper is excreted through bile and feces (>90%) and the remaining 10% is excreted through urine and skin. A considerable amount of copper excreted through bile is reabsorbed.

After copper is absorbed, ionic copper (Cu^{++}) is bound to albumin and transcuprein in portal blood and transported to the liver. Some amount of Cu^{++} also reaches the kidney and other tissues. In the liver, copper is bound to proteins, most of it to ceruloplasmin and small amounts to metallothionein and other proteins like albumin, which is released into circulation. From there, it reaches other tissues. Cells contain "chaperone proteins" in the cell membrane. These are believed to bind copper and transfer it to the intracellular compartment.

Functions of Copper

Most copper is tightly bound with different metalloproteins due to which it participates in structural and catalytic activities. There are about 2 dozen Cu-containing enzymes, which play roles in cell respiration, energy utilization, the immune system, neural behavior, bone health, blood chemistry, and antioxidant and energy production. Copper is an intermediate in oxidation–reduction reactions and serves as a cofactor for some metalloenzymes. It is also involved in gene transcription. Table 7.3 summarizes the requirement of copper for different functions.

Constituent of metalloproteins: Ceruloplasmin or ferroxidase is a protein that participates in conversion of ferrous iron (Fe^{++}) to ferric (Fe^{+++}) in order to bind with transferrin. It contains 6–7 copper atoms and is made by the liver. Another metalloprotein is hephaestin, present in the intestinal villi and is believed to facilitate the transport of iron from enterocytes into the circulatory system. In its absence, iron is retained in the intestinal cells. Hephaestin is involved in metabolism and homeostasis of iron and copper. Copper-containing enzymes are important for metabolism of catecholamines. Copper is a part of enzymes involved in dopamine synthesis and for hormones such as thyroid-releasing hormone, corticosteroid-releasing hormone, gonadotropin-releasing hormone, gastrin, cholecystokinin, vasopressin, and others.

Table 7.3: Essentiality of copper for human health.

Brain and nervous system	Brain development, maintenance of brain health throughout life, communication between nerve cells, synthesis of neurotransmitters, formation and maintenance of myelin
Epithelial and connective tissue	Maintenance of healthy skin, connective tissue, wound healing, formation of melanin
Cardiovascular and circulatory system	Structural integrity and function of heart and blood vessels, growth of new blood vessels, circulating cells (structure and function)
Immune system	Effective and healthy immune response formation of WBC Antioxidant defense against reactive oxygen species

Energy metabolism: Cytochrome (C) oxidase is an important copper-containing enzyme involved in oxidative phosphorylation (electron transfer in mitochondria within the cell). This enzyme generates an electrical gradient that is necessary for ATP production by mitochondria. Superoxide dismutase (SOD) also participates in cell respiration and energy utilization process.

Connective tissue formation: Lysyl oxidase is another copper-containing enzyme involved in the reaction that initiates the process of cross-linking, which stabilizes elastin and collagen. Collagen is important since it confers the rigidity and mechanical strength to bone and the biomechanical competence of bone depends on collagen. Lysyl oxidase is also required for proper functioning of the heart (others include cytochrome-C oxidase, cytosolic superoxide dismutase, and dopamine beta-monooxygenase).

Antioxidant defense: Superoxide dismutases (SODs) are important enzymes for removal of toxic free radicals particularly the superoxide radical in ECF and plasma. Excess free radicals are responsible for lipid peroxidation in cell membranes. Ceruloplasmin is another antioxidant, which scavenges hydrogen peroxide and other free radicals and prevents lipid peroxidation and DNA degradation.

Blood coagulation: Factor V, which is involved in blood clotting, contains copper. Similarly, copper interacts with Factor VIII and plays an important role in normal blood coagulation.

Immune system and inflammatory process: Clinical reports and evidence from experimental studies suggest that copper deficiency is associated with increased risk of infection. In severe copper deficiency, changes have been observed in the phenotypic profiles of immune cells in blood, bone marrow as well as lymphoid tissues. The number of lymphocytes and phagocytic cells were reduced. Also, secretion of proinflammatory cytokines, like interleukin (IL)-1, IL-6, tumor necrosis factor-α, has been found to be reduced.

Neurological functions: Copper is present throughout the brain and mostly in the basal ganglia, hippocampus, cerebellum, and numerous synaptic membranes. Copper is essential for normal development of the brain in early life and other neurological functions throughout life such as synthesize myelin for insulation of nerve cells and neurotransmitters to facilitate communication between nerve cells and exchanging nerve impulses. Copper deficiency was associated with altered neuropathology and behavioral changes.

Iron matabolism: Normal iron metabolism and RBC formation require adequate copper status.

Recommended Intake of Copper

ICMR-NIN (2020) has given 1.7 mg/day as the acceptable intake for adults. Requirements are increased by heat, infections, injuries, strenuous exercise, and smoking.

Food Sources of Copper

Rich sources are liver, kidney, shellfish, and oysters. Nuts, especially walnuts, whole grains are good sources. Chocolates and other foods contain small amounts of copper and consumption of a well-balanced diet generally fulfills copper requirements. Maize products, wheat, potato, cabbage, carrot, broccoli, peas, milk, apple, and banana contain some copper. Cu content in foodstuffs differ depending on the local conditions where the foodstuffs are cultivated/grown. It is influenced by the Cu concentration of manures and fungicides used in many crops of cereals, fruit, and vegetables. Ground water, Cu pipes used in household plumbing systems, affects copper content of drinking water. Cu emissions from different industries and use of copper metal in utensils may also affect Cu intake.

Deficiency of Copper: **Causes and Consequences**
Dietary copper deficiency is often indicated by lower level of ceruloplasmin and higher levels of cholesterol, triglycerides, HDL in the serum. Its deficiency alters the lipid metabolism and increases the risk of dyslipidemia, atherosclerosis and nonalcoholic fatty liver disease (NAFLD). It can be linked to the lysyl oxidase deficiency.

Regular consumption of Western diet is characterized by high fructose and high fat may result in copper deficiency. Low copper levels are found in different organs, plasma, and tissue of persons having chronic diseases including cardiovascular disease, central nervous system, and musculoskeletal disorders.

In copper deficiency also, anemia occurs and iron accumulates in the liver since ceruloplasmin is needed to transport iron to the bone marrow where RBC synthesis occurs. Copper deficiency can result in hepatic iron overload and/or cirrhosis. On the other hand, high-iron intakes can interfere with copper absorption. High-zinc intakes (≥50 mg/day) can lead to copper deficiency, due to increased synthesis of metallothionein, which binds copper and this complex is excreted. On the other hand, high-copper intakes do not interfere with zinc metabolism. High-vitamin C intakes from supplements may impair ceruloplasmin oxidase activity, but may not affect copper absorption.

Copper deficiency is characterized by the following:
- Hypochromic anemia that does not respond to iron supplementation
- Leukopenia (less number of leukocytes in the blood)
- Neutropenia (less number of neutrophils in the blood)
- Accelerated loss of bone mineral and susceptibility to fracture
- Increased peroxidation of cell membrane
- Increased blood pressure
- Rise in triglyceride level
- Poor immunity due to depressed level of T and B lymphocytes
- Respiratory infection
- Increased number of platelets
- Abnormality in glucose metabolism
- Abnormal ECG (electrocardiogram).
- Bariatic surgery high intake of zinc

These are reversible on copper administration. Risk of atherosclerosis is increased with copper deficiency since plasma cholesterol, triglycerides, HDL, and blood pressure are elevated. Deficiency also decreases nitric oxide-induced vasodilation and increases risk of thrombogenesis. Less frequent symptoms include abnormalities in the cardiovascular and immune systems. The developing fetus and young infant in the 1st month of life are particularly vulnerable and deficiency can result in neurological abnormalities. Even marginal copper deficiency can adversely influence the brain prolonged copper deficiency and high intake of zinc may predispose the person to myelopathy catheterized by tingling, numbness and pain in arm, leg, neck, abnormal reflex loss, loss of fine motor skill in writing, etc.

Some persons have an autosomal recessive disorder in which ceruloplasmin cannot be synthesized. Individuals with this condition have low serum iron, but high amount of iron in the liver, brain, and pancreas. They develop insulin-dependent diabetes mellitus and other neurological problems. Certain chromosomal disorders, nephrosis, and celiac diseases have been observed due to reduced production of certain copper-dependent enzymes.

Menkes' syndrome: It was first described by John Menkes, an American pediatrician. It is a neurological disorder caused by a genetic mutation and is fatal. It is a genetic deficiency that affects the copper levels in the body. It is caused by mutations in the *ATP7A* gene, which impairs copper export from the intestine to many body tissues. Thus, copper accumulates in some tissues like the small intestines and kidneys, whereas other tissues like the brain will have very low copper levels. Consequently, this has adverse influence on activities of enzymes that play important roles in the structure and function of tissues/systems including the nervous system, blood vessels, bone, skin, and hair. It is characterized by neurological degeneration, mental retardation, connective tissues, and vascular defects. Sufferer of MND shows sparse and "steely, kinky hair", hypotonia, hypothermia, hypopigmentation, and convulsions. Children do not grow well, exhibit failure to thrive, and have developmental delays, intellectual disability. Symptoms generally develop during infancy and children usually die before the age of 3 years.

Consequences of Excessive of Copper
Copper is a highly reactive metal thus, excess copper causes cell damage when homeostatic mechanisms are not maintained. Cu toxicity is often associated with zinc deficiency and excessive oxidative stress. High-copper levels in many persons predispose them to mental illness.

It may occur if intakes are above 10 mg or there is prolonged exposure to foodstuffs stored or cooked in copper ware, especially if the pH is acidic or from supplements. Numerous fungicidal sprays, industrial applications use copper. Copper is toxic to many phytopathogenic species. Caution is required before any toxicity appears (64 mg intake). Marked overload in the liver leads to lipid dysregulation. Toxicity is accompanied by symptoms like epigastric pain, abdominal cramps, nausea, and diarrhea. Higher doses result in liver damage and can lead to coma and death. Copper can also function as a pro-oxidant and give rise to reactive oxygen species. Disturbances in copper metabolism are also implicated now in neurodegenerative diseases like Alzheimer's disease and Down's syndrome.

Wilson's disease: Wilson's disease was first noticed by Sir SAK Wilson in Middle East population, affecting the liver and brain. It is an inherited disorder characterized by psychiatric and behavior abnormalities such as irritability, low threshold of anger, suicidal thoughts, and deteriorating academic and work performance. In this disease, biliary excretion of copper is impaired followed by accumulation of Cu in organs like liver, kidney, and brain. The disease manifests in childhood or later, where the patient generally has liver cirrhosis, fatty infiltration, and neurological problems including difficulty in swallowing, spasms of face and muscles, depression, and emotional problems.

Cu overload decreases the dopamine level and increases the norepinephrine level. This imbalance is associated with several mental illnesses such as autism, paranoid or violent behavior, bipolar disorders, and postpartum depression. If diagnosed early, patients are treated with chelators. Zinc and vitamin C have been shown to protect the body from copper overload via inhibiting intestinal absorption and promoting excretion in the bile. Molybdenum intake has also shown protective effect.

> **Laboratory Laurel:** Though involvement of copper in AD is controversial, copper toxicity in AD brains is attributed to the oxidized form of copper ions, i.e., Cu^{2+}. Alzheimer's disease is characterized by amyloid plaques and neurofibrillary tangles (NFTs) in the brain, which indicate damage of neuronal tissues in the brain. Signs include memory loss, paranoia, loss of reasoning powers, and confusion. One of the first and most severely injured brain areas in AD is the hippocampus, which is associated with neurogenesis and long-term memory storage. Another brain region that suffers from damage in AD due to plaque pathology is the cortex, associated with functions such as argumentation, feeling, and language. High concentration of trace metals, including copper, is observed in amyloid plaques.
>
> *Bagheri S, Squitti R, Haertle T, et al. Role of copper in the onset of Alzheimer's disease compared to other metals. Front Aging Neurosci. 2018;9:446.*

Fluorine

Fluorine is the ionic form of fluoride and is a halogen. Fluorine is the 13th most abundant element. The two terms–fluorine and fluoride–are used interchangeably. Fluoride is considered as a trace element because the amount present in the human body is very small (2.6 g) and only a few milligrams are required daily for dental health. However, it is not considered to be an essential element because it is not essential for growth or for sustaining human life. Fluoride is required for bone and teeth development, as it forms hydroxyapatite with the calcium present in them.

Fluorine is a widely distributed mineral found in soil, water, and food. Fluoride enters the human body not only through food and water but also from products that contain fluoride, e.g., toothpaste. The essentiality of this element for humans is well established. Consumption of foods particularly sweets and refined foods produce acid that demineralize the tooth enamel. Fluorine reduces acid production and prevents tooth decay. On one hand, fluoridation of water is done to prevent dental caries; and on the other hand, excess fluoride in drinking water leads to fluorosis (damaged and pigmented teeth and skeleton).

Human body contains approximately 2.6 g fluorine. It is found in commonly consumed foods mainly from drinking water and tea consumption. Fluoride is soluble and is absorbed in stomach and intestines. After reaching the bloodstream, it rapidly enters the mineralized tissue, i.e., bones and teeth. Absorption is enhanced by acid pH. Fluoride from fluoridated water is absorbed completely. From food, percentage of fluoride absorbed ranges from 50–80%. About one-fourth of the fluoride that is ingested is absorbed in the stomach and the remaining is absorbed in the proximal part of the small intestine, with about 10% being excreted in feces. Fluoride absorption is adversely influenced by calcium and magnesium, whereas presence of phosphate, sulfate, iron, molybdenum, and high-fat diet improves its absorption. Fluoride that is bound to protein is not readily absorbed. Retention tends to be higher in young children with uptake by the developing skeleton and teeth. Most of the absorbed fluoride is distributed in the ECF. Within 20 minutes to an hour, peak concentrations are achieved in blood and fluoride is bound to plasma protein. Fluoride concentration in blood is not homeostatically regulated. Since most of the absorbed fluoride is excreted through urine, therefore kidneys play an important role.

In the body, major fraction (99%) of fluoride is in bone and calcified tissue, with the remaining 1% being present in soft tissues. Connective tissue also contains fluoride. Almost half of the dietary fluoride is excreted rapidly through urine and about 1/10th to 1/5th is excreted through feces. Several factors influence fluoride metabolism such as acid–base balance and if there is any disorder in the same, altitude, physical activity, hormones, renal function, genetic factors and exposure through diet, water, and other sources.

Functions of Fluorine

There is no known metabolic role for fluoride and its function is more of a pharmacologic, preventive measure.

- **Formation of tooth enamel:** Fluoride supports formation of dental enamel. It binds with hydroxyapatite and forms "fluorapatite", which is responsible for hardness of teeth. It further accelerates remineralization of tooth. One of fluoride's primary actions is cariostatic, i.e., prevention of dental caries in both children and adults. It decreases acid production by bacteria in oral plaques and prevents demineralization of teeth, which results in cavities, i.e., dental caries.
- **Support bone growth:** Similar to its role in teeth, fluoride stimulates new bone growth and leads to bone mineralization. It is said that fluoride may reduce bone mineral loss in older persons because bone in which fluoride is incorporated is more resistant to fracture.

However, there is an optimal level/limit for intake above which toxicity occurs.

Recommended Dietary Allowance for Fluoride
However, WHO has recommended 0.5–1.0 mg/L of water for good dental and bone health depending on climate.

> **Fluoridation of water:** As per WHO guideline, maximum fluoride level in water is 1.5 mg/L, at which fluorosis should be minimal.
> Bureau of Indian standards IS:10500:1991 has further reduced the safer limit of fluoride intake to 1.1 mg/L. Maximum permissible limit of fluoride in drinking water in India is 1.2 mg/L. Some states like Uttaranchal, Jharkhand, and Chhattisgarh are fluorosis endemic area. GOI has planned to reduce the fluorine level in drinking water, which is coming from industrial waste and mineral deposits. International Society for Fluoride Research (ISFR) suggested only 0.5ppm fluoride only. Ministry of Health and Family Welfare, GOI has launched National Programme for Prevention and Control of Fluorosis (NPPCF).

Food Sources of Fluoride
Fluoride is present in the environment. It is discharged into water, air, and soil. Excess of it contaminates the water and soil, leading to water and soil pollution. It usually comes from the waste water from industries particularly where aluminum is used frequently. Crops, like finger millet (Ragi), groundnut, and pulses, if cultivated in fluorine-rich soil, are rich in fluorine. Tea leaves also accumulate fluoride from soil. The amount of fluoride in tea depends on the fluorine content of tea leaves as well as water used for brewing and brewing time. Water itself is a significant source, although its content varies with geographic region. Fluoride content in plants and animal food depends on its concentration in soil, water used for irrigation, and air deposition. Most foods contain less than 0.05 mg/100 g unless they are grown in high-fluoride areas. Toothpastes and other dental products that contain fluoride may also contribute considerably to fluoride intake, especially in young children who tend to swallow such products. Marine fish consumed with bones also contributes to intake. Certain medicines and medical treatments also add fluorine in the body pesticidal sprays also contain fluorine.

Fluoride and Pineal Gland
Pineal gland is also popular as the third eye since ancient times. Now, it is considered important in relation to neurogenerative diseases and dentistry. Pineal gland is a neuronal structure in the center of brain but outside the blood–brain barrier. This gland is responsible for producing melatonin, a serotonin-driven hormone, modulating sleep-wake pattern in both circadian and seasonal cycles. Pineal gland contains as much fluoride as teeth. There is correlation with pineal calcium and pineal fluoride level. There is deposition of calcium and phosphorus in it. When pineal fluoride level is high, it replaces hydroxide and carbonate groups of HA-producing fluorapatite resulting in calcification of pineal gland. Earlier calcification of pineal gland was observed in aged population but now it is found in young population also. Studies have shown the association of calcification of pineal gland with Alzheimer's, Parkinson's, schizophrenia, tremors, anxiety, depression, eating disorders, and other mental and nervous disorders.

Defluoridation is essential. In addition to avoiding fluoride exposure, it is also necessary to avoid genetically modified foods, foods grown with pesticides, and use of MSG, artificial ingredients, and chemical preservatives. There are certain ways for reducing exposure to fluoride such as replacing fluoridated water with spring water; considering use of defluoridated toothpaste under supervision; use of foods and herbs like tamarind, alfalfa, coriander, shilajit, dark leafy greens, wheatgrass, algae, and chlorella.

Causes and Consequences of Excessive Intake of Fluoride
The level of fluorine in the body is assessed by Dean's fluorosis index (DFI) and community fluorosis index (CFI). Fluoride has a strong affinity for hard tissues and easily gets deposited in teeth and bones in the body. Excessive intake of fluoride usually comes from ground water contaminated by granite rocks and industry waste water. High-fluoride concentrations in ground water (above 1.5 mg/L) may also pose health problems such as fluorosis. **Fluorosis** is a disease characterized by deposition of fluorides in the hard and soft tissues in the body. There is discoloration of teeth and crippling disorder in the skeletal tissues. Hence, they are referred as dental fluorosis and skeletal fluorosis.

In India, high-fluoride levels in water and soil are found in certain geographical regions of UP, Assam, and Tamil Nadu. Calcium and vitamin D nutrition status exacerbate the high incidence of crippling deformities in poor residents from endemic fluorosis zones in Gujarat, Bihar, and Karnataka. The incidences are high in areas where aluminum and iron ores are present.

Intake of 0.1 mg per kg of body weight, which is only twice the recommended intake during childhood, causes dental fluorosis (mottling–white or brown spots and discoloration) of teeth (at least 10 mg/day for 10 years or more). High levels of fluorine adversely affect neurodevelopment in children. Parents need to guard against children swallowing fluoridated toothpaste. Moderate-to-severe fluorosis (both dental and skeletal) is observed in adults.

In dental fluorosis, hypomineralization of the tooth enamel occurs, which is evidenced by several visible changes in enamel and tooth discoloration. Compared to normal enamel, hypomineralized enamel is opaque and does not have luster. Severity of changes is influenced by the dose, duration of exposure, and age. If the problem is mild, the teeth may have faint white lines or specks; but when it is slightly severe, white mottled patches can be seen and in really severe cases, there is brown discoloration, the teeth are brittle and pitted, and the enamel is rough.

Hypomineralization occurs because in maturing enamel, excess fluoride ions alter the rate of enzymatic degradation of enamel matrix protein called amelogenin. Also, fluoride alters the action of the protease through decreased availability of free calcium in the enamel resulting in less than normal mineralization of enamel. Unusually, high intakes lead to abnormal calcification of bone and ligaments, the ultimate consequence being skeletal fluorosis. There are several areas in India where endemic fluorosis is a public health problem due to high amounts of fluoride in soil and therefore in the water as well as the crops grown in these areas. There are three stages of skeletal fluorosis:

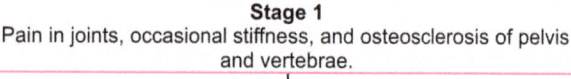

Stage 1
Pain in joints, occasional stiffness, and osteosclerosis of pelvis and vertebrae.

Stages 2 and 3
Increased osteosclerosis, calcification of ligaments, muscle wasting, hypercalcification of vertebrae, and neurological defects leading to crippling.

The development of skeletal fluorosis (a chronic condition) and its severity are influenced by how long the persons have been exposed and the amount of exposure. There is weakening of bones and high risk of wrist and hip fractures. According to the National Research Council, USA, fractures are associated with fluoride levels of 1–4 ppm. Unfortunately, fluorosis is not clinically evident in the early stages and sometimes is diagnosed as either rheumatoid arthritis or ankylosing spondylitis. Nonskeletal manifestations also occur and involve RBCs and GI mucosa. Acute poisoning has been reported to lead to nausea, vomiting, diarrhea, salivation, sweating, headaches, generalized weakness, hypocalcemia, and hypokalemia. It may also lead to cardiac arrhythmia, renal failure, and death.

Fluorine overload may result in kidney injury and nephrosis usually in case of ingestion of fluorine-containing drugs. Its symptoms can be polyuria, dehydration with hypernatremia. It also tends to suppress the thyroid function. Fluorine is apparently antagonistic to iodine. Fluoride concentration in the range of 100–200 ppm alters thyroid hormone status, i.e., increased concentration of TSH and decreased concentrations of T3 and T4, resulting in hypothyroidism.

Other adverse effects of excess fluoride include increase in size of hepatic cells, myocardial mineralization, and degeneration of the seminiferous tubules in the testes. High exposure to fluorine has been found to increase the levels of follicle-stimulating hormone and luteinizing hormone as well as decrease estrogen levels, disturb the ratio of androgens to estrogen and the ratios of estrogen receptor to androgen receptor.

Fluoride has been found to an endocrine disruptor in low doses and chronic exposure to fluoride through drinking water, when serum/plasma levels are ≥0.1 ppm, has been shown to cause insulin resistance, and impaired glucose tolerance. Blood fluoride levels have been found to be inversely associated with insulin secretion. In diabetics, fluoride exposure has been associated with reduced bone mass and bone strength.

Excess flouride may have adverse effects on the brain and affect learning, concentration, and memory. The developing brain is more vulnerable and toxicity could cause permanent damage.

Treatment: It is not just a food-based problem but a public health problem; hence, measures require community awareness and participation in solving the issue. Nalgonda technique is a popular method to minimize incidence of fluorosis by reducing the level of fluorine in underground water. This method was devised in 1960s by the National Environmental Engineering Research Institute (NEERI), Nagpur, India using lime and alum.

> **Research Glimpse:** Fluoride is often described as a "double-edged sword" as inadequate ingestion is associated with dental caries, whereas excessive intake leads to dental, skeletal, and soft tissue fluorosis. Defluoridation was the conventional and widely tested method for supplying safe water to the fluorosis-affected communities. Various techniques and materials were tried throughout the world for defluoridation of water. Defluoridation techniques can be adsorption technique.
>
> Ion exchange technique, precipitation technique, and other techniques, which include electrochemical defluoridation and reverse osmosis. Used across world and current status of defluoridation in India.
>
> *Piddennavar R, Krishnappa P. Review on Defluoridation Techniques of Water. Int J Eng Sci. 2013;2(3):86-94.*

Manganese

Manganese (Mn) is widely distributed in nature. The human body contains very small amounts, i.e., 10–20 mg. Mn is a constituent of many metalloenzymes and several enzymes are activated by Mn. However, like many other elements while it is essential, it can also be toxic.

Manganese (Mn) is absorbed in the gastrointestinal tract and then transported to organs enriched in the mitochondria (in particular the liver, pancreas, and pituitary) where it is rapidly concentrated. Mn is absorbed in the small as well as the large intestines. Mn is absorbed in the small intestine (by active transport) as well the large intestines (by passive diffusion). About 2.5% of ingested Mn is absorbed through the intestine. Changes in absorption occur in response to variations in intakes, the amount that is present in plasma and thus contribute to homeostasis. Absorption is inhibited by high intakes of calcium and phytate. Though tea contains good amounts of Mn but high content of tannin found in tea binds manganese and prevents its absorption from the gastrointestinal tract. Similarly, while the concentration of manganese in cereal grains is quite high, but phytates and fiber present in cereals limit the absorption of Mn.

Manganese is taken to the liver (vulnerable organs like pancreas and pituitary) from where it is transported to other tissues in a bound form—the protein to which Mn is bound is transferrin or α-2 macroglobulin and albumin. Mn and Fe share transferrin for transport, thus Mn uptake and distribution may be linked to iron status. High Fe intakes may compete for binding and absorption sites and thus decrease Mn absorption. On the other hand, if Fe intakes are low, Mn absorption increases. Mn is not excreted much through urine but through feces. Its homeostatic regulation occurs through hepatobiliary excretion. In blood, Mn is transported bound to plasma ceruloplasmin. Besides this protein, other proteins may serve as ligands such as albumin, transferrin, beta globulin, and transglutaminase, very small amount of Mn in either plasma or tissues is present in the free form. Most of the cellular Mn is present in the mitochondria and some amount in the nucleus and golgi apparatus. Golgi apparatus may have an important role in preventing accumulation of Mn in mitochondria and thereby impairment of mitochondrial function. Manganese is biologically active in two oxidative states Mn^{2+} and Mn^{3+}. Mn^{3+} is the form found in the enzyme manganese SOD, the oxidative state that binds to transferrin, and the form that may interact with Fe^{3+}.

Functions of Manganese

Manganese is important for growth, development of bone and connective tissue, reproduction, and central nervous system, energy metabolism, immunological function, reproductive hormone function, blood clotting, as well as regulation of cellular energy. Since it is either an integral part of certain enzymes or acts as cofactor, it plays role significant in the following:

Constituent of metalloenzymes/synthesis and activation of enzymes: Mn is a constituent of several metalloenzymes such as superoxide dismutase, arginase, phosphoenolpyruvate decarboxylase, and glutamine synthase, which play significant roles in growth and development, immune response, ATP production, and blood sugar homeostasis. It is involved in synthesis and activation of numerous enzymes such as oxidoreductases, transferases, hydrolases, lyases, isomerases, and ligases. It is also a cofactor for enzymes involved in neurotransmitter synthesis and metabolism.

Activation of vitamin B_{12}: B_{12} that is ingested is metabolized before it can serve as a cofactor. The enzymes involved in this process specifically require Mn.

Defense against free radicals: Superoxide dismutase (SOD) is a Mn-containing enzyme, present in the mitochondria that protect against oxidative stress. Mn SOD catalyzes conversion of superoxide radicals to hydrogen peroxide, which is then acted upon by other antioxidant enzymes; hence, it also helps to prevent lipid peroxidation in cell membranes.

Nitrogen metabolism: Mn is a cofactor for the enzyme arginase that is involved in urea synthesis. Mn may also be important for production of nitric oxide by microglia. Mn is also a cofactor of enzymes involved in bradykinin degradation and those involved in intracellular signaling and processing. It activates the enzyme glutamine synthetase, which converts glutamine to glutamate that is required for synthesis of the neurotransmitter gamma aminobutyric acid (GABA). It is involved in acceleration of protein synthesis, in hematopoiesis. Another enzyme activated by Mn is arginase, which is necessary for urea cycle.

Carbohydrate metabolism: It is essential for glucose metabolism and gluconeogenesis. Enzymes specifically activated by Mn are pyruvate carboxylase, phosphoenolpyruvate carboxykinase (both important for gluconeogenesis), and glycosyltransferases. It helps in synthesis and secretion of insulin, thus it provides protection in metabolic syndrome. Mn is a component or activator of some enzymes, mostly antioxidants, and plays an important role in metabolisms of carbohydrates and lipids.

Lipid metabolism: Enzymes involved in lipid metabolism and specifically activated by Mn are farnesyl pyrophosphate synthetase (cholesterol synthesis) and phosphatidylcholine synthase.

Formation of connective tissues: Glycosyltransferase is an enzyme activated by Mn and is involved in syntheses of mucopolysaccharides, which are important components of connective tissue. Mn is also necessary for proteoglycan synthesis. Proteoglycans are required for bone and cartilage formation. Mn is needed to activate the enzyme prolidase that has a role in collagen formation. If there is prolidase deficiency, wound healing is adversely affected. Thus, Mn is important for wound healing.

Brain development: Mn is required for brain development and cellular homeostasis besides having a role as cofactor for numerous enzymes as well as in neurotransmitter synthesis. It is likely to be necessary for astrocyte function also.

Other functions: Mn is necessary for enzymes involved in synthesis of compounds necessary for formation and maintenance of cartilage and other connective tissues. Mn also has a role in metabolism of sulfate and in apoptosis. Mn metabolism and homeostasis are linked to that of Fe because both are bound and taken up by transferrin and the divalent metal transporter-1. Also, Mn binds to mucin at the same site where ferric ions are bound. This binding to mucin stabilizes the ions and prevents their being precipitated in the gut lumen. Mn and Fe also have similar affinities for mobilferrin, a cytoplasmic protein, which acts as an intermediate between the iron bound to transferrin and the incorporation of iron into hemoglobin. Consequently in iron deficiency, Mn absorption increases in the gastrointestinal tract.

Recommended Acceptable Intake for Manganese

ICMR-NIN (2020) has suggested the acceptable intake for manganese to be 4 mg/day for Indian adults.

Food Sources of Manganese

Manganese (Mn) is naturally found the earth's crust, rocks, soil, water, and food. In nature, it does not occur in pure state but as oxides, carbonates, and silicates. Mn is also used in many types of industries such as steel, batteries, etc. It is also present in drinking water. Whole wheat, rice, pineapple, spinach, sweet potato, seeds, nuts, almonds, red wine, ginger, and black tea are good sources. Meat, fish, poultry, and egg contain low amounts of Mn.

Deficiency of Manganese: Causes and Consequences

Low levels of manganese in the body can infertility, bone malformation, weakness, and seizures. Mn deficiency tends to alter cell membrane permeability and results in mitochondrial dysfunction or disorder, and finally causes MetS or metabolic diseases. Deficiency will increase oxidative stress and increase in the production of ROS, which are linked to the development of insulin resistance, T2DM, and obesity. Mn competes for iron (Fe) transporters by inhibiting divalent metal transporter-1 (DMT1), binding with Fe, and disrupting the homeostasis of, cobalt (Co), lead (Pb), mercury (Hg), nickel (Ni), zinc (Zn) and cesium (Cs) in cells. Mn deficiency may also result in adverse effects on growth, birth defects, reduced fertility, impairment in bone formation, and alterations in metabolism of the three macronutrients.

Normally, Mn deficiency does not occur unless the diet is deliberately made deficient. In individuals who were seen to have Mn deficiency, there was dermatitis, slow growth of hair and nails, decrease in serum cholesterol and clotting proteins, while serum calcium and phosphorus as well as alkaline phosphatase activity were elevated.

Deficiency has been found to impair activities of osteoblasts and osteoclasts, suggesting that it may be important for healthy joints and bones. Animal studies showed that Mn deficiency adversely affects skeletal development resulting in enlarged joints, shortened limbs, twisted legs, stiffness, and lameness. In experimental studies on humans, fine scaly erythematous rash has been observed. In a child on long-term TPN, demineralization and poor growth were observed that were corrected by manganese supplementation. Mn deficiency may contribute to several diseases. Low Mn levels and low intakes have been associated with elevated plasma glucose concentrations. Manganese supplementation has been found to improve lymphocytes and SOD activity. Many diseases have been linked to low Mn concentrations in serum, e.g., epilepsy, Down's syndrome, and osteoporosis, but it is not clear what is the role of this element in these.

Consequences of Excessive Intake of Manganese

Since Mn is being widely used in many industries and medical activities, thus human bodies, particularly the brains, are at high risk of Mn toxicity. It is now considered as a common environmental contaminant. Miners, welders, and steel makers are at high risk. Mn accumulation is also associated with reproductive and developmental effects that may result in impaired fertility, impotence, and libido in males.

At typical dietary intakes, no ill effects have been observed so far. However, exposures at workplace or very high intakes have been associated with impaired motor activity (tremors). It interferes with iron absorption and affects the central nervous system. Mn can be inhaled at the workplace. Additives to petrol contain Mn that can be inhaled and taken up by olfactory neurons and transmitted to brain. Elevated Mn concentrations may be neurotoxic. Toxicity has been observed in workers exposed to high amount of Mn dust and inhalation. In China, such workers suffered from psychosis, hallucinations, and symptoms similar to Parkinson's disease.

Chromium

Chromium (Cr) is a transition element. It occurs in many valence states, the most common being Cr^{3+} and Cr^{6+}. Chromium is required in trace amounts but the amount needed for optimal health is not well defined. Cr is found primarily in two forms—(1) trivalent (chromium 3^+), which is biologically active and found in food, and (2) hexavalent (chromium 6^+), a toxic form that results from industrial pollution. In its trivalent form (Cr^{3+}), chromium is necessary for metabolism of carbohydrates as well as lipids and nucleic acids. In biological systems, Cr^{3+}, is the most stable and hence is important. It is found in food, air, and water; other forms may be present in aerosols and pollutants and can be harmful. Thus, humans are exposed to chromium through diet/food intake, inhalation as well as dermal contact.

Chromium is absorbed mainly from the jejunum and appears to be transported bound to ferritin. Extremely small amount of dietary chromium is absorbed (0.5–2%) and most of the ingested chromium is excreted in feces. Absorption tends to be lower as intakes increase. Absorption is influenced by the presence of other factors in the diet. Ascorbic acid increases absorption whereas phytate decreases it. Some medications have also been found to alter absorption. Cr^{6+} is reduced to Cr^{3+} by hydrochloric acid in the stomach. Absorption is apparently not influenced by age, however, insulin-dependent diabetics have been found to absorb twice to four times the chromium absorbed than by healthy individuals. Very small amounts are stored in the human body. The half-life of all tissue stores is estimated to be 100 days. Chromium is concentrated in various organs like liver, kidney, testes, spleen, and bone. Chromium is largely excreted through urine and small amounts are lost through sweat and bile. Urinary losses in diabetes are reportedly higher than in healthy individuals.

Functions of Chromium

Several functions have been identified for Cr, but they need to be confirmed with adequate research evidence.

Carbohydrate metabolism: Chromium is an integral part of glucose tolerance factor (GTF), which potentiates insulin action. It has been proposed that trivalent Cr is the cofactor for a biologically active molecule that potentially enhances the effects of insulin on target tissues. Studies have shown that chromium stimulates glucose uptake. This is probably through the action of chromodulin [or low-molecular-weight chromium-binding substance (LMWCr)], a peptide that contains chromium. The mechanism of action could be more than one: (a) chromium moves into the cell and its binding to apochromodulin is stimulated when insulin binds to its receptors. Chromodulin then possibly binds to insulin receptors and upregulates insulin signaling molecules resulting in increased translocation of the glucose transporter-4 (GLUT4) from the cytosol to the cell membrane. (b) Chromium inhibits the activity of negative regulators of insulin signaling, thereby improving insulin sensitivity. (c) Cr reduces insulin clearance and inhibits insulin degradation. (d) Cr reduces oxidative stress and inflammation and thus has a positive effect on insulin resistance.

Chromium promotes oxidative metabolism of glucose as well as synthesis of fatty acids in adipose tissue and decreases glycosylated hemoglobin (HbA1c) an indicator of the extent of blood glucose control. However, it is not clear whether diabetics who do not have chromium deficiency would benefit from consuming high amounts of chromium.

Growth: Malnourished children who were given a supplement containing chromium showed better growth than a group given a supplement without chromium. In patients given total parenteral nutrition, weight loss was ameliorated when

chromium was included in the TPN solution. It has been suggested that chromium may increase lean body mass.
- **Lipid metabolism:** Research evidence suggests that chromium decreases serum total cholesterol and raises HDL.
- **DNA transcription:** Binding of chromium to DNA appears to promote RNA synthesis.
- **Other functions:** Chromium may be important for increasing serum immunoglobulin in stressful conditions. It may be beneficial in conditions of trauma and those persons who lose chromium in urine when they exercise strenuously. Chromium is found to increase lean body mass and thereby could enhance athletic performance.

Recommended Acceptable Intake
ICMR-NIN (2020) has recommended that the acceptable intake for chromium for Indian adults is 50 µg/day.

Food Sources of Chromium
Whole grains, pulses, Brewer's yeast, nuts, wheat germ, green leafy vegetables, dried basil, broccoli, black pepper, cinnamon, raisins, honey, dairy products, cheese, dark chocolate, and mushrooms are good sources of chromium. Cooking in steel utensils can provide additional amounts of the metal, especially if some acidic/sour substances are cooked. Meat, poultry, fish, and dairy products are not good sources.

Vitamin/mineral supplements contain chromium. Specific supplements of chromium picolinate are also available which contain about 200-600 ug chromium per tablet.

Deficiency of Chromium: Causes and Consequences
Deficiency may limit the action of insulin and adversely affect cellular response to insulin, metabolism of carbohydrates, protein and lipids. Chromium-deficient diets may raise the total cholesterol, and lower utilization of stored fat.

In animals, weight gain is reduced and chromium depletion resulted in higher fasting blood glucose compared to rats given chromium chloride supplement. In humans given TPN, supplements decrease the requirements of insulin and improved glucose tolerance. Chromium losses may be increased during infection, acute exercise, pregnancy, and lactation as well as physical trauma and stress.

Chromium deficiency also manifests as neuropathy, encephalopathy, and impaired immune response. Chromium supplementation has been reported to reduce peripheral neuropathy. As age advances, the levels of chromium in hair, sweat, and blood decrease significantly. It is also low in gestational diabetes, as suggested by a study from south India.

Consequences of Excessive Intake of Chromium
Due to its association with carbohydrate metabolism, the use of chromium has been explored for weight management and the use of chromium picolinate as a supplement has increased, although there is no strong scientific evidence to support their use.

Hexavalent form of chromium (Cr^{6+}) is a toxic and environmental pollutant. There is evidence that Cr^{6+} is a strong oxidant. Therefore, chromium can produce hydroxyl radicals. Cr^{6+} enters the cells more readily than the trivalent form. Although Cr^{6+} is readily reduced to Cr^{3+}, chromium adducts with DNA are formed, resulting in genetic alteration and mutations. The hexavalent compound has been found to be mutagenic. Among industrial workers exposed to Cr^{6+} compounds (even dermal exposure), various health problems have been observed including allergic dermatitis, skin lesions, and increased incidence of lung cancer.

Molybdenum

Molybdenum-dependent enzymes are involved in the carbon, nitrogen, and sulfur cycles and play an important role in determining the health of the ecosystem.

Molybdenum (Mo) is an essential and ubiquitous element and is present in trace amounts (less than 1 microgram of wet tissues) bound with various enzyme molecules. It exists in many oxidation states but the most stable are 4^+ and 6^+. About half of the body, Molybdopterins are a class of cofactors in Mo-containing enzymes is present in liver; other tissues adrenal glands, kidney and bones. In food and water, Mo is present as soluble molybdates like and are rapidly absorbed by passive diffusion, over a wide range of intakes (even up to doses of 1 mg). It is possible that there is a high-affinity transporter that is involved in Mo absorption. Mo is probably absorbed from the stomach and proximal intestines (although not much is known about the mechanism of Mo absorption). About 90% of Mo may be absorbed. Sulfate inhibits its absorption. In blood, Mo is bound to the protein α2-macroglobulin. Molybdenum in conjunction with a pterin called molybdopterin (a unique pterin) is part of a large group of enzymes that have a role in transferring oxygen either to or from physiological molecule. Molybdenum combines with molybdopterin to form the molybdenum cofactor, essential for the activities of the enzymes xanthine oxidase, aldehyde oxidase, and sulfite oxidase. A major fraction of ingested Mo is excreted in urine, although the kidneys reabsorb a considerable proportion.

Molybdopterin is catabolized to urothione, which is excreted through urine. The amount of urothione reflects the amount of molybdopterin synthesized in the body. Urinary excretion is probably important for homeostatic regulation of Mo. As dietary intake increases, urinary excretion also increases, and when intake is low, urinary excretion decreases. Some Mo is also excreted through bile. Not much Mo is stored and in most of the tissue, Mo is probably associated with molybdoenzymes. In blood, Mo is believed to be present in the form of Mo^{6+} and a small amount is bound to α2-macroglobulin. Some Mo is present in RBCs where it is mostly bound to protein.

Functions of Molybdenum
Molybdenum is a part of many enzymes responsible for catalyzing redox reactions. Many of these enzymes also contain other prosthetic groups such as flavin adenine dinucleotide or heme.

These enzymes are involved in the metabolism of aromatic aldehydes and the catabolism of sulfur-containing amino acids and heterocyclic compounds, including purines, pyrimidines, and pteridines. The molybdenum atom is part of the Mo cofactor at the active site of four enzymes in humans: sulfite oxidase, xanthine oxidoreductase, aldehyde oxidase, and mitochondrial amidoxime-reducing component. At the active site of the molybdoenzymes, Mo is present in its biologically active form—an organic molecule known as molybdenum cofactor. In these, Mo is linked to a pterin forming molybdopterin as the cofactor. It is mainly involved in redox functions where it acts as a cofactor in metalloenzymes and flavin-dependent enzymes particularly xanthine oxidase and xanthine dehydrogenase including enzymes that are involved in:

- Conversion of sulfite to sulfate by sulfite oxidase, which is needed for metabolism of the sulfur-containing amino acids methionine and cysteine.
- Hydroxylation/oxidation of various purines, pyrimidines by xanthine oxidase, which catalyzes the degradation of nucleotides to uric acid (uric acid is an important antioxidant). Aldehyde oxidase is important for hydroxylation reactions.
- Synthesis of taurine from cysteine.
- Stabilizing the glucocorticoids.

Food Sources of Molybdenum
Molybdenum is present in almost all food sources in the form of soluble molybdates. It can be obtained from whole cereal grains, legumes, nuts, milk and milk products, and organ meats like liver. Large proportion of Mo intake is accounted by cereals and cereal products. Presence of molybdenum in food depends on the presence of the mineral in the soil. Molybdenum is more available from water than from solid foods. Black tea inhibits Mo absorption considerably.

Recommended Intake
Overall, there is insufficient scientific evidence but in some countries an adequate intake has been proposed. In Europe, it is 65 µg/day for adult men and women as well as pregnant and lactating women.

Deficiency of Molybdenum: Causes and Consequences
Deficiency of molybdenum is rare or observed when the diet contains antagonistic elements like copper, sulfate, and zinc. It has been seen in a patient maintained for a prolonged period on total parenteral nutrition (TPN). This patient had elevated levels of methionine, uric acid, hyperuricemia and low sulfate excretion. The patient also exhibited mental disturbance progressing to coma. Supplementation with Mo improved the condition. Low dietary intake of Mo could compromise the ability to metabolize and detoxify some xenobiotic compounds.

Genetic deficiency of the Mo cofactor has been found to occur, although rarely. Infants exhibit failure to thrive and have seizures. These infants had elevated levels of urinary sulfite, hypouricemia, and there was loss of white matter in the brain. The lifespan of individuals with genetic deficiency of the Mo cofactor is short, with most dying in infancy or early childhood. In experimental studies, severe deficiency led to development of xanthine kidney stones. Also metabolism of toxic sulfite to nontoxic sulfate compounds was impaired.

Consequences of Excess Intake of Molybdenum
High-dietary intakes of molybdenum may be associated with altered purine metabolism. Intakes in milligrams can result in gout. In animals, intakes exceeding 5 mg/kg of body weight resulted in reproductive failure. Other signs of toxicity in animals were anemia, diarrhea, osteoporosis, discoloration of hair, and joint abnormalities. Many of these are also seen in copper deficiency. In humans, intake of 540 mg/day was found to increase loss of copper through urine. Hence, the tolerable upper intake level has been set at 2 mg/day.

Excess intake of molybdenum can interfere with iron and copper absorption. Molybdenum can form compounds with copper (thiomolybdates) in the intestines, which are poorly absorbed. Moreover, it alters affinity of copper to be incorporated into ceruloplasmin and increases copper elimination. The symptoms of molybdenum toxicity are generally similar to those of copper deficiency.

Ultratrace Elements

Ultratrace elements play key roles in many biochemical processes in the body. They participate with many enzymes as cofactors and facilitate conversion of substrate molecules into specific end products. Some elements participate in oxidation reduction reactions in order to generate and for utilization of metabolic energy and are also involved the chemical transformation of molecules. Some of them have structural roles and impart stability to biological molecules.

The elements having regulatory roles are important in binding of molecules to receptor sites on cell membranes and alter the ionic nature of membranes to control transport of molecules in and out of the cell. They are also involved in gene expression and formation of certain proteins.

Ultratrace elements are those, which are required in amounts less than 1.0 mg per day. Ultratrace minerals include arsenic, boron, cadmium, nickel, silicon, and vanadium. Their physiological roles are not yet defined hence their RDA but their deficiency has been found responsible for certain degenerative diseases. Many of these elements have been reported to have toxic effect when taken in large amount. Ultratrace elements are not always obtained from dietary sources, but they may take enter the body from external exposure like industrial waste, air and water pollution, etc.; many of them are heavy metals that can cause heavy damage to the system.

Arsenic
Studies on animals suggest that arsenic may have beneficial effects in ultratrace amounts. Arsenic is semi-metallic in nature. It is present in the earth's crust and is widely distributed throughout the environment in the air, water, and land; however, its concentration varies from place to place. It is also present in high concentration in ground water in different countries. Humans are exposed to arsenic through contaminated ground water, foods, drugs, cigarette smoke, fossil fuels, etc. It can easily be present in food and organ meats and seafoods (mussel) are particularly rich in it. Excess has toxic effects in terms of cancers and skin lesions.

Arsenic is well absorbed by the body from both organic and inorganic sources. From intestines, it easily reaches the liver and other tissues. It is bound to sulfhydryl group of protein and usually found in skin, hair, and nails. It is largely excreted through urine.

Functions of Arsenic
- It is involved in metabolism of methionine, arginine, and taurine.
- It plays a role in phospholipid synthesis.
- It is antagonistic with selenium and iodine and tends to inhibit the iodine uptake by the thyroid.

Deficiency of Arsenic
It can impair the metabolism of methionine by diminishing the activity of S-adenosylmethionine (SAM). Growth deficits and abnormal reproduction have been observed in some animal species. To date, there is no evidence of deficiency in humans.

Toxicity: Besides natural drinking water containing high levels of arsenic, man-made sources such as mining, metal smelting and burning of fossil fuels contribute sufficiently to arsenic contamination of air, water, and soil. Coal-fired power plants, burning vegetation and volcanic activity and use of arsenic-containing pesticides contaminate the environment.

Arsenic in the form of arsenic trioxide, if 0.76–1.95 mg is ingested, can be fatal. Chronic exposure of arsenic concentration less than 0.05 mg/L is found to cause skin diseases, neurological and cardiovascular system disorder, and skin, kidney, and lung cancer and its elevated concentrations in drinking water may result in increased incidence of abortions and stillbirth. WHO (2018) reports that exposure to arsenic in utero and early childhood is linked to negative impacts on cognitive development and increased deaths in young adults. It is highly toxic in inorganic form.

Boron

Earlier, boron was found to be important for growth and development of vascular plants, marine algae, and some bacteria. Scientific evidence suggested and boron was unknowingly being consumed by human beings in drinking water and foods. It is found to be essential for human health. It affects bone growth and central nervous system function, alleviates arthritic symptoms, facilitates hormone action, and is associated with a reduced risk for some types of cancer.

Boron is a nonmetallic element, naturally found in soil, water, and food. Research evidence shows that it is essential for higher animals and therefore it is probably an essential element for humans. Boron from food is readily and completely absorbed (>90%) through the human gut and distributed in body water, blood and soft tissues, and excreted in urine in the form of boric acid. The half-life of boron is approximately 21 hours. Higher amounts of boron are found in bones, thyroid gland, and spleen. However, boron does not appear to accumulate in tissues even when intakes exceed average normal intakes.

Its role in plants possibly include: cell wall synthesis, lignification, sugar transport, ascorbate metabolism, and DNA synthesis. The possible functions in humans need to be established but its deficiency has given clues that boron performs significant roles.

Functions of Boron
Boron is reported to influence the formation and/or activity of substances that are involved in numerous biochemical processes such as S-adenosylmethionine, diadenosine phosphates, and nicotinamide adenine dinucleotide (NAD). It also forms complexes with phosphoinositides, glycoproteins, and glycolipids that affect cell membrane integrity and function.

In various animal models, it has been observed that boron is necessary for embryonic and fetal development, growth, and maturation. Molecules like S-adenosylmethionine (SAM) and diadenosine phosphates contain boron. Other possible functions include:

- Boron appears to be essential for growth. It improves mineralization of bone and retention of mineral in bone. Also, it may be necessary for wound healing by possibly promoting release of proteins and proteoglycans. In animals, it has been shown to have an anti-osteoporotic effect.
- Appears to be important for immune function.
- It may have a role in carbohydrate (glucose) metabolism, possibly through influencing either insulin production or insulin sensitivity.
- It may be important for brain composition, brain function, and cognitive processes such as attention, memory, and psychomotor skills.
- It may have a role in cell membrane function—influencing cellular response to hormones transmembrane/cell signaling or movement of anions and cations across membranes.
- Diadenosine phosphates are boron binders that are signal nucleotides and involved in platelet aggregation and neuronal response.
- Boron acts as a competitive inhibitor for some important enzymes and through this is possibly involved in metabolic regulation, e.g., inflammatory immune processes, metabolism of reactive oxygen species.
- It may be involved in metabolism and utilization of calcium, copper, and magnesium, possibly reduces the rate of excretion and increases serum calcium levels.
- It may be involved in triglyceride metabolism.
- It may be involved in hormone action such as enhancing beneficial effects of estrogen on bone, increasing effectiveness of insulin and 1,25-dihydroxyvitamin D.
- In animals, it has been shown to be anti-inflammatory, antioxidant, antineoplastic, anticoagulant, and to have hypolipidemic effects.
- Supplementation with boron was found to improve serum 17β-estradiol and testosterone levels in menopausal women.

Food Sources
Food sources of boron are apple, citrus fruits, nuts, and legumes (most foods of plant origin including leafy vegetables). It is also found in wine and beer.

Deficiency of Boron

Natural boron deficiency in humans is rare except where soil is deficient in boron. Low-boron intakes also result in impaired bone health and immune response. Some reports indicate that there is reduced alertness, memory, and psychomotor skills. Deficiency may increase vulnerability to vitamin D. Since it is associated with calcium metabolism and estrogen, it may increase the urinary excretion of calcium and magnesium in postmenopausal women. Therefore, there may be increased risk of osteoporosis in case of boron deprivation.

In animal studies, feeding a very low boron diet resulted in brain electrical activity changes consistent with similar to changes that occur in general malnutrition and lead toxicity. Very low boron intakes were also associated with poorer performance on tasks of motor speed and dexterity, attention, and short-term memory.

Consequences of Excess Intake of Boron

Information on toxicity is limited to case reports of poisoning. Chronic intake of 1 gram or more daily may adversely influence appetite, resulting in weight loss. Higher intakes may result in nausea, vomiting, headache, diarrhea, hypothermia, and restlessness. The kidneys may be affected.

Cobalt

Cobalt is widespread in natural environment and is frequently used in numerous industries, medicine, and nuclear power plants. Cobalt is an essential trace element for the human body and occurs in organic and inorganic forms. The organic form is a necessary component of vitamin B_{12} (hydroxocobalamin) and plays a very important role in forming amino acids, some proteins to form the myelin sheath of nerve cells, and synthesizing certain neurotransmitters. Its excess or deficiency will influence these unfavorably.

Activity of certain metalloenzymes is dependent on cobalt as a cofactor. The cobalt content of foods has not been studied much; however, nuts, potatoes, and bread appear to contain some amounts. Varying amounts (7-37%) are retained by the body. Apparently, the mechanism of absorption is the one that is involved in iron absorption. Binding of cobalt to mucin in the intestines improves the uptake of the metal. Low-iron status may increase cobalt uptake. In blood, most of the cobalt is bound to transferrin. Most of the ingested cobalt is excreted in feces.

Cobalt may be part of an oxygen sensor. This oxygen sensor which contains heme (called hypoxia-inducible factor 1 or HIF-1), stimulates production of erythropoietin.

Deficiency of cobalt can disturb the vitamin B_{12} synthesis, thus cause anemia and hypofunction of thyroid and increase the risk of developmental abnormalities and failure in infants. And excess can increase the action of thyroid and bone marrow, which might, in turn, lead to overproduction of erythrocytes, fibrosis in lungs, and asthma.

Very little is known about storage and requirements and about consequences of low intakes or deficiency; however, intakes of 6-8 mg/day for prolonged periods of time were found to be associated with pericardiomyopathy. Acute intake of ≥ 100 mg has been found to cause lowering of blood pressure, nausea and vomiting, diarrhea, loss of appetite, goiter, and hyperlipidemia. High levels of cobalt in tissues may be carcinogenic.

Cadmium (Cd)

The major source of cadmium is from weathering of rocks and the lava that is deposited from volcanic eruptions. Cadmium cannot enter our body through the skin. Cadmium compounds are found in air, earth crust, and water. It is inhaled from the atmosphere. There are many cadmium containing articles of daily use such as fungicides and fertilizers, nickel-cadmium batteries, fabric dyes, ceramic (pottery) and glass glazes, and welding or electroplating metals. High exposure can damage the vital organs like heart, liver, and kidney and it can be fatal.

In persons who smoke, tobacco contributes to cadmium uptake because tobacco plants accumulate cadmium from the soil. However, for nonsmokers, the major source is diet. Intakes of persons residing in nonpolluted areas are barely 10-40 micrograms in a day, whereas intakes of persons in polluted areas may be much higher going up to about 100's of micrograms daily.

Minute amount of cadmium has been found in body tissues, mainly in liver and kidney and body fluids (approximately 30 mg). However, cadmium is a heavy metal, which may enter the body and interact with zinc and other trace elements.

Recent observations have shown that it is associated with hypertension. Cadmium is available in most foods thus deficiency is uncommon. Excess of zinc and copper can interfere with the absorption of cadmium or vice-versa. Excess cadmium can also produce hypochromic microcytic anemia similar to iron deficiency, hypertension, and injury to reproductive organs among males.

Nickel

Nickel (Ni) is mostly combined with oxygen or sulfur as oxides or sulfides that occur naturally in the earth's crust.

Nickel has been found in body tissues in traces. In animals, Ni deprivation was found to change carbohydrate and lipid metabolism. Lack of Ni adversely influenced activities of enzymes involved in converting glucose to pyruvate and that were active in the citric acid cycle. Circulating thyroid hormone concentrations were lower in Ni deprivation. It has beneficial effects on bone in terms of bone strength and composition. It may alleviate B_{12} deficiency.

It is found in nuts, legumes, grains and vegetables, seafoods, and sea salt. However, only a small percentage (<10%) is absorbed. In iron deficiency, absorption is higher, as also during pregnancy and lactation. In blood, Ni is bound to serum albumin. The thyroid and adrenal glands contain relatively high concentrations of Ni. Most of the Ni is excreted via feces.

Silicon

Silicon is bound to glycosaminoglycans and has an important role in the formation of cross-links between collagen and proteoglycans. It is present in all body tissues, but the tissues with the highest concentrations of silicon are bone and other connective tissues including skin, hair, arteries, and nails.

Scientists have been interested in silicon because it has beneficial effects on collagen and formation of glycosamines and thus may be important for bone formation and maintenance, wound healing, and even cardiovascular health. Although it has not been shown to be essential human beings, it may be essential for plants. The human body contains approximately 1.5 mg of silicon. Most of it is present in rigid connective tissue like the trachea and aorta, lymph nodes, and bones. Higher amounts of silicon are present in those zones of the bone where growth occurs.

In food, silicon is mostly present as silica, an insoluble polymer and silicates. Sources of silicon include whole unrefined grains, fruits, and vegetables that have a high fiber and water content as well as beer. Hard water is a better source than is soft water.

Bioavailability of silicon depends on the chemical form in which it is present in foods. Silica and silicates like aluminum silicate are hardly absorbed; whereas in case of orthosilicic acid, a much higher proportion of the dose is absorbed. From foods, it is estimated that about 10–40% (depending on the food) of the silicon present is absorbed. It is probably absorbed in the proximal small intestine. Absorption may be lower in older persons. Estrogen may enhance absorption. Absorption and urinary excretion determine the amount of silicon present in blood and may be responsible for homeostatic regulation.

Silicon is stored in bones, connective tissue, and in lymph nodes. It is excreted through urine (probably in the form of magnesium silicate). Excess intakes are rapidly disposed of through urine. If renal function is compromised, silicon concentrations in blood rise.

To date, essentiality of silicon in human beings has not been established. However, from the research evidence, it appears that silicon may have certain health benefits. Binding with aluminum to form aluminum silicate and preventing the absorption of aluminum that is potentially harmful. It may affect formation and structure of collagen, binding of macromolecules to cell receptors, and may be important for bone health. Deficiency results in impaired bone growth and adverse influence on collagen synthesis.

> **Laboratory Laurel:** To develop the food composition database for silicon, 365 food items commonly consumed in Korea were analyzed, using inductively coupled plasma-atomic emission spectrometry following microwave-assisted digestion for silicon content. Further dietary silicon intake was recoded of 400 healthy Korean adult males aged 19–25 using the 24-hour recall method. This study also examined the association of silicon intake with bone status of men. Clinical markers reflecting bone metabolism used were serum total alkaline phosphatase, N-mid osteocalcin, and type 1 collagen C-terminal telopeptide concentrations. Silicon intake of the subjects was recorded to be 37.5 ± 22.2 mg/day. Major contribution of silicon was cereal and cereal products (25.6%), vegetables (22.7%), beverages and liquors (21.2%), and milk and milk products (7.0%). Silicon intake correlated positively with age, weight, energy intake, protein intake, calcium intake, and alcohol intake. After adjusted for age, weight, energy intake, protein intake, calcium intake, alcohol intake, smoking cigarettes, and regular exercise status, daily total silicon intake was
>
> *Contd...*

Contd...

> not correlated with calcaneus bone density and the bone metabolism markers, but silicon intake from vegetables was positively correlated with serum total alkaline phosphatase activity, a bone formation maker. Hence, silicon from vegetables has positive relationship with bone formation of young adult males.
>
> **Choi MK, Kim MH. Dietary silicon intake of korean young adult males and its relation to their bone status. Biol Trace Elem Res. 2017;176(1):89-104.**

Breathing of silicon particles from the environment may cause "Silicosis". Silicosis refers to the formation of small, typically round nodules in the lungs of people exposed to crystalline silica dust. Silicosis is a potentially fatal, irreversible, progressive, and untreatable fibrotic lung disease caused by prolonged inhalation and deposition of respirable crystalline silica. It can be assessed by serum copper level, which is raised in cases of silicosis. It is an age-old occupational disease caused by inhalation of silica dust, commonly found in workers of mine, blasting, stone grinders, ceramics, and paddy milling. It is characterized by inflammation and formation of nodules and lesions in the lungs (since collagen synthesis is induced in the lungs). Symptoms are shortness of breath, fever, and bluish skin. It often misdiagnosed as pulmonary edema or tuberculosis. It can be prevented by water spray and dry air filtering.

Vanadium

Vanadium is a naturally occurring element and widely found in soil, air, and water. It is released in environment via industries such as steel manufacturing and ceramics, oil refineries, and power plants. In general, it cannot be destroyed in the environment. It can only change its form or become attached or separated from airborne particulates, soil, particulates in water, and sediment.

Vanadium is a transition element present in tooth enamel, bones, liver, and body fat. It is a bioactive element although its essentiality still remains in question. Vanadium has been shown to have insulin-mimetic action. Vanadium selectively inhibits tyrosine phosphatases. Therefore, vanadium has insulin-like actions at the cellular level. Studies on animals and humans have shown that vanadium treatment lowered plasma glucose and increased peripheral utilization of glucose, hepatic glucose production was reduced. It also stimulates cellular proliferation and differentiation, and affects phosphorylation and dephosphorylation. It is useful for formation or function of bone and connective tissue. This element is present in the form of vanadate, which is present in ECF. In intracellular space, it is present as vanadyl. Most of the body content of vanadium is present in bone. Organs like kidney, spleen, liver, testes, and lung also contain vanadium. Most of the vanadium is excreted through urine.

Seafoods contain higher concentrations of vanadium as compared to the meat from land animals. Other foods have much low concentrations of vanadium. However, it is ingested also through tap water. Shellfish, mushroom, and herbs like parsley are rich sources. Foods processed in steel-containing vanadium or stored in such containers may pick up vanadium during processing or storage. In terms of food chain, vanadyl sulfate and sodium metavanadate have been used in dietary supplements.

Elevated levels of vanadium are found in patients with bipolar disorders, mania, and depression. Vitamin C is reported to protect the body from the damage caused by excess of vanadium.

> **Research Glimpse:** There are many varieties of black, green, white, and oolong teas sold in tea bags, which were used in this study. Testing of toxic element was performed—(i) tea leaves, (ii) tea steeped for 3–4 minutes, and (iii) tea steeped for 15–17 minutes. All brewed teas were found to have the lead with 73% of teas brewed for 3 minutes and 83% brewed for 15 minutes and the level of lead observed in the samples is unsafe during pregnancy and lactation. Aluminum levels were also more than recommended guidelines in 20% of brewed teas. No mercury was found at detectable levels in these samples. Teas were found to contain several beneficial elements such as magnesium, calcium, potassium, and phosphorus. However, manganese was found in excess in some black teas. There was contamination by heavy metals to the levels considered unsafe. It is suggested to have some public health warnings or industry regulation to protect consumer safety.
>
> *Schwalfenberg G, Genuis SJ, Ilia Rodushkin I. The Benefits and Risks of Consuming Brewed Tea: Beware of Toxic Element Contamination. J Toxicol. 2013;2013:370460.*

Lead (Pb)

Lead is a heavy element that has been used for centuries because it possesses some important physico-chemical properties, e.g., softness, malleability, ductility, poor conductibility and resistance to corrosion. However, because it is not degradable and is so widely used, it accumulation in the environment poses considerable health hazards. Exposure is likely to be occupation related particularly in those related to leaded gasoline, industrial processes like smelting of lead and its combustion, pottery, boat building, lead based painting, lead containing pipes, battery recycling, grids, arm industry, pigments, printing of books, among many others. Globally use of lead is discontinued in many countries although it is still used in industries dealing with car repair, battery manufacture and recycling, refining, smelting. At population level exposure is through contaminated fruits and vegetables, and lead from water pipes.

> Lead is highly toxic as it affects almost every organ in the human body, particularly the nervous system and has greater impact on children than on adults. Studies have shown adverse effects on cognitive performance because it acts as a calcium analogue interfering with ion channels. Infants are affected even by low levels of lead and this could contribute to behavioral problems, learning deficits. Lead poisoning also causes microcytic anemia in many cases because it prevents heme synthesis. It also has effects on the renal and reproductive systems. The authors have written about techniques for treating lead toxicity as well.
>
> *Wani AL, Ara A, Usmani JA. Lead toxicity: a review. Interdiscip Toxicol. 2015;8(2):55-64.*

RAPID FIRE

1. What is the difference between major minerals and trace and ultratrace elements?
2. What is the role of calcium in bone bank?
3. What is the importance of ratio of calcium and phosphorus in the body?
4. What are the functions of magnesium?
5. Why is iron deficiency anemia a public health problem?
6. What is role of zinc in prevention of infection and gene expression?
7. Comment on fluoride poisoning.
8. What are three different stages of iron deficiency?
9. Which minerals have a role in bone?
10. Which minerals are important for immunity?
11. Which minerals function as antioxidants?
12. What is the role of boron in the body?
13. What do you mean by silicosis?
14. Comment on arsenic in relation to human health.
15. Comment on lead toxicity.

EXERCISE

1. Find out the calcium, iron, and sodium intake of 10 people around you. Calculate the value and comment on their nutritional status.
2. Find out the 20 food sources rich in zinc, magnesium, and potassium of each and calculate the amount of food, which can fulfill the RDA for these three nutrients.
3. Suggest 5 recipes each, which can improve the bioavailability of calcium and iron.

SUGGESTED READING

1. Bakirdere S, Orenay S, Korkmaz M. Effect of boron on human health. Open Mineral Process J. 2010;3:54-59.
2. Bassett JHD, Williams GR. Role of Thyroid Hormones in Skeletal Development and Bone Maintenance. Endocr Rev. 2016;37(2):135-87.
3. Bellad A, Kapil R, Gupta A. National guidelines for prevention and control of iron deficiency anemia in India. Indian J Community Health. 2018;30(1):89-94.
4. Benton D. Selenium Intake, Mood and Other Aspects of Psychological Functioning. Nutr Neurosci. 2002;5(6):363-74.
5. Brown KH, Hess SY. International Zinc Nutrition Consultative Group technical document no. 2. Systematic Review of Zinc Intervention. Food Nutr Bull. 2009;30(1):S3-186.
6. Burkhead JL, Lutsenko S. The role of copper as a modifier of lipid metabolism of lipid metabolism. InTech Open Science: Open Mind. 2013;39.
7. Delange F, Hetzel BS. The Scientific Basis for the Elimination of Brain Damage due to Iodine Deficiency. In: Hatzel BS (Ed). Towards Global Elimination of Brain Damage Due to Iodine Deficiency. New Delhi: Oxford University Press; 2004. p. 151.
8. Dey S, Giri B. fluoride fact on human health and health problems: Review Med clin Rev. 2015, 2:2.
9. Dinca L, Scorei R. Boron in human nutrition and its regulations use. J Nutr Ther. 2013;2:22-9.
10. DiNicolantonio JJ, O'Keefe JH, Wilson W. Subclinical magnesium deficiency: a principal driver of cardiovascular disease and a public health crisis. Open Heart. 2018;5(1):e000668.
11. Godt J, Scheidig F, Grosse-Siestrup C, et al. The toxicity of cadmium and resulting hazards for human health. J occu med toxicol. 2006;1:22.
12. Gupta CP. Role of Iron (Fe) in Body. IOSR–JAC. 2014;7(11):38-46.
13. Hatfield DL, Berry MJ, Gladyshev VN (Eds). Selenium. Its Molecular Biology and Role in Human Health, 3rd edition. Berlin, Germany: Springer Science + Business Media; 2012.
14. Hess SY, Lonnerdal B, Hotz C, et al. Recent advances in knowledge of zinc nutrition and human health. Food and Nutrition Bulletin. 2009;30(1 Suppl):S5-11.
15. ICMR (2010) Nutrient Requirements and Recommended Dietary Allowances for Indians, A Report of the Expert Group of the Indian Council of Medical Research.

16. Ilich JZ, Kerstetter JE. Nutrition in bone health revisited: A story beyond calcium. J Am Coll Nutr. 2000;19(6):715-37.
17. Institute of Medicine (US) Panel on Dietary Antioxidants and Related Compounds. Dietary Reference Intakes for Vitamin C, Vitamin E, Selenium, and Carotenoids. Washington (DC): National Academies Press (US); 2000.
18. Institute of Medicine (US) Panel on Micronutrients. Dietary Reference Intakes for Vitamin A, Vitamin K, Arsenic, Boron, Chromium, Copper, Iodine, Iron, Manganese, Molybdenum, Nickel, Silicon, Vanadium, and Zinc.
19. Kiremidjian-Schumacher L, Stotzky G. Selenium and immune responses. Environ Res. 1987;42(2):277-303.
20. Kohlmeier M. Nutrient Metabolism. Food Science and Technology, International Series. London; Academic Press: 2007. pp. 693-9.
21. Kotecha PV. Micronutrient malnutrition in India: let us say "no" to it now. Indian J Community Med. 2008;33(1):9-10.
22. Logan AG. Dietary sodium intake and its relation to human health: A summary of the evidence. J Am Coll Nutr. 2006;25(3):165-9.
23. Longvah T, Ananthan R, Bhaskarachary K, et al. (2017). Indian Food Composition Tables. National Institute of Nutrition (Indian Council of Medical Research) Department of Health Research, Ministry of Health and Family Welfare, Government of India, Hyderabad. [online] Available from http://www.indiaenvironmentportal.org.in/files/file/IFCT%202017%20 Book.pdf. [Last accessed July, 2019].
24. Ministry of Health and Family Welfare, Government of India. Addressing Iron Deficiency Anaemia among Indian Adolescents—12 by 12 Initiative. New Delhi, India: Ministry of Health and Family Welfare; 2007.
25. Mitra1 SR, Mazumder DN, Basu A, et al. Nutritional factors and susceptibility to arsenic-caused skin lesion in West Bengal, India. Environ Health Perspect. 2004;112(10):1104-9.
26. Nielsen FH. Is boron nutritionally relevant? Nutr Rev. 2008;66(4):183-91.
27. Nutrient Requirements of Indians, Recommended Dietary Allowances, Estimated Average Requirements, A reports of the Expert Group, 2020, Indian Council of Medical research, National Institute of Nutrition, Department of Health Research, Ministry of Health and Family Welfare, Government of India.
28. Nutrition International, ICCIDD, AIIMS (New Delhi) and Kantar, 2019. India Iodine Survey 2018-19 National Report, New Delhi, India.
29. Papp LV, Lu J, Holmgren A, et al. From selenium to selenoproteins: synthesis, identity, and their role in human health. Antioxid Redox Signal. 2007;9(7):775-806.
30. Pettifor JM Vitamin D &/or calcium deficiency rickets in infants and children: a global perspective. Indian Journal of Medical Research (2008) 127:245-9.
31. Pfeiffer CC, Mailloux R. Excess copper as a factor in human diseases. J Orthomol Med. 1987;2(3):171-82.
32. Raju SM. Nutrition and Biochemistry for Nurses. New Delhi: Jaypee Brothers Medical Publishers (P) Ltd. 2010.
33. Sarvar R, Bant DD. Clinical assessment of micronutrient deficiencies among children (1-5 years) enrolled in anganwadis of old Hubli slums, Karnataka, India. IJCMPH. 2017;4(2):598-602.
34. Steggerda FR, Mitchell HH. Variability in the calcium metabolism and calcium requirements of adult human subjects. J Nutr. 1946;3: 407-22.
35. Teucher, Olivares, Cori. Enhancers of iron absorption: ascorbic acid and other organic acids. International Journal for Vitamin and Nutrition Research. 2004 Nov 1; 74(6):403-19.
36. Trailokya A, Srivastava A, Bhole M, et al. Calcium and calcium Salts drug corner. J Assoc Physicians India. 2017;65:100-3.
37. Washington (DC): National Academies Press (US); 2001.
38. Watt DL. The nutritional relationship of selenium. J Orthomol Med. 1994;9(2):111-7.
39. Weaver CM. Calcium. In: Bowman BA, Russell RM (Eds). Present Knowledge in Nutrition, 9th edition. Washington DC: International Life Science Institute; 2006. pp. 373-82.
40. World Health Organization. (2000). Chapter 6.12: Vanadium. Air Quality Guidelines, 2nd edition. [online] Available from http://www.euro.who.int/__data/assets/pdf_file/0016/123082/AQG2ndEd_6_12vanadium.PDF. [Last accessed July, 2019].
41. World Health Organization. Assessing the Iron Status of Populations, 2nd edition. Geneva, Switzerland: World Health Organization; 2007.
42. World Health Organization. Global Health Risks: Mortality and Burden of Disease Attributable to Selected Major Risks. Geneva, Switzerland: World Health Organization; 2009.
43. World Health Organization. World-Wide Prevalence of Anaemia, 1993 to 2005. Geneva, Switzerland: World Health Organization; 2008.
44. Zimmermann MB. The role of iodine in human growth and development. Semin Cell Dev Biol. 2011;22:645-52.
45. Zubillaga MB, Salgueiro MJ, Caro RA, et al. The role of zinc in growth and development of children nutrition. Nutrition. 2002;18(6):510-9.

CHAPTER 8

Water, Electrolytes and Acid-Base Balance

KEY CONCERNS
- How is water distributed in the body?
- What is fluid balance and how is it regulated?
- How much fluid is lost and how much should be consumed?
- What is dehydration and how can it be prevented?
- What is electrolyte balance?
- What is the role of different electrolytes?
- What is acid-base balance?

KEY CONCEPTS
- Distribution of fluid in the body
- Electrolytes and their role in biological system
- Causes and consequences of high/low levels of electrolytes
- Acid-base balance and buffer system in body fluids
- Causes and consequences of deviation in acid-base balance
- Thirst mechanism
- Dehydration and water intoxication

INTRODUCTION

Water is a universal biological solvent. It is the fluid in which all life processes occur and determines all physiological processes. It is a vital nutrient without which the human body can survive for only some days whereas without food the body can survive for weeks. It is a critical component of the body being the most abundant molecule/major constituent in the body, present both within and outside cells, in all tissues and organs, making it one of the most important chemical compounds. It participates actively in biochemical reactions, provides form, structure, and turgor to the cells and helps in stabilizing body temperature. It is present in blood, saliva, bile, digestive juices, urine, and perspiration. The amount of water varies in different parts of the body. Blood contains 85–90% of the body's water. It provides the medium for transport and allows exchange of molecules between cells, interstitial fluid, and capillaries. It maintains the blood volume, and is critical for blood circulation. Muscles, brain, and other organs also contain water, which is vital for their normal functioning and maintaining the internal environment of the body in a "constant" state (homeostasis). Due to its role as a carrier of nutrients to cells and removes waste products, it is very important for homeostasis.

All organs, tissues, and systems require water, i.e., they need to be adequately hydrated to function effectively. Water participates in metabolic reactions and is important for growth. As a macronutrient, water is involved in all hydrolytic reactions carried out in the body. Water is also produced in the body during oxidative metabolism of the macronutrients.

Water performs several important functions some of them are shown in Figure 8.1.

- It is a solvent for the innumerable solutes, lipoproteins, and other biological compounds within and outside the cell. It has unique properties and is a highly interactive molecule.

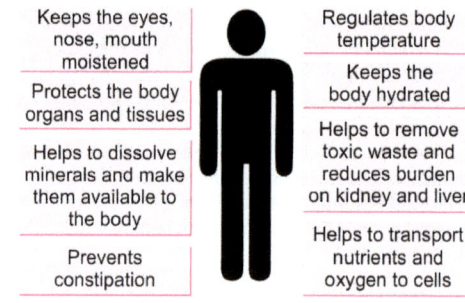

Fig. 8.1: Functions of water.

- It maintains structural and functional capacity of every cell.
- It keeps blood and other body fluids in liquid state so that they can flow.
- It carries nutrients and oxygen to cells.
- It helps to eliminate byproducts and waste products from the body.
- It participates in all chemical reactions.
- It helps to form the structure of macromolecules like proteins, glycogen.
- It regulates body temperature through evaporation in the form of sweat.
- It keeps mucous membranes moist particularly in lungs and respiratory tract, mouth, and the intestinal tract.
- It acts as a lubricant and cushions the joints (in the form of synovial fluid).
- It aids in digestion and prevents constipation.
- It quenches thirst.
- It works as a moisturizer to improve the skin's texture and appearance.
- It serves as a shock absorber inside the eyes, spinal cord, and in amniotic sac surrounding the fetus during pregnancy.
- It helps to dilute any potentially harmful or toxic substances in the bladder and removes them through urine.

- It is very important for thermoregulation because it has a large heat capacity and capacity for vaporization of heat. Therefore, the body can lose heat when ambient temperature is higher than body temperature, i.e., perspiration or sweat is evaporated from the skin, helping the body to efficiently lose heat.

COMPONENTS OF BODY FLUIDS

The body does not contain pure plain water. Body fluids consist of water in which ions (electrolytes) and other substances are present. Total body fluid is referred to as total amount of body water (TBW). Total body water consists of two compartments—fluid inside the cell and fluid outside the cell. These compartments are separated by cell membranes through which the contents inside the cell and outside the cell can be exchanged by various transport mechanisms. Fluids present in the two compartments are intracellular fluid (ICF) and extracellular fluid (ECF).

Total Body Water

In a healthy adult with body weight of about 70 kg, the total body water is about 40 L, i.e., about 55–57% of the body weight, in which (as a thumb rule) 2/3 will be ICF and 1/3 will be ECF.

> **Laboratory Laurel:** The study was carried out to determine the relationship between TBW, extracellular water (ECW) and intracellular water (ICW) with overall and central adiposity on young adult girls (n = 348, 18–24 years). Body water components (TBW, ECW, and ICW), indices of overall obesity including body mass index (BMI), body fat percentage (%BF), fat mass (FM), and central obesity including waist-to-hip circumference ratio (WHR) were measured by Body Composition Analyzer after fasting for at least 12 hours. There were significant positive correlations between WHR, FM, and %BF with body water compartments including TBW, ECW, and ICW. It is a simple low-cost and quick technique to measure overall and central obesity.
>
> *Mehdizadeh R. Relationship between body water compartments and indexes of adiposity in sedentary young adult girls. Braz J Biomotricity. 2012;6(2):84-92.*

Total body water is the largest part of the fat-free mass (FFM). The composition of proportion of different body fluids is shown in Figure 8.2.

Total body water varies from person to person and is greatly influenced by age, gender, skeletal muscle mass, and body fat content. The change in TBW is directly proportional to the change in body weight (BW) indicating the relationship of body fat and body water. In certain cases, TBW is found to be higher in obese individuals as compared to normal subjects, but the ratio of TBW:BW is lower in obese than normal.

Total body water decreases with increasing age. A newborn baby's body contains approximately 75% water, which declines with age owing to increase in adipose tissue. Newborn infants and young children have a higher amount of extracellular fluid compared to adults. A premature infant's body contains even more water (90%) than a full-term infant (70–80%). In the first 6 months of life, total body fluid as a percentage of body weight decreases and by the 2nd year of life, the percentage of body water is close to adult values. Adult proportions are generally reached in the teenage or adolescent years. During adolescence, 2/3 of TBW is present in ICF. The body of an adult male has about 63% water whereas the adult female body contains 52% water. Muscle is associated with water to a larger extent than is fat; hence, persons who have more muscle or lean body mass will have more body water. Males have more lean body mass; hence, water content in the male body is higher than in the female. Women have less water in their bodies because the proportion of body fat is higher than in the male body. Obese persons and older persons have less water in the body. Percentage of ECF and ICF at different ages is shown in Figure 8.3.

Body water can be calculated by using different formulae. The simplest way is to multiply body weight by a factor of 0.6. This is used because about two-thirds of body weight is comprised of water. Watson's and Hume–Weyer's formulas are different for males and females.

Watson's formula as shown below can be used to calculate body water. **For males:** Total Body Water (TBW) in liters = $2.447 - 0.09156 \times \text{age (y)} + 0.1074 \times \text{height (cm)} + 0.3362 \times \text{weight (kg)}$

For females: TBW in liters = $-2.097 + 0.1069 \times \text{height (cm)} + 0.2466 \times \text{weight (kg)}$

Another is the Hume–Weyers formula:
TBW-H (for males) = $(0.194786 \times H) + (0.296785 \times W) - 14.012934$

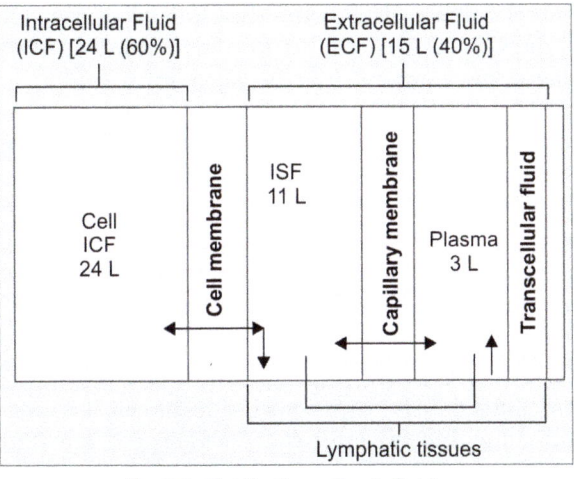

Fig. 8.2: Distribution of body fluids.

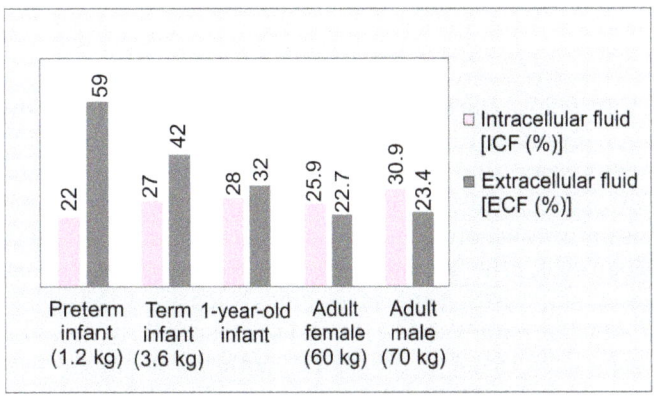

Fig. 8.3: Distribution of body fluids (ICF and ECF) in different age groups.

TBW-H (for female) = (0.344547 × H) + (0.183809 × W) − 35.270121

Where H (height) is in centimeters and W (weight) is in kilograms

A third formula is the Chertow formula:
TBW-C = H × (0.0186104 × W + 0.12703384) + W × (0.11262857 × M + 0.00104135 × A − 0.00067247 × W − 0.04012056) − A × (0.03486146 × M + 0.07493713) − M × 1.01767992 + D × 0.57894981

Where:
- A = Age in years
- H = Height in centimeters (cm)
- W = Weight in kilograms (kg)
- M = Male (Yes = 1, No = 0)
- D = Diabetes (Yes = 1, No = 0)

The Chertow formula differs from the other two, because in that, there is no separate formula for males and females and it takes into account whether the person is diabetic or not.

Ratio of ECF and ICF varies throughout the life. The ratio is higher during developmental stages and this variation corresponds with changes in cellular growth, muscle mass, level of hydration, nutritional status, and renal function (urinary output). Clinically, the ratio is altered in case of liver failure, nephrotic syndrome, protein loss, and enteropathy.

Intracellular Fluid

Fluid present inside the cells, i.e., in the cytosol or cytoplasm, is called intracellular fluid (ICF) and constitutes about 40% of total body weight. It constitutes approximately 60–62.5%, i.e., two-third of total body water, i.e., 25 liters. This fluid is quite stable because it is tightly regulated by hormones. It largely contains potassium, organic anions, and proteins. Its composition is maintained and regulated by the body. Role of ICF is critical because:
- It is a solvent for various molecules
- It is the medium in which all metabolic reactions occur within the cell
- It plays an active role in various cellular reactions
- It sustains cellular integrity.

If this fluid content falls, the cell will not be able to perform normal cellular activities and if there is too much water inside the cell, then cell could burst and be destroyed.

Extracellular Fluid

All the fluids, which are present outside the cells of the body, are collectively called extracellular fluid (ECF). About 1/3 body's water is ECF and about 20% of it is found in plasma. Since plasma in the blood travels throughout the body, it is the means of transporting a wide range of compounds as well as blood cells, proteins, clotting factors, electrolytes, nutrients, gases, and wastes. Since many fluids, such as cerebrospinal fluid (that bathes the brain and spinal cord), lymph, the synovial fluid in joints, the pleural fluid in the pleural cavities, the pericardial fluid in the cardiac sac, the peritoneal fluid in the peritoneal cavity, and the aqueous humor of the eye, are found outside the cell, they can be considered a part of ECF. Extracellular fluid constitutes 37.5% of total body water amounting to approximately 15 liters or 21.4% of body weight. Its composition is often affected by external influences.

Extracellular fluid plays a significant role in maintaining homeostasis in the internal environment. It is very important that the amount and composition of ECF be constant, so that cells, and, in fact, the entire body can function normally. Homeostatic mechanisms monitor and regulate the composition of ECF, the osmotic pressure, and pH, which in turn depend on the functioning of circulatory, respiratory, renal, alimentary, nervous, and endocrine systems.

Extracellular fluid is largely composed of:
1. Interstitial fluid
2. Plasma
3. Transcellular fluid.

Interstitial Fluid

Cells are separated by a selectively permeable cell membrane. The cell membrane not only helps to regulate exchange of material in and out of the cell but also allows movement of gases, nutrients, and waste material between capillaries. Interstitial fluid is the liquid found in interstitial or tissue spaces, between the cells or in the interstices of all body tissues, i.e., it surrounds and bathes all cells. It contains electrolytes, amino acids, sugars, fatty acids, coenzymes, hormones, neurotransmitters, salts as well as waste products. Its composition varies in different tissues in different areas of the body. It contains lymph and works in association with the lymphatic system. The ionic composition of interstitial fluid determines the concentration of ions in ECF and ICF. It essentially serves as a buffer against changes occurring in plasma volume that is influenced by water and fluid intake and can vary quickly and easily. It reduces any variations in the composition of plasma caused by absorption from the intestine or by intravenous infusion. The volume of interstitial fluid is about thrice that of intravascular fluid (IVF).

Plasma or Intravascular Fluid

It is very important since it is essential for maintaining organ perfusion (passage of fluid), transporting oxygen and nutrients to cells. Besides this, it helps in transferring hormones, cytokines, and neurotransmitters, all of which play a role in communication between organs and tissues. It is constituted mostly by water (93%) and contains dissolved proteins such as albumin, globulins and fibrinogen, glucose, clotting factors, minerals like calcium, sodium, and magnesium in ionic form, bicarbonate, and chloride as well as hormones. It plays a very important role in intravascular osmotic effects, i.e., keeping electrolyte levels in balance as well as protecting the body from infection.

Transcellular Fluid

Transcellular fluid is not present inside the cell. It is the water contained within the epithelial-lined spaces, constituting about 2.5% of total body water. It includes digestive juices, ocular fluid, and mucus, and cerebrospinal fluid, and fluid in the synovial, pericardial, pleural, and peritoneal cavities. It is also referred as the third space and many a times is not used in calculation of fluid requirement. It is a small amount of fluid (approximately 1–2 liters) present in the body.

WATER BALANCE

Water enters the body through food and drink and exits via kidney, lungs, and skin. Water balance is determined by the amount that is consumed and the amount lost. When water intake is in equilibrium with water output, the body is said to be in water balance. Besides water intake from external sources, body also produces some water as a result of biological reactions, e.g., the metabolism of protein, fat and carbohydrate and this is called metabolic water. Table 8.1 shows the amount of water intake and water output reflecting water balance.

The body maintains water balance because the kidneys, gastrointestinal tract, lungs, and skin excrete water in varying amounts, the total amount being similar to the amount that has been ingested/consumed. In healthy individuals, water balance is observed when a person drinks about 1.5 liters or 8–10 glasses of water per day and the person has normal urine output.

Water Intake

The body obtains water from dietary sources (foods and beverages). Water is required for the body's normal physiological activities such as respiration, sweating, and urination; hence, it is necessary to constantly supply water to the body to replenish the water that was lost.

Liquid Foods

It is recommended that about 6–8 glasses of water or about 2.5 liters should be consumed every day. It can include just plain potable water, or water in the form of beverages and other liquid foods like milk. Water is consumed as such. However, there is a wide variety of fluids people consume such as buttermilk, tea, coffee, cocoa, lemonade, soups, soft drinks (both aerated and nonaerated), fruit and vegetable juices among others. All of these contribute to water intake, i.e., input. Water is also consumed in curries or gravies.

Table 8.1: Water intake and output in the body.

Water intake		Water output	
Sources	Amount (mL)	Sources	Amount (mL)
All liquids consumed	1,500 (60%)	Sensible loss: • Urine • Feces	1,500 (60%) 100 (4%)
All solid foods	750 (30%)		
Metabolic water	200–300 (10%)	Insensible loss: • Skin • Lungs	900 (36%)
Total	**2,500**		**2,500**

> Nowadays, safe and clean water is a matter of concern. Wide varieties of equipment are available to purify the water. Many people purchase bottled water especially when they travel or are away from their homes for long hours. Bottled water is usually made by removing the dissolved solids (or deionizing) through reverse osmosis (RO) or ion exchange process. Mineral water is also bottled. Such water contains some minerals similar to spring water from natural streams. Bottled water of commercial different brands are available at different prices. Sometimes, spices, herbs, fruits or some vegetables are infused in water for different health purposes.

Solid Foods

The body also obtains water from the solids we eat. Almost all foods inherently contain water (remember water is present in all living matter). This water is measured as moisture content. The higher the water content, the faster foods spoil. Foods containing high amount of moisture or water content (75–95%) are "perishable foods". These include milk, fruits, and most vegetables particularly green leafy vegetables. Fruits and vegetables contain about 70–96% water and milk and milk products contain 80–85% water or moisture. Some foods contain less moisture (5–15%) and are called "nonperishable foods". Examples of nonperishable foods are cereals and cereal products like rice flakes, puffed rice, flours; pulses and legumes; and nuts and oilseeds. Even meat and chicken have considerable amount of water.

Metabolic Water

It is water produced when food is metabolized in the body, e.g., glucose (carbohydrate) after undergoing oxidative metabolism yields carbon dioxide, water, and energy. Fat and protein also release some water during oxidation. Oxidation of carbohydrate, protein, and fat produces approximately 15, 10.5, and 11.1 g of metabolic water/100 kcal of metabolizable energy, respectively. This water represents 5–10% of the body's water utilization. Per 100 kcal, the amount of water produced is about 10–14 mL, contributing a total of approximately 200–300 mL/day. Athletes may generate higher amounts of metabolic water, i.e., 500–600 mL/day due to oxidation of macronutrients. Metabolic water is the water that is produced as an end product of the energy containing molecules, i.e., protein, fat and carbohydrates. In many animals including humans, metabolic water is only a small part of total body water. However, in some animals that reside in dry lands, e.g., kangaroo, rats, metabolic water is very important because they thrive and survive on metabolic water and do not have to drink water.

> **Metabolic water from 100 g of the nutrient:**
> Fat: 100 mL water
> Carbohydrate: 55 mL water
> Protein: 41 mL water

Water Output

On an average, the human body loses approximately 2.5 liters of water in a day. Water loss, which is not visible and cannot

be easily measured, is referred as "insensible" loss. It occurs through lungs (exhalation during respiration) and skin (perspiration). "Sensible water loss" occurs through urine and feces. Water loss normally occurs through:
- **Urine** formed by the kidneys
- **Feces** through the gastrointestinal tract called (sensible loss)
- **Perspiration** evaporated from the skin as well as through water expired from the lungs or (insensible or invisible water loss). Insensible water loss is continuous, that a person is usually not aware of and is unnoticed.

Lungs

The amount of insensible water loss through small water droplets in exhaled air is 250–350 mL/day. For physically active persons, 2–5 mL water is lost from respiratory tract during each minute of strenuous exercise. Respiratory loss through lungs is more at high altitude. It has been estimated that breathing cold, dry air during rest can increase respiratory water losses by approximately 5 mL/hr. In the same environmental conditions, if a person undertakes stressful physical exercise, the respiratory water loss is higher (approximately 15–45 mL/hr).

Skin

Water loss through perspiration varies greatly. In hot humid climates or when we exercise or are physically active, we lose water through perspiration. Approximately 1–2 liters of urine is lost during a 24-hour period in a sedentary adult. Through skin, water is lost by insensible perspiration, and is approximately 450 mL per day in temperate climate. However, environmental temperature and relative humidity also influence water loss through skin as well as lungs. Water loss through feces (gastrointestinal tract) is about 200 mL/day. Thus, a sedentary adult, on average, will lose approximately 2–3 liters in a 24-hour period.

"**Sensible water loss**" is visible and is easy to measure. It occurs through urine, sweat, and feces. Daily urine output/excretion is approximately similar to the amount of free fluid consumed. Hence, it is possible to assess water balance by comparing the amount of oral liquid intake to the urine output in a given period of time. Urine volume, i.e., output varies from 800 mL/day to 1,500 mL/day. Healthy older adults tend to have higher urine output because their bodies are not able to concentrate urine as efficiently as healthy young adults. Urine volume can be reduced by physical exercise (person loses water through perspiration) and climate. Thus, lifestyle and environmental conditions have a significant impact on an individual's water loss. On an average, an adult loses about 2.6 liters (L) per day by the above routes only, maximum by urine. Water loss is influenced by environment and health status. Only a small amount is lost through feces and about 900 mL is lost through skin and respiratory tract. Water losses are influenced by various factors such as climate and environmental temperature, exercise, and health status. The loss is generally less in hot, humid weather and greatest

Table 8.2: Water output under different conditions.

Routes of water output	Normal temperature	Hot weather	Prolonged exercise
Sensible loss			
Urine	1,400	1,200	500
Water in feces	100	100	100
Skin (perspiration)	100	1,400	5,000
Insensible loss			
Skin	350	350	350
Respiratory tract	350	250	650
TOTAL	**2,300**	**3,300**	**6,600**

Source: Mahan LK, Arlin M. Krause's Food Nutrition & Diet Therapy, 11th edition. Philadelphia: WB Saunders Company; 2007.

in cold weather where the inspired air contains less moisture or at higher altitudes.

Table 8.2 shows water output at different environmental temperatures and during exercise. Water loss increases when the internal body temperature rises through activation of the sweat glands. In a hot environment, when a person exercises, rate of perspiration increases, leading to higher amount of water loss. However, when excessive perspiration occurs, there can be risk of dehydration and an increase in osmolarity of ECF. Sweat is hypotonic as compared to ECF or plasma, therefore intense sweating will result in more fluid loss than electrolyte losses. (If a person loses about 4 liters of sweat, only 4% of extracellular sodium is lost.) When electrolyte loss occurs, fluid will be drawn from the intracellular compartment into the extracellular compartment (ECF) because there is increased extracellular fluid osmolarity. Therefore, during endurance exercise, it is recommended that sportsmen should consume hypotonic drink. Fluid losses increase during fever (due to sweating), during vomiting and diarrhea (through the gastrointestinal tract).

Under normal conditions, 7–9 liters of digestive juices and other extracellular fluids are secreted daily into the gastrointestinal tract. Most of this is entirely reabsorbed in the ileum and colon. Only about 100 mL is excreted in the feces; however, it constitutes approximately 70% of fecal matter. With diarrhea or vomiting, water loss can increase to as much as 1,500–5,000 mL. Because this volume of reabsorbed fluid is about twice that of the blood plasma, excessive gastrointestinal fluid losses through diarrhea can have serious consequences, especially for the very young and the elderly. Fluid loss can also occur through vomiting, hemorrhage, burns, diuretic ingestion, etc.

Regulation of Water Balance

Water balance is required for optimum functioning of the body and it can be achieved by adjusting intake through thirst response and urinary output, which is under hormonal control. Within a 24-hour period, water balance is regulated within 0.2% of body weight in a healthy individual at rest.

Water balance of the body is crucial because changes in the total body water or in any compartment can disturb homeostasis and affect health. At all times, the body maintains the balance between the amount of ECF and ICF because survival and function of cells depends on it. If too much water enters the cells, the cells might rupture. On the other hand, if ICF is little, the cell cannot survive without sufficient water.

There is continuous exchange and mixing of fluids in the body. This exchange of fluids is regulated by osmotic and hydrostatic pressures. Under normal circumstances, osmolality of all body fluids is almost equal. However, a change in the solute concentration of any compartment results in net flow of water in order to restore balance. Thus when osmolality of ECF increases, water is drawn out of the cell and vice-versa; when ECF osmolality decreases, water moves into the cell.

Kidneys play an important role in maintaining water balance through excretion of urine. In general, a healthy adult produces about 1.5 liters of urine daily, on average. However, this volume depends on a person's hydration level. As long as the kidney is functioning normally, a minimum volume of urine (approximately 0.5 liters) is produced in order to maintain body functions. Through urine, the kidney excretes approximately 100–200 milliosmoles of solutes. These are essentially salts and water-soluble waste products—creatinine, urea, and uric acid. All of these are metabolic waste. If minimum amount of urine is not produced then the metabolic waste cannot be effectively removed from the body, which is an undesirable situation as it has adverse effects on health.

> Osmolality is maintained—approximately 280–300 milliosmoles.
> Osmolality is the ratio of solutes in a solution to a volume of solvent in a solution.
> Thus, in case of plasma, osmolality is the ratio of solutes to water in blood plasma.

Urine volume is adjusted by the kidney, if the body contains too much fluid. If a person consumes a large amount of fluid, within about 30 minutes, urine is produced (known as diuresis). The peak is reached after about 1 hour of ingestion and normal amount of urine production will occur after approximately 3 hours, by which time–fluid balance should have been established.

When blood volume decreases, two effects occur:
i. There is a decrease in blood pressure that is detected by baroreceptors in the aortic arch and the carotid arteries in the neck. Signals reach the heart to alter the rate and strength of its contractions, so that this will compensate for the decrease in blood pressure.
ii. The hormonal system in the kidney, known as the renin–angiotensin system, increases production of the hormone angiotensin II. This hormone has two effects—(i) it increases the feeling of thirst, and (ii) it stimulates the release of aldosterone, a hormone secreted by the adrenal glands. Aldosterone increases reabsorption of sodium by the kidney.

Water is reabsorbed along with the reabsorbed sodium into blood. Also, a person feels thirsty and responds by drinking water. To conserve water, the hypothalamus of a dehydrated person sends signals via the sympathetic nervous system to the salivary glands in the mouth. This results in a decrease in watery, serous output, the saliva becomes thicker and less in amount. These changes in secretions result in a "dry mouth" and the sensation of thirst.

> **Homeostasis** means the maintenance of nearly constant internal environment in the body. Internal environment is the ECF in which the cells live. ECF contains nutrients, ions, and other substances necessary for the survival of the cells. Internal environment ensures the gain in fluids and loss of fluids. In deficiency stage, there is increase of ADH and aldosterone, which support retention of water in the body. In this state, kidney tubules resorbs the water and urine output is reduced. Conversely, when fluids are in excess, secretion of these hormones is suppressed, followed by less retention of water and subsequently urine output is increased. It is a dynamic process, but ensures the proper functioning of the body.
>
> "When blood volume becomes too low, plasma osmolality will increase due to a higher concentration of solutes per volume of water. Osmoreceptors in the hypothalamus detect increased plasma osmolality and stimulate the posterior pituitary gland to secrete ADH."
>
> Homeostatic mechanisms regulate water/fluid balance not only by responding to changes in ECF and plasma volume but also to changes in osmotic concentrations. Increase in plasma osmolality also triggers thirst and release of ADH.

Thirst is a behavioral response characterized by "the desire to drink by both physiological and behavioral cues, resulting from deficit of water" through which people replenish their fluid losses during short-term periods (several hours). Thirst plays a significant role in maintaining the homeostasis of body fluids. Generally, thirst is signaled by the mouth becoming dry because saliva production decreases.

The thirst response involves hormonal and neural inputs. Since osmolality of ECF and ICF is approximately equal, any change in ECF affects the ICF, thus osmolality needs to be strictly regulated, which is under hormonal control. Water intake is regulated by osmoreceptors in response to increased ECF osmolarity.

A person feels "thirsty" usually when there are changes in plasma **osmolality** besides changes in plasma volume. When there is less body fluid or a person is dehydrated, there is an increase in the osmolality of ECF. Blood osmotic pressure increases. This stimulates osmoreceptors in the hypothalamus and the thirst center in the hypothalamus is now further activated. The osmoreceptors in the hypothalamus monitor the concentration of solutes (osmolality) of the blood.

When blood becomes more concentrated, blood osmolality increases above the normal and the hypothalamus transmits signals, triggering a need to drink water through conscious awareness of thirst. Normally, the person will respond by drinking water. The thirst center in the hypothalamus is the primary regulator of water intake. Besides the hypothalamus, there are receptors in the heart and large blood vessels, which also control the sensation of thirst.

Similarly, when the mouth becomes dry (salivation is suppressed), impulses or signals are sent to the thirst center in the hypothalamus, which stimulates the person to drink water or some fluid.

Less blood volume (hypovolemia) also stimulates thirst. Water intake raises the blood volume and dilutes the concentrated body fluids, thereby maintaining water balance.

> **Osmoreceptors** are specific sensor cells in the hypothalamus in the brain. They respond to cellular dehydration to initiate neural mechanisms that generate thirst sensation. They detect the changes in osmotic pressure and the plasma osmolarity (concentration of solute dissolved in the blood).
>
> When the osmolarity of blood changes (it is more or less dilute), water diffusion into and out of the osmoreceptor cells changes. That is, the cells expand when the blood plasma is more dilute and contract with a higher concentration.
>
> When the osmoreceptors detect high plasma osmolarity (often a sign of a low blood volume), they send signals to the hypothalamus, which creates the biological sensation of thirst. Osmoreceptors also stimulate vasopressin (ADH) secretion, which starts the events that will reduce plasma osmolarity to normal levels.
>
> **Osmolarity** is the milliosmoles of solute **per liter** of the solution. Osmolarity deals with the volume of body fluid, which is regulated by sodium and water. Osmolarity is controlled by renal control of water retention and excretion via thirst mechanism. The concentration of ions like sodium determines osmolarity.
>
> **Osmolality** is the milliosmoles of solute **per kilogram** of the solution. Plasma osmolality is measured for the concentration of various substances like glucose urea or electrolytes per kg of plasma.

Antidiuretic hormone (ADH) and aldosterone are two main hormones, which are involved in water/fluid balance. The hypothalamus of a dehydrated person stimulates by the posterior pituitary gland to secrete antidiuretic hormone (ADH). ADH, also called vasopressin, is a hormone responsible for increasing water reabsorption in the collecting ducts of the kidney nephron. This effectively dilutes the plasma. Besides, increased water absorption in distal collecting duct of the kidney, urine volume is reduced and concentration of urine is increased.

Aldosterone is a corticoid hormone and a part of renin–angiotensin system. It is secreted by the adrenal glands that regulate the balance of sodium and potassium and thus brings water-balance levels in the body. It is important to note that the kidneys normally filter approximately 180 liters of plasma in a day but excrete only about 1.8 liters of urine. However, there is a lag period, between reduction in body water and thirst. Sensations of thirst are controlled by receptors in the hypothalamus, heart, and large-blood vessels.

When water balance is restored, water ingestion is curtailed or stopped. There are stretch receptors in the stomach that monitor blood volume. Drinking fluids distend the stomach whose stretch receptors send nerve impulses that inhibit the thirst center. Also, water is absorbed into ECF through walls of the stomach and small intestine. Thus, thirst and drinking adequate amount of water help to restore and maintain homeostasis and the osmotic pressure of ECF comes back to normal. Similarly, there are stretch receptors in the atria of the heart. These are activated by a larger than normal volume of blood returning to the heart from the veins. These stretch receptors inhibit ADH secretion through the action of antinatriuretic peptide (ANP), a hormone. ANP is also known as atrial antinatriuretic factor or ANF. Besides these, moistening of the mucosa in the mouth and throat provides feedback signals and inhibits thirst.

When there is excess water, ECF becomes less concentrated (i.e., there is a decrease in osmotic pressure). Osmoreceptors in the hypothalamus detect this decrease. The hypothalamus sends signals to the posterior pituitary to decrease its release of ADH. In turn, the kidneys decrease their water reabsorption. This results in increased urine output and ECF volume returns to normal. Stretch receptors in the atria of the heart are activated by a larger than normal volume of blood returning to the heart from the veins. These inhibit ADH secretion, because the body wants to rid itself of the excess fluid volume. The third hormone that influences water balance is aldosterone that is secreted by the adrenal gland. Aldosterone acts on the kidneys to retain sodium and water and thus causes an increase in the ECF.

Other important factors that influence fluid balance are:
1. Concentration of electrolytes in blood particularly sodium
2. Capillary blood pressure
3. Concentration of protein.

Sodium has a strong affinity for water and has a very important role; in fact it has a central role in fluid and electrolyte balance. Wherever sodium moves, water follows. If sodium concentration in the blood increases, volume of the blood also increases and vice versa. Sodium concentration in blood also influences the arterial blood pressure.

Role of kidneys in fluid balance: Kidneys play a key role in fluid balance. The major role of the kidneys is to produce urine. While performing this function, kidneys regulate the body's electrolytes (e.g., sodium, potassium, calcium, magnesium, etc.), fluid balance, and acid–base balance and eliminate some waste products that have been produced by the body during metabolic processes. When normal fluid volume is restored, dehydration is relieved. Renin secretion from the kidney and angiotensin II decreases. Role of kidney in fluid balance is shown in Figure 8.4.

Dehydration appears to alter cardiovascular, thermoregulatory, central nervous system, and metabolic functions. When dehydration exceeds 2% of the body weight there may be alterations in metabolic functions of one or more body systems that seriously affect performance during endurance

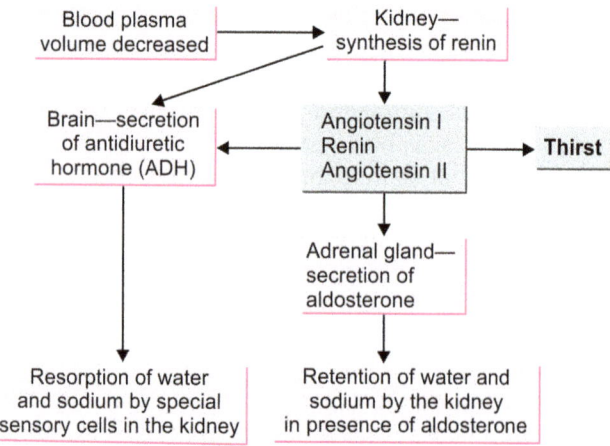

Fig. 8.4: Role of kidneys in fluid balance.

exercises. These performance decrements are accentuated by heat stress. Dehydration also increase the risk of infections.

Kidneys contribute to regulating water balance by adjusting and regulating the concentration of urine. Some amount of water is excreted daily. This water carries the waste products out of the body. This is known as "obligatory water excretion" and is generally 500 mL per day. Obligatory water loss is also called minimal water loss. This loss is through excretion of water/urine, which is the medium for getting rid of the waste products of metabolism. The amount of electrolytes and urea present determines the volume of obligatory water loss. However, urine volume increases if a person drinks more water. The excess water that is excreted is termed as "facultative" excretion. The amount of facultative losses varies within the same person and between two persons depending on the fluid intake and extent of losses from skin, lungs, and gastrointestinal tract. As urine volume increases, urine also becomes dilute.

Kidneys get rid of fluid when there is an excess and conserve fluid when there is a deficiency. Thus, the kidney helps to prevent both dehydration and fluid retention. When the volume of plasma or effective circulating plasma is increased, there is decrease in the blood pressure. This is sensed by kidneys, which synthesize and release an enzyme renin. Renin travels through the bloodstream, binds to an inactive plasma protein, angiotensinogen, and converts it to angiotensin I. As angiotensin I passes through the lung and other capillaries, an enzyme called angiotensin-converting enzyme, or ACE, converts angiotensin I to angiotensin II. Angiotensin II circulates through the bloodstream and when it reaches the adrenal gland, it stimulates the adrenal cells to release the hormone aldosterone. Angiotensin II also constricts the blood vessels that help to increase the blood pressure.

A decrease in blood volume and the resultant decrease in blood pressure further stimulate the sympathetic nervous system. Sympathetic nerves in the kidney release neurotransmitters that stimulate the smooth muscle cells to constrict. This results in decreased blood flow into and through the kidney and ultimately reduces urine formation ensuring that less water leaves the body.

Essentially, the kidneys respond to water needs, which are as follows:
- If water needs are more or body water volume is less, the kidneys will excrete less urine or vice versa.
- When plasma ADH levels are low, the kidneys become less permeable to water, they reabsorb less water and a larger volume of urine is excreted.
- In contrast, when ADH levels are high, the urine is concentrated and urine volume is relatively lower.

WATER IMBALANCE

Water imbalance implies that there is a disturbance in the water balance wherein either water loss exceeds intake or vice versa. It can occur in either dehydration or water intoxication.

Dehydration

Dehydration is a condition wherein output (excretion) is far above (in excess of) the amount of water/fluid consumed, i.e., there is either too little consumption of fluid and/or excessive loss that is not replaced. Consequently, the body contains less water than it should. It is defined as 1% or more weight loss caused by loss of body fluid. It is defined as 1% or more weight loss caused by loss of body fluid. Loss of water can occur with or without loss of other components in body fluids.

> **Dehydration** is a condition which occurs when losses (excretion) are far more (in excess) than the amount of water/fluid consumed because losses are high or fluid intake is inadequate or both. It adversely affects the cognitive and motor control.

Dehydration may result from depletion of pure water and mixed type (depletion of both water and electrolytes). Vomiting and diarrhea are two common problems that place a person at risk of dehydration. Endurance athletes are likely to lose considerable fluids through perspiration when they are running long distances. If not attended to, dehydration can be a medical emergency and even increase risk of death. It can be acute or chronic, due to excessive loss of water and/or inadequate rehydration.

Pure water depletion occurs when water intake is inadequate and there is no parallel loss of electrolytes in the secretions of the body. Pure water depletion is observed in a person who is too ill or weak to drink enough to satisfy the water requirements or in cases of coma, or has difficulty in swallowing. It may also happen, if a person is in an arid or desert region and has no water to drink. Even if water intake is stopped, the obligatory water loss continues, there is some minimum excretion of urine to get rid of the metabolic load. Hence, the body water stores get depleted. At the same time, the concentration of electrolytes rises in the ECF, which becomes hypertonic. In order to correct this imbalance, water flows from the ICF to the ECF, resulting in a reduction in ICF and intracellular dehydration.

Mixed water and electrolyte depletion occurs when there is loss of body fluids containing sodium and chloride on the one hand and there is inadequate free intake of water on the other hand. In contrast to pure water depletion, the ECF is hypotonic in the initial stages. If water loss continues, then the loss of water exceeds the loss of the electrolytes, making the ECF hypertonic. In this, both ECF and ICF are reduced.

Causes of Dehydration

Dehydration occurs due to either inadequate intake and/or excessive loss such as:
- *Poor intake of water and fluids* due to loss of appetite/thirst during illness, nausea, sore throat, or mouth sores

Excessive losses due to:
- Increased sweating due to hot weather, high humidity, dry air (air conditioning), exercise or fever
- Diarrhea
- Vomiting

- Blood loss during burn or injury
- Excessive fluid loss through urine usually during diabetes and kidney disease
- Use of diuretics
- Burns because fluid seeps into the damaged skin and the body loses water.

However, thirst sensation may be blunted in some individuals like the elderly or small children who may not voice or may not be able to express their needs. Children may not speak about their need if they are engrossed in activities they love. Also during illness, children may refuse to eat and/or drink while losses occur due to fever, vomiting, and/or diarrhea. Infants and children are at greater risk of being dehydrated because their bodies are smaller, they weigh less, the turnover of water and electrolytes in the body is more, ECF proportion is higher. Similarly, there are people who lose considerable amount of fluid through perspiration, e.g., sportspersons, people who work long hours in the hot sun. Such individuals are at risk of dehydration.

In infants, sunken fontanelles are an indication of dehydration. Dehydration can be life-threatening particularly during infancy and childhood. In the elderly who have physical illness, dehydration is associated with adverse effects on mental function. Dehydration can be mild, moderate, or severe depending on how much of the body fluid is lost or not replenished. When dehydration is severe, it is a life-threatening condition and should be considered an emergency. In severe cases, the person may go into coma (become unconscious). When the body loses more than 5% of the total body water, it has clinical consequences. Eventually, urination stops and kidneys fail to remove body's waste products. The condition is life-threatening, if body water loss is 15%. Table 8.3 summarizes the signs and symptoms in different dehydration conditions.

- Water is the driving force of nature
- Water day is celebrated on March 22nd every year
- Water is life and clean water means health

Clinical Signs of Dehydration

Once the degree of dehydration has been determined, it is necessary to calculate the fluid requirements for rehydration. Depending on the type of dehydration, i.e., isotonic or hypotonic, this can be calculated using the Holliday–Segar method.

Clinical signs include increased thirst, dry mucous membranes, and decreased urine output.

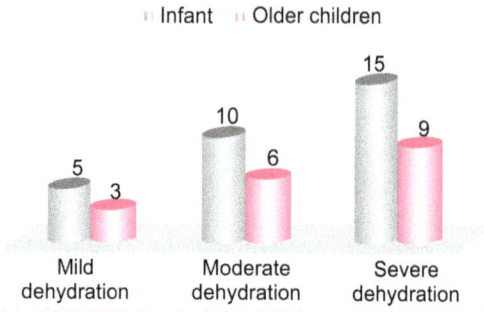

Fig. 8.5: Levels of dehydration in children.

Dehydration can be classified as mild, moderate, or severe and each of these is characterized by specific clinical signs as well as different levels of dehydration in infants and children in Figures 8.5 and 8.6 respectively.

The *rehydration phase* is divided into three types: Phase I is the emergency phase, following which there are two phases, the first 8 hours are designated as Phase II and the next 16 hours are said to be Phase III. Depending on the phase, fluid volume to be administered is decided. Experts have given recommendations for rehydrating the elderly as well.

When rehydrating a patient, it is important to pay attention to the electrolyte content as well as the carbohydrate content. Thus, tea, fruit juice, milk, carbonated beverages/soft drinks, and sports beverages may not be suitable as they do not contain appropriate amounts of the necessary electrolytes and some of them may contain excess sugar. Therefore, they should not be used for oral rehydration. The only exception is that infants who are breastfed should continue to receive mother's milk, if they have diarrhea.

Recommendations for calculating fluid requirements for rehydrating the elderly are as follow:
A formula used to calculate fluid requirements for older people is:

100 mL fluid per kg BW for first 10 kg
50 mL fluid per kg BW for next 10 kg
15 mL fluid for each after 20 kg BW

Patient weight	<30	35	40	45	50	55	60	65	70	75	80	85	90	95	100	105
Fluid requirements (liters/day)	1.7	1.7	1.8	1.9	2.0	2.0	2.1	2.2	2.3	2.3	2.4	2.5	2.6	2.6	2.7	2.8

Woodward M. Guidelines to Effective Hydration in Aged Care Facilities. Medical Director, Aged & Residential Care Services Heidelberg Repatriation Hospital. 2013.

Table 8.3: Signs and symptoms of isotonic, hypertonic and hypotonic dehydration in different conditions.

Isotonic	Hypertonic	Hypotonic
- Net salt and water loss are equal - Generally, salt is lost isotonically from GI tract, e.g., during diarrhea ECF volume is reduced - Treatment to be done with isotonic salt solutions, e.g., ORS prescribed by WHO	- Loss of water is in excess of loss of salt - Caused by inadequate water intake and/or excessive water loss - Insufficient intake may be due to lack of water, defective thirst, impaired consciousness - May be due to osmotic diuresis or diabetes insipidus - Exercising in a hot climate can also be a cause	- Loss of salt is in excess of water loss - Caused by loss of gastrointestinal fluid and water that are used to replace contains less Na and K compared to body fluid that was lost - Reduced osmolarity of plasma results in ECF moving into intracellular compartment and increases cell volume despite the reduction in ECF - Treatment is with hypertonic saline in order to restore osmolarity and then isotonic saline to compensate for ECF loss

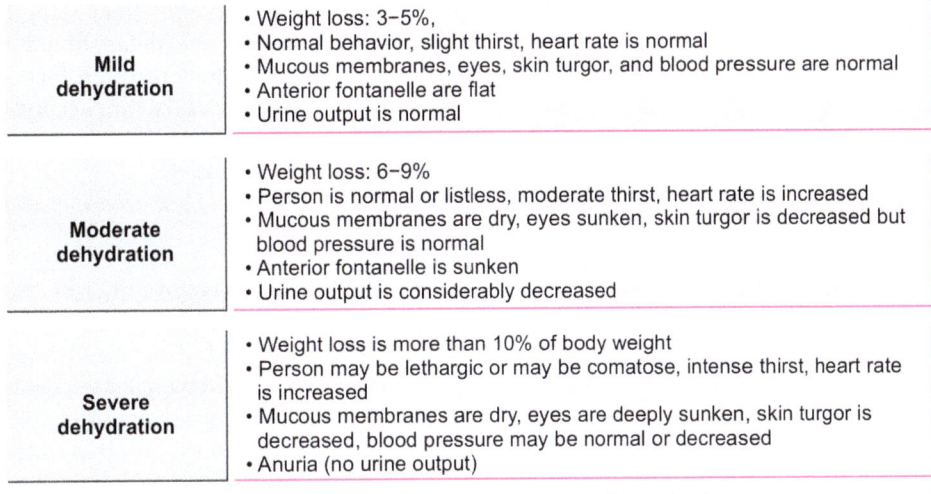

Fig. 8.6: Clinical signs of dehydration at different levels.

Laboratory Laurel: A randomized, open-label, controlled, 12-month trial at a clinical research center (years 2013–2016) was carried out on 163 healthy women (mean age 35.7 years) with recurrent cystitis (≥3 episodes in past year) who were drinking <1.5 L of fluid daily and 140 were assigned to water group or control group (water but no additional fluids). They were assessed for daily fluid intake, urinary hydration, and cystitis symptoms at baseline, 6- and 12-month visits using monthly telephone calls. There were 1.7 cystitis episodes in water group compared with 3 in the control group. Overall, there were 327 cystitis episodes, 111 in the water group and 216 in the control group. The mean time interval between cystitis episodes was 142.8 and 84 days, respectively, with a difference in means of 58.4 days. Participants in the water group had more urine volume and low urine osmolality. Increased water intake is an effective antimicrobial-sparing strategy to prevent recurrent cystitis in premenopausal women at high risk for recurrence who drink low volumes of fluid daily.

Hooton TM, Vecchio M, Iroz A, et al. Effect of Increased Daily Water Intake in Premenopausal Women with Recurrent Urinary Tract Infections: A Randomized Clinical Trial. JAMA Intern Med. 2018;178(11):1509-15.

Laboratory Laurel: In several epidemiologic studies, environmental exposure, dietary habits, and genetic factors cause kidney stone disease (KSD) worldwide. Physicians recommend high water intake (>3 L daily) to prevent KSD. In this study, 1,266 patients with kidney stones from West Bengal, India were selected and drinking water collected and analyzed for pH, alkalinity, hardness, total dissolved solutes, electrical conductivity, and salinity. As many as 53.6% of the patients consumed <3 L of water daily. All water samples were found to be suitable for consumption. Control and case water samples did not show any statistically significant alterations in the studied parameters. It is not the quality of water, rather the quantity of water consumed that matters most in the occurrence of KSD.

Mitra P, Pal DK, Das M. Does quality of drinking water matter in kidney stone disease: A study in West Bengal, India. Investig Clin Urol. 2018;59(3):158-65.

Individuals who consumed greater than approximately 2.5 L/day of fluid have been reported to have a 49% lower risk of bladder cancer than individuals who consumed less than approximately 1.3 L/day. It was also noted that the risk of bladder cancer was reduced by 7% for every addition of 240 mL (1 cup) in daily fluid intake. However, several other studies have failed to demonstrate an overall association between fluid intake and bladder cancer risk.

Prevention of Dehydration at Home Level

Maintaining water, fluid, and electrolytes balance is the key to prevent dehydration. Simply, either the fluid intake should be increased in case of low fluid intake or the loss of water from the body be reduced, which may occur in sickness or increased use of diuretics. In any case, water loss needs to be replaced. In mild or moderate dehydration, giving adequate fluids can reverse the situation. However, severe dehydration requires urgent medical attention. During diarrhea/vomiting, along with water, some electrolytes or minerals are also lost, which need to be replaced instantly otherwise, it can be a threat to health or life.

Composition of WHO ORS (Oral Rehydration Solution)	
Sodium chloride:	2.6 g
Trisodium citrate dihydrate	2.9 g
Potassium chloride:	1.5 g
Glucose:	13.5 g
Water:	1 L
Total weight of formula is 20.0 g	

Since water in the biological system also carries some electrolytes like sodium (Na^+), potassium (K^+), etc., they also need to be replaced along with water during dehydration.

During diarrhea, use of revised WHO-ORS formula has been advised. At household level, one glass of boiled and cooled water in which 1 teaspoon sugar and a pinch of salt are dissolved can be used to replace water and electrolyte loss. In addition to ORS, other liquids like "nimbu pani" with a pinch of salt, thin buttermilk with a small pinch of salt and sugar, coconut water, light black tea with sugar, and a little lemon juice can also be given. Herbal tea can also be included particularly when there is restriction of salt or sugar. It helps to improve taste and inclination to drink fluids. Often jug is kept near the patient to drink water throughout 24 hours. However, after sometime, the water becomes unpalatable, impregnated with plastic flavor (if stored in a plastic container), and it is preferable that this liquid should

WATER INTOXICATION

Water intoxication is a condition when water intake is excessively high and body is not able to handle the excess water load. Water intoxication increases intracellular fluid volume and dilutes body fluids. Drinking excessive amount of plain water leads to hyponatremia, i.e., low concentration of sodium in the blood because the intestines rapidly absorb water and the osmolality of ECF is reduced. The condition can occur during exercise when novices may drink too much water during endurance events without realizing the hazard. It may also occur in renal insufficiency where urine output is reduced. When excess water is given after surgery, trauma or any condition leading to loss of salt and water, ADH and kidney may not be able to respond.

Most cells can adapt and adjust to small changes but if the situation prolongs, cells can become distorted and normal cell function may be disrupted. Compared to dehydration, water intoxication is rare. Early warning signs are somewhat similar to dehydration and include nausea, muscle cramps, disorientation, slurred speech, and confusion. Many athletes drink more water because they think they are dehydrated. Unfortunately, water alone will increase the problem of hyponatremia.

Symptoms of water intoxication are:
- Headaches
- Restlessness
- Confusion
- Change in personality
- Blurred vision
- Cramps (and eventually convulsions)
- Swelling of the brain
- Coma and in extreme cases death.

Requirements for Water and Fluids

- The human body does not have any provision to store water. Therefore, water that is lost in the day has to be replaced on a daily basis. Requirements for water as recommended by ICMR-NIN (2020) are shown in Table 9.1A in Chapter 9.
- Under normal conditions, the requirement for water is 1 mL per kcal for adults or 35 mL per kg of body weight.
- Requirement for infants is higher, i.e., 1.5 mL/kcal or 150 mL/kg. Children require 50–60 mL per kg. Water intake must maintain adequate hydration of the body. Water requirements depend on the environmental temperature (heat) and humidity, physical activity, altitude (respiratory loss is more).

An additional 360 mL/day is required for each degree centigrade of temperature rise. More water may be required by physically active people, children, in hot and/or humid environments, and breastfeeding women. High intake of protein may increase need for water since the end product of protein metabolism is urea, which is excreted through urine. Similarly, carbohydrate intake can also influence need for water. High intake of dietary fiber in food also may influence water requirements since dietary fiber binds water and there will be more water loss through feces. When estimating water intake, one must take into account not only the water consumed, but also beverages like tea, coffee, soft drinks, fruit juices, butter milk, etc.

ELECTROLYTES AND ELECTROLYTE BALANCE

Body fluids contain some minerals, which are important electrolytes required for normal functioning of the body. These are present inside the cell and the space around the cell and the blood. Ratio of these electrolytes in each compartment is very critical. Electrolytes are inorganic salts, all acids and bases, and some proteins whereas nonelectrolytes include glucose, lipids, creatinine, and urea.

Electrolytes are charged particles. An electrolyte is a chemical substance (either a salt or acid or base) that gives ions when they are dissolved in water. Solutions made with these substances conduct electricity or electrolytes are the substances, which undergo dissociation when dissolved in water or liquid to produce conductivity. Generally, the term electrolyte is used to refer to electrically charged minerals.

Positively charged ions are called **cations** such as sodium (Na^+) and potassium (K^+); and negatively charged ions are called **anions** such as chloride (Cl^-). The presence of charged ions facilitates conductance of an electrical current through an aqueous solution. This makes it possible to measure brain activity (EEG) as well as heart (ECG) and other muscles (EMG) by placing electrodes on the body surface. Electrolytes have greater osmotic power than nonelectrolytes. The major electrolytes present in the human body are:

Cations (positively charged ions)	Anions (negatively charged ions)
Sodium (Na^+)	Chloride (Cl^-)
Potassium (K^+)	Bicarbonate (HCO_3^-)
Calcium (Ca^{++})	Phosphate (PO_4^-)
Magnesium (Mg^{++})	Sulfate (SO_4^-)

Electrolytes are present both inside the cell or in intracellular fluid (ICF) and outside the cell or in extracellular fluid (ECF) and play major roles in maintaining the homeostasis in the body. Each fluid compartment of the body has a distinctive electrolyte composition. Electrolytes are important because they are vital to health, and act as chemical messengers in the body. They carry electrical impulses from the nerves to control all tissue functions and movements. Concentrations of individual electrolytes influence cell functions. An imbalance of any of the electrolytes can lead to serious disruptions in physiologic function. Many bodily processes are highly dependent on them, primarily heart and nerve function, muscle coordination and control, and maintenance of the body's fluid levels. Electrolytes determine the chemical and physical reactions of body fluids and are involved in a number of regulatory processes. They have important functions in vital physiological processes:

- Maintenance of body fluid osmolarity and fluid balance: Concentrations of the electrolytes, especially that of sodium, affect water/fluid balance and influence the distribution of body fluids among the different body fluid compartments by controlling osmosis.
- Regulation of nerve function (conductivity of nerves)
- Regulation of acid–base balance.
- Regulation of muscle function (contraction of muscles).

On account of these physiological functions, electrolytes play a critical role in sustaining life. In case of diarrhea and dehydration, electrolytes are lost and extensive losses are life-threatening. Therefore, they have to be replaced. Maintenance of normal electrolyte concentrations is an important aspect of medical treatment and dietary management of several diseases, e.g., diarrhea to kidney diseases. Sports drinks are also designed to maintain normal electrolyte balance.

Electrolytes in Body Fluids

Some electrolytes are present primarily outside the cell (ECF), whereas others reside predominantly within the cell (ICF). In ECF, sodium is the chief cation and chloride is the major anion, whereas intracellular fluids have lower concentrations of sodium and chloride, and potassium is the chief cation with phosphate being the major anion. Also present are Mg^{2+} and SO_4^{2-}. These electrolytes are essential minerals in some biochemical reactions. Cations are responsible for nerve and muscle irritability and anions are responsible for body fluid and hydrogen ion balance. Diet is the major supplier of these ions. However, some are byproducts of metabolic reactions.

> ECF contains more cations—Sodium and Calcium; **ECF—155 mEq/L;**
> ICF contains more anions—Potassium, Bicarbonates and Phosphates;
> **ICF—202 mEq/L**

All electrolytes are present in ECF and ICF. However, the total cations are the same as the total anions in each compartment, which needs to be maintained for electrolyte balance. This balance is called **"electroneutrality"** of the solution (A solution having equal number of positively charged particles and negatively charged particles is stable). Concentrations of ions are expressed as milliequivalents per liter.

Electrolyte concentration directly affects water balance but concentrations of individual electrolytes affect cell functions as shown in Table 8.4.

Cationic electric charges must equal anionic charges both outside and inside the cell. The anions within the cell are largely polyvalent and too large to penetrate the plasma membrane. The sole cation to which the plasma membrane is permeable, and which is present in sufficient free concentration to neutralize fixed anions, is potassium.

Intracellular metabolism also plays an important role. Net synthesis or degradation of cell proteins results in changes in the intracellular fixed ions, thereby leading to an increase or decrease in cell volume. When hypoxia occurs, the glucose metabolism shifts to anaerobic glycolysis and lactic acid is the end product. Due to this, there is a reduction in the intracellular pH which in turn has indirect effects, since this acidity needs to be neutralized to maintain normal pH in the cell.

Electrolytes, particularly sodium, help the body to maintain normal fluid levels in these compartments because how much fluid a compartment contains depends on the concentration of electrolytes in it. If the electrolyte concentration is high, fluid moves into that compartment. If the electrolyte concentration is low, fluid moves out of that compartment. To adjust fluid levels, the body can actively move electrolytes in or out of cells. Thus, having electrolytes in the right concentrations, i.e., electrolyte balance is important for maintaining fluid balance among the compartments. Any change in the amount of one ion can influence other ions.

The ECF and ICF are separated by semipermeable membranes and there is continuous exchange between the fluid compartments. There is continual interchange of substances present between ISF and plasma. This exchange occurs through pores that are present in the capillary membrane. The presence of these pores makes the capillary membrane highly permeable. Since there is continuous exchange between plasma and ISF, their composition is

Table 8.4: Balance of electrolytes present in extracellular fluids (ECF) and intracellular fluids (ICF) and their functions.

Positively charged electrolytes (cations)	ECF (mEq/L)	ICF (mEq/L)	Functions
Sodium (Na^+)	142	10	Fluid balance and osmotic pressure Nerve conduction, active cellular transport Formation of mineral apatite of bone
Potassium (K^+)	5	150	Neuromuscular excitability (transmission of electrical impulses along nerves and cell membranes) Acid–base balance
Calcium (Ca^{++})	5	2	Blood clotting, bone mineralization
Magnesium (Mg^{++})	3	40	Enzyme activity
Total	**155**	**202**	
Negatively charged Electrolyte (anions)			
Chloride (Cl^-)	103	2	Fluid balance and osmotic pressure
Bicarbonate (HCO_3^-)	27	10	Acid–base balance
Proteins	16	57	Osmotic pressure
Phosphate (HPO_4^-)	2	103	Energy storage
Sulfate (SO_4^-)	1	20	Protein metabolism
Organic acid	6	10	Support acid–base balance
Total	**155**	**202**	

Adapted from: Rolfes SR, Pinna K, Whitney E. Understanding normal and clinical nutrition, 8th edition. Belmont, CA: Wadsworth Cengage Learning; 2008.

similar, except for the presence of large proteins in plasma. These large proteins are not able to pass through the capillary membrane and remain in the blood/plasma. Therefore compared to plasma, ISF has low protein concentration.

Water moves between ICF and ECF according to osmotic gradient. Hence, water will flow into that compartment which has higher osmolyte concentration. This process of flow is called osmosis. When fluid flows from one compartment to another, some force is necessary to stop the flow of solvent across a membrane. Osmotic pressure is the amount of force pressure necessary. Any alterations in osmolarity are rapidly and effectively dealt with in order to maintain the osmolarity of body fluids.

In a normal healthy person, osmolarity of the body fluids is 275-295 Osmol/L. The body contains about 60 mEq of Na per kilogram of body weight on an average, most of it being present in ECF and only 3% is present in the cells (ICF). About 70% of total body Na is readily exchangeable. Among the electrolytes, Na^+, K^+, Cl^-, and HCO_3^- are of major importance in terms of their content contributing to serum osmolality. The sodium cation participates in regulating both osmotic and electrolyte balance; chloride, however, is a passive participant in the process. About 90-95% of the osmotic pressure in ECF is provided by sodium and its anion. In ICF, the major ions are potassium and phosphate.

> **Osmosis** is the flow (diffusion) of water and/or ions through a semipermeable membrane from areas of higher concentration to areas of lower concentration. It is a fundamental process in all biological systems.
> **Osmolytes** are ions affecting osmosis.
> **Osmotic force/pressure** is usually exerted by sodium (Na^+), which controls the flow of solvent across a cell membrane. It is directly proportional to the number of particles in solutes, but is not related to the charge.
> When two fluids differing in solute concentration are separated (present in 2 compartments) by semipermeable membrane, water will flow from low solute concentration to the compartment with high solute concentration. The flow may be stopped or even reversed by applying external pressure on the volume of higher concentration. This is known as osmotic pressure.
> Osmotic pressure is expressed as osmolarity or osmolality and is measured in **osmoles (Osm) or** milliosmoles (mOsm).
> 1 **osmole** is the number of particles (molecules) in 1 gram molecular weight of undissociated solute.
> Osmolarity of a simple solution is equal to the molarity times the number of particles per molecule (molar concentration per unit volume of water). It is a simple count of the number or **osmolality** is a measure of the moles (or osmoles) of solute per kilogram of solvent expressed as: mol/kg, molal or m.

Osmotic pressure is dependent on the number of particles of the solute rather than weight of the particles and it is not related to the ionic charge.

Measurements of osmolar concentration are often expressed in **osmolarity. Osmolarity** is a measure of the osmoles of solute per liter of solution (the concentration per unit weight of water or fluid). A capital letter M is used to abbreviate units of mol/L. Osmolarity is a measure of the osmotic pressure exerted by a solution across a perfect semipermeable membrane, which allows water to pass freely but completely prevents movement of solute; compared to that exerted by pure water. Osmolarity is dependent on the number of particles in solution but independent of the nature of the particles.

Osmole is similar to the mole, i.e., molecular weight of 1 g nondissociable or nonionic molecule. When it is used for dissociable or ionic substances, which contribute to the osmotic pressure, the term osmole is used. For example, one mole of nonionic solute (glucose or urea) cannot dissociate. Hence, the osmolarity of the solution is **1 Osm/L**. Similarly, albumin gives a solution with an osmolarity of 1 Osm/L.

One mole of any solute, which can dissociate into 2 ions, will give a solution with an osmolarity of 2 Osm. Example, if 1 mole of sucrose was added to one liter of water, the osmolarity would be 2 Osm/L. Note that it does not matter, which is the molecule. If 1 mole of NaCl was dissolved in 1 liter of water, it would produce a 1 mol/L NaCl solution with an osmolarity 2 Osm/L because NaCl dissociates into Na^+ and Cl^- (two particles) in solution.

In clinical practice/laboratories, osmolality is measured using an osmometer. The normal osmolality of extracellular fluid is 275-295 mOsmol/kg. Alternatively, osmolarity is usually calculated. The calculation is derived from measured Na^+, K^+, urea, and glucose concentrations.

The calculation for osmolarity is:
Osmolarity = 2 (mmol/L Na+) + 2 (mmol/L K+) + mmol/L Glucose + mmol/L Urea
Or
2 (mmol/L Na+) + mmol/L Glucose + mmol/L Urea

Osmotic pressure (mm Hg) = 19.3 × Osmolality (milliosmoles/liter)

If blood glucose levels are normal then one can estimate osmolality approximately as:
$$2 \times \text{the sodium level}$$

When osmolality is reduced, i.e., <275, the situation is considered as "fluid overload" and when the value exceeds 295, it is considered as "dehydration".

Since osmolality of ECF and ICF is approximately equal, osmolality indicates concentration of substances inside the cell, which otherwise cannot be measured. Any change in ECF affects the ICF. Osmolality of blood increases with dehydration. If a hyperosmolar solution is consumed by a patient, it would tend to cause water to move out of the cell. Changes in ECF osmolality have a great effect on ICF osmolality. They can cause problems with normal cell functioning and volume.

Osmolarity is controlled by renal control of water retention and excretion via thirst mechanism. In normal individuals when osmolality in the blood increases, it will stimulate secretion of antidiuretic hormone (ADH). This results in increased water reabsorption, more concentrated urine, and less concentrated blood plasma. On the other hand, low-serum osmolality will suppress the release of ADH, consequently there is decreased water reabsorption and plasma becomes more concentrated. Small changes in plasma osmolality (increase of 2-3%) make a person feel the need to drink some fluid.

On the basis of osmolarity, fluids are classified into 3 categories:
1. **Isotonic solution:** Isotonic solutions have the same osmolarity as the body fluids. For patients, administration of isotonic solutions such as normal saline, Ringer's lactate, and 5% glucose D (5%W) will not change osmolarity. However, administration of isotonic solutions increases total body water.
2. **Hypertonic solution:** When concentration of water and salts in ECF is higher than the concentration in ICF, the ECF is hypertonic. In this condition, water comes out of the cell and the cell tends to shrink and die. Sometimes hypertonic fluids such as 5% glucose/dextrose and normal saline or 5% glucose/dextrose and Ringer's lactate solution may be administered to patients. Such fluids having higher osmolarity than the body fluids are used to increase intravascular osmolarity by shifting intracellular and interstitial fluids.
3. **Hypotonic solution:** When concentration of salts in a solution on one side of the membrane is lower than on the other side of the membrane, the solution with lower concentration of salts is known as hypotonic. Fluids have less osmolarity than the body fluids and contain <5% glucose or 0.3% sodium in water. Examples of fluids used for patients are: 0.45% saline, 2.5% dextrose, and 0.33% saline. Thus, when concentration of water in ECF is higher and salt is lower than in ICF, the ECF is hypotonic. In this condition, water moves from ECF inside the cell and decreases intravascular osmolarity. Hypotonic solution is used for cellular dehydration.

> **Research Glimpse:** It is known that lack of adequate fluid replacement (hypohydration) and excessive intake (hyperhydration) can compromise athletic performance and increase health risks. It is also necessary to improve drinking behavior and needs some recommendations. In this regard, The National Athletic Trainers' Association (NATA) has published a new position statement, "Fluid Replacement for the Physically Active." https://www.nata.org/NR10062017
> - Importance of maintaining Fluid Balance and Regulation
> - Importance of Maintaining Euhydration (optimal total body water content as regulated by the brain)
> - Fluid Replacement
> - Beverage Additives
> - Hydration Assessment.
>
> *McDermott BP, Anderson SA, Armstrong LE, et al. National Athletic Trainers' Association Position Statement: Fluid Replacement for the Physically Active. J Athl Train. 2017;52(9):877-95.*

Electrolytes of Extracellular Fluids

Sodium (Na^+) is the major cation and chloride (Cl^-) is the major anion in the extracellular fluid (ECF). These contribute maximum amount of electrolytes and play significant roles in fluid balance and osmotic pressure. Sodium controls the volume of the ECF and fluid movement across compartments. Other electrolytes are also necessary for their respective roles.

> - If ECF osmotic concentration increases, ECF is hypertonic compared to ICF. Consequently, water moves from inside the cells to ECF.
> - If ECF osmotic concentration decreases, the ECF becomes hypotonic and water will move from ECF into cells.

In a normal healthy individual, variations in salt (NaCl) intake do not affect the osmolarity of ECF. Most common problems with electrolyte balance are caused by imbalance between gains and losses of sodium ions. Any change in the diet can influence the electrolyte balance, but drastic changes are reflected by symptoms like muscle cramps, twitching, and cardiac contraction.

Electrolytes of Intracellular Fluids

Potassium (K^+) is the major cation and phosphate (HPO_4^-) is the major anion in intracellular fluids (ICF). Potassium along with small amount of magnesium and sodium exerts the osmotic pressure in ICF. Mg^{++} is associated with energy release. Another predominant anion in ICF is bicarbonate (HCO_3^-), which greatly influences acid–base balance in the body. Ions of ICF maintain the ionic strength inside the cell and cellular functions. K^+ participates in active transport. Although potassium imbalance is not very common, if it occurs, it can be dangerous.

Total body potassium (K) is approximately 53 mEq/kg body weight. Most of it is present within cells and almost all, i.e., 92% is exchangeable. Only 2–3% of K is present outside the cells.

Role of Interstitial Fluid in Electrolyte Balance

In the ionic composition of the interstitial fluid (ISF) and plasma, the two compartments of ECF are almost the same, although plasma is separated from interstitial fluid by the capillary wall (wall of blood vessels). The major difference between the two is that plasma contains more protein than does the interstitial fluid.

Plasma proteins influence the shift of water from one compartment to another. They are colloids and cannot pass easily through capillary membranes. Consequently, they are concentrated within the blood vessels. These proteins (albumin, immunoglobulins, and fibrinogen) are osmotically active; and a concentration gradient is created across the capillary membrane. Being solutes, they exert pressure, which is known as **colloidal osmotic pressure (COP) or oncotic pressure,** i.e., they encourage osmosis and draw water toward them.

> Colloid is a term that refers to large molecular weight particles, usually more than 30,000 that are present in a solution. In plasma, proteins are the major colloids.
>
> Oncotic pressure or colloid osmotic pressure is formed by colloid particles dissolved in solution. In plasma, proteins are responsible for oncotic pressure. Plasma protein level is 65–85 g/L.

Capillary blood has a high content of plasma proteins; therefore, it has a high oncotic pressure of 25 mm Hg. Oncotic pressure is important for fluid balance and movement of fluid across the capillaries, from the intravascular to the interstitial compartments. Thus, plasma COP helps to maintain the blood volume in vascular compartment. Albumin is the major plasma protein contributing to COP. Low-plasma COP is linked to increased mortality in critically ill patients.

Besides COP, another force that regulates the exchange of fluid between plasma and tissues is hydrostatic pressure.

Hydrostatic pressure is the force exerted against the capillary wall. It is more in the arterial end of capillaries (30 mm Hg) than at the venous end (20 mm Hg), whereas in the interstitial space, the hydrostatic pressure is 0 mm Hg. Hydrostatic pressure in capillaries influences the blood pressure and rate of flow from plasma to interstitial fluid. This pressure tends to push fluid out of capillary into ISF as capillaries are permeable to water and electrolytes but not plasma proteins.

Hydrostatic pressure drives fluid out of plasma and drives fluid into lymphatic vessels. Hydrostatic pressure is important because when this pressure builds up inside the capillary, it causes filtration and forces fluids and solutes (including nutrients) out. Thus, tissues get the nutrients required. This happens at the arterial end of capillaries. Toward the venous end, hydrostatic pressure is less than oncotic pressure, hence along with fluid, waste products are drawn into the capillary. Osmotic pressure causes the return of fluid to plasma and regulates movement into and out of cells. Simply put filtration occurs in the first half of the capillary and reabsorption occurs in the latter half.

> **Oncotic pressure** is the "PULLING" force.
> **Hydrostatic pressure** is the "PUSHING" force.
>
> If COP is higher than hydrostatic pressure, water is drawn from interstitial fluid (ISF) to plasma and fluid will leave the capillaries. Conversely, if hydrostatic pressure is higher than oncotic pressure, fluid will leave the capillaries.
>
> When there is an increase in blood pressure, hydrostatic pressure increases, resulting in more fluid moving out of capillaries into the tissues.

Under normal conditions, fluids are balanced. However, excessive accumulation of fluid in interstitium/interstitial tissues (also called edema) can occur due to four reasons:
- Increased hydrostatic pressure in vessels (including sodium and water retention)
- Increased vascular permeability
- Decreased plasma osmotic pressure, or
- Decreased lymphatic effectiveness.

The walls of the capillaries are fragile. The capillary membrane can be disrupted due to various reasons. Also, permeability of capillary membrane is increased due to increased hydrostatic pressure. This results in abnormal accumulation of interstitial fluid (ISF). For example, **ascites** is abnormal accumulation of fluid in peritoneal cavity of abdomen. Similarly, there can be accumulation of fluid in lungs. This is known as **pulmonary edema**. Edema most commonly occurs in the feet and legs, which is referred to as **peripheral edema**. The swelling is the result of the accumulation of excess fluid under the skin in the spaces within the tissues.

Excessive accumulation of interstitial fluid is generally viewed as detrimental to tissue function because edema formation increases the diffusion distance for oxygen and other nutrients, which may compromise cellular metabolism in the swollen tissue. For the same reason, edema formation also limits the diffusional removal of potentially toxic byproducts of cellular metabolism. These are especially important problems in the lungs, where pulmonary edema can significantly impair gas exchange. Edema can also occur when plasma protein levels are low either due to decreased synthesis of plasma albumin or due to increased loss. In either case, the hypoproteinemia results in decreased oncotic pressure and thereby cause retention of fluid.

Increases in capillary permeability, e.g., due to allergic reaction or inflammation can also cause edema. **Edema** refers to a clinical condition with an abnormal accumulation of tissue fluid or interstitial fluid or body cavities in the body.

Electrolyte Balance

Electrolyte balance refers to the balance between gains and losses of all electrolytes (ions) respiratory. Electrolyte balance exists when the intake of electrolytes from various sources equals the output of all electrolytes. It primarily involves balancing the rates of absorption across the digestive tract with rates of loss through kidneys, sweat glands, and defecation. The body's electrolyte content will rise, if dietary intake is higher than loss from kidney through urine and from skin through sweat, and will fall, if losses exceed gains. It must be remembered that water is gained or lost by osmosis; hence, there is a very close relationship between electrolyte and fluid balance. However, the mechanisms of regulation of the two are different and the effects of imbalance also differ.

In body fluids, the concentration of anions and cations is balanced. Hence, the entry or exit of a cation is necessarily accompanied by that of an anion, with the aim of maintaining electrical neutrality. Generally, when Na^+ ions enter a cell, in exchange K^+ ions exit the cell in order to maintain the net charge. Water itself is a neutral molecule, it has a "zero" charge. However, the hydrogen ions in water have a slight positive charge while the oxygen has a negative charge. The structure of the water molecule enables it to dissolve mineral salts. Water molecules can interact with anions as well as cations. Cations like Na^+ will be attracted toward the negative charge of oxygen, while the positively charged hydrogen atoms in the water molecule are attracted toward the negatively charged chloride ions.

Water in ICF and ECF does not remain confined to these compartments. Water and some solutes pass freely through the membranes that are semipermeable. Generally, water will move from an area or compartment that has a low concentration of solutes (dissolved substances) into one where the solute concentration is higher, until the solute concentration in both compartments is equal. The total number of cations is 155 mEq/L with a similar number of anions, so that normally, electroneutrality is maintained at all times. The body pools of the potassium and phosphate ions are related to total body proteins. Hence, changes in body protein are accompanied by changes in these ions. When protein is lost during any catabolic process, these ions are also lost. In contrast, when protein is accrued in tissues, as in anabolism, there is positive balance of both ions.

Hormonal Control of Electrolyte Balance

Since ECF plays a critical role in determining cell function and survival, its volume, composition, and osmolality are highly regulated. Hormonal control is important in maintaining

serum concentrations of sodium and potassium. Mainly two or three hormones are involved:
1. Antidiuretic hormone (ADH) or vasopressin
2. Aldosterone
3. Parathyroid hormone.

Antidiuretic hormone (ADH): It is secreted by the pituitary gland and acts on the kidney to control the amount of water in the body. When osmolarity of blood plasma is increased or there is low blood (arterial) pressure, ADH is secreted to regulate the plasma volume and maintain the blood pressure. ADH facilitates renal reabsorption of water while allowing excess sodium to be excreted in urine. It reduces the osmolarity of the blood. This is important because of the appropriate amount of water that is necessary for proper functioning of the cells, tissues, and organs.

Aldosterone: Aldosterone is a steroid hormone secreted by the adrenal cortex and functions in step with the help of other hormones. When osmolarity falls, aldosterone promotes reabsorption of sodium from renal tubule and promotes excretion of potassium in urine; hence, potassium is not conserved in the body. (Low carbohydrate may accelerate the loss of potassium from the body, profuse sweating, and also increases the loss.)

Parathyroid hormone: Parathyroid hormone is indirectly involved through its effects on calcium and phosphate.
Kidney is the main organ, which controls the volume and composition of water and electrolytes in the ECF and ICF. Kidneys play a role in keeping the ECF volume constant by changes in the amount of Na⁺ excreted. Besides the kidneys, the gastrointestinal tract plays a vital role:
- The minerals are absorbed from the foods ingested in the large intestine
- The minerals are secreted by the gastrointestinal tract into digestive juices and bile. Considerable amount of the secreted minerals are reabsorbed in the large intestine.

Under normal circumstances, the body is able to maintain fluid and electrolyte balance. However, vomiting, diarrhea, heavy sweating, burns, and wounds can lead to considerable fluid and electrolyte losses specifically sodium and chloride.

Electrolytes

Sodium

Sodium is a major cation present in extracellular fluid (ECF), the normal range being 135–145 mEq/L. It accounts for 90–95% of the solutes in ECF and contributes almost all of ECF solute concentration. Some amount is present in dissolved substances in interstitial fluid as well as in intracellular fluids (ICF). Plasma constitutes about 20% of ECF, thus sodium also determines the intravascular fluid volume. Sodium is essential for normal cellular metabolism and maintaining homeostasis. It is also found in various intestinal secretions such as bile, pancreatic juice, as well as in bones; however, the sodium in these fluids is less exchangeable.

Under normal conditions, its concentration does not vary by more than 5 mEq/L and greater variations can seriously affect some physiological functions. Sodium intake through salt and salt-containing foods varies widely among individuals on day-to-day basis. Body has the mechanisms to deal with the fluctuations in sodium intake. Sodium ions are absorbed by intestinal epithelium, with the amount of sodium absorbed being influenced by the sodium intake. The rate of sodium uptake across digestive tract is directly proportional to dietary intake. In most healthy individuals, excess is excreted in urine, feces, and sweat, and the process is regulated by sympathetic nervous system. If sodium concentration is lower than normal, it is conserved by the kidney. If losses exceed intake, ECF content of sodium declines and changes in sodium concentration are corrected by ADH. Kidneys play a critical role in sodium balance. Renal sodium excretion is regulated by the active transport system across the cell membrane.

Sodium is responsible for creating ionic difference across the cell membrane. It can pass through the pores in the cell membrane. Sodium is transported by active transport using the sodium pump (Na/K ATPase pump). Sodium ion affects the permeability of the muscle and nerve cell membranes and aids in nerve impulse conduction as well as muscle contraction. It also plays a significant role in acid–base balance.

When energy intake is high, plasma insulin level is also high, which further increases the Na⁺ resorption and consequently increases the blood pressure. Kidney regulates the blood pressure through the renin angiotensin system, which is responsible for Na⁺ retention and vasoconstriction of blood vessels. When sympathetic nervous system is hyperactive, it increases the arterial pressure.

The relationship between sodium intake and blood pressure was recognized a century ago and is now well established in ecological, epidemiological, and experimental human studies.

Estrogen also causes retention of water and sodium, leading to weight gain and bloating. Thus during menstruation and conditions when estrogen level is high, such symptoms are observed.

Sodium Imbalance

Imbalance may occur not only due to low-salt intake but also due to loss of sodium from the body along with water (during excessive perspiration, diarrhea, vomiting, etc.). Major losses occur via the alimentary canal rather than through skin. Changes in ECF Na⁺ content do not produce lasting changes in concentration because in a normal healthy person, there will be corresponding water gain or loss. "Water goes where the salt is". Thus, there will be changes in the volume and composition, i.e., total amount of ECF, but osmotic concentrations may not alter, since the body has homeostatic mechanisms to regulate electrolyte concentrations and balance. The Na⁺ regulatory mechanism allows changes in ECF volume but keeps sodium concentration stable. Changes in sodium concentration or small changes in water balance are corrected by ADH.

Changes in plasma sodium affect plasma volume and blood pressure. Loss of sodium is always accompanied by the loss of water and retention of salt, along with retention of water. When Na⁺ losses exceed intake, the ECF volume will decrease due to increased water loss either because fluid is shifted to the ICF in or through excretion, thus maintaining osmotic concentration. Generally, if there are large changes in ECF volume, they are caused by sodium imbalance. Retention of large amount of sodium leads to fluid retention and reduction in salt in the diet can have impact in reducing the edema. Excess salt in the body also increases sensation of thirst, which helps to normalize the Na^+ level because of dilution effect. On the contrary when plasma Na^+ level reduces, it has adverse effects. Low-sodium level in plasma and ECF is called **hyponatremia.** High-sodium level in blood plasma is called **hypernatremia.** It usually occurs when renal functions for sodium excretion are disturbed. Hypernatremia can occur in elderly for various reasons such as impaired thirst mechanism, some medication like discriminate use of anti-diuretic medicines. The causes, symptoms of sodium imbalance, and the treatment are shown in Table 8.5.

Potassium

Potassium is a major cation in intracellular fluid (ICF), 98% of potassium in the human body is in ICF. Very little is present in ECF. Normal serum potassium concentration is 3.5–5.0 mEq/L, whereas the intracellular concentration is 120–125 mmol/L. K^+ works opposite Na^+, and when Na^+ enters the cell, K^+ shifts out to maintain a balance of cations across the membrane, thus maintaining the electrolyte balance on both sides of the cell membrane.

Besides its role in maintaining osmotic equilibrium, potassium also aids in maintaining acid–base balance and is essential for transmission and conduction of nerve impulses, normal cardiac rhythm, and for contraction of skeletal and smooth muscles. It is absorbed from the small intestine and is excreted in urine and feces. Kidney regulates its level in body fluids under the influence of aldosterone hormone.

Potassium ion concentrations are not as closely regulated as sodium. When there is a shift of ECF to ICF or there are abnormal losses of potassium in urine, serum potassium level falls and the condition is known as *hypokalemia* (<3.5 mEq/L). During diarrhea, potassium is lost along with sodium and there is need for adding potassium in therapeutic treatment. Since kidney regulates cation excretion, therefore with the use of diuretics, potassium is excreted along with sodium.

Changes in pH affect K^+ balance. When there is acidosis, hydrogen ions accumulate in the ICF. In order to maintain the balance of cations across the membrane, K^+ shifts out into ECF and serum potassium concentration is increased. Thus, potassium retention occurs when pH falls. However, under certain circumstances, potassium levels can be elevated above the normal level. This condition is called **hyperkalemia** [>5 mM (mmol/L) of plasma], which is not only caused by acidosis but also by kidney disease, excessive consumption of potassium-rich foods, aldosterone deficiency, and sodium depletion. Aldosterone, insulin, and catecholamines influence serum potassium levels. Potassium ion excretion increases when its concentrations in ECF rise, when aldosterone is secreted or when pH rises. The causes, symptoms, and the treatment have been shown in Table 8.6.

Chloride

Chloride is a principal anion in ECF accompanying sodium, and is present in gastric juice, pancreatic juice, bile, and cerebrospinal fluid. It is a component of hydrochloric acid present in stomach. Chloride ion has a role in water balance, regulation of osmotic pressure, and acid–base balance. It is completely absorbed in the intestine and excreted (lost) in urine, sweat, and stomach secretions. Cl^- loss is similar to Na^+ loss. Salt is a major source of chloride and Cl^- level is controlled indirectly by ADH and by processes that increase or decrease renal absorption of Na^+.

Chloride is absorbed in the GI tract in order to balance its losses in urine and sweat. Under normal pH conditions, 99% of chloride is reabsorbed. If there is acidosis, fewer chloride ions are reabsorbed. The normal concentration of chloride in serum is 98–108 mmol/L. Increases or decreases in chloride can significantly influence health and can be fatal. **Hypochloremia,** i.e., decreased chloride, may occur during metabolic alkalosis or when there is prolonged or heavy sweating; persistent vomiting, low salt intake, use of diuretics as well as due to kidney disease or disease of adrenal glands. **Hyperchloremia** occurs during diarrhea, in certain kidney disease or if the parathyroid glands are overactive. Hypochloremia results in muscle spasms and coma and

Table 8.5: Causes and manifestation of sodium (Na^+) imbalances.

Hyponatremia: Low plasma sodium level <130 mmol/L	Hypernatremia: High plasma sodium level >150 mmol/L
Causes Excessive intake of water, e.g., in athletes who drink plain water, and electrolyte losses are not replaced Excessive exercise and sweating Severe vomiting/diarrhea High fever Chronic renal failure Addison's disease ECF depletion Major burns Congestive heart failure	**Causes** Excess intake of salt or processed foods with high salt and additives containing sodium Inadequate water intake Diarrhea and/or vomiting wherein fluid and sodium intake is inadequate vis-à-vis requirements Excessive sweating Burns Renal disease Use of diuretics Adrenal tumors
Symptoms Headache, nausea, vomiting, diarrhea, abdominal cramps, muscle tremors, twitching, weakness Severe hyponatremia can cause confusion, seizures, and coma. Even mild hyponatremia can cause confusion in the elderly. There could be respiratory distress from fluid overload	**Symptoms** Thirst (a major symptom) High blood pressure Confusion, agitation Dry, sticky mucous membrane Excess weight gain Increased muscle reflex activity, increased body temperature, mental impairment, irritability, and coma
Treatment Increase in salt intake or isotonic saline given intravenously	**Treatment** Drinking plain fluids can reduce the solutes in plasma and excess water can excrete out. Reduction in salt in the diet and use of diuretics can help but in certain cases, medical help is required

Table 8.6: Causes and manifestation of potassium (K+) imbalance.

Hypokalemia (Low serum K+ level in ECF) (<3.5 mEq/L)	Hyperkalemia (High serum K+ level) (>5.5 mEq/L)
Causes Low intake of food rich in K+ Increased loss of potassium due to diarrhea, vomiting High aldosterone levels	**Causes** K+ shifts out of cells Cell trauma in Fever, burns, injury Excessive intake of K+ Acute or chronic renal failure (decreased renal excretion) Diuretic therapy Insulin deficiency
Symptoms Decreased neuromuscular excitability, leg cramps, irritability, smooth muscle atony, drowsiness, confusion, distension and abnormal heartbeat (cardiac dysrhythmia) Muscle weakness Decreased reflexes Respiratory arrest Coma	**Symptoms** Tingling of fingers and lips, intestinal cramps, nausea, diarrhea Muscular weakness Loss of muscle tone Apathy, confusion Cardiac arrest
Treatment Replacement with potassium through food or drugs, if required, can help the situation	**Treatment** Low intake of food rich in potassium Medical support Dietary supplements like calcium gluconate, sodium bicarbonate

generally occurs with hyponatremia often due to persistent vomiting.

Calcium

Calcium is the most abundant ion in the body. It is a positively charged ion present in both ICF and ECF. However, calcium ions (Ca^+) are primarily extracellular cations. Serum calcium level represents free calcium, in ionic form, and is not bound to proteins. Calcium ions are maintained within a narrow range, the normal plasma concentration being 2.3–2.6 mmol/L. Ca^+ is helpful in muscle contraction, blood clotting, hormone secretion, digestion, glycogen metabolism, and bone mineralization. Ca^{2+} level is regulated by parathyroid and calcitriol. Parathyroid hormone (PTH) raises the blood Ca^{2+}. PTH is secreted by the parathyroid gland, which senses a decrease in serum Ca^{2+} levels. Under normal conditions, parathyroid hormone brings back the serum calcium level to normal by: Increasing resorption of calcium from bones into blood, increasing excretion of phosphorus in urine, and increasing formation of vitamin D in the kidney. Vitamin D stimulates absorption of calcium from the gastrointestinal tract. In contrast, calcitonin (CT) decreases blood Ca^{2+} by acting in a manner that is opposite to the action of PTH.

Homeostatic imbalances result in either hypocalcemia or hypercalcemia. **Hypocalcemia** is when the serum-free calcium ions falls below 4.4 mg/dL, or the total serum calcium is less than 8.8 mg/dL. Hypocalcemia can result from hypoparathyroidism (low parathyroid hormone), if production of the biologically active form of vitamin 1,25-dihydroxyvitamin D is low, low levels of plasma magnesium, and from elevated phosphate levels. This excess forms a complex with the free serum calcium. Hypocalcemia can cause depression, muscle spasms/cramps, and convulsions. It can occur during infection in the blood and other tissues (sepsis), diarrhea, use of diuretics, abnormal bone formation, malignancies, and interference with availability of parathyroid hormone, vitamin D and hypothyroidism. Dietary calcium, calcium supplements, essential fatty acids, vitamin D, and lysine improve the calcium absorption and reduce its loss in urine.

Hypercalcemia occurs when the free calcium ion concentration is above 5.2 mg/dL or total serum calcium above 10.4 mg/dL. This happens when bone is broken down (resorbed) at an abnormally fast rate, which results in increased serum calcium and serum phosphate. This results in fatigue, confusion, nausea, vomiting, cardiovascular symptoms, and coma; and if it is prolonged, abnormal calcium deposition can occur, e.g., deposition of calcium phosphate in kidneys leading to renal stones. Other symptoms are cardiac dysrhythmia and perhaps cardiac arrest, if the calcium level becomes too high. Hypercalcemia is not common but can occur in cancer patients, bone disorders, where bone calcium is released into the blood, and if there is excessive production of parathyroid hormone.

Phosphorus

Phosphorus is the major anion in cells/ICF and exists as phosphate (PO_4). Plasma phosphate level is 1.7–2.6 mmol/L. In soft tissues, PO_4 is mainly found in the intracellular compartment as an integral component of several organic compounds like ATP, nucleic acids, and phospholipids. Phosphate (PO_4) has an important role as a buffer in body fluids. Its level is regulated by PTH and calcitriol. Phosphate concentrations shift in the opposite direction from calcium concentrations and symptoms are usually due to the related calcium excess or deficit. Blood phosphate levels are regulated by the amount excreted by kidneys. When blood phosphate ion levels decrease, the kidneys reabsorb phosphate more efficiently and loss of phosphate reduces, thus raising phosphate ion levels. Conversely when phosphate level is raised, more of it is filtered out by the kidney and excreted in urine. Any imbalance in serum level can result in *hypophosphatemia* or *hyperphosphatemia.*

Hypophosphatemia occurs in clinical settings when serum phosphate concentration is low [<2.5 mg/dL (0.81 mmol/L)]. It is caused by alcoholism, burns, chronic starvation, diuretic use, Cushing's syndrome, hypomagnesmia, and hyperparathyroidism. Clinical features include muscle weakness, bone pain, osteomalacia, bleeding disorders, anemia, metabolic acidosis, respiratory failure or heart failure. Seizures and coma can also occur. Hyperphosphatemia occurs in serious metabolic disorders like chronic renal failure, hypoparathyroidism, and metabolic or respiratory acidosis, hypocalcemia, and when serum phosphate (PO_4) concentration >4.5 mg/dL. Symptoms of hyperphosphatemia are increased neuroexcitability and muscle cramps.

Magnesium

Magnesium ion (Mg⁺) is the second most abundant intracellular electrolyte (mainly found in ICF) and is a cofactor for enzymes. It is an essential element in nucleic acid and DNA chemistry. Normal plasma concentration is 0.8–1.3 mMol/L. Under normal conditions, it is well regulated but the capacity of the kidney to reabsorb Mg is limited. Any excess is generally removed through urine. When serum/plasma Mg level is low, the reabsorption of Mg increases. When serum magnesium level rises, the condition is known as hypermagnesemia [serum magnesium levels is >25 mM (60 mg/dL)]. Although rare, it is seen among clinically ill patients particularly in patients with renal failure. It is often caused by excessive intake of antacids and laxatives containing Mg. Symptoms are nausea, vomiting, muscle weakness, hypotension, and reduced respiration. Diuretics are often prescribed to get rid of excess magnesium.

Hypomagnesemia occurs when serum magnesium levels fall below 0.8 mM. **Hypomagnesemia** is rare but can occur due to malnutrition, alcoholism, use of some diuretics, which increase urinary Mg loss, kidney dysfunction and if the intestines are not functioning well and Mg absorption is compromised. Chronic alcoholism is the most common cause of hypomagnesemia, partly due to poor diet. Magnesium levels below 0.5 mM (1.2 mg/dL) cause serum calcium levels to decline. Some of the symptoms of hypomagnesemia, including twitching and convulsions, actually result from the concurrent hypocalcemia. Hypomagnesemia can also result in hypokalemia and thereby cause cardiac arrhythmias. Symptoms include irritability, muscle weakness, tetany, and convulsions.

ACID–BASE BALANCE

Acid–base balance refers to maintaining the pH of blood and body fluids. There are many naturally occurring acids, which are essential for several biological processes. For example, hydrochloric acid present in the stomach helps in digestion of food; uric acid is one of the end products of metabolism, whereas blood, bile, and many body fluids are alkaline (basic) in nature. Regulation of acid–base balance is critical in all metabolic processes of the human body. Lung and kidney are major regulators of acid–base balance. The overall acid–base balance is maintained by controlling the H⁺ concentration of body fluids, especially of ECF.

Many dietary components like protein, chloride, phosphorus, sodium, potassium, calcium, and magnesium affect the pH/acid–base balance. The human body has inherent buffering systems to deal with changes occurring in the pH of body fluids.

> **Acids:** Those, which release H⁺ into solution.
> **Bases:** Those, which remove H⁺ from solution.
> **Buffers:** These resist changes in pH by removing H⁺, if it is added and if H⁺ is removed, buffer replaces the H⁺. Buffer systems are either weak acids or bases or their salts that prevent drastic alterations in the pH of body fluids.
>
> *Contd...*

Contd...

> "An acid–base buffer is a solution containing two or more chemical compounds that prevents changes in hydrogen ion concentration when either acid or base is added to the solution." —Guyton
>
> Acid–base balance can be defined as homeostasis of the body fluids at a normal arterial blood pH ranging between 7.35 and 7.45.
>
> Despite variations in metabolism, diet, and environmental factors, the body's acid–base balance, fluid volume, and electrolyte concentration are maintained within a narrow range.

Acid–base balance is the state of homeostasis of the body fluids at a normal blood pH. The pH of systemic arterial blood is 7.35–7.45. The pH of venous blood and interstitial fluid is 7.35, whereas pH of intracellular fluid is 7.0. Any deviation of even up to 0.05 in pH can have drastic and sometimes devastating effects on the body. When pH decreases, it is called **acidosis (pH below 7.35)** and when the pH increases, it is termed **alkalosis (pH rises above 7.45)**. Regulation of acid–base balance is critical because enzymes are sensitive to pH and cellular metabolism depends on enzymes. Also, structure and function of proteins, permeability of cell membranes, distribution of electrolytes, and the structure of connective tissue are largely governed by pH of the surrounding body fluids. Hence, alterations in pH affect the entire body's systems and can lead to serious problems such as coma, cardiac failure, and circulatory collapse.

> **Research Glimpse:** Several studies have indicated that even a mild decrease in extracellular pH increase proteolysis. Hence, protein breakdown is reduced by correcting acidosis particularly in patients with end-stage renal disease (ESRD) and advanced predialysis chronic kidney disease (CKD). Muscle protein degradation is observed in healthy individuals without kidney disease on administration of ammonium chloride to lower the pH from 7.42 to 7.35. Short-term effects of acid–base balance on protein metabolism have long-term effects on skeletal muscle mass. Some studies revealed that the treatment with oral sodium bicarbonate for 2 years also improved mid-arm circumference and increased serum albumin in patients with stage 4 CKD. Individuals with serum bicarbonate <23 mEq/L suffer more physical disability or lack of endurance as compared with those who had serum bicarbonate ≥23 mEq/L.
>
> Abramowitz MK. Acid-Base Balance and Physical Function. CJASN. 2014;9(12):2030-2.

Normal pH of arterial blood and most body fluids is slightly alkaline, with the exception of gastric juice and urine. The pH of gastric juice is 0.9–1.2 due to the presence of HCl and the pH of urine is about 6.0 because it tends to excrete acid. The hydrogen ion concentration or pH of the blood and body fluids is critically essential for the following reasons:
- Sustains life
- Maintains homeostasis
- Optimizes the enzymatic reactions
- Maintains metabolism in the body
- For denaturation and digestion of proteins
- For structure and function of proteins
- For permeability of cell membranes
- For maintaining electrolyte balance
- For normal renal functions
- Ion-binding properties and structure of connective tissue
- Bone mineral mass

- Preserves skeletal muscle mass
- Physical gait and physical functions
- Tissue interstitial acidity.

Main Sources of Hydrogen Ions

Hydrogen ions are byproducts of tissue metabolism such as CO_2, H_2O, organic acids, carbonates, and lactate. These can be obtained exogenous and endogenous sources:

Exogenous sources: Foods containing organic acids and medicines/drugs can be a source of acid generation. A variety of organic acids are consumed through diets such as citric acid, malic acid, tartaric acid, acetic acid, and lactic acid, which are easily metabolized in the system and do not have any significant effect on pH. However, some acids like benzoic acid and quinic acid, which are found in foods like plum and cranberry, are not metabolized in our body to produce CO_2 and water. These acids bring changes in hydrogen ions in the blood and are excreted in urine (increase acidity of the urine). Orange juice in spite of having acid pH (3.7) has alkalizing effect because it contains citrate, which is converted into carbonic acid and then to CO_2 and H_2O. CO_2 goes out of the body via lungs and H_2O via kidney. Generally with a normal diet, about 50–100 mEq of H+ per day is generated mostly from metabolism of some amino acids. Sulfur-containing amino acids like cysteine and methionine yield sulfuric acid and metabolism of lysine, arginine, and histidine produces hydrochloric acid.

Endogenous sources: Acids are produced inside the body only during biochemical reactions or metabolic processes. Some of the metabolic processes are glucose metabolism, incomplete fatty acid oxidation, oxidation of amino acids containing sulfur hydrolysis of phosphoproteins, and nucleic acids. Commonly produced acids are carbonic acid, lactic acid, uric acid, ketoacids, phosphoric acid, and sulfuric acid. Anaerobic metabolism of glucose gives lactic acid, phosphorus-containing proteins on breakdown give phosphoric acid, and incomplete fatty acid oxidation yields organic acids and ketone bodies and transportation of carbon dioxide as bicarbonate releases hydrogen ions. Alkali-containing foods like citrate and metabolism of amino acids, e.g., aspartate and glutamate lead to alkali production and offset the daily acid load but the net effect is daily acid addition.

Phosphoric and sulfuric acids are produced during oxidation of proteins. These are instantly combined with bicarbonate buffer to minimize the pH change in the blood and eventually are excreted in urine. Excess intake of protein often increases the bicarbonate requirement and lowers the pH of urine. Protein from milk does not have marked effect on pH of urine due to the presence of calcium.

Carbonic acid: Carbon dioxide (CO_2) is a metabolic end product, which is eventually breathed out via lungs. Metabolism of fats and carbohydrates produces about 15–20 mL of carbon dioxide daily. Before CO_2 can be eliminated by lungs, the CO2 is taken up by the red blood cells. Here, it reacts with water and carbonic acid (a weak acid) is formed. The enzyme required for this reaction is carbonic anhydrase.

$$CO_2 + H_2O \longrightarrow H_2CO_3$$

Within cells, carbonic acid again dissociates into hydrogen and bicarbonate ions that are pumped out of the cells into plasma. In the alveoli of lungs, bicarbonate re-enters the RBCs and the bicarbonate is converted into carbon dioxide, which the lungs get rid of, when a person breathes out/exhales.

Besides carbonic acid, there are other acids that influence the pH. These are derived from protein metabolism, sulfate-containing foods from diet (which give rise to H_2SO_4) and phosphates-yielding phosphoric acid ($H_2PO_4^-$). These are mainly responsible for the daily acid load that needs to be get rid of by the kidneys.

Lactic acid: Lactic acid is produced by anaerobic metabolism (when the body is not getting enough oxygen) of glucose. Normally, lactic acid is transported from cells to the liver, where it is converted into glucose. This process is extremely useful when a person is doing intensive physical activity including endurance sports. However, if production of lactate (lactic acid) overwhelms the body's buffering systems, it accumulates in muscles and results in stiffness of the muscles as well as lactic acidosis.

Ketoacids: Ketones or ketoacids are produced by incomplete oxidation of fatty acids in the liver. These ketones are soon converted into CO_2 and water under normal conditions. During starvation or low carbohydrate intake, excessive ketones are produced leading to more hydrogen ions in the blood, reducing the blood pH, i.e., acidosis. Kidney helps to throw them out but in diabetes or renal disease, build-up of ketones is of concern.

Phosphoric acid: Phosphoric acid is produced when phosphorus-containing substances and nucleic acids are metabolized.

Sulfuric acid: Sulfuric acid is produced from sulfur-containing amino acids.

Hydrochloric acid: Hydrochloric acid is produced from amino acids, i.e., arginine, lysine, and histidine.

Increased intake of protein may not always increase endogenous acid excretion capacity because additional alkali loads may compensate for the protein-related increase in acid production. Protein itself helps to improve the renal capacity to excrete net acid by increasing the endogenous supply of ammonia, which is the major urinary hydrogen ion acceptor.

> Phosphoric and sulfuric acid are produced during oxidation of proteins. These are instantly combined with bicarbonate buffer to minimize the pH change in the blood and eventually excreted in urine. Excess intake of protein often increases the bicarbonate requirement and lowers the pH of the urine. Protein from milk does not have marked effect on pH of the urine due to the presence of calcium. Acid is also produced by chlorine ion but it is often present in association with basic sodium ion, so it does not cause much problem.

Mechanisms to Maintain Acid–Base Balance

Body fluids contain many elements in ionic form, which determine the pH of the body fluids. Different body fluids like blood, saliva, urine, etc. have different pH. Blood pH is 7.35–

7.45 (slightly alkaline) and urine pH is around 6.4 (slightly acidic) under normal circumstances.

The human body has its own regulatory mechanisms to maintain the pH, which normally occurs via kidney and lungs. Slight variations in pH of the body fluids and blood can have marked effects on the body and cause acidosis or alkalosis. Acidosis is an increase in the hydrogen ions (H^+) in body fluids (pH 6.8–7.35) and alkalosis means loss of H^+ from the body (pH 7.45–7.9). Alteration beyond the normal range of pH in either direction affects all body systems. If these alterations are not tackled in time, many serious consequences may occur such as coma, cardiac failure, and circulatory collapse. If the pH of blood goes below 6.0 or is greater than 8.0, there is high risk of death.

Hydrogen ions are present in ECF and ICF. Under normal conditions, total ions in both ICF and ECF remain constant due to buffering produced by kidney or blood during metabolism. Regulation of hydrogen ions is essential for electrolyte balance, enzymatic activity, and thereby normal body functions. Deviations in pH can damage proteins and therefore disrupt metabolism. The ability of hemoglobin to carry oxygen would also be adversely affected. The body has various ways of handling disturbance(s) in pH and there are many compounds and buffer systems, which are involved in regulating fluctuations in acid-base balance/body pH. The lungs and kidneys play very important roles in regulating acid-base balance. The lungs are able to eliminate carbon dioxide but only kidneys can get rid of metabolic acids such as phosphoric, uric, and lactic acids, and ketones and prevent metabolic acidosis. Thus, the ultimate regulator of acid-base balance is the kidney.

There are chemoreceptors in the body (peripheral and in the central nervous system), which control changes in blood pH. Hydrogen ion concentration is regulated sequentially by the body:
  i. Chemical buffer systems, which act within seconds of any disturbance in pH.
  ii. Respiratory center (located in the brainstem), which acts within 1–3 minutes and
  iii. The kidneys/renal system, which takes longer, i.e., hours to days for pH changes to occur.

The buffer systems in ICF and ECF are shown in Figure 8.7.

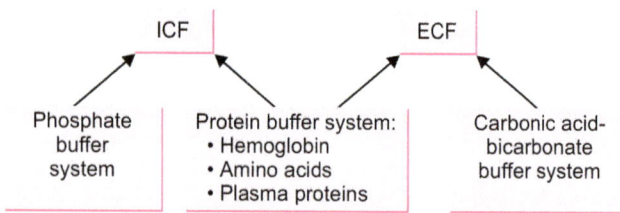

Fig. 8.7: Buffer systems in ICF and ECF.

Chemical buffer systems can neutralize either acids or bases but they are by themselves unable to get rid of the excess acids or bases. This is done by either the lungs (only carbon dioxide) or the kidneys, which play a major role.

Buffer Systems

Different types of buffer system:
- Bicarbonate buffer
- Phosphate buffer
- Ammonia buffer
- Electrolyte buffer
- Fat buffer
- Hormone buffer
- Water buffer

Extracellular buffers: In the blood, there are pairs of Buffer systems like bicarbonate and carbonic acid, phosphates, hemoglobin—oxyhemoglobin and plasma proteins. Among these, the role of bicarbonate in ECF is significant because it is the first line of defense. However, its action is temporary.

Bicarbonate buffer: The bicarbonate ions act as a buffer to maintain normal pH levels of blood/ECF. Bicarbonate buffer is a mixture of carbonic acid (H_2CO_3) and sodium bicarbonate ($NaHCO_3$) in the same solution. Carbonic acid is a very weak acid for 2 reasons:
1. It instantly dissociates into CO_2 and water resulting in high concentration of dissolved CO_2
2. Having weak concentration of acid. It is the principal buffer because carbonic acid is readily available and lungs and kidney can easily adjust with the ratio between carbonic acid and the base, like bicarbonate.

This buffer system is considered to be very effective because of the large amounts of bicarbonate in the body and its ability to excrete the CO_2 formed via respiration.

Carbon dioxide, which is an end product of metabolism, combines with water and is converted into carbonic acid (H_2CO_3) and bicarbonate. Hydrogen from carbonic acid is used to maintain pH and the remaining carbonate is reabsorbed in the kidney. This bicarbonate enters the ECF and combines with sodium and forms sodium bicarbonate ($NaHCO_3$). Thus, pH of ECF is maintained in the ratio of $NaHCO_3:H_2CO_3$ as 20:1. pH of ECF is 7.4 (range is 7.35–7.45).

$$CO_2 + H_2O \leftrightarrow H_2CO_3 \leftrightarrow H + HCO_3$$

Carbon dioxide + Water ↔ Carbonic acid ↔ Hydrogen + Bicarbonate ion

This bicarbonate ion combines with Na to give sodium bicarbonate.

$$HCO_3 + Na^+ \leftrightarrow NaHCO_3$$

Bicarbonate + Sodium ↔ Sodium bicarbonate

As carbon dioxide levels increase, pH decreases and when the carbon dioxide levels decrease, pH increases. When the pH is normal, ECF contains 1 part carbonic acid to 20 parts bicarbonate. When there is more base, carbonic acid combines with the base, resulting in production of bicarbonate and water. The normal range for serum bicarbonate is 22–30 mmol/L. This system can function only when the respiratory system and control centers are working normally.

Disruptions in the normal bicarbonate level may be due to diseases that interfere with respiratory function, kidney diseases, metabolic conditions, or other causes. This system is limited by the availability of bicarbonate ions/bicarbonate reserve. Metabolism of the amino acid methionine produces the acid H_2SO_4 that needs to be neutralized. This is done by sodium bicarbonate as shown in the equation below.

$$H_2SO_4 + 2NaHCO_3 \rightarrow Na_2SO_4 + 2H_2CO_3 \rightarrow 2CO_2 + 2H_2O + Na_2SO_4$$

Sodium bicarbonate reacts with H_2SO_4, a strong acid to form H_2CO_3, a weaker acid. Carbonic acid then dissociates into CO_2 and H_2O. The CO_2 produced is then excreted by the lungs and the Na_2SO_4 is excreted by the kidneys.

Phosphate buffer: It helps to maintain pH of the blood, which is maintained by the kidneys. Its effect is similar to that of the bicarbonate system. It works in ICF and urine and involves sodium dihydrogen phosphate (NaH_2PO_4), a weak acid and sodium monohydrogen phosphate (Na_2HPO_4), a weak base.

$$NaOH + NaH_2PO_4 \longleftrightarrow Na_2HPO_4 + H_2O$$
$$Na_2HPO_4 + HCl \longleftrightarrow NaCl + NaH_2PO_4$$

Hydrogen ion of the blood passes through kidney, disodium hydrogen phosphate (Na_2HPO_4) is converted into sodium dihydrogen phosphate (NaH_2PO_4) and excreted. Sodium is exchanged for H^+, thus kidney reduces the acidity in body fluids.

Proteins as buffers: Plasma proteins as well as intracellular proteins are the most abundant and powerful buffers. Some amino acids have free organic acid groups, i.e., carboxyl groups that function as weak acids. The amino group in amino acids allows the amino acid to function like a weak base. Protein molecules are amphoteric, i.e., they function as both acids and bases. The basic and acidic groups act as either H^+ acceptors or donors, respectively, if H^+ is added or removed. Intracellular proteins are important because they limit pH changes within cells.

Hemoglobin plays an important role in buffering H^+ ions. In fact, role of hemoglobin is important because it binds both CO_2 and H^+. Deoxygenated hemoglobin has the strongest affinity for both CO_2 and H^+; therefore, its buffering effect is strongest in the tissues. Not much CO_2 is produced in red cells. Hence, the CO_2 produced by the tissues passes easily into the RBC cell via a concentration gradient. In the red cells, carbon dioxide either combines directly with hemoglobin or combines with water to form carbonic acid. The CO_2, which binds directly with hemoglobin, combines reversibly with terminal amine groups on the hemoglobin molecule to form carbaminohemoglobin. In the lungs, the CO_2 is released and passes down its concentration gradient into the alveoli.

Ammonia buffer: Ammonia is released from the catabolism of certain amino acids such as glutamine in the kidney (cells of proximal convoluted tubule). Metabolism of one molecule of glutamine gives rise to two ammonium ions and two bicarbonate ions. The bicarbonate ions are moved to blood, whereas the ammonium ions are excreted in urine.

Electrolytes as buffers: Sodium and potassium are cations. Hence, if cells take up hydrogen ions, these result in the passage of Na^+ and K^+ ions out of cells to maintain electroneutrality. However, this process can affect potassium balance.

> **Acid–base balance systems in blood:**
> - Carbonic acid-bicarbonate buffer 53%
> - Hemoglobin–oxyhemoglobin 35%
> - Plasma proteins 7%
> - Phosphate buffers 5%

ROLE OF LUNGS AND KIDNEYS IN MAINTENANCE OF ACID–BASE BALANCE

Lungs

Lungs are important because they excrete carbon dioxide and therefore control the production of carbonic acid. The respiratory system of acid–base balance is a physiological buffering system. A large volume of carbon dioxide has to be excreted, at least 12,000-13,000 mmol per day. Deep breathing reduces the amount of CO_2 in the body and thus the level of carbonic acid in blood and tissues. When blood levels of sodium bicarbonate are reduced, excess CO_2 is expelled from lungs, thereby restoring the ratio of acid and base. When H^+ concentration is high, increased respiration (hyperventilation) can help to bring the pH up from 7.0 to 7.2-7.3 in approximately 1 minute.

> - Increased H^+ causes immediate hyperventilation. Hyperventilation (deep or more rapid breathing) expels carbon dioxide and decreases CO_2 levels in blood.
> - Also increased H^+ later increases renal secretion of $[H^+]$ and $[NH_4]$
> - Hypoventilation (shallow breathing) increases CO_2 levels
> - Decreased H^+ later decreases renal secretion of $[H^+]$ and $[NH4^+]$

When the CO_2 levels increase or pH decreases, the respiratory center in the brain senses this change and stimulates lungs to increase the respiration rate and depth. As a result, more carbon dioxide is exhaled from the lungs. Exhalation of carbon dioxide occurs within minutes of an imbalance in pH, but this cannot completely correct serious imbalances.

Kidney

In order to maintain acid–base balance, the kidney is required to perform some important tasks:

1. Reabsorption and conservation of filtered bicarbonate
2. Excretes the daily acid load. The kidney does this very effectively by hydrogen secretion, bicarbonate reabsorption, and excretion of hydrogen ions with urinary buffers (titratable acids and ammonium).
3. Helps regulate blood pH by excreting H^+ and resorbing HCO_3^-
4. When urine is acidic, HCO_3^- combines with H^+ to form $H_2CO_3^-$.

Reabsorption and conservation of filtered bicarbonate: Reabsorption and conservation of bicarbonate are done in order to ensure that its amount in the blood is not reduced. In a day, approximately 4,000–5,000 millimoles of bicarbonate are filtered through the kidneys. From this, about 85–90% bicarbonate is reabsorbed and returned to the bloodstream where sodium combines with bicarbonate to form sodium bicarbonate.

Carbonic acid is formed in the filtrate in the kidney. This carbonic acid dissociates to release carbon dioxide and water. The carbon dioxide then diffuses into the kidney tubule cells, where it triggers secretion of hydrogen ions. For each hydrogen ion secreted, a sodium ion and a bicarbonate ion are reabsorbed by cells of the proximal convoluted tubule. As a consequence of all of these actions, bicarbonate disappears from the filtrate at the same rate that it enters the peritubular capillary blood. The rate of H^+ secretion increases as body fluid pH decreases or as aldosterone levels increase. An increase in PTH reduces bicarbonate reabsorption.

Kidneys also generate new bicarbonate ions: This is done by two mechanisms involving renal excretion of acid via secretion and excretion of hydrogen ions or ammonium (NH_4^+) ions. In the event of acidosis, kidney generates new bicarbonate ions to neutralize the excess hydrogen ions. The new bicarbonate ions go into blood and an equal amount of hydrogen ions are excreted in urine. It must be remembered that there is a limit for the urine to become acid. The minimum attainable pH of urine is 4.0–4.5.

Besides lungs and kidneys, bone plays an important role in buffering acids. When excess H^+ ions are taken up by bone, the Na^+ and K^+ ions on the surface are exchanged in order to maintain the pH. Further, there is some amount of dissolution of bone mineral in order to release buffering compounds such as $NaHCO_3$, $CaHCO_3$, and $CaHPO_4$. It is estimated that about two-fifths of an acute acid load is buffered by bone. Therefore, chronic acidosis affects bone mineral and consequently diseases such as rickets, osteomalacia, and osteopenia can develop.

Disorders in Acid–Base Balance

Under some circumstances, pH of blood/plasma or body fluids can be disturbed. When blood pH decreases below 7.35, it is called **acidosis** and when the blood pH increases above 7.45, it is termed **alkalosis**. The body's response to this kind of imbalance is called compensation. In acidosis, there is a rise in acid level in body fluids. In acidosis, there is depression of central nervous system through decreased synaptic transmission leading to weakness. In severe cases, it can result in disorientation, coma, and death. Alkalosis has the opposite effect that is overexcitability of the central and peripheral nervous system, with the person showing symptoms like numbness and lightheadedness, spasm, loss of consciousness, and death.

Disorders in acid–base balance arise when there is an increased load of acidic or alkaline metabolites or deviation in blood pH, which cannot be normalized easily by buffer systems and other excretory processes in the body. There are mainly four types of acid–base imbalance and occur in different pathophysiological conditions.
1. Metabolic acidosis
2. Metabolic alkalosis
3. Respiratory acidosis
4. Respiratory alkalosis.

Metabolic acidosis: Under normal conditions, tissue metabolism produces 12,500 mEq acid per day. This acid is in the form of CO_2, which is expired from the lungs during breathing. If the body fails to completely oxidize sugar (carbohydrate/glucose) to CO_2, it results in accumulation of lactic acid that cannot be expired from the lungs but causes metabolic acidosis.

There is decreased acid excretion or increased acid production resulting in a decrease in systemic pH, i.e., 7.21 (as measured in blood or plasma), which occurs either because the H^+ ion concentration has increased or the concentration of bicarbonate has decreased. In other words, either acid production is more or alkali loss is increased or the kidneys are excreting less amount of acid. Severe metabolic acidosis can occur when the contractility of the heart is impaired. Lactic acidosis occurs when plasma lactic acid concentrations are elevated as in case of excessive exercise. Acidosis can also be due to excessive amount of ketoacids due to incomplete oxidation of fats, for example in starvation, severe diarrhea, or uncontrolled diabetes. In case of ingestion of toxins and poisoning (methanol or ethylene glycol) or drugs like aspirin, there can be excessive loss of alkali. Metabolic acidosis can also occur, if a person is consuming a high fat and low carbohydrate diet. Another cause is renal failure. Other causes are prolonged fever, less production of bicarbonate as in pancreatitis, due to excessive loss of bicarbonate in severe diarrhea, or intestinal obstruction. Maintaining the acid–base balance is one of the most strongly regulated variables in human physiology. In order to maintain homeostasis, there is a need to balance the ingestion/production of H^+ and the effective removal of these ions from the body.

> **Research Glimpse:** Increased dietary acid load tends to increase in H^+ and decrease in $HCOO_3^-$. Low-grade metabolic acidosis is a condition where there is slight increase in phosphorus and proteins) and low consumption of food-containing bases (rich in potassium, calcium, and magnesium) lead to acid–base balance changes. Prolonged, chronic, and low-grade metabolic acidosis can predispose to metabolic imbalances such as kidney stone formation, increased bone resorption, reduced bone mineral density, and the loss of muscle mass, as well as the increased risk of chronic diseases such as type 2 diabetes mellitus, hypertension, and nonalcoholic hepatic steatosis. Hence, western dietary patterns of most countries are being considered responsible for increasing incidence of noncommunicable diseases. Appropriate supply of protein and consumption of fruit and vegetable intake can bring balance, if intakes do not exceed the daily recommendations.
>
> *Carnauba RA, Baptistella AB, Paschoal V, et al. Diet-induced low-grade metabolic acidosis and clinical outcomes: A review. Nutrients. 2017;9(6):538.*

Metabolic alkalosis: This can occur if a person has prolonged vomiting due to which there is excessive loss of gastric acid, or if a person is on diuretic therapy or suffers from constipation. Metabolic acidosis can also occur, if a person consumes too much of antacids. In clinical conditions, massive blood transfusion can also lead to metabolic alkalosis.

Respiratory alkalosis and acidosis: Impairment of the respiratory system causes an imbalance, i.e., respiratory acidosis or respiratory alkalosis. The latter can be a result of hyperventilation or in asthma or fever. Respiratory acidosis occurs when a person's breathing is shallow (decreased ventilation) or a person has diseases such as chronic obstructive pulmonary disease (COPD), pulmonary fibrosis, pneumonia, emphysema, or cystic fibrosis. The level of carbonic acid in plasma increases.

Detrimental Effects of Disturbances in Acid–base Balance

Effects of metabolic acidosis can be acute or chronic. The important effects are on cardiac contractility and cardiac output. When blood pH decreases from 7.4 to 7.2, catecholamine levels increase, as a result there can be an increase in the cardiac output. However, when blood pH falls below 7.1–7.2, there is a fall in cardiac output. In acute metabolic acidosis, mental confusion and lethargy occur. Immune response can be impaired and cellular energy production can be compromised.

In chronic metabolic acidosis, the musculoskeletal system is affected. It can produce or exacerbate pre-existing bone disease. There is muscle degradation leading to muscle loss, and growth retardation in children. Glucose tolerance can be impaired because of interference with the actions of insulin. Other effects are reduced albumin synthesis and possibly accelerated progression of chronic renal failure.

In metabolic alkalosis, plasma bicarbonate levels rise. Whenever plasma bicarbonate levels rise above 24 mmol/L, the excess bicarbonate is excreted by the kidney, quite promptly. Metabolic alkalosis can occur, if there is chloride deficiency (the ability of the kidney to excrete bicarbonate is impaired) or there is potassium depletion such as due to vomiting, ingestion of bicarbonates, carbonates, acetates, citrates, and lactates found in total parenteral nutrition solutions, excessive consumption of antacids, use of diuretics, hypercalcemia, excess of aldosterone secretion. Adverse effects of alkalosis include decreased myocardial contractility, arrhythmias, decreased cerebral blood flow, confusion, and neuromuscular excitability.

Diet and Acid–base Balance

Diet can affect acid–base status and what a person eats can influence the acid–base load. The daily net acid load's magnitude (in part by influencing systemic acid–base status) has been shown to induce renal losses of calcium, magnesium, and nitrogen and adversely affects numerous endocrine functions. It is possible to estimate the acid load of individual foods or diets by calculating the Potential Renal Acid Load (PRAL). PRAL gives an estimate of the production of endogenous acid that exceeds the level of alkali produced for a given amount of food. The concept of PRAL calculation is based on physiology and it takes into account that rates of intestinal absorption of different minerals and sulfur-containing amino acids differ and that the amount of sulfate obtained from metabolism of proteins also differs. This method has been validated in healthy adults under controlled conditions. It has been shown that acid load (net acid production) and renal net acid excretion can be reliably estimated from diet composition.

There is evidence that a high-dietary acid load is a risk factor for hypertension. It may be attributed to the increase by the pituitary stimulus for ACTH synthesis followed by production of cortisol and aldosterone. Or, intracellular potassium reduction is compensated by elevated sodium levels, consequently blood pressure rises. Hence, higher intake of fruit, vegetables, and some specific nutrients (i.e., potassium and magnesium) are advocated to lower the hypertension risk.

---

pH is the measuring unit of acidity or alkalinity of an aqueous solution. To understand the same, it is of paramount importance to understand the dissociation of water. Pure water can be dissociated into H^+ and OH^-. In 1 liter of pure water, there are 0.0000001 (1×10^{-7}) grams of H^+ and the same amounts of OH^- are present (1×10^{-7}). Since pure water is neutral, value of H^+ will fix the value of OH^-. Increase in the value of one will lead to decrease the value of other. It is clear that there is possibility of 14 numerical values only, thus pH scale ranges from 1–14 only, which is a whole number. P is written in small letter, which stands for potential, and pH is potential of hydrogen ion concentration. Since it is measured in logarithm, **pH is negative log of hydrogen ion concentration.** pH scale ranges from 1 to 14. Solutions with pH 7.0 are neutral.

The H^+ concentration in the solution denotes acid and **OH^- denotes alkali.**

H^+ concentration or acid pH depiction ranges from 0 to 7 and 7 is considered neutral and 7–14 is considered base or alkali.

If H^+ concentration is more or more H^+ is added to the solution, it will be acidic. At pH 6.0, it will contain 10-fold more H^+ ions as compared to a solution with pH 7.0.

If base is added to the solution to change, the H^+ concentration will correspondingly reduce and numerical value will increase toward 7.0, at pH 8.0, there are 10-fold less H^+ ions and the solution is basic in nature.

pH of the body fluids and blood is assessed in decimal points as even a minor change in pH can lead to major change in the metabolic reactions.

Milliequivalent (mEq) is the unit of measurement used for electrolytes in a solution. It is based on the number of ions (cations and anions) in solution determined by their concentration in a given volume.

The relationship of mEq to milligram of an ionized substance in solution can be calculated as follows. When calculating equivalent of the ionized substance, the molecular weight and valence of the substance are taken into account.

One equivalent is 1 mole, i.e., the gram molecular weight of a specific substance, with the molecular weight being divided by the valence of the same.

Example: $1 \text{ Equivalent of Na} = \dfrac{23 \text{ g (atomic wt of Na)}}{1 \text{ (valence of Na)}} = 23 \text{ g}$

(1 mEq Na^+ = 23 mg)

$1 \text{ Equivalent of Ca} = \dfrac{40 \text{ g (atomic wt of Ca)}}{2 \text{ (valence of Ca)}} = 20 \text{ g}$

(1 mEq Ca^{++} = 20 mg)

Conversion of mEq to mg and mg to mEq:

$$\text{mEq} \times \dfrac{\text{atomic weight}}{\text{valence}} = \text{mg} \quad \text{OR} \quad \dfrac{\text{milligrams}}{\text{atomic weight}} \times \text{valence} = \text{mEq}$$

RAPID FIRE

Water

1. How much is the total water present in the body and how much is divided in different compartments?

2. Where will you find ECF?
3. How do ECF and ICF differ?
4. What do you mean by water balance?
5. Name the hormones, which are involved in thirst mechanism.
6. What is obligatory water loss and how much is it?
7. What do you mean by metabolic water?
8. What is dehydration?
9. What is edema?
10. What is ORS and its composition?

Electrolytes

1. What is the major difference between ICF and ECF?
2. What do you mean by osmolarity/osmolality?
3. What is the major difference between hypotonic and hypertonic?
4. What is the role of aldosterone in electrolyte balance?
5. What is the difference between facilitated diffusion and active transport?
6. What are the major sources of acid in the body?
7. What are the mechanisms to maintain acid–base balance?
8. What is the difference between respiratory and metabolic acidosis?
9. What is hyperkalemia and its symptoms?
10. What measures can be taken to reduce acidity?

EXERCISE

1. Under what physiological conditions do you feel thirst—explain with a diagram?
2. Why water balance is necessary and what are the components of water intake and output?
3. What measures you will take during dehydration and edema and why?
4. Define role of electrolytes in ECF and ICF in maintaining homeostasis.
5. Discuss the conditions, if sodium, potassium, and phosphates are in excess in ECF or ICF.
6. Explain the role of carbonic acid in maintaining acid–base balance.

SUGGESTED READING

1. Anna E Stanhewicz, W Larry Kenney. Determinants of water and sodium intake and output. Nutrition Reviews. 73 (suppl 2), 2015;73–82
2. Alpers DH, Stenson WF, Bier DM. Manual of Therapeutics, 4th edition. London: Lippincott Williams & Wilkins; 2002.
3. Austin C. Water: Guidelines for nutritional support. Nutri Supp Ser. 1996;6:27-9.
4. Buskirk ER, Puhl SM. Body Fluid Balance. Exercise and Sport. New York: CRC Press; 1996.
5. Chaffee E, Lytle IM. Basic Physiology and Anatomy, 4th edition. Philadelphia: JB Lippincott Company; 1980. pp. 500-17.
6. Chidester JC, Spangler AA. Fluid intake in the institutionalized elderly. J Am Diet Assoc. 1997;97:23-31.
7. Farell DH, Bower L. Fatal water intoxication. J Clin Pathol. 2003;56(10):803-4.
8. Food and Nutrition Board. Dietary Reference Intakes for Water, Potassium, Sodium, Chloride and Sulfate. Washington, DC: Institute of Medicine, The National Academies Press; 2005.
9. Frassetto LA, Lanham-New SA, Macdonald HM, et al. Standardizing Terminology for Estimating the Diet-Dependent Net Acid Load to the Metabolic System. J Nutr. 2007;137:1491-2.
10. Gayton AC. Textbook of Medical physiology, 5th edition. Toronto: WB Saunders Company; 1981.
11. Girvent M, Franch G, Stiges-Serra A. Water and Electrolytes. In: Gibney MJ, Ellia M, Ljungqvist O, Dowsett J (Eds). Clinical Nutrition. Oxford, United Kingdom: Blackwell Publishing; The Nutrition Society. 2005. pp. 441-56.
12. Guyton AC, Hall JE. Chapter 25. Textbook of Medical Physiology, 9th edition. Philadelphia: WB Saunders; 1996. pp. 297-308.
13. Hill LL. Body composition, normal electrolyte concentrations, and the maintenance of normal volume, tonicity, and acid–base metabolism. Pediatr Clin North Am. 1990;37(2):241-56.
14. Hume R, Elspeth Weyers E. Relationship between total body water and surface area in normal and obese subjects. J Clin Pathol. 1971;24:234-8.
15. Institute of Medicine (IOM). Dietary Reference Intakes for Water, Potassium, Sodium, Chloride, and Sulfate. Washington, DC: National Academies Press; 2004.
16. Johnson LR. Chapter 1. Essential Medical Physiology. New York: Raven Press; 1992.
17. Joshi VD, Nandedkar AN, Mendhurvar SS. Anatomy and Physiology for Nursing and Healthcare. New Delhi: BI Publications. 2006. pp. 31-47.
18. Kraut JA, Madias NE. (2010). Metabolic Acidosis: Pathophysiology, Diagnosis and Management: Adverse Effects of Metabolic Acidosis. Medscape Education. [online] Available from www.medscape.org/viewarticle/718583_6. [Last accessed July, 2019].
19 Longvah T, Ananthan R, Bhaskarachary K, et al. Indian Food Composition Tables National Institute of Nutrition, (Indian Council of Medical Research) Department of Health Research, Ministry of Health and Family Welfare, Government of India, Hyderabad (2017).
20. Lumen. Water Balance. [online] Available from https://courses.lumenlearning.com/boundless-ap/chapter/water-balance/. [Last accessed July, 2019].
21. Mahan LK, Arlin M. Krause's Food Nutrition & Diet Therapy, 11th edition. Philadelphia: WB Saunders Company; 2007.
22. Nutrient Requirements of Indians, Recommended Dietary Allowances, Estimated Average Requirements, A reports of the Expert Group, 2020, Indian Council of Medical research, National Institute of Nutrition, Department of Health Research, Ministry of Health and Family Welfare, Government of India.
23. Orten JM, Neuhans OW. Human Biochemistry, 10th edition. New Delhi: BI Publications; 1982. pp. 524-90.
24. Paradiso C. Fluids and Electrolytes, 2nd edition. Philadelphia: Lippincott, Williams and Wilkins; 1999.
25. Remer T, Dimitriou T, Manz F. Dietary potential renal acid load and renal net acid excretion in healthy, free-living children and adolescents. Am J Clin Nutr. 2003;77:1255-60.
26. Remer T, Manz F. Estimation of the renal net acid excretion by adults consuming diets containing variable amounts of protein. Am J Clin Nutr. 1994;59:1356-61.
27. Remer T, Manz F. Estimation of the renal net acid excretion by adults consuming diets containing variable amounts of protein. Am J Clin Nutr. 1994;59:1356-61.
28. Scialla JJ, Anderson CA. Dietary acid load: A novel nutritional target in chronic kidney disease? Adv Chronic Kidney Dis. 2013;20:141-9.
29. Seifter JL, Chang HY. Extracellular Acid-Base Balance and Ion Transport between Body Fluid Compartments. Physiology (Bethesda). 2017;2(5):367-79.
30. Sembulingam K, Sembulingam P. Essentials of Medical Physiology, 4th edition. New Delhi: Jaypee Brothers Medical Publishers (P) Ltd.; 2006.
31. Swaminathan M. Handbook of Food & Nutrition (Volume I). Bangalore, India: Bappco Publication; 2002.
32. Wang Z, Deurenberg P, Wei Wang W, et al. Hydration of fat-free body mass: review and critique of a classic body-composition constant. Am J Clin Nutr. 1999;69(5):833-41.
33. Watson PE, Watson ID, Batt R. Total body water volumes for adult males and females estimated from simple anthropometric measurements. Am J Clin Nutr. 1980;33(1):27-39.
34. Woodward M. Guidelines to Effective Hydration in Aged Care Facilities in Aged & Residential Care Services. Heidelberg Heights, Australia: Heidelberg Repatriation Hospital; 2013.
35. World Federation of Societies of Anaesthesiologists. Update in Anaesthesia: Acid–Base Balance Pharmacology, Issue 13, Article 12. Oxford, UK: WWW implementation by the NDA Web Team; 2001.

CHAPTER 9

Recommended Dietary Allowances and Dietary Guidelines

KEY CONCERNS
- How much I should eat to be healthy?
- Are there any recommendations, which can help me to choose and plan my diet?
- How much energy (calories) and other nutrients do I need?
- What is the meaning of RDA, DRI, %DV, etc.?
- How can I easily calculate the nutrient content present in the food I eat?
- How to assess the nutritional information on the label printed on food packages?
- Are there any examples to guide me in planning a diet, which I can enjoy and which provides adequate nutrition for my body?

KEY CONCEPTS
- RDA: Its uses and limitations
- Food guide pyramid: MyPyramid
- Food groups
- Understanding nutrient composition tables
- Meal planning: Nutritionally adequate diets
- Sample diet
- Daily value: Nutritional information on labels
- Nutrient density

Cooking is an Art, Diet is a Culture, Nutrition is a Science.
—*Dr Rama Vaidya*

INTRODUCTION

Dietary recommendations provide the keys for healthy eating patterns. These are based on strong scientific research evidence about the needs and requirements of the healthy population of a country. Recommendations for nutrients are then translated into suitable dietary guidelines that are practical and help people to select and include accessible and affordable healthy foods. Guidelines also emphasize the importance of physical activity to ensure good health and well-being and provide protection from chronic diseases.

Knowledge about nutrition needs to be used and it is important to give guidelines about the intake of various nutrients on a daily basis. Most countries have set standards and made recommendations about intakes of major nutrients that should be consumed by healthy persons in order to maintain optimal function and promote good health. These guidelines and recommendations are made by expert groups at both international and national levels. None of these recommendations are arbitrary. When making these recommendations, experts consider available scientific evidence and as more research is conducted, new evidence/information comes to light; expert groups revise their recommendations and guidelines periodically.

Optimal dietary requirements are those levels of dietary intakes of nutrients that are most likely to ensure that the individual will attain optimum potential nutritional status for:

- Normal body functions including/adequate productivity
- Freedom from infection, i.e., resistance to disease
- Prolonged and good quality of life
- Optimal development of fetus in utero and successful outcome of pregnancy
- Adequate milk production for a baby's needs
- Optimal growth and development (including achieving learning potential) throughout infancy, childhood, and adolescence
- Repair of body tissues
- Combating stress, malnutrition and pathological conditions.

Appropriate nutrition requires all nutrients, carbohydrates, lipids, proteins, minerals, vitamins, and water that are taken in adequate amounts and in the correct proportions. Many nutrients require the presence of other nutrients, if they are to fulfill their roles within the body. Each nutrient is required at a certain level. However, the amount recommended will always exceed the precise needs because the body's biological processes are not 100% efficient in utilizing and converting the nutrients in the diet. Thus, some fundamental concepts in recommended allowances are:

- **Basal requirement:** It is the minimum level of nutrient intake that should be able to maintain the desired level of nutriture in the body so that the body can optimally function without any deficiency or excess. It should be in accordance with various life stages, physiological state and gender of the individual.
- **Requirement for storage:** It is the level of nutrient intake that allows the body to maintain body tissue reserves. The

reserve provides a supply of nutrient that can be mobilized without detectable impairment of function.
- **To prevent nutritional inadequacy:** After fulfilling basal requirements and sufficient reserves of nutrients the body the given recommendation may leave only 2.5% risk of nutritional inadequacy. In this case each nutrient consumed as per RDA will maximize the health and well-being and avoid infectious and non-communicable diseases.

Evolution of RDAs

During the Second World War, it became necessary to know the amount of food rations that should be supplied to the army to protect and preserve the soldiers' health and stamina. Therefore, it was essential to know the daily requirement of the food, which would supply all the necessary nutrients for maximum health and efficiency. Before that, during the late 19th and 20th centuries, the role of nutrition in increasing productivity and economic enhancement began to be appreciated in Britain, USA, and Europe, and there was interest in feeding adequate diets at low cost to industrial workers, soldiers, working classes, and even prisoners. In the 1930s, the League of Nations Health Organization perceived the need to address nutritional status and highlighted the need for centralized nutrition policies and that the nutrition of the people needed to be supervised. In order to achieve this, it formed committees to determine the nutritional requirements of human beings, how to assess the requirements and how to measure them and how these requirements could be met. The Technical Committee of the League of Nations met in 1935 and 1936. The Committee published a report and proposed the first international tables for energy and protein requirements by age and sex. Following this, the United States set up the RDAs in the 1940s.

The first set of guidelines called Recommended Dietary Allowances (RDAs) was given in the United States, by the Food and Nutrition Board of the National Research Council in 1941.

Recommended daily requirements or allowances/amounts (RDAs) were defined and specific recommendations for energy and eight nutrients namely protein, iron, calcium, vitamins A and D, thiamine riboflavin, niacin, and ascorbic acid were listed. The aim was to "provide standards to serve as a goal for good nutrition". It also included a "margin of safety". The RDA was designed to provide better nutrition to civilians and military personnel, for food rationing during the war and guidance for the government agencies "to direct citizen's nutritional intake also taking food availability into account". In 1943, in the USA, the "basic seven" food guide was issued in order to provide a format that would be useful to the population at large. In this, it was recommended that the following foods should be consumed regularly—green and yellow vegetables, oranges, tomatoes and grapefruit, potatoes and other vegetables, fruits, milk and milk products, meat, poultry, fish, eggs, dried peas and beans, bread, flour and cereals, butter, and fortified margarine. The guide also used exchanges, so that if it was not possible to consume fruits because they were not easily available, vegetables could be considered as alternatives. In 1946, the recommendations included a National Food Guide that also gave information about recommended servings from each food group. This was done, so that it was easier for people to understand how they could obtain their requirement of each nutrient. In the UK, the first standards were published in 1950 by the British Medical Association. Similarly, many countries began to establish their own nutrient recommendations and guidelines. Food and Agricultural Organization (FAO) was joined by the World Health Organization (WHO) in the effort to "acquire the greatest possible degree of accuracy in assessing the calorie and nutrient requirements of human beings in the 1950s"; and in 1981, these two world organizations were joined by the United Nations University (UNU). During all these years, the focus of their efforts progressed and evolved to addressing several objectives such as planning and procurement of food supplies for the armed forces as well as for civilians, and evaluating the adequacy in meeting national nutritional needs. Since then from time to time, the Expert Committees have met and reviewed requirements for different nutrients.

At global level and similarly in many countries at national level, these committees regularly and periodically review evidence provided by new research on nutrient requirements and have made recommendations. Also, the number of nutrients for which recommendations were made, has increased over the years to include protein, energy, vitamin A and carotene, vitamin D, vitamin E, vitamin K, thiamine, riboflavin, niacin, vitamin B6, pantothenic acid, biotin, vitamin B_{12}, folate, vitamin C, antioxidants, calcium, iron, zinc, selenium, magnesium, and iodine. New scientific information for each nutrient is reviewed and recommendations are provided for different groups or categories—infants, children, young and older adults, and pregnant and lactating women. With evidence emerging about the needs of older adults and elderly, these are also being addressed.

In case of energy, requirements were defined in terms of the intake required to balance the energy expenditure in order to maintain body size and body composition. Given the rising prevalence of overweight and obesity, expert groups also recommend the level of necessary and desirable physical activity that is considered to be compatible with long-term good health and social desirability.

More recently, expert groups in different parts of the world recognize that there are several levels when the concept of optimal nutrition is to be considered. These levels are:
- Prevention of deficiency symptoms this level was traditionally used to establish reference nutrient intakes
- Optimizing body stores of a nutrient
- Optimizing some biochemical or physiological function
- Minimizing a risk factor for some chronic diseases
- Minimizing the incidence of diseases.

For example, in the USA, the reference value for calcium is given considering the amount needed for optimizing bone calcium levels. This is a shift from the way that calcium requirements were traditionally calculated in terms of preventing deficiency symptoms. These concepts may well be adopted in the future, after experts agree on the best approach for selecting criteria for setting reference standards for micronutrients, i.e., minerals and vitamins. An example of establishing a reference standard for optimizing a biochemical function is a level of folic acid that would minimize the plasma levels of homocysteine, a potential risk factor for cardiovascular disease. Another example is the level of zinc to optimize cell-mediated immunity. In the same manner, giving a reference standard for sodium may be done for optimizing a risk factor for a disease, i.e., a level of intake that would be compatible with minimizing hypertension. A reference standard could be given for the level of n-3 polyunsaturated fatty acids (PUFAs) to lower plasma triacylglycerols (TAGs). An example for a reference value to minimize the incidence of a disease could be the amount of folic acid to minimize the population burden of neural tube defects.

In India, a Nutrition Advisory Committee of the Indian Research Fund Association [now **Indian Council of Medical Research (ICMR)**] made the first attempt in 1944 to design Recommend Dietary Allowances for Indian population based on their typical habitual Indian diets. These recommendations were made for energy, protein, iron, calcium, vitamin A, thiamin, ascorbic acid, and vitamin D. Later allowances for energy were revised in 1958 by this Committee, based on approaches used by the FAO Committee, and the characteristics of Indian Reference man and woman were established. This is because three important characteristics influence nutrient requirements—sex/gender, age, and body weight. Some of the characteristics of the reference man and reference woman were redefined in Figure 9.1.

RECOMMENDED DIETARY ALLOWANCES (RDA)

"Recommended allowances for nutrients are amounts intended to be consumed as part of a normal diet."

> **"Recommended Dietary Allowance" (RDA) is defined as "the intakes of nutrients derived from the diet by an individual for maintenance of normal physiological functions, growth and wear and tear."** It is the amount of daily requirement for energy and several other nutrients based on age, sex, physical activity, and physiological status, which will enable the person to maintain various essential physiological and biochemical functions as well as for wear and tear and to maintain good health. A requirement for a nutrient is the amount of the nutrient that must be consumed by an individual in order to avoid its deficiency as indicated by clinical, physiological, and biochemical criteria. Requirements for the same nutrient differ from one individual to another and are notably so in case of energy.

Recommended Dietary Allowance (RDA) is a set of national standards for quantities of major nutrients to be obtained from food/diet by healthy persons in order to meet the physiological needs of the body. They are given for different nutrients based on body weight, categorized by age, sex, and level of physical activity, and physiological status. The age groups included are: infants, preschool children, school-age children, adolescents, adult men, and adult women as well as pregnant and lactating women.

Many countries rely on the Food and Agriculture Organization (FAO) and the World Health Organization (WHO) to establish and disseminate dietary allowances. Others use their own country reports as the basis of their standards. Revisions need to be made as new knowledge becomes available through scientific evidence about the public health and clinical significance of too little and

Characteristics	Reference Woman	Reference Man
Age (years)	19-39	19-39
Weight (kg)	55	65
Height (m)	95th centile values of heights	95th centile values of heights
BMI (kg/m^2)	18.5-22.9	18.5-22.9
Physiological status	Non-pregnant and non-lactating, free from disease	Free from disease
Occupational activity level	8 hours/day (480 minutes)	(sedentary, moderate or heavy activity)
Sleep	8 hours (480 minutes)	
Light – moderate activities (personal care, household work and leisure)	4-6 hours sitting and moving	4-6 hours sitting and moving
Exercise for health and well being	Minimum of 20 minutes of exercise daily and at least 150 minutes per week	

Fig. 9.1: Characteristics of the reference man and woman.

too much intake. Such information may be specific for a particular country.

> "Recommended Dietary Allowances refers to the daily dietary nutrient intake level that is sufficient to meet the nutrient requirements of nearly all, i.e., 97–98 percent of healthy individuals in a particular life stage and gender group. This is derived from the EAR as the mean plus 2 standard deviations (SD) of the distribution of requirements. The term is used to primarily evaluate individual diets. *The RDA is inappropriate for dietary assessment of groups as it is the intake level that exceeds the requirement of a large proportion of individuals within the group."*
>
> **Indian Council of Medical Research-National Institute of Nutrition. Nutrient Requirements and Recommended Dietary Allowances for Indians. New Delhi: ICMR; 2020.**

Recommended Dietary Allowances are not intended to indicate individual requirements or therapeutic needs related to a particular disease, nor they are applicable to sportsmen, astronauts, etc. These values for energy and different nutrients are intended to serve as a reference in order to meet the known nutritional requirements of the majority, i.e., 95% of the country's population. RDAs are estimates and suggested average values for intakes per day, such that the requirements of all individuals in a given population will be met. In order to do this, the Expert Group adds a margin of safety since there is variation between individuals and diets and cuisines vary tremendously especially in India.

RDA ascertains the quantity of the nutrients to be consumed but it does not reflect the food source of the nutrient. Dietary guidelines like "Food Pyramid" of "My Plate" give information about the type and quantity of food to be consumed for maintaining health. Nutrient composition tables provide the information regarding the quantity of each nutrient in individual foods.

Recommended allowances are issued by Expert groups in each country. These are Food and Nutrition Board of the Institute of Medicine, National Academy of Sciences in the US and Indian Council of Medical Research - National Institute of Nutrition in India. Issues of safety, quality and adequacy of food supply are also addressed; hence other terms are being used in addition to nutrient requirements. The Institute of Medicine, USA uses the approach known as Dietary Reference Intakes (DRIs): The DRIs represent a category for four different reference values used to assess human health and nutritional well-being. These are—(1) Estimated Average Requirement (EAR), (2) RDA, (3) Adequate intake (AI), and (4) Tolerable Upper Intake Level (UL). These four reference values have been recommended in India by the ICMR-NIN in 2020.

These are explained in the document on Recommended Dietary Allowances and Estimated Average Requirements. EAR for different nutrients is given in appendix.

Estimated Average Requirement (EAR)

In the latest recommendation in 2020 by ICMR-NIN, nutrient requirements are presented as EAR in addition to RDA. The equivalent term for this is average nutrient requirement (ANR) and refers to the average daily nutrient intake level estimated to meet the requirements of half of the "healthy" individuals, i.e., 50% in a particular life stage and gender group/in a given demographic group (i.e., age/sex/reproductive status). This term is used to evaluate populations or groups. (The term—"apparently healthy"—refers to the absence of disease based on clinical signs and symptoms of micronutrient deficiency or excess and normal function as assessed by laboratory methods and physical evaluation). Note that EAR is the nutrient intake level estimated to meet nutrient requirements of 50% of healthy individuals in a particular gender and life stage group whereas RDA is that level of nutrient intake that is sufficient to meet nutrient requirements of 97–98% of that a particular gender and life stage group. Also, EAR is to be used to evaluate population of groups as RDA indicates an intake level that is likely to be greater than the requirement of a large proportion of persons in that in a particular gender and life stage group. As per the ICMR-NIN (2020) RDA-EAR guidelines, RDA = average intake (mean) + 2 standard deviation (SD) of the distribution of requirements.

Unlike the past, it is now recommended that we do not have a single value. EAR should be used when there is need to evaluate population nutrient intakes. RDA should be used to set safe nutrient intake for the individual.

Recommended Nutrient Intake/Recommended Dietary Allowance (RNI/RDA)

It is the average daily dietary nutrient intake level sufficient to meet the nutrient requirement of nearly all (97–98%) healthy individuals in a particular life stage and gender group/demographic group. This is derived from ANI/EAR as the mean plus 2 standard deviations (SD) of the distribution of the requirement. The RDA is inappropriate for dietary assessment of groups, as it is the intake level that exceeds the requirement of a large proportion of individuals within the group. This is especially true in case of energy.

Recommended nutrient intake (RNI) is equivalent to the term recommended Dietary Allowance (RDA) and refers to the daily dietary nutrient intake level sufficient to meet the nutrient requirements of nearly all (97–98%) healthy individuals in a particular life stage and gender group. This is calculated as: ANR plus 2 Standard Deviations of the distribution of requirements. If the SD is not known, a value based on each nutrient's physiology can be used and in most cases a variation in the range of 10–12.5% can be assumed. Even though these requirements are specified for a healthy population, they can be used to assess and plan diets in clinical setting(s) by modification or adjustment of these requirements for the disease process (as for example HIV infection) and for nutrient metabolism, as there are no other standards. In case of micronutrients, because there is considerable variation in the micronutrient intakes of persons, daily requirement refers to the average intake over a period of time.

Adequate Intake (AI)

This is the recommended average daily intake of a nutrient that is recommended based on observed or experimentally determined approximations of nutrient intakes that are assumed to be adequate, by group/groups of apparently healthy people. This approach is used when sufficient data are not available to determine an EAR or RDA. In the Indian context, it is referred as acceptable intake.

Upper Nutrient Level/Tolerable Upper Intake Level (UNL/TUL)

It refers to the highest average daily nutrient intake level that is likely to pose no risk of adverse health effects to almost all individuals in the general population. As intake increases above the UL, the potential risk of adverse effects may increase.

Tolerable upper intake level is the "maximum level of habitual intake from all sources of a nutrient or related substance judged to be unlikely to lead to adverse health effects in humans. An adverse effect is a change in morphology, physiology, growth, development, reproduction, or lifespan of an organism, system, or (sub)population that results in an impairment of functional capacity, an impairment of capacity to compensate for additional stress, or an increase in susceptibility to other influences". TUL becomes relevant in the present scenario as many foods are now being fortified, particularly because risk of adverse effect of excess intake should be minimized. ICMR-NIN (2020) has given the TUL for different nutrients such as protein, calcium, magnesium, iron, zinc, iodine, niacin, vitamin B^6, folate, vitamin C, A and D.

Lower Reference Nutrient Intake (LRNI)/Lower Threshold Intake (LTI)

It refers to a value derived from the ANR/EAR. This value is calculated as the ANR/EAR minus 2 standard deviations (SD) of the distribution of requirement. This value is sufficient to meet the needs of the bottom 2% of individuals. However, different countries have used a different cut off such as 5–10% to evaluate nutrient insufficiency, although the concern is that these values would set a very low expectation of the individual nutrient intake adequacy level. Besides these, a term acceptable macronutrient distribution range (AMDR) is also used.

Acceptable Macronutrient Distribution Range (AMDR)

Besides the above four terms, AMDR is used. It refers to an appropriate range of usual macronutrient intakes that is associated with a reduced risk of chronic diseases but, at the same time, provides adequate intakes of essential nutrients. It is usually expressed as a percentage of energy, with lower and upper limits.

Specific ranges for desirable intakes of sources of energy, namely—carbohydrates, protein, and fat, are given, where the intakes are expressed as a percentage of energy intakes. The AMDRs have been recommended such that the range for each macronutrient is one that will provide adequate intakes of essential nutrients while the risk of chronic disease is reduced. The AMDRs have also been established for essential fatty acids and polyunsaturated fatty acids. The AMDRs are as follows: carbohydrates should supply 45–65% of total energy intake; protein should give 10–35% and fat 20–35% of total energy intake.

Besides looking at adequacy of nutrients, one concern is that when nutrients are consumed in excess of requirements, there may be adverse health effects. Therefore, it becomes important to define the highest level of intake at which no adverse effects of biological significance have been observed so far. This is designated by the term NOAEL (No Observed Adverse Effect Level). In the same way, LOAEL (Lowest Observed Adverse Effect Level) designates the lowest intake at which adverse effects have been observed. Adjustments are then made using certain factors in order to define reference doses.

The United States Food and Drug Administration (FDA) defines a "good source" of a nutrient as one serving of food containing 10–19% of the Recommended Dietary Allowance (RDA) or Adequate Intake (AI) for that nutrient.

Another relatively new approach for deriving nutrient requirements is optimal intakes. In this approach, it is necessary to select or establish the function of interest and the level of desired function, and it is essential that there is a plausible relationship between the selected function to the specific nutrient of concern and its function should be to promote health and/or prevent disease. An example is the adequate level of calcium intake for adolescents and young adults that has been given by the Expert Committee in the USA and is based on scientific evidence that peak bone mass increases until about 24 years of age and calcium intakes during this period should support the building up of peak bone mass.

Basis of Recommended Dietary Allowances

Expert groups clearly recognize and explicitly state that besides age, gender, and physical activity, there are day-to-day variations in the diet consumed, hence, there will be differences in the nutrient intakes. The presence of antinutritional factors and the bioavailability of nutrients, depending on the source of the nutrient, will influence how much of a nutrient should be consumed. Such variations have been taken into account when recommending the amount or level of a nutrient to be consumed. Expert groups make recommendations for a population. Also when setting the RDA, expert groups generally give a higher level for each nutrient, so that majority of the population will remain healthy and active and will not suffer from deficiency of the nutrient under consideration. It is also important to remember that the given nutrient's requirement is easily fulfilled by the diets commonly consumed in a given population, provided the diets are varied, i.e., a variety of foodstuffs are included in the daily diet. When a person is consuming the recommended amount of nutrient(s) then his/her chances of being at risk of an inadequate intake is <2.5%.

> **Research glimpse:** It is established that daily requirement of nutrients is important and comparison of intake with these is a diagnostic tool for the individual/clinical level, and at the population level. However, these are often used incorrectly. Hence, "recommended daily intake" or the RDA is conceptually used and that is the intake at which the risk of deficiency in the individual is minimal. Nutrients interact with each other and requirements are influenced by the physiological state. There is need to consider the multiple interactions that occur when food is prepared and eaten, or within the body with multiple deficiencies, or with the environment when infections occur. Thus, it is quite possible that designed interventions will fail. This is particularly relevant to the need to define specific (single) nutrient deficiency and provide single nutrient remedies through supplementation and fortification. The recommended values differ from country to country and can range from a single value for a population to four different values that define a "lower reference intake", an "average requirement", a "recommended intake" for individuals from a specific population, and an "upper tolerable intake". Authors have also given many other parameters to understand nutrient intakes in Indian context.
>
> *Swaminathan S, Raj R, Thomas T, et al. RDA for Indians-what more do we need, and do these fit requirements? Bull Nur Found India. 2015;36 (4):1-5.*

Factors taken into Consideration while Establishing the Recommendations

The following factors are taken into consideration:

> **Factors considered while making recommendations**
> - Physiological and biochemical functions and metabolism of the nutrient
> - Environment and climate
> - Dietary intake patterns
> - Different life stages, i.e., age, gender, physiological state, and individual variations
> - Basal requirements
> - Safe intake levels
> - Tolerable upper intake levels
> - Toxicity
> - Stress, illness, smoking, and trauma
> - Socio-cultural and economical status within the community

Age: As a person grows from infancy through childhood and adolescence into adulthood, there are significant changes in body size, body weight, and body composition that entail an increase in requirements for energy and other nutrients. During the periods of growth and in altered physiological state like pregnancy and lactation, nutritional demands are proportionately higher than at other stages/periods in life. The velocity of growth is significantly higher during infancy as compared to any other stage of growth. Also, nutrient requirements relative to the body size are higher as compared to the adult. Thus, energy requirement one year old child is 85 kcal/g/day and at the age of 17 years it is 45 kcal/kg body weight/day.

With regard to other nutrients there is accretion of protein and calcium resulting in expansion of the body tissues and enhancing the bone mineral mass. Protein requirement of an adult woman is 45.7 g/day while boy of 16-18 years need 55.4 g/day. While calcium needs of both adults and 13-15 year adolescent boys and girls are same, i.e., 1000 mg/day calcium. This indicates the significant role of nutrients corresponding to the biological and metabolic functions at tissue, cellular and molecular level in different life stages. Increase in energy requirements not only corresponds to the body weight but also to the physical activities and physiological status. In old age there is increased demand for water due to decrease in thirst mechanism and for dietary fiber to preserve gut health and for prevention of chronic diseases. In post-menopausal women, calcium demands are higher to overcome the reduced bone mass.

Sex: Both males and females naturally vary in their body weight, body composition, and basal metabolic rate; hence, the nutritional requirements of men and women for the same nutrient are different. Requirement for energy is not only associated with energy expenditure but is also influenced by body composition that is under hormonal influence, e.g., women require less energy (kcal) than men because women have comparatively smaller body size, lower body weight, and different body composition as well as lower basal metabolic rate (BMR). Men have more muscle mass for the same body weight than women who have more body fat. Muscle is metabolically more active, thus, the energy requirements for both the sexes are different, even if the age is similar. Requirements for B-vitamins will also differ, since their requirements depend on the energy intake. Further, in adolescent girls and women during reproductive age, the menstrual cycle that occurs every month involves loss of iron due to which they have higher RDA for iron.

Physiological state: Different stages of the life cycle are characterized by different rates of growth and development. Stages, when rate of growth and development are rapid, necessitate a higher supply of nutrients to meet the needs. Infancy, adolescence, pregnancy, and lactation are periods of growth. There is tissue deposition and the basal metabolic rate is also higher than at other periods. This increases nutrient requirements. Some nutrients assume special importance at certain life stages, e.g., folic acid before and in early pregnancy. Some but not all nutrients are required in higher amounts by the pregnant woman to provide for her own needs and that of the developing fetus. Thus, nutrient requirements are calculated in order to ensure that during pregnancy the fetus will develop well and during infancy, in fact in the first 2 years of postnatal life, the child will be well nourished enough to lay down different types of tissues such as neural, brain, muscle, enzyme systems, liver, bone, and connective tissue. Similarly, during lactation, milk production places demand for energy as well as other nutrients except iron are increased during lactation. Requirements for infants and children must focus on growth and development, while for adults, nutrients are required for maintenance of body weight and prevention of nutrient depletion of nutrient from the body (maintenance of acceptable range of nutrient-related parameters in blood and tissues is necessary).

During adolescence, the second period of rapid growth, the rate of growth, is higher than in the school years there are dramatic changes in body composition owing to hormonal changes, affecting the nutritional needs. Nutritional requirements of this age group are associated with sexual maturity rather than age itself. With maturation, nutrients needs may vary because of metabolic response. As people age, activities generally reduce in intensity, thus energy requirements of the elderly are less than in young and middle-aged adults. However, the body requires much more care and maintenance, therefore, their micronutrient requirements do not alter. Absorption may also be less in old age particularly that of vitamin D, calcium, and vitamin B_{12}, which affects their nutrient requirements.

Bioavailability of nutrients: Bioavailability indicates the amount of a nutrient that is absorbed in the intestine from the diet and is available to the body for its biological purpose(s). Bioavailability of the nutrient governs the normal functioning of the organ, e.g., iron, which is essential for several biochemical and physiological functions. Various factors, such as food source, food matrix, food additives and response of nutrient in the biological system as well as nutritional status of the individual and the physiological state of the person affect the bioavailability of the nutrients. For example, iron from animal sources such as meat is well absorbed as compared to plant sources. The bioavailability of iron varies from 5% to 15%. But addition of vitamin C in food matrix enhances iron absorption from spinach. On the contrary, presence of phytates, tannins, oxalates hinders the absorption of iron, therefore it is advocated to avoid tea and coffee (as they contain tannins) along with the consumption of iron-rich foods. For protein, protein quality and protein digestibility are considered. Needs for water soluble vitamins are associated with energy needs and cannot be stored in the body but fat and calcium can be stored in the body. Excess or deficient intakes also affect response of the nutrients used by the body. The bioavailability of certain nutrients is increased in certain biological states such as pregnancy and in a person having nutrient deficiency disorder. Absorption is increased in presence of other nutrient, e.g., presence of vitamin D enhances the calcium absorption. Germination process enhances the bioavailability of zinc and iron.

Individual variability: No two persons are the same. There are genetic, geographical, cultural, and social differences within a single age or gender group. Hence, a single RDA may not provide similar benefits to all. This variability in the requirement of a given nutrient between persons is taken into account when setting reference standards and establishing the RDA. Hence, experts give a safe level of intake in order to ensure that majority, i.e., 97.5% of the population will remain healthy.

Throughout the world, a very wide variety of food is cultivated and consumed through diverse cuisines. Within one's socioeconomic and sociocultural milieu, every person needs to select those foods that will fit into the budget and meet the nutritional requirements easily. The RDA gives the guidelines about the nutritional requirements and provides the basis for individuals to plan their diets and select appropriate foods to ensure the fulfillment of their nutritional needs.

Physical activity: Sedentary workers require less energy and B-vitamins because they do not undertake much muscular activity whereas moderate and heavy workers, whose physical activity is more, require higher amounts of some nutrients. As the intensity and duration of intense physical activity increase, requirements for energy and some vitamins also increases.

Other considerations: RDA is generally applicable to healthy persons under normal conditions. It does not cover special nutritional needs arising from metabolic disorders, chronic diseases, injuries, premature birth, other medical conditions, and drug therapies. A special or different set of nutritional advice is given under special conditions to communities or individual basis. Some nutrients are not stored in the body, e.g., most of the B-complex vitamins, whereas some like vitamin A and B_{12} can be stored. Hence for those nutrients that are stored, recommendations are made to ensure that stores of the nutrient can be built and maintained. Also toxicity of the nutrient should be prevented as in case of fat-soluble vitamins (A and D) and water-soluble vitamins (niacin and vitamin B_6). Pharmacological requirement is often different from the physiological requirements.

Uses and Applications of RDA

RDA is used for various purposes:
- For setting nutrient intake goals and developing food-based guidelines, evaluating adequacy of intakes by individuals and populations.
- For evaluating and planning diets for groups in institutions, e.g., old persons' homes, prisons, hostels, armed forces, and mid-day meals.
- For planning national food supplies, food distribution, and trade.
- For planning food aid for developing regions of the world and for emergency situations such as famine relief.
- For food product development, nutritional labeling, and nutrition and health claims regarding products by industry
- Development of nutrition policies, and food regulations
- For advocacy, health and nutrition promotion/education, evaluating nutritional quality and density of foods, production of micronutrient-rich foods, and food fortification.

Policy Decision

RDA can be used at various levels as a basis by policy makers and government to non-governmental organizations and official bodies.
- To develop guidelines to prevent nutritional deficiency nutritional programs and provides the basis for arranging the food supplies for national food programs like Public Distribution System (PDS) and other schemes like Midday Meal Scheme as well as national nutritional supplementation programs such as Integrated Child Development Scheme (ICDS).
- It helps governments to identify nutrient needs for the population and specific subgroups or target groups within

the population and make informed decisions about food policy. It is used as the basis for making decisions about provision of food supplements, food supplies through the public distribution system (PDS).
- Similarly, it may be used by non-governmental organizations when making decisions about food supplementation in public nutrition and health programs.
- It helps to determine the adequacy of food and nutrient intake by the population of the country. Also, it is used by nutritionists and health professionals to evaluate and determine the extent to which dietary intakes of groups are adequate or otherwise and whether there is overconsumption.
- It provides guidelines for policy planners for selecting the strategies to design any intervention program to combat nutritional deficiency, depending on the type of food baskets for different populations.
- It is used as a guideline map to monitor the food shortages and surpluses, when policy makers or industry make decisions about food fortification, legislation related to food supply, make decisions about import or export of food items to feed the national population or to provide subsidies to farmers or to producers, i.e., food industry.
- It helps to plan for the buffer stock of foods, which may be used in unprecedented events or emergencies, and to ration the quantity and quality of food in food aid programs providing relief to vulnerable groups and people during emergencies including natural disasters such as earthquakes, floods, or man-made disasters such as war torn areas.

Basis for Diagnosis

By comparison of individual or group intakes with the RDA, it can help in diagnosis of (for individuals, communities, and populations):
- Degree of malnutrition
- Level of undernutrition, overnutrition, and micronutrient deficiencies
- Assessment of nutritional deficiencies like anemia.

Assessment and Planning of Institutional Feeding Programs/Rations

It helps to evaluate and plan the quantity of rations and to plan menus for institutional feeding in hostels, hospitals, canteens, as well as for programs such as, supplementary feeding programs and thus to provide nutritionally adequate diets or food supplements.

Educational Purpose

- It provides guidelines to understand the essential nutritional requirements for energy and other nutrients as per physical activity, physiological status, age, and sex.
- It helps in identifying and selecting the food items that are good sources of different nutrients as per the requirements.
- It can be used for advocacy and nutrition education.
- It provides a framework for guiding different people and for research purposes.

Food Product Development and Food Labeling

It also helps the food industry to design and develop many nutritious food products, nutrient-rich recipes, and dietetic foods, which meet the health needs of specific groups, e.g., fiber biscuits and cookies, sugar-free sweets, nutribars, muesli, and other dietetic foods or foods for clinical conditions such as low-phenylalanine products for patients with phenylketonuria, ketogenic foods, and diets. Nutrition facts given on food products also provide percent daily value based on RDA.

Compare the nutrient composition of a food product: It helps to compare the nutrient composition of a food product (either calculated values or results of chemical analysis for nutrient content in the given food products). This may be expressed as the proportion of the daily requirement fulfilled by the food under consideration. Thus, it is helpful to food industry for nutritional and labeling of foods and/or to make specific nutritional or health claims. It helps consumers to interpret and evaluate information on food labels making the information on nutrient content more meaningful. This, in turn, should help the consumer to choose the foods in accordance with their needs yet receive more nutritional value for the price paid.

Clinical Significance

- It helps to evaluate the diets of patients and assess the nutritional adequacy of the diets.
- It helps in designing and preparing customized meal plan for patients, and selection of appropriate foods and menus for undernourished, overnourished, and people with special needs in health.
- There are some limitations that must be borne in mind when using RDAs.

Limitations of RDA

1. Nutrient intakes are recommended only for healthy and well-nourished persons and not for undernourished, obese, or sick people.
2. Although energy requirements are recommended according to the age, sex, and activity pattern, they cannot be used for an individual because they are given for the population groups. Individual requirements vary widely on the basis of body surface area, BMR, and energy expenditure, which depends on the type, intensity, and duration of physical activity. Further, energy requirement of an individual also varies from day to day.
3. It is assumed when the RDA for one nutrient is set, that intakes of other nutrients are adequate.
4. There are differences between individuals (inter-individual) in their nutrient requirements.
5. Experts recommend that infants should be exclusively breastfed in the first 6 months after birth. There are difficulties in making recommendations for non-breastfed and partially breastfed infants, largely due to the considerable differences in the compositions of mother's (human) and cow's or buffalo's milk as well as in the availability of several nutrients.

6. RDA tables and nutrient composition tables are not easily available to the common man. Hence, people do not have knowledge about these. Many persons also do not know how to use these tables.
7. There are tremendous agroclimatic and varietal differences in the nutrient content of each food item. Also, loss of nutrients during processing and post-harvest handling is difficult to assess. There are innumerable food combinations in different cuisines. These make the task of assessing their nutritional contribution difficult. Nutrient content of many commercial food products and food preparations is not available. Therefore, it is difficult to relate all of them to the RDA. There is a risk of excessive consumption of one or more nutrient(s), especially fat and deficit(s) in intakes of other nutrient(s).

> **Research Glimpse:** Nutrient requirements were defined for the purpose of evaluating diets of individuals and populations. Several countries, including India, have provided recommendations over the years. In India, the ICMR recommendations have a single value for a particular population group; while in other countries, up to 4 values have been reported. Currently, the commonly used definitions are for the average nutrient requirements, recommended nutrient intake or dietary allowances, and the upper nutrient/tolerable upper limit. From these requirement values, not only the risk of inadequate intakes can be calculated (using the probability approach) but the risk for excessive intakes that cross the upper limit can also be determined. With the increase in consumption of packaged foods and fortification, there needs to be clarity on the upper limit of nutrients, particularly those that are stored in the body (e.g., iron) to prevent toxicity. Measurement of accurate daily requirement of the individual is very difficult under controlled conditions or under various physiological states. There may be certain daily losses to maintain the balance.
>
> *Swaminathan S, Mani I, Thomas T, et al. Recommended dietary allowances-facts and Uncertainties. Proc Indian Natn Sci Acad. 2016;82(5):1555-63.*

Recommended Dietary Allowances for Various Nutrients

The recommended dietary allowances given by the Indian Council of Medical Research - National Institute of Nutrition (ICMR-NIN, 2020) are shown in Table 9.1A for energy, protein, carbohydrates, fats, dietary fiber, water, and some important minerals. In Table 9.1B recommended intakes for some crucial water soluble and fat soluble vitamins are given in Appendix 4 gives the Estimated Average Requirement (EAR).

Besides RDA, dietary standards are given for recommending food intakes, which will help to meet requirements for energy and other nutrients, against which food/dietary intakes can be evaluated. The concept of dietary standards was initially established when nutrient deficiencies were observed as public health problems. Later, dietary guidelines were intended to support active lifestyle, reduce chronic diseases, and help persons make food choices to meet nutrient requirements. The food guide pyramid is also used to help planning of a diet. In Australia and New Zealand, a term "Suggested Dietary Target" is used to indicate a daily average intake from foods and beverages for certain nutrients that may help in the prevention of chronic disease. In India Dietary Guidelines are issued by the ICMR-NIN for health and well being of the Indian population at large.

DIETARY GUIDELINES

Nutrition is important for life. While recommendations are given for the various nutrients, this cannot be easily understood by the lay person because recommendations are given in terms of nutrients, the language is very technical and is not easily understood by those who are not from this field. However, recommendations made in terms of foods are better understood since human beings think about consumption of foods on daily basis rather than in terms of nutrients. Dietary guidelines have been published in this country and elsewhere. Dietary guidelines are based on current scientific knowledge regarding diet and health. These are issued to provide guidance and advice on foods, food groups, and dietary patterns by helping persons choose appropriate foods that can promote overall health and well-being, protect the body, as well as prevent chronic diseases. They are given for representative individuals or population.

Dietary guidelines or food-based dietary guidelines are intended to serve as a basis for public food and nutrition, health, and agricultural policies. They are also useful for nutrition education to foster healthy eating habits and lifestyles.

Food Guide Pyramid

The Food Guide Pyramid is used as a visual food guide in order to enable individuals to understand the recommendations for dietary guidelines and put them into practice. It is a helpful tool for selecting food items necessary to design a balanced diet. It also suggests the number of servings to be included in the daily diet. Individual variations can easily be understood and practiced.

> **Food guide pyramid** is a tool that helps make healthy food choices to stay healthy and active. The design of the pyramid itself indicates the relative contribution of different food groups which the individual must use to have variety, balance, and moderation in the diet to lead a healthy life.

The Food Guide Pyramid was published by the United States Department of Agriculture in 1992. The pyramid depicted four food groups. In 2005, MyPyramid was designed for the Dietary Guidelines for American as shown in Figure 9.2. Each color represented specific food group such as orange color for grains; green color for vegetables, red color for fruits, yellow for oils and fats, blue for dairy and purple for meat, poultry, egg, fish, nuts, seeds and beans. The person climbing the steps symbolizes the slogan "steps to a healthier you".

My Plate has now been introduced by the US Department of Agriculture in 2011 to replace the MyPyramid and was unveiled by Michelle Obama. My plate as shown in Figure 9.3 consists of the five food groups. The plate is divided into four sections namely grains, fruits, vegetables, and protein foods. Dairy is depicted in a glass on the side of the plate. My Plate is based on the US dietary food guidelines. It is displayed on

Table 9.1A: Recommended dietary allowance (RDA) for energy, and other key nutrients Indians (2020).

Group	Category of work	Body weight (kg)	EAR (EER) (kcal/g/day)	Water (mL)	Protein (g/day)	Fat (g/day)	Carbohydrates (g/day)	Dietary fiber (g/day)	Calcium (mg/day)	Iron (mg/day)	Zinc (mg/day)	Magnesium (mg/day)	Iodine (µg/day)
Men	Sedentary	65	2110	3150	54	25	130	35.7	1000	19	17	385	150
	Moderate		2710	4050		30		34.8					
	Heavy		3470	5200		40		32.9					
Women	Sedentary	55	1660	2500	45.7	20	130	29.7	1000	29	13.2	325	150
	Moderate		2130	3200		25		28.5					
	Heavy		2720	4100		30		19.0					
Pregnant and lactating women	II trimester	+10Kg	+ 350	3700	+9.5	30	175	30.8	1000	40	14.5	385	250
	III trimester				+22.0								
	Lactation 0-6 months		+600	4100	+16.9	30	200	32.5	1200	23	14.0	325	280
	Lactation 7-12 months		+520		+13.2	30							
Infants	*0-6 months	5.8	550	n.a.	8.1	-	55	n.a.	300	-	-	30	100
	6-12 months	8.5	670		10.5	25	95			3	2.5	75	130
Children	1-3 years	11.7	1010	1500	11.3	25	130	10.6	500	8	3.0	135	90
	4-6 years	18.3	1360	2050	15.9	25	130	16.6	550	11	4.5	155	120
	7-9 years	25.3	1700	2550	23.3	30	130	19.9	650	15	5.9	215	120
Boys	10-12 years	34.9	2220	3300	31.8	35	130	25.1	850	16	8.5	270	150
	13-15 years	50.5	2860	4200	44.9	50	130	28.0	1000	22	14.3	355	150
	16-17 years	64.4	3320	4500	55.5	40	130	31.9	1050	26	17.6	405	150
Girls	10-12 years	36.4	2060	3050	32.8	45	130	22.5	800	28	9	255	150
	13-15 years	49.6	2400	3500	43.2	35	130	25.3	800	30	11	325	150
	16-17 years	55.7	2500	3700	46.2	35	130	25.6	800	32	12	335	150

There is no RDA for energy. There is EAR=Estimated average requirement; EER =Estimated energy requirement *AI=Acceptable intake, n.a.=Not available; ICMR_NIN (2020).

Table 9.1B: Recommended dietary allowance (RDA) for energy, and vitamins for Indians (2020).

Group	Category of work	Body weight (kg)	EAR (EER) (kcal/day)	Thiamine (B1) (mg/day)	Riboflavin (B2) (mg/day)	Niacin (B3) (mg/day)	Pyridoxine (B6) (mg/day)	Folate (B9) (mg/d)	B12 (µg/day) (mg/day)	Vitamin C (mg/day)	Vitamin A (mg/day)	Vitamin D (µg/day)
Men	Sedentary	65	2110	1.4	2.0	14	1.9	300	2.5	80	1000	600
	Moderate		2710	1.8	2.5	18	2.4					
	Heavy		3470	2.3	2.2	23	3.1					
Women	Sedentary	55	1660	1.4	1.9	11	1.9	220	2.5	65	840	600
	Moderate		2130	1.7	2.4	14	1.9					
	Heavy		2720	2.2	3.1	18	2.4					
Pregnant and lactating women	II trimester	+10 kg	+350	2.0	2.7	+2.5	2.3	570	+0.25	+15	900	600
	III trimester											
	Lactation 0-6 months		+600	2.1	3.0	+5	+0.26	330	+1.0	+50	950	600
	Lactation 7-12 months		+520	2.1	2.9		+0.17					
Infants	*0-6 months	5.8	550	0.2	0.4	2	0.1	25	1.2	20	350	400
	6-12 months	8.5	670	0.4	0.6	5	0.6	85		27		
Children	1-3 years	11.7	1010	0.7	0.9	7	0.9	110	1.2	27	390	400
	4-6 years	18.3	1360	0.9	1.3	9	1.2	135	1.2	32	510	600
	7-9 years	25.3	1700	1.1	1.6	11	1.5	170	2.5	43	630	600
Boys	10-12 years	34.9	2220	1.5	2.1	15	2.0	220	2.5	54	770	600
	13-15 years	50.5	2860	1.9	2.7	19	2.6	285	2.5	72	930	600
	16-17 years	64.4	3320	2.2	3.1	22	3.0	340	2.5	82	1000	600
Girls	10-12 years	36.4	2060	1.4	1.4	14	1.9	225	2.5	52	790	600
	13-15 years	49.6	2400	1.6	2.2	16	2.2	245	2.5	66	890	600
	16-17 years	55.7	2500	1.7	2.3	17	2.3	270	2.5	68	860	600

There is no RDA for energy. There is EAR=Estimated average requirement; EER =Estimated energy requirement; *AI=Acceptable intake, n.a=Not available; ICMR_NIN (2020).

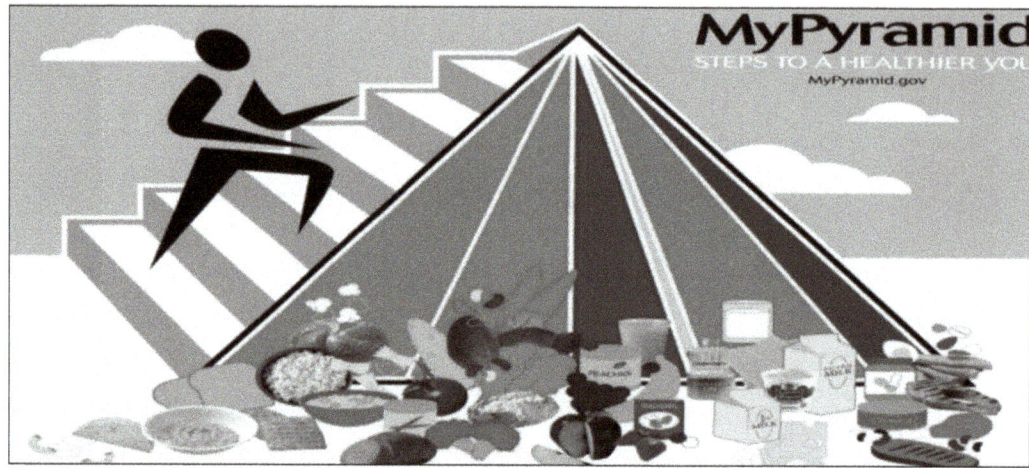

Fig. 9.2: MyPyramid is from USDA (2005) is designed on the basis of 2000 kcal depicting different food groups along with the number of servings in different bands. It also symbolizes need for physical activity by showing the person climbing the steps signifying the slogan "Steps to a Healthier You".

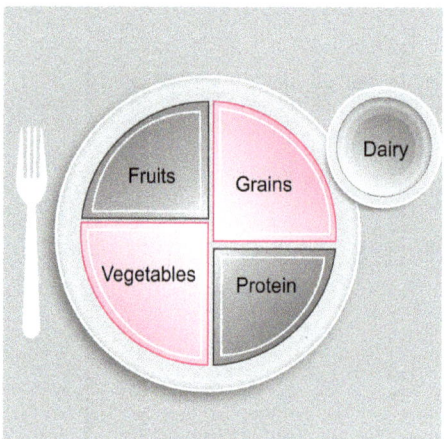

Fig. 9.3: My plate.

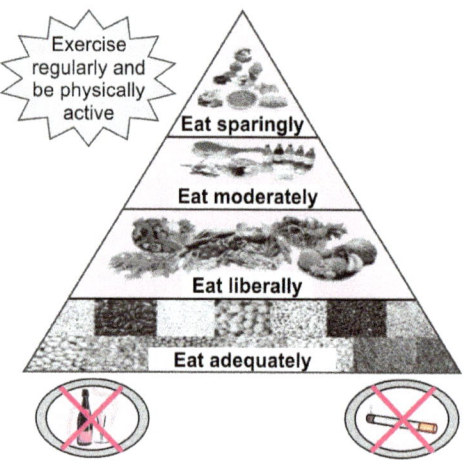

Fig. 9.4: Food pyramid.

food packaging and is used in nutrition education. The grains section is approximately 30%, vegetables section is 40%, fruits 10%, and the protein, which is represented by dairy, is about 20%. Additional/supplemental messages are given such as "Make half your plate fruits and vegetables", "Switch to 1% or skim milk", "Make at least half your grains whole", and "Vary your protein food choices". Portion control is recommended along with reduction in intakes of sodium and sugar. My plate has been considered as a good and fairly simple guide, and convey its concept easily.

FOOD GUIDE FOR INDIANS

The National Institute of Nutrition, India made recommendations in 2003 in the form of steps or a ladder, signifying the steps to good health. These guidelines are depicted as a pyramid with four bands in Figure 9.4. The shape of the pyramid is deliberately used to easily convey, which foods should be given more emphasis.

Foods shown at the base or the **first band** are to be included in larger amounts and form the base of a well-balanced diet—**"EAT ADEQUATELY".** It indicates that cereals and pulses are the foundation of a healthy diet. These provide the maximum amount of nutrients like energy, protein, certain vitamins, minerals, and fiber required in the diet. Pulses and nuts are comparatively cheap source of essential fatty acids, iron, and protein and they do not contain any cholesterol and saturated fatty acids.

Second band indicate **"EAT LIBERALLY".** It implies the need for consumption of adequate amounts of fruits and vegetables, as they are good sources of fiber, vitamins, minerals, and phytochemicals, which are essential for good health but low in fat. This group can easily provide variety to the diet, being rich in color, texture, and shapes and sizes.

Foods represented in the **third band** are protein-rich foods. Amount of these foods to be consumed is indicated by **"EAT MODERATELY".** Vegetarians can choose pulses and non-vegetarians can choose egg, meat, and fish. Besides protein, non-vegetarian foods are rich in iron, cholesterol, and different kinds of fatty acids. For example, meat is rich in saturated fatty acids and cholesterol, and consumption of these foods in excess can be harmful. Hence, it is essential to take care not to consume too much fat from these foods. Fish provide essential fatty acids particularly omega-3 and consumption of fish 2–3 times a week is healthy. The foods from this group should be consumed in moderation, as excess can be taxing to both digestion and the pocket.

Foods shown at the top indicate **"EAT SPARINGLY".** Narrow size of this band clearly indicates the importance of caution in the food selection and the amount of food consumption. This group includes fats, oils, sugar, and sweets as well as processed foods, ready to eat snacks, etc. All these add taste to the food but excess is not healthy and increases risk of disease.

Other signs are **"SAY NO"** to alcohol and smoking, as they have adverse effects on health.

Special sign is included for physical activity. If food and nutrients are essential for the body, so is exercise.

The ICMR-National Institute of Nutrition (2018) has designed a healthy "My Plate for the day" that beautifully depicts what constitutes a healthy diet. It depicts the need to include a minimum of eight food groups to help achieve a balanced diet and obtain the required macro- and micronutrients. My plate of the day is shown in Figure 9.5. As can be seen in the figure half of a meal should be constituted by vegetables and fruits, the next major constituent should be cereals and millets, followed by pulses and milk/curd.

Benefits of regularly consuming foods as per My Plate for the day are:
- Enhancement of immunity and resistance to infections
- Maintainance of good gut microflora
- Prevention of diabetes, cardiovascular diseases, heart attacks, strokes and numerous other diseases
- Attaining appropriate alkalinity to reduce inflammation and the risk of formation of kidney stones
- Prevention of insulin resistance and maintenance of appropriate insulin sensitivity and glycemic index
- Assurance of adeqaute intake of fiber and redice episodes of constipation
- Prevention of environmental pollution and toxins like heavy metals and pesticides.

Consumption of proportion of food groups indicated in the plate helps prevent macronutrient and micronutrient malnutrition (hidden hunger).

The proportion indicated in the plate ensures adeqaute intake of vitamins, minerals, bioactive compunds, functional foods, antioxidants, etc.

No vitamin or mineral supplements will provide the adequacy of all nutrients that can be met from from this model plate.

Routine consumption of certain nutrients as supplemnts will interfere with absorption of other nutrients.

Micronutrients from food are better absorpbed and more bioavailable than vitamins and minerals supplemnets/tablest/capsules/fortification.

A complete diet as indicated in the model plate provides many unknown sunstances/nutrient that cannot be met from the supplements or fortified foods.

The Dietary Guidelines developed by the National Institute of Nutrition give dietary goals as well as guidelines. These guidelines are given for different age groups.

Benefits of consuming foods daily as per "My Plate" are:
- Maintenance of a state of positive health and optimal performance in populations at large by maintaining ideal body weight.
- Ensuring adequate nutritional status for pregnant women and lactating mothers.
- Improvement of birth weights and promotion of growth of infants, children, and adolescents to achieve their full genetic potential.
- Achievement of adequacy in all nutrients and prevention of deficiency diseases.
- Prevention of chronic diet-related disorders such as diabetes, cardiovascular diseases, heart attacks, strokes and several other diseases.
- Enhancement of immunity and resistance to infections.
- Maintenance of good gut microflora that will have beneficial effect.
- Help to attain appropriate alkalinity that will help to reduce inflammation and the risk of formation of renal stones.
- Prevention of insulin resistance and improving insulin sensitivity.
- Maintenance of the health of the elderly and increases life expectancy.
- Assurance of adequate intake of fiber, improving bowel function and thereby reducing constipation.
- Prevention of harmful effects of environmental pollution and heavy metals and pesticides that are toxic.

Dietary Goals

The FAO has also issued dietary guidelines for different countries including India, which are same as given in **"Dietary Guidelines for Indians" 2011**. These consist of 15 key points that are as follows:
1. Eat a variety of foods to ensure a balanced diet.
2. Ensure provision of extra food and healthcare to pregnant and lactating women.
3. Promote exclusive breastfeeding for 6 months and encourage breastfeeding till 2 years.
4. Feed home-based semisolid foods to the infant after 6 months.
5. Ensure adequate and appropriate diets for children and adolescents both in health and sickness.

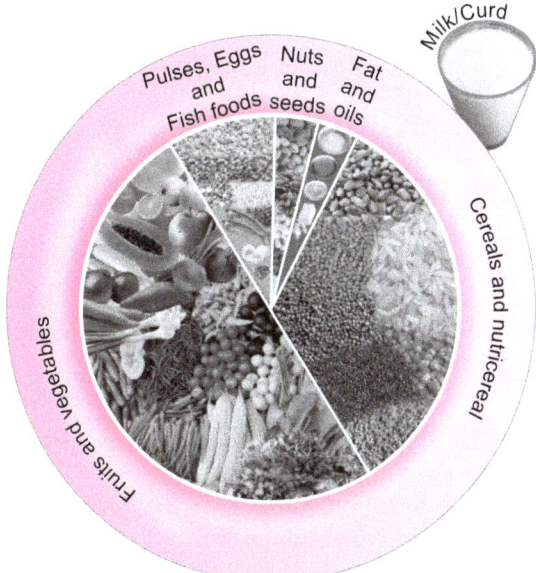

Fig. 9.5: My plate of the day.

6. Eat plenty of vegetables and fruits.
7. Ensure moderate use of edible oils and animal foods and very less use of ghee/butter/vanaspati.
8. Overeating should be avoided to prevent overweight and obesity.
9. Exercise regularly and be physically active to maintain ideal body weight.
10. Use salt in moderation/restrict salt intake to minimum.
11. Ensure the use of safe and clean foods.
12. Practice right cooking methods and healthy eating habits.
13. Drink plenty of water and take beverages, especially sugar-sweetened and carbonated beverages in moderation.
14. Minimize the use of processed foods, rich in salt, sugar, and fats.
15. Include micronutrient-rich foods in the diets of elderly people to enable them to be fit and active.

WHO has also given 5 key points for healthy diet along with the rationale for these.

Five Key Points for Healthy Diet by WHO

1. Breastfeed babies and young children:
- From birth to 6 months of age, feed babies exclusively with breast milk (i.e., give them no other food or drink), and feed them "on demand" (i.e., often as they want, day and night)
- At 6 months of age, introduce a variety of safe and nutritious foods to complement breastfeeding, and continue to breastfeed until babies are 2 years of age or beyond.
- Do not add salt or sugars to foods for babies and young children.

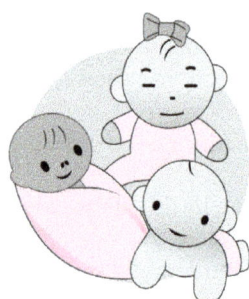

Why?
On its own, breast milk provides all the nutrients and fluids that babies need for their first 6 months of healthy growth and development. Exclusively breastfed babies have better resistance against common childhood illnesses such as diarrhea, respiratory infections, and ear infections. In later life, those who were breastfed as infants are less likely to become overweight or obese, or to suffer from noncommunicable diseases, such as diabetes, heart disease, and stroke.

2. Eat a variety of foods:
Eat a combination of different foods, including staple foods (e.g., cereals such as wheat, barley, rye, maize or rice, or starchy tubers or roots such as potato, yam, taro or cassava), legumes (e.g., lentils, beans), vegetables, fruit, and foods from animals sources (e.g., meat, fish, eggs, and milk)

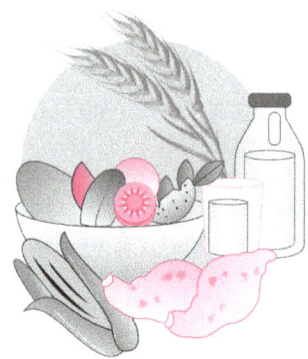

Why?
Eating a variety of whole (i.e., unprocessed) and fresh foods every day helps children and adults to obtain the right amounts of essential nutrients. It also helps them to avoid a diet that is high in sugars, fats, and salt, which can lead to unhealthy weight gain (i.e., overweight and obesity) and noncommunicable diseases. Eating a healthy, balanced diet is especially important for young children's and development; it also helps older people to have healthier and more active lives.

3. Eat plenty of vegetables and fruits:
- Eat a wide variety of vegetables and fruits.
- For snacks, choose raw vegetables and fresh fruits, rather than foods that are high in sugars, fats, or salt.
- Avoid overcooking vegetables and fruits as this can lead to the loss of important vitamins.
- When using canned or dried vegetables and fruits, choose varieties without added salt and sugars.

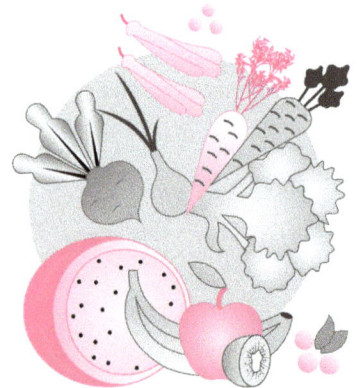

Why?
Vegetables and fruit are important sources of vitamins, minerals, dietary fiber, plant protein, and antioxidants. People whose diets are rich in vegetables and fruit have a significantly lower risk of obesity, heart disease, stroke, diabetes, and certain types of cancer.

4. Eat moderate amounts of fats and oils:
- Use unsaturated vegetable oils (e.g., olive, soy, sunflower, or corn oil) rather than animal fats or oils high in saturated fats (e.g., butter, ghee, lard, coconut, and palm oil)

- Choose white meat (e.g., poultry) and fish, as they are generally low in fats, in preference to red meat.
- Eat only limited amounts of processed meats because these are high in fat and salt.
- Where possible, opt for low-fat or reduced fat versions of milk and dairy products.
- Avoid processed, baked, and fried foods that contain industrially produced trans-fats. It is important to read the nutrition label on processed food products and then make decisions about whether to consume the food or not.

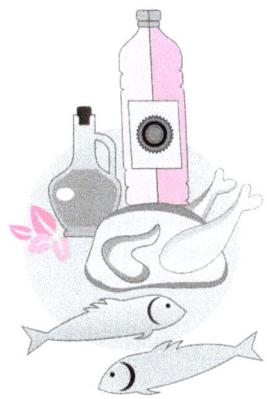

Why?

Fats and oils are concentrated sources of energy, and eating too much fat, particularly the wrong kinds of fat, can be harmful to health. For example, people who eat too much saturated fat and trans-fats are at higher risk of heart disease and stroke. Trans-fats may occur naturally in certain meats and milk products, but the industrially produced trans-fats (e.g., partially hydrogenated oils) present in various processed foods are the main source.

5. Eat less salt and sugars:
- When cooking and preparing foods, limit the amount of salt and high-sodium condiments (e.g., soy sauce and fish sauce)
- Avoid foods (e.g., snacks) that are high in salt and sugars
- Limit intake of soft drinks or soda and other drinks that are high in sugars (e.g., fruit juices, cordials and syrups, flavored milks and yogurt drinks)
- Choose fresh fruits instead of sweet snacks such as cookies, cakes, and chocolate.

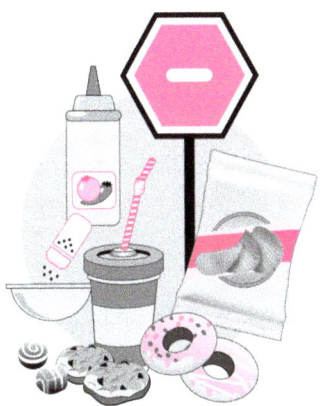

Why?

People whose diets are high in sodium (including salt) have a greater risk of high blood pressure, which can increase their risk of heart disease and stroke. Similarly, those whose diets are high in sugars have a greater risk of becoming overweight or obese, and an increased risk of tooth decay. People who reduce the amount of sugars in their diet may also reduce their risk of noncommunicable diseases such as heart disease and stroke.

FOOD GROUPS

Nutrition is essential for health. It is an everyday phenomenon. In order to achieve good health and physical efficiency, theoretical knowledge needs to be translated into practice. Most people do not have access to food composition tables and hence need guidelines for selection of foods and the appropriate amounts to be consumed. It is the responsibility of nutritionists and dieticians to convey this knowledge to the lay public, in a simple manner. Hence, various food items, which are commonly consumed, are classified into "food groups" based on the major nutrients present in them as well as based on main functions of the body.

Each food group thus is able to provide nearly sufficient nutrients to sustain good nutritional status. The US Department of Agriculture had devised the 7-food group plan in 1943. This was followed by the 4-food group plan in 1956 and 11-food group plans in 1964. Conventionally only 4-food groups were followed, namely: 1. Cereals, millets and pulses, 2. Vegetables and fruits, 3. Milk, milk products, egg, meat and fish and 4. Oils, fats, nuts and oil seeds. Indian Council of Medical Research and National Institute of Nutrition (ICMR-NIN) has devised 3-food group plan and 5-food group plan.

> **Food groups** is a nutritional classification of foods. It categorizes the foods in different groups depending upon their functions, relative types of food, and nutritional contribution. It helps the diet planner to plan a nutritionally adequate diet for the individuals in a given condition. It helps to achieve nutrient intake in accordance with RDA. It also serves as a tool for nutrition education, counseling, and food labeling.

> **Uses of food groups**
> - To enable people to select appropriate food items.
> - To help to design a balanced diet.
> - To provide variety in taste, texture, and nutrients in diet.
> - To assess diet and identify shortcomings in terms of foods that is underemphasized in the diet.
> - To help persons during nutritional counseling.
> - To design or assess nutrition labels.
> - To make nutrition policies and monitor nutrition programs.

Three-food Group Plan

Three-food group plan is based on the functions of food. It is easy to learn, understand, and practice. Meal planning is more convenient using the three-food group plan. In most cases, food selection on the basis of this "3-food group plan" easily fits into dietary practice followed in the most parts of the country like "roti, dal, sabji" or "dal–bhat and bhaji". It becomes easy to add at least one food item from each group in almost every major meal. It is also useful from consumer point of view or for the community. The three-food group is shown in Table 9.2.

Five-food Groups

Each food group provides some nutrients and would help to meet the nutritional requirements or the RDA. The Expert Group of Indian Council of Medical Research (2011) has also given five food groups along with nutrients supplied by each group, which has been given in Table 9.3.

On the eve of the centenary year of Indian Council of Medical Research and National Institute of Nutrition, released "My plate for the Day to prevent hidden hunger and protection from diseases". It also ICMR-NIN (2018) advocated dietary guidelines to follow with the theme of 'empowering nation through nutrition". The benefits of consuming the food as per "My plate" which represents the foods portions that provides 2000 kcal and 60 g proteins. The My plate includes 270 g cereals; 90 g pulses, 300 g milk/curd, 300 g vegetables; 100 g fruits, 20 g nuts and seeds and 27 g fats and oils. Eggs/fish/meat can substitute pulses. Prescribed amount of vegetables may be consumed either in cooked form/salad. Prefer fresh fruits (avoid juices) and use different varieties

Table 9.2: Food groups on the basis of functions of food (3-food groups).

Food groups	Foods included in each group	Nutrient supply by each food group
Energy-rich foods	Whole grain cereals, millets Vegetable oils, ghee, butter Nuts and oilseeds Sugars	**Major nutrient: Carbohydrates** Protein, fiber, calcium, iron, B-complex vitamins Fat, essential fatty acids, fat-soluble vitamins Proteins, vitamins/minerals Simple sugar
Body-building foods	Pulses, nuts, and oilseeds Milk and milk products Meat, fish, and poultry	**Major nutrient: Protein** Carbohydrates, invisible fat, B-complex vitamins Calcium, vitamin A, riboflavin, vitamin B_{12} B-complex vitamins, iron, iodine, and fat
Protective foods	Green leafy vegetables Other vegetables and fruits Egg, milk and milk products, and flesh foods	**Major nutrient: Vitamins and minerals** Antioxidants, fiber and other carotenoids Fiber, sugar, and antioxidants Protein and fat

Source: Indian Council of Medical Research (ICMR). Dietary Guidelines for Indians—A Manual. Hyderabad, India: National Institute of Nutrition; 2011.

Table 9.3: Food groups on the groups basis of contribution of nutrients (5-food groups).

Food group	Food groups	Foods included in each group	Nutrient supply by each food group
I	**CEREALS, MILLETS, AND PULSES**		
	Cereals and millets	Wheat, rice, bajra, jowar, corn, ragi, wheat flour, puffed rice, flaked rice (poha), vermicelli, noodles, bread	Energy, carbohydrates, protein, iron, thiamin, niacin, fiber
	Pulses	Bengal gram, black gram, green gram, red gram, lentil (whole as well as dal), cowpea, peas, rajmah, soybeans, dry beans	Energy, protein, iron, calcium, B-vitamins invisible fat, fiber
II	**VEGETABLES AND FRUITS**		
	Roots and tubers	Onion, potato, yam, sweet potato	Starch, fiber
	Green leafy vegetables	Amaranth, spinach, drumstick leaves, coriander leaves, fenugreek leaves, etc.	Carotenoids (precursor of vitamin A), invisible fats, riboflavin, folic acid, calcium, iron, fiber
	Other vegetables	Carrots, brinjal, lady finger, pumpkin, gourds, beans, capsicum, cauliflower	Invisible fats, carotenoids, riboflavin, folic acid, calcium, iron, fiber
	Fruits	Mango, guava, papaya, orange, sweet lime, water melon	Vitamin C, carotenoids, fiber
III	**MILK AND ANIMAL FOODS**		
	Milk	**Milk:** Milk, curd, skimmed milk, cheese, paneer, khoa	Protein, fat, vitamin B_2, calcium
	Animal foods*	Meat, fish, egg, poultry	Protein, fat, essential fatty acids, vitamin A, D, and E, and minerals
IV	**FATS AND OILS, NUTS AND OIL SEEDS**		
	Fats and oils	Butter, ghee, hydrogenated fat (vanaspati), vegetable oils like soybean, mustard, sunflower groundnut, coconut Almonds, cashew nuts, figs, dates, pistachio	Energy, fat, essential fatty acids Essential fatty acids, oils, vitamins and minerals
V	**SUGAR, JAGGERY, HONEY**		
	Sugar, jaggery, honey	Sugar, jaggery, honey Jams, jellies, soft drinks Cakes, sweets, and sugar-laden desserts	Energy, carbohydrates High fructose

Note: *For nonvegetarians, one serving of pulse can be substituted with one serving of egg/meat/chicken/fish.
Source: Gopalan et al & Rao et al. Nutritive value of Indian Foods. 2004.

of cooking oils, vegetables, fruits, nuts, etc., to obtain a variety of phytonutrients, vitamins, minerals and bioactive compounds.

USE OF FOOD COMPOSITION TABLES

Knowledge of the nutritional composition of foods is extremely important for the study of human nutrition and its application in daily life. Knowing the nutritive value of different foods is essential for planning and providing appropriate diets for individuals at different stages of the life cycle and for groups of persons. It is also the basis for application in the treatment and management of disease. Thus, planning of diets for different people depends on this information.

Food composition tables (FCTs) are repositories of values for the food composition that is nutritionally relevant. FCTs are used in routine health practice as well as for nutrition research. These values of foods are useful in nutritional surveillance, consumer nutrition appraisal, nutrition labeling of foods, understanding the etiology of disease prevalence, clinical settings, dietetic counseling, planning menus, meal planning, and dietary guidelines—recommendations and even to estimate intake of toxic and non-nutritive components as well as to assess environmental impact of foods. In India, nutrient profiling of foods began almost a century ago and the food composition tables were published in 1937, 1951, 1971, and 1989 and now in 2017.

Since nutritional disorders are public health concerns in India since ages, the food composition tables are useful in activities directed toward prevention and control of malnutrition. The Indian Council of Medical Research (ICMR) earlier known as Indian Research Fund Association (IRFA) along with National Institute of Nutrition (NIN) has broadened the perspective of nutrient analysis in the new IFCT, 2017. Economic liberalization and globalization has led to tremendous changes in the food and nutrition scenario not only in India but worldwide. In India, the National Institute of Nutrition, Indian Council of Medical Research (ICMR) published the **Indian Food Composition Tables (IFCT, 2017)**. National Institute of Nutrition has made an app called "Nutrify India now". The app provides information on nutritive value of foods in 17 different Indian languages. The App has the facility to monitor one's the energy balance, between calories consumed and also the one's energy expenditure.

The latest repository gives mean values and standard deviations, as well as giving values for many more nutrients as well as fatty acid composition, etc. In the new updated IFCT (2017), values for bioactive substances like polyphenols have been included.

This database lists food items, which are categorized according to the food group, e.g., cereals, pulses, etc. Within each group, items are listed alphabetically with a serial number. The local name in different languages and the scientific name/botanical name of each food item according to serial number are given in the Appendix I. It must be noted that the values given are for raw food items. Photographs of individual food items are also included in the database, so that visual identification is easy. Values for cooked foods are not given. The National Institute of Nutrition updates the database as and when they have analyzed more foods or foods already included for nutrients that had not been previously included.

The following tables are given, which provide the nutrient composition in 100 g edible portion of the food items.
- Table 1: Proximate principles and dietary fiber
- Table 2: Water-soluble vitamins
- Table 3: Fat-soluble vitamins
- Table 4: Carotenoids
- Table 5: Minerals and trace elements
- Table 6: Starch and individual sugars
- Table 7: Fatty acids profile
- Table 8: Amino acid profile
- Table 9: Organic acids
- Table 10: Polyphenols
- Table 11: Oligosaccharides, phytosterols, saponins, and phytates
- Table 12: Fatty acid composition of edible oils and fats

An example from Table 1 given in the book IFCT (2017) is shown in Table 9.4, where it indicates the proximate principles, which includes the nutritive value for moisture content, crude protein, fat, total fiber (soluble and insoluble), and ash (total mineral). The total of these 5 components is subtracted from 100 and the value for carbohydrates is obtained by difference. Further, the value for energy is given in kilojoules (kJ) that has been converted, as seen in Table 9.4 and Appendix 1, calculated from the calorific values for carbohydrates + fat + protein (i.e., 4, 9, 4 kcal/g). The table also indicates the unit of measurement for individual nutrients as well as the number of decimal points.

Table 9.4: Nutrient composition as given in the book IFCT (2017).

S.No.	Food item	Moisture (g)	Protein (g) (N×6.25)	Fat (g)	Minerals (g)	Total Fiber (g)	Carbohydrates (g)	Energy (kcal)
A019	Wheat flour (whole)	11.1	10.57	1.53	1.28	11.36	64.17	320
A018	Wheat flour (refined)	11.34	10.36	0.5	0.76	2.76	74.27	351

Source: Longvah T, Ananthan R, Bhaskarachary K, et al. (2017). Indian Food Composition Tables. National Institute of Nutrition, (Indian Council of Medical Research) Department of Health Research, Ministry of Health and Family Welfare, Government of India, Hyderabad.

Limitations of Food Composition Tables

Food is essentially biological material, and there are innumerable natural variations in the amounts of different nutrients due to several factors such as soil composition, climate, seed variety, agricultural practices, harvesting and storage, transport conditions, methods of processing (time, temperature), use with other ingredients during preparation/processing as well as the type of packaging. Different technologies are used in food processing and these may have varying influence on food composition. Different technologies that will help to retain vital health components in the food are being developed, but some of them are still in experimental stages. However, these technologies can help to reduce nutrient losses, but still there are considerable differences in nutrient content from plate to plate of the same food item. Hence, the nutritive values of raw foods do not fully reflect what the actual intake of a nutrient is. There are many nutrients that are easily destroyed when a food is exposed to air or heat. Vitamin C, folic acid, and thiamine are most sensitive to loss under different environmental conditions. However, analyzing all the variety of foods in a country like India, with tremendous regional variations and unique cuisines is a mammoth task and is time consuming and extremely expensive.

Nowadays, there are many software-based databases for cooked foods. It must be remembered that these databases are essentially calculated values based on the National Institute of Nutrition's database.

MEAL PLANNING FOR NUTRITIONALLY ADEQUATE DIETS

Let us understand the meaning of different terms used in meal planning.

> **Meal:** The number of food preparations planned, prepared, and consumed at one time in a day is called meal. Usually, breakfast, lunch, and dinner are considered meals, whereas evening tea and snacks are not.
>
> **Diet** includes meals, snacks, and beverages consumed in a day. Diets are of different type based on the nature (vegetarian and nonvegetarian); region (North Indian and South Indian) and purpose (normal, therapeutic, sports, etc.).
>
> **Meal planning** is the thought process given prior to purchase and preparation of the food items to be used in a specific meal. It focuses on the nutritional requirements, skill to cook, and food preferences, etc.
>
> **Diet planning** includes the planning of different meals including beverages and snacks for the whole day. Diet planning should specifically be directed to meet the requirements of specific needs of the person or a group of persons.
>
> **Balanced diet** is one which includes the foods from at least 3–5 food groups in a meal in adequate amounts and proportions. It should provide all the required nutrients for a given person. The diet should also satisfy hunger and taste as well as food preferences.

Diets should be healthy, nutritionally adequate, and socially, culturally, and personally acceptable and also provide some safety net to prevent nutrient deficiency or excess and onset of disease. Adequate and balanced diets promote health and well-being. Different people perceive "healthy diet" differently but it is essential in each and every life stage. It must support growth and development during pregnancy, infancy, childhood and adolescence, milk synthesis during lactation, and maintain a good state of health and wellbeing in adulthood as well as protect from illness in each life stage. It is necessary to adhere to balanced meals and knowledge about the principles will help individuals to adopt healthful dietary practices and consume balanced meals most of the time. Even when snacks and beverages are chosen for consumption between mealtimes, the person will try and choose wisely and not go overboard, just for the attractive appearance, taste, and flavor. A family may consist of people of different age groups and activity levels; hence, it is rather difficult to meet the demands and tastes of each and every member. Again, knowledge of the basic principles of meal planning will help to manage and provide a balanced diet for everyone.

Traditionally, Indian meals were balanced and each meal included the foods from at least 3–5 food groups in a meal in adequate amounts and proportions. Whether the meal was served in a thali like in Maharashtra, Gujarat, or in North India, or on a banana leaf in south India, different preparations were included to provide balanced meals. This tradition is continued in some communities or on special occasions. It signifies the freshness, pure, economical and use of locally available material as well as prevents use of synthetic material and pollution of environment.

Balanced diet is one that contains adequate proportions of carbohydrates, fats, and proteins, along with the recommended daily allowances of all essential minerals, vitamins, (nutritionally adequate) and health-promoting substances.

Balanced diet means that the meals a person consumes in a day, i.e., in a 24-hour period, i.e., major meals like lunch, dinner as well as snacks, will "provide all the nutrients in required amounts and proportions". Such a diet will fulfill the nutritional requirements as per the recommendations given by experts according to age, gender, physiological state, and physical activity. At the same time, diets should satisfy the hunger and sensory appeal. The word "balanced" means that planning a meal is an art not only from the point of view of taste, texture, and visual appeal but more importantly from the nutritional perspective. One should not consume too much (more than what the body needs) or too little (less than what is required) of any food or food group.

It should generally provide 50–60% energy from carbohydrates (preferably complex carbohydrates), 10–15% energy from protein and 20–30% from oils and fat. It should be noted that this includes visible fat/oil used in cooking and butter applied to bread, ghee applied to chapatti/roti, and the invisible fat that is inherently present in foods like meat, nuts, and oilseeds, etc. Besides this, a balanced diet will supply the micronutrients and other constituents in food like dietary fiber, antioxidants, and other phytochemicals that protect the body and are important for maintaining optimal health.

Meal Planning

Meal planning is the thought given prior to purchase and preparation of the food items to be used in a specific meal. The following issues need to be thought about or addressed for a making good meal plan.
- What to serve?
- How much to serve?
- How much to spend?
- Where to shop?
- How much to buy?
- How to prepare food?
- How to serve meals, at what time?

> **Meal planning:** Meal planning is a simple exercise, which involves applying the knowledge of food, nutrient requirements, and individual preferences to plan adequate, acceptable meals. It is a skill, which improves with practice.

Aims of Meal Planning are to:
- Fulfill the nutritional needs of an individual or members of a group.
- Use money's worth to make appropriate food choices and get the best nutritional value vis-à-vis cost.
- Invest on nutrient-rich/nutrient-dense food items rather than energy-dense foods.
- Help in the purchase, preparation, and service of appropriate food items.
- Help to economize on time, labor, and fuel.
- Provide variety in the diet through proper selection of foods.
- Make meals appealing and palatable by proper selection of food in terms of color, texture, and flavor.
- Cater to individual preferences and yet provide adequate nutrients in meals.
- Wastage is minimized and at the same time, leftovers are better utilized.
- Pre-preparation required for food preparation and service can be made in advance.

Steps in Meal Planning

1. Meal planning starts with the thinking of a person's age, sex, physical activity, meal time, or group of people and the occasion. It can be done for one or few meals or one full day from morning to night.
2. Three major meals (breakfast, lunch, and dinner) and 1–3 small meals/snacks (mid-morning, evening tea/snack, and bedtime) can be planned for one full day. The number of snacks depends on the age, work schedule, and physiological status as well as state of health, if any member of the family has some acute or chronic health problem.
3. A gap of 2–3 hours should be kept between main and small meals and of 4–6 hours between 2 main/major meals.
4. Try to schedule the breakfast before 8–10 am, lunch before 2–3 pm, and dinner before 8–9 pm. The meals, which coincide with circadian rhythm of the body, are likely to have less adverse or harmful effects on the body.
5. Use the food pyramid/food groups or the MyPlate as a guide for selection of foods.
6. Each main meal should contain one to two items from each food group like energy providing, body building, and protective food groups. The fourth food group of fat/sugar would be included to prepare the food and should be used in moderation.
7. If the individual has a 3-meal pattern (major meals), each meal should contribute approximately one-third of the nutritional requirements. If a person has more than 3 meals per day, one-third of the requirement should be consumed in the breakfast. The rest of the day's requirement is to be distributed among the different meals.
8. For a minor/small meal, even a single food preparation, cooked or raw like fruit or a healthy beverage (not carbonated beverages or soft drinks that contain only sugar) may be sufficient. Take care that none of the meals especially minor meals or snacks are calorie-rich/energy-dense, which is often the case. Here, preference should be given to nutrient-dense foods, i.e., foods that have good amount of protein and micronutrients.
9. Consider the monthly income (money spent on food), availability of food in season, and food preferences of the individual(s) while selecting the food item(s).
10. Write the menu plan for each meal giving the name of the food preparation along with quantity in household measures.
11. Make a table for representing food preparations in each meal, main food ingredients used in each food preparation, and amount of each food ingredient. Columns can further be added for calories and other nutrients to be calculated.
12. For calculation of nutritive value for selected nutrients, refer to the book "Indian Food Composition Tables (2017)" published by the National Institute of Nutrition (NIN).
13. Food selection should be done in a way that the food preparation/meal gives variety in color, flavor and taste, and texture. It should also suit the daily routine/pattern of the individual and occasion.
14. Basic meal plan does not include infants and persons who have any health problem or disease that requires special diets or dietary modifications and/or restrictions.

The number of servings including amount of food per serving, as per the dietary guidelines by NIN (2011) to be included from different food groups for different individuals as per ICMR-NIN (2011), shown in Table 9.5.
- One serving of a pulse/legume can be exchanged for one nonvegetarian food.
- Pregnant and lactating women need to include extra nutrient supply as per RDA.
- Elderly persons should ensure that their fat/oil intake in a day does not exceed 20 g.
- Even other persons should not consume more fat/oil than the amount recommended.
- Elders should consume at least 200–300 mL of milk and about 400 g vegetables in a day.

Table 9.5: Portion size and number of portions suggested for different individuals.

Particulars	Cereals and millets (30 g)	Pulses (30 g)	Milk and milk products (100 mL)	GLV/Other vegetables (100 g)	Roots and tubers (100 g)	Other vegetables (100 g)	Fruit (100 g)	Sugar (5 g)	Fat (5 g)
	Number of Portions								
Men									
Sedentary worker	12.5	2.5	3	1	2	2	1	4	5
Moderate worker	15	3	3	1	2	2	1	6	6
Heavy worker	20	4	3	1	2	2	1	11	8
Women									
Sedentary worker	9	2	3	1	2	2	1	4	4
Moderate worker	11	2.5	3	1	2	2	1	5	5
Heavy worker	16	3	3	1	2	2	1	6	6
Children									
Preschool child (1–3 years)	2	1	5	0.5	0.5	0.5	1	3	5
Preschool child (4–6 years)	4	1	5	0.5	1	1	1	4	5
School-age child (7–9 years)	6	2	5	1	1	2	1	4	6
Adolescent girl (10–12 years)	8	2	5	1	1	2	1	6	7
Adolescent boy (10–12 years)	10	2	5	1	1	2	1	6	7
Adolescent girl (13–15 years)	11	2	5	1	1	2	1	5	8
Adolescent boy (13–15 years)	14	2.5	5	1	1.5	2	1	4	9
Adolescent girl (16–18 years)	11	2.5	5	1	2	2	1	5	7
Adolescent boy (16–18 years)	15	3	5	1	2	2	1	6	10

Source: Dietary Guidelines for Indians—A Manual. Hyderabad, India: National Institute of Nutrition, Indian Council of Medical Research; 2011.
Note: Amount of the foodstuff in grams per portion is indicated in parentheses under each foodstuff.

- Adequate water should be consumed to avoid constipation and dehydration.
- Leafy vegetables should be consumed regularly (at least 3-4 times in a week).

DAILY MEALS

Breakfast

Breakfast is the first meal of the day and is very important from the nutritional point of view. Literally, it means breaking the fast, because it is eaten after a gap of 8-10 hours after consuming a meal (dinner) on the previous night. It is said to be adequate if it contains the main food groups namely, energy giving, body building, and protective foods and provides approximately one-third of the day's RDA. It will boost the energy level and help to maintain it throughout the day and prevent physical and mental fatigue.

Ayurveda prescribes *dincharya*. Western scientists have started looking into the cohesion of nature, sleep wake cycle and impact of food on the biological systems. Circadian rhythm encompass the functioning of the body's internal clock with the clock in the nature (that involves sunrise to sunset and night). Breakfast is the first meal of the day but for the people who work till late night and wake up late and do not eat at appropriate times of the day, are at risk of lifestyle disorders that are likely to adversely effect the body. Such persons must be careful about their food choices and the time of eating food.

Skipping breakfast or eating a breakfast that is inadequate in quantity or quality can increase risk of undernourishment and prompt the person to overeat later in the day. Lack of knowledge about its importance, lack of time to prepare breakfast, and lack of appetite in the morning are some of the reasons for the skipping or consuming inadequate breakfast.

Traditional breakfast preparations eaten in India are healthy and should be consumed. While selecting breakfast food preparations, care must be taken that it includes sufficient protein, complex carbohydrates, vitamins, minerals as well as some fat and fluids to feel satiated till lunch. Breakfast containing more simple carbohydrate and fat may soon give the hunger pangs. That often leads to high calorie intake in rest of the day. Nowadays, many ready-to-eat breakfast cereals are available in the market, which can be eaten as such or need addition of only milk or fruits/fruit juice for example corn flakes, muesli, but care should be taken to avoid those containing sugar. Other breakfast food items, which are nutritious, can be consumed singly or in combination as follows:

Breakfast solid food preparations: Plain paratha with curds/milk, stuffed paratha, chapati, bhakri or rotla, porridge/dalia, omelette or boiled or fried egg, lapsi, idli/dosa (with sambar or chutneys, dhokla, muthia, upma, uttapam, poha, chilla/pudla, thepla, vermicelli, bread, sandwiches. Depending upon the dish, nutritional value can be enhanced by adding sprouts, vegetables, nuts, milk, seeds or fruits etc.

- **Beverages:** Milk plain, tea/coffee/fruit juice/lassi/smoothie, etc.
- **Accompaniments:** Raw fruits, chutneys, etc.
- **For nonvegetarians:** Egg preparations, chicken sandwich, etc.

Lunch

It is the second major meal and includes staple foods. It needs to provide one-third of the RDA for the individual. It is most influenced by the work schedule of the person and the facility and availability of the arrangement for the meal service. Some people consume lunch at home; some eat lunch in canteens in their organization/place of work. Some carry packed lunch or some eat in restaurants. Most people like to have a complete meal at lunch time. It is often a balanced meal, if it is well planned. It is usually consumed between 1 pm and 3 pm. However, it may vary and will be influenced by individual needs and preferences. The type of food preparation is also governed by the individual preference and the types of preparations and meal services available. If not eaten, work performance and behavior may be affected. Technically, this meal should contain all food groups and provide variety, on a daily basis. The following food items can be included:

- **Cereals:** Chapati/phulka/bhakri/paratha/rice/khichdi/pulao/biryani/bread/thepla
- **Pulses:** Dal/sambar/chole/rajma/usal/other pulse preparations
- **Vegetables:** These preparations can be based on a single selected vegetable (e.g., bhindi bhaji/sabji) or a combination of two vegetables (methi aloo/aloo matar) or more than 2 vegetables (mixed vegetables, e.g., vegetable korma). These vegetables can be prepared dry or in a curry form using variety of preparation methods. Selected vegetables should be local, seasonal and fresh.
- **Salads:** Salads with one or more vegetables, e.g., tomato and cucumber slices, carrot or radish sticks, some green leafy vegetables can be chopped into it, sprinkle with some roasted seeds or salad dressings, lemon juice, etc. to enhance flavour and nutrient content onion, with pulses like sprouted moong/chana. Fruits are used as such.
- **Milk products:** Plain curd/yogurt, butter milk, raita, custard, kheer, ice cream, other milk preparations. Post lunch drinking thin butter milk, plain or seasoned with a pinch of roasted cumin, carom seeds asafoetida, are good options for better digestion.
- **Egg/meat/fish preparations** (one portion of this can be eaten instead of one portion of a pulse preparation), e.g., fish curry, mutton curry, mutton curry, prawn pulao.
- **Sweet preparations** or desserts can also be included occasionally but should not be eaten daily. Small amount of fennel seeds/mishri/coconut or a fruit may satisfy the post meal sweet craving.
- **Accompaniments:** Some people prefer to have raw onion and green chili, some prefer papad and pickle. Those who include pickle and papad should consume only small amounts as both items are rich in sodium. Also, it is better to have roasted papad than fried papad.

Many people go out to work and carry lunch, which is popularly known as packed lunch.

Packed food: It has certain limitations, which necessitate modification in food preparation and serving style. The following points should be considered for designing a packed food/lunch:

- It is better to have dry foods—gravy preparations or beverages may spill during travel or they may require special containers.
- It may not be possible to have a large variety of foods. Variety may require additional preparation in the morning, or additional or many containers and there may not be enough time or a proper place to eat all the different varieties.
- Temperature of the food preparation needs to be considered. Very hot food or foods, which require refrigeration if packed, may spoil if it is eaten much later in the day. Certain hot preparations may not be palatable or may become soggy, e.g., noodles, dosa.
- Packed lunch should preferably contain food preparations which are attractive, palatable or can be shared within the peer group.
- Age of the person should be considered.
- Portion size is important. Nutrient density of the packed meal is also crucial.
- It is important not to include biscuits, chips, and noodles in a packed lunch.
- Packed lunch should consist of a cereal preparation, vegetables, a pulse preparation and a fruit.

Snacks

After a hard day's work, a person often feel exhausted by evening and may need replenishment of energy for the rest of the day. Snacks are usually eaten for relaxation or enjoyment. Many a time, they may be eaten because the person is attracted, although he/she may not be hungry and has the appetite to consume such foods.

A snack should be nutritious and should not replace a meal. Many of the popular snacks provide "empty calories" or are energy-dense. Such snacks should be avoided. Snack consumption often leads to overeating and overconsumption, which may lead to different types of diseases including obesity. Snacks can be eaten at any time of the day, such as mid-morning, as most of the snacks energize the person. They also have a "feel good" factor. Following preparations are often used as snacks:

- **Freshly prepared snacks** such as sandwiches, pakoras, bhajia, cutlets, kachoris, samosa, batata vada, and vada pav can be some of the breakfast items and also eaten as evening snacks. Frankie, chat items (aloo chaat, tikki, bhel puri, pani puri, ragda pattice), dabeli, cholebhature, fruit chat, pav bhaji, noodles, momos, chaps, litti chokha, missal pav, dhokla, khandvi, dal vada, medu vada, dahi vada, appams.
- **Snacks having long shelf life:** Dal moth, mathri, chakli, chivda, sev, gathiya, khakhra, and namakpara. If sweet preparations like laddo, barfi, panjiri, sweet biscuits, cake, etc. are eaten, they should be eaten sparingly.
- **Beverages:** Tea/coffee/fruit juice/lassi/milk shake/nimbu pani/jal jeera/mocktails/soft drinks/thandai/kanjee.
- **Indian sweets** eaten along with major meal or as such and as per occasion, e.g., gulab jamun, halwa, barfi, rasgulla, laddoos, gujiya/karanji, malpua, rabdi, basundi, kheer/payasam, ghevar, jalebi, kulfi, and imarti. A lot of varieties are available in the market. Indian sweets although energy dense and high in fat also supply protein rather than mostly carbohydrates.

Note: All fried, salty, and sweet foods (particularly ultra processed and packaged) should be eaten in small amounts and only occasionally. It is preferable to consume steamed and shallow fried preparations. Fruits with milk can also be consumed during snack time rather than choosing fried preparations.

Dinner

Generally, it is similar to lunch in terms of composition because it is one of the major meals of the day. However, some people prefer light dinners, whereas some families have heavy dinners. Dinner timings also vary widely depending upon the duty hours of family members. Food preparations included in this meal are generally more appetizing since dinner is generally eaten at home with the family, in a relaxed manner. Many persons usually consume packed lunch, which is limited in terms of nutritional quality. They need to pay adequate attention to the nutritional quality of their dinner. It is very important that persons/families must guard against consuming heavy, deep-fried, and rich food items. Dinner should provide the remaining 1/3rd of the day's energy and nutrient requirements. At the same time dinner must be easy to digest to avoid gastric and sleep disturbances.

It is important not to eat dinner after 9–10 pm. It is better that there is a gap of 2–3 hours between dinner and going to bed. Some people consume some food late at night. These foods should preferably contain some protein and some carbohydrate like milk, so that it will help the persons to relax and sleep well. Chocolates, biscuits, desserts, and ice creams should be avoided late at night.

Table 9.6: Sample menu providing approximately 2,000 kcal.

Meal	Food preparation	Quantity consumed in household measures
Breakfast (8–9 am)	Milk	1 large glass
	Vegetable poha	1 bowl
	Mint coriander chutney	1 teaspoon
Lunch (1–2 pm)	Chapati	2–3
	Rice	½ bowl
	Chana dal with dudhi or lauki	1 bowl
	Vegetable stir fry	1 bowl
	Plain curd or butter milk seasoned with roasted jeera, dried mint	1 bowl or 1 medium glass
Evening snack (5–6 pm)	Idli	2–3
	Sambhar, chutney	1 bowl, 1 tablespoon
Dinner (8–10 pm)	Chapati	2–3
	Palak paneer curry	1 bowl
	Vegetable salad/seasonal fruits	1 bowl/1 fruit

Research Glimpse: There is accumulating evidence that suggests that circadian desynchrony, defined as when physiological processes are out of alignment with internal clocks, may be a contributing and modifiable factor in the development of type 2 diabetes. Almost all living organisms display circadian rhythms that cycle within a 24-hour period. Disruption of circadian rhythms from shifting the light/dark cycle or from genetic manipulations often results in metabolic disturbances such as obesity, impaired glucose tolerance, and reduced lifespan in mouse models. In humans, shift workers are at high risk for metabolic disorders. However, it is not the only cause but other factors also influence. Shift workers often belong to lower socioeconomic status, smoke, drink alcohol, and consume high-fat foods. There is evidence that small shifts in meal timing (such as skipping breakfast, or eating erratically, without consistent daily meal times) negatively impact glycemic control and lipid metabolism. This may help to understand the advocacy about change in lifestyle or adherence to meal times.

Hutchison AT, Wittert GA, Heilbronn LK. Matching meals to body clocks—Impact on weight and glucose metabolism. Nutrients. 2017;9(3):E222.

The menu items, chosen for the different meals, depend upon the culture in various regions of India. An example is given in Table 9.6. Several sample menus for different caloric contents are given in Dietary Guidelines for Indians (2011) and new RDA reference of ICMR-NIN (2020).

PERCENTAGE OF CONTRIBUTION OF DIFFERENT NUTRIENTS

When planning a balanced diet, it is recommended that the diet should provide 50–60% of total calories from carbohydrates preferably complex carbohydrates, approximately 10–15% from proteins and 20–30% from fats. The amount of fat includes both invisible fat (that which is inherently present in various foods) and visible fat/oil (that which is used for cooking or added/applied, e.g., butter on bread, ghee on chapatti). The example given below is a calculation of percent energy obtained from the three macronutrients:

1. **Protein:** 70 g × 4 kcal = 280 kcal divided by 2,000 = 0.14 multiplied by 100 = 14%
2. **Carbohydrate:** 317.5 g × 4 kcal = 1,270 divided by 2,000 = 0.635 multiplied by 100 = 63.5%
3. **Fat:** 50 g × 9 kcal = 450 divided by 2,000 = 0.225 multiplied by 100 = 22.5%

DAILY VALUE (DV)

Percent Daily Value (DV) is given in the Nutrition Facts label as a guide to the nutrients supplied by one serving of food. For example, if the label mentions 15% for calcium, it means that one serving provides 15% of the calcium you need each day.

The DVs are based on a 2,000-calorie diet for healthy adults. Even if your diet is higher or lower in calories, you can still use the DV as a guide. For example, it tells you whether a food is high or low in a specific nutrient:

- 5% or less of a nutrient is low.
- 20% or more of a nutrient is high.

> Daily value is the recommended intake of a nutrient based on a 2,000 kcal or a 2,500 kcal diet.
>
> Percent DV is the percentage recommended intake (DV) of a specific nutrient provided by a serving of the food.

How to decode your daily value or nutrition facts on the food package?
- Look at the serving size
- Look at the calories
- Look at %DV
- It is always advisable to try and get more of fiber, calcium, iron, vitamins, and less of sodium, saturated fats, and fats.

Consuming a nutritionally adequate diet requires knowledge of nutrient composition of foods. Most processed foods have information about the nutritional content of the food "Nutrition Facts". Often the label specifies the content per 100 g of the food and may also give in addition, the amount of nutrients supplied by one serving of the food. However, for convenience and better understanding by consumers, manufacturers in the food industry also give information on daily values. The daily values were created essentially to provide consumers with a base or benchmark for comparing various foods and to be able to comprehend the nutrient contribution of that food when reading labels giving the nutritive value on the package.

Daily value gives the consumers an idea about the contribution of key nutrients toward fulfilling requirements. The percent DV tells us how much of a given nutrient a single serving of an individual packaged food or dietary supplement contributes to one's daily diet. For example, if the DV for a certain nutrient is 300 mg and a packaged food or supplement has 45 mg in one serving, the %DV for that nutrient in a serving of the product would be 15%. One way, a food processor/manufacturer may give information is to express the percentage of RDA for a specific nutrient that is fulfilled by the food under consideration. More commonly, however, manufacturers express it as a percentage of "daily value".

The US Food and Drug Administration (FDA) have recommended the use of daily value on food labels. Daily values are expressed on the basis of 2,000 kcals and sometimes 2,500 kcals as well. "The US FDA has established four sets of Daily Values (DVs) for labeling of foods and dietary supplements—adults and children 4 years and older, children 1 through 3 years, infants 1 through 12 months, and pregnant and lactating women. Daily values comprise two sets of reference values for reporting nutrients in nutrition labels—the Daily Reference Values (DRVs) and the Reference Daily Intakes (RDIs). In order to avoid confusion especially among consumers, the single term "Daily Value" is used to designate both the DRVs and RDIs. With the DV, we are able to compare different products for their nutritional value and this will enable the consumers to choose more nutritious foods. DVs are based on the reference caloric intake of 2,000 calories for adults and children aged 4 years and older, and for pregnant women and lactating women.

In India, amendments are done by the FSSAI in Food Safety and Standards (Labeling and Display) Regulations and in the new version of 2019, some salient information is given in the section on Nutritional Information.

Nutritional Information means the declaration of calories, which is obtained from fats, saturated fat, trans-fat, cholesterol, sodium, carbohydrates, dietary fiber, sugars, protein, vitamin A, vitamin C, calcium, and iron present in the product. The calories are mentioned on all the product labels.

Besides necessary information about the product, the food label must provide "Nutritional Information" or "Nutritional facts". Nutritional values on the label are given for 100 g or 100 mL or per serving of the product and that shall contain information for the following:

i. Energy value in kcal;
ii. The amounts of protein, carbohydrate (specify quantity of sugar), and fat in gram (g);
iii. The amount of any other nutrient for which a nutrition or health claim is made: That where a claim is made regarding the amount or type of fatty acids or the amount of cholesterol, the amount of saturated fatty acids, monounsaturated fatty acids and polyunsaturated fatty acids in gram (g), and cholesterol in milligram (mg) shall be declared, and the amount of trans-fatty acid in gram (g) shall be declared in addition to the other requirement stipulated above;
iv. Wherever numerical information on vitamins and minerals is declared, it shall be expressed in metric units;
v. Where the nutrition declaration is made per serving, the amount in gram (g) or milliliter (mL) shall be included for reference beside the serving measure".

In case where "trans-fat free" is indicated, it implies that the amount of trans-fats present is less than 0.2 g per serving of food and the claim "saturated fat free" may be made in cases where the saturated fat does not exceed 0.1 g per 100 g or 100 mL of food, e.g., Label for edible oils or blended oil must reflect the process.

However, it is not necessary to provide the nutritional information specified for ready-to-eat and other food products for raw agricultural commodities, like, wheat, rice, cereals, spices, spice mixes, herbs, condiments, table salt, sugar, jaggery, or non-nutritive products, like, soluble tea, coffee, soluble coffee, coffee–chicory mixture, packaged drinking water, packaged mineral water, alcoholic beverages or fruit and vegetables, processed and prepackaged assorted vegetables, fruits, vegetables, and products like, pickles, papad, or foods served for immediate consumption such as served in hospitals, hotels or by food services vendors or *halwais*, or food shipped in bulk, which is not for sale in that form to consumers. Further, declaration regarding Food Additives and source of food and veg or nonveg in terms of green and red dot in square is suggested. A cross thin border indicates the food is not for human consumption.

The label provides printed information on the percentage contribution made by the macronutrients, i.e., carbohydrate, fat, and protein to the 2,000 kcals. Thus, the consumer can calculate the percentage of the 2,000 kcals consumed, based on the different foods consumed and the percentage daily value supplied and the number of servings consumed. Information on daily value is useful also for comparing different foods, to identify foods that are good sources of a specific nutrient as well as to make decisions based on price vis-à-vis the nutritive value of the food. Understanding daily values can help the consumer make healthful choices.

Daily value is expressed in percentage to find out the percentage of a given nutrient in comparison to specified RDA for that nutrient for an individual. It instantly indicates whether there is too little of a nutrient or the food is a good source of the nutrient. Daily value is generally given for processed foods and the information is generally printed on food package. However, it is important to remember that daily values are general standards, whereas individual requirements may be either more or less than the daily value specified on the label.

Percent daily value gives a unit of measure for one serving and sometimes for 100 g of the product. % DV is a means of evaluating the nutrient contribution vis-a-vis the total amount present in the food and allows us to compare different foods. For some nutrients like vitamins, daily values are recommended based on a 2,000 kcal or 2,500 kcal diet. For cholesterol and saturated fat, DVs represent the upper limit, which should not be exceeded. Although DV is calculated on the basis of 2000 kcal, it must be borne in mind that most people may not require 2000 kcals per day. An example for some nutrients and nutrition facts is shown in the box.

How to calculate %DV?

Total fat : $8.6/65 \times 100 = 13.2\%$
Saturated fat : $3.7/20 \times 100 = 18.6\%$
Carbohydrates : $14.5/300 \times 100 = 4.8\%$

This indicates that the product is high in fat and low in carbohydrate.

NUTRITION FACTS*
Serving size: 1 ounce (28 g)
Amount per serving

Calories	148	Calories from fat—77 kcal	
		% Daily value	
Total fat	8.6 g	13.2%	
Trans-fats		0%	
Saturated fats	3.7 g	18.6%	
Cholesterol	0 mg	0%	
Sodium	164.4 mg	6.9%	
Total carbohydrate	14.5 g	4.8%	
Dietary fiber	1.8 g	7.2%	
Sugars	1.6 g		
Protein	3.2 g		
Vitamin A	0%	Vitamin C	0%
Calcium	2.1%	Iron	3.3%

Not a significant source of vitamin A, C, calcium, and iron.
*Percent daily value is based on a 2,000 calorie diet. Your daily values may be higher or lower depending on your calorie needs.

Daily value may also be used for a component or many components, which has/have an impact on health, for example, content of saturated fats and content of trans-fats. It is recommended that the amount of saturated fats consumed should be less than 10% of energy (kcals) consumed.

Unfortunately in India, most consumers are not aware of the meaning of daily value and do not read labels much, before they purchase processed foods. Also, many small scale manufacturers do not have enough knowledge about the RDA for Indian population. There is a need for concerted efforts to be made to create awareness about these important aspects that are relevant to health.

NUTRIENT DENSITY

A nutrient-dense food will be a good source of healthy nutrients, but has relatively low amount of calories. Nutrient density means how much of a specific nutrient is present in one serving or 100 g of foodstuff or a food preparation. This concept can be used to assess the contribution of a particular food in relation to the RDA and the energy consumed. Nutrient-dense foods generally provide several nutrients in varying quantities but fewer calories. Also, the relative cost of food in terms of nourishment is high. Foods that contain vitamins, minerals, complex carbohydrates, lean protein, and healthy fats, e.g., fruits and vegetables, meats, eggs, peas, beans, and nuts are considered nutrient-dense foods because they are rich sources of nutrients, besides most of them having a high antioxidant value but, at the same time, they possess much lower amount of calories. The simplest way of expressing nutrient density is to express nutrient density as per gram or per 100 grams of the food or per 1,000 kcals of the food. One way of expressing nutrient density is INQ or index of nutritional quality.

Similarly, we can calculate energy density of foods. Energy density is the amount of kilocalories provided by foods per gram or per 100 grams. Lower energy density foods will provide fewer calories per gram or per 100 grams. Low energy density foods generally have a higher water content, e.g., soups, dal, foods like rice, pasta, vermicelli, etc. that absorb water during cooking. Also many foods are naturally high in water, such as fruits and vegetables. The amount of fiber in foods also influences the energy density. More amount of fiber will reduce energy density as is found in case of fruits and vegetables. Nuts and oilseeds are more energy dense than are whole pulses and legumes. High-energy density foods tend to include foods that are high in fat and have a low moisture/water content, for example biscuits and confectionery, wafers, almonds, walnuts, groundnuts, butter, oil, ghee, and cheese.

Energy density is calculated by dividing the calories provided by the weight of the food, which can be 100 g or weight of a portion. The density of different foods can be compared. Foods can be classified as very low-energy density, low-energy density, medium-energy density, or high-energy density, which is shown in Table 9.7.

Uses of Nutrient Density or Index of Nutritional Quality (INQ)

- As a tool for nutrition education and consumer education.
- Can become the foundation of dietary recommendations and guidelines.
- Helps persons to select correct foods easily to fulfill daily requirements.
- Useful in dietary management of obesity and other diseases.
- Deficiency of a nutrient in a foodstuff can be easily detected.
- Deficit in nutrient intakes can be detected.
- Helpful in strategy planning and policy making.

Research Glimpse: **Nutrient profiling** is the technique of rating or classifying foods on the basis of their nutritional value. Foods that supply relatively more nutrients than calories are defined as nutrient dense. Nutrient profile models calculate the content of key nutrients per 100 g, 100 kcal, or per serving size of food. These rigorous scientific standards were applied to the development of the **nutrient-rich foods (NRF) family**. First, the NRF models included nutrients to encourage as well as nutrients to limit. Second, NRF model performance was repeatedly tested against the **Healthy Eating Index (HEI)**, an independent measure of a healthy diet. HEI values were calculated for participants in the 1999–2002 NHANES. **Models based on 100 kcal and serving sizes performed better than those based on 100 g.** Formulas based on sums and means performed better than those based on ratios. The final NRF 9.3 index was based on 9 beneficial nutrients (protein, fiber, vitamins A, C, and E, calcium, iron, potassium, and magnesium) and on 3 nutrients to limit (saturated fat, added sugar, and sodium). Higher NRF 9.3 scores were associated with lower energy density and more nutrient-rich diets. The nutrient density of foods can be a useful tool for consumer education and can also become the foundation of dietary recommendations and guidelines.

Drewnowski A, Fulgoni VL. Nutrient density: principles and evaluation tools. Am J Clin Nutr. 2014;99(5 Suppl):1223S-8S.

Laboratory laurel: The Indian Migration Study (IMS) is a sib-pair study nested within the larger Cardiovascular Disease Risk Factor Study (CVDRFS) in industrial populations from 10 companies across India (n = 19,973 for the questionnaire survey, n = 10,442 for biochemical investigations). The participants included urban migrants, their rural siblings, and urban residents (n = 6555, mean age: 40.9 years) from Lucknow, Nagpur, Hyderabad, and Bangalore. Dietary information was collected using validated interviewer-administered semi-quantitative food frequency questionnaire. Other information gathered was standard of living index (14 parameters), tobacco, alcohol, physical activity, medical histories, as well as blood pressure, fasting blood and anthropometric measurements were collected. Nutrient databases were used to calculate nutrient content of regional recipes. Vegetarians ate no eggs, fish, poultry, and meat. Multivariate linear regression was used to compare the macro- and micronutrient profile of vegetarian and nonvegetarian diets. Results showed that the vegetarians (32.8%) consumed greater amounts of legumes, vegetables, roots and tubers, dairy and sugar, while nonvegetarians had a greater intake of cereals, fruits, spices, salt, fats, and oils. Vegetarians had a higher socioeconomic status, and were less likely to smoke, drink alcohol, and engage in less physical activity. Multivariate analysis showed that vegetarians consumed more carbohydrates ($\beta = 7.0$ g/day), vitamin C = 8.7 mg/day, and folate ($\beta = 8.0$ mcg/day) and lower levels of fat ($\beta = -1.6$ g/day), protein ($\beta = -6.4$ g/day), vitamin B_{12} ($\beta = -1.4$ mcg/day) and zinc ($\beta = -0.6$ mg/day). Overall, Indian vegetarian diets were found to be adequate to sustain nutritional demands according to recommended dietary allowances with less fat. Lower vitamin B_{12} bioavailability remains a concern among vegetarians.

Shridhar K, Dhillon, PK, Bowen L, et al. Nutritional profile of Indian vegetarian diets—the Indian Migration Study (IMS). Nutr J. 2014;13:55.

The **Index of Nutritional Quality (INQ)** is a method of quantitative and qualitative analysis of single foods, meals, and diets, which has special significance in assessing clinical nutritional problems. The INQ is a ratio of the nutrient-to-calorie content of foods, which may be calculated by computer and printed as bar graphs and tabular data. The number of nutrients and the nutrient standards used for analysis are flexible parameters, which may be varied for each clinical situation. Illustrative examples include INQ analysis of simple foods, an institutional house diet, the diabetic exchange list, and the diagnostic evaluation of the dietary intake of a hospitalized patient.

Calculation of Index of Nutritional Quality (INQ)

INQ = Amount of nutrient intake in 1,000 kcal ÷ recommended allowance of that nutrient in 1,000 kcal

If the INQ value is more than 1.0, the food is considered to be a good source.

Table 9.7: Foods classified on the basis of energy density.

Category of foods based on energy density	Amount of kilocalories per gram of food	Examples
Very low-energy density foods	Less than 0.6 kcal/g	Fruits like melons, vegetables like gourd vegetables
Low-energy density foods	0.6–1.5 kcal/g	Most types of fruit and vegetables, low-fat soup, low-fat curd or yogurt, skim milk, boiled rice
Medium-energy density foods	1.5–4 kcal/g	Dal, rice with dal/sambar, potato curry/sabji/sabjis containing potato/pulses/nuts like coconut/gingelly seeds/peanuts
High-energy density foods	More than 4 kcal/g	Biscuits, wafers, chocolates, butter, ghee, oil, mayonnaise

INQ = % of the recommended intake for the particular nutrient present in "X" amount of the food ÷ % energy requirement provided by the food.

If the INQ value is >0.9, the food source is said to be adequate in the given nutrient.

Nutrient density is a quantitative measure to compare the nutritional quality of a single food or food combinations relative to the recommended dietary intake. INQ may also be calculated as:

INQ= Amount of nutrient per 100 g / RDA for the nutrient under consideration ÷ energy per 100 g population average for energy intake.

If INQ value is between 2 and 6, the food is said to be a good source.

For example = nutrient density or INQ of protein from egg for a sedentary male

One egg is of 50 g and contains 6.7 g protein and 87 kcal
Adult man's RDA for protein is 60 g and for energy is 2,320 kcal

INQ =

$$\frac{\text{Ratio of protein content of egg in relation to RDA for protein}}{\text{Ratio of energy content of egg in relation to RDA for energy}}$$

$$\text{INQ} = \frac{6.7/60.0 = 0.1117}{87/2{,}320 = 0.0375} = 2.97$$

Hence, egg is said to be a good source of protein.

Foods of low-nutrient density, which provide energy in considerable amounts, are known as "empty calorie foods". Some examples of such foods are wafers, cola beverages, carbonated soft drinks, chocolates, etc. If these foods are not consumed in moderation, a person is at risk of putting on weight, becoming obese and has a high risk of developing other health problems. There are some foods, which may contain other important nutrients but are energy dense. These foods also need to be consumed in moderation.

Most of the indicators described in the preceding section are quantitative. These indicators generally require using the nutritional composition tables that give values or amounts of various nutrients present per 100 grams of edible portion of a particular food. These values are then used to calculate these indices as well as to quantify the nutrient intakes of individuals based on the amount and type of foods consumed. Individual foods or the entire day's diet can then be evaluated for adequacy of nutrients according to the recommended daily intakes or allowances and any lack/excess of nutrient that may be seen can then be corrected accordingly.

However, it is worthwhile to examine diets from qualitative perspectives that include dietary patterns, and the variety of foods included.

Across the world, nutritionists and health professionals are working on developing tools and indicators to assess diet quality especially in relation to the risk of different diseases and mortality in different populations. Many methods have been developed, with some examining the intake of nutrients, some look at food groups, and some use a combination of both. Among the various tools, the most popular ones are the Healthy Eating Index (HEI), the Diet Quality Index, the Nutrient Rich Score, the Healthy Diet Indicator, the Mediterranean Diet Score, and the Diet Diversity Score.

Healthy eating index: This uses a scoring system wherein the scores range from 0 to 100. The higher score, indicates that the diet or eating pattern or foods selected are in line or accordance with the key dietary recommendations given in the Dietary Guidelines for Americans. It measures diet quality but does not include quantity. It is a valuable tool for monitoring changes in diet patterns. The Healthy Eating Index was introduced in 1995 by the United States Department of Agriculture's (USDA) Center for Nutrition Policy and Promotion. In 2015, a new version of the Healthy Eating Index was introduced. It has been designed to align with the 2015-2020 Dietary Guidelines for Americans. In the original version, five food and nutrient groups, i.e., grains, vegetables, fruits, milk and dairy products, and meats, and each group could receive a score ranging from 0 to 10 based on the number of servings consumed from each group. Diet variety and some nutrients like total fat, saturated fat, cholesterol, and sodium, are also assigned scores varying from 0 to 10 points. The higher the score, the better the diet quality.

A 9-component Alternate Healthy Eating Index (AHEI) was designed to target food choices and macronutrient sources associated with reduced chronic disease risk. It was also developed based on dietary guidelines and the food guide pyramid proposed by the US Department of Agriculture (USDA) and emphasizes the consumption of plant foods and unsaturated oils.

The overall HEI-2015 score has 13 components that reflect the different food groups and key recommendations. Diet quality index (DQI): Originally, this index was developed to assess the intake of eight food groups and the recommendations of the Committee on Diet and Health of the National Research Council Food and Nutrition Board and of the United States government. The DQI has been revised several times DQI-aI, DQI-aII, DQI-R, and DQI-I (International). It has been used to find out the association between diet quality and morbidity and mortality. This helps in finding the link between nutrition and diet. Diet quality indicators that have been used are energy, energy density, total fat (%kcal), saturated fat (%kcal), cholesterol, sodium, fiber, calcium, simple sugars, fruits and vegetables, and dairy products.

Mediterranean diet score (MDS): "Mediterranean Diet" refers to the dietary pattern found in areas that produce olive oil in this geographic region. This diet pattern has come into focus because scientific evidence from the 1960s clearly indicates that Mediterranean populations had lower incidence of cardiovascular diseases compared to populations that consumed a "Westernized diet". Characteristically, the Mediterranean Diet contains olive oil, the main source of lipids, nonstarchy vegetables, legumes, whole grains, and fruits, including nuts; moderate intake of poultry and fish (depending on proximity to the coast); low intake of whole milk and dairy products and red meats; and low-to-moderate intake of wine as the main source of alcohol during the meals. Over time, other foods have been incorporated because more information regarding the traditional Mediterranean diet of reference has become available, which included less typical foods such as eggs, animal fats, margarine, beverages with added sugar, cakes, pies, cookies, and sugar. The MD score varies from zero, signifying minimum adherence to the traditional Mediterranean diet, to 9, meaning maximum adherence. Variations of the MDS are available such as the Mediterranean Dietary Pattern Adherence Index (MDP), Cardioprotective Mediterranean Diet Index (CARDIO), the Mediterranean Diet Quality Index (Med-DQI), and Mediterranean-Style Dietary Pattern Score (MSDPS). Many research studies have used these indices to examine the association between adherence to the Mediterranean Diet and risk of noncommunicable diseases.

The **Healthy diet indicator:** In 1990, the World Health Organization published international dietary guidelines for prevention of chronic diseases. Following this, the healthy diet indicator (HDI) was developed to quantify whether diets were aligned to these guidelines. If a person's intake was within the recommended borders, this variable was coded 1; and if the intake was outside these borders, it was coded 0, e.g., a polyunsaturated fatty acid intake of 3–7%, energy was coded as 1, and an intake below 3 or higher than 7 as 0. The HDI was calculated as the sum of 9 dichotomous variables (range 0–9).

A single food alone will not provide all nutrients; therefore it is essential to consume a variety of foods, i.e., to have diversity in the diet. Dietary diversity is the number of different foods or food groups consumed over a given reference period. Dietary diversity will help in having balanced diets and improving health outcomes, besides ensuring intakes of important micronutrients other essential functional components like fiber and antioxidants, which are protective in terms of preventing chronic/noncommunicable diseases.

RAPID FIRE

1. Define reference men and reference women.
2. Define RDA and its significance.
3. Name 3- and 5-food groups.
4. What are the dietary guidelines for Indians?
5. What do you mean by different remarks and signs given in Indian food pyramid?
6. Name four major factors, which affect RDA.
7. Define EAR, DRI, and TUL.
8. What are the steps you will follow in meal planning?
9. What do you mean by % daily value and nutrient density?
10. List the various scores or diet quality indices used. Explain for any four how the diet quality is assessed.
11. Name any four indicators used to assess nutritional quality.

EXERCISES

1. Find out your own nutrient requirements (energy, 3 macronutrients, 3 vitamins, and 3 mineral). Plan a menu for your tiffin box.
2. Plan a sample menu for a family (a man and a woman who is pregnant also) and one 4-year-old child.
3. Collect 10 food packets, write nutrition facts label on them, and assess them from nutrition point of view for different nutrients and %DV on them.
4. Calculate the nutrient density for 5 nutrients for milk and bread as per RDA of a 12-year-old girl.

SUGGESTED READING

1. Das JK, Rehana A, Kent LS, et al. Women's and adolescent nutrition: physiology, metabolism, and nutritional needs. Ann NY Acad Sci. 2017;1393:21-33.
2. Dietary Guidelines for Americans for Americans, 8th Edition; 2015-2020.
3. Dietary Guidelines for Indians—A Manual. Hyderabad, India: National Institute of Nutrition, Indian Council of Medical Research: ICMR; 2010.
4. FAO/WHO/UNU, Expert Consultation on Protein and Amino Acid Requirements in Human Nutrition. WHO Technical Report Series No.935, 2007
5. Food Safety and Standards Authority of India. (2018). Food Safety and Standards (Labelling and Display) Regulations. [online] Available from: https://currentaffairs.gktoday.in/tags/food-safety-and-standards-labelling-and-display-regulations-2018. [Last accessed August, 2019].
6. FSSAI. Draft Guidelines for making available Wholesome and Nutritious Food to School Children; 2015.
7. Gopalan C, Ramasastri BV, Balasubramanian SC, et al. Nutritive value of Indian foods. Hyderabad, India: National Institute of Nutrition, Indian Council of Medical Research; 2007.
8. Greenfield H, Southgate DAT. Food Composition Data. Production, Management and Use. Chapman and Hall, London: CEC Agro-Industrial Research; 1992.
9. Guerrero MLP and Pérez-Rodríguez FDiet Quality Indices for Nutrition Assessment: Types and Applications. 2017. DOI: 10.5772/intechopen.69807.
10. https://foodsafetyhelpline.com/fssai-drafts-the-new-labelling-and-display-regulations- 2019.
11. https://poshan.outlookindia.com/story/poshan-news-my-healthy-plate-for-the-day/348589
12. https://www.nin.res.in/downloads/My_plate_for_the_day.pdf.
13. Leitzmann C. Adequate diet of essential nutrients for healthy people. [online] Available from: http://www.eolss.net/sample-Chapters/C10/E5-01A-06-01.pdf. [Last accessed August, 2019].
14. Longvah T, Ananthan R, Bhaskarachary K, et al. Indian Food Composition Tables National Institute of Nutrition. Hyderabad, India: (Indian Council of Medical Research) Department of Health Research, Ministry of Health and Family Welfare, Government of India; 2017.
15. Murphy SP. Dietary standards in the United States. In: Bowman BA Russell RM (Eds). Present Knowledge in Nutrition, 9th edition, volume II. Washington, DC. International Life Sciences Institute; 2006. pp. 859-75.
16. Nutrient requirements and Recommended Dietary Allowances for Indians. New Delhi, India: ICMR; 2011.
17. Nutrient Requirements of Indians, Recommended Dietary Allowances, Estimated Average Requirements, A Reports of the Expert Group, 2020, Indian Council of Medical Research, National Institute of Nutrition, Department of Health Research, Ministry of Health and Family Welfare, Government of India.
18. Qadeer I, Ghosh SM, Arathi PM. (2018). Shifts in Recommended Dietary Allowances in India: The Undercurrents of Political and Scientific Logic. [online] Available from: http://csdindia.org/wp-content/uploads/2018/06/Shifts-in-Recommended-Dietary-Allowances-in-India-Prof-Imrana.pdf. [Last accessed August, 2019].
19. Shetty P. Assessing Human energy requirements. Towards National Nutrition Security, Silver Jubilee Symposium (Nov 29–Dec 1st 2004). New Delhi, India: Nutrition Foundation of India: 2004. pp. 93-100.
20. Sorenson AW, Wyse BW, Wittwer AJ, et al. An index of nutritional quality for a balanced diet. New help for an old problem. J Am Diet Assoc. 1976;68(3):236-42.
21. Source: http://www.nal.usda.gov/fnic/DRI//DRI_Energy/21-37.pdf.

22. Source: ICMR. Dietary Guidelines for Indians, A Manual, 2nd edition. Hyderabad, India: National Institute of Nutrition. 2011.
23. Swaminathan M. Advanced Textbook on Foods and Nutrition. Volume II. Bangalore, India: Bappco: The Bangalore Printing and Publishing Co. Ltd.; 2006.
24. Taylor CL, Albert J, Weisell R, et al. International Dietary Standards: FAO and WHO. In: Bowman BA, Russell RM (Eds). Present Knowledge in Nutrition, 9th edition, Volume II. Washington, DC: International Life Sciences Institute; 2006. pp. 876-87.
25. WHO. A healthy diet sustainably produced. information sheet; 2018.
26. World Health Organization/Food and Agriculture Organization (WHO/FAO). A model for establishing upper levels of intake for nutrients and related substances. Report of a Joint FAO/WHO Technical Workshop on Nutrient Risk Assessment. Geneva: WHO/FAO; 2006.
27. Younger KM. Dietary reference standards. In: Gibney MJ, Vorster HH, Kok FJ (Eds). Introduction to Human Nutrition. The Nutrition Society Textbook Series. Oxford, UK: Blackwell Publishing; 2002.

10

CHAPTER

Food Exchanges

KEY CONCERNS
- What are food exchanges, food groups, and serving size?
- What is the role of food exchanges in meal planning?
- How much is one serving size of each food group?
- How is the standardization of recipes done?

KEY CONCEPTS
- Food exchanges given by national and international bodies
- Role of food exchanges in meal planning
- Serving size and standardization of serving size

INTRODUCTION

Diet and nutrition are crucial in promotion and maintenance of good health in each life stage. Both are equally important during illness, particularly in chronic diseases. Once noncommunicable diseases like diabetes and hypertension set in, it is essential to make dietary modifications for the rest of one's life irrespective of age, sex, socioeconomic status, and geographic region. Food habits differ from one community to another, between countries and from one region to another within a country. However, nutritional requirements are similar for specific age, sex, and health condition, within the same country. Nobody would like to eat a monotonous diet for a long time even if he or she is prescribed some dietary modifications or restrictions.

Human beings have an inherent desire to have variety of foods in their diet and even when a person is ill, he/she would like to eat foods as per their liking. Dietary changes during short illness are usually manageable, but in chronic diseases like diabetes, cardiovascular or kidney disease, etc., people find difficulty to accept changes in their regular dietary pattern especially if there are drastic changes in their diets. Dieticians/medical nutrition therapists have grouped or categorized commonly consumed food items and food preparations, so that a healthy as well as sick person can have variety, enjoy his/her food, and still meet the nutritional requirements.

It promotes eating appropriate foods and speeds up the recovery because patients often neglect foods that them but are not of their liking. Therefore we need to offers alternatives that will help them obtain good nutrition through eating healthy foods. This can be done by exchanging the food item with similar nutrient profile, e.g., rice for wheat and curd or cheese for plain milk.

The food exchange system is useful in planning different meals not only for normal healthy individuals but also for sick persons. As the name suggests, food exchanges provide alternative choices of foods with similar nutritional composition. Foods from different regions and cultures can easily be accommodated by varying the quantity of food, substituting ingredients and method of cooking.

FOOD EXCHANGES

Everyone requires a nutritionally adequate diet but everybody is not aware of his/her nutritional requirements. To a certain extent, dietary guidelines help them select the foods necessary for a balanced diet. Since, it is often difficult to fulfill one's needs as well as the desire for eating variety of foods; the food exchange system was developed to help overcome this challenge.

In 1950, the American Diabetes Association and American Dietetic Association and the United States Public Health Service collaboratively developed a system of listing foods to help diabetic persons to select foods from a given food basket, monitor portion size, as well as monitor and maintain nearly consistent intakes of calories, carbohydrates, protein, and fat. In India, the National Institute of Nutrition, Indian Dietetic Association (IDA), and other academic institutions have recently grouped food items with specific portion size. The list is called "food exchange".

Food exchange list is an appropriate tool for effective nutrition education, intended for improving nutrition knowledge, attitudes, and dietary behaviors both at individual and community levels. The meal planning food exchange list, formulated in 1950, is a tool that allows the dietitian/patient interchange of foods within a particular food group, so as to provide flexibility and ensure better adherence to the dietary regime in relation to the management of disease. The food exchange list has undergone five revisions to keep pace with the current developments in food, nutrition, and its relationship to health and is still considered the most appropriate tool for management of noncommunicable disease like diabetes mellitus and cardiovascular diseases (CVD).

> A **food exchange** is listing of the foods in one group with specified amount of food (weight/volume). Foods in a given group have similar content of a given nutrient, i.e., similar amount of carbohydrate or fat or protein as the other foods included in the list.

This amount is generally acceptable in the form of approximate consumable portion size and it is convenient to assess the nutritional value. The specified amount of a food is considered as its serving size, although the amount in a serving differs from one food item to another. Multiples and/or fractions of the serving size can be used in planning diets as per the requirement of the individual. Many a times household measures are used, how much they are equivalent in grams and mL is shown in Figure 10.1.

Importance of Food Exchanges in Meal Planning

Food exchange system is based on principles of good nutrition and still encourages and facilitates the consumption of a wide variety of foods of the individual's own choice. It is an educational tool, which helps individuals to eat more balanced diets. Exchange means substitution. If a nutritionally appropriate food is not preferred or not available then another food with similar nutritional content can be chosen instead.

Foods are categorized in different food groups. An exchange system works on the standard amounts of different foods that provide similar nutrient(s) content and calories or same nutrients and different quantity of different food items, e.g., 25 g of barley or oats or 1 chapati will provide 80 kcal and 1–3.5 g protein and to obtain 40 kcals from fruits, either 20 grapes or ½ of a big apple can be selected. Sometimes, it is also necessary to restrict or add a particular food depending upon the health or disease condition and then another food can replace the food that needs to be restricted.

Foods planners can select, mix, and match foods from each exchange list, as per food preferences and cost, and still have equivalent nutritional value. It is usually used in dietary management for weight control, diabetes, and other conditions.

The requirements for total calorie and other nutrients must be assessed first from the RDA table given in Table 9.1A. This is applicable to healthy persons. In case of persons with some disorder or disease condition(s), the estimation of energy requirement is done differently. Variety and moderation are necessary for balanced and palatable meals. Food exchanges are handy tools that help to simplify diet planning. Food exchanges help to:

- Maintain the quantity of food, and provide a balanced meal.
- Provide the required amounts of macronutrients including energy.
- Break the monotony in the meals, provide variety and flexibility in the diet, and make the diet interesting.
- Regulate the nutrient intake particularly carbohydrates by diabetic person and protein by cases with kidney transplant, sports, malnutrition, etc.
- Equate to real portion sizes.

> **Research Glimpse:** There is need to plan nutritionally adequate vegan diets for children, so that their requirements for growth and development can safely be met. Sometimes, it seems difficult but increased number and availability of natural and fortified vegan foods help achieve the goal for children. Food exchange methodology ensures the adequate supply of key nutrients and also accurate, reliable, and easy-to-use meal planning tools. Daily portions of each food exchange group have been calculated, so the resulting menu provides at least 90% of the Dietary Reference Intakes (DRIs) of protein, iron, zinc, calcium, and n-3 fatty acids for each age group, sex, and physical activity level. These diets do not provide enough vitamin B-12 and vitamin D; hence, fortified plant drinks, breakfast cereals, or plant protein-rich products could provide these two vitamins. This tool can be used to plan healthful and balanced vegan diets for children and adolescents.
>
> *Menal-Puey S, Martínez-Biarge M, Marques-Lopes I. Developing a Food Exchange System for Meal Planning in Vegan Children and Adolescents. Nutrients. 2018;11(1):E43.*

FOOD EXCHANGE LISTS

Food exchanges have been developed by many organizations. Here in this chapter, food exchanges (revised version) by the Indian Dietetic Association (IDA) (2018) are given. These are being practiced in many educational institutes and clinical practice.

Most food exchanges are designed on the basis of food groups. One type of exchange list is where carbohydrates or protein or fat are kept constant and approximate amount of the food/ portion size is varied. Foods which are rich in protein, are grouped as milk, meat, and nuts and oil seeds. Carbohydrate is mainly contributed by cereals, pulses, roots and tubers, and sugars. Vegetables and fruits are categorized in various ways, where calories are used as the basis for calculation.

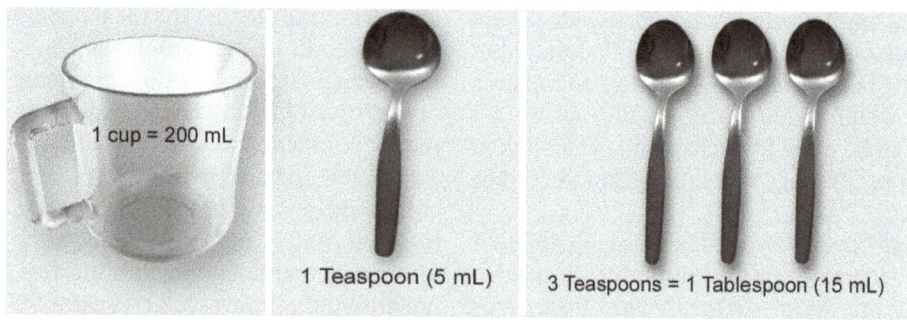

Fig. 10.1: Household measures.

Food Exchanges

Food Exchange Lists

- Cereal exchange
- Pulse exchange
- Milk exchange
- Meat/cheese exchange
- Marine exchange
- Egg exchange
- Nut exchange
- Fruit exchange
- Vegetable exchanges—group A, B, and C
- Fat exchanges
- Sugar exchanges

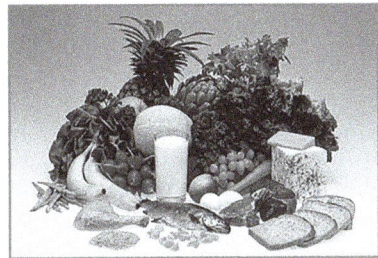

Cereal Exchanges

Cereal exchange implies that all edible foods prepared from cereals like wheat, rice, bread, etc. can be exchanged/substituted for each other. For example 1/2 cup of cooked rice will provide the similar amount of nutrients as 1 idli or one small dosa or 2 slices of bread (Table 10.1 and Fig. 10.2). For example, if 6 exchanges of cereals in a day have been prescribed, while planning a meal, the food preparations that can be included at different meals in the day are shown. On different days and different meals, different food items can be consumed. Each of following item can be exchanged with another.

For example:

Breakfast:	1 slice of bread	= 1 exchange
Lunch:	½ cup cooked rice + 1 chapati	= 2 exchanges
Evening snack:	1 idli	= 1 exchange
Dinner:	2 chapatis	= 2 exchanges

Table 10.1: Cereal exchanges.

1 cereal exchange = 13–21 g carbohydrate, 1–3.5 g protein, 80–94 kcal, fat 0–2.0 g, fiber = 1–4 g		
Food items	**Raw (g)**	**Approximately cooked weight**
Barley	25	1 C
Bread (white)	–	25 (1 slice)
Cornflakes	25 (5 tablespoons)	–
Dosa flour (dry) (cereal:pulse—4:1)	25	1 medium
Idli flour (dry) (cereal:pulse—4:1)	25	1 large
Oats	25	Depends on the recipe
Quinoa	25	Depends on the recipe
Rice flakes (dry)	25 (2 tablespoons)	1/3 C
Rice, raw milled	25 (2 tablespoons)	½ C
Vermicelli	25	½ C
Whole wheat flour	25	One chapati (medium size)
Sooji	25 (2 tablespoons)	75
Ragi flour	25 (3½ tablespoons)	75
Sago	25 (3 tablespoons)	75
Noodles	25	75
Rice, puffed/flakes	–	1 cup
Potato	100	–
Yam	75	–
Sweet potato	75	–
Colocasia	100	–
Tapioca	50	–

Millets are also consumed like cereals and now referred as nutricereals. It includes finger millet (ragi), Kodo millets (type of rice), little finger millet (sama rice), Pearl millet (bajra) and Sorghum (jowar). One millet exchange is 25 g in raw form and ½ cup in cooked form and provides 15.5–17 g carbohydrates, 2–3 g protein, 78–87 kcal, 0.5–1.5 fat and 2–3 g fiber. Consumption of millets also provide much more vitamins, minerals and several bioactive substances

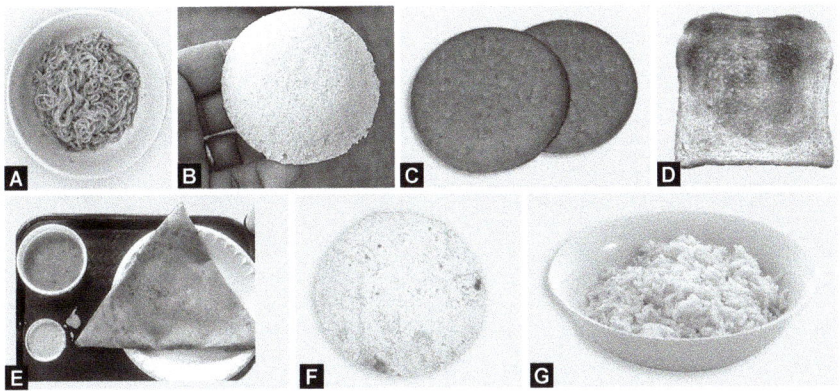

Figs. 10.2A to G: Cereal exchange items. A. 1 cup noodles; B. 1 idli; C. 2 marie biscuits; D. 1 bread slice; E. 1 plain dosa; F. 1 chapati; G. 1/2 c cooked rice.

protecting health, e.g., ragi provide extra calcium. These millets are also useful when gluten rich grains are restricted in certain health conditions.

Sago exchange: 25 g of sago provides 85 kcal and 22 g carbohydrates but no other nutrients present in other foods from cereal exchange.

Pulse Exchanges

Pulse exchange is used for any type of whole pulse or dehusked pulse (dal). Hence, two types of pulse exchanges are mentioned here because both provide different values of calories and nutrients. The same can be used for various forms like sprouted pulses or pulse flour. For an adult, usually 2–3 pulse exchanges are included. The three exchanges can be 1 cup of cooked dal, which is equal to 2 exchanges that can be given at one meal of the day and sprouts can be given in another meal (Table 10.2).

Soybean exchange is of 20 g and ½ cup of cooked portion providing 2.0 g carbohydrate, 8.0 g protein, 75 kcal, 4.0 g fat and 4.5 g fiber.

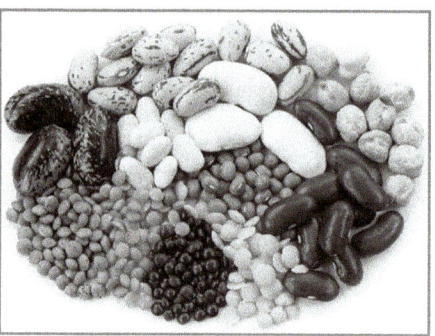

Milk Exchanges

The amount of liquid milk is different from milk powder, (Table 10.3) e.g., 100 mL liquid milk is equivalent to 28 g of skim milk powder. The importance of milk exchange lies in its low carbohydrate content and that these foods are good sources of other essential nutrients such as protein and calcium.

Table 10.3: Milk exchanges.

One milk exchange = 6.0–8.5 g carbohydrate, 4.0–6.0 g protein, 110 kcal, 6.5–7.5 g fat and no fiber		
Item	Amount (mL)	Household measure
Buffalo's milk	100	½ cup
Cow's milk	150	¾ cup
Curd (cow's milk)	185 g	<1 cup
One skimmed milk exchange = 14.0–16.0 g carbohydrate, 9.0–11.0 g protein, 100 kcal, negligible fat and no fiber		
Item	Amount (mL)	Household measure
Skimmed milk	350	1¾ cup
Skimmed milk powder	38 g	5½ teaspoons

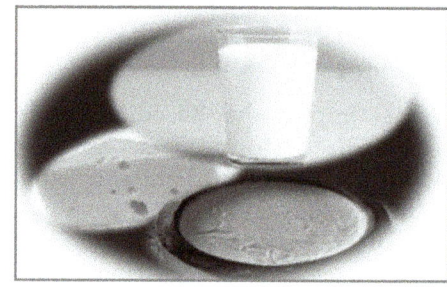

Non-vegetarian Exchange

It includes chicken and poultry and other some of the non-vegetarian foods generally consumed described in Tables 10.4 and 10.5. This exchange does not provide carbohydrate and fiber but good amount of protein and fat. In terms of energy supply it is rather same with one exchange of egg,

Table 10.2: Pulse exchanges.

1 Pulse exchange = 12–14 g carbohydrate, 5.5–6.0 g protein, 81–83 kcal, 0.0–1.5 g fat and 2–4 g fiber		
Item	Amount (g)	Household measure
Bengal gram dal	25	½ cup cooked
Black gram dal	25	½ cup cooked
Green gram dal	25	½ cup cooked
Lentil dal	25	½ cup cooked
Red gram dal	25	½ cup cooked
1 Whole pulse exchange = 10–14.5 g carbohydrate, 5.0–6.0 g protein, 69–83 kcal, 0.0–1.0 g fat and 2–6.5 g fiber		
Item	Amount (g)	Household measure
Bengal gram	25	ND
Black gram	25	ND
Green gram	25	ND
Lentil	25	ND
Red gram	25	ND

Table 10.4: Meat exchange.

1 Meat exchange = negligible; carbohydrate, 11.0–13.0 g protein, 84–91 kcal, 4.0–5.0 fat and no fiber		
Item	Amount (g)	Cooked portion
Beef, chops	65	–
Chicken, poultry, breast skinless	50	ND
Goat, chops	65	ND

(ND: not done)

Table 10.5: Marine food exchange.

Marine food exchange = negligible carbohydrate, 13.0–19.0 g protein, 85 kcal, 1.0–3.0 fat and no fiber		
Item	Amount (g)	Cooked weight
Sea crab	125	–
Mackerel	85	–
Pomfret black	69	–
Prawn small	120	–
Tuna	76	–

fish, even one exchange of vegetarian foods like nuts, pulses and cereals. Variation is found in other nutrients. One egg is equal to 50 g meat and 75 g of fish as well as 25 g of pulse or 25 g of cereals.

One egg weight approximate 50 g and is considered as one **egg exchange,** which provides negligible amount of carbohydrate, 6.6 g protein, 85 kcal, 6.5 fat and no fiber.

Vegetable Exchanges

A wide variety of vegetables is available, especially in India, with different vegetables being available in different seasons. Vegetables differ considerably in the amount (weight and volume) of edible portion (per 100 g) and nutritional content. Commonly consumed vegetables have been grouped into three: (1) group A, (2) group B, and (3) group C. Both groups include approximately 100 g of raw vegetables or ¼–¾ cup of cooked vegetables. But group A and group C provide half the calories (30 kcal) compared to group B (50–60 kcal). Group B vegetables also provide more carbohydrates, especially starch and some proteins. Table 10.6 gives the list of vegetables in groups A, B, and C. Essentially, group A consists of leafy vegetables, group B comprises roots and tubers, and group C consists of other vegetables. If a particular vegetable is not available in some seasons or in geographical area, other choices are available.

Table 10.6: Green leafy vegetables.

Group A: One green leafy vegetables exchange = 2.0–5.0 carbohydrate, 2.5–4.5 g protein, 34–36 kcal, <1.0 fat and 9.0 g fiber		
Food ingredients	Raw weight (g)	Cooked portion (cups)
Agathi leaves	50	¼ cup
Amaranth leaves	115	½ cup
Cabbage green	160	¾ cup
Cauliflower greens	100	½ cup
Coriander leaves	110	½ cup
Curry leaves	55	¼ cup
Drumstick leaves	50	¼ cup
Fenugreek leaves	100	½ cup
Lettuce	160	¾ cup
Mint	95	½ cup
Mustard leaves	115	½ cup
Radish leaves	135	¾ cup
Spinach	145	¾ cup
Group B: Roots and tuber exchange = 8.0–12.0 carbohydrate, 0.5–3.0 g protein, 48–54 kcal, <1.0 fat and 1.0–6.5 g fiber		
Food ingredients	Raw weight (g)	Cooked portion (cups)
Beetroot	140	¾ cup
Carrot (orange)	150	¾ cup
Carrot (red)	130	¾ cup
Colocasia	55	¼ cup
Onion (big)	100	½ cup
Potato (brown skin big)	75	<½ cup
Sweet potato (pink skin)	50	<½ cup
Radish (round, white skin)	160	<¾ cup
Tapioca	65	<½ cup
Yam	60	<½ cup

Contd...

Contd...

Group C: Other vegetables exchange = 2.0–6.0 carbohydrate, 0.5–4.0 g protein, 28–30 kcal, <1.0 fat and 1.5–7.5 g fiber		
Food ingredients	Raw weight (g)	Cooked portion (cups)
Ash Gourd	170	¾ cup
Beans (scarlet, tender)	70	<½ cup
Bitter gourd (ridges, long)	145	¾ cup
Bottle gourd (elongated)	270	<1½ cup
Brinjal all varieties	120	½ cup
Broad beans	100	½ cup
Capsicum (green)	185	<1 cup
Cauliflower	130	>½ cup
Cho-cho–marrow	160	¾ cup
Corn (baby)	40	<½ cup
Cucumber (elongated)	150	¾ cup
Drumstick	100	<½ cup
French bean	125	½ cup
Knol-khol	190	¾ cup
Kovai (big)	170	¾ cup
Ladies finger	110	<½ cup
Mango green (raw)	60	<½ cup
Parwar	125	<½ cup
Plantain flower	140	<½ cup
Plantain green	35	<½ cup
Plantain stem	75	<½ cup
Pumpkin (green cylindrical)	120	½ cup
Pumpkin (orange, round)	130	½ cup
Ridge gourd (turai)	230	2 cup
Snake gourd	240	<2½ cup
Tinda	200	1 cup
Tomato green	220	¾ cup
Tomato ripe, red (hybrid)	160	<1½ cup
Tomato ripe local	155	<1½ cup
Zucchini (green)	150	¾ cup

Nut Exchanges

Nut exchanges are given in Table 10.7. Since nuts are rich in protein and good quality of fat and low in carbohydrates hence they are good source of nutrients especially for vegetarians. Nuts also vary in size thus measured in different quantities.

Fruits Exchange

Fruits vary much more in their size and amount of edible portion. With the food exchange system, it is possible to get an estimate of the edible portion of watermelon that is equivalent to a specific number of grapes, e.g., one slice of watermelon is approximately equal to 20 grapes or 2 plums or ½ banana. It provides fewer calories, i.e., 40 kcal and this energy is mainly obtained from carbohydrates (simple sugars, mostly fructose). Fruits usually do not contain fat and protein, one of the exceptions being avocado 4 grams of fat (Table 10.8).

Table 10.7: Nut exchange.

Group nuts exchange = 1.0–4.0 carbohydrate, 1.0–4.0 g protein, 83–87 kcal, 6.0–9.0 fat and 1.0–2.0 fiber		
Food ingredients	Raw weight (g)	Quantity
Almond	14.0	12 numbers
Cashew	14.5	6 numbers
Coconut Kernel, fresh (grated)	21.0	4 teaspoons
Groundnut	16.0	20 numbers
Pistachio	16.0	24 numbers
Walnut	13.0	5 numbers

Table 10.8: Fruit exchange.

One fruit exchange = 40 calories, 10 g carbohydrates		
Item	Rounded of weight (g)	Size/numbers
Apple	70	½ big
Apricot (dried)	15	–
Avocado (fruit)	25	–
Banana (poovan)	40	½ medium
Banana (ripe red)	40	–
Cherries	70	–
Custard apple	40	1 medium
Dates (processed)	15	2 numbers
Fig	50	–
Gooseberry	170	–
Grapes (seeded, green)	75	18–20 numbers
Grapes (seeded, black)	70	–
Guava pink flesh	90	–
Guava white flesh	125	1 medium
Jackfruit ripe	50	3 numbers
Jambu ripe	70	12 numbers
Lime (sweet pulp)	150	–
Litchi	75	–
Musk melon (orange flesh)	175	4–5 slices
Orange	110	1 medium
Papaya, ripe	170	4 thin long slices
Pear	110	1 medium
Pineapple	100	1 thick slice
Plum	70	5 numbers
Sapota	60	½ big
Strawberries	170	–
Tamarind pulp	15	3 teaspoons
Watermelon	200 g	1 big slice

Regional variations are seen in terms of the size and shape of the food ingredients particularly fruits. Since there are many recipes and methods to cook the food, hence, the quantity of cooked food is an approximate quantity.

Fat Exchanges

One gram of all types of fat/oil provides 9 kcal and each fat source can be taken as 10 g in one fat exchange. Butter gives only 72 kcal/10 g due to presence of moisture in it. Rest of the edible fats and oils gives 90 kcal/10g. However, because of their physical nature, their amount in household measures may vary, e.g., 3 teaspoons of oil will be equal to 2 teaspoons of solid fat like ghee. One exchange of fat in terms of household measure of 2 teaspoons that is equal to 10 g. It is same for butter, cows ghee, hydrogenated oil and cooking oil. It provides 8–10 g fat, 72–90 kcal. There is no carbohydrates, protein or fiber in it.

Sugar Exchange

It includes honey, jaggery and refined sugar. Since sugar is simple carbohydrate and one gram carbohydrate gives 4 kcal. One teaspoon of sugar contain 5 grams sugar hence using one teaspoon of sugar add 20 kcal and no other nutrients. Jaggery and honey contain some moisture and other nutrients. Hence one sugar exchange provides 16-20 kcal.

The **American Dietetic Association and the American Diabetes Association (2003)** has given simplified exchange lists, where they have categorized foods into three main groups: 1. Carbohydrate group; 2. Meat and meat substitutes group; 3. Fat group.

One serving in the group of starches contains 80 calories, 15 grams (g) of carbohydrates, 3 g of protein, and 1 g of fat. Beans, peas, and lentils are starches, but they are counted as one starch plus one lean meat exchange. The serving sizes vary because of the variety of foods. Each serving in the fruit group has 60 calories, 15 g of carbohydrates, and no protein or fat. Vegetables provide 25 calories, 2 g of protein, 5 g of carbohydrates and no fat. Vegetable serving sizes are 1/2 cup cooked and 1 cup of raw vegetables. Salad greens are considered as a free food that can be eaten any time. Sweets and desserts are allowed as long as they are eaten with a meal, so they do not cause a large spike in blood sugar. Table 10.9 gives the amount of nutrients including kilocalories from different foods in each group.

Carbohydrate group: This includes exchange lists for starches, nonstarchy vegetables, and other carbohydrates. The starches list includes exchanges for bread, cereal, peas, beans, and lentils (pulses and legumes), starchy vegetables, soups, crackers and snacks, and other starches.
1. When selecting from foods from this group, it is wise to choose starch-containing foods with little fat.
2. If starchy foods are prepared with fat, it is important to note that such a preparation is to be counted as one starch and one fat serving.
3. Other starches are the less nutritious foods and it is advised that a person use them occasionally as part of a planned meal or as a snack.

Table 10.9: Nutrients including kilocalories from different foods in each group.

Groups/Lists	Carbohydrate (g)	Protein (g)	Fat (g)	Energy (kcals)
Carbohydrate group				
Starches	15	3	0–1	80
Fruit	15	–	–	60
Milk				
Fat-free/low fat (1/2–1% fat)	12	8	0–3	90
Reduced fat (2% fat)	12	8	5	120
Whole	12	8	8	150
Other carbohydrates	15	Vary	Vary	Vary
Nonstarchy vegetables	5	2	–	25
Meat and meat substitutes				
Very lean	–	7	0–1	35
Lean	–	7	3	55
Medium-fat	–	7	5	75
High fat	–	7	8	100
Fat group	–	–	5	45

Source: American Dietetic Association; American Diabetes Association. Exchange Lists for Weight Management and Exchange Lists for Meal Planning. 2003.

4. It should be noted that pulses and legumes are regarded as meat substitutes because of their protein content.
5. Foods included in this list are normally considered for carbohydrate counting.
6. Fruits include fresh, frozen, canned, dried fruits and fruit juices. It is advisable to consume whole fruits since they are a source of fiber. When selecting fruit juices, care should be taken to select those that do not contain added sugar. If fruits canned in sugar syrup are used, the juice from the can should be completely drained. Also, fruits canned in heavy syrup should be avoided.
7. Many processed and packaged foods such as breakfast cereals, fruit juices, and other foods contain sugar. It is important to study the label information and note the amount of sugar present. This should be taken into account and the serving size should be adjusted accordingly.
8. Different types of milk are available. Other milk products like cheese, paneer, and khoa will be considered as meat substitutes because of the protein content.
9. Other milk-based foods such as ice cream, condensed milk, fruit yogurt, milkshakes, thandai, sweetened curds, and Indian sweets like barfi are to be considered in the carbohydrate group because of the sugar content. Note: Many of these are likely to be concentrated sources of carbohydrate, fat, perhaps saturated fat and trans fat; hence, the portion size should be selected accordingly.
10. Baked food items, such as cakes, cookies, nankhatai, biscuits, and pastries, contain refined flour, have saturated fat, and are likely to contain trans fats.
11. All foods mentioned in points 8–10 are likely to contain simple carbohydrates and less amount of fiber. In contrast, cereals (except rice) and millets will supply complex carbohydrates.
12. Starchy vegetables like potato, sweet potato, colocasia root, tapioca, yam, green peas, corn, plantain (raw banana), corn, mixed vegetables with corn, plantain, and pumpkin are separately listed.
13. Items such as sugar-free puddings, sherbets, some cakes, noodles, and pancakes are included in the carbohydrate group in the "other starches" list.
14. Nonstarchy vegetables include vegetables such as beans, broccoli, beets, cabbage, cauliflower, celery, carrot, cucumber, brinjal, green onion/onion stalk, lady finger, capsicum, radish, lettuce, spinach, tomato, turnip, water chestnut, pumpkin, zucchini, and gourd vegetables.
15. All sweets and desserts, including cakes, chocolates, puddings, are listed under "Other Carbohydrates". These should be consumed occasionally.
16. Various preparations are made in India using different combinations, which include cereal and vegetable, vegetable and pulse, or such vegetables with potato. Sometimes, high amount of oil may be used. Hence, the portion size for carbohydrate group and fat group should be calculated accordingly.
17. Products that are labeled as sugar-free may contain a nutritive sweetener or an artificial sweetener/sugar substitute. The carbohydrate and calorie content of these should be taken into account.

Meat and Meat Substitutes

The milk category is subdivided according to the amount of fat (0–8 g) and calories (100–160). Otherwise, one serving has 12 g of carbohydrate and 8 g of protein. Each serving in the meat category is about 1 ounce and provides 7 g of protein, but this group is also subdivided into lean (0–3 g of fat and 45 calories), medium-fat (4–7 g of fat and 75 calories) and high-fat (8 or more g of fat and 100 calories) proteins.

- Although meat, fish, and poultry are good sources of protein, at the same time, meat and poultry are high in fat, particularly saturated fat, and they also contain cholesterol and no fiber.
- For vegetarians, pulses and legumes are good meat substitutes. In contrast to meat and meat products, they do not contain saturated fat or cholesterol but contain fiber.
- Milk and milk products are good substitutes for meat.
- It is wise, therefore, to trim the fat from meat (use lean meat).
- Some processed meats or meat products, soy products or seafood, especially if the preparation contains bread, flour, etc. may contribute some carbohydrate to the diet if they are consumed in large amounts.
- It is advisable to consume high-fat protein food sources not more than three times in a week.
- Fat should be removed from the meat before cooking.

Fat Group

- One exchange is based on a serving size containing 5 g of fat and provides 45 kcalories.

- All fats/oils are high in calories; hence, it is advisable to limit the number of servings.
- Nuts and seeds, like melon seeds, sunflower seeds, pumpkin seeds, and gingelly seeds, contain considerable amount of fat.
- The fat composition of nuts and seeds is beneficial for health. Also, they provide a number of other important nutrients.
- Other foods such as peanut butter, salad dressings, sesame paste (tahini), avocado, olives, mayonnaise, coconut fresh and dry, dairy creamer, margarine, bread spread, cheese spread, and nut butters/paste all contain fat and hence the portion size should be calculated accordingly.
- When selecting oils/fats, it is advisable to choose those containing MUFA and PUFA instead of saturated fats/hydrogenated fats.
- Besides these visible sources, it is very important to remember that many foods contain invisible fat.
- Many processed and ready-to-cook and ready-to-eat foods, sweets, and savouries contain hidden fat.
- Many sugar-free food items like sweets do contain considerable amount of fat.
- Many foods are labeled as "low-fat" or "fat-free". For such foods, the label information must be checked.

Free Foods

According to the American Dietetic Association and American Diabetes Association, "A free food is any food or drink contains less than 20 kcals or less than 5 grams of carbohydrate per serving". Foods such as diabetic jam should be limited to 3 servings per day and should be spread over the entire day, rather than consuming them all at one time because it can raise the blood sugar level. However, for foods without a serving size, e.g., diet soft drinks, can be consumed whenever desired (Table 10.10).

In 2008 the American Dietetic Association and the American Diabetes Association has published a practical guideline entitled "Choose your foods: Exchange lists for diabetics".

Food exchange groups now includes, (1) Carbohydrates, (2) Meat and meat substitute, (3) Fat, (4) Free foods, (5) Combination foods, (6) Fast foods and (7) Alcohol.

Choose your foods was published by the American Dietetic Association and the American Diabetes Association in 2008 for diabetics.

The booklet was developed through an online survey of 14,000 members of the American Dietetic Association and American Diabetic Association. The basic philosophy of these guidelines more or less is the same as the previous editions. It is intended to be used as a basis for nutrition education materials. It includes carbohydrate counting, weight management, and also helps students to learn about diabetes meal planning.

Color codes as seen in the book cover have been used to separate food groups. Brown color represents starches, orange represents fruits, blue is for milk, green is for vegetables, red for meat and meat substitutes, and yellow is for fats (Fig. 10.3).

Table 10.10: List of free foods.

Foods with defined serving size	Foods without defined serving size
Non-dairy creamer (2 T powder)	Sugar-free chewing gum
Fat-free cream cheese (1 T)	Carbonated or mineral water
Fat-free mayonnaise (1 T)	Club soda
Reduced fat/low-fat bread spread (1 T)	Sugar-free diet soft drinks
Fat-free/low-fat salad dressing (1 T)	Black coffee without sugar
Whipped Toppings—Regular (1 T)—Fat free (2 T)	Black tea without sugar
Sugar-free hard candy—1 piece	Jal-jeera
Light jam or jelly (dietetic, sugar free)—(2 T)	Seasonings
Unsweetened cocoa powder (1 T)	
Ketchup (1 T)	
Soy sauce (1 T)	
Yogurt (2 T)	
Salsa (¼ cup)	
Chutneys (1 T)	

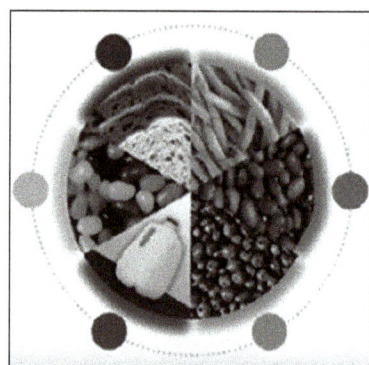

Fig. 10.3: Chose your foods: Exchange lists for diabetes.

It is aimed at helping both type 1 and type 2 diabetics to meet the following goals:
- Achieve and maintain blood glucose close to the normal range
- Have a lipid profile that decreases the risk for vascular disease
- Maintain normal blood pressure or it should be close to normal.

The booklet includes specific guidelines:
- Fiber intake should be close to the recommended adequate intake—14 g/1,000 kcal.
- Saturated fat intake should be limited to <7% of total caloric intake.
- Trans fat intake should be minimum.
- Sodium intake should be <2,300 mg/day.

Specific recommendations have been included to increase the use of fruits, vegetables, whole grains, legumes, low-fat dairy products and lean meat.

Some of the changes include:
- The "starch + fat" category has been deleted from the starch list.
- A "dairy-like products" category (e.g., soy and rice milks, smoothies) has been added to the Milk List.
- Leafy greens have been moved to the free foods list from the nonstarchy vegetable list.
- Very lean meats have been integrated into the lean meat list, and a new category has been added to the meats and meats substitute group, the plant-based protein list.
- Several lists (sweets, desserts and other carbohydrates, combination foods, and fast foods) have been subdivided for ease of use.
- An alcohol list has been added to provide adults who choose to drink with information (in alcohol equivalents) about calories and carbohydrates.
- High-sodium foods and foods that are good sources of fiber have been flagged to bring these to the attention of users.
- Sodium: If a food contains >480 mg sodium/serving or if a main dish/meal contains >600 mg/serving, it is flagged.
- Good sources of fiber are flagged: To be classified as a good source, the food should provide 10–19% of the dietary reference intake for fiber and if a food contains more than 3 g fiber per serving, it is flagged.
- Similarly, starch with added fat is flagged.
- Carbohydrate choices are based on the fact that foods included in the starch, fruit, and milk lists of carbohydrate group contain similar amount of carbohydrate, i.e., approximately 15 g and provide approximately 80 kcal/serving and therefore these foods can be interchanged, although attention should be paid to some nutrients like calcium that are provided by milk but not by other foods.
- Some adults consume alcohol. On daily consumption it should be taken care as it contributes the calorie intake. However, if it is occasional intake, its calorie consideration may be avoided.

Carbohydrate Counting

Carbohydrate (carb) counting is a good strategy for nutritional management of diabetes mellitus. It is well established and helps improve glycemic control and maintain blood glucose control near normal. It helps improve the metabolic profile and thus to reduce the risk of developing diabetes complications and to improve the quality of life. Patients can be taught how to evaluate the carb content of a food/meal and exchanges. Carb counting facilitates adherence to prescribed diets while allowing flexibility in choosing a variety of foods.

Carbohydrate counting was first created in Europe in 1935 and was later recommended worldwide, in 1995, by the American Diabetic Association. Importance is given to the amount of carbohydrate intakes, although it must be borne in mind that conversion of 100 g of carbohydrate can vary from as little as 15 minutes to 2 hours. Carb counting can be used by both type 1 and type 2 diabetic patients.

It is essential for the patient to know the amount of carbohydrates that he/she can consume at each meal and based on the carb count, they can choose the foods. Carb counting can be basic or advanced. Whether the basic counting or advanced carb counting method is used depends on the patient's lifestyle, daily routine, and whether he/she is on insulin. Carb counting is absolutely necessary for those using insulin pump. One can also use both methods simultaneously. Figure 10.4 and Table 10.11 give the salient points of basic and advanced carb counting methods.

A four-step process is followed:

Step 1: Calculate the total carb intake allowed per day [based on the calculation: 50–60% of total energy intake should be supplied by carbohydrate, 15–20% from protein (1 g per kilogram of body weight) and 25–40% is to be obtained from fat].

Step 2: Count the total carbs in grams or carb choices (1 carb choice is equivalent to 15 g of carbohydrates)

Step 3: Distribute the day's total carbs between the meals consumed in a day

Step 4: Plan the list of foods as per the carb equivalents.

> For patients on insulin, the insulin : carb ratio should be borne in mind. 1 unit of insulin is needed to metabolize 15 g of carbohydrate.

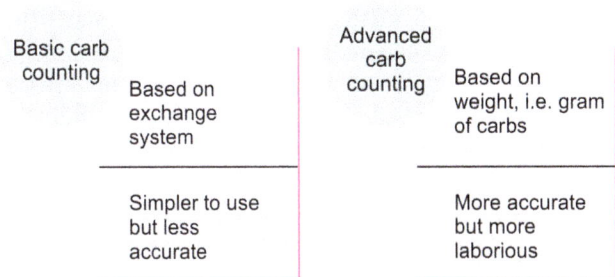

Fig. 10.4: Basic and advanced carb counting.

Table 10.11: Methods of basic and advanced carb counting.

Basic carb counting	Advanced carb counting
Foods are divided into groups	Based on the nutritive value database
1 carb choice is equivalent to 15 g carb per serving	The basic steps are similar to those used in basic carb counting
Can substitute foods within groups or between groups	To do this, information is required about pre- and postprandial blood glucose monitoring. It is necessary to know the insulin sensitivity factor and meal bolus
Helps to have more diversity in terms of food choice	The advantage is that the insulin dose can be administered according to the carb content in the meal
The figure of 15 grams per carb choice is not very rigid, it can vary between 8 g and 22 g of carbohydrate	Allows flexibility according to the patients' mealtimes, appetite, and variability in exercise and physical activity regimes
More useful for patients with type 2 diabetes, those who are not on insulin	Suitable for persons on insulin, i.e., type 1 diabetics
—	Can estimate how much fast-acting insulin is required, need to know about basal rate and bolus rate

Intake of fiber and protein needs to be taken into account:
- Fiber decreases absorption of carbohydrates. Therefore, while doing meal planning, the fiber content of the recipe/preparation must be calculated and this should be subtracted from the total carbohydrate content of the recipe.
- About 35–60% of protein is converted to glucose. The carbs equivalent in the protein must be calculated and taken into account when counting carbs.

Portion Size and Serving Size

Portion is the amount of food a person chooses to eat at one sitting, whether it is a meal or a snack or beverage. It depends upon the liking or availability and can vary, especially in commercial food establishments. Thus in some food outlets/restaurants, the size of a burger or a vada or samosa can be much bigger than in other places. Similarly, one may consider two slices of bread with cheese or two slices of bread with tomato and cucumber as one portion. But the size of the slices may vary considerably. Also in some cases, one portion could be made with three slices of bread. Unlike serving size, there is no standard portion size; it varies from person to person or from one food service to another.

"Food portion size can be defined as the actual amount of food that is placed on the plate, reflecting the choice of the consumer, restaurant, or food producer, or the amount of food or drink normally eaten or drank at the time of consumption" (Benton, 2015). It is not only the size of portion an individual consumes in one sitting but also the subsequent changes in the meal size and meal frequency. Large portion often results in high-food intake, high-energy intake, increased BMI, and obesity. However, the trend of eating large size of vegetable portion size can be beneficial. It is not always directly related to appetite and hunger. It can be the habit or accessibility to, particularly favorite foods, sweet, and alcoholic beverages, ready-to-eat snacks particularly when eating out.

> **Laboratory Laurel:** In view of high prevalence of obesity and evidence of increase in the food portion size consumed in developed countries and in developing countries, this study was done in Brazil. The data from the National Dietary Survey of 24,527 individuals for 2 days of food record aged over 20 years was used. Six beverages were selected such as soft drinks, 100% fruit juices, fruit drinks, alcoholic beverages, milk, and coffee or tea. The investigators examined the association between portion size and excess weight using Poisson regression, adjusted for age, sex, income, and total energy intake. Coffee and tea were found to be the most frequently consumed beverages in Brazil, followed by alcoholic beverages (524 mL), then by soft drinks (270 mL), 100% fruit juice, fruit drink, and milk was consumed in large portion sizes. The researchers observed that intake of alcoholic beverages and soft drinks was positively associated with excess weight. The authors highlighted that this needs to be addressed as an issue for public health intervention and consumption of large portions should be discouraged.
>
> *Bezerra IN, Alencar ESD. Association between excess weight and beverage portion size consumed in Brazil. RSP (Rev Saude Publica). 2018;52:21.*

Serving Size

Serving size is the amount of food or drink, which can be measured in terms of weight, volume or number, e.g., one slice of bread or one cup of milk. The amount in a serving is standard and defined. Serving size has been designed after assessing portion sizes from food consumption surveys to have a convenient measuring size with desired nutrient content. **One serving size is the amount of raw or cooked food set for each food exchange list or food group.** One serving size for cereals will be different from one serving size of milk. Within one exchange list, serving size can differ, e.g., one serving of liquid milk is 150 mL and one serving of paneer is only 30 g. It serves as a guide to understand and use the food pyramid, food exchange lists, and nutritional facts on labels. It plays a significant role in meal planning and calculation of nutrient content in a given meal. By varying the serving size, desired nutritional value can easily be obtained. On the basis of serving size, many nutritious recipes have been standardized, which further add value in meal planning for specific dietetic meals and food product development for food industry.

> **Serving size = Reference Amounts Customarily Consumed (RACC).**
> *Source:* US Food and Drug Administration
> One serving size is the amount of raw or cooked food set for each food exchange list or food group.
> Portion is the amount of food a person chooses to eat at one sitting or at one time.

Standardization of Serving Sizes and Recipe

Standardization is a process by which a product is developed in such a manner that it produces same results on repeated production. In nutrition and menu planning, standardization is done to suit the requirements of the user and the use of standardized recipe is desirable to maintain the precise amount of nutrients and consistency in quantity and taste, texture, and appearance.

It is a written formula for producing food preparation anytime, anywhere. Standardization is repeated, if any changes in the ingredient or the process are made in the original or basic recipe. During standardization, attention is paid to the following:
- Selection and weighing of ingredients including water
- Preparation (if applicable)
- Preparation time for different steps
- Cooking methods
- Temperature
- Equipment (if any special equipment used)
- Yield of the final product in terms of weight and measures (volume or number).

> **Use of Standardization**
> - Quantity and quality of final product are predetermined.
> - Amount of individual ingredients is known.
> - Procurement of individual ingredients is easy and convenient.
> - Nutritional value of the ingredients or the full recipes can easily be assessed and computed.
> - Ready to use for future reference.
> - Helps in meal planning and determining portion size.
> - It can be tried by new enthusiasts.
> - Useful in dietetic clinics.

RAPID FIRE

- What do you mean by food exchange?
- Mention the carbohydrates provided by cereal, pulse, meat, and vegetable group C.
- What is difference between milk exchange and meat exchange?
- What is new name for food exchange given by American Dietetic Association?
- What is the difference between portion size and serving size?
- How much is included in each food exchange in one serving?
- What is difference in the serving size if you take liquid milk or milk powder and why?
- Name the association who has initiated food exchange.
- How many exchanges are required for fat and sugar for a healthy adult?
- What is difference between vegetable exchange A and B?

EXERCISE

- Plan the number of exchanges of each food in 2,000 kcal diet for a healthy vegetarian adult woman.
- How will you utilize the exchange list for a nonvegetarians and diabetic person?
- How many calories and protein will be provided in a meal comprised of exchanges—4 cereals, 2 pulses, 2 (1 + 1) vegetables, 2 fats, and 1 milk.
- Standardized 2 recipes and each should utilize 2 exchanges of whole grain cereals, 1 exchange vegetable A or B, 1 fat exchange, and 1 milk exchange.

SUGGESTED READING

1. Bajaj M. Diet Metrics: Hand Book of Food Exchanges. 2019. Notion Press
2. Benton D. Portion size: what we know and what we need to know. Crit Rev Food Sci Nutr. 2015;55(7):988-1004.
3. Ex Rx.net. Food Exchanges. [online] Available from: http://www.exrx.net/Nutrition/FoodExchanges.html. [Last accessed August, 2019].
4. Geil PB. Choose Your Foods: Exchange Lists for Diabetes: The 2008 Revision of Exchange Lists for Meal Planning. Diabetes Spectrum. 2008;21(4):281-3.
5. Indian Dietetic Association (IDA). Clinical Dietetic Manual, 2nd edition. New Delhi, India: Elite Publishing House; 2018. pp. 271-81.
6. Raghuram TC, Pasricha S, Sharma RD. Diet and Diabetes. Hyderabad, India: NIN, ICMR; 1997.
7. Salis S. Diet in Diabetes Simplified. Your Personal Diabetes Nutrition Coach. Notion Press. 2020.
8. Salis S. Nutrition Basics and A Quick Guide to Carbohydrate Counting. Medtronic. 2018.
9. Seth V, Singh K. Diet Planning through Health and Disease: A practical Manual. New Delhi, India: Phoenix Publishing House Pvt Ltd.; 2001.
10. The Diabetic Exchange List (Exchange Diet), https://diabetesed.net/page/_files/THE-DIABETIC-EXCHANGE-LIST.pdf
11. Wheeler ML, Daly A, Evert A, et al. Choose Your Foods: Exchange Lists for Diabetes, Sixth Edition, 2008: Description and Guidelines for Use. J Am Diet Assoc. 2008;108(5):883-8.

CHAPTER 11

Nutrition and Dietary Considerations at Different Life Stages

KEY CONCERNS
- What are the changes that occur at different stages of the life cycle?
- What are the nutritional requirements at each life stage?
- What are the nutritional and dietary considerations while feeding young children?
- What are the reasons for differences in dietary recommendations for different age groups?

KEY CONCEPTS
- Physiological changes, nutritional requirements, dietary considerations, dietary guidelines in the following life stages:
  - Pregnant and lactating mothers
  - Infants and toddlers
  - Preschool children
  - School children
  - Adolescents
  - Adults
  - Elders

"All the World's a Stage
And all the men and women merely players
They have their exits and their entrances
And one man in his time plays many parts
His act being seven ages"
Shakespeare wrote in "As You Like It"

Human life is a continuum. It begins in the mother's womb, with the fertilization of the ovum. From the size of a pinhead, the fertilized ovum develops into an embryo and then a fetus. The fetus grows and develops at an amazing rate during the 9 months in utero until birth. The small human baby which weighs about 3 kg on average, grows, develops, and matures into adulthood. From conception until death, life is a process of continuous change, with growth, maturation, decline, and death being a part of this natural process.

Nutrition plays a very important role throughout life for growth, development as well as maintenance of good health and quality of life in adulthood and old age. Poor nutrition even prior to conception and during pregnancy has important implications for health in later life. Throughout life, new cells are formed, they mature, carry out specific functions, die, and are replaced by new ones. All of this requires nutrition. Thus, nutrition is an everyday phenomenon. A cell that is being formed today cannot wait for a supply of nutrients in the next few days.

Adequate supply of energy and nutrients is essential for metabolic and cellular functions, skeletal growth, and development of vital organs like brain, heart, liver, and kidney. Nutrient deficiencies in childhood lead to growth retardation that ultimately compromises body size, development, maturation and functional capacity, and increases risk of morbidity in the short term and in the long term, even in adult life. In adults, malnutrition compromises performance and productivity, increases risk of morbidity with adverse consequences on quality of life, and has tremendous economic implications. At different stages of the life cycle, there are different concerns and should be taken care of if and when they occur (Table 11.1).

Table 11.1: Concerns at different stages of life.

Ages	Issues of concern
Infancy	Birth weight Breastfeeding concerns Complementary feeding Ensuring optimal growth and development (first growth spurt during postnatal life) Failure to thrive Preventing undernutrition/ morbidity/ mortality
Preschool years	Ensuring normal growth and development Formation of good food habits Preventing malnutrition/ morbidity/ mortality
School years	Ensuring normal growth and development Establishment of good food habits Preventing obesity
Adolescence	Ensuring normal growth and development (second growth spurt) Preparing girls for motherhood Ensuring adequate bone mass Preventing undernutrition/overweight and obesity
Adulthood	Nutrition and productivity Nutrition during pregnancy and lactation Maintaining good metabolic health and prevention of obesity and chronic noncommunicable diseases Promoting good quality of life
Older age	Maintaining muscle mass and bone mass and density Preventing cognitive decline Ensuring adequate food and nutrient intake and preventing undernutrition Preventing morbidity Managing chronic disease(s) Ensuring good quality of life

GROWTH

Growth is a term often used interchangeably with the term development. Both phenomena are important, interdependent, and interrelated physiological processes. Growth generally takes place during the first 2 decades of life, but development continues thereafter (Fig. 11.1). Growth is a continuous phenomenon that begins with conception and stops at the end of adolescence, i.e., it ceases with maturity. Normal growth is an indicator of good health and deviation from normal growth is indicative either of malnutrition or some pathological conditions including hormonal problems. Periodic assessment and monitoring of growth and development facilitates early detection of growth faltering or any symptoms of disorder or disease. Good nutritional status is essential for supporting growth and development and maintaining the required pace in infants, children, and adolescents. Both hyperplasia (increase in number of cells) and hypertrophy (increase in size of the cells) processes need adequate supply of all nutrients as well as energy. During rapid rates of cell division, adequate supply of nutrients required for DNA and RNA synthesis should be ensured.

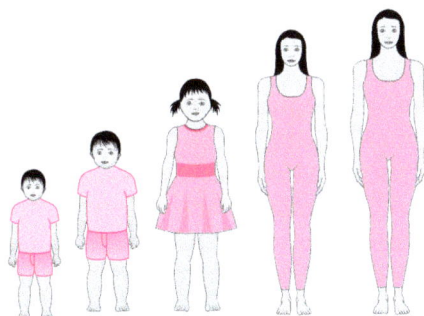

Fig. 11.1: Different stages of growth.

Characteristics of growth
- It is fundamental in fetal life and during childhood and and adolescence. Growth is at highest rate in these life stages.
- Growth is characterized by hyperplasia and hypertrophy.
- It is sequential from general to specific.
- It is characterized by physical changes such as increase in body size, alteration in body shape and tissue composition.
- It can be measured quantitatively in terms of height, weight, bone size, and dentition
- Growth rates vary in different ages and stages of life.
- Growth patterns of boys and girls are distinctly different during puberty.
- Between 2 and 6 years the brain increases to 90 percent of its adult weight.
- Growth of left hemisphere (important for language skills) levels off between 3 to 6 years.
- Right hemisphere (important for spatial skills, e.g., drawing and recognizing shapes) develops gradually over childhood and adolescence.
- Growth rate is rapid during the prenatal, neonatal, infancy and adolescent stages, but is slower during childhood.
- Physical growth ceases with maturity at adulthood.

DEVELOPMENT

Development is a lifelong phenomenon with some organs reaching maturity fairly early in life and others may take several years. For example, development of the central nervous system continues into adulthood, ossification of the skeleton continues until around 25 years of age whereas kidneys mature by 40 weeks of gestation. The brain completes its development by 3–5 years of age. Sexual maturation takes place in adolescence, although physiological and hormonal changes related to puberty may start at 6–8 years of age. There are critical periods in development and these are vulnerable to environmental insults. If the opportunity for development at that particular stage and age is bypassed, it may not occur at a later stage. Development proceeds from the simple to the complex. Development is:

1. An increase in the complexity of function and progression of skills.
2. It enhances the capacity and skills of a person to adapt to the environment.
3. The pattern of development in all humans is similar, although the rate may vary among different persons.
4. Functional maturity of different organs and parts of the body is achieved at different ages.

Principles of development
- Development is continuous—even after maturity, personality continue to develop in different dimensions.
- Development is gradual, e.g., the child learns to crawl before the child learns to walk.
- Development is sequential. It occurs in two directions:
  1. Cephalocaudal sequence: Growth from head to legs and not vice versa.
  2. Proximodistal sequence: It occurs from center to periphery. The child first tries to hold the body before regulating motor skills of the fingers.
- Rate of development varies person to person—at puberty girls develops faster than boys.
- Development proceeds from general to specific, e.g., child can wave his/her arms and legs first before they can hold any object.
- Most traits are correlated in development, e.g., a child learn to speak along with socialize with others.
- Growth and development are the product of both heredity and environment.
- Development is predictable, e.g., central incisor teeth will erupt musch before the molar teeth.
- Development brings about both structural and functional changes—first the organ forms before it functions in fetus and later also.
- There is a constant interaction between all factors of development—all physical, mental, language, motor development occurs at the same time but at different rate.

When a child is reasonably well nourished and has not been burdened much by disease, typically growth is rapid during infancy, slows down during childhood, until the adolescent when second growth spurt starts. Normal growth is a reflection of overall health and nutritional status. Different phases of human growth are shown in Figure 11.2.

The human body changes in size, proportion, and composition as it grows. During periods of growth, the rate of cell turnover in all organs and tissues and thus the whole body, is slanted toward cell formation than the breakdown of cells. However, once the person has reached maturity, i.e., adulthood, the rate of cell turnover is in equilibrium (state of maintenance). With aging, the rate of cell breakdown

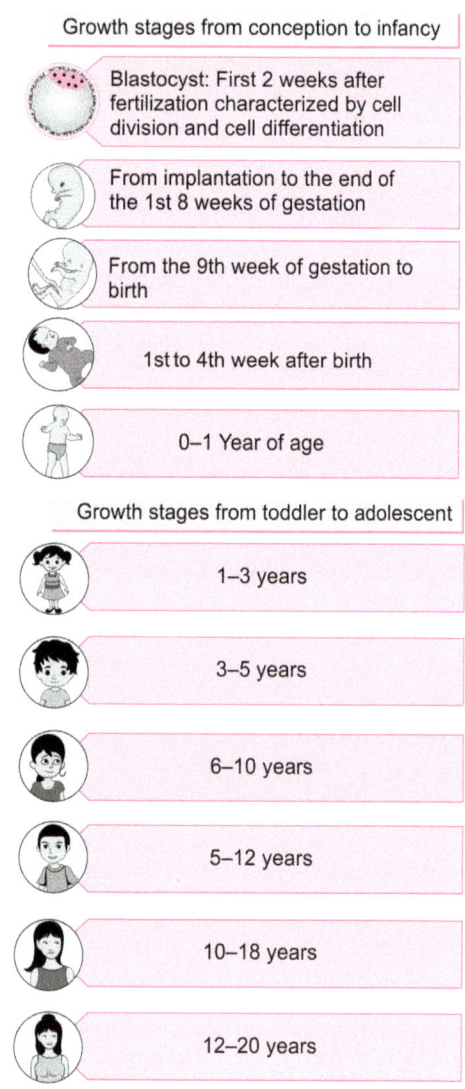

Fig. 11.2: Phases of human growth through the life cycle.

exceeds the rate of formation. This is reflected a decline in various physiological functions (called senescence). Growth is genetically predetermined but is substantially affected by nutrition, chronic systemic disease, hormones, emotions, and other environmental factors.

Understanding the normal patterns of growth is important, to be able to assess whether a child is growing normally and if not, it enables early detection of pathological deviations, i.e., whether the growth is compromised due to undernutrition or due to a metabolic disease or some disease or hormonal deficit. Some salient characteristics of growth from infancy through adolescence are:
- The highest rate of growth is in fetal life, infancy, and adolescence.
- During infancy, growth in the first 6 months is more rapid than in the second half of the 1st year.
- In childhood, rate of growth is slower than in infancy and early childhood.
- Between 2 and 10 years of age, children grow at a steady pace. Children are expected to gain approximately 2–3 inches in height and 2 kg/5 lbs per year.
- Between 9 and 15 years of age, there is a final growth spurt at puberty.
- At 8–9 years, girls' rate of growth is higher than boys until about 13 years of age. Girls begin to have more adipose tissue than boys.
- Between 2 and 6 years, the brain increases to 90% of its adult weight.
- Growth of left hemisphere of the brain (important for language skills) levels off between 3 and 6 years.
- Right hemisphere of the brain (important for spatial skills, e.g., drawing and recognizing shapes) develops gradually over childhood and adolescence.

Preconception Period

Couples often plan their baby, but a large percentage of pregnancies in India are unplanned. There is often great concern during pregnancy but the pre-pregnancy period is of great importance for two major reasons: (1) this period is when the foundation can be laid for the forthcoming pregnancy and (2) most women only learn about onset of their pregnancy after 1 or 2 months of missing their periods. The preconceptional period is very crucial as it lays the foundation of pregnancy. Consumption of a wide variety of nutritious foods is essential as it ensures healthy pregnancy and outcome. During preconceptional period, fulfillment of all the nutrient requirements, especially, DHA, iron, iodine, calcium, folic acid, and vitamin D is very important. Females on restricted diets, underweight, undernourished as well as overweight/obese mothers, smokers, adolescents, and mothers with multiple pregnancies are at a higher risk of having unfavorable pregnancy outcomes like miscarriage and abortions. Healthy diet and lifestyle are two major determinants of healthy pregnancy outcome. As such, there is now strong scientific evidence that obesity during preconceptional period can affect the weight gain during pregnancy, birth weight of the offspring, and cause alterations in glucose metabolism of the offspring which can result in impaired glucose tolerance and cardiometabolic risk, later in adulthood.

THE FIRST 1000 DAYS

The first 1000 days of life include the time between time of conception and second birthday of the child (280 days of pregnancy + 365 days of first year of life + 365 days of second year of life). It is a window of opportunity to establish the foundations for optimum growth and development across the lifespan. The right nutrition and care during the first 1000 days determines survival of the child, his or her ability to grow and mature and gain good health and wellbeing. Optimal nourishment in first 1000 days will contribute to the stability and prosperity of the society and nation.

Maternal prenatal nutrition and the child's nutrition in the first 2 years of life (1000 days) are crucial for a child's neurological development and lifelong mental health. Fetal brain growth accelerates during the second half of pregnancy, and the rate of growth remains high during the 1st year of life with continued growth for the next several years. Although all nutrients are necessary for brain growth, key nutrients that support neurological development include protein, zinc, iron, choline, folate, iodine, vitamins A, D, B_6 and B_{12}, and long-chain polyunsaturated fatty acids particularly the essential fatty acid, arachidonic acid, and omega-3 fatty acids.

Failure to provide the key nutrients during this critical period of brain development may result in lifelong deficits in brain function despite subsequent nutrient repletion. After birth, nutrition continues to be important for the child's mental, physical, and social growth and development. Under nutrition in first 1000 days may result in lower IQ, less success in schools and work place and dysregulation in behaviour.

The developing brain requires iron during embryonic and fetal period as well as infancy up to 3 years of postnatal life. Iron is required for proteins that regulate myelin production, neurotransmitter synthesis, and neuronal energy production. These processes in turn support speed of processing in the brain, as well as behaviors, emotion, learning and memory. In a review of 21 studies, 19 studies were found to have reported impaired mental, motor, socioemotional, or neurophysiologic functioning in infants with iron deficiency anemia compared to infants without iron deficiency anemia.

PREGNANCY AND FETAL DEVELOPMENT

Pregnancy is perhaps one of the most crucial stages in life, since it lays the foundation for the future of the child.

It is also a critical phase for the woman herself. All of the processes that occur during pregnancy or embryonic and fetal development are highly orchestrated, with very precise coordination. Poor nutritional status prior to and during pregnancy has serious and long-term effects and there is a risk of maternal morbidity, early/preterm delivery, and low birth weight. Prenatal development comprises three periods:
1. Periconceptional period: 0–2 weeks of pregnancy
2. Embryonic period: 2–8 weeks of pregnancy
3. Fetal period: 9 weeks to term

These stages essentially refer to stages of development of the embryo/fetus. In general for all purposes, pregnancy is divided into **three trimesters**, the duration of each being 12–14 weeks (Table 11.2). Therefore, the **first trimester** includes both the periconceptional and the embryonic period. The **second trimester** begins from week 13 or 14 until the end of week 26 and the **third trimester** is from week 27 until term, i.e., delivery. Based on gestational age, the average length of a pregnancy is 40 ± 2 weeks. Generally, the term gestational age is used to express the age or duration of pregnancy and is calculated from the last normal menstrual period. Major changes that occur in the mother and the developing fetus are summarized in Table 11.3.

The three developmental periods and their characteristics are:
1. **Periconceptional period:** Starts with the fertilization of the ovum by the sperm and formation of the zygote. After fertilization, there is rapid division of cells that together form a blastocyst. At about 2 weeks of gestation, the

Table 11.2: Typical features of pregnancy in three trimesters.

	I Trimester	II Trimester	III Trimester
Typical features of pregnancy in three trimesters			
Periods in each trimester	Conception to 12 weeks	13–28 weeks	28–40 weeks (birth)
Fetus in womb (in utero)			
Approximate length (inches) and (weight) of the fetus by end of trimester	2.5" (30 grams)	12" (1.0 kg)	20" (2.7–3.0 Kg)
Approximate weight gain (kg)	0.6–1.0	3.0–3.5	6.0–8.0
Gestation weight gain (g/day) based on 10 kg	17	60	54
Protein deposition (g/day)	0.0	1.3	5.1
Fat deposition (g/day)	5.2	18.9	16.9
Increased calorie requirement (kcal/day)	85	280	470
Increased protein requirement (g/day)	0.5	9.5	22
Crucial nutrients needed in each trimester	Docosahexaenoic acid (DHA), iron, calcium, folic acid, vitamin D, protein	DHA, iron, calcium, folic acid, vitamin D, vitamin A, vitamin B_6, choline, vitamin B_{12}, protein	DHA, iron, calcium, copper, zinc, magnesium, folic acid, vitamin D, vitamin A, vitamin B_6, choline, vitamin B_{12}, protein

Table 11.3: Changes occurring during each trimester of pregnancy and in the fetus during intrauterine life.

Trimester	Changes occurring in pregnant woman	Changes occurring in the fetus
I trimester	Missed menstrual periods Risk of morning sickness (nausea, vomiting, heart burn) Headache Food cravings and food aversions Hormonal changes affect all organs Frequent urination, constipation Weight loss or gain	All major organs are formed Nerves and muscles begin to work Can form fist Eyelids formed to protect eyes but eyes are not formed Head growth occurs at a slow pace
II trimester	General aches and pains in back, abdomen, groin, or thigh Stretch marks may appear on abdomen, breasts, thighs, or buttocks Darkening of the skin around nipples of the breasts and sometimes other parts of body Itching on the abdomen, palms, and soles of the feet Nausea, loss of appetite, vomiting, fatigue combined with itching (need doctor's advice) Swelling of the ankles, fingers and face (need doctor's advice)	Bone marrow begins to make blood cells Taste buds appear on tongue Footprints and fingerprints are formed Hair begins to grow on head Lungs are formed, but do not function yet Sex organs begin to form, e.g., testicles and scrotum in boys and uterus and ovaries in girls
III trimester	Enlargement of breast and nipples (preparation for lactation) of belly button may be present The baby drops or moves lower in the abdomen Breathing may become difficult Heartburn Difficulty in sleeping	The protective waxy coating (vernix) develops Body fat increases Baby is getting bigger and has less space to move around Movements are less forceful Baby's organs are capable of functioning on their own Baby may turn into a head-down position for birth

blastocyst implants itself into the inner lining of the uterus, i.e., the endometrium. Nutritional status of the mother is important because cell division and the nutrients required for the blastocyst are supplied by the mother's body. Folic acid is crucial in this stage to prevent neural tube defects. The onset of several malformations and pregnancy-related disorders, i.e., congenital abnormalities, fetal loss, miscarriage, insufficient fetal growth, premature birth, and preeclampsia, may indeed occur during this period.

2. **Embryonic period:** Most women are not even sure that they are pregnant at this stage. The cells of the blastocyst continue to divide rapidly and also begin to differentiate. This stage is critical because organogenesis occurs, i.e., formation of the different organs and tissues begin. There is rapid growth, and the baby's main external features begin to take form. It is during this critical period (most of the first trimester) that the growing baby is most vulnerable to adverse influences. Since the embryo receives all nutrients directly from the mother, good maternal nutrition is imperative for prenatal development. Maternal diet and body composition affect the growth of the developing embryo. Energy, protein, riboflavin, niacin, vitamin B_6, folate, vitamin B_{12}, vitamin A, zinc, and manganese are all important. Poor maternal nutrition can cause metabolic and hormonal changes in the mother. Deficiency of folic acid can interfere with embryonic development and deficiency of other nutrients can lead to congenital abnormalities in the fetus. Deficiency of riboflavin adversely affects skeletal formation; vitamin B_6 and manganese deficiencies may cause neuromuscular problems and lack of vitamin B_{12}, niacin, folate, and vitamin A may lead to defects in central nervous system.

Besides these, other adverse influences are alcohol, certain prescriptions and recreational drugs, infections like rubella or cytomegalovirus as well as X-rays or radiation therapy.

3. **Fetal period:** Most of the organs have formed by the beginning of the fetal period. This period is critical because rapid growth and development of functional capacity of the various organs occurs. The embryo and fetus grow from weighing less than a milligram to a baby weighing about 3 kg. It is extremely important to recognize that this rapid fetal growth and development can occur only if there is a continuous and adequate supply of nutrients. By the end of the second trimester, the nerve cells in the brain have finished dividing and the maximum number has been achieved, the fetus' own immune system begins to function and weight gain starts to increase by the 6th month of pregnancy, as fat is deposited in the fetal body.

Undernutrition leads to a range of adaptive responses such as redistribution of blood flow in the fetal body and changes in the production of fetal and placental hormones which control growth. These responses may include changes in placental transport function, an area about which we need to know a lot more than we presently know. Even without changes in overall fetal body size, the growth of certain organs such as the heart and kidney can be altered.

The term "critical period" is used because when an organ is being formed, if it is exposed to any insult, the process is disrupted or growth and development of the organ may be limited/compromised in an attempt to adapt. Critical periods are the periods when rapid cell division occurs. Different tissues undergo rapid cell division at different timings in utero. For example, long bones develop in the second trimester and kidney matures during the weeks immediately before birth. At different stages of fetal life, different organs are formed and they mature, hence the impact of nutritional deficiency/deficiencies or even excesses, depends (a) on the stage of pregnancy and which organs were vulnerable and (b) the severity of the deficiency or magnitude of excess. The level of nutrient intake can alter the gene expression of the fetal genome and predetermine the lifelong consequences. This phenomenon is also termed as fetal programming.

Functions of the Placenta

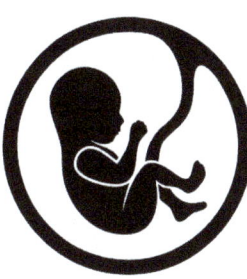

The placenta is a temporary organ formed during pregnancy. It provides an essential link between the mother and the fetus. The maternal body supplies nutrients to the fetus, through special life support systems—the placenta, amniotic fluid, and the umbilical cord.

The placenta is connected to the fetus by the umbilical cord. At full term, the placenta measures about 7 inches in diameter and weighs approximately 1 kg. The formation and functional maturity of the placenta, i.e., its capacity and its size are critically essential, because it affects the growth and development of the fetus and the survival of the fetus and the birth weight and survival of the newborn. The placenta is metabolically active and matures throughout pregnancy and it synthesizes several amino acids and hormones. The placenta is rich in blood vessels and performs the following vital functions:

- It transfers oxygen and nutrients from the mother's blood to the fetus via the umbilical vein.
- It picks up carbon dioxide and metabolic waste products from the fetus (via the two umbilical arteries) and transfers them to maternal blood, to be got rid of by the mother's body (kidney and lungs).
- It produces hormones that are important for the maintenance of pregnancy including estrogen, progesterone, and human chorionic gonadotropin.
- Nutrients are transferred across the placenta through different transport mechanisms.

Thus, the placenta is the "fetal supply line". However, harmful substances can cross the placenta and mothers need to avoid alcohol, drugs, smoking, etc. during pregnancy to ensure that the fetus is protected from these.

In order that fetal growth and development is well supported, besides formation of the placenta, the mother's body undergoes tremendous changes physiologically and metabolically. These changes and adaptations occur in such a fashion, as to create a suitable environment for fetal growth, delivery, and lactation.

Physiological Changes During Pregnancy

Gestational Weight Gain

Pregnancy entails an increase in body weight. Two components contribute to this weight gain: (a) health and weight of the fetus, amniotic fluid as well as placenta and (b) increase in maternal tissues comprising by enlargement of the uterus, increase in blood volume and ECF, development

Table 11.4: Total weight gain and rate of weight gain as recommended by Institute of Medicine, USA (2009).

Prepregnancy weight status as per BMI	Recommended total weight gain range (kg)	Recommended rates of weight gain in second and third trimester kg/week*
Underweight (< 18.5)	12.5–18	0.51 (0.44–0.58)
Normal (18.5–24.9)	11.5–16	0.42 (0.35–0.50)
Overweight (25–29.9)	7–11.5	0.28 (0.23–0.33)
Obese (>30)	5–9	0.22 (0.17–0.27)

*It is assumed that weight gain in first trimester is 0.5–2 kg

Source: Institute of Medicine (IOM). Weight gain during pregnancy: re-examining the guidelines. Washington: National Academy Press; 2009.

of the breasts, and deposition of adipose tissue. Generally, in a well-nourished mother, body weight is increased by about 8–12 kg in 9 months of pregnancy. Most of the weight gain occurs in the second and third trimesters.

Gestational weight gain is influenced by environmental factors like food and nutrient intake, level of physical activity and exercise, energy balance and medical condition (if any). Low gestational weight gain increases the risk of intrauterine growth retardation and mortality of the fetus or neonate. If the mother is thin and undernourished, she may need to gain more than the 12 kg weight; whereas, mothers who are overweight need to gain less than 12 kg weight (Table 11.4).

Low or high weight gain may have different effects on the offspring and the woman herself. Underweight and undernourished mothers frequently give birth to low birth weight babies, who have suffered intrauterine growth retardation (IUGR) and at high risk of premature delivery, poor birth outcome and prenatal mortality. Mothers who have high weight gain deliver heavier babies who may be predisposed to obesity and associated disorders. Infants of mothers with gestational diabetes are at high risk of childhood metabolic syndrome (central adiposity, insulin resistance, and hypertension) because such neonates have higher fat mass and alter glucose metabolism.

There is increase in fat mass, total body water, and muscle mass thus increasing the body weight. The rate of nutrient (fat and protein) deposition varies in different trimesters which also govern the fetal development and maternal weight gain.

Increase in Blood Volume

There is about 45–50% increase in blood plasma volume compared to nonpregnant state. Also, there is formation of red blood cells (RBCs). In the third trimester, red cell mass has increased by about 15–20% in order to facilitate oxygen and nutrient supply to the fetus and for newly formed maternal tissues. Because the increase in plasma volume is more than the increase in red cell mass, there is a natural fall in the hemoglobin level (by 1–2 mg/100 mL). Expansion of blood volume and growth of maternal tissues requires substantial amount of protein and other important nutrients. It is also necessary for maintenance of pregnancy.

Increase in Hormone Levels

Several hormonal changes occur, which are mentioned below:

- Soon after implantation, there is a rise in serum chorionic gonadotropin hormone. This hormone is important for maintaining the corpus luteum for the first 2 to 2½ weeks of pregnancy. A corpus luteum is a mass of cells that is formed in ovary, after the ovum has been discharged and is responsible for the production of the hormones in early pregnancy. The corpus luteum secretes estrogen and progesterone until the placenta develops enough to take over their production.
- Placental lactogen which stimulates lipolysis antagonizes the action of insulin and probably has an important role in ensuring that the fetus has a continuous supply of energy-yielding compounds like glucose. It also promotes breast development and after delivery, it disappears from maternal circulation.
- Steroid hormones estrogen and progesterone. They are secreted by the placenta after 8–10 weeks of pregnancy.
- Progesterone stimulates maternal respiration, relaxes the smooth muscles especially of the uterus and GI tract, breast development, and inhibits milk secretion during pregnancy.
- Estrogen stimulates growth of the uterus, enhances uterine blood flow, and may promote breast development.

Development of maternal tissues: Maternal tissues include uterine tissues, breast tissue, adipose tissue, as well as blood and extracellular fluid. Mammary glands (breasts) develop in preparation for forthcoming lactation. During pregnancy, there is deposition of fat (adipose tissue) around the pelvic region.

Increased oxygen demand: Since the oxygen demand is increased for tissue development, it results in increased oxygen carrying capacity of blood. Eventually, it may slightly increase the heartbeat, palpitation or blood pressure of the woman. BMR increases by 20–30%. Breathing becomes deeper and gaseous exchange in lungs becomes more efficient. Respiratory rate increases and so does the oxygen consumption. Cardiac output and heart rate increase. Blood pressure decreases in the first half of pregnancy and returns to normal in the second half.

Altered GI and kidney functions: Gastrointestinal changes occur including slower gastrointestinal motility. Renal functions are also altered in order to excrete metabolic wastes of both mother and fetus. Sodium retention increases.

Increased absorption of nutrients: Slower gastrointestinal motility is an advantage because it allows more time for absorption of nutrients. This improves absorption of iron, calcium, vitamin B_{12}, and other nutrients.

Changes in blood volume, plasma proteins, and lipids: There is increase in blood/plasma volume. Total plasma proteins particularly albumin decrease. Most of the lipids, i.e., triglycerides, VLDL, LDL, and HDL are increased.

Fetal Nutrition

Fetal nutrition is determined by a combination of maternal diet, nutrient stores, nutrient delivery to placenta, and the capacity of the placenta to transfer the nutrients. Fetal growth and development is totally dependent on the ability of the mother to nourish the fetus so that it can achieve its growth potential. This is influenced by:

i. The mother's nutrient intake, nutritional status including nutrient stores and metabolism. It is not only what she consumes during pregnancy that is important. Her nutrition and health during her childhood and adolescence determine her present health and nutritional status, her body size, and nutrient stores.
ii. The development and functioning of the placenta (a metabolically active organ).
iii. The fetus itself.

The fetus needs a steady supply of glucose, fatty acids, and amino acids that it will utilize for energy as well to synthesize the proteins and lipids that its body requires. The fetus requires glucose to be supplied since it does not have the metabolic capacity (gluconeogenesis) to synthesize glucose on its own. Similarly, essential fatty acids need to be supplied. The fetus then metabolizes these to the important eicosanoids that its body requires. Several physiological and metabolic changes occur in the mother's body to enable and ensure that the fetus receives the nutrients it needs. The fetus requires about 50 kcal/kg/day for various metabolic functions and another 40–50 kcal/kg/day for its own tissue deposition. If the mother's diet is qualitatively and/or quantitatively inadequate, it will limit fetal growth and development. It is critical that the fetus receives the appropriate nutrients in sufficient amounts as per the requirements of the stage of development.

Some effects of intrauterine nutrition are mediated by epigenetic effects of nutrients. Epigenetics describes the cellular processes that determine whether a certain gene will be transcribed and translated into its corresponding protein. It is a specific kind of metabolic programming, which occurs through DNA methylation. Food containing nutrients that can act as methyl donors, such as folic acid and choline, may be of particular interest in this regard. These epigenetic changes may have lifelong effects and even may have transgenerational consequences. This means that, for instance, effects of malnutrition during pregnancy not only affects the health of the offspring but also of the grandchildren.

> **Laboratory Laurel:** A cohort study was conducted on 1199, 5-year old Japanese children with the objective of examining the relationship between maternal fat consumption during pregnancy and behavioural problems in children. A diet history questionnaire was used to assess intakes and a strengths and difficulties questionnaire for emotional, conduct, hyperactivity and peer problems in the children. The investigators reported that higher maternal intakes of MUFA, n-6 PUFA, linoleic acid α-linoleic acid were associate with increased risk of childhood emotional problems but no such association was seen for total fat intake, SFA and n-3 fatty acids.
>
> *Korsmo HW, Jiang X, Caudill MA. Choline: Exploring the Growing Science on Its Benefits for Moms and Babies. Nutrients. 2019. 11(8): 1823.*

Factors Affecting Nutritional Status During Pregnancy

Numerous factors affect the nutritional status of the mother. These include:
- Family support
- Food availability
- Family income
- Age at menarche and conception
- Health status of the women—past and present
- Physical activity and work load
- Personal dietary habits
- Literacy level and nutrition knowledge
- Beliefs and taboos related to food and healthcare
- Smoking, alcohol or drug abuse
- Exposure to irradiation
- Access to health care services and counseling
- Parity and birth spacing.

These factors influence the food behavior of pregnant women. Food choices during pregnancy or lactation in Indian society are often dictated by family traditions or cultural beliefs or taboos. In addition, many mothers may have problems like morning sickness, nausea, and vomiting. These problems tend to modify food choices and food intake. Some women experience cravings for sour foods like lemon, pickle. The urge to eat nonfood items during pregnancy has been frequently observed in many women and this phenomenon is called **Pica.**

> **Pica** is an irresistible desire to eat nonfood items like clay, sand, wood, cement, cloth, buttons, etc. It is usually observed during pregnancy. Women also exhibit very strong attraction or rejection to some smells toward some food like oil, ghee, fruit, etc. or nonfoods like paint, etc.

Nutritional Requirements During Pregnancy

Nutritional status of the mother before and during pregnancy is most critical for optimal growth and development of the fetus. Maternal nutrition greatly influences not only fetal nutrition but also is a determinant of the child's nutritional status, growth and development after he/she is born. Maternal nutrient supply to fetus begins with conception and determines the rate of growth, body composition, and gestational age of the fetus.

Nutritional requirements are increased to support fetal growth as well as development of the supporting system, i.e., the placenta as well as to support maternal metabolism and development of maternal tissues to support pregnancy and fetal growth as well as preparation for lactation. Hormones play a large role in directing the nutrients toward the uterus and placenta so that they are transferred to the developing fetus which is solely dependent on the mother. Continuous supply of nutrients via placenta affects fetal growth, placental transport. The placenta utilizes, produces essential and nonessential amino acids for regulating gene expression, cell signaling, antioxidant responses, immunity, and neurological functions. Body can synthesize nonessential amino acids only when enough energy and suitable forms of nitrogen and carbon are available.

Nutritional requirements during pregnancy are different in the three trimesters and vary with age, body weight, body size, dietary pattern, and nutritional status of the mother during her adolescence and prepregnancy period. During pregnancy requirements for energy, protein, iron, iodine, folate and other key nutrients are higher than nonpregnant women. However, requirements for calcium and vitamin D remain the same in normal and pregnant women.

Energy: Energy cost of pregnancy (kcal) relates to the energy deposited in the form of tissue deposition and increase in BMR. It is much higher in the second and third trimesters. Deposition of protein and fat in the fetus is higher in the second trimester as compared to the first and third trimesters. This deposition entails extra energy needs to support growth of the fetus, placenta, and other associated maternal tissues as well as to fulfill the increased metabolic demands of the pregnancy. Considering the body weight of reference women, i.e., 55 kg under normal health conditions, there is 10–12 kg total gain in weight during pregnancy. Calorie needs also increase correspondingly with increase in weight gain in three trimesters of pregnancy. Variation in the requirement may depend upon many factors such as nutritional status, body composition, and psycho-socio-cultural factors. Physical activity level further alter the energy requirements.

ICMR-NIN (2020) has retained the previous recommendation of 350 kcal/day in addition to RDA for energy for non-pregnant women performing different activity levels. However, on the basis of gestational weight gain (GWG), of 10 kg and 12 kg, additional energy requirements in 1st trimester would 70, 85 kcal/day; in 2nd trimester would be 230 and 280 kcal/day and in 3rd trimester it would be 390 and 470 kcal/day respectively. The average needs in 2nd and 3rd trimester would be 310 and 375 kcal in 10 and 12 kg GWG respectively. Hence, it is essential to learn that eating for two or consuming excessive amount of energy from the beginning of pregnancy is not required at all. Figure 11.3 gives the requirements in three trimesters for different levels of physical activities.

Protein: Additional protein during pregnancy needs special attention particularly during third trimester. Efficiency of conversion of dietary protein into fetal, placental, and maternal tissues is about 70%. It can be achieved by additional intake of 9.5 g/day and 22 g/day protein in second and third trimester respectively. Inadequate intake of protein results in poor pregnancy outcome (low birth weight and length). Similarly, high intake of protein affects fetal development.

	Sedentary work	Moderate work	Heavy work
Non-pregnant woman	1660	2130	2720
Pregnant woman	2010	2480	3070
Lactating woman (first 6 months)	2260	2730	3320
Lactating woman (6–12 months)	2180	2650	3240

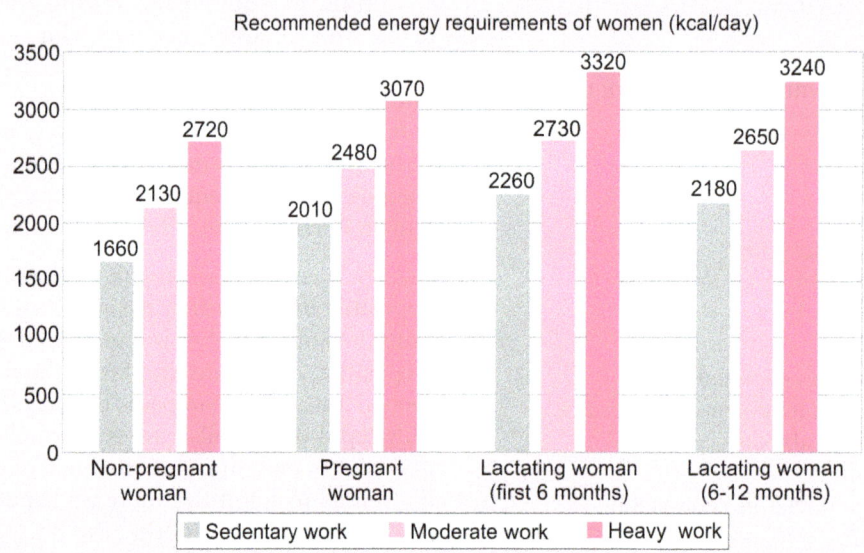

Fig. 11.3: Energy requirements for non-pregnant, pregnant and lactating women.

Protein needs are increased to maintain the body reserves and replace the increased turnover in this period. The ratio between energy and protein is also important. Extra protein is required to support the expansion of blood volume and protein deposition in fetus, uterus, and placenta and breasts. Protein is required for cell formation, formation of enzymes, hormones, antibodies, muscles, collagen, and many body tissues including skin, blood, bones, etc. Positive nitrogen balance and supply of all essential amino acids particularly lysine, methionine plays a pivotal role in growth and development. It is essential that the mother consumes proteins of good biological value. Protein quality is also of great importance. Foods having PDCAAS (Protein Digestibility Corrected Amino Acid Score) close to 1 are of good quality, signifying that these food sources can provide all the essential amino acids. PDCAAS level of cereals and pulses are lower. Thus, addition of milk or egg or meat to either cereal or pulse along with combination of cereal and pulse is recommended to improve protein quality and improve PDCAAS. Protein supplements during pregnancy are not advisable.

Glycine requirement is high in late pregnancy and it becomes a conditionally essential amino acid. Insufficiency of glycine may produce adverse effects. Intrauterine fetal programming and adverse effects of qualitatively and/ or quantitatively inadequate diets have been shown to increase risk of disease(s) in adulthood. Intrauterine growth retardation (IUGR) in infants may not show growth retardation during childhood period but can result in shorter, lighter, and weaker adolescents. Therefore, the concept of ensuring good preconceptional nutrition is of great concern. The WHO in 2007 increased the protein requirement in the third trimester to 31 g and stated that this should be obtained from high quality protein sources. The type and quality of protein affects gene expression especially the gene associated with IGF-I (Insulin Growth Factor) and its binding protein which plays a role in protein synthesis and body composition. In children whose protein intake was restricted, decrease in nitrogen balance, and decrease in IGF-I concentration as well as IGF-I binding proteins has been reported.

Fat: Fat is one of the energy-yielding nutrients which contributes not only to fulfilling the energy requirements of the pregnant woman but is also deposited in fetus and maternal tissues. It is not just the amount of fat but the quality of fats is extremely important, than just the total amount for fetal development of brain and retina and infant growth. It is necessary to ensure that the relative proportion of polyunsaturated fats (n-3: n-6 ratio) is adequate and particular attention needs to be paid to ensure that maternal intake of n-3 fatty acids is adequate [essential fatty acids and their derivatives such as arachidonic acid (n-6), and DHA (n-3)]. DHA and long chain polyunsaturated (LCPUFA) are crucial to the fetus because it is involved in visual and neural function as well as neurotransmitter metabolism. It is accumulated in utero and is predominantly provided to the fetus through placental transfer. The amount supplied is dependent on maternal diet as the human body is not efficient at converting ALA to DHA. They are part of the structural lipids of all cell membranes and also for formation of steroid hormones and for the synthesis of eicosanoids like prostaglandins. Incorporation of n-3 fatty acids is several times faster than other fatty acids like linoleic acid and α-linolenic acid. Omega-3 fatty acids also play a role in determining the length of gestation, maturation of many organ systems including brain and eye and preventing perinatal depression. The percentage of calories to be obtained from fat is not different from that of nonpregnant women, i.e., it should supply 20–35% of total energy intake. According to the World Association of Perinatal Medicine Dietary Guidelines Working Group, pregnant women should consume 100–200 mg DHA per day, to support optimal pregnancy outcome.

Laboratory Laurel: A cohort study was designed to find out the relationship between maternal fat consumption during pregnancy and behavioral problems in 1199 Japanese children aged 5 years of age. Diet history questionnaire was used for dietary intake of mothers and Strengths and Difficulties Questionnaire was used for studying emotional and conduct related problems, hyperactivity and problems with peer group. Higher maternal intake of monounsaturated fatty acids, α-linolenic acid, ω-6 polyunsaturated fatty acids, and linoleic acid during pregnancy were independently associated with an increased risk for childhood emotional problems. However, no relationships was found between maternal intake of total fat, saturated fatty acids, ω-3 polyunsaturated fatty acids, eicosapentaenoic acid, docosahexaenoic acid, arachidonic acid, or cholesterol, and the ratio of ω-3 to ω-6 polyunsaturated fatty acid intake during pregnancy and any of the outcomes.

Miyake Y, Tanaka K, Okubo H, et al. Maternal fat intake during pregnancy and behavioral problems in 5-y-old Japanese children. Nutrition. 2018;50:91-6.

Laboratory Laurel: Maternal mental health (MMH) especially postpartum depression (PPD) poses adverse consequences for women, their offspring and families. Intake of long-chain PUFA, especially DHA and EPA, has been associated with a range of mental health outcomes. It tends to improve fluidity of cell membrane and neurotransmitter function in the brain and influences MMH, but there is limited evidence of an association of PPD with n-3 fatty acids.

Ramakrishnan U. Fatty acid status and maternal mental health. Matern Child Nutr. 2011;7(s2): 99-111.

Micronutrients

Supply of micronutrients from the periconceptional period throughout pregnancy is crucial. Requirements for most vitamins and minerals are increased. Adequacy of iron, folate, and vitamin B_{12} is very crucial at the time of conception and throughout pregnancy for RBC production and sustained cell division for enlargement of uterus, growth of placenta and fetus Their requirements are shown in Figure 11.4.

Folic acid: Role of folic acid begins before conception. Folic acid plays a significant role in cell division and maturation of red blood cells (as a methyl donor for DNA and RNA synthesis). Thus, folate is necessary for normal metabolism, reproduction, and development. During the periconceptional period of pregnancy, adequate intake of folic acid is crucial for the mother to start pregnancy with good folate status. Folate is essential for closure of the neural tube during embryogenesis, in the first 28 days after conception, much before a woman learns about her pregnancy. Neural tube defects are common complex congenital malformations. Neurulation is a fundamental event in embryogenesis that culminates in the formation of the neural tube, which is the precursor of the brain and spinal cord. Closure of the neural tube is very important for maintaining brain development and for the initial formation of the skull. Hence, ensuring good folate status by ensuring adequate intake is imperative 1 year before or at least from the moment a woman is trying to conceive until 12 weeks of pregnancy and thereafter as well. WHO advises that a weekly iron folate supplement be given to chronically anemic population. Every day one tablet containing 500 µg of folic acid along with iron (60 mg elemental iron) is given to pregnant women for 180 days under Anemia Mukt Bharat (2019). Deficiency of folic acid increases the risk of birth defects such as cleft palate and lip, spina bifida, congenital and cardiovascular defects, poor fetal growth, and preterm labor. In deficiency, blood homocysteine levels (an indicator of CVD) are increased. According to ICMR (2020), folic acid requirement is increased from 220 µg to 570 µg in pregnancy. 1 µg of food folic acid is equal to 0.5 µg of synthetic folic acid taken on empty stomach or 0.6 µg folic acid with meal. Chemical form of folic acid is different. Folate from natural food sources consists of formyltetrahydropteroylglutamates. Folic acid used in supplements is pteroylmonoglutamic acid. However higher dose of supplementation need further studies. It should be obtained from food sources or supplements to ensure normal growth and maturation.

Vitamin B_{12}

Like folic acid, B_{12} is required for normal cell division, cell differentiation and for development and myelination of the

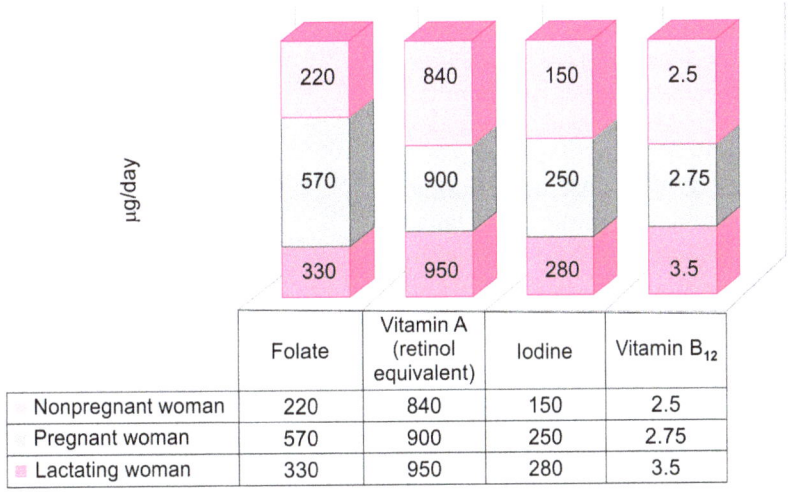

	Folate	Vitamin A (retinol equivalent)	Iodine	Vitamin B_{12}
Nonpregnant woman	220	840	150	2.5
Pregnant woman	570	900	250	2.75
Lactating woman	330	950	280	3.5

Fig. 11.4: RDA for Folate, vitamin A, iodine, B_{12} during pregnancy and lactation (for EAR refer Appendix 4).
Source: (ICMR-NIN, 2020)

central nervous system. Deficiency of this vitamin is linked to higher risk of several adverse outcomes of pregnancy such as spontaneous abortion, delivering an infant who is small for gestational age or has been subjected to intrauterine growth retardation, low birth weight, pregnancy-induced hypertension, neural tube defects, and preterm delivery. Children born to B_{12}-deficient mothers also have higher risk of adverse health outcomes, developmental abnormalities, and anemia. B_{12} is concentrated in the fetus and stored in the liver which is used during the first few months of postnatal life, provided maternal intakes are adequate. In infants with moderate and severe B_{12} deficiency, demyelination and brain atrophy has been reported. It is a nutrient of concern, because its food sources are all animal sources with the exception of milk and milk products. It is also synthesized in healthy gut as well as during fermentation of some plant foods.

Vitamin B_6
Vitamin B_6 is important for several metabolic processes and development of nervous system via biosynthesis of neurotransmitters. Vitamin B_6 is found to be effective in prevention of nausea in the first trimester. It improves maternal and perinatal outcomes. It plays a significant role in prevention of preeclampsia, preterm births, and birth defects. RDA for vitamin B_6 is 2.3 mg/day during pregnancy (ICMR-NIN, 2020).

Vitamin B_2
Vitamin B_2 (riboflavin) is required for metabolism of carbohydrates, proteins, and fats and release of energy for the formation and functioning of the skin, lining of the digestive tract, blood cells, and other vital organs in the fetus. Energy is critically required for cell division and development and later by the fetus, as it becomes active.

Vitamin C
Additional 15 mg/day of vitamin C has been suggested during pregnancy hence a pregnant woman would require 80 mg/day vitamin C. It will not only prevent scurvy in young infants but also saturate the immune cells (neutrophils) with ascorbic acid and limits its excretion.

Vitamin D
Vitamin D has several important functions in the body, especially in bone metabolism. Besides this, it has been found to promote insulin action and secretion, modulate immune function, and is important for lung development. It therefore has the potential to play an important role in the development of the fetus. The conversion of 25(OH)D to 1,25(OH)$_2$D during pregnancy is different from nonpregnant women. The fetus depends fully on maternal 25(OH)D supplies. 25(OH)D readily crosses the placenta and it is activated into 1,25(OH)$_2$D by fetal kidneys. Vitamin D deficiency has been linked to increased risk of preeclampsia, gestational diabetes mellitus, preterm birth, and other conditions. Inadequate exposure of the mother to the sun increases risk of vitamin D deficiency in the infant and has an effect on the immune system and bone development. Vitamin D is also important for maintaining maternal calcium homeostasis. Vitamin D deficiency in the mother has been reported to be associated with maternal osteomalacia and neonatal hypocalcemia, tetany, and hypoplasia of teeth enamel. Poor vitamin D status of the mother may also be associated with lower bone mass in the child. However, vitamin D supplementation for pregnant women is not recommended by the World Health Organization.

Vitamin A
Vitamin A requirements are increased during pregnancy. RDA for vitamin A is 900 μg/day to meet the requirements for growth, cell differentiation, formation of epithelial lining, and immune system as well as vision. However, excessive consumption of retinol particularly from supplements is not advisable during pregnancy since it is teratogenic.

Vitamin E
Vitamin E is an antioxidant and hence protects against oxidative stress. Vitamin E deficiency has been linked to placental aging, vascular endothelial injury, development of preeclampsia, abruptio placentae, abortion, and increased risk of intrauterine growth restriction and premature rupture of membranes, premature birth as well as in disorders common to preterm infants such as chronic lung disease and necrotizing enterocolitis.

Vitamin K
Deficiency of vitamin K can lead to hemorrhage in pregnant women and especially in newborns, since this vitamin is needed for formation of prothrombin that has a role in blood coagulation. Women who are on anticoagulant therapy are at greater risk.

Iron
Iron is a nutrient of concern during pregnancy because this mineral is required for fetal growth and development. RDA for iron increases from 29 mg/day to 40 mg/day for expansion of blood volume, synthesis of maternal organs, storage of iron in the fetal liver and loss of iron through blood loss at the time of delivery. It is involved in formation of iron-containing compounds like hemoglobin (important for transporting oxygen to the developing fetus), myoglobin, and certain enzymes. Iron is also required for neurological development. It supports synthesis of neurotransmitters, plasticity and influences the language, cognitive, and motor skills not only in young children but also in school children, adolescents, and in adulthood. During the last trimester, the fetus accumulates considerable amount of iron that will be used in the first 6 months of postnatal life (when the baby is breastfed and milk is a poor source of iron). Maternal anemia during pregnancy is associated with reduced birth weight, perinatal, maternal and infant mortality as well as higher risk of premature delivery. Iron deficiency can lead to neurological defects. Although absorption of dietary iron is increased during pregnancy, it may not be sufficient to meet the increased demand. Hence, iron supplements are generally recommended to improve the pregnancy outcome. However, excess iron may increase the risk of oxidative stress, lipid peroxidation, and impaired glucose metabolism as well as gestational hypertension.

Iodine
During pregnancy, iodine is required for the production of fetal thyroid hormones (as the fetal thyroid begins to function

only around the 12th week of gestation), requirement is 250 µg/day. It is also essential for growth, formation, and development of organs and tissues as well as metabolism of glucose, proteins, lipids, calcium and phosphorus, and thermogenesis. Iodine deficiency increases the risk of spontaneous abortion, perinatal mortality, birth defects, and neurological disorders. Maternal deficiency of iodine during pregnancy results in fetal hypothyroidism that can cause mental retardation (cretinism). Deficiency in later stages of pregnancy has less severe impact than in the early part of pregnancy. WHO has stated that iodine deficiency is a preventable cause of brain damage. Thus, adequate intake of iodine is important for development of the fetus. Use of iodized salt can prevent iodine deficiency to large extent.

Calcium

Calcium requirement is 1000 mg/day which is same as normal woman as well as during pregnancy owing to increased absorption in pregnancy. Maternal absorption is increased in correspondence to the fetal demand. The fetus requires calcium, most of which is deposited during the third trimester. Maternal turnover is also increased. Thus, adequate maternal intake is required, not only to supply adequate calcium to the fetus but also to maintain maternal bone reserves.

Zinc

Zinc is also important for structural, metabolic, and immune functions that include cell growth, development, and differentiation. It also supports brain development. Its retention increases with the progress of pregnancy. Zinc is important for nucleic acid metabolism, participates in DNA synthesis (thus is important for protein synthesis), and formation and stabilization of enzymes. Hence, its requirement is also increased during pregnancy. Zinc deficiency has been linked to abortion and stillbirth, preterm delivery, fetal neural tube defects, intrauterine growth retardation, and low birth weight. Zinc supplementation during pregnancy has been found to improve birth length. Zinc deficiency also alters circulating levels of a number of hormones associated with the onset of labor, and because zinc is essential for normal immune function, deficiency may contribute to systemic and intrauterine infections, both major causes of preterm birth. Low birth weight and prematurity are significant risk factors for neonatal and infant morbidity and mortality. It has been hypothesized that zinc supplementation may improve pregnancy outcomes for mothers and infants. UNICEF recommends that antenatal supplements including zinc, iron, and folic acid be given to pregnant women in developing countries because they are likely to have low dietary intakes of these micronutrients. According to the WHO, there are no harmful effects of zinc supplementation, but the public health benefit of zinc supplements to pregnant women appears to be limited.

Magnesium

Magnesium is an important mineral and its requirement increases during pregnancy from 325 mg to 375 mg/day. Many studies indicate that women from lower socioeconomic background have low magnesium intakes. Although studies are limited, there may be a link between magnesium inadequacy and preeclampsia during pregnancy. However, there is limited evidence to make a case for providing magnesium supplementation during pregnancy. But mothers should be advised to consume magnesium-rich foods during pregnancy.

Copper

Copper is essential for embryonic development. Plasma copper concentrations significantly and progressively increase during pregnancy and return to normal after delivery. This increase relates to the synthesis of ceruloplasmin, due to altered levels of estrogen. Dietary deficiency can result in structural abnormalities and increased risk of cardiovascular disease. Severe copper deficiency can lead to reproductive failure and early embryonic death. The role of different nutrients and the consequences of deficiency of nutrients are explained in Table 11.5.

Impact of Nutritional Deficits on Fetal Growth

Nutritional challenges exerted by maternal nutrient intake during fetal development influence fetal growth, birth weight, fetal survival and more importantly have long-term implications in terms of functional, metabolic capacity and the risk of chronic, non-communicable diseases in later life of the offspring. Single nutrient deficiency is uncommon and multiple nutrient deficits in intrauterine environment is one of the major causes of intrauterine growth retardation (IUGR). Generally, the fetus adapts to the nutritional imbalance by metabolic structural and functional changes. In response to maternal undernutrition and inadequate nutrient supply, the production of hormones and sensitivity of various tissues to these hormones is altered, blood flow is redirected and growth slows down. It alters the rate of growth and development of the fetal organs and tissues. Nutrients are diverted to some important organs such as the brain at the expense of other organs (liver, pancreas and muscles). These organs are compelled to adapt. These adaptations may permanently alter the structure and functions of the various organs. The fetus requires glucose for energy and low glucose concentrations will slow down fetal growth and development.

Fetal changes in the womb
- Reduction in cell mass
- Changes in the structure of the tissue or organ at micro level
- Altered endocrine system and resetting the hormone production
- Alteration in lipid metabolism
- Effects on protein utilization
- Increased amino acid oxidation
- Increased lactate oxidation
- Decreased glucose oxidation due to inadequate supply
- Decreased supply of methyl donor for DNA synthesis
- Altered cardiac function
- Redistribution of blood flow
- Ultimately this is reflected in smaller body size.

Thus, any nutritional imbalance brings profound changes in maternal and fetal metabolism and physiology. Impact of fetal undernutrition persists throughout life.

Accumulating evidence indicates that epigenetic changes occur in response to maternal diet and environmental

Table 11.5: Role of nutrients during pregnancy.

Critical nutrients	Role in pregnancy	Effect of deficiency
Protein	Cell division, DNA synthesis, expansion of blood volume Formation of hormones, enzymes and antibodies	Increases risk of maternal insulin resistance, preterm birth, and IUGR Reduced growth of placenta and the fetus Protein energy malnutrition Growth retardation
Fats	Provision of energy Deposition of adipose tissues	Lower gestational weight gain Fetal growth may be impaired
Fatty acids (omega-6 and omega-3)	Support fetal growth particularly of brain and eye	Impaired brain development Impaired visual acuity Behavioral deficits may not be reversed with postnatal supplementation
Folic acid	Methyl donor for methylation and DNA synthesis Cell division Development of fetal heart, brain, spinal cord, and placenta	Impaired cell growth and cell division Risk of neural tube defects Risk of megaloblastic anemia Risk of cancer later in life
Vitamin A	Cell differentiation during cell growth Development of healthy bones, teeth and eyes, etc.	Fetal growth retardation Low birth weight
Vitamin B_6	Participates in gluconeogenesis Synthesis of heme and neurotransmitters Plays a role in decreasing homocysteine level	Affects fetal brain development and response to the immediate environment
Riboflavin	Coenzyme involved in metabolism of methionine and homocysteine Metabolism of amino acids, lipids and glycogen as one carbon unit provider	Abnormal protein synthesis Impaired cell division Elevated homocysteine level in the blood Inadequate fetal stores increases risk of postnatal deficiency Negative consequences on developing brain, possibly demyelination, abnormal pigmentation, hypotonia, enlarged liver and spleen, sparse hair, food refusal, anorexia, failure to thrive, and diarrhea
Vitamin C	For formation of collagen, connective tissues, cartilage, muscles, and the lowest layer of skin	Poor pregnancy outcomes such as low birth weight, preeclampsia Poor fetal brain development—affect learning
Iron	*Placenta formation* Formation of neurotransmitters Synthesis of heme Production of blood cells Transport of oxygen to cells Formation of iron dependent enzymes	Depleted blood volume Low hemoglobin level Anemia Maternal hypoferriemia Irreversible changes in some of the brain functions of fetus
Zinc	Structural and regulatory functions as coenzymes Neurotransmission, maturation	Impaired DNA/RNA synthesis and cell division Low birth weight Infectious disease
Iodine	Normal brain development and maturation Regulate metabolic rate (BMR)	Impaired blood cells, impaired functioning of nervous system, physical and mental growth retardation
Calcium	Maintain maternal bone reserves and to improve neonatal bone density during lactation	Growth retardation Low bone density
Vitamin D	Calcium metabolism Bone development	Several disorders of calcium metabolism in both the mother and her infant, including neonatal hypocalcemia and tetany, infant hypoplasia of tooth enamel, and maternal osteomalacia
Choline (Betaine is a precursor of choline)	Involved in methylation (donation of methyl group) to homocysteine to form methionine Formation of memory part in hippocampus (brain part) Formation of acetylcholine Normal membrane functions	Deficiency may increase homocysteine level, which is not desirable in pregnancy, which may increase the risk of preeclampsia, premature birth even maternal and neonatal deaths

conditions (stress) and contribute to the 'fetal origins of several adult metabolic disorders,' i.e., development and progression of diseases (non-communicable linked to inflammation) such as rheumatoid arthritis, metabolic disorders (obesity, type 2 diabetes), cardiovascular disease, and cancer. These are rooted in perturbations that have occurred in utero during pregnancy and/or postnatal life. Evidence suggests that the metabolic phenotype is shaped and this may be across generations affecting lifelong risk. These adaptations are manifested in poor insulin secretion, reduced growth of β cells, insulin resistance (IR), glucose intolerance (GI), hypertension (HT), non-insulin dependent diabetes mellitus (NIDDM) and altered lipid metabolism, in adult life. Both maternal undernutrition as well as obesity has adverse influence. If the mother is diabetic, high glucose concentrations also have an adverse effect on growth of the embryo.

Low Birth Weight Babies

As defined by the WHO, low birth weight (LBW) is a weight at birth less than 2,500 g (5.5 pounds). The baby can be LBW either as a result of being born preterm (PT) (before 37 weeks of gestation) or due to small gestational age (SGA), i.e., less than the 10th percentile of weight for age or both. In developing countries including India, LBW and SGA are generally due to intrauterine growth retardation. In India, 25–30 % of babies are low birth weight (LBW). Of these 60% are attributable to fetal growth restriction, while the remaining 40% are born preterm, constituting a quarter of the global burden of preterm births (Fig. 11.5). Preterm babies are at a higher risk of neonatal mortality, as well as increased risk of post-neonatal mortality. They also have a risk of being stunted and suffering long-term neuro-developmental impairment during childhood. Preterm birth increases risk of mortality and LBW is associated with early growth retardation postnatally, infection, developmental delays as well as risk of death in infancy and childhood.

The term "small-for-date" is used for those infants whose development potential has not been fully achieved in utero. Such babies also suffer long-term developmental sequelae such as problems with learning and behavior, as their neurological development may be affected. Malnutrition has adverse effects on brain and neurological development because the brain develops in utero and its development is completed in the first few years of life itself. There is a link between socioeconomic status and birthweight and it can be improved by better maternal nutrition resulting in better outcome of pregnancy.

Barker and his team in 1992 put forward the concept of "thrifty phenotype" to describe the association between fetal and infant malnutrition and the risk of development of NCDs in later life. Such infants develop under constraints of limited nutrient(s) supply and development of some tissues could occur at the expense of others. For example, brain growth will be supported at the expense of truncal growth, the growth of skeletal muscle, the development of abdominal organs (liver, pancreas, kidneys), and some parts of the vascular network. These alterations may lead to permanent changes in the structure and physiology of many tissues, leading to reduced functional capacity in later life. Onset of disease could be triggered more readily by "stressors" even if better nourishment is provided. For example, undernutrition during infancy results in low pancreatic beta cell mass, increasing the risk of type 2 diabetes and the metabolic syndrome later in life. Obesity in later life exacerbates the condition.

Reasons for LBW are multiple and interdependent; some of them are as follows:
- Low prepregnancy weight of the mother
- Insufficient weight gain during pregnancy particularly during second trimester
- Insufficient nutrient intakes particularly of protein, amino acids, and micronutrients in first trimester and energy and other nutrients in third trimester
- Anemia and poor compliance with iron supplementation
- Low maternal education
- Inadequate availability, access to, utilization of healthcare services and resources, i.e., lack of adequate prenatal care
- Cultural beliefs regarding food intake in pregnancy and food fads
- Strenuous activity outside home during third trimester when energy intake is inadequate
- Smoking and alcohol consumption
- Depletion of nutrients due to closely spaced pregnancies
- Malaria
- Maternal vascular diseases, maternal diabetes, elderly primigravidae
- Twin or multiple fetuses
- Desire of some women to look fashionable and slender aggravates the undernourishment leading to low birth weight child.
- Short maternal stature is related to infant size (reflects chronic undernutrition if it is not genetic) rather than paternal stature.

Pregnancy in Special Conditions

There are certain situations in pregnancy during which the woman is at high risk. The causes of these may be physiological and many a times, social/cultural and environmental. Examples of situations that are challenging are: teenage pregnancy, gestational diabetes, high blood pressure, preeclampsia (pregnancy-induced hypertension), and if the woman has eating disorders or other chronic conditions. Teenage pregnancy is common in a social system where girls are married before they reach puberty or unmarried young girls due to several other reasons are sexually active and become pregnant. Dietary intake of such high-risk teenage girls is often deficient in nutrients. They are also ignorant of requirements during pregnancy and complications. Some conditions that pose challenges are briefly discussed.

Teenage/Adolescent Pregnancy

Teen pregnancy refers to pregnancy during adolescence or under the age of 18 years. Adolescence is characterized by sexual maturation and growth spurt due to which nutritional requirements of the adolescent girl's body increases. If she is pregnant, the need for nourishing her fetus and her own

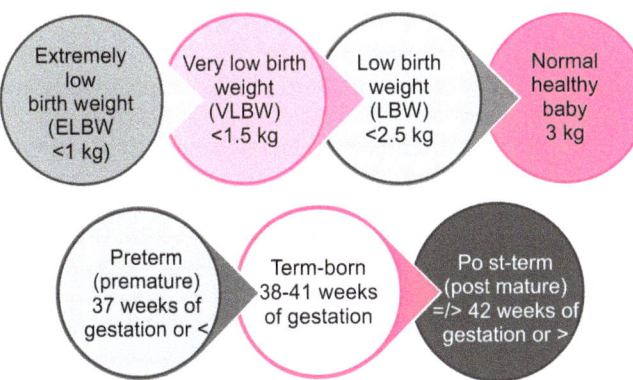

Fig. 11.5: Birth weights of ELBW, LBW, and normal healthy infants; weeks of gestation—preterm, term and post-term.

requirements for her own growth spurt and for the various physiological changes that usually occur during pregnancy together, will increase her nutrient requirements, which will be more than that of an adult pregnant woman. Thus, the nutrients that she consumes have to be shared by her body as well as the fetus. Hence, pregnant adolescent girls have to face a dual edged sword, i.e., meeting their own physiological needs and the nutritional demands of the fetus, which is often practically difficult to meet. The girls are usually not financially independent and are not allowed to make their own decisions. Education level is often low at this age. Medical (prenatal) care may not be available/accessible. Poor environmental support and high physiological requirements result in poor pregnancy outcome such as miscarriage, abortions, low birth weight, congenital defects, high morbidity, and high mortality.

Gestational Diabetes Mellitus

Gestational diabetes mellitus (GDM) is glucose intolerance during pregnancy (gestation). The diabetes may be preexisting or may develop during pregnancy. In case of the latter, blood glucose levels usually return to normal after childbirth. However, there is a high risk of developing type II diabetes both in mother and the child later in life. It also increases the risk of premature delivery. It is common in obese women who generally have insulin resistance. High maternal weight gain during pregnancy also predisposes to GDM. Blood glucose should be monitored daily since tight control is beneficial. Regular monitoring of blood pressure is also important. Dietary management is important for women who have diabetes and help from a qualified dietician should be sought. Nutrient requirements are individualized especially for energy and protein. Artificial sweeteners should be avoided. Gestational diabetes increases risk of caesarean delivery and macrosomia in the offspring.

Obesity and Pregnancy

The prevalence of obesity is rising in our country. This is of concern because obesity increases risk of several health problems many of which are serious concern—gestational diabetes, preeclampsia (high blood pressure), sleep apnea (this leads to fatigue and increases the risk of high blood pressure, preeclampsia, eclampsia, and heart and lung disorders). Also, risk of pregnancy loss and birth defects like neural tube defects (NTDs) is higher. Obesity also makes ultrasound examinations difficult to carry out in terms of visualizing the baby's anatomy. There is risk of the baby being macrosomic, which in turn increases risk of the infant being injured during birth and/or caesarean delivery. For women who are extremely obese, gaining less than the recommended amount or losing weight during pregnancy might lower the risk of having a baby whose weight is greater than the 90th percentile for gestational age (large for gestational age).

Also, a baby born to an obese mother is at risk of becoming obese in later life. This is partly due to genetic influence and that the infant very likely is exposed to an obesogenic environment that will accelerate the process of fat gain early in life. Obese children would also become at risk for type II diabetes.

Even if a mother is obese, she should not try to lose weight during pregnancy. What is important that great care should be taken to avoid excessive weight gain. Studies indicate that losing weight or gaining too little weight during pregnancy can increase the risk of preterm birth or that the baby is small for gestational age and having a baby whose weight is less than the 10th percentile for gestational age (small for gestational age). There is also risk of stillbirth. An obese mother may be recommended to gain less weight during pregnancy than a mother with normal BMI. It is generally advisable that an obese woman should first lose weight and then conceive in order to avoid the problems associated with obesity.

> **Research Glimpse:** Our gut microbial communities are resilient, i.e., they are capable of maintaining a stable and balanced state, although there could be alterations in the gut environment, diet, etc. This resilience is very important in terms of humans achieving and maintaining optimal health. Loss of microbial resilience has been associated/linked to diseases such as obesity, diabetes, and metabolic syndrome. However, the role of the gut microbiota is not fully elucidated and understood, especially in terms of reasons why in some individuals co-evolved microflora do not develop resilience, setting such individuals on a path that results in poor metabolic health. This review examines the connections between the developing gut microbiota and intestinal barrier function in the neonate, infant, and during the first years of life. The authors propose that in early life the gut microflora is in a dynamic and vulnerable state and is shaped by early life events. Not only are gut microflora composition and resilience influenced, but there is also an influence on gut permeability, all of which are very important for achieving and maintaining good metabolic health and reducing the risk of diseases. The authors have suggested new potential research directions aimed at developing a greater understanding of the longitudinal effects of the gut microflora on metabolic health and potential interventions that can help to "recalibrate" infants who are "at risk" of having unfavorable gut microflora profiles.
>
> *Kerr CA, Grice DM, Tran CD, et al. Early life events influence whole-of-life metabolic health via gut microflora and gut permeability. Crit Rev Microbiol. 2015;41(3):326-40.*

Dietary Guidelines for Pregnant Mothers

In order to ensure a normal and healthy pregnancy, the mother should:

- Ensure adequate weight gain
- Eat well-balanced meals with plenty of fresh fruits and vegetables
- Increase intake of folate and iron rich foods along with vitamin C rich foods
- Include foods rich in omega-3 fatty acids, calcium, and carotenoids
- Increase intake of complex carbohydrate foods and reduce intake of free sugars and foods containing high fructose corn syrup, sugar-sweetened beverages
- Eat whole fruits instead of fruit juices
- Ensure that the RDA for protein is met by good quality protein sources such as egg, milk, oily fish, and pulses

- Avoid alcohol, caffeine, smoking, tannin rich foods like tea, coffee, cola beverages
- Reduce intake of salt, sugar, and refined foods
- Regularly drink 8-10 glasses of water or fluids like buttermilk (without salt) or milk
- Avoid skipping meals
- Eat small size meals at a time and eat several times a day, preferably at regular timings
- Avoid processed foods and consume freshly prepared meals
- Sedentary women should do regular exercise like walking. Before undertaking heavy exercises in a gymnasium, the mother should consult her obstetrician.

LACTATION

Lactation is the natural process of milk production by the mammary glands that are present within the fatty tissue of the breast. From the second trimester of pregnancy, the mammary glands are prepared for milk secretion under the influence of several hormones [adrenocorticotropic hormone (ACTH), growth hormone, glucocorticoids, and thyroid stimulating hormone (TSH)] especially estrogen and progesterone. Under their influence, the number of cells that produce milk increase and the ducts through which milk is transported expand. Synthesis of milk occurs in specialized structures known as alveoli. Milk is secreted when there is a stimulus, e.g., suckling by the infant. For this, there is an interaction of hormones like prolactin and oxytocin as well as reflexes of the infant, i.e., rooting and suckling reflexes are essential. When the infant suckles the nipple, signals are transmitted to the sensory nerves to the hypothalamus which then stimulates the pituitary gland to secrete oxytocin and prolactin. These hormones are carried through blood to the breasts, where oxytocin causes contraction of the myoepithelial cells of the mammary gland leading to milk ejection, i.e., milk is released into the ducts that lead to the nipple (Fig 11.6). In less than a minute after the beginning of suckling, milk begins to flow. Prolactin stimulates the synthesis of milk. Initiation of milk secretion/lactation is known as lactogenesis. Adequate lactation should provide comfort, sufficient milk supply, and lead to good infant and maternal health. Acharya Sushruta clearly enumerated factors that encourage milk ejection such as thought, sight or touch as well as physical contact of the child, but affection for the child is mainly responsible. The more the baby sucks at the breast, the greater is the stimulus for milk production. On the 3rd or 4th day after delivery, milk ejection starts. It is especially interesting that fondling of the baby by the mother or hearing the baby crying often gives enough of an emotional signal to the hypothalamus to cause milk ejection. Many psychogenic factors including anxiety and stress can inhibit oxytocin secretion and consequently depress milk ejection.

There are four stages of lactation:

1. **Stage I of lactogenesis:** During the latter part of pregnancy, the mammary glands enter this stage. The mammary gland develops the ability to secrete milk and lactose; protein and immunoglobulin are present in the fluid secreted by the gland. However, the high levels of progesterone and estrogen inhibit, lactation. Soon after delivery (parturition) progesterone levels drop and the mammary glands synthesize colostrum—a thick, yellowish nutrient-rich fluid.
2. **Stage II of lactogenesis:** This stage is around the time of parturition/delivery between days 2nd or 3rd to 8th after delivery. The mammary glands begin to secrete a large volume of milk. The placenta is detached (after delivery) resulting in a sharp drop in progesterone and estrogen levels. Several hormones like insulin, growth hormone, cortisol, and parathyroid hormone are needed to facilitate mobilization of nutrients that are required for milk synthesis and secretion.
3. **Galactopoiesis:** This is the stage where once lactation is established, it is maintained. Once lactation is initiated, the combined action of the two hormones—prolactin and oxytocin is necessary. Prolactin stimulates milk secretion. Oxytocin acts on muscle cells called myoepithelial cells that surround the alveoli and causes them to contract and forces milk out of the alveoli. Suckling by the baby or physical stimulus to the breast, stimulates the mammary gland to secrete milk and it is the most important stimulus for milk secretion (Fig. 11.7).
4. **Involution:** This occurs approximately 40 days on average after breastfeeding stops. Peptides that inhibit milk secretion build up and hence milk secretion is reduced and then ceases.

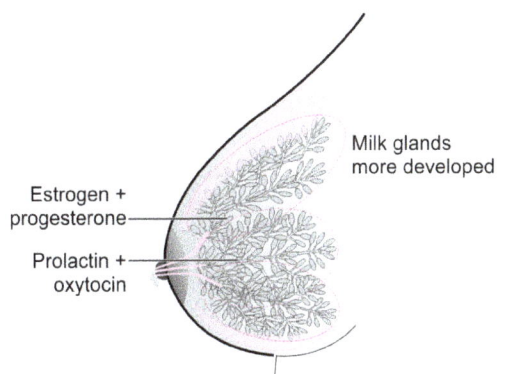

Fig. 11.6: Lactating breast structure.

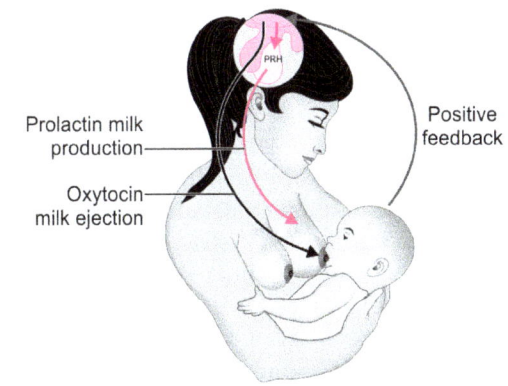

Fig. 11.7: Role of prolactin and oxytocin in lactation.

> **Advantages of lactation**
> - Ensures safe and right food for the baby
> - Ensures adequacy of food for 4–6 months
> - Strengthens mother-child bonding
> - Helps in birth spacing
> - Benefits mother's health
> - Helps involution of the uterus (go back to its original shape and size)
> - Saves money
> - Environment friendly
> - Reduces risk of vascular changes associated with future cardiovascular diseases
> - Reduced risk of cancers (breast, ovarian, and endometrial)

Factors Affecting Lactation

Lactation is an essential activity of postnatal care and nurture of the infant. It provides food for the baby, also supports the mother to recover fast and prevents another pregnancy. Smoking and use of drugs, pesticides, and highly flavored food or beverages are harmful to the baby because most of them are lipid soluble and easily transferred through the breast milk. Following factors have strong influence on lactation:

Endocrine functions: Lactation is controlled by adequate release of hormones like oxytocin, prolactin and which can be affected by physiology and external stressors.

Dietary factors: In India, it is believed that use of galactogogues has positive effect on lactation. Many of the galactogogues are nutrient-dense that would supply essential nutrients to the mother.

> In Ayurveda, the Acharyas describe various treatment formulations in cases of stanyanasa and stanyakshya such as cereals, meat, cow's milk, sugar, curd and use of desired things cure stanyakshya. Happiness, absence of sorrow, anger, fear, and excessive walking influences the lactation. Use of stanyajanandravya (drugs capable of increasing amount of milk) as decoction of roots of Viran, Shalli, Shshthika, Ekshuvalika (*Saccharum officinarum*), Darbha (*Imperata cylindrical*), Kusha (*Desmostachyabi pinnata*), Kasha (*Saccharum spontaneum*), Gundra, Itkata, Katrina, Pestledtila (*Sesamum indicum*), Iashuna (*Allium sativum*), fish, sringataka (*Trapa natans*), vidarikanda (*Pueraria tuberosa*), madhuka, alabu are also used for stanyajanan. Satavari (*Asparagus racemosus*) along with milk is also recommended.

Psychological factors: Willingness of a mother to breastfeed the baby is crucial for milk flow. Some mothers do not want to feed their babies for variety of reasons. Some are confused whether they will be able to breastfeed and many do not know how to position the baby. Many mothers think that if the baby cries, it is because he/she is hungry and try to turn toward readily available baby foods. One good indication is how frequently the baby wets its diapers and the weight gained by the baby is an important indicator. Under most circumstances, even in a hot climate, the baby can thrive on solely breast milk. Mothers who have problems and new mothers should seek advice regarding breastfeeding. Nowadays, well-trained lactation counselors are there to help mothers. Breastfeeding Promotion Network of India (BPNI) is an organization that is doing a great deal in this area.

Sociocultural factors: In some communities, certain taboos and beliefs are strongly linked to lactation presumably in favor of both the mother and the baby. However, most of them lack scientific evidence, e.g., colostrum is bad and should not be given to child. Child should not be exposed to open air/sun and kept inside at least for 40 days.

Nutritional Requirements of the Lactating Mother

The lactating mother requires adequate nutrition to enable synthesis of breast milk. Generally, mothers produce more milk in the first 6 months when the baby is fed only milk. Upon giving solid or liquid food including water during breastfeeding, milk secretion may tend to decrease. Nutritional requirements of lactating mothers are estimated based on the volume of milk secreted and its composition. DHA supports psychomotor development in the 1st month of life via breast milk.

Energy: During the first 6 months postpartum, energy cost of milk production is estimated to be 573 kcal/day. This is added to the energy requirement for nonpregnant women. The RDA for sedentary women is 1660 kcal/day. Hence the lactating mother would require 2260 kcal/day in first 6 months. After 6 months when the volume of milk decreases, the additional requirement also decreases to 520 kcal/day. Food sources of energy are important. Energy dense food needs to be replaced by nutrient dense foods like nuts, milk, pulses (egg and fish if nonvegetarian), would be better choices.

Protein: Protein requirement is increased to meet the needs for milk synthesis. The quality of protein is very important because high quality protein can support the synthesis of milk protein. Also, during exclusive breastfeeding, RDA for protein is increased by 16.9 g/day in the first six months and 13.2 g/day later, if breast milk still represents a substantial proportion of the infant's diet.

Fat: Fat is the major source of energy for the infant and human milk (hind milk) is rich in fat. Some amount of fat is also mobilized from adipose tissue of the mother to the infant through milk. Presence of essential fatty acids particularly DHA and long chain fatty acids in maternal diet is crucial for brain development. Hence, selection of fat source(s) is crucial. Visible fat in the form of ghee or butter may fulfill the energy requirement, but they do not provide the EFA required. Invisible sources of fat containing n-3 fatty acids are useful.

Vitamins: Requirement for folic acid is lower as compared to pregnancy as shown in Figure 11.4, because there is no cell division. However, RDA for vitamin A is significantly 950 mg/day. Requirements for thiamine, riboflavin, and niacin correspond with energy needs. RDA for vitamin C is high, i.e., 115 mg/day.

Minerals: RDA for calcium during lactation is increased to 1200 mg/day while iron requirements are decreased to 23 mg/day. Infant stores iron in the body from the mother during pregnancy, that is sufficient for 6 months of life only. This is because while the mothers are breastfeeding, generally there will be amenorrhea and thus the mothers will not have any losses through menstruation. Requirements for some trace minerals are also higher.

Dietary Guidelines for Lactating Mother

- A well-balanced diet should be consumed by mothers ensuring that all the nutrient requirements are met through appropriate food selection.
- Since a lactating mother's energy requirements are much higher than a pregnant woman's, she needs energy-rich foods.
- She often feels hungry, hence food selection in each meal should be such that it supplies nutrient dense foods such as nuts or high protein foods, which will also provide micronutrients.
- Since she does not need extra fat, she is not required to consume very high amounts of fat but inclusion of foods containing EPA/DHA and LCPUFA is important.
- She can have frequent meals, i.e., five to six times a day.
- Mothers should emphasize whole grains, nuts and seeds, fruits and vegetables, and safe dairy products.
- Add some galactagogues in the diet, e.g., adding extra *Jeera* in the seasoning (*See* box).
- Fluid intake should be adequate.
- Mothers who are keen to lose weight should refrain from using fad diets. Breastfeeding itself can help the mother to lose weight. Also, regular moderate physical activity is good for the mother's health.
- Feeding immediately after exercise is not advisable, since there may be some lactic acid in the milk if the mother has undertaken vigorous exercise.
- It is advisable to avoid alcohol, caffeine, smoking, and self-prescribed drugs since some medicines can be transferred through breast milk.

> Traditionally in India, the breastfeeding mother is also served special foods. These special foods are called **Galactogogues**. Galactogogues are considered to be special foods which tend to improve breast milk secretion and enhance well-being and recovery of the mother. Such foods are relatively rich in nutrients including energy and also may have some medicinal value. Commonly used galactogogues are *methi* seeds, fennel seeds, cumin seeds, dill seeds (*suva*), *tulsi* seeds, garden cress seeds (*halim*), poppy seeds (*khuskhus*), garlic, edible gums, *ajwain*, dry ginger (*sonth*), coriander seeds, etc. Different communities from different regions make a variety of preparations like *kheer*, porridge, *laddoos*, *burfi*, *halwa*, *panjeeri*, sprinkles, and decoctions like herbal teas. Sometimes, they are included as a part of major meals or snacks.

Ayurveda advises the breastfeeding mother to consume warm, easily digested foods. Spices that help in digestion are advised, e.g., cumin, fennel, fenugreek, ginger, turmeric, black pepper, garlic, dill, and coriander. The mother is advised that she consume plenty of vegetables, pulses like *mung* and lentils, soaked figs, dates, rice *kheer*, whereas she should avoid dry and cold food, raw vegetables, leftover food, fried food, foods that are difficult to digest as well as stimulants like coffee, black tea, chocolate, and alcohol.

BREASTFEEDING

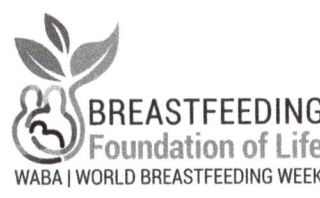

Infant demand is perhaps the most important factor in the regulation of milk production. Maternal nutrition and other factors do not play a large role in regulation of milk production. Similarly, the size or shape of the breasts does not affect much. However, the amount of milk produced depends on infant demand and suckling. If water or milk or any other fluid or foods are introduced, the rate of milk production decreases in proportion to the amount that has been fed to the infant. For successful breastfeeding, the attitude of the mother and proper positioning of the baby are very important. Even the thought of feeding the baby or hearing its cry can stimulate milk secretion. On the contrary, unwillingness to feed the baby, anxiety, stress, or fatigue reduces milk production.

Recommendations for Breastfeeding

The World Health Organization (2018 revised) and the Ministry of Women and Child Development (Food and Nutrition Board, Government of India, 2006) have made recommendations for Infant and Young Child Feeding (IYCF). Many mothers may require and should receive practical support to enable them to initiate and establish breastfeeding and manage common breastfeeding difficulties. The Optimal and Appropriate Infant and Young Child Nutrition Practices and Strategies (2016) are as follows:

- **Initiation of breastfeeding immediately after birth preferably within 1 hour.** All mothers should be supported to do so. This can be facilitated by early (as soon as possible after birth) and uninterrupted skin-to-skin contact between mothers and infants should be facilitated and encouraged.
- **Exclusive breastfeeding for the first 6 months,** i.e., first 180 days with no other milk, food, drink or water being fed to the infant, unless it is medically indicated otherwise.
- Mothers may need coaching on how to continue giving breast milk, by expressing breast milk and its storage, if they are separated from the baby for any length of time.
- If expressed breast milk or other feeds are medically indicated for term infants, feeding methods such as cups, spoons, or feeding bottles and teats may be used during their stay at the facility.
- **After baby completes 6 months, introduction of optimal complementary feeding should be practiced** preferably with energy dense, homemade foods.
- Appropriate and adequate complementary feeding from 6 months of age while continuing breastfeeding.
- Breastfeeding should be continued minimum for 2 years and beyond.
- Mother should practice responsive feeding by communicating (talking, singing), maintain eye contact with baby, look into the eyes, touch, and caress the baby while feeding.

- Mothers should be supported to recognize their infants' cues for feeding, closeness and comfort, and enabled to respond accordingly to these cues with a variety of options, during their stay at the facility providing maternity and newborn services.
- In addition, WHO Growth Charts are recommended for monitoring growth.
- For preterm infants who are unable to breastfeed directly, non-nutritive sucking and oral stimulation may be beneficial until breastfeeding is established.
- If expressed breast milk or other feeds are medically indicated for preterm infants, feeding methods such as cups or spoons are preferable to feeding bottles and teats (recommended, moderate-quality evidence).

Besides this, recommendations and strategies have been advised for facilities providing maternity and newborn services. They should have a clearly written breastfeeding policy that is routinely communicated to staff and parents. The health facility staff who provide infant feeding services, including breastfeeding support, should have sufficient knowledge, competence and skills to support women to breastfeed. Facilities providing antenatal care should counsel pregnant women and their facilities about the benefits and management of breastfeeding. Access to ongoing support and appropriate care should be planned for and coordinated for parents and infants when being discharged from the facility.

Prelacteal Foods

In India, there is a tradition of giving nonmilk foods and liquid, e.g., honey/sugar or glucose solution/cow's urine/"*janamghutti*", etc. These foods called "Prelacteal foods" should not be given because they can be a source of infection for the delicate newborn whose immune system is still immature. The best practice is to put the baby to the breast immediately within an hour of the delivery. Human milk is unique and highly nutritive fluid with immunologic and growth-promoting properties that nature makes to suit the requirements, growth pattern, and the physiological maturity of the human infant.

The composition of animal milk suits the requirements of their young. Mammalian milk including human milk is species-specific. Health experts strongly recommend that the baby should be given colostrum. Human milk is unique because its composition changes as the baby grows to meet the changing needs of the baby during growth and maturation. For example, "Colostrum" or early milk, i.e., milk secreted in the first few days after delivery has lower concentrations of fat than mature milk but higher concentrations of protein and minerals.

It is thicker than mature milk, yellowish in color, and is rich in essential nutrients and numerous anti-infective factors. Gradually, milk changes in composition. Mature milk is produced usually after 21 days. Besides changes during the first 3 weeks, composition changes within a single feed. Milk that is secreted at the beginning of the feed has a lower fat content and as the infant continues to breastfeed, the fat content increases during the several minutes of the feed. Milk secreted at the beginning of the feed is known as fore milk and that secreted toward the end of the feed is called hind milk. The higher fat content of hind milk is thought to give satiety to the infant.

Colostrum

Colostrum is the first form of breast milk and it should be given within an hour after birth. Colostrum is a yellowish thick fluid, rich in protein, immunoglobulins, and electrolytes. The yellowish color is attributed to the high concentration of carotenoids such as α-carotene, β-carotene, β-cryptoxanthin, lutein, and zeaxanthin. Major proteins are casein, lactoferrin, α-lactalbumin and immunoglobulin (IgA), and amino acids such as lysine, leucine, isoleucine, valine, arginine, and threonine in higher concentration. Antibodies provide protection from infection throughout life.

Human Milk Bank

India had a tradition of wet nurses who breastfed infants who were not or could not be fed by their biological mothers for various reasons. *Acharya Vagbhata* advised for arrangement of two wet nurses in situations where the own mother was unable to breast feed the baby. Examination of wet-nurses (including physical, physico-psychological qualities) has been described in Ayurvedic literature, so that breastfeeding results in proper growth and development in child. *Acharya Charaka* says that wet-nurse should be young, modest, nonaddict, similar in *desha*, affectionate to the child, free from diseases, *jivitvatsa* (having alive child), having adequate amount of breast milk, etc.

Often there is need for milk substitute. Some mothers are unable to breast feed and in a few unfortunate cases, the mother may not be living. In 1980, WHO and UNICEF made the joint statement "Where it is not possible for the biological mother to breastfeed, the first alternative, if available, should be the use of human milk from other sources".

In the modern era, milk banks serve to provide human milk to infants who are deprived of breast milk from their own mothers. Human milk banks should be made available in appropriate situations. In India, the first Milk Bank was established by a neonatologist Dr Armida Fernandez in 1989 at the Lokmanya Tilak Municipal General Hospital (LTMGH) in Sion, Mumbai. Later, other hospitals in the country are also establishing human milk bank following certain guidelines provided by Indian Academey of Pediatrics (2014).

Human milk bank is a service for collecting, screening, processing, storing, and distributing donated human milk. It is next best to giving the infant the breast milk of its biological mother. It is not only used as infant food but also in the treatment of several infant diseases. The American Academy of Pediatrics advocates human milk since it plays a critical role in improvement in nutritional status of all babies as same components cannot be present in formula milk. Expressed maternal milk (EMM) is useful in increasing weight gain, improving protein status, and bone mineralization. Mothers, who are interested in contributing, express their breast milk and donate it to the bank, where it is screened and pasteurized in order to prevent transmission of infection to the infant. Milk is stored in containers and frozen and can be stored for approximately 3 months.

CHILDHOOD YEARS

Childhood years include the period from infancy to adolescence including puberty. The terminology of early childhood that is between 0-8 years has been used by several organizations. WHO (2020) considers early childhood as a period of physical, socioemotional, cognitive and motor development and recommends four support strategies for better improvement, i.e., (1) Response care giving, (2) Promote early learning, (3) Integrate care giving and nutrition intervention and (4) Support maternal mental health.

Since child's age is the key feature in terms of the growth, development and nutrition, care and other characteristics. In pediatrics, childhood is categorized 6 life stages, i.e., newborn or neonate (0–28 days), infancy (till 1 year), toddler (till 3 years), preschool (till 6 years), school age (till 12 years) and adolescence (till 18 years). Largely on the basis of growth and development, childhood in this section, are discussed in terms of infancy, preschool years, school age and adolescence years.

Infancy

Infancy is the period between birth up to 12 months of age/postnatal life. Early childhood is as critical a period of the life cycle as is fetal life. Many organs systems are still growing and continue to mature. The critical developmental processes include:
- Myelination of the central nervous system
- Development of immune memory
- Maturation of lungs and kidneys
- Changes in gastrointestinal system
- Changes in body composition.

Infancy is characterized by very rapid rate of growth and development. Changes in weight, height and body circumferences occur at faster rate in this age as compared to other stages of life are given in Table 11.6. Characteristically, there is rapid cell division, fast weight gain, synthesis of new cells and tissues, formation of hormones, enzymes, antibodies, and the maturation of the vital organs. The only other stage in life when such rapid growth will occur is during the adolescent/pubertal growth spurt.

Birth weight of the infant is crucial. A normal healthy infant's weight is 3.0–3.5 kg. Birth weight is an indicator of growth in fetal life, the newborn's chances of survival and future growth, development, and morbidity pattern. Immediately after birth, in the first few days, an infant normally loses about 5–10% of his or her body weight. This is due to loss of fluids and some breakdown of body tissues. By the end of the 1st week, however most infants regain this weight by 2 weeks of age and thereafter should start gaining weight and grow quickly. By the first 4–6 months, birth weight usually doubles and by 12 months, it should have tripled. Rate of weight gain indicates the adequacy of nutrition and care given to the infant.

Measurement of body weight is an easy, practical, and economical way to assess growth pattern of the infant. The baby should be weighed every month and the weight plotted on growth charts and its progress monitored. These charts are divided into percentiles. Most infants follow a consistent growth pattern and if a child changes the percentile, especially if there is a downward shift, it calls for immediate attention since the infant's growth may be slower than expected.

During the 1st year, tremendous development occurs. From having little control over their bodies, babies develop muscle control, by 6 months most infants will be able to sit upright with support. These developmental changes influence how and what the baby should be fed.

There are major achievement stages that are known as developmental milestones. These can be easily identified and are classified into three categories: motor development, language development, and social/emotional development. The sequence of achievement of milestones is the same for all babies, although the age of attainment of milestones may vary among different infants.

Like prenatal life, the first 2 years are critical for promoting optimal growth, health and development of young children, and the feeding pattern of the infant is a major determinant of growth and development as well as health during adult life. The rapid growth rate during infancy requires adequate supply of nutrients which is usually fulfilled by the mother's milk. After 4–6 months, complementary foods are given to infants for optimal growth and development and risk and occurrence of diseases.

Nutritional Requirements of Normal Healthy Infants

It is well established that infant nutrition lays the foundation of the future nutritional status of an individual, including bone health, muscle function, immune and cognitive function, rates of aging and the risk of adult CHD, diabetes, stroke, asthma, and cancer.

Table 11.6: Normal physical changes in anthropometric measurements in infancy.

Age groups	Weight	Length (cm)	Head circumference (cm)	Chest circumference (cm)
At birth	2.5-3.5/3* kg	45-55 / 50*	33-37/35*	33 cm
0-3 months	25-30 g/day	3.5 cm /month	2 cm /month	HC > CC by 3 cm
4-6 months	20 g /day	2.0 cm /month	1 cm /month	
7-9 months	15 g/day	1.5 cm /month	0.5 cm /month	
10-12 months	12 g/day	1.0 cm /month	0.25 cm /month	> 6 months to 12 months

(HC: head circumference; CC: chest circumference; *: average value)

Nutritional needs of infants are much higher than that of adults on the basis of per kilogram body weight. Recommended Dietary Allowances ICMR-NIN, 2020 for infants are shown in Tables 9.1A and B in Chapter 9 and EAR is given in Appendix 4. The table indicates that the requirement is higher for certain nutrients such as protein, vitamin B_1, B_2, B_6, iron, magnesium, and iodine when the baby is growing and touching 12 months. However, the need for vitamin A, vitamin D and vitamin B_{12} are the same throughout the 1st year of life.

Energy: Energy needs of the infant are higher than that of adults on the basis of per kg body weight. This is required for the rapid growth that occurs in the 1st year. Also, the basal metabolic rate is high and there is a need to establish energy reserves in the body. At birth, about 35% of total energy is expended by the infant's body on growth. At the end of 12 months, this has declined to 5%. In the first 6 months of life, the baby requires 550 kcal/day and 670 kcal/day in first half and second half of the infancy. The requirements are usually fulfilled by the mother's milk in the first half of infancy (6 months) and subsequently from both breast milk and complementary foods. Milk provides 65 kcal/100 mL.

Protein: RDA for protein is high in the first 6 months of life, at the rate of 8.1 g/day and gradually increased to 10.5 g/day in the next 6 months. Average protein requirement is for maintenance + deposition, i.e., growth. According to experts, breastfed infants may require relatively less protein, i.e., 10–15% lesser than infants fed cow's milk or infant milk food.

Fat: After 6 months of life infant needs to be given 25 g fat per day. The fat in mother's milk furnishes 40–50% of energy. Fat composition of mother's milk includes phospholipids, essential fatty acids, long chain fatty acids (DHA), and medium chain triglycerides which are influenced by the maternal fat intake. Human milk fat is better absorbed and supports formation of cell membranes, retina and the development of brain structure, functions, and cognition. It is also used for fat storage which provides insulation to reduce heat loss from the body and provides padding to protect vital organs. It also improves the utilization of fat-soluble vitamins. Essential fatty acids present in milk helps in regulating growth, inflammatory responses, immune function, vision, cognitive development and motor systems in newborns.

Vitamins: Vitamin requirement is high and requirements for most vitamins which are adequately met by breast milk except for vitamin D and K. Breast milk is low in vitamin D and is also influenced by vitamin D status of the mother. In such conditions, infant may require vitamin D from supplements or should be exposed to the sun for 20-30 minutes daily in the morning. Infants are often given a dose of supplemental vitamin K to prevent risk of hemorrhage.

Minerals: Mother's milk can only supply adequate amount of minerals in the first 6 months of life. The absorption of iron, zinc and calcium from mothers' milk is also better as compared to bovine milk. The proportion of calcium and phosphorus is just right to support growth and development of bones, smooth muscles, and nerves. In absence of breastfeeding, or supplement with cow's milk the ratio of calcium and phosphorus is much higher and that is much higher in buffalo's milk. It may cause excess of calcium and tax the immature kidneys. Hence animal milks are avoided. On contrary deficiency of desirable minerals may cause adverse effects on the nervous system, parathyroid, intestinal flora, and bones. After 6 months, breast milk is not sufficient, hence complementary feeding needs to introduced containing all required nutrients in sufficient quantity. Additional iron and zinc are needed for sustaining growth and to prevent infantile anemia and infection. Fluoride is also essential in infancy for development of gums and tooth enamel (but supplemental fluoride is not required).

Water and electrolytes: Mother's milk provides sufficient water and electrolytes for first few months. According to experts, extra water is not required because it can increase the risk of infection and interfere with breastfeeding. Mother's milk is low in electrolytes, hence its renal solute load is lower than that of cow's milk and reduces the burden on the still maturing kidneys.

Composition and Characteristics of Human Milk

Breast milk is the best food for the baby. Colostrum is the first form of breast milk and that should be given within an hour after birth. It is also referred as Mother's milk. The composition of mother's milk has been given above and its virtues lie in the adequate amount and proportion of nutrients needed by the infant, the passive immunity it gives to the infant and last but not the least the emotional bond that develops between mother and child.

Experts emphasize that external source of water may interfere with breastfeeding and fills the baby with non-nutritive fluid so that the baby is pacified and may not cry but the baby's nutrient needs are not met. There is no medical or nutritional value to water. Water decreases the frequency of breastfeeding, which in turn decreases the mother's milk supply. Early introduction of cow's milk may also result in gastrointestinal problems. Infants given cow's milk are more likely to have iron deficiency anemia than breastfed infants.

According to Acharya Charaka, the milk which is normal in color, smell, taste, and touch, mixes evenly and disappears, when a drop is added to water, is known as pure milk. This milk provides nourishment (*pusttikar*) and good health (*aarogyum*) to the child. Acharya Sushruta described that *sheetha* (cold), clean, free from impurities, sankhabh, sweet in taste, mixes evenly in water, not producing any froth or streaks. This type of milk provides good health, growth and development of body, and strength to the body.

Mother's milk is the best food for first 6 months and thereafter because it cannot provide all the nutrients required by the infant, it should be given along with complementary foods for ensuring optimal growth of the infant. Both breast milk and complementary foods together have a strong influence on physical, mental, and emotional development of the baby. Both have great impact on childhood as well as in adulthood in promotion of health and prevention of disease.

Composition of Human Milk

Mother's milk contains all the essential nutrients in the right proportion as well as enzymes, hormones, and growth factors and anti-infective factors necessary for the growth and development of the infant. Recent studies show that mother's milk also contains stem cells. These cells are able to cross the GI tract, and migrate into the blood of the infant, from where they travel to various organs including the brain, and become functioning cells. Volume and composition of milk markedly differ from mother to mother and the stage of lactation. A healthy mother produces on average, about 520-860 mL breast milk in 24 hours and she can nourish the infant for first 6 months on exclusive breastfeeding.

> **Advantages of mother's milk**
> - Provides nutrition tailored to infant's needs
> - Contains DHA for retina development and cognition
> - Provides immunity
> - Saves life by preventing deaths due to diarrhea and other infections
> - Improves physical and intellectual potential
> - Is the best source of food and nutrition security for the infant
> - Strengthen the bonding between mother and child
> - Helps in birth spacing
> - Benefits mother's health
> - Environment friendly
> - Is cost effective and less expensive than cow's milk or formula

Energy: Mother's milk provides 65 kcal/100 mL. Calorie content of the milk is primarily due to its fat content.

Protein: Human milk has appropriate protein content of 0.9–1.1 g/100 mL. It contains higher percentage of soluble protein in whey. The casein: whey protein ratio for cow milk is approximately 80:20 compared to human milk that has a ratio between 20:80 to 40:60 and decreases to 50:50 in late lactation. The lower casein content makes mother's milk more digestible and places less load on the immature kidney compared to cow's or buffalo's milk. Presence of lactoalbumin in its whey makes mother's milk better than other milks. Also, human milk contains lactoferrin which protects against pathogens. Lactoferrin protects the baby from *Escherichia coli* infection. Hence, exclusively breastfed babies are less likely to die from diarrhea and respiratory infection as compared to nonbreastfed babies. It also contains lipases which are important for fat digestion and growth factors.

The amino acid composition is also appropriate for the infant's needs. There are several differences between breast milk and cow's milk. The ratio of cysteine: methionine ratio is higher in human than in cow's milk. This is advantageous because the enzyme cystathionase is required to convert methionine to cysteine. Human infants' liver and brain have low levels of these enzymes and preterm infants completely lack it. Cysteine is required for development of the central nervous system. Also, taurine is synthesized from cysteine. Taurine is needed for development and function of brain and retina as well as conjugation of bile salts. Cow's milk does not contain the amount of cysteine or taurine as per the infant's requirements. Cow's milk also contains higher amounts of phenylalanine and tyrosine that the infant has limited ability to metabolize.

Fat: Fat is a major source of energy for the infant. Hind milk is rich in fat (4 g/dL) which helps to satisfy the infant. Fat content and fatty acid composition of the mother's milk is greatly influenced by the maternal diet. Human milk fat is mainly composed of 90% triglycerides and remaining are essential fatty acids, particularly docosahexaenoic acid (DHA), cholesterol, phospholipids, diglycerides, monoglycerides, glycolipids, free fatty acids, and sterols. It also contains fat-soluble vitamins (A, E, D, K). Human milk contains fatty acids with 18–22 carbon atoms that are needed for brain and retinal development. Large amounts of omega-6 and omega-3 long chain fatty acids, mostly the 20-carbon arachidonic acid (AA) and the 22-carbon docosahexaenoic acid (DHA), are deposited in the developing brain and retina during prenatal and early postnatal growth.

The presence of AA and DHA in human milk is important because infants, especially preterm infants, may have limited ability to synthesize the amounts required by their body. Studies indicate that infants who received breast milk had better visual acuity at 4 months of age and slightly better cognitive development than formula-fed infants. Also, breast milk may protect the developing neonatal brain from injury by providing all the substances and growth factors that act synergistically. This advantage is not derived from formula or cow's milk that has been fortified or supplemented with various nutrients.

Carbohydrates: Breast milk has a high lactose content that provides about two-fifths of the calories provided by breast milk to the infant. It aids calcium absorption; stimulates growth of gut flora; and supports synthesis of some organic acids and some vitamins. Organic acids tend to reduce pH in the gut and inhibit undesirable growth of bacteria and improve absorption of calcium, phosphorus, magnesium, and other minerals. Human milk also contains numerous oligosaccharides that may support the growth of lactobacilli in the infant's gut. Mature human milk contains almost 10 times higher concentration of oligosaccharides than cow's milk.

Vitamins: Mother's milk contains desirable amount of vitamin A and vitamin E (β and ϒ tocopherol); low amount of vitamin D and negligible amount of vitamin K. The amount of water-soluble vitamins like thiamine, riboflavin, niacin, etc. are closely associated with mother's diet and their utilization and secretion is affected by the energy and protein intake.

Minerals: Mineral content of mother's milk is appropriate for the infant. It has the right proportion of calcium and phosphorus, i.e., the Ca: P ratio is 2:1 whereas in cow's milk it is 1:2.6. Sodium content in human milk is also low, while the potassium content is quite high that seems to be beneficial for the infant. High mineral content may stress the immature baby and increase the renal solute load. The renal solute loads are 10 mOsmol/100 mL for breast milk, 40 mOsmol/100 mL for cow's milk, and 70 mOsmol/100 mL for skim milk. Efficiency of absorption of iron, zinc, and other minerals is better from mother's milk than from cow's milk. In spite of low iron content in the milk, bioavailability of iron from mother's milk is high due to presence of lactoferrin, which also prevents the baby being anemic.

Immunological properties: Human milk contains the immunoglobulins A, D, G, E, and M that are synthesized by cells of the mother's immune system and transported into milk. Milk contains secretory IgA (SIgA). It helps the baby to fight any infection. These are important for conferring passive immunity to the infant whose own immune system is immature, still developing and until the infant's body can begin production of its own antibodies. SIgA is important because it is not denatured by the acid in the stomach and reaches the small intestines, intact. Breast milk also contains *Lactobacillus bifidus* which also prevents the baby from several infections.

Breast milk contains transferrin and lysozyme. Transferrin binds iron and makes it unavailable to pathogenic bacteria. Lysozyme enhances the bactericidal activity of SIgA. Oligosaccharides and mucins, interferon, and fibronectin in human milk also play a role in conferring passive immunity. Besides this, breast milk contains macrophages, lymphocytes, and polymorphonuclear lymphocytes. All of these protect the vulnerable infant from gastrointestinal and respiratory infections, especially in the 1st year of life. Breastfed children suffer less from intestinal and respiratory allergy and have lower risk of autoimmune diseases.

Bioactive factors: Human milk contains numerous bioactive compounds such as epidermal growth factor, nerve growth factor, insulin-like growth factors, transforming growth factor, and interleukins. All these factors are growth modulators. Certain factors apparently have a role in gut maturation. Bioactive compounds protect the infant from infection and inflammation and contribute to immune maturation, organ development, and healthy microbial colonization.

Psychological benefit: Baby receives more sense of security, love, care, and affection during breastfeeding as compared to other feeding.

Economic benefit: Mother's milk does not incur any cost while other milks do. Besides cost of other liquid or powder milks, cost is involved in heating and formula preparation and maintenance of extra hygiene for the baby.

Other benefits: Mother's milk is sterile and for formula preparation, water needs to be sterile to prevent infection. Sterile environment minimizes the risk of contamination. Mother is also free from the special arrangements for heating the milk particularly when she is not at home and it saves fuel.

Studies show that babies who are breastfed are leaner. Babies who were formula fed consumed more formula, more energy, protein, fat, carbohydrates, and gained more weight than breastfed infants. Though cow's milk is used and considered to be good substitute for mother's milk, it should not be continued for long. Cow' milk contains beta lactoglobulin to which infants are often intolerant. The type of sugar and protein put the baby at high risk of cow milk allergy. Prolonged feeding with cow's milk can also increase the risk of tetany, late onset metabolic acidosis, milk allergy, iron deficiency anemia, dental caries, and zinc and copper deficiency.

Sometimes, the infant is given cow or buffalo's milk because the mother thinks there is insufficient production of milk. Other reasons could be lack of desire to breast feed the baby, mother's illness, etc. Mother's milk always has an edge over cow and buffalo milks and the comparison is shown in Table 11.7.

It is best to feed the infant on demand. The infant's stomach is very small and at one time the infant is not able to consume

Table 11.7: Comparison of mother, cow and buffalo milks.

Nutrients	Mother's milk	Cow's milk	Buffalo's milk	Remarks
Energy (kcal/100 mL)	65	67	117	High energy in buffaloes' milk is due to high fat content, difficult to digest
Protein (g/100 mL)	1.1 (more lactalbumin)	3.2 (more casein)	4.1 (more casein)	Animal milk has different ratio of casein to whey. Casein is higher in animal that is difficult to digest and low lactalbumin limits the immune effects. Cow's milk has lower availability of cysteine and tryptophan
Carbohydrates (g/100 mL)	7.4 (more lactose)	4.4 (less lactose)	5.0 (less lactose)	Lactose is sweet and enhances calcium absorption. Galactose from lactose supports synthesis of myelin sheath of the nerves
Lipids (g/100 mL)	3.4 (more EFA)	4.1 (more SFA)	6.5 (more SFA)	EFA supports development of the retina (eye) and nervous system while SFA are difficult to digest
Vitamins	Contains all in adequate quantity	Vitamin A is high	More vitamin A and D	Vitamins in mother's milk are fully utilized. Heating of cow or buffalo milk is necessary before use which tends to destroy some water soluble vitamins
Calcium (mg /100 mL)	28	120	210	Proportion of calcium: phosphorus is more favorable in mothers' milk. Excess calcium in other animals' milk may be difficult to be absorbed by the infant
Immunological factors	Present	Absent	Absent	Mother's milk contains immunoglobulins, lactoferrin, macrophages that act as antiviral and antibacterial agents and protect the baby from infections

(EFA: essential fatty acid; SFA: saturated fatty acid)

large amounts. As the infant grows, its stomach capacity increases but it is still much less than that of older children and adults. Therefore, infants need to be fed frequently. This practice should be continued for the first 2–3 years of life until the child's stomach capacity is comparable to that of older children and adults.

The stomach capacity on the 1st day after birth is only 5–7 mL and about 12 mL on day 2. The amount of colostrum that the mother secretes on the 1st day is about 25–36 mL. Unlike the adult's stomach, the newborn's stomach cannot stretch. Nature has made it so that the volume of colostrum is suitable for the newborn's stomach capacity. Hence, the high nutrient density of the colostrum is very useful so that the infant gets the nutrients it requires. On the 2nd day, the volume of colostrum secreted is 113–185 mL. Hence, the baby needs to be given small frequent feeds. Functional gastric capacity of infants has been estimated to be about 30 g/kg body weight.

On the 3rd day, it is about 22–27 mL (about the volume equivalent to the fist of the infant). By day 10, it has increased to 45–60 mL which is equivalent to the size of a ping-pong ball, in contrast to the adult stomach which has a capacity of about 900 mL. Measurement of the breast milk intake is not practically possible. The approximate amount of formula feed that can be given at a single feed to the infant of average weight at different ages is given in Table 11.8.

Table 11.8: Amount of formula per feed for infants of average weight at different ages.

Infant's age	Volume that can be given in one feed
2 weeks	60–90 mL
3–8 weeks	90–120 mL
2–3 months	120–180 mL
4–5 months	150–180 mL
5–7 months	150–180 mL
7–9 months	180–240 mL
9–12 months	180–240 mL

Complementary Feeding

The World Health Organization and UNICEF recommend that complementary foods be introduced around 6 months of age. Introduction of any food or liquid other than breast milk given to the infant is known as complementary feeding and this transition from breastfeeding to feeding solid foods is known as the period of weaning. Foods that are given in addition to breast milk are known as complementary foods. These foods complement breast milk in meeting the infant's nutrient requirements and do not substitute it. This coincides with other physical and motor development. Around 6 months of age, the infant puts things into her mouth and is interested in new tastes. The mouth has developed enough to enable the infant to make chewing and grinding movements, teeth have begun to erupt, and the tongue extrusion reflex has disappeared. Also amylase that is essential for digestion of starch, is now secreted by the intestines.

> WHO (2001) has also given recommendations for adequate appropriate complementary feeding. Complementary feeds should be:
> **Timely**: Foods should be introduced at the appropriate age, when the need for energy and nutrients exceeds what can be provided through exclusive and frequent breastfeeding.
> **Adequate**: Foods should provide sufficient energy, protein, and micronutrients to meet the growing child nutritional needs.
> **Safe**: Foods should be hygienically prepared and stored, and fed with clean hands using clean utensils and not bottles and teats.
> **Properly fed**: Foods given should be consistent with a child's signals of appetite and satiety, and meal frequency and feeding method are appropriate—the caregiver should actively encourage and persuade the child to consume sufficient food using fingers, spoon or allows self-feeding by the child if she is old enough.

In 2008, the European Society for Pediatric Gastroenterology, Hepatology and Nutrition recommended that "complementary feeding, i.e., solid foods and liquids other than breast milk or infant formula should not be introduced before 17 weeks and not later than 26 weeks". Early introduction of complementary solids before 4 months of age in industrialized countries has been found to be associated with increased risk of health problems like diarrhea, wheezing, and increased percentage of body fat as well as body weight. Late introduction increases the risk of undernutrition and increased risk of infections.

The aim is to introduce soft digestible foods that the infant can tolerate. The foods should be nutrient dense, in order to fill the increasing gap between nutrient requirements and the supply from breast milk. Thus, complementary foods are given for the following reasons:

- To fulfill the increasing requirements of essential nutrients and energy that cannot be met by breast milk alone
- To sustain rapid growth and development especially brain development
- Reduce chances of growth faltering, malnutrition
- Intestinal secretions may be now enough to digest foods other than milk
- To prevent energy and nutrient deficiencies
- Reduce the risk of respiratory tract infection, diarrhea, and other forms of morbidity
- Support development of good food habits
- Enhance better psychosocial, motor, and lingual development
- To gradually accustom the child to family foods.

> **Factors affecting complementary feeding**
> - Culture and religion
> - Urban and rural (including tribal) settings
> - Autonomy of the caregiver
> - Household family composition
> - Presence of alternate caregivers
> - Attitude and belief of the caregiver
> - Income, wealth, and resources
> - Mother's/caregiver's health and workload
> - Education and knowledge about nutrition
> - Psychological attachment with the baby.

Delayed and inadequate complementary feeding is commonly seen in many developing countries. It is associated with high infant mortality rate (IMR) which is attributed to increased risk of malnutrition and infection. Inadequate implies that the complementary foods are inadequate in quantity and nutritional quality. Inadequacy in energy, protein, and micronutrients can lead to growth faltering and malnutrition. Many a times watery, starchy gruels, dal water, etc. that are deficient in energy, protein, and micronutrients, are given to the child. Also, the frequency of feeding these, their consistency, and nutrient densities may be poor. At the same time, too much of a poor-quality complementary food can displace breast milk which is more nutritious and place the child at a disadvantage.

For optimal nutrition, on the one hand, it is necessary to add foods that are nutrient dense and at the same time they should be low in volume to facilitate infant feeding. It is also important to see from where the calories are coming; hence, free sugars particularly sugary drinks should be avoided. At this stage, taste preferences are shaped and these can lead to lasting attitude(s) toward food. Texture is also important because the child is learning to chew and swallow. Hard and big-sized food should be introduced only when the child can chew well and swallow.

In certain Indian communities, introduction of first semisolid or solid food to the infant is a ritual and celebrated as *"Annaprashan",* generally at 6-7 months of age. Complementary foods should be nutritious and should gradually provide a larger proportion of the infants' nutrient needs. Between 6 and 12 months, complementary foods should provide half the nutrient needs with the rest coming from breast milk. Between 12 months and 24 months, complementary foods should provide two-thirds of the nutrient requirements and breast milk provides the remaining one-third. According to the National Family Health Survey (NFHS-IV, 2017) in India only 9.6% of children aged 6-23 months, breastfed or not breastfed, had a minimally acceptable diet. This data is indicative of risk of stunting in later years.

Nutritional Composition of Complementary Foods

According to the WHO (2001), with average intake of breast milk, the complementary food must provide 200 kcal/day at 6-8 months; 300 kcal/day between 9 months and 11 months and 550 kcal/day for 12-23 months old babies. Protein and other essential nutrients should be provided as per the RDA. Energy density of complementary foods is important. It should range from 1.07 kcal per gram to 1.46 kcal per gram of the feed. The amount of energy and nutrients obtained from complementary foods depends on the amount of milk (breast milk or formula) that the child consumes. Generally, in Indian homes, cereal-based gruels are the first to be introduced. Rice, *dalia, sheera, laddoo*, rusk, bread, and porridge are common cereal preparations used for infants, with the recipe being modified to suit the infant's physiological maturity and developmental stage. Rice is generally well accepted by infants. It is sweet, easy to cook and digest, and it is easily mixed with other foods as well. However, white, milled and polished rice is a poor source of many vitamins and minerals. Wheat is another cereal that can be used, but some children are allergic to the gluten present in it. Instead other cereals like ragi, oats, bajra can be used in appropriate preparations and amount. The diet for infants may also add some sprouted or soaked cereals, legumes, and low fiber fruits with ascorbic acid can be added, e.g., mashed banana, cooked pureed apple.

Malted cereals are a good choice. During this process, amylase—the starch-digesting enzyme—breaks down starch into simple sugars making it more digestible and lowers the viscosity of the food making it easier for the infant to swallow. Malting makes the food more nutritious, digestible, and many antinutrients like phytate are reduced, thereby enhancing the availability of minerals like iron. Since the baby cannot eat and digest large amount of cereals, malting or use of ARF (see box) can reduce the volume and provide more nutrient dense feeds. Fermentation can also be used to improve the nutritional quality of the complementary feeds.

> **Amylase rich food (ARF):** It can be made at home. Wheat or any other cereal is soaked for 6-12 hours and then allowed to germinate. Germinated seeds are dried under controlled environment (37°C) and further powdered. During this process, amylase activity increases making the starch more digestible. Small amounts are added to the gruel or porridge, making them less viscous and more of the basic cereal flour can be used per unit volume.

Energy density can be increased by adding oil/fat. However, oily, fried, and high fat foods should not be given. A small amount of fat not only increases the energy content but it also enhances the palatability of the food, provides important essential fatty acids, and increases the absorption of fat-soluble vitamins. It is important to include a variety of foods and expose the baby to different textures and flavors, as food habits are formed/begin to be formed.

Micronutrient content should be improved by incorporating mashed seasonal fruits or vegetables in the meal. The snacks should be like finger foods so that the child can eat on its own and does not take much time for the mother or caregiver to prepare.

Frequency of intake of complementary foods: How frequently the infant is given feeds is equally important. Few number of feeds may not fulfill nutrient requirements and giving too many may displace breast milk. FAO, WHO, UNICEF and Indian organizations has suggested several considerations with regard to complementary feeding. Table 11.9 mentions its salient features considering recommendations of above mentioned organizations.

Consistency of Complementary Foods

The readiness or physical maturity of the infant, maturation of alimentary canal, and development of the appropriate reflexes and skills are very important. The baby should be able to hold its head and at a later stage, coordinate its hand to mouth movements. Intestinal maturation is required, especially synthesis of enzymes like amylase for digesting the starch present in the complementary foods. The baby cannot be directly fed with the family food. In the beginning, the baby is given pureed foods that are similar to milk in consistency which can be given with spoon and feeder. This is a transition period and infants soon learn to slurp. The

Table 11.9: Salient features of complementary feeding.

Age group	Amount /day	Frequency	Consistency/texture	Food choices
6-7 months	2–3 table spoons	2 times/day along with mother's milk	Well cooked, soft, well mashed but gradually increase thickness	Rice, dal gruel, vegetable, egg, fish, little oil/butter/ghee
6-8 months	½ bowl/cup of 250 mL	2–3 meals along with mother's milk	Mashed, pureed, semisolid foods, thick porridge	Rice, dal gruel, more varied seasonal fruits, vegetable, egg, fish, little oil/butter
9-11 months	1 bowl/cup of 250 mL, Liquid can be drunk using cup; pick up small pieces of food and carry them to mouth	3–4 meals + 2 small snack along with mother's milk	Finely chopped/grated (to mix in the preparation) or mashed, liquid beverages Finger foods	Cooked food fresh fruits, vegetables, cereals, pulse, dairy, egg, fish, meat (not pieces) Not spicy or sugary
12-24 months	1-2 bowl/cup of 250 mL	3–4 meals + 1–2 small snacks depending on the appetite along with mother's milk on demand	Soft solids, crispy not hard and can be from the family meal	Family food modified as per taste of the child

If not breastfed then add 1–2 cup milk per day and 1-2 extra meals every day as per nutritional status

consistency of foods should gradually change from mashed and pureed to solid as the infant gets older and her abilities develop. By 6 months, the infant is able to move its tongue from side to side and tendency to push solid food out of mouth decreases with the disappearance of the extrusion reflex. Mashed, pureed, and semisolid foods can be started at 6 months. Thin and sweet beverages must be avoided to avoid dilution of nutrient density. By 7–9 months, the infant begins to sit with support and can drink from a cup with help, pick up small pieces of food, and carry them to her mouth. By 9–10 months, infants can chew and swallow, manipulate food with their tongues and this is the time to introduce soft solids. One should start with thick porridges or gruels that are fed with a spoon and the consistency should be gradually altered so that it is pasty, making it thicker until the child eats family foods. If there is considerable delay in introducing solid foods, there may be feeding difficulties later. By 12–18 months, rotary chewing movements can occur fully, and the baby is better able to drink from a cup and the ability to feed improves. By 12 months, children are generally able to eat family foods. However, care should be taken to ensure that the foods are nutrient dense. Gradually, semi-solid and solid foods should be introduced, bite sized and then larger pieces, while ensuring that the child will not choke. Hard foods should be avoided until the child has teeth and can chew these properly. Finger foods can also be offered to them which they enjoy. This will encourage self-feeding.

> **Finger foods:** Finger foods are eaten directly with the hand without any use of spoon, fork or knife. These foods can be given when the baby begins to hold any little object or food with her thumb and forefinger and tries to put it in the mouth. This signals that the baby can gradually start self-feeding.
>
> Finger foods should be big enough for the baby to grasp (but not the size that would make her choke or push food into the nostril) and nutritious. The purpose is to allow the child to indulge in eating process and avoid choking. The food should be cut into tiny bits that the child will not choke on. For fruits like apples, it is wise to peel and discard the skin. Vegetables like carrot should be cooked so that it is easy for the baby to chew. If peas are given, they should be mashed. Any foods that are consumed by the family can be given, provided the consistency and texture is appropriate. Food pieces should not be more than half inch in length or breadth.

Sometimes, mothers may introduce fruit juice. Not more than 120–180 mL of juice should be given to infants older than 6 months of age. However, it should be avoided to the extent possible. Higher amounts can lead to excess energy intake, dental caries, diarrhea, flatulence, and abdominal cramps. Foods that can increase risk of choking or that the child may carry and push into his nostrils should be avoided, e.g., popcorn, groundnuts, grapes, and candy. Finger foods can be introduced. Canned foods should be avoided since they may harbor risk of carrying a highly pathogenic organism—*Clostridium botulinum*. Tea, coffee, cola beverages, carbonated soft drinks, and other sugary drinks should not be given. They contain many substances that interfere with nutrient absorption. Sugary drink may contain refined sugar or high fructose corn syrup that is very harmful for the body. Everyday micronutrient rich foods should be included in the meals given to the baby. Even leafy vegetables can be mashed and mixed with the food. In low income households, roti/chapatti should be soaked in dal or milk or buttermilk, mashed and given to the infant.

Choice of food: It widely varies from region to region. Primarily, it is culturally driven and similar to family tradition. Staple foods are always preferred to start with. Careful attention is needed in choice of foods. Gradually, a wide variety of foods can be introduced. It should include vitamin A-rich fruits and vegetables every day and adequate quantities of protein foods that may come from pulses, nuts, and nonvegetarian foods like egg, meat, poultry, and fish. Beans and peas should be well cooked. Children under 2 years may choke on raisins, nuts, grapes, bread, popcorn, raw vegetables, and other hard foods. Anything that is given should become soft and mushy when it is soaked.

Porridges made with staple cereals like rice, wheat flour, *ragi* flour, in milk or buttermilk or *mung* dal without spices can be first started. Gradually cooked and mashed vegetables, fruits, mashed rice, mashed *khichri*, bread soaked in dal or milk and mashed, semolina or *atta sheera*, *upma* without chilies, mashed *idli*, *dosa*, *adai*, etc. can be given. Ensure that the child is not exposed much to or bribed or fed with ready to eat packaged and processed food like chocolates, candies, cakes, chips etc. as these are HFSS (high fat, sugar and salt).

Food preparation: It is extremely important that mothers and caregivers wash their hands with soap and water before feeding the child or preparing the complementary feeds. Safe drinking water should be used and the cooking area as well as utensils should be clean. Utensils should be cleaned with soap and water and neither mud nor ash should be encouraged. The baby should be fed with *katori* and spoon which should be boiled or sterilized in pressure cooker. All raw food materials should be washed well. Unclean materials and practices will be sources of infection and cause diarrhea and respiratory infections increasing the risk of malnutrition and mortality.

Simple washing, soaking, boiling, steaming, simmering, poaching, mashing or grinding, and sauteing are enough to make infant food.

> **Research Glimpse:** Complementary foods and utensils both were found to be contaminated with bacteria like *E. coli* and other organisms. About 60–70% urban women wash utensils with hot water and detergent and > 80% rural and tribal women wash them with mud/ash and water. Delayed weaning and inadequacy of complementary foods which is further contaminated are some factors responsible for high mortality due to diarrhea and infection. Education regarding breastfeeding, weaning foods, and use of clean feeding utensils (boiling or sterilizing them in a pressure cooker) has been advocated to prevent and control malnutrition. Use of fermented milk (curd) and cereal-pulse mixture with green leafy vegetable has been suggested for ICDS and other nutrition programs. Use of chlorine tablets is suggested to make water potable.
>
> *Agarwal KN. Weaning practices in other parts of the world: case study India in Early Nutrition: Impact on short and long term health. Nestle Nutr Ins Workshops Ser Pediatr Program. 2011;68:107-15.*

Babies should be breast fed on demand and complementary foods should be given between breast feeds. Complementary food should be given before milk. Whenever the baby is given complementary foods, she should be held in a sitting position to avoid choking. Always be present when the baby is fed complementary foods. The infant should not be left unattended.

> **Laboratory Laurel:** Food protein quality, as measured by the Digestible Indispensable Amino Acid Score (DIAAS), requires the determination of true ileal digestibility of indispensable amino acids (IAAs) in children. In this study, true ileal IAA digestibility of four (rice, finger millet, *mung* bean, and egg) commonly consumed complementary foods in children aged < 2 years was assessed using the dual-isotope tracer method. It further calculated the DIAAS of complementary feeding diets and their relation to stunting in children aged 1–3 years in representative Indian rural population. Rice, finger millet and *mung* bean were intrinsically labeled with deuterium oxide (^2H_2O), whereas egg was labeled through oral dosing of hens with a uniformly ^2H-labeled amino acid mixture. True ileal IAA digestibility was lowest in *mung* bean (65.2%), followed by finger millet (68.4%) and rice (78.5%), and was highest for egg (87.4%). There was a significant inverse correlation of complementary food DIAAS with stunting in survey data ($r = -0.66$, $P = 0.044$). The addition of egg or milk to nationally representative complementary diets theoretically improved the DIAAS from 80 to 100. It is concluded that the true ileal IAA digestibility of four foods commonly consumed in complementary diets showed that the DIAAS was associated with stunting and reinforces the importance of including animal source food (ASF) in diets to improve growth.
>
> *Shivkumar N, Kashyap S, Thomas TK, et al. Protein-quality evaluation of complementary foods in Indian children 2019. The American Journal of Clinical Nutrition, 109 (5): 1319–1327.*

Guidelines for Infant Feeding Practices:
- Introduce solid foods on eruption of teeth (8–9 months) and when baby can sit and hold his head firmly.
- Avoid feeding the baby everytime he cries. Schedule the breast feed and complementary food with a gap of 2–3 hours.
- Introduce one type of food at a time in small quantity using tea spoon or special feeding cup. Infant may accept a new food after 8–10 times of trials.
- Initiate with mushy and soft foods and gradually introduce semisolid foods.
- Use fresh, seasonal, and locally available foods.
- Use safe water for drinking, cooking as well as for cleaning.
- Use baking, boiling, streaming, and to prepare baby foods instead of frying.
- Grinding (stone grinding), germination, and malting are good ways to reduce volume and increase nutritional quality, e.g., amylase rich foods (ARF).
- Use complementary feeds within 2 hours of preparation, avoid refrigeration.
- Avoid microwave heating because temperature is high in the center and cool on outer surface and it may burn or scald the tongue or mouth of the baby.
- Add about 1 teaspoon butter, vegetable oils in food preparation in a day.
- Allow the baby to take time to learn the art of eating and enjoy eating process. Do not scold the baby for spillage and mess; it may lead to food rejection or behavioral problems.
- Do not force or coax the baby to eat a particular food. Watch reactions and pay attention to unusual signs and symptoms and consult doctor.
- Never leave the baby alone or unwatched while eating to avoid putting wrong food in mouth or choking throat by food.
- Too thin consistency may dilute the nutrient intake and baby may remain hungry while too concentrated or too much food may pose digestive problems.
- Avoid foods containing artificial preservatives, colors, flavors, excess of sugar, salt, spices, and strong flavored natural foods like capsicum, onion.
- Prefer homemade food instead of commercially processed food.
- Reduce volume of food but make it nutrient dense because the child cannot eat large amounts at a time.
- Never criticize food while feeding; it leaves a negative impact on the baby.
- Inculcate good food habits by introducing right kind of food in right amount in pleasant environment. Use attractive bowls and spoons.
- Avoid feeding in front of electronic gadgets like TV, mobile, etc.
- Healthy eating habits during infancy prevent childhood obesity and other health issues.

Some Homemade Recipes of Complementary Foods

About 2-3 g roasted flax seeds or its powder should be added in the mix or in any food made for the child, e.g., chapati, porridge, etc. after 9-11 months. This is to help ensure intake of n-3 fatty acid. Following ingredients can be used in given proportion to make powder and stored in airtight jars and keep in cool and dry place. Prepare them for one week use and again make it. Roasted grains may get rancid faster than raw grain. Roasting is necessary for better cooking, taste and digestibility.

- Roasted rice: Roasted Bengal gram/roasted green gram without husk: roasted groundnut: jaggery (4:1:1:2).

- Grind each ingredient separately to a fine powder and sieve them together. The mixture can be used to prepare porridge or *laddoo*. Store it in air-tight jar.
- Bajra or ragi or wheat: dehusked green gram or Bengal gram: skim milk powder: groundnut: sesame seeds (12:3: 2:2).
- Roast cereals, pulses, and nuts separately. Grind them and mix together, sieve if necessary. Store in air-tight jar and keep it in a dry place or refrigerator to avoid rancidity from ground nut or sesame seeds. Use the mixture by mixing water or milk. It can be made sweet or salted.
- Wheat flour (9 g); green leafy vegetable (10 g); Bengal gram flour or *mung* flour (3 g); oil or butter (2 g).
- Cook and mash/puree vegetable preferably a leafy or yellow orange vegetable (e.g., amaranth or spinach). Add to flours. Knead dough. Prepare roti. Smear fat. Give baby for chewing or soak in milk/dal, mash, and feed.
- Rice (10 g); lentil (10 g); small diced potato (6 g); grated papaya (6 g); oil (5 g), *jeera, haldi,* and salt for seasoning.
- Wash everything before use. Heat oil, add seasoning and other ingredients. Cook well till soft. Serve warm.

The food square formula shown in Figure 11.8 can be used to design recipes.

Use of Infant Formulas

Under certain conditions, the mother is not able to feed the baby or the baby is not able to suckle. Under such circumstances, he/she has to be fed animal milk (breast milk from a milk bank if available, would be the best option). Infant formulas are ready-to-use milk food designed to furnish the nutritional needs of the infant. These are usually similar to breast milk in nutrient composition. These are available in the form of powders, concentrates, or liquid. In India, the Infant Milk Substitutes, Feeding Bottles and Infant Foods (Regulation of Production, Supply and Distribution) Amendment Act (2003) bans the promotional and marketing activities of baby food manufacturers, in fact all forms of promotion of baby foods for children under 2 years of age. The aim is to regulate marketing practices of manufacturers that may result in unnecessary introduction of complementary foods before 6 months of age or discourage the use of homemade complementary foods. This Act has been passed by the Government of India (GOI), in keeping with the National Policy and the Global Strategy for Infant and Young Child Feeding.

Nutrition for Low Birth Weight Babies

The baby can be LBW either as a result of being born preterm (PT) (before 37 weeks of gestation) or due to small gestational age (SGA), i.e., less than the 10th percentile of weight for age or both.

In developing countries including India, LBW and SGA are generally due to intrauterine growth retardation. Globally, 15–20% of babies are born low birth weight. According to NFHS-IV (2016), 18% of Indian infants are LBW. Preterm birth increases risk of mortality and LBW is associated with early growth retardation postnatally, infection, developmental delays as well as risk of death in infancy and childhood.

Improved care and optimal feeding of LBW babies can improve their chances of survival as well as help them grow and develop. LBW infants can be full term or preterm (PT) and/or small for gestational age (SGA). These infants differ in terms of maturity of organs and systems and hence their ability to adapt to the extrauterine or postnatal environment. Their feeding abilities differ and their fluid and nutritional requirements are also different. The following limitations are faced by LBW infants:

- Many infants may not be able to suckle and breastfeed and may need to be fed by spoon or gastric feeding.
- In the first few weeks, they may be more susceptible to illness, making feeding more difficult.
- Preterm (PT) infants have high fluid requirements because they have high insensible water loss.
- Preterm infants are likely to have low nutrient reserves since most of the nutrient stores are laid down in the last trimester of intrauterine life.
- Their gastrointestinal tract is immature and this immaturity can compromise their ability to tolerate oral feeds.
- Protein loss is considerable through urine in the form of urea and desquamated epidermal cells from skin, and unless the baby is fed, the protein losses can be high.
- Even if the child is given intravenous fluid, oral or nasogastric feeding should be initiated as early as possible (within 48–72 hours) for the PT infant's GIT to be benefited.
- Feeding orally stimulates maturation of the GIT, promotes release of gut hormones and essentially prepares the gut when the baby will be fed orally.
- If feeding is delayed, there are morphological changes such as decrease in mucosal mass and villus height, increased permeability with loss of important digestive enzymes like sucrase and lactase.

Nutritional requirements of low birth weight babies should compensate the insufficiency in body composition and meet the pace of growth. Such babies need to be fed preferably under medical supervision to reduce the risk of infection and better chances of adequate nutrient input, growth, and survival. Colostrum is very effective to meet the nutritional needs and increases the chances of survival. Energy and protein needs are high.

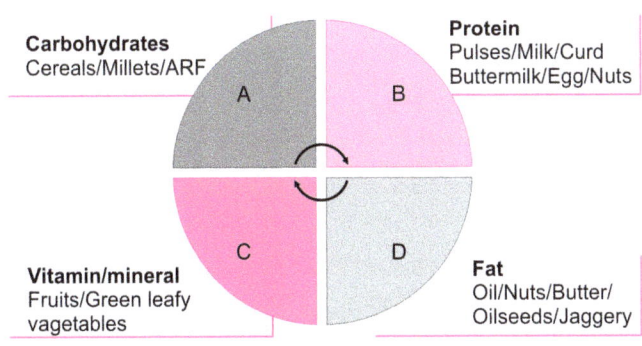

Fig. 11.8: Food formula for recipe design.

The actual feeding protocol is beyond the scope of this chapter because it is essentially a matter of clinical management to ensure survival as well as growth and development. Many infants may have to be kept in intensive care. The mode of feeding and tolerance and whether the infant is ill becomes the basis for making decisions about feeding protocols. Sick infants need to be treated. In case of healthy LBW infants (even if they are PT), the feeding of choice is mother's milk since it meets the requirements of the infant. If the baby cannot breastfeed, breast milk should be expressed by the mother. LBW infants also need iron supplements.

Monitoring growth of these infants is important. The aim should be to try and ensure that there is as little interruption in growth and development of the newborn and to provide optimal nutrition to the neonate.

Nutrition for Preterm Babies

The goal of nutritional management of the preterm infant is to provide adequate amount of nutrients that will help to ensure the growth rate and body composition of a normal healthy fetus of the same gestational age in terms of weight, length, head circumference, organ size, tissue components including cell number and structure, concentrations of blood and tissue nutrients, and developmental outcomes. Failure to provide the necessary amounts of all of the essential nutrients to preterm infants can not only result in growth failure, but can also increase morbidity and compromise brain growth that in turn would limit neurological development.

The body composition of a preterm baby differs from that of a full-term baby, with preterm babies having less lean tissue although fat mass may be similar. Proteins, minerals (calcium, iron, zinc), and electrolytes (sodium, potassium, etc.) are also two to five times less in preterm babies compared to term infants. Energy requirements are increased by 20% on the basis of body weight. However, there are some reports in the literature, that these babies have increased intra-abdominal adiposity when they achieve catch-up growth. Hence, it needs to be determined as to how nutritional management can enhance lean tissue accumulation rather than more fat in these infants.

Nutritional requirement of preterm babies is extraordinarily high and determined by the body weight, body composition, and health status. Deposition of nutrients in fetus usually occurs in the third trimester; therefore, premature or preterm baby has compromised nutrient reserves that need to be supplied from external sources. They have 50% less lean body mass (LBM) one-tenth of the body fat in comparison to the normal full-term baby. Fluid, protein, sulfur amino acids, essential fatty acids, calcium, phosphorus, zinc, vitamin K and A, sodium, potassium, and chloride are critically important for preterm babies. Preterm infants born before 32 weeks of gestation need additional vitamin D, calcium, and phosphorus until they reach term postmenstrual age.

However, a sudden increase in the nutrient supply is not well tolerated; in addition, they are at high risk of lung infections. Such babies need expert medical care for revival and survival.

Energy: Energy requirement is rather less because of low BMR and negligible movement. However, they are given energy at the rate of 105–130 kcal/kg/day.

Protein: Protein requirement is high and that can be 2.5–3.0 g/kg/day. Amino acids like cysteine, tyrosine, methionine are needed for catch-up growth and neurological development. Care should be taken not to give excessive amount of protein as that increases the load on the kidneys.

Fat: Percentage of body fat is very low in preterm baby. Docosahexaenoic acid (DHA) and arachidonic acid (ARA) are required by preterm infants to support growth and development to modulate cell growth, inter- and intracellular communication, and protein function. DHA is selectively accumulated in specific tissues like retina and brain gray matter and its depletion causes reduced visual function, cognitive and behavioral abnormalities, altered neurotransmitter metabolism, and decreased membrane protein and receptor activities.

Minerals and vitamins: Premature infants need supplementation with iron to increase hemoglobin and prevent hemolytic anemia; vitamin D to improve calcium absorption and retention for bone health and zinc for cell-mediated immunity, cognitive process, and mental development.

Fluid and electrolytes: Amount of extracellular fluid (ECF) is more in preterm than full-term babies so they are at higher risk of dehydration, electrolyte imbalance, edema, and death. Water loss is more because of their larger body surface area relative to the body weight and it occurs through skin, lungs, and urine. Preterm infants require more water at the rate of 150 mL/kg/day. Loss of water may lead to electrolyte imbalance; thus, sodium, potassium, and chloride need to be paid attention to.

In addition to nutritional support from parenteral nutrition and breast milk, **Kangaroo care** is given to the baby to support catch up growth and various biological processes. The warmth through skin-to-skin touch stimulates both mother and baby. It also helps the mother to able to secrete sufficient milk.

> **Kangaroo care:** The preterm infant is given skin-to-skin touch preferably by the mother for a few hours every day and the mother keeps the baby on her body or close to her body like a kangaroo and the body of the mother works like an incubator. Body temperature of the mother helps to regulate the body temperature of the infant. It also supports to fulfill the nutritional and immunological needs and ensures physiological and psychological warmth and bonding. Baby has better chances of adaptability and chances of survival. It also helps the mother to able to secrete sufficient milk.

Preschool Child (1 to 6 years)

During this period, maturation of organs and systems continues. Brain development is completed in this period. The adverse effects of undernutrition and other environmental insults will be manifested as functional deficits in organs and systems.

The child aged between 1 year and 3 years is termed a **toddler** and a child between 3 years and 6 years is referred as **preschooler**.

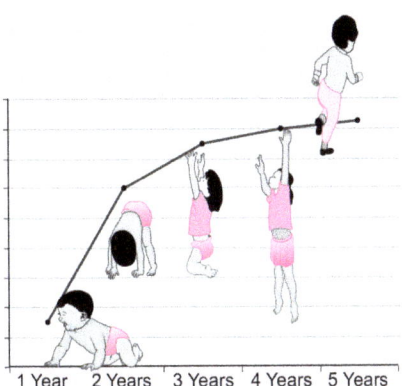

Preschool children normally grow at the rate of 2-3 kg/year in weight. If child weight is expected to be 3 times of the birth weight, then it can be 4, 5 and 7 times at 2, 3 and 7 years respectively. Annual height gain may be 12.5 cm in 2 year old toddlers and decrease to 10.0 cm and 7.5 cm in 3 year olds and 3-6 year old preschoolers, respectively. The velocity of gain in 2-year olds is about 1 cm per month, in preschoolers 3 cm per month. During the third year of life, average rate of height gain is 2-3 inches per year. Physical growth in the childhood years occurs at a steady rate and is slower compared to infancy and the child's nutrient needs correspond with these changes in growth rates.

Weech's formula can be used to determine the expected weight (kg) and height (cm) in preschool children.

Formula for weight (1-6 years):   age in years × 2 + 8
Formula for height (2-12 years): age in years × 6 + 77 cm

Though the rate of growth in preschool age is rather slow and steady as compared to infancy period, the development of all organs particularly that of the brain occurs at this age. Brain is made up of neurons which are responsible for processing of information. Structural development of brain occurs in preschool age and functional maturity comes later as the child grows and is exposed to the environment. The functioning of the brain depends upon the generation of electrical potentials through the synaptic gaps between cell bodies. The brain requires nutrients such as choline, folic acid, iron, zinc and special fats [e.g., gangliosides, sphingolipids, and docosahexaenoic acid (DHA)]. Gene expression in the brain is also affected by nutrition. During preschool period, the child acquires fundamental cognitive and interpersonal skills. The child's vocabulary, motor coordination improves, and the child is able to concentrate on tasks for slightly longer periods.

Increase in head circumference, chest circumference, and midarm circumference is good indicator of development of the brain, bones, and muscles, respectively. In addition to nutrient supply, loving care, exposure to learning stimuli, and communication play a significant role in growth and development of the child.

Monitoring of growth is essential especially between 0 years and 3 years. After this age, it is important to assess whether the child is growing well and to prevent development of overweight and obesity. This can be done by comparing the child's weight, height, and BMI with the growth charts given by the World Health Organization. Children whose BMI is below the 5th percentile, are classified as underweight. A BMI below the 3rd percentile is indicative of undernutrition. Children having BMI between the 85th and 95th percentile are overweight and above the 95th percentile, are obese. Thus, it is important that the BMI should be between the 5th and 85th percentiles. If the BMI is persistently above the 85th percentile, the parents must take care.

Between 1 and 6 years of age, there is no difference in the growth pattern of boys and girls. Physical growth and physiological maturity, episodes of illness and cognitive development are influenced by a wide variety of external factors such as feeding practices, food and nutrient supply, knowledge and attitudes of the care provider, healthcare facilities as well as availability of resources and affordability of healthcare services as well as foods.

Nutritional Requirements during Preschool Age

Preschool is a golden period of life when children grow, enjoy, and experience the external world within available resources. At the same time, it is a most vulnerable age from various angles. Fulfilling nutritional requirements is important for their physical, physiological, and psychological growth and development. Excess or deficient intake of nutrients can easily result in growth faltering, morbidity, and mortality. Deficiency of nutrients can easily result in growth faltering, morbidity and mortality as well as compromise brain development. Particular attention must be paid to micronutrient intakes. On the other hand, allowing children to eat energy dense, micronutrient poor foods could set the child on the path of overweight and obesity.

In general, growth curves of healthy children may differ for each child. Parents and caregivers should provide a diet that is appropriate for their child's age. They should offer a wide variety of foods to ensure that their child is getting enough nutrition. Overall, preschoolers need to be fed diets of high nutritional quality. Recommended Dietary Allowances (RDA) of most important nutrients for preschool children are shown in Tables 9. 1A and B in Chapter 9 given by ICMR-NIN (2020) and EAR in given in Appendix 4.

Energy: These children need energy for growth, i.e., synthesis of growing tissues (2 kcal/g of weight gain) and physical activity. BMR is higher than in adults, as the child is still growing. However, compared to infancy, the requirement is lower when it is expressed per kilogram of body weight. Adequate energy is needed to provide for the energy that is expended (the child becomes physically active as she learns to walk) and to ensure that new tissues can be synthesized. Although growth rate is slower than during infancy, the energy expended on physical activity increases with age as the child becomes more physically active. Habitual physical activity is influenced by the social and economic environment in different geographical locations which may carry forward in later years of life as well as the health status of the child. Children who are ill and/or undernourished are likely to be less active and apathetic. It has been observed that children from poor or rural communities are rather more active than their urban counterparts who have more facilities for transport and may not have enough space to play.

Protein: Protein is required for optimal growth and development of tissues and organs; and synthesis of enzymes, hormones, neurotransmitters, and antibodies. Protein should contribute about 10–20% of the total energy intake. Protein deficiency in this age may adversely affect brain development; and reduced cell replication that will be reflected by poor growth (low weight for age and low weight for height) and poor immunity. There is higher risk of morbidity.

Fat: Fatty acid composition is important for growth and development. The role of essential fatty acids in brain development is well established. After 6 months of age, fat should contribute 35% (upper limit) of total calorie intake. Attention should be paid to intake of n-3 fatty acids as well as linoleic acid. Visible fat intake should be 25–30 g/day. Very low fat diets should not be given because energy intakes and essential fatty acid intakes will be compromised. Energy density of low fat diets is likely to be too low and the diets may be too bulky for children between 1 and 3 years of age, when their stomach capacities are limited. Also, intake and/or absorption of fat-soluble vitamins as well as zinc and iron are likely to be compromised. On the other hand, when energy intake from fat exceeded 40%, it has been found to reduce intake of some trace elements. Deficiency of these important micronutrients causes a number of neurodevelopment disorders like dyslexia, ADHD (attention deficit/hyperactivity disorder), and also impairs the motor functions, independent of general ability.

Calcium: Calcium intakes should be adequate to promote skeletal development and ensure that bone mineralization occurs which have an impact on bone density in later years. To the extent possible, dairy products and other calcium-rich foods like ragi, green leafy vegetables, sesame seeds should be included in the child's diet.

Iron: Iron aids availability of oxygen to all the cells in the body including brain. Iron deficiency will deprive oxygen supply to the body and adversely affect the cognition, memory, and eventually the child's performance in school. Prolonged or severe iron deficiency may cause irreparable damage which may be attributed to reduced neurotransmitters (dopamine, epinephrine) and their receptors are also altered. Biosynthesis of several enzymes is also reduced which seriously affects the brain functions. Anemic children are more unhappy, hesitant, and fearful to interact with their environment.

It is also important to pay attention to other nutrients like vitamin C to promote iron absorption and for collagen formation and zinc for better growth and immunity—vitamin A, vitamin D, and other vitamins and minerals for growth and development and utilization of macronutrients.

> **Laboratory Laurel:** Individuals who did not suffer growth failure in the first 3 years of life completed more years of schooling, scored higher on tests of cognitive skill in adulthood, had better outcomes in the marriage, earned higher wages and are less likely to live in poor households, and for women, fewer pregnancies and smaller risk of miscarriages and stillbirths. Growth failure has adverse impacts on body size and several dimensions of physical fitness in adulthood but does not have marked effects on risk indicators of cardiovascular and related chronic diseases. These results provide a powerful rationale for investments that reduce early-life growth failure.
>
> *Hoddinott J, Maluccio J, Behrman JR, et al. The consequences of early childhood growth failure over the life course. IFPRI Discussion paper 01073. 2011.*

Guidelines for Ensuring Nutritional Adequacy in Preschool Children's Diet

Preschool age is an impressionable young age full of curiosity and imitation. It is also the age for **habit formation.** By this age, children are able to indicate, speak, and express their food choices and they often imitate the food behavior of older persons around them. Preschoolers also tend to be picky and may be unpredictable. This may be associated with the age when the child is attempting to become independent. Their rate of growth is slower than in infancy, hence they may eat accordingly. Many at this age are wary about eating new foods. This is the age for formation of good food habits and behavior. At this age, children will eat less or may not want to stop playing to eat. Hence, the mother/caregiver needs to expose them to healthy and nutritious foods. The following guidelines will help develop healthy food habits:

- Children have small appetites and should be given three meals with one to two snacks in between such as fruits, *poshtik laddoo*, milk, curd, and other varieties of snacks. Sweets and fried foods, as well as of energy rich snacks should be avoided.
- Children are sometime assertive and may either demand or reject the food to seek attention or express their food choice(s). Allow them to do so.
- Highly flavored, spicy food, and foods with artificial colors, flavors, and additives are not advisable. They cause indigestion, irritation, and other problems. If necessary, modify the seasoning in home-made foods.
- Encourage the child to eat family meals.
- Avoid bulky food in one serving size with less nutrient density, e.g., *kurmura, bhel*.
- Give unfamiliar food along with familiar and favorite food.
- Give nutritious food after play or school as they usually eat well at that time.
- Check temperature, consistency, texture, appearance, shape, and size of food. Children may prefer fruit cut into sticks or bite sized pieces rather than the whole fruit.
- Never bribe the child to eat a particular food or meal.
- Select food preparations from all food groups and include them at various meals and snacks throughout the day rather than including all in one meal.
- Train children to distinguish between unhealthy or healthy foods.

- Check their attraction and craving through advertisements or window shopping.
- Schedule meal time before the child is very hungry. Let meal time be family meal time.
- Keep dining atmosphere pleasant and comfortable.
- Use a table/chair according to child's stature.
- Use colorful, attractive, and nontoxic eating utensils for them.
- Avoid hurry during feeding or avoid leaving behind the child and letting her eat alone.
- Allow children to eat by themselves.
- Have patience with their eating process even if they make a mess and avoid scolding.
- Make meal time a story telling time and use some nutrition-related stories.
- Consider use of food jags a temporary phase. Reinforcing with emotions may make them more stubborn. Food jags are behavioral pattern of eating and children eat few self-selected items only.
- Finger foods containing nutrient dense ingredients are good for them.
- Avoid chocolates, soft drinks, refined, and sticky foods to avoid the risk of dental caries.
- Parents should not purchase or prepare unhealthy foods.
- Television should be turned off during meal times and when the child is eating.
- Children should be allowed to eat under supervision only.
- Minimize consumption of processed, ready-to-eat foods, and eating out in streets and restaurants.

Catch-up Growth

It is a phase of accelerated growth usually after a period of growth retardation or growth failure in young children (frequently observed in children below 2 years of age) and premature babies when the cause of growth retardation is removed. Catch-up growth is defined as "height velocity above the normal statistical limits for age and/or maturity during a defined period of time, following a transient period of growth inhibition." Due to illness, children often lose weight. It is essential that catch-up growth after an infection is ensured for children to maintain good nutritional status. The World Health Organization recommends that children be given one extra healthy meal for a period of 2 weeks after the onset of illness so that malnutrition is prevented.

It is frequently observed that malnourished children can catch up in growth when they receive adequate nutrition. It is associated with high velocity of increase in height, weight, and head circumference. This accelerated growth continues until the child reaches its original growth curve. The velocity may be influenced by several environmental factors particularly nutrient intake and infection or illness as well as hormonal profile. In certain cases, severely malnourished children are voraciously hungry and rate of weight gain in such children can be several times more than normal. If they are provided adequate nutrients, infant mortality can be reduced. It is not possible to know whether catch-up growth is complete for an individual child, but if final height is within the target range, it can be considered that catch-up growth has probably been completed.

Middle Childhood: School age (6–12 years)

Some children may appear to grow and mature fast while others may appear immature. This is because children grow and develop at different rates. At this age, growth rate is slow and steady but considerable changes occur in body shape, body composition, physiology, and psychology of children. It is the prepubescent period during which the body prepares itself for the second growth spurt that will occur at puberty. Environmental factors including diet and physical activity play a large role in determining weight, height, and growth. Differences between boys and girls will be noticeable around 8–9 years of age; particularly girls begin to gain weight and develop secondary sexual characteristics. The salient features of school age are:

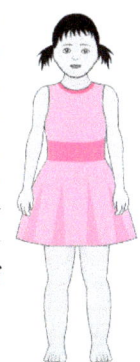

Physiological Changes

- Development of secondary sexual characteristics in girls after 8–9 years and in boys around 11–12 years.
- Girls gain relatively more adipose tissue and boys gain more of muscle or lean body mass.
- Lengthening of bones results in gain in height—lower limbs grow faster than the trunk.
- Bone mineralization occurs and bone mineral density (BMD) is higher in boys than girls.
- Blood volume expands.

There are some characteristics in behavior pattern that need to be considered when fulfilling nutritional requirements of this age group.
- They are physically active and want to explore the world.
- They can understand when they are taught.
- They may like to play and eat in groups.
- Display moodiness but at the same time like to please others.
- Like competitiveness in sports and games.
- They may like to imitate their peers.
- They may be exposed to smoking, alcohol, or substance consumption and indulge in negative behavior which must be checked and not permitted.
- They are exposed to television, messages, and advertisements on mobile phones and their food choices may be influenced by these media.

Nutritional Requirements of the School Age Child

School-age children have developed more advanced feeding skills and are able to help with meal preparation. Their nutritional requirements can be met with three healthy meals and nutritious snacks between meals.
- Many food habits, likes, and dislikes are established during this time.
- School-age children are often willing to eat a wider variety of foods than their younger siblings.
- Eating healthy snacks after school is very important.

Nutritional requirements of both girls and boys are similar till 9 years of age, but thereafter their nutritional requirements differ since there are differences in body composition and stature. Girls have slightly lower requirement for energy yielding nutrients. Differences are attributed to gender, growth rate, biological needs, and physical activity. RDA for energy and other nutrients is presented in Tables 9.1A and B in Chapter 9 and EAR in Appendix 4.

Energy: Energy requirement of a 10-year-old child is similar to or slightly more than that of an adult woman, e.g., EAR for 10-year-old girl is 2060 kcal/day and of sedentary woman is 1660 kcal/day. This energy is required for synthesis of growing tissues and metabolic and physical activities. Similarly, a 10-year-old boy requires 2220 kcal/day compared to the EAR of 2110 kcal/day for a sedentary man.

Protein: RDA for protein increases considerably over the 6–7 years duration of middle childhood (from 23.3 g/day at 7–9 years to 44.9 g/day for 13–15-year-old boys). Protein is required for tissue synthesis that occurs at puberty including bone development, expansion of blood volume, synthesis of hormones, etc. High quality of protein containing essential amino acids should be provided.

Fat: Fat should provide 25–30% of total calorie intake and the amount of visible fat consumed (from all sources) should not exceed 35-50 g/day. The source of fat should be carefully selected to ensure that the child receives the required essential and n-3 fatty acids.

Micronutrients: All micronutrients are required at this age. Attention should be paid to calcium intake to support the growth spurt during puberty and ensure adequate bone mineralization. It has been observed that intake of dairy products is linked to higher peak bone mass which is also important because it serves to maintain bone mass in adulthood. In older age, there is a physiological loss of bone with increasing age, but if the peak bone mass has been adequate, the person will still have adequate bone mass and thus will have lower risk of osteoporosis and fractures in later adult life. Adequate intakes of iron, vitamin A, folic acid, and vitamin B_{12} are required to prevent anemia. Zinc is also important for growth and immunity. Adequate intake of B-vitamins and vitamin C cannot be ignored hence sumptuous amount of colorful fresh fruits and vegetables should be added in their daily diet.

Water and electrolytes: Drinking water is essential as children often tend to play outside and tend to sweat a lot. It also requires intake of electrolytes, may be in the form of beverages. A note of caution is that children do not need to be given glucose solutions or electrolytes constantly. Normal food intake and fluids especially water or buttermilk, *nimbu pani* without salt is to be encouraged. High intake of sodium may lead to high blood pressure even in children. Consumption of highly processed food, sauces must also be checked because they contain high sodium.

Diet has a great impact on children's ability to work and think. Some studies have shown that deficiency of energy, protein, and iron reduce the physical performance and deficiencies of zinc, iodine, and folate influence the cognitive development and neuropsychological functions. Inadequacies of these nutrients even during infancy can have an impact on school performance and emotional response to stress and impair motor skills. Excessive intake of one nutrient can result in imbalance of other nutrients. Excessive energy intake can cause overweight and obesity. Sometimes, effects of excess or insufficiency may not be visible immediately but may be manifested as health problems in adulthood or in old age.

Food Behavior in School Age Children and Dietary Guidelines

School going children tend to be like their school mates and like to eat things their friends eat. This is also the age of exploration and experimentation, and children are easily swayed by media and market. However, this is the age for learning and formation of food habits which are likely to continue for the rest of life. If they are left unwatched or are cared for, given easy access to popular, tasty but unhealthy food items, they soon become the part of their food behavior. Thus, children are at high risk of developing unhealthy food habits. This can result in a wide range of health problems such as overweight, obesity, high blood pressure, insulin resistance, diabetes, and poor immunity. Street foods also increase risk of infections. This further reduces the chances of eating safe, healthy, and nutritious food. A structured eating plan with regular meals and snacks is important to establish good eating habits. Pizzas, burgers and similar foods may be given occasionally but never should be a substitute for meals. Every meal should include all five food groups. The whole family should have balanced diets and the goal should be to ensure that the child's growth and development occur normally while the child maintains a healthy weight. Parents, school, and media all together can help in this regard and bring more favorable results in developing good food habits. Some of the following measures can help in shaping the food behavior of children of this age:

- Parents and elders should set good examples of good eating habits.
- Give variety of foods rich in color, taste, and texture.
- Make sure that the child has balanced diet in all three major meals.
- Ensure that the child has a healthy breakfast (note jam is energy dense and does not contain as much fruit as claimed, it contains more sugar). Ensure that milk and fruit and a cereal are included for breakfast. Always serve breakfast, even if the child is in a hurry. Cereal can be provided as a cheese/chutney/vegetable/egg sandwich or chapatti roll.
- Ensure that the child gets adequate number of servings of fruits, vegetables, and dairy products.
- Meal timings must correspond to school timings.
- Food preparation should not interfere with their play time in recess in school.
- Parents can modify popular food items to make them more nutritious and interesting and prepare them at home, instead of restricting such foods.

- Teaching about food composition and impact of different foods on health in very scientific way may not interest them rather telling these things in interesting manner or through stories/games and activities may be helpful.
- Involve children in the selection, meal planning, and preparation of foods and teach them to make healthy choices by providing opportunities to select foods based on their nutritional value.
- Mother-to-child and child-to-child pattern of nutrition education often works well and can have profound and positive effects in coming years of life.
- Train them to know the basis of selection of foods, i.e., food groups and serving size.
- Make them understand the difference between nutrient dense and energy dense foods.
- Guide them to differentiate harmful or healthful foods and their consequences. Give examples of role models.
- Allow them to eat and enjoy social gatherings. This will improve social participation. Slowly, the child can be guided about which foods should be selected and the ones to avoid when eating outside the home. Teach them to eat small portions of energy dense or junk foods if they cannot be avoided.
- Do not force the child to eat anything because you think right.
- School feeding programs can be of great help to upgrade the health of the children.
- Food items should also be liked by peer group.
- Do not permit frequent indulgence in popular food items (junk food/beverage) and buying from vending machine or canteen.
- Do not permit munching snacks while watching TV, playing, and reading.
- Parents should provide recommended serving sizes of different foods.
- Give them nutritious snacks and beverages after play or vigorous activity because children will feel hungry. Instead of chips and other snacks like ready to eat noodles, provide them sandwiches, fruits, milk or yoghurt, or fruit milk shake/*lassi*. Avoid biscuits especially cream biscuits, *wadas*, *pakodas*, and foods that are high in energy, fat and/or sugar (Avoid HFSS foods).
- Ensure that fluid intake is adequate.
- Avoid giving them carbonated soft drinks or drinks that are reconstitutable powders that are basically containing synthetic flavors. Traditional beverages like lemonade would be preferable. Children can be easily taught to make this beverage. Instead of beverages, encourage children to drink water.
- Sugar-free drinks should be discouraged. Their acidity can cause tooth decay.
- Controlling portion sizes and eating nonprocessed foods help limit calorie intake and increase nutrients.
- Play with them before meals to encourage good food habits and boost psychological health.
- Monitor and try to control when and where the child eats foods. Provide regular daily meal times, ensure that meal times are pleasant, and that parents and other interact socially with the child and the family demonstrates healthy eating behaviors.
- Serve meals at the table, instead of in front of the television, to avoid distractions.

Laboratory Laurel: Children's diet and nutrition not only influences their current health status and scholastic performance, but it has long-term consequences in later years of life. Diet preferences and practices acquired during childhood usually persist for life. Researchers studied children aged 5–11 years, residing in Pune city for their food habits, frequency of various types of food eaten, and the preferences/dislike to various food items. About half of the children were nonvegetarians. Approximately 70% of children consumed milk daily, in spite majority of them did not like milk. Snacks, fast food, and processed foods were the most preferred food by them. Only 5% children consumed green leafy vegetables daily. Most children consumed fruits two to six times weekly. Researchers highlighted the need to "educate parents, especially in the middle and higher socioeconomic groups for correcting the dietary habits of their children to ensure their healthy and productive lives as adults".

Mukherjee R, Chaturvedi S. A study of the dietary habits of school children in Pune city, Maharashtra, India. Int J Comm Med Public Health. 2017;4(2):593-7.

Packed lunch: Selection of food preparations is very crucial issue because lunch is one of the major meals. In schools, the recess time is fairly short and within this time, the child is expected to consume her meal. This time is also used for eating, playing, and meeting friends. They are more eager to play rather than sit and spend a lot of time in eating food. Packed lunch should have the following characteristics:

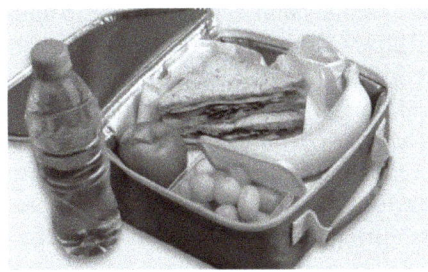

- Recipes in lunch box should be nutrient dense.
- Too many varieties should be avoided in 1 day. Varieties are preferred on different days.
- It should be attractive and some favorite item can be included, provided it does not contain too much sugar and/or fat.
- It should provide one-third of the day's requirement.
- Staple cereals, sources of good quality protein, a dairy product (if possible), and fruit/vegetable should be included.
- Packed lunch should be dry or semisolid. Avoid liquid or oily preparations to avoid spillage in school bags on books, etc.
- Food should be palatable enough even when cold or dry. For example, noodles, dosa are unpalatable when cold. Salads are not a good choice for packed lunch for school children as it gives low energy and takes time to consume. Whole fruits are a good choice rather than cut pieces. Similarly, a whole tomato can be included.

- Food should not become soggy, mushy, mixed up, or ferment in lunch box.
- It should be one complete meal rather than just a snack. Packed lunch preparations may include some cereal (preferably whole grains rather than refined flours), pulse, cooked vegetable, *paneer*/cheese, etc.
- Biscuits, cakes, chips/wafers should be avoided. The child spends many hours in school and the meal should be filling enough that the child will not feel hungry so that overfeeding occurs when the child comes home from school. Almost half a day is spent by the child in school. Letting him be hungry in school and overfeeding at home is not good.

Besides food, it is important to pay attention to physical activity pattern of children:
- Ensure that the child is involved in physically active sports outside the home every day. It improves physical activity and social interaction.
- Parents should limit children's video, television watching, and computer use to less than 2 hours daily and replace the sedentary activities with activities that require more movement.
- Children and adolescents need at least 60 minutes of moderate-to-vigorous physical activity to maintain good health and fitness and for healthy weight.

Adolescence

The World Health Organization defines adolescent age between 10 and 19 years, beginning with puberty and ending at adulthood or a transition from childhood to adulthood, and is the second phase of growth spurt after infancy. Characteristic changes occur in this period, including sharp fluctuations in physiological, hormonal, sexual organs, neurological, and behavioral changes. Up until around 7–8 years, boys and girls do not differ much in height. However, from this age onward, sexual dimorphism becomes quite evident. The second growth spurt occurs during this period and there will be changes in their physical development at a rate that is unparalleled since infancy. Adolescent girls and boys face many challenges. They long for social and economic independence, identity, and acquisition of skills in carrying out roles in various academic and vocational areas. However, adolescent age lays the foundation for adopting adult roles and responsibilities.

> **Puberty** is a process of transformation, during which a child's body is transformed into an adult body and capable of reproduction. The process is governed by surge of specific hormones which bring major changes in body size, shape, composition, and functional abilities of different organs of the body. There is growth of secondary sex characteristics like breast development, pubic hair, facial hair, etc. as well as change in voice.

Adolescence is the beginning of a productive life; hence, it is a critical life stage in life. Adequate nutrition is critical in this age, as it not only fulfills their requirements but also lays the foundation for next generation and prevents disease in adulthood. Inadequacy may result in stunting and poor bone remodeling and poor turnover of the nutrients needed for all biological functioning. There is a gain in height, skeletal size, and changes in body weight, composition, and shape. Adolescents gain approximately 15–20% of the adult's height and 50% of the adult's weight. Nutrition and growth in adolescence particularly for girls is important for achieving their potential adult stature. Women with short stature are at risk of complications in delivery, such as obstructed labor.

Physical development includes:
- **Rapid gain in height and weight:** The growth spurt in adolescence takes place over a period of 2–4 years. Generally, the period is longer for boys than girls. Girls begin their growth spurt earlier at 9–10 years of age; whereas, in boys it begins approximately 2 years later at 11 years. The maximum linear growth, i.e., increase in height, also known as peak height velocity occurs at an average age of 11.5 years in girls. The average gain in height is 5–6 cm and peak height velocity is as much as 8–10 cm/year. At this time, both will gain weight as well, although boys gain mainly muscle, whereas in girls there is gain in body fat. In girls, weight gain occurs 6–9 months prior to height gain. For example, if weight of 9 year old girl is 25 Kg then it can double to the tune of 50 Kg by the age of 15 years in healthy conditions. There are variations between different children.
- **Bone mass** doubles between onset of puberty and young adulthood. About 6 months after peak height velocity, bone growth is greatest. Adolescents gain about one-fourth of peak adult bone mass during this period. There are gender differences since boys have about 25% more bone mass than girls.
- Difference in fat mass and muscle mass and the site of where they are present and where fat is deposited determine the body shape and body contouring in both sexes. This is also governed by different sex hormones. At the end of puberty, boys will have about 13% body fat and girls about 20% body fat. By 20 years of age, young women will have 26% body fat.
- Fat deposition, particularly in girls, is relatively higher for development of adipose tissue to accommodate reproductive organs. The site of fat distribution is usually around the trunk among children and deposited intra-abdominally and subcutaneously. It may cause establishment of obesity or increased abdominal girth in children who consume more fat and do less physical activity.
- **Development of secondary sex characteristics:** During puberty, levels of several hormones increase, especially the sex steroid hormones. These hormones are responsible for the development of the secondary sex characteristics like appearance of breast, pubic hair, facial hair, etc. as well as change in voice. Testosterone stimulates muscle growth. Estrogen regulates fat mass and menstrual cycle. Estrogen also promotes bone growth.
- **Brain development:** During puberty brain develops, particularly; there is development of areas involved in regulation of behavior, emotion, perception, etc. Connections among different regions of the brain increase. The adolescent's ability for abstract thinking, planning, deductive reasoning, and processing information

increases. Cognitive development leads to increased self-awareness, self-regulation, and self-direction. Complete development occurs late in adolescence. The changes in body shape, composition, and body functioning, and increased self-awareness and independence make adolescents concerned about their own body image. Also, they are more susceptible to influences of their friends. They can understand risk but are not as good as adults at decision making. All these factors influence their food intake and lifestyle, consequently affecting their health and nutritional status.

> **Laboratory Laurel:** This study, with 170 women (15–45 years), was carried out in 4 months in Isfahan, Iran. Premenstrual syndrome (PMS) in young girls and women can cause suicide, dissociation of familial relationships, abnormalities in the daily work and interpersonal relationships in the patients, and bring about direct and indirect economic burden for the society. Subjects were divided into three groups—who were given Mg, Mg plus vitamin B_6, and placebo. PMS diagnosis in patients was made by noting the PMS symptoms daily for 2 months. Medical intervention was carried out in two menstrual cycles and the results of pre- and post-test were compared. The findings indicated that Mg plus vitamin B_6 and placebo significantly reduced the PMS symptoms, or had the greatest and the least effect on the mean score of PMS, respectively.
>
> *Fathizadeh N, Ebrahimi E, Valiani M, et al. Evaluating the effect of magnesium and magnesium plus vitamin B_6 supplement on the severity of premenstrual syndrome. Iran J Nurs Midwifery Res. 2010;15(Suppl1):401-5.*

Nutritional Requirements During Adolescents

Nutritional needs are increased compared to the school years. This is required for the growth spurt and increase in body size. Adequate intake is of utmost importance not only to meet requirements for growth and development during the pubertal period but also for good health in later years of life. Requirements for selected nutrients are given in Tables 9.1A and B in Chapter 9 and EAR in Appendix 4. Requirements for boys are higher than for girls because of differences in their growth and development. The only nutrient that is required in higher amounts by girls is iron due to menstrual blood losses.

Energy: Energy requirements are relatively very high in comparison to adults, e.g., a 14 year-old girl requires 2400 kcal/day and a sedentary woman needs only 1660 kcal/day. Adolescents need energy for growth and development as well as for play or physical activities. However, girls' requirements are approximately 500 kcal/day less than boys which may be attributed to the differences in their body size and body composition. Unfortunately many adolescent girls or even boys tend to consume less energy in order to stay/look slim and often result in health issues. Role of eating enough and eating right comes in these circumstances. Do not forget to indulge in exercise that will utilize the energy in better way.

Protein: Boys require more protein than girls for the greater lean body mass (LBM), increase in stature/body size, blood volume, and for other metabolic functions throughout adolescence. Protein is also utilized for bone development besides for the synthesis of hormones and enzymes. Deficiency of protein can lead to growth retardation and other health problems which may appear in later years of life.

Fat: Fat requirement is high during the growth spurt and in case of girls some critical amount of adipose tissue is needed for normal menstruation. Fat is utilized for energy and formation of certain body constituents. At the same time, excess intake should be prevented in order to prevent health risks.

Vitamins: Antioxidant vitamins like A, E, and C are required to face physiological stresses and strengthen body systems. Vitamin D supports skeletal growth and is needed to attain peak bone mass and achieve final adult height. If vitamin A intakes are marginal, there can be adverse effects on bone growth as well as sexual maturation. Requirement for thiamin, riboflavin, and niacin corresponds to energy requirement and requirement for vitamin B_6 is associated with protein metabolism. Folic acid requirement is high for cell division in growth phase particularly among adolescent girls for forthcoming pregnancy. Also because vitamin A is very important for immunity, insufficient intakes can make adolescents susceptible to infection. Vitamin B_6 plays an important role in heme synthesis and protein and amino acid metabolism and adequate intakes of this vitamin should also be ensured.

Minerals: Need for **iron** is high for rapid growth of tissues, transportation of oxygen to cells, and expansion of blood volume and muscle mass. Girls need more iron to compensate for the loss of iron during menstruation, both girls and boys need more iron for expansion of blood volume. Adequate **calcium** is essential for lengthening of bones, increasing bone density, and calcification. **Zinc** is a component of several enzymes and genes required for sexual maturation. Calcium absorption and deposition usually peak around menarche in girls. Bioavailability of calcium is also important and influenced by other factors like source of calcium (vegetable, dairy, or supplement), vitamin D status, intake of protein, sodium and other nutrients, and physical activity level. Puberty is the strong indicator for peripheral and axial bone mineral density.

Food Behavior of Adolescents

Adolescents are independent in making their food choices. Parents' influence may become less because they think that they are now grown up and would like to be independent. **Peer group, media, and body image** play important roles in determining their food choices. Availability of money, time, and facilities also influences the type of food they consume. Since they like to be with friends, eating out, snacking, and drinking may be indulged in by many. There are marked gender differences in food choice and all are related to their body image.

Girls gain weight rapidly during puberty and may try to lose weight by skipping meals in order to look slim and smart. In the process, they may miss out on obtaining the essential nutrients their bodies require. Occasionally, girls may become obsessed with body weight and slimness to the extent of developing eating disorders like anorexia nervosa or bulimia. Boys may indulge in energy dense and protein rich foods to increase energy, build muscles, and enhance their fitness levels.

Reasons for food choices
Convenience
Access to money
Easy access to ready to eat foods
Availability of cheaper food (snack and cola drinks)—fast foods
Discounts and free offers
Vendor facility
Canteen facility in college
Peer pressure
Advertisements and media
Foods associated with body image
Ignorance about role of food and nutrition in future health
Casual attitude
Stress on enjoyment
Clash between timings for meals, class time and other activities

Dietary Guidelines for Adolescents

- Nutritionally adequate diet is needed by adolescents; it is important that all essential nutrients be consumed as per their requirements.
- Consumption of whole balanced meal should be encouraged rather than dependency on junk food, chips, and chocolates.
- Include calcium-rich foods like milk, curd, *paneer*, cheese, sesame seeds, and green leafy vegetables
- Include iron-rich foods along with vitamin C rich foods
- Include protein-rich foods like egg, meat, dairy products, pulses, nuts, and seeds
- Include plenty of vegetables and fruits through various food preparations
- Occasionally, include tasty and popular food also in their diet.
- Discourage overeating of sweets, fried foods, ready to eat snacks, processed, and soft drinks. Foods like chocolates and ice creams should not be used as stress busters.
- Biscuits are energy dense and should not be consumed when hungry. There will be a tendency for overconsumption as they are not satiating or filling.
- Teach them to identify and consume foods that are good for health.
- Discourage indiscriminate dieting and use of fad diets.
- Encourage them to eat family food and take packed lunch/tiffin box from home.

ADULTS

At the age of 18 years, an individual is considered an adult. Growth ceases at the end of adolescence but maturation continues for metabolic activities and bone density reaches its peak at 30 years of age. There are marked gender differences in body weight, height, body composition, biological functions, and physiological needs. They are influenced by genetic as well as environmental factors like food intake and life style. Adulthood is one of the most productive years of life. Women go through pregnancy and lactation. Adulthood is the longest period in an individual's lifetime. This is the stage of longest duration because it can span 4–6 to more than 6 decades in the life of an individual. Each decade has its own characteristic considerations and it is generally divided into three stages as shown in Figure 11.9. Nutritional management at these three stages can be tailored as per the needs of the specific age group.

Early adulthood is characterized by cessation of growth and completion of maturation. This stage is characterized by numerous challenges such as making careers and meeting professional demands, settling in life, and in terms of nutrition and health, is crucial in terms of maintenance of body weight, fitness, and health. Bone density continues to develop until the middle of the 3rd decade of life and is important to prevent osteoporosis later in life. Some males may continue to grow until age 20 and with this there will be accumulation of lean body or muscle mass. Women need to pay attention to nutrition because these are the reproductive years.

Middle age is characterized by gradually slowing down of metabolism (lower BMR compared to the previous years), lower production of certain hormones, and alteration in blood and body composition. Late adulthood is characterized by reduction in blood volume and body fluids. Studies show that mobility gradually begins to decline, although it may not be noticeable in the 3rd decade of life. Body composition begins to change and persons find it difficult to lose weight while many gain weight after 40 years of age. Fatigue and digestive disturbances are frequently experienced. Hormonal changes occur—women undergo menopause and in males, testosterone levels begin to decline. This is the age when responsibilities both at home and family as well as at the workplace are the most, leaving very little time for self. Adequate food and nutrient intake, regular physical activities, daily routines, and positive outlook can delay aging and process of disease occurrence.

Late adulthood or older adults: Career may be at peak for many of individuals. Many of them would have fulfilled their family responsibilities in terms of raising children and therefore have more times for themselves. Some may have disposable incomes and indulge in activities which may not be health protective. Muscle mass and body fat decrease with age. This results in a lower metabolic rate increasing the possibility of weight gain. However, these changes can be offset by exercise. Immunity also gradually reduces, that can be further compromised if nutrient especially micronutrient intakes are poor. Bone loss and lack of exercise can also adversely influence the posture of a person.

Ability to taste and smell are gradually compromised or reduced, gastric and saliva secretions begin to decline, and problems such as constipation, indigestion, flatulence, and bloating begin to be experienced. Many persons may have

| Early adulthood of the young adult years • (20-30 years) | Middle age • (30-40 years) | Late adulthood • (45-60 years) |

Fig. 11.9: Stages of adulthood.

to manage chronic health problems such as hypertension, dyslipidemia, diabetes mellitus, arthritis, etc. If a person does not have any of these problems, the focus should be to have a nutritionally well-balanced diet and healthy life style to prevent occurrence of such problems which is termed "Compression of Morbidity". The ultimate goal should be well-being and good quality of life.

Food Behavior of Adults

Food behavior of adults is gender specific and highly influenced by family traditions and job profile. Adults in early age are still in a progressive life stage in terms of job/career and family. When they are at home, they may usually consume home prepared meals but when they are outside, they tend to eat out in restaurants or street foods or ready to eat/processed foods. Where and what the individual eats is influenced by the availability of time and money as well as whether the person is living with family or lives alone.

- Though adults prefer family food, many frequently indulge in fried and sweet snacks and consumption of beverages including alcohol. Hence, their sugar and fat intake may be excessive, and obesity, especially abdominal obesity, is seen in a considerable proportion of persons.
- Men usually stay several hours outside home due to professional demands; hence, they may largely depend upon snacks and beverages, more often than not purchased from restaurants or cafeterias or fast food joints. This may result in energy consumption in excess of their expenditure. Some studies have shown that men carry and eat less fruits at the work place in order to avoid peeling and the risk of spoilage. They may carry tiffin box to their work place.
- Dinner is usually consumed at home with family by most persons but it is often consumed late followed by sitting and working or watching television and then sleeping. Meal composition of dinner widely varies from family to family. Age of different family members, working hours, and when different members, especially the person who prepares the meal return home, often determines the composition of the meal.
- Watching news and daily soaps on television, surfing the net and computer, and mobile usage tend to restrict after dinner walks.
- Women eat poorly particularly in nuclear families because they may not cook a full meal for themselves and often consume baked or fried snacks or stay hungry. Working women may tend to carry a packed lunch but the meal is more often not balanced, with protein sources or fruits being less likely to be included. The food consumption of women in joint family is largely influenced by the family tradition and the work load in the house.
- Many persons especially those who are working, tend to skip breakfast or eat very late. Skipping breakfast has been found to be associated with obesity.
- Therefore although both men and women may eat whole meals, their nutrient intakes may not be balanced in accordance with their requirements. Deviation in nutrient intake tends to adversely influence their biological functions resulting in manifestation of chronic diseases.
- Aging and onset of disease can be delayed by following recommended nutrient intake and dietary guidelines. Regular exercise helps to a very large extent. Vigorous physical activity for half an hour, 5-6 days a week is advisable.
- Adults are at high risk of stress for various occupational and nonoccupational reasons; hence, relaxation techniques must be followed on regular basis.

Nutrient Requirements of Adults

Nutritional requirements vary with body weight, age, sex, physical activity, and the physiological state can be seen from Tables 9.2A and 9.2B in Chapter 9 and EAR in Appendix 4.

Energy: Adults require energy for maintenance and continuation of optimal metabolic and physical activities. On an average, the energy requirement for following categories is:

Healthy adult	30 kcal/kg body weight/day
Overweight	20 kcal/kg body weight/day
Underweight	40 kcal/kg body weight/day

Energy contribution from macronutrients should be 55-65% from carbohydrate; 15-25% from fat, and 10-15% from protein. Energy needs differ on the basis of physical activity pattern, e.g., sedentary men and women need much less calories than heavy workers.

Protein: Adults require protein for maintenance of biological functions and repair of tissues. They require 0.83 g/kg body weight/day. The requirement is more for sports persons, pregnant, and lactating women. Higher protein is also given in certain pathological conditions like burns, surgery, etc. Consumption of high quality protein (egg, meat, milk, and combination of pulse and cereals) can reduce the protein requirement. Choice of protein food is crucial owing its amino acid composition. Low protein is advisable in certain pathological conditions like kidney disease. Protein in middle age helps to maintain bone health and muscle mass, but excess protein can be harmful for kidney function.

Fat: Adults need fat for energy, maintenance of integrity of cell membranes; lubrication of joints, and utilization of fat-soluble substances. Sources of fat are very important due to their fatty acid composition. Adults need only 20-30 grams of visible fat, and the remaining 20 grams fat can be obtained from invisible fat sources such as nuts and seeds. Processing of fat is also critical, e.g., hydrogenated fat is harmful due to the presence of trans fatty acids. Fats from nuts and seeds are good as they contain more of essential fatty acids and fats from fried food are bad because they are often oxidized. It is better to consume few walnuts rather than few cutlets. On an average, 500 g all types/form of fats and oils per person **per month** may be sufficient. Intake of cholesterol should be controlled.

Vitamins: Thiamine, riboflavin, and niacin requirements are in accordance with energy intake and needed for basic metabolic functions. Other B vitamins and vitamin C are essentially required in adequate amounts for numerous biological functions. Vitamin C and E act as antioxidants and helpful in prevention of oxidative stress and the risk of chronic diseases.

Minerals: Calcium, iron, zinc, iodine, selenium, sodium, and potassium are of great importance because they regulate biochemical, enzymatic, and hormonal functions in the body. Adequacy of mineral intake protects cardiac and bone health in later years of life and prevents various diseases.

Dietary Guidelines for Adults

- Daily diet should include food items from all food groups.
- Each meal should provide about one-third of the daily nutrient requirement and should contain minimum of three food groups.
- Follow three meals in a day pattern, i.e., breakfast before 10 am, lunch before 3 pm, and dinner before 8–9 pm.
- Avoid frequent and *ad libitum* snack consumption.
- Reduce excessive intake of salt, sugar, fat, and refined flours.
- Avoid free sugar and replace with some amount of jaggery, honey, if otherwise restricted.
- Intake of fiber from fruits, vegetables, whole cereals including millets and pulses is essential.
- Inclusion of about 400 g of colored fruits and vegetable is advocated.
- Non-vegetarains can add fish, meat, egg 2–3 times a week in prescribed amount (50–75 g in one serving)
- Nuts like groundnuts, sesame seeds, almonds, raisins, cashew nuts, figs, walnuts, flax seeds, pumpkin seeds, sunflower seeds can be added according to one's financial resources. They are good sources of EFA and 10–30 g per day may be taken.
- Use some amount of spices like turmeric, pepper, and clove, cinnamon, nutmeg, bay leaves, fennel, cardamom, coriander, and herbs like coriander, mint, and curry leaves, basil, etc. as they are rich in phytochemicals and provide some nutrients. These substances not only provide zest to food but are also helpful in maintaining and protecting health.
- Include calcium rich foods like milk, curd, *paneer*, ragi, and sesame seeds in the daily diet.
- Addition of iron rich foods like egg, meat, GLV, pulses along with vitamin C rich foods like capsicum, cabbage, *amla*, lemon, etc. is important for ensuring adequate iron status.
- Regular consumption of yellow, orange, and red color foods adds value in health protection as they are rich source of β carotene, vitamin C, and bioflavonoids.
- Avoid ultraprocessed and packaged food as much as possible and prefer home-made simple food.
- Daily physical exercise is quintessential for nutrition and health.

OLD AGE

Aging is a natural (normal) biological process, involving cellular and physiological deterioration/decline, increasing vulnerability to disease, and decreased ability to adapt to stress because of impaired homeostasis. It occurs at different rates. Therefore, it is hard to pinpoint from which day an individual starts aging. Aging is unavoidable but deterioration of health is avoidable.

According to WHO, the age of 60 or 65 years, roughly equivalent to retirement ages in most developed countries, is said to be the beginning of old age. The UN cutoff is 60+ years to refer to the older or elderly persons. Within the elderly population, further classification can be done—oldest old (normally those who are 80+ years) and centenarian (100+ years), and even super-centenarian (110+ years).

Aging is a reflection of the sum total of care, use/misuse, or neglect of the body in previous years of life. Like any other life stage, nutrition plays a critical role in maintaining health and well-being in old age. Healthy young adults gradually become more vulnerable to injury and illness. Illnesses, infections, accidents, or traumas have a cumulative effect on health and nutritional status in later years of life. It can influence, agility, endurance, or muscle coordination and hence determine how physically active the older person is. If a person is active and has positive attitude toward life, has good health for many years, and is able to handle crisis with more composure, the quality of life of such a person is likely to be good. Physical, physiological, psychological conditions, social prestige, financial status, personal life style, family composition, and family support are some factors that drastically influence health of the elders. This is a period of critical changes in body, mind, and spirit.

Aging can be associated with changes in lifestyle and health that may affect the types of foods eaten and the nutritional status. Loneliness, boredom, depression, and worrying about the future can lead some to neglect of food intake; some persons may skip meals, and in general their dietary/eating habits may be poor. It is important to address these factors and seek ways to improve diet, even if this means asking for help from friends, family, or other community services.

Another problem that compromises food and nutrient intake is the relatively poorer financial status of the elderly. Metabolic disorders like diabetes, underweight, or overweight are often seen in this age group.

Physiological Changes in Elders

Functions of most systems and organs diminish in old age. By 70 years of age, pulmonary function, cardiac output, liver function, and kidney function are lower than the function in the young adult at 25 years. The ability to participate in physical activities changes as a person grows older, and this change is accelerated from 50 years of age and onward. Several physical and physiological changes underlie this, less delivery of oxygen to tissues of body, decreased chest wall elasticity, and less amount of blood output to supply skeletal muscles.

Body composition: There is loss of bone density and muscle mass which result in difficulty in walking and maintaining balance. Loss of muscle mass is known as sarcopenia. At the same time, the proportion of body fat increases. Thus, the ratio of fat to muscle also increases. The distribution of body fat also changes. In young persons, the fat is generally subcutaneous, whereas in the elderly it is mostly intra-abdominal and intramuscular. Waist-to-hip ratio also increases.

Many older persons have frequent aches and pains in different parts of the body and there is high risk of frequent falls and fractures. Arthritis, rheumatism, osteoporosis, and other related problems are common in senior citizens. Regular walk, mild exercise, and sun bath support bone health. Regular consumption of dairy products, ragi flour, sesame seeds, sweet lime, guava, amla, egg, etc. can fulfill the increased demands for protein, calcium, vitamin D, and vitamin C.

Muscle strength: Getting old is characterized by loss of muscle mass and muscle strength. In contrast, there is increase in percent body fat. This occurs due to poor dietary intake, lack of strength giving exercises, and thereby lack of protein synthesis in the body particularly the muscles. There is reduced voluntary muscular movement.

> **Sarcopenia** is age-related loss of muscle mass and muscle strength and function. Loss of muscle mass results in decreased muscle strength. Sarcopenia begins in the 4th decade of life but the rate of loss of muscle mass is greater after 75 years of age. It is seen more in persons who are physically inactive but occurs even in those who are physically active. Factors that contribute to sarcopenia are decreased protein synthesis and decreased hormone levels. Sarcopenia is partly reversed if a person does appropriate physical exercises particularly resistance training.

Changes in body fluids: Ratio of ECF and ICF alters, affecting kidney and cardiac functions. Some persons may have constipation or diarrhea. Loss of body fluid results in dehydration and weakness. Moisture in skin is also reduced leading to wrinkles. Regular intake of water and fluids at frequent intervals is advisable. Plain safe drinking water, soups, and juices are good. Thirst sensation is reduced, thus chances of water intake are also lessened. Dependency on thirst to drink water should be avoided. Persons who are dependent on others for feeding should be especially paid attention to.

Immune system: Adequate intake of protein, energy, vitamins A, C, E, and minerals like copper, zinc, iron, and selenium help to synthesize immune system components like antibodies, neutrophils, and T-cells. Poor nutrient intakes impair the immunity which is a cause of concern among older population, as it reduces the healing capacity on the one hand and increases the chances of infection. Sufficient intake of these nutrients can prevent the infections and speed up the healing process.

Digestive system: There is reduction in gastric juices, gastric acid, and digestive enzymes resulting in slowing down of the digestive processes. Absorption of food and nutrients is also less efficient than in younger age. **Achlorhydria** (low acid in stomach) affects digestion of protein, and absorption of vitamin B_{12} and calcium. Peristalsis also becomes slow resulting in constipation. Judicious selection of food may improve the digestion. The combination of rice, pulses, and one GLV and starchy vegetable will do better than fried fast foods. Milk, fruits, and nuts in different forms can be given to provide nutrients and improve digestion.

There is decreased secretion of saliva, therefore elders find difficulty in swallowing. Soft and soggy textured food may make swallowing easier. Also, periodontal disease may make chewing difficult. Addition of some amount of mild spices may stimulate saliva secretion. Loss of taste buds results in alteration in taste sensations. Perception of sweet taste decreases and that for bitter taste increases. Loss of taste (hypogeusia) may also occur due to zinc deficiency. In many individuals, decay or loss of teeth affects ability to chew. Eating hard and chewy food is difficult and well cooked, soft, mashed foods are preferable. In this age, sensitivity to sweet taste diminishes and that for bitter taste increases.

The digestive system is very sensitive to emotions. Many elderly persons may either not feel like eating when they are upset, i.e., either they are lonely, depressed, or worried. Some may experience a stomach upset. Regular contact with friends and relatives, through visits and telephone calls, can help prevent these problems.

It is not unusual for older people to have constipation. This is caused by changes in tissue and muscles and reduced thirst. Regular exercise, like daily walks, can help prevent constipation. Also, a well-balanced diet with adequate fiber and fluid intake also encourages normal bowel function and minimizes the need for laxatives. Laxatives should be discouraged because they interfere with absorption of important nutrients.

Metabolic rate: Energy requirement gradually decreases with age due to reduced BMR and physical activities. With age, anabolic rate reduces and catabolic rate increases leading to degeneration. Repair and regeneration of newer cells occurs at a slower rate.

Excretory system: There are marked changes in kidney function that may be due to reduced number of nephrons and reduced glomerular filtration rate (GFR). It may also be due to imbalance in water, electrolytes, and protein intake.

Circulatory system: The heart slows down and its ability to pump blood is less as compared to a young adult. Consequently, older people have less energy and stamina to work. Circulation is less, hence old persons' extremities particularly their hands and feet may be cold. Also, blood vessels lose their elasticity. In some persons, edema of extremities can occur, because blood tends to "pool" in feet and legs. The rate of RBC production is reduced resulting in poor oxygen carrying capacity. In older persons who have poor circulation, this can result in forgetfulness and poor cognition. Also, poor nutrient intakes increase the risk of anemia. There is increased pressure on the heart due to narrowed arteries resulting in cardiac problems.

Inclusion of complex carbohydrates, protein, omega 3 fatty acids, and vitamin A and C rich in the diet and exclusion of salt, sugar, refined, and processed foods and saturated and trans fats are essential for good cardiac health.

Circulatory changes also bring susceptibility to development of "little strokes", the symptoms of such episodes are headache, vision disturbances, loss of balance, confusion, and dizziness when the person stands quickly from a sitting or reclining position. It is important to consult a doctor if such episodes occur. In addition, some elderly persons may be given medications that also influence circulation. It is important to know the effects and side effects of medications that are prescribed for the older person.

Other changes: There is loss of hearing and vision. Motor control gradually deteriorates. All these changes necessitate special attention in modifying the texture of food or supplying appropriate cutlery.

Hormonal changes in old age: Among women, there is reduction of estrogen during menopause (cessation of monthly periods) and increase in prolactin may lead to fat accumulation.

Nervous system: Loss of short-term memory and disorientation are commonly observed in old age. Nerve transmission may be slower which can be improved by calcium and magnesium intake. Mental exercises and involvement also support the cognition and attentiveness.

Frailty: Many elder persons are frail. "Frailty" is considered as a distinct syndrome that either precedes or is a cause of disability. Frailty is associated with decreased resistance to stressors, as a result of cumulative decline in multiple physiological systems and makes the person vulnerable to adverse outcomes. A person is said to be frail if any three of the following five symptoms are present such as weakness, walking at slow speed, low level of physical activity, unintentional weight loss and exhaustion.

Malnutrition is one of the causes of frailty. Involuntary weight loss >10% is a specific sign of malnutrition. Other causes include atherosclerosis, cognitive impairment, and sarcopenia. Frail older adults are more likely to die, be hospitalized, or become disabled.

Factors Affecting Nutrition of Elderly People

Aging can affect the appetite and food intake which has a great impact on nutrition of the elder people. Gender differences are frequently observed. Some factors have been observed in most communities of the world to affect the nutrition of elders:

Loneliness: Eating alone often reduces the quantity as well as quality of food intake. If they are living alone, impact of loneliness on food intake worsens.

Physical disability: Elders may tend to walk slowly and with difficulty. Physical limitations such as arthritis that restrict mobility, loss of vision, impaired mental function like Alzheimer's disease, prevent them from going for shopping (groceries, vegetable, fruits etc.), eating out, and even going to the dining area within the house. Physical limitations can affect nutrition by affecting ease of obtaining and preparing foods.

Lack of knowledge about cooking: This is a problem particularly with men, when they need to stay alone and do not have any support for cooking food. Some persons may be unwilling or unable to cook. However in cities, some ready to eat foods like cornflakes, *museli*, frozen meals are available but elders may often prefer to adhere to habitual dietary patterns. For such situations, such ready to eat processed foods seldom solve the problems.

Lack of financial resources: After retirement, most elders have less disposable incomes. Hence, limited money is saved for future emergencies and may not be spent on their own food and nutrition.

Chronic illnesses: A substantial proportion of elderly persons suffers from some health problem or the other and are prescribed medication(s). Illness not only depletes the body reserves but also delays recovery. Chronic illness is a serious and unavoidable expenditure.

Mental disturbances: Depression and dementia are very common among elders for various biological, nutritional, neurological, pathological, social, and psychological reasons. With aging, short-term memory is frequently affected, especially seen in Alzheimer disease.

Social problems: Since elders are not so productive, other people even their family members tend to ignore them and their nutritional, medical, and physical needs.

Healthy eating is just as important for seniors as it is for young adults, adolescents, and children. While the emphasis is on "healthy" (being healthy and choosing healthy foods), it is also important to make eating an enjoyable and sociable activity that the older person can look forward to. To have a healthy lifestyle, a good diet should be combined with regular, moderate exercise. This can include activities such as walking and swimming. Exercise helps to regulate appetite and weight, strengthens the heart, blood vessels, lungs and bones, improves circulation and lung function, and also improves sleep.

Nutritional Requirements of Elders

Energy requirements of the elderly are generally lower than in younger and middle-aged adults for two reasons: (i) slower metabolism and (ii) relatively less amount of physical activity. On the other hand, protein requirements are higher. Adequate intake of good quality protein should be ensured in order to avoid loss of muscle mass as well as to support muscle protein synthesis. Attention should be paid to vitamin D status, calcium and phosphorus intakes as well as sodium and potassium intakes. All intakes should be according to health status and presence of disease that may necessitate dietary modifications/restrictions. Attention must be paid to musculoskeletal and cardiac fitness and health. Adequate intakes of folate, choline, vitamin B_{12}, and vitamin B_6 can help to prevent cognitive decline.

Adequate fluid intake is essential as the aged population is at risk of dehydration. According to the World Health Organization (2002), fluid requirement can be calculated as 30 mL/kg of body weight per day for adults. ICMR-NIN (2020) has increased the water/fluid requirement as compared to the adult for the reason that elders often do not sense the thirst due to its altered mechanism. Sedentary elder men and women need 2.8 and 2.55 liters water per day and with moderate active members need 3.3 and 3.0 liters water respectively. In case of any pathological situation change in water intake should be as per medical guidance.

In addition to the recognized essential nutrients, consumption of phytochemicals will have additional benefits because they have anti-inflammatory, antimicrobial, antioxidant, and antimutagenic, antiangiogenic, or hormonal properties. These properties exhibit beneficial effect in prevention of many chronic diseases like cancer and heart disease. It may not be necessary to consume large amount of supplements but consuming diverse fruits and vegetables in suitable forms, i.e., texture and consistency would be beneficial as they would provide both micronutrients and phytoactives, variety in taste, make the diet colorful, etc.

Dietary Guidelines for Elders

- Higher intakes of fruits, vegetables, nuts, dairy, fish, and whole grains may delay muscle strength and cognitive decline which is common in advanced age.
- Older persons have small appetite; hence, small, frequent and nutrient dense (especially micronutrient) foods should be included. Major meals can also be small and with few dishes. Variety of ingredients can be added in one dish only.
- Invite friends and relatives to share meals with the elderly person.
- Nourishing, digestible, easy to chew and easy to swallow foods and beverages are preferred. Milk shakes, fruit yogurt, biscuits, pancakes, idli, etc. can be good choices.
- Try to make meal platter or dining table more welcoming and attractive. Offer familiar, well-liked foods.
- When an elderly person has poor appetite or complains about digestive problem(s), it should be looked into.
- Ensure four to five serving of fruits and vegetables and cut down on fried foods, particularly those containing trans fats.
- Add full cream dairy products. The fat is easily digested, cream increases energy and calcium content of the diet. It can also facilitate the peristalsis.
- Add some amount of butter to vegetables and bread, etc. to increase energy content and enhance flavor of the diet.
- Consume fat from whole foods such as nuts, seeds, beans, and fatty fish to get high in ω-3 and ω-9 fatty acids.
- Avoid refined fats and fatty spreads.
- Emphasize healthy traditional vegetable- and legume-based dishes.
- Limit traditional fat-rich dishes and heavily preserved/pickled dishes.
- Ensure adequate intake of fluids preferable in the form of gravy in the vegetable or pulse or meat preparation, soups, and other beverages. Of course, regular and adequate intake of water is advisable, especially in hot weather. Adequate fluid intake is necessary for maintaining body temperature and functioning of digestive system. It will reduce constipation which is quite common in this age due to reduced motility of the intestine and reduced physical mobility.
- Fluid intake may be inadequate because of decreased thirst sensation and reduced ability to conserve water and because they want to avoid frequent urination. Reliance on laxatives, use of prescribed diuretics, infections, immobility, and excessive use of caffeine or alcohol put the person at risk of dehydration.
- In case of medical problems such as kidney disease, fluid intake and output should be monitored and fluid intake should be determined in consultation with the doctor.
- Some signs of dehydration are mental confusion, decreased urine output, constipation, nausea, lack of appetite, dry lips, and elevated body temperature.
- Include natural sources of fiber (nonstarch polysaccharides) such as whole grains, fruits, and vegetables to reduce constipation. It will also help in controlling blood sugar.

Nutritional Deficiencies in Old Age

Nutrition is an important determinant of health in the elderly especially those who may have any illness. Importance of nutrition has been increasingly recognized as a significant factor for persons older than 65 years of age. Malnutrition in the elderly often goes undiagnosed. Common indicators are involuntary weight loss, abnormal BMI, decreased dietary intake, and deficiencies of specific micronutrients. Presence of morbidity such as diabetes, heart disease, etc. increases the risk of malnutrition. Often the weight loss goes unrecognized, since some weight loss is expected as muscle mass decreases. Isolation and depression exacerbate the problem. Elderly population has commonly been found to have cobalamin (vitamin B_{12}) and folate deficiency. Intakes of protein and calcium may be low and vitamin D deficiency can occur since the person may not be exposed to sunshine. There may be increased risk of falls and fractures. Low vitamin D status has been linked to higher risk of decline in cognition as well as muscle strength, low moods and depression.

Low intake of B vitamins, especially folate, B_{12}, and B_6 may increase risk of low functionality, cognitive decline, heart disease, and stroke. Inadequate intake of dietary protein has been linked with poor muscle function and decline in physical capacity leading toward sarcopenia.

Lower intake of energy- and protein-rich foods for prolonged period results in PEM and older persons become frail and find difficulty in walking and maintaining balance. Intake of other nutrients like B-vitamins, iron, calcium, zinc, and electrolytes also affects the degree of malnutrition and body functioning. PEM not only affects the physical stature but also mental functioning.

Elders who have limited access to food, living alone, low income, and poor transport facilities are vulnerable to PEM. It is important that the elderly live the last stage of life with dignity and have as good a quality of life as is possible.

Exercise in Old Age

Many videos are today shared on whatsapp on how gracefully many elderly are going through this important phase of life. Almost all of these persons exercise a great deal. It is essential for them to increase muscle strength and muscle mass to maintain their functional status and independence. Certain aerobic and strength-training exercises are appropriate for individuals age 60 and older. It is crucial for elder population. Those who had not done exercise in earlier years, must undertake exercise gradually, start with lighter exercises, after discussing with their healthcare providers. Older persons can do stationary cycling regularly and strength training 2–3 days a week, with a day of rest between workouts. Before indulging in a particular exercise regime, they should be first evaluated for their ability and risks by a physiotherapist for the type of exercise, its frequency, duration, and intensity.

Besides muscle health, exercise helps a person to feel fresh, improves insulin sensitivity, and improves mood. In addition, for those who can go out of the home for exercise, it provides a great opportunity to make friends.

RAPID FIRE

1. List the three stages of pregnancy and salient features of fetal development.
2. What are advantages of breastfeeding?
3. How does preterm birth influence nutritional requirements of the baby?
4. Give guidelines for formation of good food habits in children.
5. What is catch-up growth?
6. Why is adolescence, the period of second growth spurt?
7. List the important considerations for complementary feeding.
8. What is role of nutrition in different stages of adulthood?
9. How do physiological changes in old age influence food intake of elderly?
10. What is frailty and sarcopenia?

EXERCISES

1. Differentiate between growth pattern in preschool and school age from infancy.
2. Plan two complementary recipes—one freshly prepared for feeding and one that can be stored.
3. Interview one pregnant woman + one lactating woman + elderly person. Record their food intake for previous day 24 hours. Calculate nutritive value of their one day meal and compare with RDA.
4. What dietary considerations will you suggest for school age children and adolescent?

SUGGESTED READING

1. Agarwal KN, Agarwal DK. The Growth – Infancy to Adolescence. New Delhi: BS Publishers and Distributors; 2003.
2. Ballard O, Ardythe LM. Human milk composition: Nutrients and bioactive factors. Pediatr Clin North Am. 2013; 60(1):
3. Barker DJ. The malnourished baby and infant and relationship with Type 2 diabetes. Br Med Bull. 2001;60(1):69-88.
4. Bharadva K, Tiwari S, Mishra S, Mukhopadhyay K, Yadav B, Agarwal RK, Kumar V. Human milk banking guidelines. Indian Pediatr. 2014;51(6):469-74.
5. Black MM. Effects of vitamin B12 and folate deficiency on brain development in children. Food Nutr Bull. 2008;29(2Suppl):S126-S131.
6. Bruce KD. Maternal and in utero determinants of type 2 diabetes risk in the young. Curr Diabetes Rep. 2014;14:446.
7. Cetin I, Alvino G, Radaelli T, et al. Fetal nutrition: a review. Acta Paediatrica. 2005;94(Suppl 449):7-13.
8. Cetin I, Berti C, Calabrese S. Role of micronutrients in the periconceptional period. Hum Reprod Update. 2010;16(1):80-95.
9. Coletta JM, Bell SJ, Roman AS. Omega-3 fatty acids and pregnancy. Rev Obstet Gynecol. 2010;3(4):163-71.
10. Edmond K, Bahl R. Optimal feeding of low birth weight infants: Technical review. Department of Child and Adolescent Health Development. World Health Organization. 2006.
11. ESPGHAN Committee on Nutrition, Agostini C, Decsi T, et al. Complementary feeding: A commentary by the ESPGHAN Committee on Nutrition. J Pediatr Gastroenterol Nutr. 2008;46:99-110.
12. Fruhbeck G. Overnutrition. In: Gibney EM, Elia M, Ljungqvist O, Dowsett J (Eds). Clinical Nutrition. US: Blackwell Publishing; 2005. pp 30-61.
13. Goodfellow LR, Earl S, Cooper C, et al. Maternal diet, behaviour and offspring skeletal health. Int J Environ Res Pub Health. 2010;7:1760-72.
14. Granic A, Mendonça N, Hill TR, et al. Nutrition in the very old. Nutrients. 2018;10(3):269.
15. Greenberg JA, Bell SJ, Ausdal WV. Omega-3 fatty acid supplementation during pregnancy. Rev Obstet Gynecol. 2008;1(4):162-9.
16. Gupta A, Khushwaha KP, Sobti JC, et al. Breastfeeding and Complementary Feeding. Guidelines for the Nutritional Professionals. 2001.
17. Hemlata R, Radhakrishna KV, Kumar BN. Undernutrition in children and critical windows of opportunity in Indian context. Indian J Med Res. 2018;148:612-20.
18. Hess SY, Lonnerdal B, Hotz C, et al. Recent advances in knowledge of zinc nutrition and human health. Food Nutr Bull. 2009;30(1):s5-s11.
19. Khandelwal S, Swamy MK, Patil K, Kondal D, Chaudhry M, Gupta R, et. al. The impact of DocosaHexaenoic Acid supplementation during pregnancy and lactation on Neurodevelopment of the offspring in India (DHANI): trial protocol. BMC Pediatr. 2018;18(1):261.
20. Koletzko B, Lien E, Agostoni C, et al. World Association of Perinatal Medicine Dietary Guidelines Working Group. The roles of long-chain polyunsaturated fatty acids in pregnancy, lactation and infancy: review of current knowledge and consensus recommendations. J Perinat Med. 2008;36:5-14.
21. Kurpad A. Undernutrition. Clinical Nutrition. In: Gibney EM, Elia M, Ljungqvist O, Dowsett J (Eds). US: Blackwell Publishing; 2005. pp. 63-84.
22. Martin CR, Ling PR, Blackburn GL. Review of infant feeding: Key features of breast milk and infant formula. Nutrients. 2016; 8(5): 279.
23. Morais JA, Chevalier S, Gougeon R. Protein turnover and requirements in the healthy and frail elderly. J Nutr Health Aging. 2016;10(4):272-83.
24. Morgan JB, Dickerson JW (Eds). Nutrition in Early life. England: John Wiley and Sons Ltd; 2003.
25. Pandde C, Mouzon SH. Maternal obesity and metabolic risk to the offspring: Why lifestyle interventions may have not achieved the desired outcomes. Int J Obes. 2015;39:642-9.
26. Pasricha S, Thimmayamma BV. Dietary Tips for the Elderly. National Institute of Nutrition, Hyderabad: Indian Council of Medical Research; 2005.
27. Patton GC, Sawyer SM, Santelli JS, et al. Our future: a Lancet commission on adolescent health and wellbeing. Lancet. 2016;387:2423-78.
28. Picciano MF. Pregnancy and lactation: Physiological adjustments, nutritional requirements and the role of dietary supplements. J Nutr. 2003;133:1997S-2002S.
29. Pillai R, Kurpad AV. Amino acid requirements in children and the elderly population. Br J Nutr. 2012;108 (s2):S44-S49.
30. Paul VK, Bagga A. (eds). Ghai Essential Pediatrics , 9th edition (HB 2019).
31. Recommended Dietary Allowances and Estimated Average Requirements, - Nutrient Requirements for Indians-2020. A Report of the Expert Group, Indian Council of Medical Research, National Institute of Nutrition.
32. Rosa FW, Turshen M. Fetal nutrition. Bull World Health Organ. 1970;43: 785-95.
33. Sankar MJ, Agarwal R, Mishra S, et al. Feeding of low birth weight infants. AIMS NICU Protocols. Department of Pediatrics, All India Institute of Medical Sciences, New Delhi; 2008.
34. Singh K, Verma B. Breast feeding- an Ayurveda perceptive. J Homeop Ayurv Med. 2012;1:112.
35. Thomas L, Al Saud1 NB, Durighel G, Frost G, Bell J. The effect of preterm birth on adiposity and metabolic pathways and the implications for later life. Clinical Lipidology. 2012;7:3,275-88.
36. Tiwari S, Bharadva K, Yadav B, et al, for the IYCF Chapter of IAP. Infant and Young Child Feeding Guidelines, 2016. Indian Pediatr. 2016;53:703-13.
37. Tomkins CT. Does fetal under-nutrition predispose disease in adult offspring. University of Alberta Health Sciences. 2007;4(1).

38. Tsang RC (Ed). Vitamin and Mineral Requirements in Preterm Infants. New York: Marcel Dekker, Inc; 1985.
39. WHO (2002). Complementary feeding: Report of the global consultation convened jointly by the Department of Child and Adolescent Health and Development and the Department of Nutrition for Health and Development and Summary of guiding principles for complementary feeding of the breastfed child.
40. WHO (2009). Infant and young child feeding: Model chapter for textbooks for medical students and allied health professionals.
41. WHO (2020). Improving Early Childhood Development: WHO Guideline.
42. WHO (2001). Complementary feeding—report of the global consultation: Summary of guiding principles.
43. WHO (2017). Guidelines. Protecting, Promoting and Supporting Breastfeeding in Facilities Providing Maternity and Newborn services. [online]
44. WHO. Keep fit for life: meeting the nutritional needs of older persons. Geneva, Switzerland: World Health Organization/Tufts University School of Nutrition and Policy; 2002. pp. 3-4.
45. WHO and UNICEF. (2018). Implementation Guidance- Protecting, promoting and supporting breastfeeding in facilities providing maternity and newborn services: the revised Baby-Friendly Hospital Initiative.
46. Wiens D, DeSoto MC. Is high folic acid intake a risk factor for autism?—A review. Brain Sci. 2017;7(11):149.
47. World Health Organization. Health situation and trend assessment. [online]. Available from http://www.searo.who.int/entity/health_situation_trends/data/chi/elderly-population/en/ [Last Accessed August, 2019].
48. World Health Organization. Health statistics and information systems. [online]. Available from https://www.who.int/healthinfo/survey/ageingdefnolder/en/ [Last Accessed August, 2019].
49. World Health Organization. Zinc supplementation during pregnancy. [online]. Available from www.who.int/elena/titles/zinc_pregnancy/en/ [Last Accessed August, 2019].
50. Wu G, Bazer FW, Cudd TA, et al. Maternal nutrition and fetal development. J Nutr. 2004;139(9):2169-72.

12
CHAPTER

Nutrition in Deficiency Disorders and Some Diet-related Diseases

KEY CONCERNS
- Which are the nutritional deficiency disorders of public health concern, how they can be identified and managed at community level?
- What preventive measures can ameliorate PEM, vitamin A, iodine, and iron deficiencies at national level?
- Which are the diet-related chronic diseases prevalent at global level and how can they be prevented?

KEY CONCEPTS
Etiology, prevalence, and consequences and preventive measures of the following:
- Protein-energy malnutrition (PEM)
- Anemia
- Iodine deficiency disorders (IDD)
- Vitamin A deficiency (VAD)
- Overweight and obesity
- Hypertension
- Diabetes
- Osteoporosis

INTRODUCTION

"Malnutrition" includes problems caused by nutritional deficiency disorders at one end of the spectrum (undernutrition) and diet-related chronic diseases linked to overweight and obesity (overnutrition) at the other end. Various factors are responsible for malnutrition including social, economical, political and environmental factors, most of them being preventable and modifiable. Nutritional imbalance and unhealthy eating habits/feeding practices for young children adversely influence nutritional status. Emphasis on energy-dense foods combined with physical inactivity increases the risk of diet-related noncommunicable diseases. Both undernutrition and overnutrition compromise health status, immune competence, earning capacity, well-being, and quality of life; and pose a serious threat to national economy, overall productivity, and development. Genetics, age, gender, history of infections and vaccinations, early life experiences with diet, stage in the female menstrual cycle, stress, habitual exercise levels, smoking, and alcohol consumption are linked to increasing prevalence of noncommunicable diseases like obesity, hypertension, diabetes and even cancers and autoimmune diseases.

Poor nutritional status is often ignored by adults or even those who are ill; however, it is a major contributor to increased morbidity and mortality. There is loss of lean body mass and impairment of functional capacity compromising the quality of life. Malnutrition increases the severity of illness, the length of hospital stay and healthcare costs. The current database shows that a significant proportion of the world's child population is underweight and suffers from protein and energy malnutrition (PEM) and/or micronutrient malnutrition (MNM). MNM is prevalent in both industrialized and developing countries and includes vitamin A deficiency (VAD), iodine deficiency disorder (IDD), and nutritional anemia.

Dietary inadequacy, poor nutrient utilization in the body, and lack of physical activity are among the major reasons for undernutrition. Nutrient deficiency disorders are often associated with poverty and hunger that still prevail in numerous communities worldwide. Many national and international agencies are working for combating and reducing these problems. Several policies and programs along with advancement in technology, transport, political reforms, socioeconomic status, education level, and medical science can contribute to solving this problem. In India, because of the large population, absolute numbers of persons suffering from different nutritional problems are high. Approximately, following of the children under 5 years of age are reported to be underweight, a considerable proportion is stunted and millions have vitamin A, iodine, and iron deficiencies. These deficiencies are not only common in children but also commonly found in adolescents and women of childbearing age. Hence, it is very likely that the next generation will also be afflicted. Also, it is likely that even the elderly are affected.

Many chronic diseases may have their origin in maternal (fetal) and childhood malnutrition. Physiologically and metabolically, there are alterations due to the nutritional deficits. When faulty diets and sedentary lifestyle are superimposed, they may further increase the risk of a wide range of noncommunicable diseases. People who have easy access to processed and ready-to-eat foods that are rich in fat, sugar and salt or junk food and soft drinks often consume such foods and become victims of diet-related problems.

Previously, diseases like high blood pressure, diabetes, and heart disease were associated with older age and affluence, but many epidemiological and clinical studies reveal that obesity and its associated health problems such as diabetes and high blood pressure occur in children and among the socioeconomically disadvantaged groups in both rural and urban settings.

Thus, undernutrition and overnutrition coexist in the same society in several countries including ours. Thus, India faces the double burden of malnutrition. Malnutrition is a dual-edged sword. It takes a heavy toll on people; millions of children die of diarrhea; millions become blind, millions are stunted and mentally retarded and the primary cause may be malnutrition. According to NFHS-V (2020) data of 22 states, percent of stunted and wasted children under five ranges from 22.3 to 46.5 and percent of severely stunted and severely wasted children under five ranges from 4.3 to 10.6 and 13.3 to 41.0 respectively.

PROTEIN–ENERGY MALNUTRITION (PEM)

It is a syndrome synonymous with undernutrition, there is low food intake, i.e., energy and protein intakes are insufficient and also involve deficiency of other nutrients vis-à-vis the requirements. World Health Organization (WHO) defines malnutrition as "the cellular imbalance between the supply of nutrients and energy and the body's demand for them to ensure growth, maintenance, and specific functions." Poor diets both in terms of quantity and quality are responsible for malnutrition. It commonly occurs in infants and children, adversely affecting their physical and mental development. Frequent episodes of infections often aggravate the condition to the extent of hospitalization and mortality. It can also occur in adults and elders with varying degrees of muscle wasting and energy deficits. Extreme forms of PEM are referred as kwashiorkor and marasmus.

Etiology of PEM

Causes of PEM have been grouped into categories, and under each, the causes are listed in Table 12.1. PEM can be categorized as primary protein-energy malnutrition and secondary PEM. Primary PEM generally occurs in children and elderly persons. It is caused by lack of adequate nutrient intake resulting in the functional and structural abnormalities which are often reversible with nutritional therapy.

Secondary PEM is caused by illnesses that alter appetite, digestion, absorption, or nutrient metabolism.

Prolonged duration in PEM state and unattended frequent infections or illnesses may cause irreversible changes in organ functions and growth faltering.

Effects of PEM

Numerous biochemical changes occur in PEM and these changes vary according to the degree of severity of malnutrition. PEM which affects organs and metabolic functions (including macronutrient metabolism) as well as fluid and electrolyte balance. Deficiencies of many micronutrients like vitamins A, B, iron, and zinc. The biochemical and physiological changes occurring in PEM are given in Table 12.2. These changes depend upon the timing, duration, and severity of nutritional insult.

Usually PEM is associated with young age children but it is frequently observed in older population as well. It is associated with a decline in: functional status, impaired muscle function, decreased bone mass, immune dysfunction, anemia, reduced cognitive function, poor wound healing, delayed

Table 12.1: Causes of protein–energy malnutrition (PEM).

Dietary inadequacy	Nonavailability of food Poor planning of making food available at meal times Less priority to have food and hunger pangs are ignored
Low economic status	Low income and poor purchasing power Less access to and availability of food, healthcare
Poor knowledge and attitudes	Low literacy Lack of understanding of appropriate foods and use of available food Lack of knowledge to recognize signs and symptoms Lack of knowledge about where to go in case of health problems
Insufficient care and infant feeding practices	Misconception and restriction of certain foods for child feeding Delayed and inadequate complementary feeding for young children High dilution of formula feed/animal milk and complementary foods Use of more starchy food and less of nutrient-dense foods Low BMI (<18.5) of mothers Low birth weight of the child Age - high risk in 1-3 years Birth order and birth interval delay in the initiation of breastfeeding, lack of colostrum
Infection and diseases	Frequent episodes of illness and infectious diseases like diarrhea, respiratory infection, cold, cough, measles, pneumonia, and malaria Chronic illness
Poor environment, sanitation and hygiene	Vicious circle of infection and low food intake resulting in growth faltering Measles and helminthic infections Poor access to and availability of healthcare services Lack of safe drinking water, poor sanitation and hygiene, use of unsafe water in food handling, cooking and cleaning, and poor personal hygiene Housing in high density or polluted areas with proximity to garbage heaps, drains, and open areas of defecation
Sociocultural factors	Gender bias, preference for male child and discrimination against girl child Low decision-making power of caregiver Workload of caregiver, family traditions, and composition of the family Infrastructural resources, policies and programs of government Use of services of faith healers

Table 12.2: Changes in functions of different body organs in protein–energy malnutrition (PEM).

Body organs	Changes in organ functions
Gastrointestinal tract	Flattening and broadening of the villi affecting digestive enzymes and absorption, atrophy of mucosa when food is in short supply Bacterial overgrowth due to decreased gastric acidity, reduced gut motility, Increased transit time, and impaired absorption of sugars that are utilized by intestinal microflora Poor reabsorption of bile salts Increased permeability of intestinal epithelium
Liver	Fatty liver—more so in kwashiorkor
Pancreas	Impaired production of pancreatic enzymes, the most affected being lipase followed by trypsin and amylase
Kidney	Changes in renal function—glomerular filtration rate, ability to excrete sodium, potassium, and to concentrate urine
Brain–nervous system	Notable morphological changes in brain—decrease in brain volume, number of neurons, and poor interconnectivity between nerve cells Damaging changes in intellectual potential Delay in myelination of nerve cells, development of nervous system, adverse effects on neurosensory auditory pathways Reduced motor and sensory nerve conduction velocity Poor attention and impulsiveness, diminished ability to adapt to stressful situations, susceptibility to affective disorders like anxiety, and diminished motivation and exploratory behavior

recovery from illness, higher rate of hospital admission and mortality. Persons with PEM have poor appetite, low energy levels, reduced lean body mass coupled with a decline in biological and physiological functions such as changes in cytokine and hormonal levels, fluid electrolyte regulation, delayed gastric emptying and diminished senses of smell and taste.

Changes in Protein

There is significant loss of muscle mass and reduction in total serum protein marked by low serum albumin (<35 g/L), i.e., hypoalbuminemia. Hypoalbuminemia leads to fluid retention due to oncotic pressure, leading to edema. It is also associated with reduced BMI that may result from wasting of muscles and fat. However, in kwashiorkor, edema may mask the wasting. There is reduced synthesis of visceral proteins, numerous important proteins like transferrin, ceruloplasmin, hemoglobin, and retinol-binding protein (RBP), adversely affecting their vital functions in the body. Reduced synthesis of hemoglobin is responsible for anemia and low RBP increases risk of keratomalacia. Proteins involved in the immune system are also compromised. There is remarkable reduction in alpha and gamma globulins, the types of immunoglobulin G (IgG) responsible for combating frequent infections like diarrhea, respiratory infections, etc. C-reactive proteins and cytokines are often raised in response to infection and platelet count is also reduced.

During infection, protein breakdown increases. Further loss of protein can occur from the gut, consisting of endogenous nitrogen loss and unabsorbed nitrogen, and protein from food. Total amino acid concentration in plasma is lowered. Levels of branched-chain amino acids (valine, leucine, and isoleucine) and tyrosine are particularly low in kwashiorkor. But concentrations of nonessential amino acids remain normal or may be higher.

Dietary protein quality is an important factor. Many young children receive sufficient dietary protein but the protein quality is not good. Lack of essential amino acids, poor digestibility, energy deficit, and infections are associated with stunting. Stunted children have been reported to have significantly lower serum concentrations of conditionally essential and nonessential amino acids as well as some sphingolipids compared with nonstunted children. Intake of milk and other animal foods such as egg, fish, and meat show a strong association with linear growth in children in developing countries.

> **Laboratory laurel:** Serum amino acids, glycerophospholipids, sphingolipids, and other metabolites were measured and anthropometric measurements were taken in 313 children, aged 12–59 months, from rural Malawi. There about 62% children were stunted. Stunted children had lower serum concentrations of all 9 essential amino acids conditionally essential amino acids (arginine, glycine, and glutamine), nonessential amino acids (asparagine, glutamate, and serine), and 6 different sphingolipids compared with nonstunted children. Stunting was also associated with altered serum glycerophospholipid concentrations. The authors stated that children with a high-risk of stunting may not receive may not receive adequate choline and essential amino acids choline, an essential nutrient for synthesis of sphingolipids and glycerophospholipids.
>
> *Semba RD, Shardell M, Sakr Ashour FA, et al. Child Stunting is Associated with Low Circulating Essential Amino Acids. EBioMedicine. 2016;6:246-52.*

Changes in Lipids

Fat malabsorption occurs commonly in malnutrition, which increases loss of fat in feces even on a low-fat diet. An increase in free bile acids and decrease in conjugated bile acids due to which fat is not absorbed in the gut lumen. The fatty liver of protein deficiency has been attributed predominantly to a defect in the secretion of hepatic triglycerides. Synthesis of lipoproteins is impaired, thus restricting mobilization of lipids from liver and accumulation of triglycerides associated with a reduction in hepatic phospholipids, resulting in excess of lipids in liver, i.e., fatty liver. Fatty liver is another striking feature of kwashiorkor that is not present in marasmus. Levels of essential fatty acids are lower, although the level of plasma free fatty acids is raised. The levels of phospholipids, triglycerides (TG), and cholesterol are reduced. There is loss of subcutaneous fat. Protein deficiency results in a reduction in plasma triglycerides and phospholipids.

Changes in Carbohydrates

Glycogen stores are low and rate of gluconeogenesis is also low. Hypoglycemia may frequently occur. Glucose absorption is impaired due to deficiency of disaccharidase enzymes in the intestinal mucosa. There is reduced response of insulin and fasting plasma insulin levels are generally low, resulting in impaired glucose tolerance.

Changes in Hormone Levels

Inadequate pituitary function and elevated plasma growth hormone (GH) are associated with PEM, children with kwashiorkor have higher GH concentration than marasmic children. GH stimulates lipolysis and increases the concentration of free fatty acids. It also reduces gluconeogenesis, thereby reducing oxidation of amino acids. There is reduced level of circulating insulin and thyroxin, which influences energy metabolism. Some degree of hypothyroidism is present. Low thyroid activity is an adaptation in PEM, which lowers BMR and helps to conserve some amount of energy. Plasma glucocorticoids and cortisol levels are high. Plasma level of aldosterone is high in kwashiorkor but not in marasmus.

Changes in Water and Electrolytes

In kwashiorkor, there is retention of body fluids resulting in edema. Typically, edema begins from feet and legs and extends toward upper extremities and face (termed moon face). The increase in total body water (TBW) is largely due to the increase in extracellular fluids (ECF). There is reduction in potassium, which is mostly due to loss of muscle mass, loss through stools, and inadequate intake. This may lead to dehydration after during diarrheal episodes that are common in PEM. Depletion of potassium would be higher during diarrheal episodes that are common in PEM. In contrast to potassium, sodium is retained in the body but generally there is hyponatremia. Magnesium deficiency occurs in PEM and the causes are similar to the causes of potassium deficiency. Besides inadequate intake, absorption of calcium and magnesium is inhibited by phytates. During rehabilitation, attention should be paid to dietary potassium and magnesium, since inadequate intakes will limit the synthesis of lean body mass.

Changes in Status of Micronutrients

Vitamin A deficiency often coexists with PEM. This is attributed to decreased hepatic synthesis of RBP required to transport vitamin A from liver to tissues, low intakes of vitamin A, and possible malabsorption of the vitamin. There is redistribution of iron, zinc, and copper causing their deficiencies. Zinc deficiency results in loss of appetite and growth failure (stunting). Low intake and infection contribute to zinc deficiency. Magnesium and potassium deficiencies increase the risk of mortality. Both calcium and phosphorus are decreased in PEM. Selenium deficiency influences production of free radicals by the neutrophils. Deficiency of vitamin D influences maturity of bone cells as well as immune cells.

> **Research Glimpse:** Infectious diseases in children are the major cause of morbidity and mortality in developing countries. PEM is the underlying reason for the increased susceptibility to infections and certain infectious diseases also cause malnutrition, which can result in a vicious cycle. Malnutrition and bacterial gastrointestinal and respiratory infections represent a serious public health problem. The increased incidence and severity of infections in malnourished children are largely due to poor immune function and diminished functional capacity of all cellular components of the immune system, which alters the metabolic responses.
>
> *Rodríguez L, Cervantes E, Ortiz R. Malnutrition and gastrointestinal and respiratory infections in children: a public health problem. Int J Environ Res Public Health. 2011;8(4):1174-205.*

Change in Immune Functions

Infection and infectious diseases like diarrhea and respiratory infections are frequently observed. Measles and helminthic infections increases the need for protein but reduce the absorption creating the deficiency of protein. Recurrent infections are also coupled with micronutrient deficiencies particularly zinc, selenium, copper, iron, vitamin A. This is due to several alterations in the generation of phagocytic cells, production of immunoglobulins, interferon, and other components of the immune system. Alterations include:

- Increased cytokine production
- Loss of phagocytic activity
- Reduced number of T lymphocytes and cell-mediated immunity
- There is a reduced capacity of host to produce antibodies, and concentrations of immunoglobulins (IgA, IgM, and IgG) are lower
- Interference with the production of nonspecific protective substances (antioxidants)
- Reduced resistance to bacterial toxins
- Diminished inflammatory response
- Alterations in collagen formation and wound healing
- Reduced appetite or anorexia leading further poor dietary intake.

> Cytokines are small soluble proteins/polypeptides released by various immune cells like neutrophils, basophils, eosinophils, mast cells, dendritic cells, macrophages, B cells and T cells. They act as messengers or cell signaling molecules, that function at the site of inflammation, infection or trauma. They include several interleukins (IL), tumor necrosis factor (TNF), etc. Cytokines impact growth, development, maturation, activation and life span of immune cells. They can alter the activities of the cells and that alteration can modify the expression of genes. Overreaction of body's immune response is called 'cytokine storm' that can be fatal also which is often observed during COVID-19 infection in some patients.

These changes are modulated by hormones, cytokines, and other proinflammatory mediators and are aggravated by reduced food intake; deficiencies of zinc, iron, vitamin B_6, vitamin A, copper, and selenium, deficiency of micronutrients impairs the immune response which are of great concern in infection because the deficiency of one or more of these impairs the immune response.

There are three levels of immune protection which are governed by different nutrients as shown in Figure 12.1. Periodic high-dose vitamin A supplementation, oral zinc

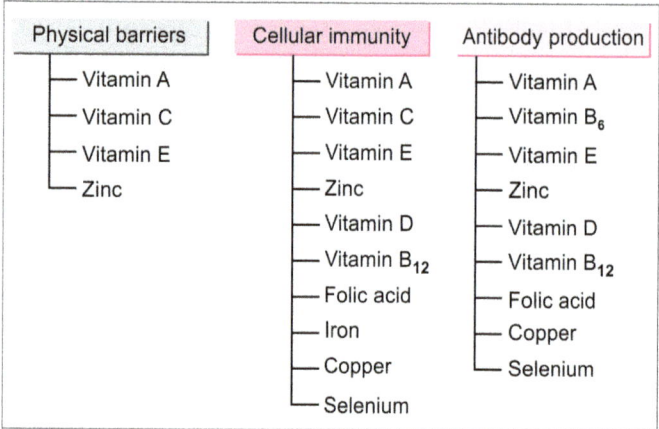

Fig. 12.1: Protective nutrients for immunity.

supplementation, and regular use of iodized salt in cooking, help to improve health status of millions of children in developing countries.

Effect on Brain Development

Protein deficiency severely affects brain development. It may reduce the weight of the brain and the number of neurons. PEM tends to influence the biochemistry of the developing brain, causing changes in myelination, development of synapses, dendritic activity, formation of learning centers, and also morphological changes in cerebral cells. Duration and severity of PEM, environmental stimulation, love and care, maternal knowledge and education of mother also influence brain development. Prolonged deprivation of protein and many other nutrients may affect children's learning skills and can leave a permanent mark on the child, which may also have long-term implications. Timing of occurrence of PEM with regard to developmental stage is important.

Maternal nutritional status during pregnancy also has critical implications for brain development and function. Deficiencies in micronutrients like folic acid, iodine, iron, zinc, selenium, copper, and magnesium and vitamins A, C, D, E, B_6, and B_{12} during the prenatal period, i.e., when embryonic and fetal development occur, have been shown to cause specific neurologic deficits. Thus, morphological and biochemical changes in PEM adversely affect functions of GI tract, brain, heart, liver, and kidney. Physical growth is delayed and decreased. Three types of Protein Energy Malnutrition—kwashiorkor, marasmus, and marasmic kwashiorkor.

Kwashiorkor

Cicely Williams coined the term "kwashiorkor" in 1930 for "sickness of the older child when next baby is born". It is predominantly due to protein deficiency, although the energy intake is also inadequate. Starchy diets (rice/cassava) may provide some calories but are deficient in protein, vitamins, essential fatty acids, and trace elements. Weight for age is between 60% and 80% of the reference median. Children with kwashiorkor exhibits nutritional edema and metabolic disturbances, such as hypoalbuminemia and hepatic steatosis (infiltration of liver cells with fat) or fatty liver.

Marasmus

Marasmus is derived from a Greek word meaning *"withering* or *to waste away"*. It is predominantly due to energy deficiency, i.e., inadequate food intake. Commonly occurs in first year of life due to lack of breast feeding, diluted animal milk introduction and lack of timely and inadequate complementary feeding. It is a form of severe starvation, characterized by muscle wasting, and absence of subcutaneous fat. Body uses all the fat stores before it uses muscles. There is wasting of groin followed by thighs, buttocks, chest and abdomen and buccal pad. Marasmic children have less than 60% of the body weight for their age, with no edema (Table 12.3). Some are anorexic and some may be very hungry but seldom tolerate large amount of food intake. Marked weakness is revealed as they cannot stand alone without help. Hypothermia (body temperature lower than normal), hypoglycemia, low heart rate, and blood pressure may be present. Complications like gastroenteritis, respiratory infection, dehydration, and eye lesions are frequent.

Marasmic Kwashiorkor

It is also a severe form of malnutrition, caused by severe deficiency of protein, energy, and other nutrients. There is

Table 12.3: Features of kwashiorkor and marasmus.

Particulars	Kwashiorkor	Marasmus
Age of occurrence	6–24 months	12–36 months
Face	Moon face	Monkey face
Chest	Narrow and backward	Rib cage is visible
Stomach	Balloon-like stomach	Touching back
Legs and hands	Edema	No edema
Skin	Lesions and pigmentation	Loose hanging skin
Hair	Brown, pluckable due to low tensile strength	Thinning, coarse
Liver	Fatty and enlarged liver	No fatty liver
Infection	Respiratory infection and diarrhea	Very frequent episodes of diarrhea
Body temperature	Normal	Below normal/subnormal
Other nutrient deficiencies	Vitamin A, all B vitamins, and Fe	All micronutrients
Appetite	Poor	Good
Water and electrolyte balance	Increased total body water and retention of sodium with hypopotassemia	No depletion unless associated with diarrhea
Plasma Proteins and other characteristics	• Reduced albumin and transferrin • Low leukocyte count • Slow wound healing • Less immunocompetence	Hypoprotinemia Low immunity

depletion of fat reserves; slow metabolism and low body temperature. It usually occurs in children aged 6–18 months, particularly those fed diluted or improperly prepared formula feeds. It may cause irreversible damage to the body. These children exhibit features of marasmus with edema and hypokalemia as well as hypoalbuminemia. For rehabilitation, it is necessary to first restore and maintain electrolyte balance, followed by inclusion of protein according to the child's ability to digest and tolerate.

In adults, PEM is associated more with loss of lean body mass and reduced albumin. Symptoms can be edema, muscle wasting, tiredness, and changes in skin, hair, and gastrointestinal responses.

ASSESSMENT OF NUTRITIONAL STATUS

Generally, assessment of nutritional status is based on anthropometric measurements, by comparing weight and height of the individual with reference standards for chronological age. Weight is an indicator of body size but is influenced by food intake as well as illness. Thus, weight reflects acute malnutrition because body weight changes rapidly due to these influences. Height reflects skeletal growth and influenced by genetic and other biological factors. Height does not reflect acute variations as weight does, but long-term malnutrition influences skeletal growth and therefore height. Therefore, height is an indicator of chronic malnutrition. Acute malnutrition is classified into severe acute malnutrition (SAM) and moderate acute malnutrition (MAM) according to the degree of wasting and the presence of edema. The classification of nutritional status is given in Table 12.4.

Basic measurements to identify the level of malnutrition
1. Weight for age
2. Height for age
3. Weight for Height
4. Mid-Upper-Arm Circumference (MUAC)

Table 12.4: Classification of nutritional status.

Indicators	Explanation
Children	
Moderate underweight	Weight for age <2 SD below the reference standards
Moderate wasting	Weight for length/height < 2 SD below the reference standards
Moderate stunting (moderate chronic malnutrition)	Length/height for age <2 SD below the reference standards
Overweight	Weight-for-length/height* or BMI-for-age >2 SD and ≤ 3 SD of the median
Obese	Weight-for-length/height* or BMI-for-age >3 standard deviations (SD) of the median

Source: World Health Organization. Guideline: Assessing and managing children at primary health-care facilities to prevent overweight and obesity in the context of the double burden of malnutrition. Updates for the integrated management of childhood illness (ICMI). 2017 pg vii.

* Weight-for-length used in infants and young children aged 0–23 months and weight-for-height used for children aged 24 months and older.

- Low weight with reference to designated age is referred as underweight
- Low height with reference to designated age is referred to as stunting
- Low weight for reference height is wasting.

MODERATE ACUTE MALNUTRITION (MAM)

Moderate acute malnutrition (MAM) is defined as a weight-for-age between -3 and -2 z-scores below the median of the WHO child growth standards or if the MUAC is between 115 millimeters and <125 millimeters. The individual may have low weight-for-height (wasting) and/or a low height-for-age (stunting). Similarly, moderate wasting and stunting are defined as a weight-for-height and height-for-age, respectively, between -3 and -2 z-scores. MM affects many children in poor countries. Children with moderate malnutrition have an increased risk of mortality.

SEVERE ACUTE MALNUTRITION (SAM)

Besides weight and height, Mid-Upper-Arm Circumference (MUAC) is also used to assess nutritional status and the degree of malnutrition. Z-scores are used to judge the nutritional status. The diagnostic criteria to identify severe acute malnutrition among children between 6 and 60 months of age is severe wasting (based on weight for height) with a z-score below minus 3 SD or mid upper arm circumference below 115 mm (11.5 cm). Presence of bilateral edema is a clinical sign, and any child between 6 and 60 months having low MUAC or bilateral edema should be immediately referred for full assessment at a treatment centre for the management of severe acute malnutrition (SAM). Z-scores are described in Chapter 13 that deals with assessment of nutritional status. SAM children often suffer from one or more of the following medical complications which need attention during treatment and rehabilitation

- Anorexia or loss of appetite
- Intractable vomiting (vomiting after every oral feed)
- High fever - Child has high body temperature, or axillary temperature > 38.5°C, rectal temperature > 39°C.
- Hypothermia - low body temperature, or axillary temperature < 35.0°C, rectal temperature < 35.5°C.
- Lower respiratory tract infection- cough with difficult breathing, fast breathing
- Severe anemia – Pale palms or unusual paleness of the skin
- Skin lesion- Child has broken skin, fissures, flaking of skin.
- Unconsciousness- Child does not respond to painful stimuli (for example, injection).
- Lethargy, not alert or drowsy, no interest in surrounding
- Hypoglycemia- often no clinical sign but the child sleeps with eyes slightly open.
- Convulsions- During a convulsion, child's arms and legs stiffen because the muscles are contracting. Ask the mother if the child had convulsions during this current illness.

Table 12.5: Measurement of Mid Upper Arm circumference (MUAC).

MUAC	Measurement in mm
Normal	Above 12.5 cm or 125 mm
Moderate malnutrition	11.5–12.5 cm or 115–125 mm
Severe malnutrition	<11.5 cm or 115 mm

Diagnosis of SAM

In children between the ages of 6 and 59 months, Severe acute malnutrition (SAM) is defined as:
- Weight/height or Weight/length < -3 Z score, using the WHO Growth Charts
- Presence of visible severe wasting
- Presence of bipedal edema of nutritional origin
- Mid- upper arm circumference (MUAC) < 115 mm (Table 12.5).

PREVENTION AND CONTROL OF PROTEIN-ENERGY MALNUTRITION (PEM)

PEM in severe or chronic cases can be life-threatening and is frequently associated with multiple organ failure. Hence, the first goal of management of acute malnutrition is the stabilization of vital functions, particularly cardiovascular function and blood pressure and acid-base and electrolyte imbalances. It can be done by nutritional rehabilitation. IAP (2013) has given a Consensus Statement of the Indian Academy of Pediatrics on Integrated Management of Severe Acute Malnutrition (SAM). It is advocated to integrate SAM treatment with other treatments at health posts, primary health centers, nutrition rehabilitation centres (NRC) district level hospitals, tertiary level centers. A full clinical examination is required in order to confirm the presence of medical complications and to determine whether the child has an appetite. Poor appetite can be risk of early mortality. It is recommended that if the child has an appetite based on the observations of the appetite test and one is clinically well (i.e., the case is not complicated) and alert should be treated as an outpatient. However, if the child has medical complications, has severe edema of fails the appetite test requires inpatient care and should be admitted and treated as in-patients? The criteria for passing the appetite test (IAP, 2013) are shown in Table 12.6.

Percent range for malnourished children under 5 years in 22 states of India as per NFHS V-2020	
Stunted	22.3–46.5%
Wasted	9.8–25.1%
Severely stunted	4.3–10.6%
Severely wasted	13.3–41.0%

Home diet may not be sufficient and nutritionally adequate to prevent deterioration and death. There are provisions for F75, F100 and Ready-to-Use-Therapeutic Food (RUTF) which brings rapid improvements in children suffering from acute malnutrition as they are taken care by the trained health care providers. Table indicates the amount of therapeutic food that should be consumed by the child in a day. The amount of RUTF to be consumed differs by the child's body weight. It is shown in Table 12.6.

Table 12.6: Criteria for appetite test (IAP, 2013) before admission and amount of feed to be given.

Body weight (kg)	Minimum amount of RUTF to be consumed for passing appetite test (mL or grams)	Amount of RUTF per day
>4	15	105–130 g/day
4–6.9	25	200–260 g/day
7–9.9	35	260–400 g/day
10–14.9	50	400–460 g/day

SAM children above the age of 6 months are transferred from inpatient to outpatient care on the basis of certain criteria:
- Child has a good appetite (eating at least 120-130 kcal/kg/d) along with micronutrients,
- No longer has edema,
- Gains weight (>5g/kg/d) on three consecutive days.

Complete anti-microbial treatment and appropriate immunization are also initiated. Besides the sufferer child, mother is also advised and trained to properly prepare and feed the child at home.

The decision to transfer the child from inpatient to outpatient care is based on its clinical condition and not on the basis of anthropometric indices such as MUAC or weight for height/length. Discharge from treatment should be done only when the child's weight for height/length is greater than minus 2 Z-score and the child has not had edema for at least two weeks or the child should have MUAC >125 mm (12.5 cm). However, it should be noted that WHO recommends that the same criterion should be used for identification of severe acute malnutrition and to assess nutritional recovery and that percentage weight gain should not be considered as a criterion for discharge. It is also strongly recommended that children with SAM should be followed up after discharge and periodically monitored so that there is no relapse.

Interventions to prevent child undernutrition:
- Reducing low birth weight by ensuring better maternal nutrition and appropriate antenatal care
- Promoting exclusive breast feeding
- Timely introduction of complementary feeding
- Appropriate nutrient-dense complementary foods
- Use of safe drinking water
- Deworming children
- Growth monitoring of children
- Ensure better hygienic conditions
- Create home environment for love and care
- Provision of community based therapeutic food(s)
- Sensitize mothers and other family members to ensure good nutrition for the growing child
- Disseminate guidelines regarding complementary feeding
- Timely adequate immunization
- Referral services to hospitals etc, in case of emergency
- Use of local traditional methods (home remedies) for minor illnesses
- Health and nutrition and elementary education.

Many of the services for preventing malnutrition are provided through Government of India's Integrated Child Development Services (ICDS). Under ICDS, each child below

5 years of age is given daily supplementary food, providing 500 kcal and 12–15 g protein. Beneficiaries as per their prescribed ration and dose are also provided supplementary nutrition (food), deworming tablets, immunization and treatment of minor illnesses; as well as iron–folate tablets. Besides children from 6–60 months beneficiaries include pregnant and lactating women and adolescent girls. All mothers are given nutrition education.

It is also necessary to ensure that food given at home is adequate enough in quantity to satisfy hunger; edible and culturally acceptable. Nutritional quality of food is extremely important and the diet should provide required energy and other nutrients. The food should be safe to consume. It is important to feed the young child frequently. Home food should not be replaced by food from Anganwadi. That is supplementary food to enhance the nutritional status of the individual beneficiary.

> Diarrhea frequently occurs in malnourished children. Dehydration can be life-threatening and hence calls for immediate action. The first-line of treatment is correction of fluid and electrolyte imbalance. Electrolytes that need replenishment usually are potassium, sodium, and chloride. At home level, ORS solution prescribed by WHO should be given. If dehydration is severe, the child should be taken immediately to a doctor/hospital for the treatment. Besides ORS, the child should be given soft foods that are easily digestible. Breastfeeding should be continued. Once the child recovers, she should be given adequate food that will ensure catch-up growth. World Health Organization-recommended rehydration solution for malnourished children (ReSoMal) for rehydrating severe acute malnourished children. Indian Academy of Pediatrics (IAP) Guidelines for the management of severe acute malnutrition has recommended use of low-osmolarity ORS with added potassium supplements or preparing ReSoMal with low-osmolarity ORS as per WHO recommendation. At several places Nutrition Rehabilitation Centers are set up to take care of SAM cases in India.

VITAMIN A DEFICIENCY

World Health Organization defines vitamin A deficiency (VAD) as "tissue concentrations of vitamin A low enough to have adverse health consequences even if there is no evidence of clinical xerophthalmia". Depletion of vitamin A stores impairs normal physiological functions. VAD adversely affects visual/ocular capacity, integrity of epithelial lining, and immunity. There is growth retardation, poor reproductive health, and increased risk of anemia. Nonspecific consequences may increase morbidity and mortality.

The VAD is a major public health problem affecting large number of preschool children, pregnant women, and breastfeeding women around the globe. It is preventable, because it generally occurs in communities where food choices and food intake are limited.

Causes of Vitamin A Deficiency

1. Inadequate breastfeeding and poor quality of complementary feeds.
2. Inadequate consumption of vitamin A-rich foods over a long period of time (months or years) mainly due to poverty, poor accessibility, perishability, and high cost of such foods and some religious concerns with regard to animal foods, which are rich sources of vitamin A.
3. Poor handling of rich food sources at various stages after harvesting, cooking/processing.
4. Ignorance about importance of vitamin A in protection of health and prevention of diseases.
5. General malnutrition and other micronutrient deficiencies.
6. Inflammatory conditions, infections, or liver disease as well as fat malabsorption.

Consequences of Vitamin A Deficiency

Insufficient vitamin A intake results in depletion of liver stores and affects various organs of the body as well as cellular functioning.

Eye

Visual cycle is interrupted and initial symptoms of VAD are blurred vision and night blindness (poor adaptation to light in dark). Lack of the vitamin interferes with formation of mucus by epithelial cells of the eye, which makes the cornea and conjunctiva and inner surface of the eyelid dry. As a result, cornea is also keratinized, and then ulcerated (keratomalacia). Progression of symptoms may lead to blindness.

Epithelial Cells in Different Organs

VAD diminishes mucus production by epithelial cells in mouth, throat, respiratory tract, urinary tract, and genital tract and increases the risk of infection. Pregnant women having VAD are at risk of urinary tract infection (UTI).

Immune System

VAD reduces immunity and increases the risk of viral, parasitic, and bacterial infections like diarrhea, respiratory infection, measles and tuberculosis.

Growth Retardation

VAD may cause growth retardation in children. If pregnant women have VAD, there is risk of intrauterine growth retardation (IUGR). Breast milk of mothers with low vitamin A stores is also low in vitamin A; hence, their children are also at risk of VAD as they are likely to have poor stores of vitamin A.

Diagnosis of Vitamin A Deficiency

Subclinical and clinical signs and symptoms are easy to diagnose. WHO has given the classification of xerophthalmia (collective form of VAD and blindness) (Table 12.7). Vitamin A deficiency is declared as a public health problem on the basis of both clinical and subclinical indicators of deficiency. Low-serum retinol (0.70 μmol/L or below) is indicative of deficiency.

Prevalence of Vitamin A Deficiency

According to WHO (2009), globally VAD is prevalent in about 40% of the population, mainly among preschool

Table 12.7: Classification of xerophthalmia.

Indicators	Symptom	Description
XN	Night blindness	Earliest symptom of VAD, impairment of dark adaptation, inability to see particularly after sunset or in poor light
X1A	Conjunctival xerosis	Dryness of conjunctiva, unwettability, loss of transparency, wrinkling, and depigmentation; eyelids may also become thick, rough, and wrinkled
X1B	Bitot's spot	Dirty white/grayish. Foamy and raised spots on the surface of the conjunctiva, generally on the outer side of the cornea. These spots are accumulation of denuded conjunctival epithelial cells
X2	Corneal xerosis	A sign of severe VAD. Cornea loses its normal, smooth, and glistening appearance, becomes dry and rough; child tend to keep eyes closed particularly in bright light due to photophobia
X3A	Corneal ulceration/keratomalacia (<1/3 of corneal surface is involved)	Ulceration of cornea. If ulcer becomes deep, it may lead to perforation
X3B	Corneal ulceration/keratomalacia (≥1/3 of corneal surface is involved)	Destruction and liquefaction of full thickness of cornea leading to prolapse of iris resulting in permanent blindness. Corneal structure melts into a cloudy and gelatinous mass. In infective conditions, eye will be red and swollen
XS	Corneal scarring	Ulcer on healing leaves a white scar that varies in size depending on the size of the ulcer. When the scar is big or positioned centrally and blocks the pupillary region, normal vision is affected
XF	Xerophthalmic fundus	Globe destroyed by advanced keratomalacia

Source: WHO. Control of vitamin A deficiency and xerophthalmia. Report of a joint WHO/UNICEF/USAID Helen Keller International/IVACG Meeting, Technical Report Series 672. Geneva: WHO; 1982.

Table 12.8: Prevalence of low-serum retinol and night blindness to define VAD as a public health problem.

Indicator and group	Prevalence criteria/cut-off level		
Low-serum retinol (0.70 µmol/L or below)			
Children 6–71 months of age and pregnant women	Mild	Moderate	Severe
	≤2 to <10%	≥10 to <20%	≥20%
Night blindness			
Children 24–71 months of age	>0% to <1%	≥1% to <5%	≥5%
Pregnant women		≥5%	

Source: WHO. Global prevalence of vitamin A deficiency in populations at risk 1995–2005. WHO Global Database on Vitamin A Deficiency. Geneva: WHO; 2009. p. 8.

children, pregnant, and lactating women. WHO (2011) has given criteria for declaring VAD as a public health problem (Table 12.8). Due to VAD, about 250,000–500,000 children worldwide become partially or totally blind every year and about half of them die due to VAD. In India, 35.4 million preschool children show subclinical symptoms and 1.8 million suffer from xerophthalmia. Presently, VAD is a public health problem only in isolated geographical pockets of the country, with wide variations in the prevalence of VAD within the states.

Prevention and Control of Vitamin A Deficiency

Multiple approaches are required at community and national levels.
1. Vitamin A supplementation
2. Food-based approach or dietary diversification
3. Nutrition and health education
4. Fortification.

Vitamin A Supplementation

A large dose of the vitamin is given in the form of pills, capsules, or syrups. Benefit of supplementation is that the specific nutrient is made available in a highly absorbable form. Supplementation is a rapid, cost-effective, and easy way of controlling deficiency. Vitamin A drops are distributed at various levels usually by the Government of India, and reached to the target group through ICDS and nongovernmental organizations (NGOs). Vitamin A drops were given to children as per WHO guidelines (2011) (Table 12.9). Coverage data reported in NFHS-V (2020) shows that majority of children aged 9-59 months have received

Table 12.9: Oral prophylactic dose of vitamin A for children 6–59 months of age (WHO Guidelines, 2011).

Target group	Infants 6–11 months of age (including HIV+)	Infants 12–59 months of age (including HIV+)
Dose	100,000 IU (30 mg RE) Vitamin A	200,000 IU (60 mg RE) Vitamin A
Frequency	Once	Every 4–6 Months
Route of administration	Oral liquid, oil-based preparation of retinyl palmitate or retinyl acetate	
Settings	Populations where the percentage of night blindness is 1% or higher in children 24–59 months of age or where the prevalence of vitamin A deficiency (serum retinol 0.70 µmol/L or lower) is 20% or higher in infants and children 6–59 months of age	
An oil-based vitamin A solution can be delivered using soft gelatin capsules, as a single-dose dispenser or a graduated spoon can be used.		

Source: WHO Guideline: Vitamin A supplementation in infants and children 6–59 months of age. Geneva: WHO; 2011.

vitamin A dose. In 22 states overall percent coverage was 44.4 to 91.9 %. These figures indicate that in some states, coverage needs to improve considerably. Besides this, it is emphasized that dark green leafy vegetables or yellow fruits and vegetables should be consumed regularly; mothers should breastfeed and not discard colostrum since it is a good source of vitamin A. If the family is nonvegetarian and can afford it, then egg yolk can be given to young children and when it is appropriate, small amount of liver can be fed. Supplementation is a short-term measure.

Food-based Approach or Dietary Diversification

Dietary intervention or food-based approach is necessary for sustained and long-lasting results. Although food-based approach is feasible, it involves many other interventions to practice dietary diversification in daily diet. Dark green leafy vegetables or yellow fruits and vegetables should be consumed regularly; mothers should breastfeed and not discard colostrum since it is a good source of vitamin A. If the family is non-vegetarian and can afford it, then egg yolk can be given to young children and when it is appropriate, small amount of liver can be fed. This entails inclusion of dark green leafy vegetables, carrots, high beta-carotene containing sweet potato, papaya, mango, palm kernel oil, egg, milk products, fish and liver in order to improve vitamin A intakes and status. This can be achieved through:

- **Horticulture approach:** Cultivation of vitamin A-rich foods in kitchen gardens is an easy and inexpensive way. Many of the foods do not require much land, e.g., mint, fenugreek, coriander leaves can be grown in small pots; they do not require much investment and expertise. Also, papaya and mango trees can be planted near residential areas or kitchen gardens. In high rise building areas or scarcity of space some green leafy vegetables, tomatoes, etc. are also grown on terrace in pots or hydroponically.
- **Poultry keeping and animal husbandry:** Poultry breeding is a good option because egg and meat products are rich sources of vitamin A. In several parts of the world, many households still prefer to keep cows or buffaloes for fresh milk for the family. Some supply it commercially to other households.

Nutrition and Health Education

It will be beneficial and effective to disseminate knowledge about vitamin A and consequences of its deficiency especially to mothers. Also, schools are a good platform wherein children can easily learn about good food sources of vitamin A and its importance. It would be good if this education is an part of School health programmes and part of children's curriculum. The messages can easily be communicated from "child to child" and "child to mother" and "mother to mother" approaches. Health education for cleanliness and hygiene can prevent many infectious diseases. Various types of audiovisual aids, multimedia, and social marketing methods can be used for health and nutrition education and make the public at large aware about vitamin A prophylaxis programs of the government and the importance of vitamin A.

Fortification

Addition of vitamin in the form of retinyl palmitate to sugar has been successful in raising serum retinol among preschool children. Other vehicles are vegetable oils, margarine, milk, and milk products. With the advancement in fortification technology, multiple nutreints have been added to single commonly consumed food(s). In recent years, biofortification has been used and golden rice is one good example of biofortified rice. Multiple fortification is also being tried and used.

National Nutrition Programme to Curb Vitamin A Deficiency

The National Prophylaxis Programme against Nutritional Blindness (NPPNB) due to VAD was started in 1970 in order to prevent nutritional blindness. In 2006, eligibility of children was broadened to the age group of 9 months to 5 years and oral prophylactic doses were revised in consultation with recommendations of WHO, UNICEF and Ministry of Women and Child Development. In 2016, the programme was renamed as National Vitamin A prophylaxis programme. Recently NITI (National Institution for Transforming India) Aayog, which formulates policies and provides technical support to the Government of India, recommended six monthly vitamin A supplementation along with other health interventions such as food-based and horticulture-based interventions, food fortification and capacity building of functionaries for elimination of VAD. The main objectives of the NPPNB are:

1. **Prevention of vitamin A deficiency:**
   i. *Promoting consumption of vitamin A-rich foods:* Promotion of regular intake of vitamin A-rich foods by all pregnant and lactating women and children under 5 years of age by increasing local production and consumption of GLV and other carotenoid-rich plant foods.
   ii. *Creating awareness about the importance of preventing vitamin A deficiency:* Awareness to be created among women for attending antenatal clinics, immunization sessions, and for women and children to be registered under ICDS program.
   iii. **Prophylactic vitamin A dosage schedule along with immunization:**
      - 100,000 IU at 9 months with measles immunization
      - 200,000 IU at 16–18 months, with DPT booster
      - 200,000 IU every 6 months, up to the age of 5 years.
2. **Treatment of vitamin A-deficient children:**
   i. All children with xerophthalmia are to be treated at health care centers.
   ii. All children having measles to be given one dose of vitamin A, if they have not received it in the previous month.
   iii. All cases of severe malnutrition to be given one additional dose of vitamin A.

Night blindness and conjunctival changes (such as Bitot's spots) and corneal xerosis/ulceration are indications for immediate vitamin A supplementation. Corneal damage due to vitamin A deficiency (changes in the normally clear central part of the eye) threatens eye-sight and it is a medical emergency. All children with clinical signs of vitamin A deficiency must be treated as early as possible.

> **Research Glimpse:** Earlier, poor Indian children used to become blind due to corneal ulceration. To tackle this public health problem, vitamin-A prophylaxis program was launched nationally in 1970 after field testing, using Bitot's spot as the clinical sign to assess the prevalence of vitamin-A deficiency. According to Indian Council for Medical Research (ICMR), prevalence of Bitot's spots among children decreased over time but, whether this was attributable to mass vitamin-A prophylaxis program is uncertain, due to other factors like wider vaccination coverage, increased breastfeeding rates, and improvement of healthcare services. Excess vitamin A has harmful effects resulting in loss of bone density and growth retardation in susceptible individuals. Food-based approach including breastfeeding along with timely measles vaccination can be a good option to tackle vitamin-A deficiency symptoms. Post-measles children should receive vitamin A in age-specific daily doses for 2 weeks + vitamin-A–rich food, like green leafy vegetables, red palm oil, liver, etc. Scientific community in India needs to consider and avoid "one size fit to all" approach, particularly to prevent harmful effects of high dose of vitamin A as well as help to utilize local health resources in India.
>
> *Bhattacharya S, Singh A. Phasing out of the Universal Mega Dose of Vitamin-A Prophylaxis to Avoid Toxicity. AIMS Public Health. 2017;4(1):38-46.*
>
> *Bhattacharya S, Singh A. Time to revisit the strategy of massive vitamin A prophylaxis dose administration to the under five children in India—An analysis of available evidence. Clin Nutr ESPEN. 2017;21:26-30.*

IODINE DEFICIENCY DISORDERS

Iodine deficiency disorders (IDDs) that adversely affect the quality of life of millions of children and adults, are one of the most preventable causes of brain damage and mental retardation in the world. Iodine deficiency can start from intrauterine extending up to adult life. IDD is a term collectively used for all clinical and subclinical symptoms of iodine deficiency. It is more of a geographical and environmental problem rather than being caused by socioeconomic reasons. IDD can be prevented by ensuring adequate intake of iodine, particularly during pregnancy. Even mild iodine deficiency during pregnancy can adversely affect neurological development to the fetus and consequent cognitive and learning abilities of the young child. Children with IDD have lower intelligence quotient. Hence, IDD impairs the human resource development and progress of the country.

Most of iodine in the body is concentrated in the thyroid gland and the remaining in mammary glands, eyes, gastric mucosa, cervix, and salivary glands. Iodine is essential for synthesis of the thyroid hormones—triiodothyronine (T3) and thyroxine (T4). It is required in all stages of life, particularly fetal life (during pregnancy) and early childhood. Normal thyroid gland contains approximately 5 mg of T4, which can maintain euthyroid status for at least 50 days. T4 and T3 circulate in the blood in bound and free forms. Major proportion is bound to the binding proteins—thyroxine-binding globulin (TBG), thyroxine-binding prealbumin (TBPA), and thyroxine-binding albumin (TBA). Binding to these proteins is important because they prevent urinary loss of iodine. The unbound forms of hormones are biologically active. In the thyroid gland, iodine is incorporated in the protein thyroglobulin. This protein is required for synthesis of thyroid hormones and is a sensitive indicator for measuring iodine status. Low circulating levels of this protein indicate long-term depletion.

When dietary iodine is not sufficient for prolonged period of time, T4 level falls while TSH level is elevated. The body tries to adapt by increasing TSH secretion by the pituitary gland, which stimulates thyroid to increase iodide uptake for synthesis of T4 and its release in adequate amount in the blood. This is done by increase in size of the thyroid gland and synthesis of thyroglobulin. Thus, in prolonged and/or severe deficiency, thyroid gland undergoes hypertrophy and hyperplasia of follicular cells, which are manifested as enlargement of thyroid gland and known as goiter.

Severe iodine deficiency not only leads to goiter formation but also adversely affects growth, development, and maturation of other tissues especially fast developing and sensitive tissues particularly brain. When the fetus is developing (especially up to trimester II of pregnancy) iodine deficiency can have devastating effects on fetal brain development. However, the damaging effects can be reversed at this stage by introducing iodine in the diet. But, if iodine deficiency continues, the damaging effects on the brain can be permanent and such children may never achieve optimal, physical, and mental level of growth. Also, there is high risk of fetal and neonatal mortality. Iodine is accumulated in the breast and transferred through breast milk, hence iodine intake by lactating mothers should be adequate.

Causes of Iodine Deficiency Disorders

Two major causes of IDD are:
1. Inadequate intake of iodine
2. Inadequate utilization of iodine

Inadequate intake of iodine can be due to low iodine content in foods that in turn depend on the iodine content of water and foods grown/cultivated in a specific region. Iodine content of foods grown in deficient soil will have low iodine content and people residing in such geographical areas are at high-risk of iodine deficiency. In several areas of the world, environmental iodine deficiency occurs that is caused when iodine present in the upper crust of earth is leached out by heavy rains, repeated flooding and glaciations.

Inadequate utilization of iodine is due to the presence of goitrogens in certain foods. Goitrogens are substances that interfere with iodine metabolism and tend to reduce iodine absorption and are also called thyroid inhibitors. Goitrogenic/antithyroid activity of certain plants (grains, vegetables, and fruits) is due to presence of cyanogenic glucosides, glucosinolates (thioglucosides), and thiocyanate, referred as cyanogenic constituents and the plants are called cyanogenic plants. Cyanogenic constituents affect the synthesis of thyroid hormones in thyroid gland either by inhibiting iodide uptake or by interfering with the activity of thyroid peroxidase (TPO). TPO is an enzyme that is important for synthesis of T4 and T3 from diiodothyronine (DIT) and monoiodothyronine (MIT).

Goitrogens are found in commonly consumed foods like spinach, cabbage, pear, peaches, bamboo shoots, broccoli, strawberry, lima beans, maize, millet, broccoli, soy and soy products, mustard, peanuts, sweet potato, and tea. Some goitrogens are also found in environment. However, the goitrogens can be largely inactivated by cooking. Drinking large amounts of tea may affect iodine absorption. Consumption of excess of goitrogenic plants may induce goiter. Recent studies indicate that cooking losses of iodine are influenced by many factors like socioeconomic status, sanitary status, and personal hygiene, contribute to IDD. Apart from iodine intake, a number of factors can affect iodine levels. Minerals like calcium, manganese, magnesium, and fluoride restrict iodine uptake by thyroid gland.

Laboratory Laurel: In this study, iodine losses were studied using different methods of cooking that included boiling, roasting, shallow frying, deep frying, pressure cooking, and microwave cooking in *namkeen dalia, chapati, paratha, poori, chole,* and *upma*. The salt used in the study was adequately iodized (>15 ppm). Minimum loss occurred during shallow frying where cooking time was 1 minute 15 seconds and maximum loss occurred during pressure cooking where cooking was done for 26 minutes only. Iodine loss ranged from 6.58% to 51.08%. Losses during boiling, roasting, deep frying, and microwave cooking were 40.23%, 10.57%, 10.40% and 27.13%, respectively. Loss of iodine was attributed to type of cooking method and time of addition of salt during cooking.

Rana R, Raghuvanshi RS. Effect of different cooking methods on iodine losses. J Food Sci Technol. 2013;50(6):1212-6.

Consequences of Iodine Deficiency Disorders

Iodine is required at every stage of life from intrauterine life to old age. Major disorders of IDD are goiter, cretinism, hypothyroidism, and hyperthyroidism. Iodine deficiency is characterized by mental impairment and physical abnormalities (congenital anomalies). Persons with IDD have low BMR, chronic fatigue, reduced immune function, weak muscles, and dry skin.

Physiological groups health consequences of iodine deficiency
- All ages goiter
- Hypothyroidism
- Increased susceptibility to nuclear radiation
- Fetus spontaneous abortion
- Stillbirth
- Congenital anomalies
- Perinatal mortality
- Neonate endemic cretinism including mental deficiency with a mixture of mutism, spastic diplegia, squint, hypothyroidism and short stature
- Infant mortality
- Child and adolescent impaired mental function
- Delayed physical development
- Iodine-induced hyperthyroidism (IIH)
- Adults impaired mental function

Infants born to iodine-deficient mothers develop cretinism. Goiter among children is reflected in low IQ and symptoms of hypothyroidism. IDD results in poor mental development and cretinism. There is stunting of physical and mental growth, sluggishness, deaf-mutism, and defective gait. The manifestations and their severity depend upon the period when IDD occurs. In early pregnancy (up to II trimester), IDD results in neurological damage to the fetus while late deficiency (III trimester) is associated with myxedematous manifestations. Children born to women with mild-to-moderate hypothyroxinemia have been reported to have neurological alterations, reduced IQ, and attention problems. Also, children exhibit abnormal bone development. Each life stage differs in the manifestation of symptoms of IDD. WHO/ICCIDD/UNICEF (2007) and FAO (2004) have listed the health consequences of iodine deficiency disorders (IDD) in different age groups (Fig. 12.2).

Goiter

It is characterized by a disproportionate increase in size and number of cells of thyroid gland resulting in enlargement of the thyroid gland, which is visible externally as a protrusion in

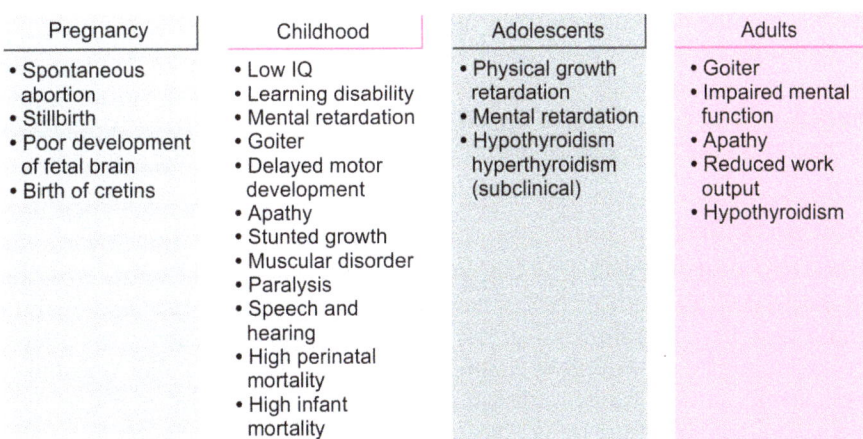

Fig. 12.2: Iodine deficiency disorder (IDD) spectrum in different age groups.

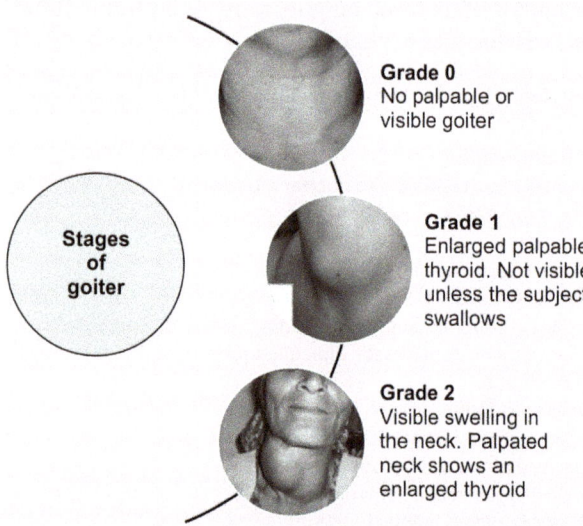

Fig. 12.3: Stages of goiter.

Table 12.10: Criteria for prevalence of iodine deficiency disorder (IDD).

Indicators	Mild	Moderate	Severe
Goiter grade 0 (%)	5.0	20–29.9	≥30
Urinary iodine excretion (μg/L) (median)	50–99	20–49	<20

Source: WHO (2014). WHO indicators for assessing iodine deficiency disorders and their control through salt iodization.

the neck region. It is a noninflammatory, nontumorous, and nontoxic condition. Interestingly, most people in endemic goiter regions do not consider IDD as a health problem except that enlarged gland in the neck is considered as a hindrance in beauty among girls of marriageable age. Most of the families are also unaware of salt iodization. Its wide prevalence in specific geographic regions is referred to as "endemic goiter", e.g., hilly regions of Uttarakhand. Women and children are most affected. WHO has given grades of goiter, which are shown in Figure 12.3.

Cretinism

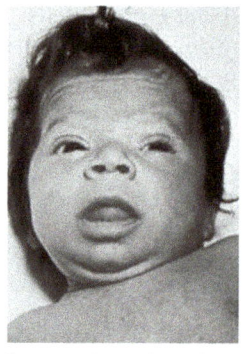

European paintings in 16th century depicted faces of cretins who were considered demons or angels, these were children who suffered from severe iodine deficiency disorders. In the 19th century, school children showed tremendous improvement in school performance after use of iodized salt. Cretinism is a form of hypothyroidism generally found in infants with severe iodine deficiency. Persons suffering from this are referred as cretins who often exhibit feeble mind and are stunted, deaf, mute, and mentally challenged. Myxedematous cretinism is characterized by thickened facial features, coarse and dry skin, swollen tongue, deep hoarse voice, and apathy. Such infants do not feed well and do not gain adequate weight, resulting in growth retardation. They do not cry much and have abnormal bone growth.

Prevalence of IDD and Use of Iodized Salt

In 2007, IDD was reported to be a public health problem in 47 countries by WHO/ICCIDD/UNICEF. UNICEF (2009) has reported that an estimated 38 million newborns are at risk of lifelong consequences of brain damage caused by iodine deficiency. Among them, 18 million were from South Asia, and 13 million out of these 18 million were from India. About 71 million people suffer from goiter and other IDD problems.

According to an IDD newsletter on "Across India, Women are Iodine Sufficient" (2015), there has been dramatic improvement in the quality and coverage of iodized salt in India in the past 10 years due to universalization of iodized salt (in production and distribution across the country). As per National Family Health Survey (NFHS)-IV (2016), 93% household use iodized salt. However, there are considerable differences in iodized salt coverage, with gaps in access, although these are gradually reducing. Among the different zones, states in the south zone, namely Andhra Pradesh, Karnataka, Kerala, Tamil Nadu, and Telangana, have below average coverage (only 62%) of adequately iodized salt. These are assessed by goiter or urinary excretion as shown in Table 12.10.

Prevention and Control of Iodine Deficiency Disorder

This requires administrative involvement at national and international levels as per the magnitude of the problem. The following ways are employed to reduce the problem of IDD:

1. Fortification
2. Universal salt iodization program
3. Supplementation
4. Nutrition education.

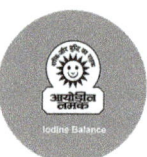 

Fortification of salt with iodine has been the most accepted method around the world for prevention and control of iodine deficiency disorders or goiter. Use of iodized salt is an effective, low-cost means of providing iodine to the public. However, losses occuring during storage, especially if the bags used for packaging do not provide a good moisture barrier. It is recommended that the lag period between manufacture and distribution, sale and consumption of iodized salt should be as short as possible, in order to obtain maximum benefits of salt fortification with iodine. Government of India has also taken the initiative for universal salt iodization and is working through the National Iodine Deficiency Disorders Control Programme (NIDDCP). The logo shown in circle is found in iodized salt in India. Recently any fortified food can easily be identified with logo of plus F.

National Iodine Deficiency Disorders Control Programme (NIDDCP): In 1962, the Government of India launched the National Goiter Control Programme (NGCP), later it was restructured in 1986 and again in 1992. Currently, the National Iodine Deficiency Disorders Control Programme is in operation with the following objectives and activities:

- Supply of iodized salt in place of common salt to the entire country
- Resurvey to assess the impact of iodized salt

- To assess the IDD magnitude in various districts in target groups [children 6-12 years and women (15-44 years) particularly pregnant women]
- Detection of goiter
- Health education and awareness activities (IEC).

The NIDDCP is executed by multiple agencies comprising the Health, Industry, and Railway Ministries of the Central Government. The Ministry of Health and Family Welfare and Directorate General of Health Services (DGHS) are responsible for the national implementation of the national program. The Salt Department, under the Ministry of Industry, is the nodal agency for production, distribution, monitoring, and quality control of iodized salt. The Salt Commissioner, in consultation with the Ministry of Railways, arranges for the movement of iodized salt from the production center to the states. The State government is responsible for distribution of iodized salt within the state either through the Public Distribution System (PDS) or through the open market. For effective implementation of the NIDDCP, a central IDD Cell is established at Directorate General of Health Services (DGHS) level. It is responsible for coordinating surveys, training, monitoring, and management of the IDD program. All the states/union territories have been advised to set up IDD Control Cell.

Under the Prevention of Food Adulteration Act (PFA Act), the level of iodization has been fixed at 30 ppm of iodine in salt at the manufacturing level and 15 ppm at the household level. To ensure exclusive use of iodized salt in endemic areas, the sale of noniodized salt is being discouraged nationally. In spite of these efforts, prevalence of IDD is still high in some districts of Himachal Pradesh, Maharashtra and Karnataka. It indicates the need for increasing awareness about the significance of iodine in health and how iodized salt should be used in order to minimize the cooking losses.

Supplementation: Initially, oral iodine solution was given as a supplement. After World War II, iodized oil was used for supplementation. Initially, the intramuscular form was used and later it was given orally. Use of oral form of iodized oil is advantageous compared to the intra-muscular form because it can be given as a single annual dose and does not require trained persons to inject. However, its limitation is that it is more expensive than iodization of salt, coverage tends to be limited and there has to be direct contact with each individual who has to be administered the iodized oil. WHO (2007) has recommended the dose of iodized oil. The single dose of iodized oil that is recommended for pregnant and lactating women, as well as women of reproductive age (15-49 years) is 400 mg/year. For children under 2 years of age, the recommended dose is 200 mg/year.

Further, the WHO has stated that children 0-6 months of age, who are exclusively breastfed, will receive iodine through breast milk, since the lactating mother will be receiving iodine supplementation. Also, if complementary food is not fortified with iodine, supplementation is required for children aged 7-24 months.

It should be noted that IDD can be eliminated, however, deficiency of iodine is related to geochemical deficit rather than social and economic factors. Therefore, in areas where there is iodine deficit in soil due to reasons such as erosion, deforestation, flooding and rivers changing course, the risk of recurrence of IDD is possible, if supplementation is slackened. Therefore, in such areas, regular monitoring is required.

NUTRITIONAL ANEMIA

Anemia is a worldwide public health issue. It is a pathophysiological problem in which production, morphology, and functionality of red blood cells (RBCs) are adversely affected. Since RBCs are responsible for delivering oxygen to tissues and cells in the body, in anemia, there is varying degrees of impairment of tissue oxygenation. Oxygen supply to tissues is a tightly controlled mechanism depending upon the rate of oxygen supply and demand. Oxygen delivery is dependent upon the blood hemoglobin concentration.

Nutritional anemia is of three types and commonly encompasses deficiencies of iron, folic acid, and vitamin B_{12} as well as other nutrients that are required for hemopoiesis (Fig. 12.4).

Hematopoiesis: It is the process by which immature precursor cells develop into mature blood cells. It occurs in liver, spleen, and bone marrow at different stages of life. Hemopoiesis begins in the 1st week of gestation and continues throughout life. This essential process is highly regulated with nutrition playing an important role. From 6-7 weeks of fetal life, bone marrow is the major site for hemopoiesis or hematopoiesis and erythropoiesis. For erythropoiesis, bone marrow requires adequate supply of several nutrients, viz. energy, protein, iron, cobalt, zinc, folic acid, vitamin C, vitamin A, vitamin B_{12}, vitamin B_6, thiamine, and riboflavin. Deficiency of any of these nutrients can compromise synthesis and result in reduction in hemoglobin concentration of blood, i.e., anemia. The role of these nutrients and the outcome of their deficiencies are shown in Table 12.11.

Classification of Anemia

Anemia is classified as microcytic, normocytic or macrocytic based on mean corpuscular/red cell volume. The commonly occurring nutritional anemias are described in Table 12.12.

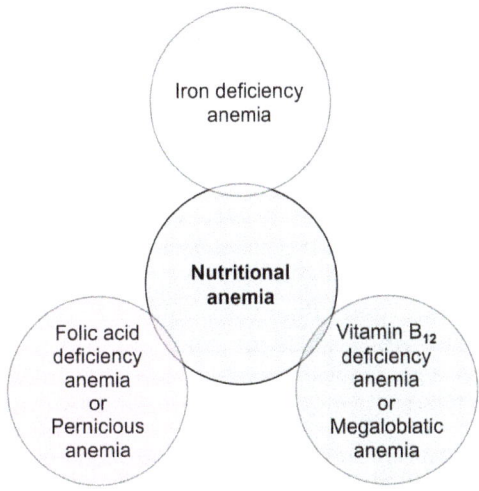

Fig. 12.4: Types of nutritional anemia.

Table 12.11: Hematopoietic nutrients, their role in hemoglobin synthesis, and consequences of deficiency.

Nutrient involved	Role in RBC or hemoglobin synthesis	Possible outcome in deficiency
Iron	Integral part of hemoglobin and support oxygen carrying capacity	Iron deficiency anemia (IDA)
Protein including all essential amino acids particularly methionine	For formation of certain proteins including: • Hemoglobin—for carrying oxygen to target tissues • Erythropoietin (EPO) is a protein hormone formed in kidney that sends signal to bone marrow to manufacture blood cells • Intrinsic factor (IF) is another protein molecule formed in digestive tract and used in the absorption of vitamin B_{12} that play an important role in formation of red blood cells • Methionine plays major role in synthesis of such proteins and is involved along with vitamin B_{12}	Reduces formation of red blood cells Reduced absorption of vitamin B_{12}
Vitamin B_{12}	Essential for the regeneration of tetrahydrofolate (THF) in folate metabolism and formation of DNA. Important for conversion of homocysteine to S-adenosylmethionine (SAM), the methyl donor which is important for DNA methylation	Pernicious anemia or megaloblastic anemia
Folic acid	Folate participates in erythropoiesis and is important for maturation of RBC, since it is a cofactor important for DNA and RNA synthesis	Macrocytic anemia
Vitamin C	Converts Fe^{+++} to Fe^{++} Releases Fe from stores	Absorption of iron is reduced
Vitamin A	Plays a role in hemoglobin synthesis	Coexists with IDA and PEM
Vitamin B_6	Involved in heme synthesis, therefore is required for erythropoiesis and regulate availability of iron from the stores	Microcytic hypochromic anemia
Riboflavin	Iron-requiring enzymes use riboflavin as flavin adenine dinucleotide (FAD) and flavin mononucleotide (FMN) are two coenzymes which are riboflavin depended participate in oxidation—reduction helps in mobilization of stored iron for synthesis/ increase the hemoglobin concentration in the blood synthesis	May alter impair iron absorption, and/or impair iron utilization for the synthesis of hemoglobin
Vitamin E	Acts as an antioxidant to prevent oxidative stress	Increased hemolysis (destruction of RBC)
Copper	Ceruloplasmin is a copper-containing protein made in the liver. It is a ferroxidase enzyme that converts ferrous to ferric iron	Hypochromic, microcytic anemia

Table 12.12: Parameters to assess status of nutritional anemia.

Hemoglobin status	Normocytic anemia — decreased hemoglobin/ hematocrit	Microcytic anemia	Macrocytic anemia
RBC	Decreased production of normal-sized red blood cells and/or increased destruction or loss of red blood cells (hemolysis)	Small, hypochromic	Larger in size
Symptoms	Usually asymptomatic associated with other morbidities ,e.g., chronic kidney disease, cancer, IBS, bone marrow disorders, etc.	Paler than usual	Restlessness, tingling in hands and feet memory problems
MCV (femtoliter or fL)	80–100	<80	>94
MCHC (picograms or pg)	>31	<31	>31
Nutrient deficiency	Early stages of iron deficiency in some individuals Other nutrients involve—protein, vitamin C and vitamin B_{12}	Iron	Vitamin B_{12} and folic acid
Other causes	Common in PEM, lack of nutrient absorption	Thalassemia/ Sideroblastic anemia	Alcoholism and liver disease Drug-induced hypothyroidism

[MCV: mean cell volume; MCHC: mean corpuscular hemoglobin concentration—average amount of hemoglobin in a single red cell (Hb/Hematocrit) hematocrit is the ratio of packed RBCs to blood volume; MCV—size of the red blood cells].

Microcytic anemia: It is also referred as microcytic hypochromic anemia. It is characterized by small red blood cells (microcytes) that are hypochromic (paler or decreased red color), i.e., paler than usual and or normal, because hemoglobin, which gives the color to red blood cells, is decreased. It generally is a consequence of iron deficiency. It is often lab tested by mean corpuscular volume (MCV).

Macrocytic anemia: The blood cells are larger in size and is caused by folate deficiency.

Megaloblastic anemia: It indicates folic acid deficiency with the presence of large, immature, and abnormal RBC.

Pernicious anemia: It Indicates deficiency of vitamin B_{12}. In this condition body is not able to produce normal healthy red blood corpuscles (RBCs). It is chronic illness and due to poor dietary intake or low absorption of vitamin B_{12}. It is often indicated by high level of MCV (macrocytic anemia).

Normocytic normochromic anemia: It is possibly due to deficiency of multiple nutrients—iron, folate, and vitamin

B_2 and B_{12}. It can also be caused by blood loss, bone marrow failure, increased plasma volume as in pregnancy or overhydration, hemolytic anemia, hypothyroidism, adrenal insufficiency, kidney diseases, liver diseases, and cirrhosis.

Iron deficiency and no anemia: In iron deficiency, there is insufficient iron in the body to maintain normal physiological functions of tissues. It can occur in the absence of anemia, if it has not lasted long enough or if it has not been severe enough to cause the hemoglobin concentration to fall below the threshold for the specific sex and age group. Although iron deficiency is the most common cause of anemia, there are other causes such as acute and chronic infections that cause inflammation.

Iron Deficiency Anemia (IDA)

Iron deficiency anemia (IDA) represents insufficient mass of RBCs circulating in the blood. There are separate threshold levels of hemoglobin in the blood for different age groups. IDA is caused by several dietary, physiological factors, and pathological conditions. Infestation/infection caused by worms also causes anemia. Some of the main causes are:
1. Low-dietary intake of iron-rich foods
2. Poor absorption of iron in gastrointestinal tract
3. Loss of iron from the body
4. Increased demand for iron
5. Low body stores of iron.

Low-dietary Intake of iron-rich foods: Food intake itself is low in many parts of the world in terms of quantity, quality, and safety. This can be due to various socioeconomic and other reasons. These are several concerns related to low-dietary intake of iron, which are as follows:
- The plant/cereal-based Indian diet is low in iron content. It also contains good amount of polyphenols (tannins) and phytate that inhibit iron absorption.
- Frequent consumption of tea, coffee with food. Tea contains polyphenols that reduce iron absorption.
- Low and infrequent consumption of animal foods like meat, egg, and liver. They contain heme iron that is better absorbed.
- Low intake of green leafy vegetables, nuts, seeds, and millets. However, some foods may contain varying amounts of oxalates and other inhibitory substances, that may reduce iron absorption.
- Non-adoption of cooking methods that can increase iron content, e.g., use of iron utensils, and/or methods to enhance iron bioavailability, e.g., using acid-containing foods or germination to reduce the phytate content.
- Low intake of vitamin C-rich foods along with iron-rich foods, which otherwise could have improved the bioavailability of iron.
- Consumption of food deficient in nutrients like protein, folic acid, vitamin B_{12}, riboflavin, pyridoxine, vitamin C, vitamin A, and copper.
- Dependency on the intake of milk and milk products particularly during the 1st year of life for nutrition but dairy foods are poor sources of iron.
- Complementary foods, which are poor in micronutrients including iron.
- Cultural taboos related to inappropriate food habits/feeding practices.
- Ignorance about right combination of foods needed to fulfill iron requirements.

Poor Absorption of Iron in Gastrointestinal Tract: Many factors influence iron absorption:
- Nutritional status including low body iron stores
- Hemoglobin level
- Physiological condition
- Rate of RBC production
- Type of dietary source of iron and the presence of iron-enhancing or -inhibiting substances
- Pathological conditions
- Use of certain medicines or drugs.

Absorption of iron from plant foods (even iron-rich) is only 5–10% whereas iron absorption from animal food sources is relatively higher. Plant foods contain phytates and polyphenols that inhibit the absorption; hence, the bioavailability of iron from these foods is low. Iron absorption is increased to 10–20% when the physiological demand is higher, e.g., in pregnancy. Evidence shows that iron absorption is enhanced in malnourished people when body stores are low. Poor absorption of iron is observed in postmenopausal women.
1. Food containing inhibitors, like tannin, etc., reduce the absorption, hence, selection and combination of food is important, e.g., *roti* should not be consumed with tea. Many persons consume tea soon after a meal; this inhibits the absorption of iron present in the meal.
2. Though milk is a poor source of iron, breast milk fulfills the baby's iron requirement in the first 6 months due to lactoferrin that is present. Lactoferrin binds iron and increases the delivery of iron to tissues and prevents its use by intestinal bacteria.
3. Usually, method of cooking does not much influence the iron content. Processing methods can influence iron availability, for example soaking, fermentation, germination, and combination of foods rich in ascorbic acid/organic acids improve the absorption.
4. Use of iron utensils for cooking tends to increase the iron content.
5. Heme iron from animal sources is better absorbed compared to nonheme iron.

Loss of Iron from the Body: Under following incidences, blood loss causes loss of iron from the body.
1. Small amount of iron (0.6 mg/day) is regularly lost through feces, bile, sweat (skin), and mucosal cells of GIT. This loss is inevitable and referred to as basal loss. Women have an additional loss during menstruation (~1.0 mg/day).
2. Infestation with worms like hookworm, which is quite common in among children in tropical countries, increases loss of iron from the body.
3. *Helicobacter pylori* infection can also cause blood loss.
4. Inflammation in any part of the gastrointestinal tract from esophagus to colon may result in blood loss. In certain

cases, there are bleeding episodes and occult blood in feces (melena).
5. Extensive loss of iron through blood loss during accidents, surgery, cuts, internal bleeding in some pathological condition. Iron is lost in burns depending upon the severity and amount of blood loss.
6. Use of nonsteroidal anti-inflammatory drugs (NASAIDs) like anti-inflammatory medicines, e.g., aspirin and antacids increase loss of iron.
7. Postpartum hemorrhage after delivery, repeated pregnancies.

Increased Demand: Iron needs are increased during periods of growth such as in pregnancy, infancy, adolescence, and during intensive exercise as well as in certain pathological conditions. Thus, iron requirement increases when either blood loss is excessive and/or the body has low iron stores.

Low Body Stores of Iron: Low stores of iron can be due to various reasons. Low intake of bioavailable iron with continuous relatively high basal loss depletes iron stores from spleen, liver, and bone marrow. Stored form of iron, i.e., ferritin, is easily mobilized for hemoglobin synthesis. According to the ICMR (1990), at birth, the body contains 270 mg of iron and there are virtually no iron stores between 6 months and 2 years. Thereafter, stores start building at 5 mg/kg body weight and need to be maintained until menarche in adolescent girls. In males, stores start building up from 15 years of age and after growth spurt is completed, iron stores in 70-kg men increase from 200 mg to 1,000 mg during 18–30 years. Iron stores are depleted first before appearance of IDA.

Indicators of Anemia

Iron is a part of hemoglobin. It is transported bound to the protein transferrin and when the intake of iron is more than the requirement, iron is stored primarily in the storage protein, ferritin. Stages of anemia have been described pictorially in Chapter 7 in iron. Generally, hemoglobin is used to diagnose anemia. Hb estimation is a relatively inexpensive method and can be done for large numbers at community level. With hemoglobin, examination of peripheral blood film can be used to diagnose iron deficiency anemia. Since iron deficiency anemia is hypochromic and microcytic, this will be reflected in the hematocrit values. Further, anemia is categorized as mild, moderate, or severe, based on the hemoglobin level. World Health Organization has given threshold values, which are shown in Table 12.13.

In severe anemia, hemoglobin level is <70 g/L and in very severe anemia, it is <40 g/L. There is also a risk of congestive heart failure. Severe anemia in pregnant women increases the risk of maternal mortality and requires medical treatment.

Hematocrit value or calculated as follows: MCV × RBC concentration. Normal hemoglobin and hematocrit values may vary with age, gender, at different stages of pregnancy, and at high altitude and by smoking.

Low hemoglobin level is not caused by iron deficiency alone. It may be caused by deficiency of the other hematopoietic nutrients. Studies have shown that vitamin A supplementation without iron supplementation in many cases increased hemoglobin levels. Also, fall in hemoglobin occurs in the third stage of iron deficiency when all the iron stores in the body are depleted. However, in order to control IDA, it is necessary to have an indicator that will reflect iron status before the iron stores are depleted. The World Health Organization (WHO, 2004) has recommended the use of serum ferritin because it is an indicator of body stores that are used wherever heme synthesis is required. Also, serum ferritin level falls much before hemoglobin decreases, so it helps to detect ID earlier.

Serum Ferritin

Body stores iron in the form of ferritin; hence, estimation of serum ferritin reflects iron stores in the body. Its concentration varies with age and sex. It is high at birth and falls by end of infancy. At 1 year of age, it again starts increasing and continues to increase in adulthood may be up to 30–39 years of age. In women, it remains relatively low until menopause when it rises. Its use is limited in pregnancy, as it falls. However, one of the limitations is that during infection and inflammation, serum ferritin level rises because it is an acute phase protein. Hence, there can be individuals who have ID but their serum ferritin may be increased and if the level is above the cut off, such a person may go undetected. The World Health Organization has given the serum ferritin concentrations that can be used to detect ID (Table 12.14).

There is one more indicator that is a good indicator of ID and is not affected by infection and inflammation like serum ferritin. This indicator is serum transferrin receptor, which helps to differentiate anemia due to iron deficiency from anemia due to chronic inflammation. This indicator is useful to differentiate chronic inflammation or infection in developing countries where the prevalence of anemia is high and the risk of malaria and other infections is also high.

Table 12.13: Hemoglobin threshold to define anemia.

Age or gender group	Hemoglobin threshold (g/dL)	Hemoglobin threshold (mmol/L)	Anemia (g/dL)	Mild anemia (g/dL)	Moderate anemia (g/dL)	Severe anemia (g/dL)
Children (0.5–5.0 years)	11.0	6.8	<11.0	10.0–10.9	7–9.9	<7
Children (5–11 years)	11.5	7.1	<11.5	11.0–11.4	8–10.9	<8
Children (12–14 years)	12.0	7.4	<12.0	1.0–11.9	8–10.9	<8
Women, nonpregnant (>15 years)	12.0	7.4	<12.0	1.0–11.9	8–10.9	<8
Pregnant women	11.0	6.8	<11.0	10.0–10.9	7–9.9	<7
Men (>15 years)	13.0	8.1	<13.0	11.0–12.9	8.0–10.9	<8

Source: WHO (2017) Nutritional anaemias: tools for effective prevention and control, p 7.

Table 12.14: Values of serum ferritin concentration indicative of iron deficiency.

	Serum ferritin (µg/L)			
	Less than 5 years		5 years and older	
	Male	Female	Male	Female
Depleted iron stores	<12	<12	<15	<15
Depleted iron stores in presence of infection	<30	<30	—	—
Severe risk of iron overload (adults)	—	—	>200	>150

Source: WHO (2011). Serum ferritin concentrations for the assessment of iron status and iron deficiency in populations, Vitamin and Mineral Nutrition Information System (VMINS). [Online] Available from https://www.who.int/vmnis/indicators/ferritin/en/.

It reflects the degree of tissue iron supply and is useful in diagnosis of tissue iron deficiency. Its synthesis is associated with reduced supply of iron to the bone marrow and increased erythropoiesis. However, one of the limitations is the high cost of the test.

Clinical Features of Anemia

- Significant pallor of tongue, nail beds, and palms (pale palmar creases suggest severe anemia)
- Fatigue, low exercise capacity (mild anemia can produce decreased exercise tolerance)
- Fissures at the corner of the mouth (angular stomatitis)
- Glossitis/painful red tongue with flattening and atrophy of papillae
- Nails become flat and later spoon-shaped (koilonychia) in severe anemia. It is rare in children <6 years of age, as hemoglobin is sacrificed to maintain tissue growth
- Iron deficiency affects mental functions, i.e., attention span, alertness, and learning; also, children become irritable.

Consequences of Anemia

Iron deficiency with or without anemia has several adverse consequences compromising human health and child development. It is also the major cause of premature births, low birth weight, and perinatal mortality. In developing countries including India where deficiencies of energy, protein, vitamin A, and zinc are high, including malaria infection, anemia worsens the problem. Iron deficiency anemia is one of the high-risk factors for global burden of disease and national productivity and a challenge to national economy. Consequences of iron deficiency include:
- Negative effects on energy metabolism
- Reduced work performance and productivity
- Increased risk in pregnancy
- Increased risk of low birth weight
- Greater risk for maternal and infant mortality in the perinatal period
- Delayed mental and physical development of children
- Changes in immune function
- Adverse effects on temperature regulation
- Severe anemia, may lead to mortality and cognitive and functional outcomes.

Prevalence of Anemia

According to WHO (2008), if prevalence of anemia is more than 5% in a community, it is considered a public health problem, when is more than 5% in a community. The WHO (2011) report indicates that globally, about 43% of children, 38% of pregnant women, 29% of nonpregnant women, and 29% of all women of reproductive age are anemic. The WHO report also states that about 42% of anemia in children is likely to respond to iron supplementation and about 50% of the anemic women would probably be cured by treatment with iron supplementation.

Anemia is prevalent in both developing as well as industrialized countries. Most affected countries are in Africa, Asia, Latin America, and Caribbean, especially South Asia, as similarly indicated. Anemia Mukt Bharat Guidelines has released the prevalence of anemia in India in 2018 as shown in Table 12.15. The Comprehensive National Nutrition Survey (2016–2018) report indicates that about 40 percent of 12–48 month old children, 24% of the 5–9 year old children, and 28% of the 10–19 year old children are anemic. As per NFHS-V (2020) in 22 States, prevalence of anemia continues to be high, since percent anemic in different groups are as follows: 6-59 months children (40.0-92.5); women of reproductive age (15-49 years) (25.8-92.8); adolescent girls (15-19 years) (31.4-96.9); pregnant women (22.2-78.1); adolescent boys (15-19 years) (5.6-75.6) and men (15-49 years) (7.8-39.6).

Prevention and Treatment of Anemia

NITI Aayog for the National Nutrition Mission has set the objectives for dealing with anemia under the banner of "Anemia Mukt Bharat". The Ministry of Health and Family Welfare, Government of India's, Intensified National Iron Plus Initiative (I-NIPI) in 2018, released operational guidelines for "Anemia Mukt Bharat".

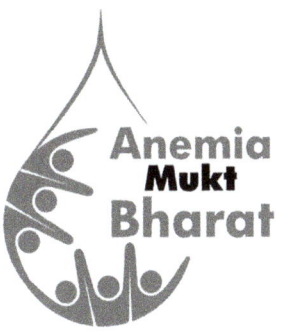

Complying with the targets of POSHAN Abhiyaan and National Nutrition Strategy set by NITI Aayog, the Anemia Mukt Bharat strategy is designed to reduce prevalence of anemia by 3 percentage points per year, between 2018

Table 12.15: Prevalence of anemia in India.

Age group	Prevalence (%) as per Anemia Mukt Bharat
Children (6–59 months)	58
Adolescent girls (15–19 years)	54
Adolescent boys (15–19 years)	29
Women of reproductive years	53
Men (15–49 years)	NA
Pregnant women	50
Lactating women	58

and 2022, among children, adolescents, and women of reproductive age. The main interventions are:
1. Prophylactic iron and folic acid supplementation
2. Deworming
3. Intensified year-round behavior change communication campaign (*Solid Body, Smart Mind*) focusing on four key behaviors:
   a. Improving compliance to iron folic acid supplementation and deworming
   b. Appropriate infant and young child feeding practices
   c. Increase in intake of iron-rich foods through dietary diversity/quantity/frequency and/or fortified foods with focus on harnessing locally available resources, and
   d. Ensuring delayed cord clamping after delivery (by 3 minutes) in health facilities
4. Testing and treatment of anemia, using digital methods and point-of-care treatment, with special focus on pregnant women and school-going adolescents
5. Mandatory provision of iron and folic acid-fortified foods in government-funded public health programs
6. Intensifying awareness, screening and treatment of non-nutritional causes of anemia in endemic pockets, with special focus on malaria, hemoglobinopathies, and fluorosis.

In addition to the above, the following also help to prevent anemia:
1. Food fortification, particularly staple foods
2. Nutrition education, and
3. Maintenance of sanitation and hygiene.

Food-based Approach: Food-based approaches can contribute tremendously to prevent and control anemia on sustainable basis, availability and consumption of iron-rich foods is essential. For this, first, there is a need to address important issues like production, preservation, processing, marketing, and preparation of food. Secondly, distribution of food is important, which includes intra-family food distribution and care for vulnerable groups. Hence, there is need to look into the resources, which can facilitate the increased cultivation of plant foods specifically legumes, iron-rich cereals/millets, green leafy vegetables, and domestication of animals/poultry to facilitate and enable increased consumption of iron. Food-based approaches should focus on:
1. Promotion of breastfeeding infants till 6 months of age and followed by complementary feeding containing iron-rich foods including enhancers of iron absorption
2. Increased consumption of animal foods such as egg, liver, meat, fish, and poultry
3. Increased consumption of vitamin C (25 mg/meal) for better absorption of iron
4. Use germination/fermentation to increase iron bio-availability by reducing the content of inhibitors like phytates, oxalates, bran, phosphates, and polyphenols/tannins
5. Production of food products rich in iron, vitamin C, and vitamin A can be encouraged
6. Use of lemon, fruits or sources of vitamin C, A or foods containing organic acids such as citric acid/malic acid/tartaric acid along with meals is advisable. Addition of sprouted pulses or meat may improve iron status of individuals.
7. Promotion of kitchen gardens for growing green leafy vegetables, vitamin C and vitamin A-rich foods like papaya, mango, guava, lemon, tomato, etc.
8. Choose food and food preparations, guava, lemon, tomato, etc. which are culturally and economically acceptable.

Fortification: Fortification of desired nutrients through commonly consumed food is a useful approach to improve iron status. It is a cost-effective and sustainable way for providing iron to large number of people. However, the technical, operational, and financial aspects and feasibility need to be studied before launching foods fortified with iron. The technique is not used for individuals but for covering large population. Fortificant should not produce any undesirable effect on sensory appeal of the final food product after cooking or storage. Various iron salts have been tried, for example ferrous sulfate, ferrous fumarate, EDTA, etc. Ferrous sulfate tends to produce organoleptic problems in stored wheat flour. Different countries are using different salts in different food products like salt, sugar, bread, soy sauce, flours, etc. In US and UK, ferrous sulfate and elemental iron and in Europe, ferric pyrophosphate and ferric orthophosphate are used. "Sprinkles" containing ferrous fumarate is also being used. Iron chelated with EDTA has better bioavailability compared to ferrous sulfate and has been used in sugar, masala, and fish sauce. Dual fortification of salt containing both iodine and iron in order to increase iron intake has been developed. Staples like wheat flour and rice are also being used for fortification with iron at Food Fortification Resource Centre (FFRC) of FSSAI.

Iron Supplements: Iron supplementation is widely used to combat anemia. It is a relatively inexpensive method for increasing iron intake and is used in prophylaxis programs like National Nutritional Anaemia Prophylaxis Programme (NNAPP) of the Government of India, at community level as well as in healthcare settings. It can be given orally and parenterally. It is commonly recommended during pregnancy and for high-risk individuals including preterm/full-term infants, preschool and school-going children, adolescents, and lactating women. It may also be used in certain diseases like cardiac problems, kidney dysfunctioning, and after surgery, where anemia often occurs.

Many formulations of iron supplements are commercially available, e.g., ferrous sulfates, ferrous gluconate, ferrous fumarate, iron dextran complex, etc. having varying amounts of elemental iron. Various interventions have used iron supplementation along with folic acid and some with both folate and zinc. Intermittent supplementation has been found to be effective and can be used instead of daily supplementation. However, some individuals experience side effects like nausea, constipation, and staining of teeth. It is important to understand that excessive dose of iron will not provide extra benefits rather it may have health hazards.

Since anemia is widespread in India, the National Nutritional anaemia Prophylaxis Programme (NNAPP) was launched in 1970 to reduce incidence of nutritional anemia among children and mothers. This program is implemented by the Ministry of Health and Family Welfare, Government of India. It is operated as part of the RCH program. Under the revised policy, the target group has been expanded to include infants 6–12 months, school children 6–10 years, and adolescents 11–18 years of age, clinically found to be anemic.

Supplementation to different target groups through this program is as follows:

- **Children 6–60 months:** 20 mg elemental iron + 100 μg folic acid (one tablet of pediatric IFA or 5 mL of IFA syrup or 1 mL of IFA drops) for 100 days, if the child is clinically found to be anemic.
- **School children 6–10 years:** 30 mg elemental iron + 250 μg folic acid for 100 days.
- **Adolescents aged 11–18 years:** 100 mg elemental iron + 500 μg folic acid for 100 days. Adolescent girls are to be given greater priority in the program.
- **Pregnant women:** One tablet of 100 mg elemental iron + 500 μg folic acid to be given prophylactically daily and if clinically anemic, 2 such tablets to be given daily for 100 days.
- **Nursing mothers and acceptors of family planning:** One tablet containing 100 mg elemental iron + 500 μg folic acid daily for 100 days.

Nutrition Education: Nutrition Education should be provided regarding anemia, its causes, consequences, and control strategy through ICDS, health services (to reach young children and their mothers), and schools (to reach children and their parents). Mothers of young children should be educated about importance of care and feeding practices, the need to include micronutrient-rich food sources in complementary foods and in the meals of all children including adolescents. Similarly, women and adolescent girls in general and particularly pregnant women should be educated about the importance of iron, the consequences of its deficiencies, and the food sources of iron as well as ways to improve bioavailability of this mineral. It is also important to educate about the role of other micronutrients especially folic acid, vitamins C, B_{12}, A and a mineral, zinc.

This program also includes health and nutrition education to improve overall dietary intakes and promote consumption of iron- and folate-rich foods as well as food items that promote iron absorption. Adequate supplies, distribution, motivation, and ultimate compliance of people determine the success of such programs.

Reduction of other Micronutrient Deficiencies

It is important to reduce the deficiencies of several micronutrients particularly because they play a role in erythropoiesis and prevention of anemia as seen in Table 12.11.

Deworming

Regular deworming is necessary to eliminate helminth infestation. Maintenance of environmental sanitation and hygiene will help to prevent infections and worm infestation. Albendazole tablet is distributed at various health centers for deworming.

Malaria Eradication

Malaria is a major world health problem. An estimated 2 billion people worldwide live in malaria-endemic areas and approximately 1 million children die each year from malaria. Malaria is caused by the parasite *Plasmodium falciparum* or *Plasmodium vivax*, the former is more virulent. During acute infection, there is an acute drop in the hemoglobin level (in chronic infection, there is a slower decrease) because RBC hemolysis occurs, circulating erythrocytes are removed and there is decreased production of RBC in bone marrow. The Government of India is implementing the National Anti-Malaria Programme that indirectly contributes to prevention of anemia.

OVERWEIGHT AND OBESITY

Changes in human diet and activity patterns have had drastic effects on our health status and overweight and obesity have emerged as major problems worldwide, affecting all socioeconomic groups. It has drastically changed body composition, body shape, and nutritional and health outcomes. In modern societies, typically diets are high in saturated fat, trans fat, refined sugar, refined flour, etc. Urbanization, affluence, and higher purchasing power have resulted in greater use of automated appliances, automobiles. Computers and now mobiles have made it much easier to obtain food easily at one's doorstep, thereby reducing physical activity, especially in cities. People staying in closed spaces (office, home, work places) tend to find excuses for less chances to walk and feel less motivated.

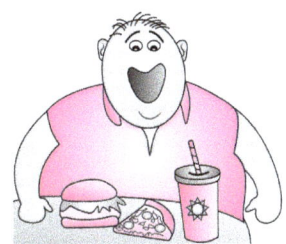

Obesity is a multifaceted health problem caused by complex interactions of genes, environment, and lifestyle. It is progressively increasing at global level, taking pandemic proportions in adults as well as in children. Overweight children often become overweight adults. It is a serious concern for health professionals and if it goes unchecked, it will influence the economy of the country as well as the social fabric. It tends to harm the person's physique, level of fitness, self-confidence, work progress and social acceptance. Besides all individual is at high risk of wide range of endocrine and metabolic diseases like PCOD in girls and women, insulin resistance, high blood pressure, digestive and dental issues including musculosketal problems. Reports indicate that it occurs in both middle- and high-income and also in low socioeconomic groups of people, with women being inflicted more than men.

According to WHO "Overweight and obesity are defined as abnormal or excessive fat accumulation that presents a risk to health. A body mass index (BMI) over 25 is considered overweight, and over 30 is obese". Extra body fat is accumulated in adipose tissue [in subcutaneous adipose tissue and in abdominal (visceral) region], which is not only a storage depot of fat but also acts as an endocrine organ due to which pathological conditions may occur.

Subcutaneous fat: It is the fat that is accumulated under the skin, and is said to be "jiggly" that is typically deposited. It is relatively less harmful. It may be indicative of low muscle mass and insulin resistance. It can cause sagging tissues and cosmetically unappealing.

Visceral or abdominal fat: It is also referred as intra-abdominal (IA) or central obesity. Typically the individual has a large abdomen or protruding belly (paunch), although the arms and legs may not have much fat. Considerable amount of fat is deposited beneath the walls of the viscera, i.e., deep within the abdominal cavity, padding the spaces between the abdominal organs.

> **Morbid or severe obesity:** "A serious health condition that results from an abnormally high body mass that is diagnosed by having a body mass index (BMI) greater than 40 kg/m², a BMI of greater than 35 kg/m² with at least one serious obesity-related condition, or being more than 100 pounds over ideal body weight (IBW)." It is crucial in bariatric treatment.

Fat cells present in adipose tissues are called adipocytes. Individual adipocytes can increase in size or volume. More numbers are drawn from preadipocytes and size of the cell regulates the metabolic activity. Visceral adipocytes are relatively smaller than subcutaneous fat cells. In addition to adipocytes and preadipocytes, adipose tissues also contain stromovascular cells, connective tissue matrix, endothelial cells, sympathetic nerve fibers, and macrophages, which may participate in their functionality.

Visceral fat is biochemically and metabolically different from subcutaneous fat. Location of adipose tissue in the body determines the endocrine behavior of the fat. Adipocytes release certain cytokines (cell signaling proteins) that are called adipokines. Enlarged fat cells release more amounts of adipokines. To date, over 50 types of adipokines have been identified. These adipokines not only regulate body weight homeostasis, but also are associated with inflammation, insulin resistance, diabetes, atherosclerosis, and some forms of cancer. Some examples of adipokines are leptin, interleukins 6, 8, and 10, TNF-α, TGF-β, angiotensin II, etc. There is often a low-grade inflammation in obesity, which may be due to infiltration of macrophages.

The increased level of interleukin 6 stimulates the liver to synthesize and secrete C-reactive protein (CRP) which is biomarker of inflammation. It is predisposing factor associated with the obesity-induced diseases such as atherosclerosis, metabolic syndrome, insulin resistance, and diabetes mellitus. It is also associated with development of psoriasis, depression, cancer, and renal diseases.

In obese persons, adipocytes become insensitive to the action of insulin resulting in greater breakdown of triglycerides resulting in high level of circulating free fatty acids. Obesity is the most common metabolic and nutritional diseases. It may lead to potentially life-threatening complications and substantial reductions in life expectancy. It has been established that there are chances of early origin of obesity in the prenatal period (fetal stage), maternal undernutrition that may influence development and increase the risk of and predispose a person to adulthood obesity and associated disorders.

Overweight and Obesity in Adults

Obese adults are either continuing the obesity from younger age or developed by energy imbalance, poor lifestyle, some pathological reason, or use of certain drugs. Body weight reflects nutritional status and the imbalance between energy intakes (diet) and expenditure (lifestyle). Variation in body weight is attributed to age, gender, physiological status, changes in food intake, stress, exercise, and other environmental factors. Racial, ethnic, demographic, socioeconomic, and lifestyle factors also markedly influence the body weight in a group of people. Gain in body weight reflects changes in body composition due to deposition of excess fat, muscles, and/or water retention that affect metabolic functioning.

How can we determine if a person is overweight or obese? Internationally, reference values are different from those for Asians and Indians, because they are more vulnerable to metabolic problems at a lower BMI in 2018, For adults, WHO defines overweight and obesity as follows: overweight is a BMI greater than or equal to 25; and obesity is a BMI greater than or equal to 30. In Asian cut off BMI is lower than WHO cut off, i.e., BMI < 23 is for overweight and <25 for obesity due to higher rate of obesity related morbidities and mortality. According to Indian Consensus Group (for Asian Indians residing in India) guidelines (2009) a BMI of ≥23 kg/m² and ≥25 kg/m² as overweight and obese, respectively. According to NFHS V (2020) the percentage of adult women and men with BMI more than 25 kg/m² is 11.5–36.3 and 13.9–45.3 respectively.

Waist circumference is also an indicative measure of central adiposity that is not indicated by BMI. Therefore, besides estimating BMI, it is worthwhile to measure waist circumference and waist-hip ratio (WHR). The NFHS V (2020) indicates that the percentage of adult men and women in 22 states of this country is quite high,.i.e., 13.9–45.3% and 44.1–87.8% respectively. Waist circumference (WC) is frequently used for assessment of the degree of overweight and obesity, specifically abdominal obesity. It can be used in large and varied population including bedridden patients as it is simple to measure using a standardized measuring tape. Cut off values for WC given by the Centers for Disease Control (CDC) are given in Table 12.16.

Other methods can be used, e.g., skinfold thickness, magnetic resonance imaging (MRI), and dual energy X-ray absorptiometry (DEXA), bioelectric impedance, which reveal amount and distribution of fat in different parts of the body including subcutaneous and visceral fat with varying degrees of precision, but also require technical skill and special instruments. These assessment methods are briefly described in Chapters 5 and 13.

Table 12.16: Cut off values for waist circumference (cm).

Classification	Male	Female
Not overweight	<94.0 cm	<80.0 cm
Pre-obese	94.0–101.9 cm	80.0–87.9 cm
Obese	102.0 cm	>88.0 cm
Indicative of abdominal adiposity	≥90 cm	≥80 cm

Factors Affecting Overweight and Obesity

At certain stages of the lifecycle, weight gain is desirable because it signifies growth. For example, during infancy, childhood, adolescence, and pregnancy is physiological gain. Also, an undernourished/underweight person needs to gain weight. However, at all stages of the life cycle including these stages, every individual must take care to maintain desirable body weight since excess gain (above the desirable level) increases the risk of overweight and obesity and its associated diseases. Imbalance between energy intake and expenditure is a major factor leading to weight and fat gain. However, there are many genetic, physiological/endocrine, psychological, and environmental factors that contribute to the problem.

Genetic factors: Several genes have been found to influence the phenotype and have a role in obesity, especially onset in early life. Genetic causes can be divided into: (a) monogenic causes—caused by a single gene mutation that involves leptin, (b) syndromic obesity that is either associated with neurodevelopmental abnormalities and malformations of other organs or systems, and (c) polygenic obesity—several genes together have an effect—it is said that their effect is "amplified" in an obesogenic environment (one that contributes to weight gain).

Physiological Factors

Food acquisition (orexia) is the primary aim of all living organisms including humans for survival and wellbeing. Food preferences and eating patterns may be influenced by physiological demand. Body has a signaling system to acquire food through appetite and hunger and this mechanism is regulated by the hypothalamus and neurons in the brain to ensure that there is sufficient food intake for survival. Satiety is another signal of sufficiency. However, humans quite often eat more than required. The human body conserves energy for future use when food may be in short supply. Intake of food is not necessarily in tune with body needs and can be influenced by sight, smell, and thought of food, social circumstances, and emotional state. In many cases, eating behavior is dysregulated.

Neurological and Endocrine Factors

Neurological and endocrine factors may alter body composition and metabolism, leading to obesity. Appetite is regulated by the hypothalamus in the brain, influencing neurons, such as "anorexigenic" and "orexigenic" neurons that inhibit or stimulate appetite respectively, and affect the rate of macronutrient oxidation. It is influenced by hormonal signals, eventually bringing about physiological alterations in hunger, satiety, and energy metabolism. Appetite is associated with desire to eat and in most cases is influenced by cognitive experience like sight and smell of food. Sometimes even thought or talk of food may also provoke eating.

When a person feasts, the excess of carbohydrate, fat, and protein eaten is converted to fat that is deposited in adipose tissue. In almost all societies, availability of affordable, processed foods, rich in energy and fat and low in fiber, has increased, resulting in overconsumption of energy-dense foods. Combined with sedentary lifestyles, this has precipitated overweight and obesity in a considerable proportion of the population including children. Several factors govern food intake:

Eating habits and eating patterns: These include taste preferences of the individual, interest, mood/emotional factors, time of eating, skipping meals especially breakfast, dietary restraint, and cultural and societal norms. Eating patterns include portion size, variety in the diet, eating frequency, eating regularity, snacking, skipping meals, consumption of energy-rich beverages/snacks/fast foods that are low in fiber and other nutrients, eating out, eating more on festivals, holidays, social gatherings, parties, etc.

Food composition: This is an important consideration because it determines the nutrient and energy intake. Among the three macronutrients, protein provides greater satiety. The type of carbohydrate consumed influences physiological aspects of overweight and obesity. Simple sugars provide instant energy and make the food tasty but if not utilized for physical activity, they are soon converted into fat and promote weight gain. Increasing intake of low-glycemic foods (complex carbohydrates), fiber-rich foods, fruits, and vegetables as well as water in the diet are more filling and help to reduce energy intake. However, consuming low-energy foods or skipping meals in order to reduce energy intake lowers the metabolism. Low BMR is also responsible for weight gain. This reduction in BMR needs to be offset by increasing physical activity.

Food cravings: At times, a person may have very strong irresistible desire/craving to eat a particular food item. Generally, people like chocolates, cakes, sweets, cold drinks, chips/wafers, etc., but they are all obesogenic.

Social and Environmental Factors

High disposable incomes, greater exposure to processed foods through varied marketing strategies, have created an "obesogenic" environment at home, in the work place, malls, specialty food outlets, and recreational places. Obesogenic environments that promote eating and reduce physical activity are supported by the following changes that have occurred:

1. Increased modernization, urbanization, and "mallinization" have increased the availability of vast variety of foods.
2. Promotion of food products by popular celebrities (TV characters and sportsmen) often encourage to buy and eat the same food product.

3. Change in social and family structure: There are more nuclear families having one or fewer number of children. They are exposed to more than required amount of food.
4. The number of social gatherings like birthday parties has increased in which children also participate. Usually, foods served in these gatherings are rich in fat and energy resulting in consumption of energy-dense food and more amount of food.
5. Energy-dense foods are colorful, flavorful, and tasty but are generally not satiating.
6. Marketing strategies such as "buy one get one free", free coupons, jumbo size, extra portion for the same price, and value for money contribute to overconsumption. Most of these are ultraprocessed foods that provide convenience in terms availability, accessibility, storability, and ease of preparation and consumption, but they are energy dense.
7. Both parents work and there is no one to cook food for family. Hence, children may rely on energy-dense foods that are stored at home or purchased from outside. Examples of easily accessible foods and cheap foods are bread, biscuits, butter, chips, noodles, puffs, pastries and cakes, and cola drinks. Street foods are unhealthy from point of view of composition and hygiene.
8. Children love to eat sweet food items which are rich in calories.
9. Persons who snack in front of TV/while working with computer tend to eat more.
10. Skipping meals leads to compensatory increase in hunger and high intake of energy-dense foods or excess food consumption for energy deficit.
11. When jumbo sized food portions are offered, people tend to consume the whole portion even if they are not hungry rather than "wasting" the food.
12. Lack of emphasis on mindful eating of healthy foods for various reasons.
13. High price of healthy foods like milk and milk products, fruits and vegetables, and whole grains and pulses may further limit their consumption.
14. Cheaper foods are rich in empty calories coming from hydrogenated fats, refined oil, high fructose corn syrup. They are high in salt or sodium and packed in packing materials suggested to be endocrine disruptors.

Reduced physical activity: It is more common in urban areas, especially in metropolitan cities due to:
1. Sedentary lifestyle due to excess television viewing, excessive use of computer, internet surfing, and social media (Facebook, Twitter, Instagram, etc.).
2. Large disposable incomes encourage persons to buy more luxurious and comfortable items that tend to reduce physical activity, leading to reliance on automated transport for daily travel, people prefer to use lifts and escalators instead of using stairs.
3. Lack of interest and/or time to participate in the games or do exercise.
4. In cities, lack of playgrounds, which are safe and nearby the house, and lack of sidewalks/pavements, which restrict opportunity to walk.

Psychological Factors

Obesity is associated with psychological problems. Overweight persons may be victims of bullying by colleagues/peers and feel guilty or unable to handle the situation. This may lead to sadness, loneliness, nervousness, and depressive behavior, adversely affecting their self-esteem, school grades in children and work performance in adults. Many individuals seek comfort and indulge in eating (overconsumption) high-fat and high-sugar foods when they are unhappy/stressed.

Laboratory Laurel: 230 working women were studied for the impact of eating behavior on health risks using the 3-Factor Eating Behavior Questionnaire 18 and burnout using the Bergen Burnout Indicator 15, at baseline and after 12 months. Body weight, percent body fat, weight change, and burnout were measured. Women who experienced burnout had higher scores for emotional and uncontrolled eating. The study indicated the importance of treating burnout and eating behavior first in the treatment of obesity.

Nevanpera N, Hopsu L, Kuosma E, et al. Occupational burnout, eating behavior, and weight among working women. Am J Clin Nutr. 2012;95(94):934-43.

Guidelines for Preventing Obesity

Obesity can be prevented or treated by regulating food and energy intake, and physical activity. This entails behavioral modification to achieve both, and training for it takes considerable time to bring positive changes in the attitude toward healthy eating and daily activities. Expertise of nurses, nutritionists, psychologists, physicians, and social workers is needed. Key messages for preventing obesity are:
1. Consume well-balanced diet, drink plenty of water, and ensure adequate intake of micronutrients and proteins.
2. Include wholegrain foods, fresh fruit, and vegetables for fiber, which provide fullness and limit excessive eating.
3. Any obsession or compulsion in food selection and eating behavior needs to be strictly controlled. Help of professional counselor should be sought, if psychological issues are involved.
4. Restrict consumption of ultraprocessed foods and energy-dense foods, as these are often rich in sugar, fat, and salt, contain refined flours; soda and monosodium glutamate (MSG) may increase water retention. Thus, avoid eating very sweet, salty, or oily foods especially at night.
5. Instead of whole milk and curd, use skim milk and buttermilk.
6. Regular vigorous exercises for 30–45 minutes and diet regulation and control are of great help. Sleeping during daytime should be avoided at all costs.
7. Practice ways to destress like yoga, meditation, music, and dance or start a creative hobby.
8. Join a group who is participating in a similar weight loss regimen, it motivates and helps to maintain the routine.
9. Avoid overenthusiasm while losing weight. Have patience. It is long process for good results.
10. Follow maintenance diet after desired weight loss otherwise there may be yo-yo effect and weight may rebound.

11. Persons with problem like diabetes, heart disease, and hypertension should undertake any weight loss program under medical supervision.
12. Look nutrition fact labels for the source of calories and % daily values. Many a times a healthy ingredient is advertised but amount of that is minimum and maximum calories are coming from hydrogenated fats.
13. Pay attention to packaging material, supply chain or storage time and conditions
14. Prefer seasonal, fresh and local food to include in the diet
15. Enhance flavor in the meal by slow cooking method, adding culinary spices and herbs
16. Follow food plate goal or food pyramid recommended by your nation
17. Consult dietician or nutritionist and follow the advice by your health profession on physical activity.

Since increasing prevalence of obesity in childhood and during adolescents is a global concern with regard to health in their future, it is briefly discussed.

Childhood Obesity

Childhood obesity has become a global public health problem. In India, NFHS V (2020) data shows that 1.9–13.4 percent of children under 5 years of age are overweight. The causes of childhood obesity are primarily due to energy imbalance as is seen among adults. A child (6–10 years) with a BMI greater than the 85th percentile but less than the 95th percentile is considered "overweight" and a child having a BMI greater than the 95th percentiles for age and sex is considered obese. The same applies to adolescents. BMI for children is age and sex specific. It differs between girls and boys due to the differences in body fat. Standards in terms of percentiles have been given by the WHO, the Centers for Disease Control and Prevention, and the American Academy of Pediatrics. In India, standards have been given by Khadilkar and coworkers that are also recommended by the Indian Academy of Pediatrics. The percentile ranking on the charts indicates the relative position of the child's BMI and nutritional status. Children can be categorized as underweight, healthy weight, overweight, and obese.

For Children Under 5 Years of Age

Overweight is weight-for-height greater than 2 standard deviations above WHO Child Growth Standards median; and obesity is weight-for-height greater than 3 standard deviations above the WHO Child Growth Standards median.

Childhood obesity may be an outcome of a many factors that have a role in weight regulation such as genetics, developmental influences ("metabolic programming", or epigenetics), and environmental factors. Metabolic programming begins in utero and and is influenced numerous environmental factors. Eating behavior and the habit of indulging in physical activity that determine body weight and BMI are influenced by the home and school environment. After infancy, children grow, become independent, and are influenced by peers and media. However, in the early years of life, parental food choices influence their eating patterns. Parents/guardians are the role models for children's food intake and health outcomes. In certain cases, children do not get enough homemade food or balanced diet as per their needs for their growth and development. They are dependent upon external food supply and they are unaware of the health consequences of processed and packaged foods particularly ultraprocessed foods that tend to be high in fat, trans fat, sugar, and salt and are energy dense. Children may lack knowledge about healthy foods except fruits, but they often do not like to carry these and peel by themselves. Also, fruits are fairly expensive. On the other hand, they are attracted by the popular, attractive, and tasty food items that are sold at relatively low prices at small shops located on street corners and even food courts in malls. Consequently, many children become victims of childhood obesity and other undesirable health outcomes. Obesity increases the risk of children being teased, which can have negative psychological implications. Consequently, they perform poorly academically and suffer from other problems such as depression, low self-esteem, and low confidence. Parental or external influences also affect their type and duration of physical activity behavior.

Promoters of Childhood and Adolescent Obesity

- Allowed to eat *ad libitum*
- Addition of sugar, butter, cheese, jam, and peanut butter to persuade the child to eat family foods
- Irresistible appearance, taste, and flavor
- Prefer jumbo size of favorite foods
- Lack of regular meal timing
- Skip breakfast and other major meals and compensatory eating of junk foods
- Easy accessibility of favorite foods in and outside home
- Abundant stock of energy-dense food stored in refrigerator or cupboard
- Exciting advertisement of fast foods and popularity of the particular food or brand
- Frequent visit to shopping malls, movies, and social gatherings
- Gifts, treats, or rewards of sweets and chocolates
- Lack of parental knowledge about nutrition and preparation of healthy foods
- Lack of parental acceptance in early years about the child's ability to regulate its energy intake and coercing child to empty the plate
- Both parents are working or single parent—working and staying alone, parental indulgence
- Parents themselves may be poor role models
- Use of food to relieve child's boredom or as punishment and reward or when child is emotionally upset
- Parents allow children to eat snack in front of television or video or computer screen
- Parents provide sedentary life—comfort travel, desk work for homework, and reading
- Inadequate sleep
- Excessive viewing of TV, use of computers and mobiles.

Laboratory Laurel: Accumulation of fat mass in obesity resulting from hypertrophy and/or hyperplasia is associated with adipose tissue dysfunction in adults. 171 lean and obese children (0–18 years) were studied for clinical characterization of adipocytes. Obese children had higher number and larger-sized adipocytes in early childhood compared to lean children. There was decreased basal lipolytic activity and significantly enhanced stromal vascular cell proliferation, as well as increased macrophage infiltration, and formation of crown-like structures, in adipose tissue of obese children aged ≥6 years, as well as high-sensitivity C-reactive protein levels. Clinically, adipocyte hypertrophy was not only associated with serum leptin levels, but also highly and independently correlated with Homeostatic Model Assessment of Insulin Resistance (HOMA-IR), a marker of insulin resistance.

Landgraf K, Rockstroh D, Wagner IV, et al. Evidence of early alterations in adipose tissue biology and function and its association with obesity-related inflammation and insulin resistance in children. Diabetes. 2015;64(4):1249-61.

Research Glimpse: Leptin plays a significant role in controlling appetite, food intake, and weight control. A MEDLINE search of papers published between 1994 and 2016 indicated a relationship between leptin levels and pediatric obesity. Leptin directly interacts with the hypothalamus for energy balance regulation. Leptin can be a good biomarker for predicting childhood obesity. Also, there is interrelationship among insulin, lipoproteins, exercise, and growth hormone.

Alamri NS, Alzein EH, Jareedan TWA, et al. Leptin as a Potential Biomarker for Childhood Obesity. EC Paediatrics. 2017;3(5):435-46.

Consequences of Childhood Obesity

Obesity in childhood/adolescence increases the risk of developing chronic noncommunicable health problems at an early age. There are several consequences, some of which may occur in the short-term and some may be manifested later in life.

Nutritional imbalance: Consumption of energy-dense foods increases intake of empty calories while the child is deprived of other vital nutrients like protein, calcium, and iron causing nutritional imbalance and risk of nutrient deficiencies.

Hampers proper growth and development: Deprivation of nutrients has adverse effects on growth and maturation.

Further decrease in physical activity: They are less active, less curious, and less responsive to extracurricular and competitive activities in school.

Poor academic performance: It is likely that they are poor performers in academics also.

High risk of adulthood obesity: Childhood obesity increases the risk of adulthood obesity.

Dental caries: Eating more sugar causes dental caries.

Behavior problems: Children tend to become either aggressive or depressed. Other behavioral problems are observed in obese children.

Chronic diseases: Obese children are at high risk of impaired glucose tolerance and diabetes mellitus, hypertension, cardiovascular diseases, orthopedic diseases, and cancer in the long-term.

Other problems: Sleep problems, early puberty/menarche, eating disorders such as anorexia and bulimia, skin infections, asthma, and other respiratory problems have been observed in obese children.

Overweight and Obesity in Adolescence

Overweight and obesity are defined for children aged between 5–19 years. Overweight is BMI-for-age greater than 1 standard deviation above the WHO Growth Reference median; and obesity is greater than 2 standard deviations above the WHO Growth Reference median.

Childhood obesity predisposes to obesity in adolescence. Overweight and obesity in adolescents can result in a broad range of adverse health effects in them. During adolescence, the individual goes through the second growth spurt, which includes several hormonal and metabolic changes. Some hormones play a role in regulating hunger as well as satiety. There is a strong relationship between economic status and obesity. Lifestyle choices such as long hours spent on studying because of academic pressures, use of computers and mobiles (screen time) all lead to inactivity and snacking and munching while doing so, all contribute to obesity. Food behavior includes consuming unhealthy foods/diets that promote weight gain and are poor in fiber and important micronutrients. Adolescents tend to be influenced by media, advertisements, celebrity physique, and peer groups. They can become easy victims of their "halo effect". They may try several products, supplements, and meal replacements to look beautiful or handsome/have a "perfect" body that may make them end up with undesirable consequences. Unfortunately, they ignore parents, elders, and even medical advice. Bulimia, an eating disorder, depression, desire to be thin, peer pressure, stress, lack of sleep and/or poor sleep health, deficiency of nutrients like vitamin D, PCOS (polycystic ovarian syndrome), hormonal imbalance, skipping meals, overeating at social gatherings and irresistible desire to eat chocolates, sweets, and confectionary items also contribute to development of obesity.

Research Glimpse: Globally, prevalence of childhood obesity is rising. The International Association for the Study of Obesity (IASO) and International Obesity Task Force (IOTF) estimated that about 200 million school children are either overweight or obese. There is difficulty in assessing childhood obesity because cut-off given by WHO and IOTF for Asian Indian adults is not applicable for children and adolescents. Hence, age- and gender-specific normograms of BMI are used. Data was collected from 16 of the 28 States in India from 1981 to 2013. Prevalence of obesity was higher in northern states as compared to south India. Pooled data after 2010 showed prevalence of 19.3% childhood overweight and obesity, which was 16.3% in 2001–2005. This rising trend was seen not only to higher socioeconomic groups but also in the lower income groups where underweight still remains a major concern.

Ranjani H, Mehreen TS, Pradeepa R, et al. Epidemiology of childhood overweight and obesity in India: A systematic review. Indian J Med Res. 2016;143(2):160-74.

Prevention of Childhood Obesity

The Indian Academy of Pediatrics (IAP, 2004) has given strategies for preventing and also treating the childhood obesity. These are:
a. Reduced calorie intake
b. Increased activity levels
c. Decreased sedentary behavior
d. Family involvement
e. Behavioral changes.

However, it is important to remember that limiting calorie intake of growing children can result in decreased velocity of linear growth and therefore may be harmful. Reducing the food intake may also result in inadequate intake of certain important nutrients like iron, calcium, zinc, and vitamins A, C, and E. High degree of dietary control, particularly by parents, may increase the risk adverse psychobehavioral pattern, which may reduce the beneficial effect of treatment. If really necessary, intervention should begin after 3 years of age and before adolescence.

Ways to Curb Obesity in Children and Adolescents

For parents and caretakers:
1. Parents need to be role models for healthy food habits and create anti-obesogenic environment at home.
2. Establish daily meal timings and train them to eat at least one major meal with the whole family.
3. Monitor that the child does not skip meals including breakfast.
4. Never use food as a reward.
5. Never encourage them to give orders for home delivery of fast foods.
6. Engage them in learning and cooking nutritious foods for the child.
7. Arrange for children to have healthy foods in parents' absence.
8. Avoid storing energy-dense foods at home.
9. Give them healthy packed lunch from home rather than money to buy food from outside.
10. Use whole grains, vegetables, and fruits. Encourage children to eat fruits and vegetables. Encourage whole fruit rather than fruit juice consumption.
11. Involve them in food-associated activities like food purchase, organizing utensils or food in respective places, reading food labels as per their age.
12. Encourage them to participate in school extracurricular/sports activities. Divert time spent on watching TV to physical activities.
13. Walk and play with them in house or outside whenever possible.
14. Reduce use of motor vehicles.
15. Monitor their fluid intake. Teach children to drink water instead of sweetened or carbonated beverages.
16. Monitor and restrict time spent in TV viewing, computer use, and sitting.
17. Regularly monitor body weight, blood pressure, lipid profile, and any nutritional deficiency.
18. Reach out to gather information about nutritional composition of food products and their health effects.
19. Train the child to respect health aspects of meals rather than look for fun/taste.
20. Pay attention to child's indulgences in food choices and eating behavior.
21. Teach children to eat at meal times and define non-eating times, i.e., "eating-free" in the day.

For schools
1. Ensure that foods sold in the school canteen or vending machine are nutritious and not energy dense. Ultra-processed foods like chips should not be allowed.
2. Fruits should be made available in the school.
3. Keep watch on the content of packed lunch.
4. Persuade parents to keep nutritious and digestible food in the lunch box.
5. Try to organize one meal in school, if possible, like mid-day meal/school lunch.
6. Increase awareness in parents and children with regard to the consequences of poor dietary habits and inactivity.
7. Promote health and nutrition education through curricular and extracurricular activities.
8. School should not permit promotional activities for unhealthy foods.
9. Focus on all-round development plus physically fitness and socially and emotionally readiness to face challenges in future.

Media
1. Depiction of nutrition and growth, if shown with their role model, may have better influence.
2. Health messages can/should be entertaining, story based, and related to their lives.
3. Whenever necessary, statutory warning should be emphasized.
4. Avoid target marketing of obesogenic foods and beverages.
5. Responsible advertising and scheduling of advertisements.
6. No advertisements of empty calorie and junk foods particularly during children's programs.

Policy Level
FSSAI has launched a campaign "Eat Right India" for reducing consumption of HFSS foods (high fat, high salt and high sugar)

Parental support, a healthy home and school environment can go a long way in preventing obesity in children and adolescents. Home is the first exposure where the child learns eating and forms the food habits. Restricting sedentary behavior like TV viewing, video games, or internet surfing and encouraging outdoor play are beneficial. Involvement of children in food activities like cleaning, selecting, and stirring under supervision helps in developing good food habits and satisfaction. School is the place where children receive knowledge that is imprinted in their minds. Providing nutrition knowledge and promotion of physical fitness for health and well-being can do wonders in curbing childhood obesity. FSSAI has also launched the "Yellow Book" in view of Safe and Nutritious Foods (SNF) @ Schools initiative.

DIABETES

According to WHO (2018), 422 million people had diabetes and among them 69.2 million are living in India. Thus, diabetes has now become a global epidemic. India is said to have the highest prevalence and it is estimated that 98 million people may have type II diabetes by 2030. WHO declared diabetes as the seventh leading cause of death in 2016. Almost half the deaths occurred before the age of 70 years owe to diabetes. Diabetes is a major cause of blindness, kidney failure, heart attacks, stroke, and lower limb amputation. Prevalence of diabetes has risen by 64% across India over the last two to three decades, according to the Indian Council for Medical Research, Institute for

Health Metrics and Evaluation, and the Public Health Foundation of India (2017). Percentage of women and men with blood glucose level (BGL) greater than 140 mg/dL or taking medicine to control blood sugar, as per NFHS V (2020) is 6.7–24.8 and 8.0–27.6 among 22 states. Prevalence is higher in urban than in rural areas, and among higher socio-economic sectors (SES). However, in urban areas of some of the relatively more affluent states, diabetes is more prevalent among the lower SES. Diabetes affects both men and women and now the prevalence of diabetes in children is increasing. Millions of people are likely to be prediabetic or suffer from insulin resistance and other co-morbidities of heart, liver, kidney and bones. Demographic and nutrition transition has brought drastic changes in dietary patterns and lifestyles, with one of the consequences being diabetes. With such large numbers being affected by this serious and chronic disorder, the country and its economy face tremendous challenges.

Diabetes mellitus is an endocrine/metabolic disorder caused by absolute or relative deficiency of insulin. Insulin is produced by the beta cells of the pancreas and is required for glucose to enter the cell (binds to receptors on cell membranes) and be utilized. Insulin regulates many metabolic processes in the body, but in case of diabetes that control is lost resulting in several problems. Hyperglycemia or high blood glucose level is by abnormalities in the metabolism of carbohydrates, and often that of lipids cholesterol and protein.

Diabetes is a silent disease in the beginning and is often not diagnosed for months and years together. It can be well managed by adequate, appropriate in quality and quantity and timely food, exercise, and medication (FEM). However, if it is not treated in time and blood sugar is not kept in tight control, it can progressively cause many complications affecting feet, eyes, heart, and kidneys. The American Diabetes Association (2018) has classified diabetes into four clinical classes as shown in Table 12.17.

Type I Diabetes

Type I diabetes, also known as insulin-dependent diabetes mellitus (IDDM), was previously known as juvenile diabetes. It usually occurs in children and young adolescents, although it can occur in all age groups. It is caused by the absolute deficiency of insulin hormone due to autoimmune disorder that destroys pancreatic beta cells, which produce insulin. Though its cause is not well understood, there can be genetic predisposition. Type I diabetes is caused by complex interaction between genetics, the immune system, and environmental factors. The immune system may be stimulated or triggered by some factor in the environment to produce antibodies. Normally, antibodies protect the human body and its organs by helping to resist "foreign agents". Antibodies recognize the organs and do not attack them, however, in autoimmune disorders, antibodies, i.e., autoantibodies, attack and destroy own cells in the body. Autoantibodies gradually destroy insulin-producing cells and this may remain unnoticed for some time. When majority of β-cells have been destroyed and insulin production is very low/ceases, then symptoms of type I diabetes appear. Blood glucose level constantly remains high (>110 mg/dL).

Since insulin is required for glucose uptake by cells, without it the cells compensate by utilizing protein and fat for energy production. As a result, there is rapid weight loss. Use of large amount of fats for energy results in the formation of ketones that accumulate and can be detected in urine. If the situation is not corrected, it can lead to ketoacidosis, i.e., blood pH is in acidic range, and the situation can be life-threatening. Other symptoms are polyuria (frequent urination), polydipsia (increased thirst), and polyphagia (increased hunger) as well as fatigue. Another life-threatening situation in type I is hypoglycemia (<70 mg/dL). High blood glucose level for a prolonged period without aid of insulin can be harmful and life-threatening. Hence, in type I diabetes, insulin replacement therapy is a must and needs to be started quickly. It can be given in the form of insulin injections or insulin pumps under medical supervision. Patient requires lifelong exogenous insulin for survival.

Type II Diabetes

Type II diabetes is also called non-insulin–dependent diabetes mellitus (NIDDM) because it does not require insulin therapy. However, the name, NIDDM, is not used since some patients require insulin to control diabetes. It is generally found in adults but can occur in all age groups. It is due to insulin resistance that is inability of insulin receptors to respond to insulin. Most persons with type II diabetes have normal or elevated level of insulin (hyperinsulinemia).

Prediabetes

"Prediabetes" is a term used for individual who does not meet the criteria for diabetes but have high blood sugar

Table 12.17: Types of diabetes.

Type 1 diabetes	Type 2 diabetes	Gestational diabetes mellitus (GDM)	Other specific types of diabetes
• Due to autoimmune β-cell destruction • Absolute deficiency of insulin hormone • Usually appear in childhood or early adulthood	Due to progressive defect in β-cell insulin secretion on the background of insulin resistance	Diabetes diagnosed during second or third trimester of pregnancy. It is not clearly overt diabetes. Fasting plasma glucose 5.1–6.9 mmol/L or 1-hour post-load plasma glucose ≥ 10.0 mmol/L or 2-hour post-load plasma glucose 8.5–11.0 mmol/L	It occurs due to other causes such as genetic (defects in β-cell function), pancreatic disease (cystic fibrosis or pancreatitis) secondary to other diseases, medical conditions or due to medication or drug induced (used during treatment of HIV/AIDS or organ transplantation). These forms of diabetes are frequently characterized by onset of hyperglycemia at an early age (generally before age 25 years). They are referred to as maturity-onset diabetes of the young (MODY) and are characterized by impaired insulin secretion with minimal or no defects in insulin action

to be considered as normal. Their HbA1C is between 5.7–6.4% (34–47 mnol/mol). It is an intermediate condition between normalcy and diabetes. There is impairment of insulin responsiveness to carbohydrate from exogenous and endogenous sources. Hence, there is impaired fasting glucose (IFG) and impaired glucose tolerance (IGT). Rapid urbanization and societal and professional influences may predispose IGF and IGT. Prediabetes predisposes individuals to diabetes and CVD.

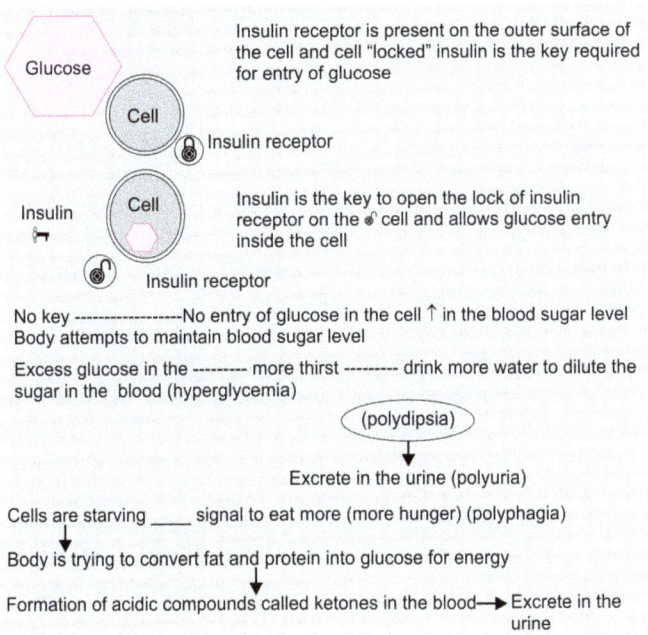

Risk factors for prediabetes
- Overweight or obese
- First-degree relative with diabetes
- History of CVD, hypertension, low HDL cholesterol level (less than 35 mg/dL), high triglyceride level (250 mg/dL)
- Women with polycystic ovary syndrome
- Physical inactivity
- Other clinical conditions associated with insulin resistance (e.g., abdominal obesity, acanthosis nigricans).
- Regular testing as recommended by the experts is advisable.

Insulin Resistance

Insulin stimulates receptors of the cells of the tissues particularly muscle cells for glucose uptake and provide energy. This capacity differ from person to person that affects their energy levels. Cell receptors do not respond to insulin the state is referred as insulin resistance. The body produces insulin but does not utilize it properly. Muscle, fat and liver cells do not respond well to insulin. Body produces more insulin for normal functions of these cells. Hence insulin levels are high in the blood and indicative of insulin resistance. As a result pancreas continue to secrete insulin. Insulin-resistant persons, therefore, have high plasma insulin levels. Insulin resistance (IR) preceed diabetes and commonly found in persons with abdominal obesity, hypertension, dyslipidemia and type 2 diabetes. Weight loss can improve insulin sensitivity and reduce insulin levels. Insulin resistant people often observed with Acanthosis nigricans (dark skin lines or patches forming on the groin, armpits, and the back of the neck) and Polycystic ovary syndrome (PCOS) characterized by irregular menstrual cycles, infertility, and periods that cause pain.

IR can be assessed by HOMA-IR stands for Homeostatic Model Assessment of Insulin Resistance. It can be obtained by HOMA-IR Blood Code Calculation

Insulin (uIU/mL (mU/L) X Glucose(mg/dL) = HOMA-IR
The HOMA-IR calculation requires US standard units. To convert from international SI units:
Insulin: pmol/L to uIU/mL, divide by (÷) 6
Glucose: mmol/L to mg/dL, multiply by (x) 18
Healthy Range: 1.0 (0.5–1.4)
Less than 1.0 means you are insulin-sensitive which is optimal.
Above 1.9 indicates early insulin resistance.
Above 2.9 indicates significant insulin resistance.

In case of insulin resistance or insulin insufficiency, there may be deposition of visceral, hepatic, and intramyocellular fat, which may increase the production of free fatty acids; cytokines, thereby increasing the inflammatory condition. Oxidation and oxidative stress is also increased in absence of glucose utilization.

Currently, prevalence of insulin resistance is rising. Insulin resistance is when cells in your muscles, body fat, and liver start resisting or ignoring the signal given by insulin, i.e., even when insulin is present, glucose does not bind to the receptors and does not enter the cells. It remains in circulation, resulting in elevated blood sugar/blood glucose levels. Many factors play a role in insulin sensitivity including genetics, aging, and ethnicity, but the driving forces behind insulin resistance are excess body weight, excess percent body fat, particularly visceral fat, lack of exercise, smoking, and poor sleep health including inadequate sleep or short sleep duration. Initially, as insulin resistance develops, the body tries to compensate by producing more insulin. However, if this situation continues, the pancreatic beta cells are unable to keep pace and meet the demand for more and more insulin and ultimately get worn out. Insulin resistance often has been found to exhibit lipid triad: (1) high levels of plasma triglycerides, (2) low levels of HDL, and (3) the appearance of small dense low-density lipoproteins (sdLDL). This lipid triad may indicate the risk of atherosclerosis.

Gestational Diabetes

It is characterized by elevated blood glucose level during pregnancy and is usually diagnosed in the second or third trimester. Many a times, blood glucose level returns to normal after delivery, but risk of having diabetes is increased in such women. Genetic predisposition, age and ethnicity, and maternal obesity are risk factors for GDM. Reduction in prepregnancy/preconceptional weight, i.e., having a BMI and percent body fat close to desirable range, can reduce the chances of GDM. Medical Nutrition Therapy (MNT) is helpful to control blood glucose level and ensuring healthy pregnancy. Exercise under guidance can be good adjunct therapy along with MNT. Care is needed to avoid ketosis; hence, extreme calorie restriction is not advisable; rather distribution of carbohydrate along with enough protein and micronutrients are important for achieving good pregnancy outcome. Energy requirements need to be fulfilled for necessary pregnancy weight gain but excess weight gain and postprandial hyperglycemia should not occur. Tight glycemic control is critical and postpartum glycemia should be monitored regularly.

Diagnostic Criteria for Diabetes

In a healthy individual, insulin helps to normalize the blood sugar level, which is maintained within the range of 70–100 mg/dL, at all times. When blood sugar level is elevated, it is known as hyperglycemia. Blood sugar level can fall below normal and is called hypoglycemia.

Table 12.18: Diagnostic criteria for blood sugar levels for normal persons and in prediabetes and diabetes.

Parameters	Normal blood sugar level	Prediabetes	Diabetes
Fasting Plasma Glucose (FPG) (mg/deciliter)	<100	100–125	>126
After 2 hours of 75 g glucose load or random plasma glucose in a symptomatic patient	<140	140–199	>200
Glycated hemoglobin (Hb A1c)	<6.0	5.7–6.4	≥6.5
Fasting: Fasting Plasma Glucose (FPG); (fasting for 8 hours with no calorie intake) 2-h PG (Plasma glucose): (2 hours glucose load with 75 g glucose with anhydrous form as per WHO) The unit—mmol/L—can also be used			

Source: American Diabetes Association (2020) Standards of Medical Care in Diabetes -2020. The journal of Clinical and applied Research and education Diabetes care 42(suppl 1): s12.

Chawla R, Madhu SV, Makkar BM, Ghosh S, Saboo B, Kalra S, On behalf of the RSSDI-ESI Consensus Group. 2020.

RSSDI-ESI Clinical Practice Recommendations for the Management of Type 2 Diabetes Mellitus 2020.

Hyperglycemia—when blood sugar level is >200 mg/dL (random)

Hypoglycemia—when blood sugar level is <70 mg/dL (random)

HbA$_{1c}$ and its significance: Glycosylated hemoglobin is formed when glucose residues bind to free amino terminals in α- and β-chains of hemoglobin. Glycosylation is a continuous process occurring throughout the 120-day lifespan of RBCs and depends upon plasma glucose concentration. Since the lifespan of RBC is 120 days, HbA1c value reflects the degree of blood glucose control during the previous 3 months. Normal HbA1c level is 4–6%. High HbA1c indicates poor glycemic control or there is risk of diabetic complication(s). Sometime, HbA$_{1c}$ test results may be misleading in case of anemia and use of supplements of vitamin C and E. High-cholesterol levels, kidney/liver disease may also affect the test. It may remain high even if blood glucose level returns to normal. However, a combination of diet, exercise, and medication can help to control blood glucose as well as glycosylated hemoglobin levels.

A1C test has greater advantage over fasting plasma glucose and oral glucose tolerance test (FPG and OGTT). it is more convenient and does not require fasting state. There is a requirement of taking two readings consequently to confirm the test, e.g., it is 7% in first and 6.8 in next then it confirms the presence of diabetes.

Hormonal Control of Blood Sugar

Blood sugar is under neuroendocrine control, regulated by many hormones and neurotransmitters. Hormones help to stabilize and maintain the appropriate concentration of glucose in the blood in physiological range, at all times. The hormones involved in regulation of blood sugar level are:

> Hormones involved in regulation of blood sugar level.
> 1. Insulin
> 2. Glucagon
> 3. Epinephrine
> 4. Glucocorticoids

Insulin: Insulin is the major hormone regulating the blood sugar levels. It is produced by the β-cells of the islets of Langerhans in the pancreas. It is released whenever blood glucose level is elevated after ingestion of food, primarily carbohydrate intake. Presence of carbohydrate in the duodenum causes release of gastrointestinal hormones, which increase the sensitivity of the β-cells to increased glucose concentration. Glucagon-like peptide-1 (GLP-1), a hormone, is secreted from the lower gut and is related to the secretion of insulin. It is a hormone that is mainly produced in enteroendocrine L cells of the gut and is secreted into the blood stream when food containing fat, protein hydrolysate and/or glucose enters the duodenum.

Insulin facilitates the entry of glucose into the cell by binding to specific receptors on the cells for glucose uptake from circulation and promotes utilization of glucose by the cell for energy production, and thus decreases blood glucose levels. Its role is more significant in skeletal muscles, liver, heart (vascular smooth muscle cells), kidney, adipose tissues, and brain because insulin is required for glucose to enter these cells. It also promotes the conversion of glucose into energy stores in the form of glycogen in muscles and liver and fat in adipose tissues (anabolic function of insulin). When blood glucose level returns to normal or falls further, insulin production ceases. The action of insulin is opposed by other hormones like glucagon, epinephrine or adrenaline, and norepinephrine, which play important roles in glucose homeostasis.

> **Research Glimpse:** Insulin resistance (IR) is a predisposing factor and best indicator of future diabetes. Insulin sensitivity in the peripheral tissues is decreased. Oxidative stress plays a key role in IR. It also has direct roles in development and progression of many chronic diseases, such as type II diabetes. Due to increased supply of glucose when carbohydrate intake, particularly refined carbohydrate/sugar, is high, mitochondria have more substrate available to make ATP. Thus, the mitochondria produce more of their natural byproduct of oxidative stress, i.e., ROS. This increased ROS damages the cell, proteins, lipids, etc. and induces further oxidative stress leading to inflammation. There is a link between inflammation, insulin resistance, and obesity. Free fatty acids (FFAs) are abundant in obesity and cause cellular dysfunction, especially in the mitochondria, which further result in impaired glucose utilization. Excess adipose tissue secretes cytokines, named adipokines, that are responsible for chronic inflammation. Chronic inflammation is a cause of many degenerative diseases including neurodegenerative diseases and heart disease. Because excess fat is the cause of these inflammatory problems, it is important to maintain a healthy weight, particularly healthy body composition. Visceral fat is strongly linked to metabolic syndrome and oxidative stress. Imbalance in utilization of fat and protein favors damaged protein accumulation over its degradation. Antioxidants improve insulin sensitivity, thus antioxidant vitamins like ascorbic acid (vitamin C) and tocopherols (vitamin E) have therapeutic role in neutralizing the oxidation being done by the radical. Ascorbic acid showed significant amelioration of oxidative stress and improvement in insulin sensitivity in muscle tissue.
>
> *Samantha H, Hsu WH. The etiology of oxidative stress in insulin resistance. Biomed J. 2017;40(5):257-62.*

Glucagon: It is produced by the alpha cells of islets of Langerhans in the pancreas and its action is antagonistic to insulin. Glucagon is secreted in response to low-blood glucose concentration, e.g., during fasting or starvation. It helps in raising blood glucose level by increasing the rate of glucose release from liver by stimulating glycogenolysis, i.e., breakdown of glycogen to glucose. At the same time, it inhibits glycogen synthesis in the liver. Glucagon does not act on muscle to release glucose because muscle cells lack glucagon receptor. It also enhances triacylglycerol degradation resulting in ketone bodies formation. It tends to induce hunger that generally makes a person eat and raises the blood glucose level (BGL). The cyclic actions of insulin and glucagon help to maintain the BGL. Glucagon and insulin ratio is crucial for maintaining blood sugar level. Ketone bodies and fatty acids serve as substrates to meet energy requirement.

Epinephrine: The effect of epinephrine on the liver is similar to that of glucagon. It is a stress hormone produced by the adrenal glands. It stimulates rapid breakdown of glycogen in liver to yield glucose and increases blood glucose level. It also inhibits insulin-mediated uptake of glucose by cells. Epinephrine secretion increases during stress, thereby helping to meet the extra demand for energy. In stressful conditions, more glucose is released from the liver. At the same time, there is a rise in growth hormone and cortisol levels. As a result, muscle and fat become less sensitive to insulin and more glucose is released in the bloodstream raising the BGL. Therefore, it is difficult to control BGL in stressful conditions in diabetics. Epinephrine also increases breakdown of body fat during fasting. During intense exercise, epinephrine promotes degradation of muscle glycogen and eventually the lactate levels in blood can increase.

Glucocorticoids: They are steroid hormones produced by the adrenal cortex. Cortisol is one of the hormones, which stimulates the liver to produce glucose from glycogen and from amino acids. It helps to maintain BGL and counteracts the action of insulin. It works during starvation or when glucose supply is not enough or when blood glucose level is low. Prolonged action of cortisol in stress leads to high blood sugar level.

Growth hormone: It is secreted by the anterior pituitary gland. It raises the blood glucose level by increasing the synthesis of glucose by the liver.

Main Causes of Diabetes

Heredity and aging are considered to be predisposing factors for diabetes; however, poor dietary pattern and physical inactivity are important factors driving the diabetes epidemic globally. Major causative factors are given in Figure 12.5. Other causes could be:

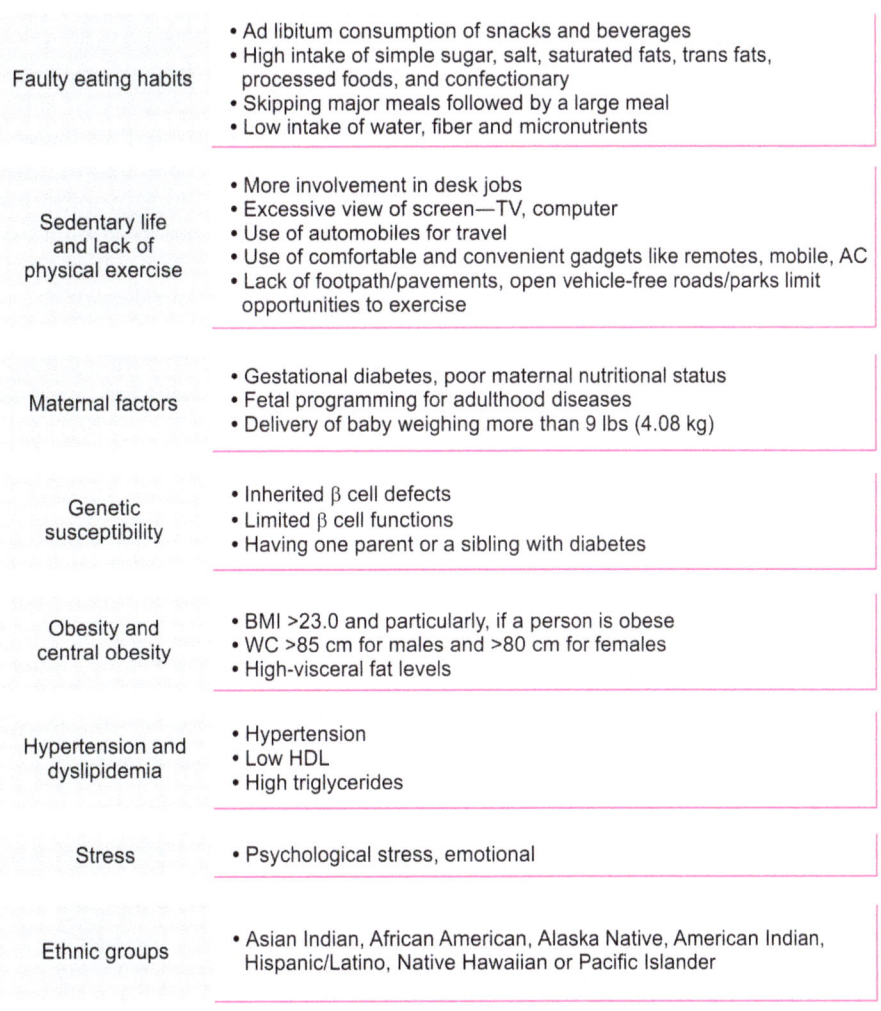

Fig. 12.5: Major causative factors of diabetes.

Genetic mutations: Monogenic diabetes is caused by mutations in a single gene that compromise the ability to produce insulin, e.g., neonatal diabetes and maturity-onset diabetes of the young. In cystic fibrosis, there is scarring of the pancreas that prevents the pancreas from making enough insulin. In hemochromatosis, excess iron is stored in the body. If the condition is not treated, the buildup of iron can damage the pancreas as well as other organs.

Hormonal problems: If excess of some hormones is produced by the body, it can result in insulin resistance and diabetes, for example—Cushing's syndrome in which too much cortisol is produced; acromegaly, which is caused by excess production of growth hormone; or hyperthyroidism when thyroid gland produces too much of thyroid hormone.

Damage to pancreas: Damage to pancreas can be caused by pancreatitis, pancreatic cancer or trauma, damaging the beta cells that are then unable to produce insulin in sufficient amounts, the consequence being diabetes. Removal of damaged pancreas also leads to diabetes as the beta cells are lost.

Medications: Some medications can either harm the beta cells or interfere with insulin's action. Examples are niacin, some diuretics, psychiatric drugs, some drugs prescribed for seizures, drugs prescribed for treatment of HIV, glucocorticoids that are prescribed to reduce inflammation for patients with rheumatoid arthritis, asthma, ulcerative colitis or lupus, and immunosuppressants that are prescribed for preventing rejection of a transplanted organ.

Health conditions: Polycystic ovary syndrome (PCOS) and acanthosis nigricans, depression also, increase the risk of diabetes.

Risk factors for gestational diabetes include overweight and obesity, too much weight gain during pregnancy, and/or a family history of diabetes.

Metabolic syndrome is a disorder (previously known as syndrome X) characterized by elevated fasting blood glucose, dyslipidemia, obesity, and high blood pressure. It is a cluster of conditions associated with insulin resistance. It is defined as having three or more of the following:

Abdominal obesity:

Waist circumference	≥85 cm for males and ≥82 cm for females
Fasting triglycerides	≥150 mg/dL
Fasting blood glucose	≥100 mg/dL
HDL cholesterol	<40 mg/dL for males and <50 mg/dL for females
Blood pressure	≥130/85 mm Hg

Persons with metabolic syndrome are at greater risk for developing type II diabetes and cardiovascular diseases (CVD).

Complications of Diabetes

Over a period of time, diabetes progressively leads to impairments and dysfunctioning of various organs, especially if blood glucose is not tightly controlled. These complications can occur in both type I and type II diabetes. These complications are a result of the effect of hyperglycemia on blood vessels, nerves, and organs.

Consequences of uncontrolled diabetes:

Increased risk of:
- Impairment in hearing
- Impairment in eyesight—diabetic retinopathy may lead to blindness
- Foot ulcers—risk of limb amputation—gangrene
- Peripheral neuropathy—loss of sensation in the nerves of extremities
- Kidney dysfunctioning—kidney failure
- Cardiovascular disease and stroke

There is overproduction as well as underutilization of glucose in hyperglycemia. Glucose is synthesized but not utilized by the liver and glucose uptake by muscles and adipose tissues is drastically reduced. In uncontrolled diabetes, glucose is excreted by the kidneys. Along with glucose, water is excreted and this loss of water can lead to dehydration. Hence, patients often complain of feeling thirsty or the need to drink water (polydipsia) and that a large volume of urine is excreted (polyuria).

In long-standing diabetes, there is slow development of many pathological conditions such as abnormalities in small arteries (microangiopathy—diabetic retinopathy and nephropathy) and abnormalities in large arteries (macroangiopathy—coronary heart disease and peripheral vascular disease) and diabetic neuropathy. These conditions involve organs where insulin is not required for entry of glucose and glucose levels are increased in these organs. Organs included are brain, peripheral nerve tissues, kidney, intestine, lens, and red blood cells and get affected by uncontrolled or long-standing diabetes.

When sugar levels are high in urine, urea and creatinine in plasma are good indicators to identify renal function. Urinary protein excretion (proteinuria) above 300 mg/day is indicative of diabetic nephropathy. Microalbuminuria is another sensitive test for the same.

Comorbidities are common in diabetes. These include hypertension, obesity, and dyslipidemia. Hence, during management, treatment for these morbidities along with diabetes is necessary.

Dietary Management of Diabetes

Management of diabetes is central to regulate the blood sugar level and prevent its complications. Diet and drugs as well as exercise play a critical role in diabetes. These are some of the principles of dietary management of diabetes and preventing its complications. Following the prescriptions given by the physician is essential, especially for persons on insulin therapy. Similarly, adhering to dietary prescriptions given by the dietitian is important.

Goals to be achieved by diabetics

Obesity	by 10% maintain normal BMI
Blood pressure	130/80 mm Hg
LDL	<100 mg/dL
HDL	>50 mg/dL
Triglycerides	<150 mg/dL
HbA1c	<7.0

1. Maintain desirable body weight if overweight or obese, attempt to reduce 5% at a time
2. Maintain tight control of blood sugar level and regularly monitor blood sugar level
3. Maintain regular timings for meal
4. Eat small servings at a time including wide range of foods
5. Consume 8–10 servings of fruits and vegetables
6. Follow 5–6 meal pattern rather than 2–3 large-size meals in a day
7. Consume nutrient-dense food, as they tend to prevent food craving and satisfy hunger
8. Consume complex carbohydrates rather than simple sugar in every meal/snack
9. Use the concept of glycemic index and glycemic load in selection of carbohydrate containing food.
10. Total carbohydrate intake of the day should be 50–55% of total calories, protein should contribute 15–20% of the calories (unless kidney function is impaired), and 25–30% should be supplied from fat.
11. Divide carbohydrate intake in different meals. Total carbohydrate distribution can be—25% in breakfast, 30% in lunch, 30% in dinner, and 15% in evening tea.
12. Use fiber-rich food that contains dietary fibers @14 g/1,000 kcal (Emphasize soluble fiber).
13. Use carbohydrate counting especially for those who are on insulin.
14. Add sufficient fat but low-fat diet is more favorable. Select fat sources that contain more of MUFA, PUFA, and EFA.
15. Saturated fat intake should be <7% of total calories.
16. Minimize intake of *trans* fat, as it helps to lower LDL cholesterol and increase HDL cholesterol.
17. Include protein food sources of high biological value. Consumption of high-quality protein delays blood sugar rise and supports synthesis of enzymes, hormones, and neurotransmitters, which can delay progression of disease and other cellular damage.
18. Reduce salt intake (sodium preferably should be ≤1,500 mg)
19. Add sufficient vitamins E, C, B_6 and zinc, chromium, and magnesium are crucial in diabetes. Also, include foods that provide antioxidants such carotenoids and flavonoids.
20. Snacks can be roasted Bengal gram, peanuts, nuts, and fresh whole fruits like apple, pear, berries, peaches, papaya, watemelon, muskmelon in a given amount, etc. rather than fried or confectionary items.
21. Maintain blood lipid profile, kidney profile within expected range.
22. Maintain regular pattern of exercise such as yoga, walking, and comfortable in gym under supervision (foot care is important).
23. Limit alcohol consumption to a moderate amount (one drink per day or less for adult women and two drinks per day or less for adult men).
24. Improve the quality of life by adopting good food habits, daily regimen of exercise, enough sleep, rest, and work. High stress may be detrimental.
25. Besides diet and physical activity behavior therapy also support achievement of target goal.

Foods to be avoided in diabetes	Foods to be restricted in diabetes	Foods to be used freely in diabetes
Glucose, sugar, honey, all sweets, chocolates, and candies	Potatoes, yam, arbi, sweet potatoes, mangoes, grapes, bananas, alcoholic beverages, fried foods, parathas, pooris, pakoras, mathris, deep fried foods, dry fruits, cakes, and pastries	Green leafy vegetables, tomatoes, cucumber, all gourd vegetables, e.g., *dudhi*, ash gourd, pumpkin, ridge gourd, cabbage, cauliflower, French beans, capsicum, bitter gourd, pointed gourd, cluster beans etc. Radish, soup, buttermilk, tea, and coffee without sugar

Hypoglycemia

Hypoglycemia is defined as a measurable glucose concentration <70 mg/dL (3.9 mmol/L). It is a threshold for neuroendocrine responses to falling glucose in people without diabetes. According to the American Diabetes Association (2018), there are three levels in hypoglycemia:

Level-1 hypoglycemia in hospitalized patients is defined as a measurable glucose concentration <70 mg/dL (3.9 mmol/L) but ≥54 mg/dL (3.0 mmol/L).

Level-2 hypoglycemia [defined as a blood glucose concentration <54 mg/dL (3.0 mmol/L)]. It is the threshold at which neuroglycopenic symptoms begin to occur and require immediate action to resolve the hypoglycemic event.

Level-3 hypoglycemia is defined as a severe event (<40 mg/dL) and characterized by altered mental and/or physical functioning that requires assistance from another person for recovery.

Hypoglycemia is experienced particularly in type I diabetes/stress, trauma, illness, or surgery. Hypoglycemia is very common in self-monitored individuals having type I diabetes marked by plasma glucose concentration of ≤70 mg/dL. However, in severe cases, it can be <40–50 mg/dL, which urgently requires medical treatment. Symptoms of hypoglycemia are shakiness, dizziness, sweating, hunger, clumsiness, and sudden behavior change. Hypoglycemia can impair judgment, behavior, and performance of physical tasks. Immediate attention and medication are essential. It can occur due to the following reasons:

- During or after strenuous exercise or indulging in excessive work or exercise than usual
- Delay or omission of a snack or main meal
- Eating insufficient carbohydrate or food
- Overdose of insulin or when insulin is at peak
- Overindulgence in alcohol followed by low-food intake
- Administration of excessive medication/surgery.

Hypoglycemia can be frightening as well as life-threatening. Mild hypoglycemia can be present when an individual feels shaky, is unable to concentrate and very irritable, and may cry for no reason. In severe hypoglycemia, the person may be more confused and may also need assistance from others. There may be risk of falling and accidents. It is necessary to instruct family members, friends, and schools or colleagues at the work place to give some carbohydrate-containing foods in such situations. Foods can be any of the two to three glucose biscuits or 3/4 cup orange juice or soft drink/a handful of raisins/six hard candies/toffees/two teaspoons of sugar or honey/1 cup skim milk. Basically, there is need for quick supply of glucose in the body to restore blood glucose level. Further medical advice needs to be sought.

Management of diabetes in different conditions is difficult. Dietary management including some nondietary management, physical exercise, relaxation, education and prescribed medication provides some support to deal with and lead an active and productive life. This will delay or minimize the complications. Lifestyle interventions and counseling work satisfactorily; however, medical advice and interventions cannot be ignored.

- Diabetes is chronic.
- Diabetes is degenerative.
- Diabetes is dreadful only when complications are difficult to handle.
- Diabetes does not require hospitalization unless linked with complications.
- Diabetes does not require any sick leave.
- Diabetes is manageable with daily regimen of simple diet, prescribed drugs, exercise, and sleep/relaxation.

Carbohydrate Counting

Carbohydrate counting is a technique for managing blood glucose levels. It is widely used in planning a meal when carbohydrate intake needs to be monitored and controlled as in case of diabetes and obesity. In this procedure, instead of calculating the total kilocalories, the amount of carbohydrate is calculated. One carbohydrate serving is equal to 15 grams of carbohydrates. By keeping track of the amount of carbohydrates a person eats and setting a maximum limit on the total amount of carbohydrates to be consumed, he/she can keep blood glucose levels in the target range. Carbohydrate counting can help a diabetic person to choose what and how much to eat and match one's insulin requirements with the amount of carbohydrate that is eaten and/or consumed through beverages. It is valuable for persons with diabetes especially those who are on insulin or who use insulin pump or for those persons who find it difficult to control their blood glucose. Overall, it may be used more by type I (insulin-dependent) diabetics who do self-monitoring of blood glucose regularly and frequently. For many people with diabetes, it can be effective for managing the condition. Once the person has mastered this, it will lead to better blood glucose control, greater flexibility, and freedom of lifestyle. It is an approach that requires time and effort with guidance from a diabetes healthcare professional. In order to do it successfully, the person has to learn all about carbohydrates, understand portion sizes, know the exchange list well, learn how to adjust carbohydrate intake to the insulin, and be willing to spend time (and be able) to do the required mathematical calculations as well as being dedicated to monitoring blood glucose levels frequently. Hence, persons interested in carbohydrate counting should consult a dietitian.

Carbohydrate counting is a method used to manage blood sugar level by dietary means. It provides more options in the diet. In this method, food items are so chosen so that the desired amount of carbohydrate in the meal can be obtained. It is useful for diabetic people. In the food exchange list, carbohydrate content of each food group is given. Small amount of sweets can also be adjusted within the selected range of carbohydrate in the meals in a day.

Carbohydrate counting can be taught to persons once they have become very familiar with exchange lists and are consuming healthy balanced diets, and can control their blood glucose. At this stage, this will help them to plan their diets by focusing on the carbohydrates consumed. Those who monitor blood glucose regularly and keep a record of blood glucose as well as the type and amount of carbohydrate eaten, the insulin dosage or the oral hypoglycemic agent are likely to benefit substantially.

HYPERTENSION

Hypertension is the term used to indicate high blood pressure. Blood pressure is a measurement of the force exerted by blood on the arterial walls as the heart pumps blood and it circulates through the circulatory system. Blood 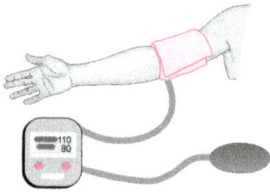 pressure readings (measured using a sphygmomanometer) are usually given as two numbers (written as 120/80 mm Hg):
- Systolic blood pressure—120 mm Hg
- Diastolic blood pressure—80 mm Hg.

Systolic blood pressure is the top/first number that measures the pressure when the heart contracts and diastolic blood pressure is the bottom/second number, which measures pressure when the heart relaxes.

The heart contracts with each beat, followed by constriction of arteries and a rise in blood pressure, thereafter the heart relaxes between two beats. Systolic blood pressure measures the pressure when the heart contracts and diastolic blood pressure measures pressure when the heart relaxes between two consecutive heart beats.

Hypertension is a pathological condition in which either systolic or diastolic or both are elevated. When a person's blood pressure is ≥140/90 mm Hg most of the time, he/she is said to have high blood pressure/hypertension. If the blood pressure is ≥120/80 mm Hg but less than 140/90 mm Hg, the condition is called prehypertension. Prehypertension predisposes a person to develop high blood pressure (HBP).

2020 International Society of Hypertension Global Hypertension Practice Guidelines issued the following guidelines for categorizing blood pressure:
- **Normal:** Less than 130/85 mm Hg;
- **High-normal:** Systolic 130–139 *and* diastolic 80–89 mm Hg;
- **Grade I:** Systolic between 140 and 159 *or* diastolic between 90 and 99 mm Hg;
- **Grade II:** Systolic equal or more than 160 *and* diastolic equal or more than 100 mm Hg;

- Prevalence of hypertension is high enough to be of concern in India, as per figures reported in NHFS-V (2020) for 22 states. Percentage of women with elevated blood pressure is 15.7–34.5 and for men the prevalence is 15.4–41.6.

Causes of Hypertension

In most cases, there is no known cause for hypertension and this is known as essential hypertension. High blood pressure (HBP) can be a result of another medical condition or some medications. This is known as secondary hypertension, which can be due to chronic renal disease, disorders of the adrenal gland such as Cushing's syndrome, preeclampsia in pregnancy, and hyperparathyroidism.

Heredity and advanced age play a role in increasing the risk of hypertension. High intake of sodium increases the risk of high BP, as many commonly consumed foods like chips, pickles, papads, sauces, etc. contain good amount of sodium. Low intake of magnesium, calcium, and potassium may alter the ratio of sodium to these minerals and increase the risk of HBP. Frequent intake of alcohol and cola beverages aggravate the problem.

Stress increases the risk of high BP. There are many physical, psychological, and environmental stresses, which can contribute to the occurrence of high BP. Physical stress can be due to overwork and intense exercise beyond the capacity of the body for a long period. Psychological stress may include emotional issues lingering over a period of time. Environmental factors might be related to the side effects of certain medicines, financial issues, surroundings, lack of movements where the person is residing like noise, gas, etc. Overweight and obesity and diabetes and their associated disorders are often associated with hypertension. With prevalence of obesity in younger age groups including children, the risk of hypertension also increases.

Consequences of High Blood Pressure

Initially, the person whose BP is high feels very restless, may exhibit trembling, complain of a headache and confusion and pounding in chest or neck. When blood pressure remains high for a longer period, the arteries become less flexible, harder, and narrowed. Less blood flows and risk of damage to the inner lining of arteries increases. More cholesterol and fat tend to get deposited inside the arterial wall, which further reduces the blood flow. The heart is not relaxed enough between two beats and the heart needs to work harder to pump the blood for the body. As a result, diastolic blood pressure also increases. High diastolic blood pressure increases the risk of cardiovascular disease (CVD) that may be due to the damage caused in heart muscles or blood vessels. HBP can also cause plaque in the arterial wall to break away from the arterial wall. This ruptured plaque can act like blood clot and cut off the blood flow. Persistent hypertension may damage the functioning of heart that can be fatal. In case of high blood pressure, less waste is filtered from the blood, because of adverse effect on kidney function.

Persistent HBP, when untreated or uncontrolled for a long period of time, may lead to several serious complications like atherosclerosis, ischemic heart disease, heart failure, stroke, and kidney problem. These problems get worsened when high blood pressure is present along with the diabetes. It tends to be the major cause of hospitalization and deaths in the world.

Measures to Reduce High Blood Pressure

Since high blood pressure seriously affects physical, physiological, professional, personal, and economical life of the person, it is advisable to take some judicious measures like simple dietary changes and modifications in the lifestyle in order to prevent the onset of hypertension, control it and minimize its associated risks. Dietary and lifestyle modification are found useful for preventing and controlling high BP:

Dietary Modifications

- **DASH (Dietary Approaches to Stop Hypertension):** DASH diet has been found to be a good approach. It is an eating plan that emphasizes consumption of fruits, vegetables, and low sodium, low-fat dairy foods, low amounts of saturated fat, total fat, and cholesterol to reduce blood pressure. The DASH diet includes whole grains, poultry, fish, and nuts. It employs reduced amounts of fats, red meats, sweets, and sugared beverages. It includes the foods rich in potassium, calcium and omega 3, and magnesium.
- **Reduce sodium intake:** Common salt is sodium chloride. 1 g salt contains 400 mg sodium. WHO advocates that sodium intake of more than 2 g/day and low potassium intake is a risk for hypertension. People with hypertension can have 1500 mg. Many food additives like cooking soda, baking soda, and ajinomoto are basically sodium salts. Pickles, papad, and sauces contain salt as preservatives. Cheese, processed food, and salted snacks such as biscuits, chips, popcorn, instant noodles, instant soups, canned foods, etc. contain considerable amount of sodium because salt is used in their preparation for taste and preservation. It is not advisable to add salt to food at the table while eating. It is advisable to restrict or totally avoid consumption of foods containing high salt or sodium. Use of potassium salt or low-sodium salt instead of common salt is beneficial.
- **Ensure adequate intake of calcium, magnesium, and potassium:** It can be done by inclusion of low-fat dairy products except cheese to add calcium; green leafy vegetables for magnesium. Fruits and vegetables are rich in potassium such as bananas, watermelon, potatoes, tomatoes, oranges, sweet lime, leafy vegetables, milk, soya bean, and almonds. Eating three to six servings of these foods would ensure sufficient potassium intake and regulate blood pressure.
- **Increase intake of PUFA:** Foods rich in omega-3, EPA, and DHA like fish oil are found to attenuate pathogenesis of renin-dependent hypertension.
- **Reduction in intake of sugar and simple carbohydrates:** Though it does not directly affect the BP but it increases risk of overweight/obesity and many preparations usually contain more salt and fat.

- **Addition of herbs** like coriander, mint or garlic or lemon juice improves the taste and flavor and reduces the need to add more salt.

Lifestyle Modification

- Low-intensity physical exercise like brisk walking for about 30 minutes daily.
- *Relaxation*: Relaxation techniques like breathing exercise, listening favorite music and friend and indulging in hobbies.
- *Yoga practice*: Perform yoga daily under guidance.
- *Behavior modification*: Avoidance of hyper-reactivity, anger, rage, yelling, and acceptance of present situation.
- Maintain normal body weight preferably having BMI 18.5–23.0 kg/m² for adults.
- Limit alcohol intake and smoking.
- Eat regularly at the same time everyday.
- When feeling change in BP, measure the BP, relax and review reasons, and follow remedial measures soon.
- Learn the art of managing time and overcome the habit of procrastination.

OSTEOPOROSIS

Osteoporosis is a metabolic bone disorder resulting from an imbalance of bone remodeling due to the rate of bone resorption being higher than the rate of bone formation. Metabolic bone disease is a term that covers several bone abnormalities caused by many disorders/conditions, e.g., osteomalacia in adults, rickets in children osteitis fibrosa cystica, and Paget's disease of bone. This gives rise to low bone mass and deterioration in its microstructure leading to pain and inflammation. According to WHO (2003), "Osteoporosis is a systemic skeletal disease characterized by low bone density and microarchitectural deterioration of bone tissue with a consequent increase in bone fragility". Since the bones become fragile and porous, they may break easily. In the early stages, osteoporosis is asymptomatic (hence is known as 'silent thief') and is not diagnosed, but becomes clinically evident when the person suffers from a fracture. It is a silent disease like dyslipidemia and hypertension, but is a major cause of high morbidity and disability particularly in elder population. If a person takes steps to keep the bones healthy, the risk of developing osteoporosis can be reduced.

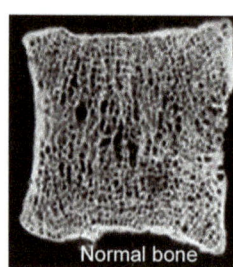 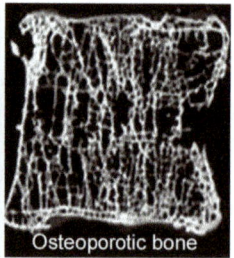

Normal bone   Osteoporotic bone

Osteoporosis can be classified into primary (Type I) and secondary (Type II) osteoporosis. Primary/type I osteoporosis is associated with aging in both sexes due to degeneration of both trabecular and cortical bones. It occurs in women soon after menopause (postmenopausal osteoporosis) and in men during and after middle-age. Poor dietary habits, nutritional deficits, and lack of exercise during the growing years limit the bone density even at younger age. Such habits continue into adulthood.

However, women, particularly postmenopausal women, are at much higher risk due to their low peak bone mass. Around menopause, women have lower estrogen level, due to which they are at relatively higher risk. Secondary osteoporosis may set in due to certain medications or certain medical conditions like hyperparathyroidism.

Peak bone mass is usually attained around 30 years of age and is largely associated with adequate intake of calcium and vitamin D along with sufficient exercise for building up of reserves. Thereafter, there is gradual loss of bone mass that is accelerated at menopause in case of women. The loss is approximately 0.6% in the 60–69-year age group; it increases to 1.1% among 70–79-year-old women, with a further increase to 2.1% per year in those above 80 years of age. Thus, the risk of fractures increases progressively with age and is associated with significant morbidity.

Risk Factors for Osteoporosis

Nutritional factors, physical exercise, age, gender, and lifestyle factors predominantly influence the bone density. Several genetic and environmental factors determine bone health and bone mass. People of all races and ethnicity are prone to osteoporosis and fractures. However, various studies have shown that Asians have lower bone mass and blacks have more bone mass than whites. Prolonged use of some medication can increase bone loss, such as oral or high-dose inhaled corticosteroids, thyroid hormone replacement, and aromatase inhibitors. Complications of osteoporotic fractures, particularly at the vertebrae and hips, can increase the risk of mortality.

Some risk factors are unchangeable or unmodifiable whereas some are modifiable:

Unchangeable risk factors	Changeable or modifiable risk factors
Race/ethnicity (white/Asian descent)	Diabetes
Sex/gender	Tobacco use
Age	Anorexia nervosa, calcium intake, vitamin D status
Family history	Sedentary lifestyle
Body frame size (smaller frame, thin-boned frame tends to be associated with higher risk)	Excessive alcohol consumption
Hormonal factors, e.g., lower level of sex hormones, i.e., estrogen in postmenopausal women, testosterone levels in men, excess thyroid hormone, overactive parathyroid or adrenal glands	Physical exercise such as resistance exercise increases bone mass
Dietary factors including low calcium intake throughout life especially during accumulation of peak bone mass, eating disorders, conditions associated with malabsorption of nutrients	Increase dietary calcium intake, improve vitamin D status, treatment of pathological conditions
Medical: Long-term use of corticosteroids, treatment for cancer, immobility	Use of some drugs or antacids which increases urinary calcium excretion

Symptoms of Osteoporosis

There are typically no symptoms in the early stages of bone loss. But once your bones have been weakened by osteoporosis, you might have signs and symptoms that include:
- Back pain, caused by a fractured or collapsed vertebra
- Loss of height over time
- A stooped posture
- A bone that breaks much more easily than expected or fracture.

Causes of Osteoporosis

In some cases, spinal fractures can occur even if you have not fallen. The bones that make up your spine (vertebrae) can weaken to the point of crumbling, which can result in back pain, lost height, and a hunched forward posture.

Nutritional Factors

Adequacy of nutrient intake sustains muscle strength and reduces the risk of falls and fractures. Intake of calcium and vitamin D before and during puberty is crucial because maximum growth and development of bones occur by 30 years of age. Bone mass has been found to be positively associated with energy and protein intake. These nutrients not only build up the bone reserves, they also maintain the bone mass, prevent occurrence of osteoporosis, and are useful in the treatment of osteoporosis. During the process of bone formation, collagen secretion occurs and hydroxyapatite is formed, which require adequate supplies of calcium, phosphorus, protein, vitamin C, and vitamin K. Deficiency of any one of these nutrients restricts the process of bone formation and adversely affects bone density. The following nutrients have important roles in bone health and prevention of osteoporosis:

Calcium deficiency: Calcium is critical for bone formation. Its intestinal absorption requires parathyroid hormone (PTH) and vitamin D, i.e., D3. Calcitriol (D3) improves calcium absorption particularly in prepubertal and postpubertal periods in women, but is less effective in postmenopausal women. In postmenopausal years, PTH level increases due to low-estrogen level, resulting in bone loss. Calcium intake reduces PTH activity.

Blood calcium level and parathyroid hormone (PTH) are also very critical in maintaining bone density. Low-blood calcium level tends to increase PTH, which results in osteoclast activity (resorption of bone). In order to maintain blood calcium level, calcium is withdrawn from bone bank and bones become weak and porous.

Low-estrogen level reduces the response of osteoblasts (formation of bones) to PTH. It is advocated that calcium (500 mg) and vitamin D (700 IU) supplements may reduce the risk of fracture and improve BMD. Calcium supplements may be advised by physicians, if calcium intake is low. Calcium malate has been found to be better absorbed as compared to calcium citrate or calcium carbonate. However, high dose of malate reduces absorption of other minerals like zinc and magnesium. Excessive use of vitamin D supplement may induce calcification of soft tissues (kidney). Calcium absorption is reduced in case of milk alkali syndrome, anemia, constipation, and consumption of foods containing oxalates and phytates like spinach, sesame seeds.

Absorption of calcium is crucial and the body's ability to absorb calcium and other minerals is largely influenced by availability of HCl in the stomach. HCl secretion reduces with age, thus calcium availability is reduced. It is important that as a person ages, calcium intakes must be adequate. If dairy products are being used as a source, they should be low-fat dairy products. If supplements are used, care should be taken that intake is not excessive. The Health and Medicine Division of the National Academies of Sciences, Engineering and Medicine, USA previously known as the Institute of Medicine has recommended that total calcium intake including both dietary sources and supplements should not exceed 2,000 mg per day for persons above 50 years of age.

Adequacy of vitamin D status is important, particularly in persons who are house bound and/or those who are not exposed enough to sunlight. For such individuals, it is possible that the physician prescribes a vitamin D supplement.

Excess of phosphorus: Most foods are rich in phosphorus excess. Ratio of calcium to phosphorus is important to be effective. If there is imbalance in the Ca:P ratio, phosphorus stimulates PTH secretion. Thus, it is essential to consume calcium-rich foods like milk or curd with meals or other foods to maintain bone health.

Magnesium deficiency: More than 50% of the body's magnesium is present in bone tissue. It serves as a cofactor for several enzymes and is useful in bone cellular functioning and bone fluids. Low magnesium in the body deter the absorption of calcium and make vitamin D supplementation less effective for bone health.

> Phosphoric acid from soft drink is a cause of bone loss even in teenagers particularly when calcium supply is inadequate. Also, soft drinks may replace milk intake in diets of young persons.

Vitamin K: Vitamin K plays an important role in formation of osteocalcin, which is a bone-specific protein (Gla protein) made by osteoblasts and needed for maturation of bones. Serum osteocalcin is released into the circulation from the matrix during bone resorption and, therefore, is considered a marker of bone turnover and indicates risk of hip fracture. Vitamin K is also found in most foods. However, vitamin K2 rich foods like nat to or fermented vegetables are more effective in bone health. Optimal intake helps in maintaining calcium homeostasis, bone health, and reduction in risk of fractures.

Protein: Adequate protein (1 g/day) is required for bone formation. Positive effect of protein on bone health is linked with adequate intake of calcium during growth period during childhood and adolescents. Earlier, high-protein intake and animal protein were associated with increased urinary loss of calcium. However, it is also related to the type of protein and amino acid composition. It has been estimated that for a 10-g increase in dietary protein, urinary calcium increases by 16 mg. However, "western type" diet may be another factor. Other nutrients found in the protein sources, e.g., phosphorus, potassium, calcium, and phytoactives, such as isoflavones, antioxidants, salt, oxalate, phytates, and caffeine, can influence the effects of animal and plant food sources of protein. Increasing intake of purified protein, both plant and animal sources, increases renal net acid excretion leading to increased urinary calcium. Protein replenishment in patients with hip fracture can improve not only BMD, but also muscle mass and strength. Good quality protein intake along with good amount of calcium and vitamin D intake is beneficial for bone health.

Other nutrients: **Fluoride** is incorporated into hydroxyapatite, and increases the hardness of bones. **Copper** is needed for cross-linking of collagen and elastin molecules. **Manganese** is required for biosynthesis of mucopolysaccharides in bone matrix formation. **Vitamin C** plays a role in formation and maturation of collagen. **Zinc** is present in enzymes needed for collagen synthesis and osteoblast activity. **High-sodium** intake along with low-calcium intake increases the risk of osteoporosis because it may increase urinary calcium loss. It is not always the same case as linked with body mass index also.

> **Research Glimpse:** Boron is essential for the growth and maintenance of bone; improves wound healing; and impacts the body's use of estrogen, testosterone, and vitamin D along with other functions. Boron supplementation reduced the daily urinary excretion of calcium in women by 44% and increased vitamin D levels. It improves absorption of magnesium and deposition in bones. The mineral has been to be protective against osteoarthritis (OA) with intake of usually 3–10 mg/d. Low-boron level was found in femur heads, bones, and synovial fluid of OA patients compared with individuals without OA.
>
> *Pizzomo L. Nothing Boring about Boron. Integr Med (Encinitas). 2015;14(4):35-48.*

Isoflavones

Genistein and other isoflavones have estrogen-like activity and may be important for bone health. Inadequate nutrient intakes may not be always the cause for low BMD but utilization of nutrients is also important. Intake and utilization are often limited by aging, smoking, caffeine and alcohol consumption, diabetes, chronic renal failure or gastrointestinal malabsorption, all of which can contribute to pathogenesis of osteoporosis.

> **Research Glimpse:** Bone metabolism is affected by mechanical, genetic, and environmental factors and plays a major role in osteoporosis. Though influence of environmental pollution on the occurrence of osteoporosis is still not clear, pollutants containing heavy metals could affect bone mass. In this study, 65 osteoarthritic patients underwent for biopsies to identify heavy metals accumulation in bone tissues. Bone head biopsies were studied by BioQuant-Osteo software, scanning electron microscopy, and energy dispersive X-ray microanalysis. Lead, cadmium, and chromium accumulation were observed. This study sheds new light on the pathogenesis of osteoporosis, as these elements could play a role in the development of osteoporosis at cellular/molecular and epigenetic level.
>
> *Scimeca M, Feola M, Romano L, et al. Heavy metals accumulation affects bone microarchitecture in osteoporotic patients. Environ Toxicol. 2017;32(4):1333-42.*

Physical Activity

Besides good nutrition, regular physical exercise is very important for building bone and also helps to prevent bone loss. Physical activity and exercise across the lifespan help to preserve bone health. Physical exercise is effective in stimulating osteogenesis, i.e., formation of bone-forming cells. Stresses from muscles contraction and maintaining body weight in upright position against the pull of gravity also stimulate osteoblast function.

Two types of exercise affect bone and muscle strength. These are weight-bearing and aerobic exercises, e.g., walking, climbing stairs, jogging, skipping rope, running, and Tai Chi. Weight-bearing exercises increase bone remodeling and strength and can help to limit the progress of bone loss. They affect mainly bones in the legs, hips, and lower spine. Walking and running are easy to do. Balance exercises like Tai Chi help to reduce the risk of falls especially as a person gets older. The other types of exercises are strength and resistance exercise. These exercises help to strengthen the muscles and bones in the arms and upper spine. These are done with load (weight lifting) and without load (swimming and cycling). These stimulate specific sites in the body and tend to improve muscle mass and bone density.

Exercise intensity is also important. Health outcome of various exercises depends upon FITT (Frequency, Intensity, Time, and Type). Also, one should combine strength training exercises with weight-bearing and balance exercises. Targeted bone loading exercises favorably affect the bone health and helpful in prevention and treatment of osteoporosis. It is important to remember that discontinuing in exercise can reverse its beneficial effects. Exercise is beneficial regardless of the age when the person starts exercising, but starting early enough when a person is young and continuing to exercise throughout life are most beneficial. Exercises like swimming, cycling, and exercising on machines are beneficial for cardiovascular health but do not have much benefit for bone health.

> **Laboratory laurel:** This cross-sectional study was done on 2,401 older patients at the Geriatric Center, University College Hospital, Ibadan. Sociodemographic characteristics, anthropometric indices, and physical and lifestyle habits were assessed. Point prevalence of osteoporosis was 56.9% (males = 43.7% and females = 65.8%). Factors significantly with osteoporosis were increasing age, female sex (the odds of having osteoporosis with yearly increase in age was 6.9%), lack of formal education, lack of engagement in occupational activities, and living with relatives/friends. Other significant factors were receiving social support from relatives/friends, nonparticipation in sporting activities at younger ages, prolonged use of medications for peptic ulcer disease, and hospitalization on or after the age of 60 years and asthenic build.
>
> *Alonge TO, Adebusoye LA, Ogunbode AM, et al. Factors associated with osteoporosis among older patients at the Geriatric Centre in Nigeria: a cross-sectional study. South African Family Practice. 2017;59(3):1-7.*

Lifestyle Factors

Sedentary lifestyle is commonly associated with poor dietary habits, low nutrient intake, and lack of physical exercise. Alcohol consumption, smoking, and caffeine intake through coffee and cola consumption further deteriorate the osteoporotic condition because they limit the intestinal absorption of calcium. Also, menstrual dysfunction and anorexia in young girls have been shown to be associated with low bone mass.

Prevention and Control of Osteoporosis

Osteoporosis is a noncommunicable disease and is an inevitable episode of aging. However, osteoporosis and fractures are not directly linked with aging or low BMD as fractures can occur in otherwise normal persons. Elder persons are at greater risk and often suffer from other compounding factors, which can increase the chances of falls and fractures. These may be poor eye sight, diabetes, and renal disorders.

> **Laboratory laurel:** The investigators assessed prevalence of osteopenia and osteoporosis among 1,022 Saudi men aged ≥50 years and identified factors associated with osteoporosis/osteopenia. Anthropometric parameters and biomarkers were measured. Bone densitometry was assessed using dual X-ray absorptiometry (DEXA) to measure BMD levels. A structured questionnaire was used to assess sociodemographic and lifestyle factors. Prevalence of osteopenia was 40.7% and that of osteoporosis was 9.3%. Factors significantly associated with osteopenia were low educational level and low BMI, and factors significantly associated with osteoporosis were old age, low BMI, smoking, and a family history of fragility fractures.
>
> *Mohammed J, Farsi A, Merdad LA, et al. Osteoporosis, Osteopenia and their Associated Risk Factors among Saudi Males. Int J Osteoporosis Metab Disord. 2018;11(1):14-22.*

Depression, poor dietary intake, and poor orientation and arrangement of furniture in the home can cause falls and fractures in elders and others.

Nutritional strategies are important because they are well tolerated, effective, and easily modifiable. Following the guidelines given below on a regular basis, from childhood, during adolescence, and particularly in old age, may reduce the risk of osteoporosis and fractures. These may also be helpful in dealing with osteoporosis along with medical treatment.

- Regular consumption of milk and milk products
- Regular intake of foods rich in calcium, protein, and vitamin K
- Avoid smoking and cola drinks
- Regular exposure to sun to ensure adequate vitamin D status
- Regular exercise to maintain integrity of bone tissues and BMD
- Regular checkup of BMD after the age of 50 or 60 years.

Group education for making behavioral change with regard to lifestyle has been found to affect significant positive impact on making healthy decisions and improve bone health and other aspects of life. With advancement in medical science, some anabolic therapies are being found useful in improving the bone density.

> **Laboratory laurel:** This systematic review and meta-analysis evaluated the effects of dietary protein intake alone and with calcium, with/without vitamin D (Ca ± D) on bone health measures in adults. Sixteen randomized controlled trials and 20 prospective cohort studies that had focused on the effects of "high-versus-low" protein intake or synergistic effect of calcium with/without vitamin D with dietary protein on bone health outcomes were reviewed. The reviewers stated that there was moderate evidence to suggest that higher protein intake may have a protective effect on lumbar spine (LS) bone mineral density (BMD) compared with lower protein intake (net percentage change: 0.52%; 95% CI: 0.06%, 0.97%, I2: 0%; n = 5) but no effect on total hip (TH), femoral neck (FN), or total body BMD or bone biomarkers. There was limited evidence in relation to the effect of protein with Ca and/or D on LS BMD, TH BMD, or forearm fractures. For FN BMD and overall fractures, there was no conclusive evidence vitamin D. The authors concluded that "current evidence shows no adverse effects of higher protein intakes. Although there were positive trends on BMD at most bone sites, only the LS showed moderate evidence to support benefits of higher protein intake" and "high-quality, long-term studies are needed to clarify dietary protein's role in bone health".
>
> *Shams-White MM, Chung M, Du M, et al. Dietary protein and bone health: a systematic review and meta-analysis from the National Osteoporosis Foundation. Am J Clin Nutr. 2017;105(6):1528-43.*

RAPID FIRE

1. Give your view on dual burden of malnutrition.
2. What is the role of protein and vitamin A in PEM?
3. Differentiate kwashiorkor and marasmus on any four major characteristics.
4. What is dose of vitamin A given in prophylaxis program?
5. Define hematopoietic nutrients and name them.
6. Which nutrient deficiencies are related to nutritional anemia, name them?
7. Define hemoglobin, ferritin, and transferrin and one function of each.
8. Define goiter and goitrogenic substances.
9. What is the difference between overweight and obesity in terms of BMI?
10. What roles school, parents, and media can play in curbing the childhood obesity?
11. Suggest four foods which can be included and four foods which need to be excluded in case of hypertension.
12. Name the organization of which guidelines are followed internationally for assessing hypertension and diabetes.
13. What are the goals to maintain in diabetes and if not what are the risks?
14. What is hypoglycemia and how will you manage it in emergency?
15. Give list of nutrients important to prevent osteoporosis.

EXERCISE

1. Find the 15 children having PEM, vitamin A deficiency, and anemia in your living area based on clinical features.
2. Meet 15 persons having at least two diseases like obesity, diabetes, osteoporosis, and hypertension. Find out the cause and effect on their life and what changes they have made in their diet and exercise pattern in their daily routine.

3. Design a guideline for preventing 4 diet-related diseases in adults and 2 in children.
4. Suggest 4 Government programmes to your community to improve their nutritional status.

SUGGESTED READING

1. Abstracts of the 2nd Joint Meeting of the European Calcified Tissue Society and The International Bone and Mineral Society. 25-29 June 2005, Geneva, Switzerland. Bone. 2005;36 (Suppl) 2:S103-479.
2. Agarwal KN, Saxena A, Bansal AK, et al. Physical growth assessment in adolescence. Indian Pediatr. 2001;38(11):1217-35.
3. Alamri NS, Hussain AH, Alzein EH, et al. Leptin as a Potential Biomarker for Childhood Obesity. EC Paediatrics. 2017;3(5):435-46.
4. American Diabetes Association. Classification and diagnosis of diabetes: standards of medical care in diabetes. Diabetes Care. 2019;42(Supplement 1):S13-S28.
5. American Diabetes Association. Diabetes care in the hospital: Standards of medical care in diabetes—2018. Diabetes Care. 2018;41(Suppl 1):S144-S151.
6. Benedetti MG, Furlini G, Zati A et al. The effectiveness of physical exercise on bone density in osteoporotic patients. BioMed Res Int. 2018;2018:1-10.
7. Benjamin C. Management of protein-energy malnutrition—An update. J Pediatr Gastroenterol Nutr. 1998;27(2):243.
8. Berkey CS, Rockett HR, Field AE, et al. Sugar-added beverages and adolescent weight change. Obes Res. 2004;12(5):778-88.
9. Bhave S, Bavdekar A, Otiv M. Recommendations:-IAP National Task Force for Childhood Prevention of Adult Diseases: Childhood Obesity. Indian Pediatrics. 2004;41(6):559-75.
10. Bhor N. (2018). A Call for Development of a Growth Standard to Measure Malnutrition of School-Age Children. Working Paper No. 11 Research Area: Development Azim Premji University. [Online] Available from https://azimpremjiuniversity.edu.in/SitePages/pdf/APU-181951-Working-Paper-Series-11-21.05.2018.pdf. [Last accessed September, 2019].
11. Black RE, Laxminarayan R, Temmerman M, et al. Reproductive, Maternal, Newborn, and Child Health: Disease Control Priorities, 3rd edition (Volume 2). Washington (DC): The International Bank for Reconstruction and Development/The World Bank; 2016.
12. Bull FC et al. Guidelines on Physical Activity and Sedentary Behaviour World Health Organization, 2020.
13. Capacci S, MazzocchiM, Shankar B, et al. (2013). The triple burden of malnutrition in Europe and Central Asia: a multivariate analysis FAO Regional Office for Europe and Central Asia: Policy Studies on Rural Transition No. 2013-7. [Online] Available from http://www.fao.org/3/CA1810EN/ca1810en.pdf. [Last accessed September, 2019].
14. Cederholm T, Jensen GL, Correia MITD, et al. GLIM criteria for the diagnosis of malnutrition—A consensus report from the global clinical nutrition community. Clin Nutr. 2019;38(1):1-9.
15. Chawla R, Madhu SV, Makkar BM, Ghosh S, Saboo B, Kalra S. On behalf of the RSSDI-ESI Consensus Group. RSSDI-ESI Clinical Practice Recommendations for the Management of Type 2 Diabetes Mellitus 2020.
16. Food and Agriculture Organization of the United Nations. (2006). The double burden of malnutrition case studies from six developing countries. FAO nutrition paper 84. [Online] Available from http://www.fao.org/3/a0442e/a0442e00.pdf. [Last accessed September, 2019].
17. Gulati S, Anoop Misra A. Sugar intake, obesity, and diabetes in India. Nutrients. 2014; 6(12): 5955-74.
18. Gupta Jain S, Puri S, Misra A, et al. Effect of oral cinnamon intervention on metabolic profile and body composition of Asian Indians with metabolic syndrome: a randomized double-blind control trial. Lipids Health Dis. 2017;16(1):113.
19. Gupte S, Gupte RK, Gupte R. Iron deficiency anemia: Management and prevention in children. JK Science. 2001;3(4):160-5.
20. Hetzel BS. (1993). The Prevention and Control of Iodine Deficiency Disorders—Nutrition. [Online] Available from http://www.unscn.org/layout/modules/resources/files/Policy_paper_No_3.pdf. [Last accessed September, 2019].
21. Hochkogler CM, Hoi JK, Lieder B, et al. Cinnamyl isobutyrate decreases plasma glucose levels and total energy intake from a standardized breakfast: A randomized, crossover intervention. Mol Nutr Food Res. 2018;62(17):e1701038.
22. https://www.cdc.gov/nccdphp/dnpao/growthcharts/who/recommendations/development.htm
23. https://www.nhp.gov.in/national-vitamin-a-prophylaxis-program_pg
24. Hypertension Study Group. Prevalence, awareness, treatment and control of hypertension among elderly in Bangladesh and India: a multicentric study. Bull World Health Organ. 2001;79(6):490-500.
25. ICCIDD, UNICEF, WHO. Assessment of iodine deficiency disorders and monitoring their elimination: A guide for programme managers ,3rd edition. Geneva: World Health Organization; 2007.
26. IC HEALTH supported by Ministry of Health And Family Welfare, Government of India and World Health Organization. National Cardiovascular Disease Database, Sticker No. SE / 04/ 233208. [Online] Available from http://www.searo.who.int/india/topics/cardiovascular_diseases/NCD_Resources_National_CVD_database-Final_Report.pdf. [Last accessed September, 2019].
27. Icmr Guidelines for Management of Type 2 Diabetes 2018, Indian Council of Medical Research.
28. IDF Clinical Practice Recommendations for managing Type 2 diabetes in Primary Care I. International Diabetic Federation 2018.
29. Indian Academy of Pediatrics. Consensus Statement of the Indian Academy of Pediatrics on integrated management of severe acute malnutrition. Indian Pediatr. 2013;50: 399-404
30. International Diabetes Federation. (2009). IDF Diabetes Atlas, 4th edition. [Online] Available from https://www.idf.org/e-library/epidemiology-research/diabetes-atlas/21-atlas-4th-edition.html. [Last accessed September, 2019].
31. International Osteoporosis Foundation. (2017). Exercise Recommendations. [Online] Available from www.iofbonehealth.org/exercise-recommendations. [Last accessed September, 2019].
32. Iseme RA, Mcevoy M, Kelly B, et al. Is osteoporosis an autoimmune mediated disorder? Bone Rep. 2017;7:121-31.
33. Jaghsi S. Relation between vitamin K and osteoporosis. In: Barbeck M, Rider P, Kacarevic ZP, Jung O, Rosenberg N (Eds). Clinical Implementation of Bone Regeneration and Maintenance. DOI: 10.5772/ intechopen. 89656.
34. Jha RM, Mithal A, Malhotra N, et al. Pilot case control investigation of risk factors for hip fractures in the urban Indian population. BMC Musculoskelet Disord. 2010;11:49.
35. Jolly JJ, Chin KY, Alias E, et al. Protective effects of selected botanical agents on bone. Int J Environ Res Public Health. 2018;15(5):963.
36. Kapil U. Massive Dose Vitamin A Supplementation (MDVAS) to Children in India: is there enough evidence to continue the programme? Bull Nutr Found India. 2018;39(2):1-4.
37. Kapur D, Agarwal KN, Agarwal DK. Nutritional anemia and its control. Indian J Pediatr. 2002;69(7):607-16.
38. Kapur D, Sharma S, Agarwal KN. Dietary intake and growth pattern of children 9-36 months of age in an urban slum in Delhi. Indian Pediatr. 2005;17:351-6.

39. Keramat A, Mithal A. Risk factors for osteoporosis in urban Asian Indian women presenting for a preventive health checkup. 2nd Joint Meeting of the European Calcified Tissue Society. Geneva; 2005.
40. Khadilkar VV, Khadilkar AV. Revised Indian Academy of Pediatrics 2015 growth charts for height, weight and body mass index for 5-18-year-old Indian children. Indian Journal of Endocrinology and Metabolism. 2015; 19(4) 470-6.
41. Kotecha PV. Nutritional anemia in young children with focus on Asia and India. Indian J Community Med. 2011;36(1):8-16.
42. Kuczmarski RJ, Ogden CL, Grummer-Strawn LM, et al. (2000). CDC growth charts: United States Advance data from vital and health statistics. No. 314 National Center for Health Statistics.. [Online] Available from https://www.cdc.gov/nchs/data/ad/ad314.pdf. [Last accessed September, 2019].
43. Kurpad AV, Swaminathan S, Bhat S. IAP National Task Force for Childhood Prevention of Adult Diseases: The effect of childhood physical activity on prevention of adult diseases. Indian Pediatr. 2004 ;41(1):37-62.
44. Lawrence JP, Brands NW, Daniel SR, et al. Dietary approaches to prevent and treat hypertension: a scientific statement from the American Heart Association. Hypertension. 2006;46(2): 296-308.
45. Lobstein T, Baur L, Uauy R; IASO International Obesity Task Force. Obesity in children and young people: A crisis in public health. Obes Rev. 2004;5 (Suppl) 1:4-104.
46. Manarym M, Solomons NW. Public health aspects of undernutrition. In: Gibney MJ, Margetts BM, Kearney JM, Arab L (Eds). Public Health Nutrition. UK: Blackwell Publishing and The Nutrition Society; p. 179.
47. Mangano KM, Sahni S, Kerstetter JE. Dietary protein is beneficial to bone health under conditions of adequate calcium intake: an update on clinical research. Curr Opin Clin Nutr Metab Care. 2014;17(1):69-74.
48. Mendoza-Salonga A. Nutrition and brain development. SA Fam Pract. 2007;49(3):40-2.
49. Ministry of Health and Family Welfare, Government of India. (2016). Final Report of National Family Health Survey. [Online] Available from https://dhsprogram.com/pubs/pdf/frind3/frind3-vol1andvol2.pdf. [Last accessed September, 2019].
50. Ministry of Health and Family Welfare. (2006). Vitamin A and IFA supplementation. [Online] Available from http://motherchildnutrition.org/india/pdf/mcn-vitamin-a-ifa-supplementation.pdf. [Last accessed September, 2019].
51. Ministry of Women and Child Development, Government of India. (2011). Report of the working group on nutrition for the 12th five year plan (2012-2017). [Online] Available from http://planningcommission.gov.in/aboutus/committee/wrkgrp12/wcd/wgrep_nutition.pdf. [Last accessed September, 2019].
52. Ministry of Women and Child Development, Government of India. (2012). ICDS and Nutrition in the Eleventh Five Year Plan (2007–2012) Sub Group Report, Working Group on Development of Children for the Eleventh Five Year Plan (2007–2012). [Online] Available from http://wcd.nic.in/wgicds.pdf. [Last accessed September, 2019].
53. Mishra A. Ethnic-Specific Criteria for Classification of Body Mass Index: A Perspective for Asian Indians and American Diabetes Association Position Statement. Diabetes Technology & Therapeutics. 2015;17(9):667-71.
54. Mohan V, Ranjit Unnikrishnan R. Precision diabetes: Where do we stand today? Ind. J .Med. Res. 2018;148(5):472-5.
55. National Nutrition Monitoring Bureau (NNMB). Hypertension & diabetes among adults and infant & young child feeding practices - report of third repeat survey, NNMB technical report no. 26. Hyderabad: National Institute of Nutrition; 2012
56. National nutrition monitoring bureau, nnmb technical report no. 26, Diet and nutritional status of rural population, prevalence of hypertension & diabetes among adults and infant & young child feeding practices, report of third repeat survey national institute of nutrition indian council of medical research hyderabad, 2012
57. Nieves JW. Osteoporosis: the role of micronutrients. Am J Clin Nutr. 2005;81(5):1232S-9S.
58. Onis MD, Blossner M. WHO global database on child growth and malnutrition. WHO. 1997. [Last retrieved on 2010 Oct 01]. Available from: http://whqlibdoc.who.int/hq/1997/WHO_NUT_97.4.pdf.
59. Qaseem A, Wilt TJ, Kansagara D, et al. Hemoglobin A1c targets for glycemic control with pharmacologic therapy for nonpregnant adults with type 2 diabetes mellitus: A guidance statement update from the American College of Physicians. Ann Intern Med. 2018;168(8):569-76.
60. Raj RK, Krupad AV. Nutrition in obesity and diabetes. New Delhi and Philadelphia; Jaypee Brothers Medical Publisher Pvt Ltd.; 2015.
61. Reddy V. Protein energy malnutrition. In: Bamji MS, Krishnaswamy K, Brahmam GNV (Eds). Textbook of Human Nutrition, 3rd edition. New Delhi, India: Oxford and IBH Publishing Co. Pvt. Ltd. 2009. pp. 265-80.
62. Riddle MC (Eds) American Diabetes Association Standards of Medical Care in Diabetesd 2020, Volume 43, Supplement 1.
63. Rubha S, Vinodha R. Effects of protein energy malnutrition on peripheral nerve conduction in children. Int J Med Res Health Sci. 2015;4(4):768-70.
64. Saklayen MG. The Global Epidemic of the Metabolic Syndrome. Curr Hypertens Rep. 2018;20(2):12.
65. Salis S. Diet in Diabetes Simplified: Your Personal Diabetes Nutrition Coach. Notion Press. 2020
66. Samir Dalwai, Panna Choudhury, Sandeep B Bavdekar, RupalDalal, Umesh Kapil, AP Dubey, Deepak Ugra, Manohar Agnani, HPS Sachdev. Consensus Statement of the Indian Academy of Pediatrics on integrated management of severe acute malnutrition. Indian Pediatr; 2013, 50:399-404
67. Sekhar Kar S, Sekhar Kar S. Prevention of childhood obesity in India: Way forward. J Nat Sci Biol Med. 2015. 6(1): 12–17.
68. Semba RD, Shardell M, et al. Child stunting is associated with low circulating essential amino acids. 2016;6:246-52.
69. Semba RD. The rise and fall of protein malnutrition in global health. Ann Nutr Metab. 2016;69:79-88.
70. Sixth report on the world nutrition situation: Progress in Nutrition. United Nations Standing Committee on Nutrition, Geneva, Switzerland. http://www.fao.org/3/a-as211e.pdf.
71. Unger T, Borghi C, Charchar F, et al. Clinical Practice Guidelines 2020 International Society of Hypertension Global Hypertension Practice Guidelines.
72. Utter J, Neumark-Sztainer D, Jeffery R, et al. Couch potatoes or French fries: Are sedentary behaviors associated with body mass index, physical activity, and dietary behaviors among adolescents? J Am Diet Assoc. 2003;103(10):1298-305.
73. Vijayaraghavan K. National control programme against nutritional blindness due to vitamin A deficiency: Current status & future strategy. Ind J Med Res. 2018. 148(5): 498-505
74. Welsh JA, Cogswell ME, Rogers S, et al. Overweight among low-income preschool children associated with the consumption of sweet drinks: Missouri, 1999-2002. Pediatrics. 2005;115(2005): 223-29.
75. WH Dietz Jr, Gortmaker SL. Do we fatten our children at the television set? Obesity and television viewing in children and adolescents. Pediatrics. 1985;75(5):807-12.
76. White JV, Guenter P, Jensen G, et al. The Academy Malnutrition Work Group; The ASPEN Malnutrition Task Force; The ASPEN

Board of Directors. Consensus Statement: Academy of Nutrition and Dietetics and American Society for Parenteral and Enteral Nutrition: Characteristics recommended for the identification and documentation of adult malnutrition (undernutrition). J Parenter Enteral Nutr. 2012;36(3):275-83.
77. WHO. (1996). Indicator for assessing Vitamin A deficiency and their application in monitoring and evaluating intervention programmes. [Online] Available from http://www.who.int/nutrition/publications/micronutrients/vitamin_a_deficieny/WHONUT96.10.pdf. [Last accessed September, 2019].
78. WHO. (2004). WHO Scientific Group on The Assessment of Osteoporosis at Primary Health Care Level, Summary Meeting Report Brussels, Belgium, 5-7 May 2004. [Online] Available from https://www.who.int/chp/topics/Osteoporosis.pdf#targetText=According%20to%20the%20WHO%20criteria,a%20diagnostic%20and%20intervention%20threshold. [Last accessed September, 2019].
79. WHO. (2011). Serum retinol concentrations for determining the prevalence of vitamin A deficiency in populations, WHO/NMH/NHD/MNM/11.3, Vitamin and Mineral Nutrition Information System.
80. WHO. Child growth standards. Acta Pediatr Suppl. 2006;450:5-101
81. WHO. Global prevalence of vitamin A deficiency in populations at risk 1995–2005. WHO Global Database on Vitamin A Deficiency. Geneva: WHO; 2009.
82. WHO. Guideline: Updates on the management of severe acute malnutrition in infants and children. Geneva, World Health Organization; 2013 (http://www.who.int/nutrition/publications/guidelines/updates_management_SAM_infantandchildren/en/).
83. WHO. Guideline: Vitamin A supplementation in infants and children 6–59 months of age. Geneva: World Health Organization; 2011.
84. WHO. Obesity: preventing and managing the global epidemic. Report of a WHO Consultation (WHO Technical Report Series, No. 894). Geneva: World Health Organization; 2000.
85. WHO. Waist circumference and waist-hip ratio: report of a WHO expert consultation. Geneva, 2008.
86. WHO child growth standards and the identification of severe acute malnutrition in infants and children: A joint statement by WHO and UNICEF, 2009.
87. WHO Physical status: the use and interpretation of anthropometry. Report of a WHO Expert Committee. WHO Technical Report Series 854. Geneva: World Health Organization; 1995
88. World Health Organization, Classification of Diabetes Mellitus, ISBN 978-92-4-151570-2; 2019.
89. World Bank Report. (2007). India's Undernourished Children: A Call for Reform and Action. [Online] Available from http://siteresources.worldbank.org/. [Last accessed September, 2019].
90. World Health Organization. (2001). Iron Deficiency Anaemia: Assessment, Prevention and Control. A guide for programme managers.
91. World Health Organization. Global prevalence of vitamin A deficiency in populations at risk 1995-2005. Geneva: WHO; 2009
92. Yadav K, Pandav CS. National iodine deficiency disorders control programme: Current status and future strategy. Indian J Med Res. 2018;148(5):503-10.
93. Yajnik CS. The lifestyle effects of nutrition and body size on adult adiposity, diabetes and cardiovascular disease. Obes Rev. 2002;3(3):217-24.
94. Yakoob MY, Bhutta ZA. Effect of routine iron supplementation with or without folic acid on anemia during pregnancy. BMC Public Health. 2011;11(Suppl 3):S21.

13
CHAPTER

Assessment of Nutritional Status

> **KEY CONCERNS**
> - What is nutritional status?
> - How can it be assessed?
> - Are there specific tools and techniques to assess nutritional status?
> - Will they help in identifying health problems or nutritional deficiencies?
> - Will it be helpful in nutritional and medical treatment process and aid in patient recovery?
> - Are there specific tests for different nutrients and for pediatric/geriatric populations?
>
> **KEY CONCEPTS**
> - Nutritional status and nutritional screening
> - Stages at which nutritional disorders occur
> - Methods of assessing nutritional status:
>   - Nutrition screening
>   - Nutritional assessment
>   - Anthropometric measurements
>   - Biochemical tests
>   - Clinical symptoms
>   - Dietary intake
>   - Use of electronic tools.
> - Assessment methods for pediatric, geriatric, and hospitalized populations.

Optimal nutritional status is critical for optimal functioning of the body, maintaining and promoting good health and physical performance, having a good immune response, and preventing both infectious and noncommunicable diseases. Overall, good nutritional status helps us achieve a sense of well-being and is very supportive in treatment of diseases and response to medical therapies. Nutrition is a major determinant of health for all human beings but particularly in pediatric and geriatric populations, both in hospital and community settings. Changes in physiological function lie along a continuum and are influenced by several factors such as age and sex, dietary intake as well as psychological and environmental factors. Dietary pattern reflects the habitual intake of food and is often used to assess nutritional risk. Undesirable physiological changes distinctively impinge on the nutritional status of the person. Nutritional screening and nutritional assessment can help to identify the changes occurring in the body and provide the information required for timely and adequate interventions.

NUTRITIONAL STATUS

Nutritional assessment is more detailed and takes a longer time. Generally, assessment involves doing more tests than are used for nutrition screening. It consists of a detailed examination of metabolic, nutritional, or functional variables by a trained dietitian with expertise or a nurse with expertise in nutrition. It gives more in-depth information although it costs more. The goals of nutrition assessment are to determine whether children are growing well and their development is normal, to establish the nutritional status of the person, to determine whether the person is at risk of undernutrition or is overweight/obese, to provide the guidelines for nutrition therapy based on which the nutrition plan is developed, and to monitor the impact of nutrition therapy.

Nutritional status tells us about the current health status of a person or a group of people which is an outcome of nutrient intake and utilization of nutrients. Any change in dietary input, physical activity and state of health or disease may alter the nutritional status and can disturb the functioning of the body at cellular and molecular levels.

Malnutrition is essentially either undernutrition or overnutrition that can result in suboptimal body function. Malnutrition can occur if nutrient intakes are not in accordance with the requirements of the body, i.e., either inadequate intakes and/or excessive losses occur or in some cases, intakes of specific foods may be more and that of other foods are less than required resulting in adverse consequences. Nutrient requirements and nutritional status are influenced by:

- **Stage of life cycle:** Nutrient needs are higher during periods of growth, i.e., infancy, adolescence, pregnancy, and lactation and any deficit or excess in nutrient intakes has an effect on nutritional status of the individual.
- **State of health:** Nutrient needs tend to be higher during illness/disease, e.g., fever, stress, trauma, injury, smoking, aging, medications, abuse of drugs, interactions with other nutrients, competition between nutrients, and nutrient deficiencies.
- **Changes in** transport, pH changes, availability of carrier molecules, e.g., carrier proteins, changes in storage and processing, excretion of nutrients, e.g., increased gastrointestinal motility, and changes in renal function.

Assessment of nutritional status is, thus, important both in community and clinical settings. In case of children, it is important because they are in different stages of growth and development. It is equally important for the geriatric population as they may be fragile, sensitive, and are at risk of suffering multiple nutritional problems as well as diseases. Assessment is crucial in hospitalized patients, particularly critically ill patients for whom monitoring at regular intervals not only helps in diagnosis and interpretation but also their treatment and recovery. Usually, body weight is measured because it is easy and is inexpensive, but body weight by itself cannot give information about either deficiencies or excess of nutrients, particularly proteins, lipids, vitamins, and minerals, nor does it reflect the changes in physiological function and pathological processes.

For diagnosis of nutritional status, nutrition screening and nutritional assessment are done. Both facilitate the regular screening followed by assessment and support early recognition of deficiencies/excesses and pathological conditions, appropriate nutritional prescriptions, aid in speedy recovery, and reduce the duration of hospital stay. Nutrition screening is done before nutritional assessment and it is essentially rapid. Table 13.1 explains the difference between nutrition screening and nutritional assessment.

Table 13.1: Differences between nutrition screening and nutritional assessment.

Nutrition screening	Nutritional assessment

• She/he is the first step of identifying the person who may be malnourished or at risk of malnourishment
• If the person is malnourished, then nutritional assessment is carried out
• If person is at risk of malnourishment, then it is rescreened and decision is taken accordingly
• She/he is a rapid and simple method
• She/he is conducted in community and hospital
• She/he is carried out by a nursing staff or community healthworker
• She/he estimates and focuses on the:
  ➢ Recent weight changes (loss)
  ➢ Current BMI
  ➢ Recent food intake
  ➢ Disease severity.
• She/he is done using one of the following tools:
  ➢ Malnutrition Universal Screening Tool (MUST) at community level
  ➢ Nutritional Risk Screening (NRS) in hospital setting
  ➢ Mini nutritional assessment (MNA) for the elderly
  ➢ Subjective global assessment (SGA).
	• She/he includes actual body measurements and other parameters
	• She/he clearly indicates the level/grades of malnutrition
	• She/he is a long and complex process
	• She/he is carried out by dietitians, nutritionists, or staff in healthcare practice
	• She/he is long and complex process
	• She/he includes many assessment methods such as:
	  ➢ Anthropometric measurements
	  ➢ Biochemical methods
	  ➢ Clinical signs
	  ➢ Dietary intake.
	Each method has different indicators depending upon the needs and facilities it carries out.
	It is also carried out for:
	• Individuals
	• Group of people (selective population) in community as well as in clinical settings.

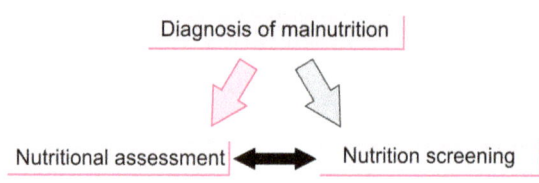

Nutrition Screening

According to the American Society for Parenteral and Enteral Nutrition (ASPEN, 2018) nutrition screening is defined as—a process to identify an individual who may be malnourished or at risk for malnutrition to determine if a comprehensive nutrition assessment and appropriate intervention are indicated. It identifies the characteristics known to be linked with nutritional problems. Nutrition screening facilitates a positive health outcome by early detection and timely intervention for the nutritional problems associated with many disease conditions. It also broadens the collaborative efforts of the healthcare team.

Nutrition screening is required both in hospitals and at community level. It is fairly concise and not expensive. This is done using rapid and simple methods/tools/tests to identify people who are either malnourished or at risk of malnutrition and based on the screening results, decision can be made whether there is a need for more detailed assessment. At community level, screening can be done even by trained healthcare or community level service providers, e.g., Integrated Child Development Services (ICDS), growth monitoring of children is done by trained Anganwadi Sevikas. However, the service providers should be well-trained. Usually, standardized training is provided as per national policy and guidelines and the requirements of specific programs. The service providers are required to fill in recording formats and adhere to reporting mechanisms as decided by the authorities. Generally, nutrition screening can include weight measurements, measuring mid-upper arm circumference, and perhaps bilateral pitting edema. Questions are generally asked related to recent illnesses, food intake, appetite, and hunger.

> **Main Aims of Nutrition Screening**
> Recent weight loss
> • Body mass index (current)
> • Recent food intake
> • Disease severity
> Nutrition screening, as is usually followed in hospital patients, is dealt with later in this chapter in the section on assessment of hospitalized patients.
> 1. Malnutrition universal screening tool (MUST) at community level
> 2. Nutritional risk screening (NRS) in hospital setting
> 3. Mini nutritional assessment (MNA) for the elderly.

In hospitals, nutrition screening should be done generally upon admission or within the first 24–48 hours, and it may be done by the nursing staff. The methods used should be sensitive enough to identify all patients who are malnourished or who are at risk. Based on the observations, an action plan must be thought of and a defined course of action must be carried out. For nutrition screening, tools are used to detect whether the patient is at risk or has protein energy malnutrition, to determine whether this likely to worsen especially whether the disease will worsen this state, i.e., lead to deterioration in nutritional status. The focus is on the following:

Nutrition Screening and Nutritional Assessment

According to the British Dietetic Association (2012), "nutritional assessment is the systematic process of collecting and interpreting information in order to make decisions about the nature and cause of nutrition-related health issues that affect an individual".

> **Nutrition Assessment:** A comprehensive approach to identifying the nutrition-related problems that uses a combination of the following: medical, nutrition, medication and client histories; nutrition-focused physical examination; anthropometric measurements; and biomedical data/medical diagnostic tests and procedures (ASPEN, 2018).

Nutritional status is a complex interaction of internal or constitutional factors and external environmental factors. Internal or constitutional factors include age, sex, nutritional behavior, physical activity, and diseases and external environmental factors are food safety, cultural, social, and economic circumstances. Nowadays, pollution, plastic, radiation, medical procedures, and drug interaction also affect the nutritional status.

Nutritional screening and dietary assessment are not confirmatory methods to estimate nutritional status. These methods depend upon the skill of the interviewer, training, and cooperation of the subject. Hence, biochemical and clinical methods are used along with these methods. Several factors, which influence the choice of assessment method and their interpretation, are shown in Figure 13.1.

Purpose of Assessing Nutritional Status

In order to maintain good health, it is important to assess nutritional status of individuals and of groups/communities. The purpose of assessing nutritional status is to:
- Identify individuals or populations who are either malnourished or at risk of being malnourished
- Identify nutritional deficiencies and excesses
- Based on the findings, to plan and develop strategies/programs, to address the gaps/needs, and improve the situation.
- Nutritional status affects the patients' response to illness. Especially in children, growth and development in children is compromised by poor nutritional status as well as medical illness, e.g., accurate estimation of protein, energy, and other nutrients will enable taking decisions about treatment that can help slow down the catabolic state which is very high during traumatic stage or surgery.
- In clinical medicine, it is important to identify the malnourished patients because besides medical intervention, there is a need for early nutritional intervention in order to: (i) prevent the patient from becoming malnourished by effecting dietary modifications or changes, (ii) monitor patients' progress and track the effectiveness of the dietary intervention, and (iii) do referral wherever necessary.
- It has been observed that with a weight loss of 10% or more, the risk of adverse outcomes is greater, and hospital stay is likely to be prolonged. In lean and healthy persons, it has been reported that when weight loss exceeded one-third, the risk of mortality was greater. Malnourished persons not only have longer hospital stays but their recovery is slower, they are more susceptible to developing complications, and overall are at risk of higher morbidity and mortality.
- To monitor nutritional status when there are shifts or changes in policy in public nutrition and health.

For nutritional status assessment, the **Triple A cycle** model (a three-step process) given by the UNICEF can be applied (Fig. 13.2). Analysis of the problem is contextual. For example, in young children who are undernourished, it is important to identify practices that might be causing infection, reason(s) for poor intakes, etc. The results of nutritional assessment determine the course of action. Action could include developing and establishing appropriate nutrition care plans that include nutrition education and counseling and if necessary other support including referral to food security, resources required, etc.

> Most chronic diseases which improve over time, when appropriate nutritional therapy/intervention is provided, start with metabolic or biochemical changes. Functional interpretation of laboratory data is important because changes can be identified earlier. Medical nutrition therapy or any other required treatment can be initiated.

Nutritional status is a continuum from being well-nourished at one end to being overtly malnourished at the

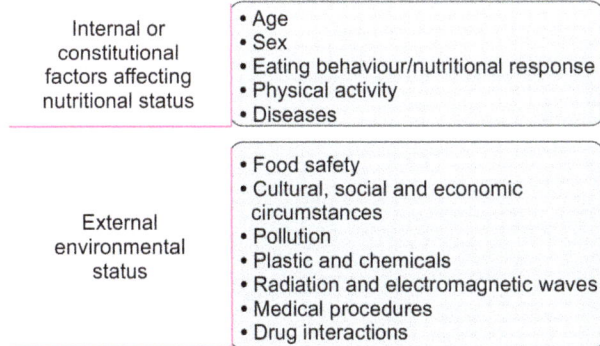

Fig. 13.1: Factors influence the choice of assessment method and their interpretation.

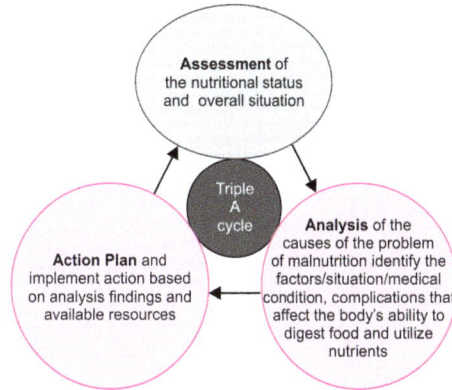

Fig. 13.2: Triple: A cycle model.

other (Table 13.2). There are stages in between and at each stage, nutritional status assessment may need a different approach or method (Figs. 13.3A and B).

However, no single measurement can give the information required to make a judgment. Therefore, a combination of different measurements is used. Whatever the methods applied, it is important to ensure their accuracy and precision. The method or test must be specific to the nutritional state and should be sensitive to changes in nutritional status. Also, to the extent possible, the test or method should be easy to apply and reproducible.

> The sensitivity of the test reflects the probability that the screening test will be positive among those who are diseased. In contrast, the specificity of the test reflects the probability that the screening test will be negative among those who, in fact, do not have the disease.
>
> **Specificity:** It is known as true negative rate. The test/method must correctly identify a healthy person, i.e., one who does not have the condition.
>
> **Sensitivity:** It is known as true positive rate. The test/method must correctly detect a person who is having the particular condition he/she is being tested for.

Almost every nutrient has an indicator and/or specific criteria and a normal range which has an upper and lower level/concentration or cut-off point. It is important that objective measurements of nutritional status be used for nutritional screening as well as for nutritional assessment.

Components of medical history are necessary before either screening or detailed assessment: Whether it is screening or detailed assessment, it is important for the nutritionist/dietitian to study the medical history and take note of salient issues, which are usually obtained from the medical record(s) that includes:
- Illness both present and past, both acute and chronic.
- Duration of current illness, symptoms.
- Therapies and medications—attention should be paid to medications prescribed, because many medications interact with nutrients.
- Whether the person is taking any nonprescription or over-the-counter medication (self-medication). This should be noted for both allopathic and traditional systems of medicine.
- Also, it is important to note hospitalizations in the past, operations/surgeries, for children history of past growth

Table 13.2: Continuum of nutritional status.

Stages of Health	Changes occurring in the body during loss of health	Changes occurring at cellular and molecular level in the body	Possible tests to be performed in different stages
I	Well-nourished	Normal physiological changes continue	Assess dietary intakes, physical activity, and quality of life They are generally adequate
II	Malnutrition	Impaired absorption/increased nutrient loss/inadequate intakes	Assess dietary intakes, physical activity, and quality of life
III	Depletion of body stores, tissue levels Decreasing deposits/stores	Wastage of protein and fat Decreased visceral protein synthesis Increased protein degradation	Initial biochemical alterations but no overt symptoms Need to rely on case records (medical)
IV	Impaired cellular function, alteration in biological, physiological, and biochemical function	Decreased cell mass	Initial biochemical alterations but no overt symptoms Need to rely on case records (medical)
V	Capacity of cells and tissues, organs to function normally compromised Anatomical and functional changes	Organ dysfunction	Specific test, if available
VI	Clinical signs	Decreased immune defense and inflammation	Can detect dietary deficiencies, biochemical abnormalities Early stages of disease
VII	Overtly malnourished	Increased infections, other pathological conditions	Clinical signs and symptoms Diagnosed pathology Tissue damage Organ failure

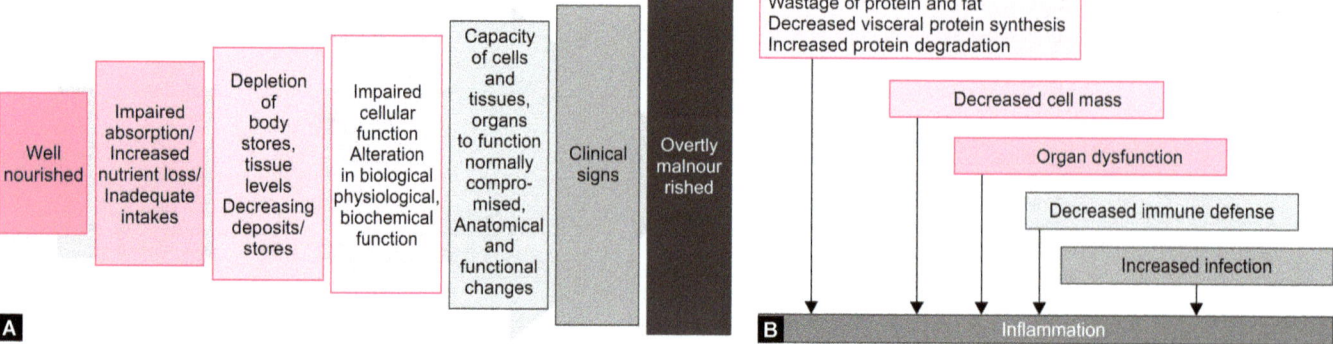

Figs. 13.3A and B: Continuum of nutritional status.

patterns if available, onset of puberty, and developmental history including feeding abilities/problems with feeding.
- Functioning of systems must be reviewed especially for children, oral motor function and dental development should be looked into.
- There is need to take note of the family's social and cultural background especially issues/areas related to diet, hygiene.
- Presence of gastrointestinal symptoms such as vomiting, diarrhea, constipation, and gastroesophageal reflux should be noted.

Methods of Nutritional Assessment

Methods of nutritional assessment can be direct or indirect and each method includes suitable applications (Fig. 13.4).

Indirect Methods

Indirect methods are used to identify community health or nutritional status. Indirect methods are food balance sheets that are used to study national food availability and household consumption and expenditure surveys that essentially measure household food consumption. The following variables are generally used to reflect the nutritional influences on the population of a community or a country/national level:
- Ecological variables including crop production
- Economic factors like per capita income, population density, and social habits
- Vital health statistics particularly infant and under-5 mortality and fertility indices.

This information is generally obtained through surveys. The objectives of these surveys are:
- To provide inputs for national accounts or consumer price index
- To measure poverty
- To obtain food consumption data that may be used to assess food security or vulnerability and diet diversity
- To plan and monitor food-based nutritional interventions. To determine the needs and priorities for feeding programs, food production, food storage and transportation, food enrichment, and nutrition education that is socioculturally relevant
- To serve as a basis for community development programs
- To stimulate food industries to produce nutritious foods at affordable cost
- To provide a basis for food policies
- To create awareness and consciousness among government, health professionals as well as lay persons
- To help support the findings related to morbidity (including noncommunicable diseases), mortality, anthropometry, and biochemical tests.

However, it must be remembered that care needs to be taken not to assume that food consumption is equal among household members. Also, this data does not specifically reflect intakes of specific groups, nor it is adequate to identify vulnerable age groups like preschoolers, etc.

Direct Methods

Direct methods are usually performed on individuals or a group of people having similar conditions. For convenience, they are mnemonically planned as A, B, C, and D as shown in Figure 13.4. These methods use anthropometric measurements, biochemical and clinical indices, and the food consumption, nutrient intake, and eating patterns (Table 13.3).

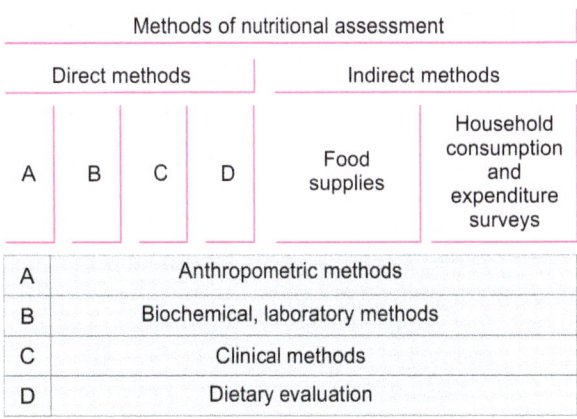

Fig. 13.4: Methods of nutritional assessment.

Table 13.3: Components of nutritional assessment.

Anthropometric measurements	Biochemical analysis	Clinical evaluation	Dietary history and current intake
Body mass index Usual adult weight Recent weight changes Skinfold measurement	Complete blood count Protein status Lipid profile Electrolytes BUN/creatinine	Physical examination Chronic conditions Current health status Oral health and dentition Medication use and polypharmacy	Food preferences and food habits Cultural or religious food habits Meal frequency Lack of control over food selection and choices Fluid intake Alcohol intake Special diets Vitamin/mineral/botanical supplement use Current intake compared to current nutritional needs Chewing and/or swallowing problems Functional limitations that impair independence with eating Cognitive changes affecting appetite and ability to feed self Physiological changes that affect the desire to eat

ANTHROPOMETRIC MEASUREMENTS

Anthropometry is the study of measurement of the human body in terms of the dimensions of bone, muscle, and adipose (fat) tissue. Anthropometric measurements are quantitative, noninvasive, relatively inexpensive, and easy to do. They can be used to assess health as well as growth and development in case of children and adolescents, and can assist in selecting appropriate treatment options, if the anthropometric indicators suggest that health and well-being are at risk. They are used to assess and predict performance, health and survival of individuals, and reflect the economic and social well-being of the population. Applications include the prediction of who will benefit from interventions, identifying social and economic inequity, and evaluating responses to interventions. There are several advantages of using anthropometry but there are some limitations as well. These are given in Table 13.4.

Anthropometric measurements can also be used as a baseline for physical fitness and to measure the progress/improvement (growth), especially in terms of body composition and size vis-à-vis sports performance of athletes. Each type of sport requires appropriate body size and composition and these can be used to monitor and ensure that the athletes/sportspersons stay in peak physical shape.

For anthropometric measurements, whole body measurements are generally taken. The core elements or most commonly taken measurements are height and weight, based on which body mass index is calculated. Weight and height are routinely measured in children in order to assess their nutritional status and to determine whether their growth is appropriate for age. Anthropometric measurements and indicators include:
- Body weight
- Body height
- Body girth (circumferences)—head circumference, chest circumference, mid-upper arm circumference, waist circumference, and hip circumference
- Length of extremities—knee to heel, arm length
- Ratios of body circumference—waist-hip ratio
- Ratio of weight and height—weight for height, waist-to-height ratio.

> Anthropometry can be categorized as:
> - **Physical (static) anthropometry**—addresses basic physical dimensions of the body.
> - **Functional anthropometry**—is concerned with physical dimensions of the body relevant to particular activities or tasks.
> - **Newtonian data**—yields body segment mass data and data about forces that can be exerted in different tasks/posture.

- Other examples of functional tests include:
  - Thiamine deficiency can be detected in urine, but measurement of the enzyme transketolase in red blood cells will be a more accurate indicator of its severity.
  - Measurement of serum folate, RBC folate, and serum B_{12} are static tests. Functional tests for macrocytic anemias are:
    - **Homocysteine:** Folate and B_{12} are needed to convert homocysteine to methionine; high homocysteine may mean deficiencies of folate, B_{12}, or B_6.
    - **Methylmalonic acid:** Methylmalonic acid measurements can be used along with homocysteine to distinguish between B_{12} and folate deficiencies (↑ in B_{12} deficiency).
    - **Schilling test:** Radiolabeled cobalamin is used to test for B_{12} malabsorption.
- **Protein status:** Static indicators have been described in the section on biochemical indicators of muscle activity and/or muscle mass. However, muscle activity or muscle strength can be assessed as a functional indicator of muscle

Table 13.4: Advantages and limitations of anthropometry.

Advantages/merits or strengths	Limitations
Methods are precise and accurate, provided standardized techniques are used Procedures use simple, safe, and noninvasive techniques	If there is more than one person doing measurements, need to take care of interobserver errors
Equipment required is relatively inexpensive, portable, and durable, and can be made or purchased locally	Equipment is available with fairly wide range of sensitivity and accuracy. Some expensive but accurate equipment is not easily portable
Relatively unskilled personnel can perform measurement procedures, once they are well-trained	Persons should be well-trained and there should be minimum intraobserver error. For example, when a child is weighed or its length is measured for monitoring its growth, a small measurement error can result in large errors in growth charts. Error of three-fourths inch can lead to 25% error in the growth chart plotting
Information is generated on past nutritional history	Methods are unable to pinpoint the principal cause(s) of undernutrition, as the poor nutritional status may be the result of factors such as repeated insults owing to infections and poor care in children
Methods can be used to quantify the degree of undernutrition (or overnutrition) and provide a continuum of assessment	Methods are unable to distinguish the effect of specific nutrient deficiencies (e.g., zinc deficiency) that affect growth in children due to inadequacy of food in general
Methods are suitable for large sample sizes	–
Methods can be used to monitor and evaluate changes in nutritional status over time, seasons, generations, etc.	Methods are not highly sensitive to detect changes in nutritional status following inadequacy of food over short periods of time
Methods can be adapted to develop screening tests to identify those at high risk	Anthropometry is associated with relatively higher costs and organization is required to obtain representative and quality data for the purpose of estimating numbers of undernourished

mass. This is because muscle activity is directly related to cell energy function which is less in a malnourished person and improves when a person is nutritionally rehabilitated.

Muscle strength can be assessed in active form and passive form.

Active form: The strength of specific muscle is measured, e.g., apprehension activity.

Passive form: Muscle contraction and relaxation in response to different electrical intensities is measured, e.g., muscle contraction of the adductor pollicis in reaction/response to an electrical stimulus to the ulnar nerve.

Body Weight

Body weight is a measure of overall nutritional status. Body weight is the total sum of weight of the bones, muscles, body fat, and total body water. It can fluctuate on daily basis due to variations in food and water intake, excretory products, i.e., urine and feces as well as exercise. Beside voluntary weight loss, dehydration and disease can reduce body weight as can water retention, i.e., edema, both of which can occur in malnutrition and disease.

By itself body weight does not give much information, unless it is examined in relation to age, sex, and height/length. It should be measured in kilograms or pounds, using a digital or beam balance scale. For children who are not able to stand alone or independently on the scale (generally up to approximately 24 months of age), a pan version of the scale is used. If children do not cooperate at all, an adult should stand on the scale with the child and then the child should be handed over to someone else and the adult is weighed alone. Weight of the child is calculated as the difference between the weight of adult + child and adult alone.

Weight should be measured in light or minimal clothing (footwear should be removed, as also outer garments). In case of infants, there should be no diaper. Prior to each measurement, the scale must be zeroed and it should be calibrated at least on a monthly basis using a known range of weights and checked for accuracy. The persons should be positioned in the center of the scale. Weights are generally recorded to the nearest 0.1 kg (100 g) for children and adults and to the nearest 0.01 kg (10 g) for infants. Spring balances should not be used as they are not accurate. Weighing scales (like all anthropometric equipment) should be maintained properly, keeping them free from debris, dirt, etc. and should be placed at a distance from drafts or motors that create vibration or air currents. It is important to ensure that the scale is not overloaded.

Percent Ideal Body Weight: Nutritional status can be judged also by percent ideal body weight which can be used to classify the degree of overnutrition or undernutrition. In children, percent ideal body weight can be used as a clinical goal during nutritional rehabilitation. Percent ideal body weight (IBW) can be calculated as follows:

$$IBW = Actual\ weight/Standard\ body\ weight \times 100$$

ICMR NIN (2020) has given the body weight for persons of different age groups and genders.

An adult may be said to be malnourished if the body mass index is < 18.5 kg/m².

In clinical settings, the percent of usual body weight loss that is involuntary is an indicator of nutritional status and nutritional risk.

Percent weight loss = Previous weight–Current weight/ Previous weight × 100

The classification for interpretation of IBW is:
- >200% IBW—morbid obese
- >120% IBW—obese
- 110–120% IBW—overweight
- 90–110% IBW—normal range
- 80–90% IBW—mild wasting
- 70–80% IBW—moderate wasting
- <70% IBW—severe wasting.

If weight loss is very high, the risk of postoperative mortality is increased. A child who has lost 5% or more weight in the previous one month can be considered to be at nutritional risk (Table 13.5).

Weight loss assessment is worthwhile because it is inexpensive and a simple screening tool. The limitation/disadvantage of using weight loss by itself is that it is difficult to obtain accurate patient history and to get accurate premorbid weight of the person and the duration over which the patient lost weight. At best, one gets an estimate. Serial weight measurements, if available, are more accurate. Generally, a ≥6% preoperative weight loss is considered to be serious because it is associated with increased postoperative complications and even death. Weight loss can be considered in combination with BMI. For persons less than 70 years of age, BMI < 20 kg/m² can be used as a cutoff and for persons ≥70 years, the BMI cut off should be <22 kg/m².

Length/Height/Stature

Height or stature is the distance from the top of the head to the sole of the feet. Length is measured in supine position for young children below 24 months, and for bedridden patients as they cannot stand. Height/length is an indicator of long-term nutrition and can reflect chronic undernutrition particularly stunting (although stunting may be caused by problems such as growth hormone deficiency). Accurate measurement is essential to calculate CHI (creatinine height index) and BEE (basal energy expenditure) from Harris–Benedict equation. It is also required to calculate BMI.

- Height is measured with a stadiometer or an anthropometric rod. If these are not available, then a standardized, nonstretchable tape can be fixed to a smooth wall, taking care that the wall has no skirting.

Table 13.5: Interpretation of involuntary weight loss for nutritional assessment.

Time period	Severe loss (percent of body weight)
1 week	>2%
1 month	>5%
3 months	>7.5%
6 months	>10%
Postoperative	(≥20%)—high risk of mortality

- Ask the person to remove his/her footwear or shoes, all bulky clothing especially headscarves to ensure the person, especially a child is standing in the correct position. It should be ensured that any objects on the head, e.g., clips, hair ornaments, or plaits/braids should be removed first.
- Ask the person to stand with his/her heels together, ensuring that the body weight is evenly distributed on both legs. For children, it should be ensured that they stand in the right position.
- Ask the person to look straight, so that head is perpendicular to the body. Particular attention needs to be paid to the chin. The person should be so positioned that the back is straight, feet are flat on the floor, shoulder blades, and buttocks and heels touch the stadiometer's vertical backboard/scale or the wall. If the person especially a patient is not able to have all three points of contact on the vertical backboard, then at least the heels and buttocks must touch it. The feet should be facing outward at a 60-degree angle. In case a patient has some defect, e.g., genu valgum, the feet should be separated so that the knees do not overlap, while the person does not lose balance and maintains contact between the knees.
- Arms should be allowed to hang loosely at the sides with the palms facing the thighs.
- Once the person is appropriately positioned, the horizontal bar of the stadiometer should be lowered until the hair is compressed to the crown of the head. The headboard should be level at right angles to the tape fixed on the stadiometer and the feet are still touching the floor. The person who is measuring should ensure that his/her eyes are level with the indicator. If necessary, a small stool should be used to ensure that the person taking the measurement is at eye level.
- Height is read to the nearest 0.1 cm. The individual should be asked to step away and the measurement should be done again. The two measurements should be within half a centimeter of each other. If they are not, the entire procedure should be repeated.

Length measurement: Recumbent or supine length is measured for infants and young children below 24 months of age, those who cannot or will not stand straight or even patients who are unable to stand, or children who measure less than 30 inches, or children who weigh less than 20 lbs. For recumbent or supine length, two persons are required, especially when children are to be measured.

Method: With parent's or assistant's help, lay child down on the board; ensure that the child is placed in the center of the board and that the head should be touching the fixed headboard.
- The child's body should be straight in line with the headboard, shoulders and buttocks flat against the surface.
- The parent/assistant should hold the child's head gently against the headboard with child's eyes looking straight up.
- The person doing the measurement should gently press the child's knees with his/her left hand to fully extend the child's legs to full length.
- With the right hand, the sliding piece at the foot of the scale is to be moved, till it is firmly (at right angles) against the child's feet. Ensure that the toes are pointing straight upward.
- Remove the child and repeat the entire procedure.

If child does not cooperate, ask the parent/caregiver to soothe the child, wait patiently until the baby is calm enough to be measured. Try using toys to distract the baby. As is done for standing height, the two readings are to be compared. The difference between the two readings should not exceed one-fourth of an inch or half a cm. If the difference is greater, the procedure needs to be repeated until the difference between the two readings is within the permissible limit. The new reading should be recorded. In case the child has not been cooperative, this should be noted.

It is important to remember that length (supine length) overestimates height by approximately 0.5–1.5 cm, therefore for children when serial measurements are made for growth monitoring, it is essential to record the method of measurement.

For children who have physical constraints or are nonambulatory, alternative measures should be used. Upper arm length and lower leg length have been found to be reliable and valid indicators of stature in children. For taking these measurements, sliding calipers and anthropometer should be used and measurements should be recorded to the nearest 0.1 cm.

Ratio of weight and height: By relating weight to height, one is able to make judgments about nutritional status. Different indicators are used to assess nutritional status:

Adults—body mass index (*see* Fig. 5.5 in Chapter 5).

Children—height for age, weight for age, and weight for height/length.

Z-scores (WHO standards—2006) and Standards are given by the Indian Academy of Pediatrics.

Software anthro plus (WHO) can be used to calculate Z-scores.

Currently z scores are used for assessing child nutritional status. At individual level, z-score or the standard deviation score is considered to be the most appropriate indicator for malnutrition, particularly in children. The z-score expresses the anthropometric value of interest as the number of standard deviations or z-scores above or below the median or mean value. Use of Z-score cut off points overcomes the shortcomings of using percentage of growth deficit as an indicator. Z-score calculates the difference between the actual measurement and the age and sex matched reference population divided by the standard deviation (SD) of the reference, and is calculated by the formula:

$$\text{Z-score} = \frac{\text{Observed value for the individual} - \text{median value of reference population}}{\text{(STD deviation) SD value of reference population score}}$$

Z-score is an index of severity for health and nutrition problems and the larger the value of the z-score, the greater the dispersion from the mean or median value and values below the mean or median values i.e., negative z-scores

Table 13.6: Indicators for classification of nutritional status.

Indicators	Explanation
Children	
Underweight	Weight for age <2 SD below the international standards
Wasting	Weight for height <2 SD below international standards
Stunting	Height for age <2 SD below international standards
Adults	
Chronic Energy Deficiency (CED)	Body mass index (weight (Kg)/Height (m)^2 <18.5

indicate undernutrition and vice versa. It helps to categorize individuals according to the degree of severity of malnutrition. It also suggests whether intervention for the community is required or not. A z-score below minus 2 indicates moderate malnutrition and below -3 SD is indicative of severe malnutrition (Table 13.6).

Z-score is recognized as the best for analysis and for presentation of anthropometric data. It has several advantages compared to other methods. It is independent of gender and age. Besides using it at individual level, it can be used to calculate summary statistics like mean and standard deviation for a population.

Height is an age-independent measure. Low height for age is termed as stunting, low weight for age is designated as underweight, and low weight for height, below the reference standards for age and gender is wasting. Weight for height is more useful in classifying the nutritional status. Currently for children 0–6 years of age, the WHO standards are recommended, wherein different categories/grades of nutritional status are given as standard deviation or z-scores. The World Health Organization's software AnthroPlus is freely available for calculation of z-scores and nutritional status assessment. For older children, standards given by Khadilkar and coworkers that have been adopted by the Indian Academy of Pediatrics can be used. For children, there is no fixed BMI value for diagnosing obesity. Instead, BMI percentile should be used for interpretation. However, even when BMI is used, it should be used with caution if the person has edema or has a high tumor burden. This is also applicable to pregnant women or in athletes with large muscle mass.

Circumference Measurements

For all circumference measurements, a flexible, nonstretchable standardized tape should be used, having a least count of 1 mm. Body circumferences are also measured, i.e., waist, hip, limbs, e.g., mid-upper arm circumference. These are important because they can indicate whether the person has increased risk for noncommunicable diseases such as cardiovascular disease, type 2 diabetes mellitus, etc.

Head circumference (HC): The tape should be placed at the maximum distance around the head, above the eyebrows, ears, and occipital prominence. The tape should be tightened until it fits snugly, ensured that it lies flat against the head, is parallel on both sides, and the frontal occipital circumference measurement is to be recorded to the nearest 0.1 cm. Head circumference essentially reflects head growth that occurs most rapidly in the first 3 years postnatally. It can be used as part of nutritional assessment for children up to 3 years or up to 5 years, especially for those who are at nutritional risk. However, HC is not as sensitive indicator as are weight and height because under conditions of nutritional stress, brain growth is preserved to the extent possible. It cannot be used as an indicator of nutritional status for children with hydrocephalus, microcephaly and macrocephaly.

Mid-upper arm circumference (MUAC): This is generally measured on the left arm. This is a good indicator of nutritional status and is generally used for young children and infants (Table 13.7). It may also be useful to assess nutritional status of pregnant women.

Method:
1. The arm should first be flexed at a 90-degree angle, with hand facing toward body and arm upward.
2. Use a simple nonstretchable standardized measuring tape and the point where the measurement is to be made should be marked—at the midpoint between the lateral tip of the acromion and the olecranon (tip of the elbow and tip of the shoulder).
3. The infant/child should be held upright or made to stand upright and the arm can then be relaxed by the side. A flexible, nonstretchable tape is then placed perpendicular to the long axis of the arm, round the arm and then tightened without squeezing or pinching the arm and recorded to the nearest 0.1 cm. MUAC should

Table 13.7: Interpretation of measurement in mid-upper arm circumference (MUAC).

Measurement in MUAC (millimeters or centimeters)	Color representation in MUAC tape	Indication of nutritional status	Remarks
Children			
<11.0 cm (110 mm)	Red color	Severe acute malnutrition (SAM)	Child should be referred immediately for treatment
11–12.5 cm/110–125 mm	Orange or red color	Moderate acute malnutrition	Child should be referred immediately for supplementation
12.5–13.5 cm/125–135 mm	Yellow color	At risk of acute malnutrition	Caregivers should be counseled and child followed-up through growth monitoring
>13.5 cm/135 mm	Green color	Well-nourished	–

Source: WHO child growth standards and the identification of severe acute malnutrition in infants and children A Joint Statement by the World Health Organization and the United Nations Children's Fund, 2009.

be measured three times (in triplicate) and the average should be calculated.

Its advantages are that it is age independent, requires little equipment, and is very inexpensive. It is a good indicator of nutritional status and is recommended for children between 6 months and 59 months of age. It is recommended for assessment of acute energy deficiency in adults during emergency situations. The major determinants of MUAC are arm muscle and subcutaneous fat both of which are important for survival during starvation. Compared to weight and height indices, MUAC is not influenced by localized edema, e.g., bipedal edema or ascites. It is a sensitive indicator of tissue atrophy than is body weight. For children, the cutoffs for classification according to degree of undernutrition are as follows:

Mid-upper arm circumference (MUAC) may also be used for adults. For adults including women who are nonpregnant, nonlactating as well as pregnant and lactating women, the MUAC cutoffs are given in Table 13.8.

Table 13.8: Assessment criteria for MUAC (adults).

	Moderate acute malnutrition	Severe acute malnutrition
Adult males	>224–<231 mm	<224 mm
Adult females	>214–221 mm	<214 mm

Source: Holland D. (2011). HTP v 2 Module 6: Measuring malnutrition: individual assessment of acute malnutrition. [online] Available from https://www.ennonline.net/htpv2module6.

In older population and ill patients, MUAC is a helpful indicator of malnutrition (normal : 23 cm in males, >22 cm females).

Advanced technologies like ultrasound are available; however, waist and hip circumferences are useful for assessing regional especially abdominal adiposity. Abdominal adiposity has been linked to metabolic syndrome, cardiovascular disease, stroke, and diabetes mellitus.

Length of extremities: Length of extremities such as upper leg length, upper arm length is measured. Studies have shown that the length of extremities is related to chronic diseases. Shorter upper leg length has been shown to have a higher prevalence of metabolic syndrome and shorter upper arm length has been found to be associated with a higher prevalence of diabetes mellitus.

Upper arm length is measured from shoulder to elbow. The measurement is done in a different manner for infants and children between 2 years and 18 years of age. For children who are up to 24 months old, the arm is first to be bent at a 90° angle and the length is measured from superior lateral surface of the acromion to the inferior surface of the elbow. For older children, the child should be asked to allow the arm to hang freely in a relaxed position at the side. The distance between the lateral surfaces of the acromion to the tip of the radius is measured.

Lower leg length is measured as knee to heel length for infants aged 0–24 months. For older children aged 2–18 years, calf length is measured. For infants, the leg is to be bent at a right angle at the hip, knee, and ankle and the superior surface of the knee to the heel is measured. For older children, the leg is to be first crossed over the opposite knee and then the medial tip of the tibia to the distal tip of the medial malleolus is to be measured. For both these measurements, the right leg/right side should be measured. If there is abnormality in both extremities, then the one that is least affected should be measured.

Additionally, skinfold thickness and body composition can be measured. Body composition measurements are done to estimate the amount of adipose tissue, muscle, and bone. Changes in body dimensions and anthropometrics and body dimensions reflect the overall health and welfare of individuals and populations. If needed, body composition should be measured. For children, it may be relevant for the physician to assess sexual and skeletal maturation.

SKINFOLD MEASUREMENT

Skinfold measurement is done to obtain an idea of the amount of subcutaneous fat and based on these, using some equations, total body fat can be calculated. Detailed methods for measuring skinfold thickness are given in books on nutritional assessment. One of the easiest measures is the triceps skinfold since the triceps is easily accessible.

Method of triceps skinfold (TSF) measurement:
- Person should be standing upright and arm should be relaxed at the side.
- The midpoint of the upper arm should be marked over the center of the triceps muscle on the back of the arm.
- The person taking the measurement should lift the skinfold with his/her thumb and index finger about 1 cm above the marked point.
- The caliper is then placed at the marked point and kept for 4 seconds. The caliper is not to be released before then, because it can pinch. The measurement is recorded to the nearest mm and the caliper is then removed.
- The procedure is to be repeated twice (readings are taken in triplicate) and the average of the three readings is calculated.
- TSF can be compared with standards given by the WHO.
- If MUAC has been measured, upper arm muscle area and fat area can be calculated to estimate the upper arm muscle area and fat area because they are clinical indicators of total body stores of muscle and fat.

MAMC = Midarm muscle circumference (MAMC), an indicator of muscle mass can be calculated from MUAC and TSF, using the following formula:

$$MAMC = MUAC\ (cm) - \pi \times TSF\ (cm)$$

Standard for MAMC: Males 25.3 and females 23.2

Percent of standard = (Measurement for the person/standard) × 100

Grades of malnutrition: >90% mild deficit, 60–90% moderate deficit, and <60% severe deficit.

Body Composition

While BMI is useful, it has its limitations, and it does not reflect the amount of lean body mass or body fat. In many acute and chronic diseases, nutritional assessment requires information about body fat and lean body mass. In some cases, knowledge about bone health is also required. This entails assessment of body composition which is noninvasive. Body composition is generally done by bioelectric impedance analysis (BIA) although the gold standard is dual-energy X-ray absorptiometry (DEXA). Many methods of measuring body composition are given in Chapter 5.

- **DEXA:** This is an indirect low-radiation measurement of bone mineral density. DEXA scans can be done for lumbar spine, hips as well as the whole body in adults. In infants, children, and adolescents, measurements are done on the lumbar spine and whole body. Although, in clinical settings, it is mostly used for the assessment of bones, whole-body scans give information about body composition, i.e., fat-free mass, fat mass, and percent body fat, as well as bone mineral content. Advantages of DEXA are the precision, and short time required. Although radiation is used, the dose is very small. Values are compared with reference values for healthy persons, specific for age and sex. One limitation is that measurement in younger children has to be done while they are asleep, or sedation may be required. Results for bone mineral content and bone mineral density are assessed using a z-score/standard deviation score, which compares the individual with the reference database. A z-score of 0 is the mean, i.e., similar to the 50th percentile of the reference data, with +1, +2, −1, and −2 representing plus and minus 1 and 2 standard deviations from the reference mean. The limitations are lack of appropriate reference datasets, especially for diverse ethnic groups. Another limitation is that DEXA gives a two-dimensional assessment of three-dimensional structures, including bone.

  Due to its high cost, DEXA is not routinely used for body composition; however, it is very useful in clinical settings to monitor persons who have poor bone mineral density. For such individuals, scans every 6–12 months may be recommended after the baseline assessment. Persons who have values in the low normal range but with risk factors may need testing every 1–2 years. Persons at risk are those suffering from chronic illness such as inflammatory bowel disease, cystic fibrosis, celiac disease, children who have poor growth, persons with reduced physical activity, and those receiving medications like corticosteroids, or anticonvulsants.

- **Air displacement plethysmography:** This is a newer method for assessing body composition; it is safe, rapid, and noninvasive. The person is required to either sit or lie down (depending on the equipment used) in a closed chamber with as little clothing as possible. The estimates of body composition are reliable and valid but these instruments are not available in all clinical settings.

Biochemical Indicators

Biochemical tests that are used as biomarkers for different nutrients are objective, quantitative and relatively more accurate in indicating the specific nutrient (s) status in an individual. Levels may not reflect nutrient present at tissue level. Biochemical tests can detect nutrient deficits long before anthropometric measures are altered and clinical

Table 13.9: Static and functional tests.

Static tests	• Measurement of circulating levels of nutrients in blood or urine • Assume that the biochemical tests reflect either total body content or measure levels of nutrient in biofluids or tissues—the one most sensitive to depletion • Thus, the test may identify the presence of a nutritional problem
Functional tests Provide a measure of the biological significance of a nutrient	• Measure the effect, or lack there of, how body uses that particular nutrient • Superior indicator of severity • For example, changes in activity of specific enzymes, e.g., alkaline phosphatase for zinc • Physiological performance in vivo, e.g., immune competence, taste acuity for zinc, dark adaptation for vitamin A, muscle function, grip strength • Concentrations of specific blood components—Ferritin or Transferrin receptors for Fe, RBP for vitamin A

signs and symptoms appear, i.e., they can detect subclinical nutrient deficiency, which is an important advantage. Generally nutrient status is assessed by measuring various enzymes or enzyme activities and/or other metabolites present in samples of blood, urine, other body fluid or body tissues. Biochemical tests can be grouped into two general categories: static tests and functional tests that are also referred to as direct and indirect tests as shown in Table 13.9.

Static tests: Static tests measure the nutrient or its metabolite in the blood, urine, or body tissues, e.g., serum levels of albumin, calcium, or vitamin A.

Functional tests: Functional tests indicate the final outcome of a nutrient deficiency and the impact of one or more nutrient deficiency on the physiologic process(es). It reflects the alteration or failure of the tissue or organ to function optimally. Deficiency of one nutrient in one tissue may impact the other that is dependent on that nutrient for optimal performance. Functional tests are of thus biologic importance. The drawback of such tests is their non-specificity; they may indicate general nutritional status and do not conclusively indicate any specific nutrient deficiency. However, they are used in many pathologic conditions, such as metabolic profiles. Impairment of immune status resulting from protein energy malnutrition and other nutrient deficits may be indicative of deficiency of multiple nutrients.

The objectives of using biochemical indicators or laboratory indices are:

- To detect marginal nutritional deficiencies particularly when diet histories are not available or are unreliable. They are useful especially before overt clinical signs of disease are seen.
- To supplement or enhance other studies, e.g., dietary assessment—community studies among specific population groups, to pinpoint nutritional problems, or modalities that the results have suggested or failed to reveal.

What are the specimens that are generally used?
- Serum: The fluid from blood is allowed to coagulate and clot containing blood cells is removed
- Plasma: Blood is centrifuged with anticoagulants, and the fluid that is separated is plasma
- Erythrocytes: Red blood cells
- Leukocytes: White blood cells
- Other tissues: Scrapings and biopsy samples
- Urine: Random samples or timed collections
- Feces: Random samples or timed collections
- Less common: Saliva, nails, hair, and sweat.

Precautions to be taken while sample collection
- The collection of samples of blood and urine needs to be preplanned and coordinated.
- It is important to select the appropriate laboratory, and arrange to reach samples with deterioration or spoilage. The analytical laboratory should have facilities for colorimetry, spectrophotometry, fluorimetry, chromatography, flame and atomic absorption spectrophotometry, and microbiological assay because each test is done differently and requires different equipment/instruments.
- The laboratory should be supervised by a qualified person, the test should be performed by a well-trained analyst, and advice should be obtained before determining which tests should be undertaken and how the data are to be interpreted.
- One condition may be due to different nutrient deficiencies and therefore the appropriate test needs to be selected.

Instructions to the patients before blood sampling: Before doing anything, patient should be instructed and prepared as follows:
- Patient should come for phlebotomy (giving the blood sample) generally after 8–10 hours of fast. She/he should be advised to have light meal the evening before, refrain from smoking, drinking tea/coffee, and avoid physical exertion before the test. Each of these conditions can alter the concentrations of blood analyses significantly. Every time overnight fast before blood collection may not be required.
- However, the patient can take her/his daily medication with water as prescribed.
- The time of day that samples are to be obtained may influence the findings, particularly if this is done shortly after the individual has eaten or taken a vitamin supplement.
- Optimally, blood samples should be taken in the morning before breakfast or any food or drink is consumed.
- For urinalysis, the optimal sample is a total 24-hour collection. If this is not possible, the best sample is the first upon arising.
- When that is not feasible, compromises must be made, and considered in interpreting the data. The best compromise would be to obtain samples at least 2–3 hours after the last meal. Ideally, all samples are to be collected under the same circumstances.
- Subject should be seated for at least 15 minutes prior to venipuncture. Preferentially, patient should be lying down comfortably in relaxed manner, when blood is taken. Venipuncture should be done without prolonged tourniquet application.

Laboratory methods are used to study the status of different nutrients, levels of blood lipids such as cholesterol and triglycerides, glucose, and various enzymes that are implicated in heart disease, diabetes, and other chronic diseases. Some laboratory tests are used to measure markers of inflammation and some as indicators of organ function, e.g., hepatic function. Many factors influence the interpretation of blood tests are described in Figure 13.5.

Medical	Behavioral	Physiological
Disease	Physical activity	Homeostatic regulation
Inflammation	Dietary habits	Circadian rhythms
Trauma	and food intake	Diurnal variation
Malignancy	Smoking	Endocrine variation
Weight loss	Alcohol	Interaction between
Hydration status	Drug abuse	nutrients
Constitutional	**Technical**	**Pharmacological**
Age	Contamination	Drugs/medications
Sex/gender	Sampling errors	
Genetics	Accuracy and precision	
	Sensitivity of test	
	Specificity of test	

Fig. 13.5: Factors influencing interpretation of blood tests.

Commonly used tests include albumin, prealbumin for assessing nutritional status and C-reactive protein (CRP) is used as a marker of inflammation. Tables 13.10A and B list some of the biochemical markers used and their concentrations.

Evaluating nutritional status by laboratory methods is a more objective and precise approach than community assessment, dietary methodology, or clinical assessment methods. For most of the tests, biological tissues, i.e., blood and/or urine is used. The tests generally evaluate specific biochemical functions that depend on adequate supply of the nutrient of concern under scrutiny. However, one problem is that the interpretation of laboratory data is often difficult and does not necessarily always correlate with either clinical or dietary findings. Another limitation is that status for all nutrients cannot be studied.

Often, laboratory values will be obtained suggesting marginal or acute deficiencies when the patient appears clinically normal, since clinical signs usually occur only after prolonged inadequate intake of nutrients. An example is hemoglobin. Low hemoglobin levels indicate anemia, but low hemoglobin is seen only when the body iron stores are depleted. Thus, depending on the nutrient, the person may be in various stages of depletion and, if this state continues, will become ill. Also, isolated nutrient deficiencies are uncommon. Generally, a deficiency in one nutrient can be considered an almost certain indicator of other nutritional inadequacies; these too should be rigorously investigated.

Let us take anemia as an example:
By definition, for diagnosis of anemia the amount of hemoglobin in red blood cells is considered and the size of the RBCs is also taken into account. Anemia is defined

Table 13.10A: Selected biochemical markers used to assess protein status.

Biochemical parameters	Explanation	Concentration in blood/body fluid	Significance
Albumin	Albumin is synthesized in the liver. It is also present in skin, mucosa and viscera. It is related to the disease severity. It is responsible for plasma colloid oncotic pressure. Hence short-term fasting can increase the plasma albumin level.	Plasma: Normal – 3.5-5.5 g/dL Moderate visceral protein depletion – 2.8-3.5 g/dL Severe protein depletion < 2.8 g/dL	Hypoalbuminemia in hospitalized conditions can indicate diminished synthesis, loss, liver disease or infection
Pre-albumin	It is also called transthyretin. It is produced by the liver. It has key role in transport protein. It carries thyroxine and transport retinol.	Normal – 15.7-29.6 mg/dL Mild visceral depletion–10-15 mg/dL Moderate depletion 5-10 mg/dL Severe depletion <5 mg/dL	Sensitive indicator Falls with protein deprivation and rises with refeeding. But values may fall in infection and certain medications can raise the values
Transferrin	Transferrin is synthesized in liver and is responsible for iron absorption and transportation.	Serum - Normal 170-250 mg/dL Mild visceral protein depletion–150-170 mg/dL Moderate depletion 100-150 mg/dL Severe depletion <100 mg/dL	Values are decreased in extreme liver disease, post surgery, trauma or infection
Retinol binding protein (RBP)	Binding protein for vitamin A	~60 mg/L – normal >60 mg/L – in uremia, alcoholism <60 mg/L – in malnutrition, malabsorption, vitamin A deficiency, cirrhosis, infection, severe stress	Responds quickly to nutritional support, reflects recent dietary intake but is not sensitive to adapted starvation Can be used to follow up but is not useful for patients with renal disease

Table 13.10B: Functional tests for assessment of protein status.

3-methyl histidine (3MH)	3MH is an amino acid found in actin and myosin in muscle tissue. Histidine residues when not recycled are excreted in urine.	Normal – 3.63-69.27 µmol/mmole of creatinine in millimole	Values outside the range are indicative. Outside range is indicative of muscle protein degradation. Useful in sports
Creatinine	It is a waste product. Produced from creatine during muscular activity. Creatine is a natural compound made in the liver and transported in the muscles. It can be tested in blood as well as in urine analysis	Normal serum creatinine = 0.6-1.1 mg/dL for women; 0.7-1.3 mg/dL for men Creatinine clearance 88-128 mL/min for women 97-137 mL/min for men	Value can be high in people with high intensive muscular work. It is high in case of kidney malfunctioning.
C-reactive protein (CRP)	It is a protein made in the liver and released in the blood in response to inflammation. Inflammation is the response to protect the body when it is injured or infected.	Clinically normal range is 0-3.0 mg/L	It is a marker of inflammation in the body. It is raised in case of infection, inflammation, autoimmune disease, heart and liver diseases, arthritis and trauma.
Hemoglobin	It is a protein in RBCs containing iron. It helps to transport oxygen to all the cells of the body.	13.5-17.5 g/dL men 12.0-15.5 g/dL women	These values may differ for children depending upon the blood volume. Values are decreased in case of anemia.
Urea	Urea is the breakdown product of proteins or amino acids. It is released into the blood, then taken to the kidney from where it is excreted out in the form of urine.	Blood Urea Nitrogen is tested as BUN. Urea is about double the value of BUN. BUN 10 mg/dL = 21.4 mg/dL To convert BUN to urea Multiply BUN (mg/dL) by 0.357 = urea (mnol/l) Normal serum/plasma urea = 2.5-7.8 mmol/L Normal serum/plasma BUN = 7.0-22 mg/dL	The values indicate kidney functions. It indicates urea production and kidney clearance. Values may be high in aging or age related activities.
Insulin growth factor I (IGF-I)	Affects growth hormone secretion	Median serum **IGF-I level** was 374.1 ng/mL at the age of 18. The serum **IGF-I level** decreased to 180.1 ng/mL at the age of 35–39, further decreased to 92.7 ng/mL at ages older than 70	Marker of nutritional status lower serum IGF-I is indicative of growth retardation and zinc deficiency
Serum orosomucoid (ORM)	Glycoprotein, acute phase protein secreted from liver and adipose tissues	Normal - 0.55-1.05 g/L Malnutrition -<0.55 g/L Inflammation >1.05g/L	Low level- impaired liver function and loss of protein High level – due to high fat intake ORM relates to BMI

as a hemoglobin concentration below the 95th percentile for healthy reference populations. Anemia is not a disease but a symptom of conditions including extensive blood loss, excessive blood cell destruction, or decreased blood cell formation due to a variety of reasons, with nutritional anemias being caused by deficiencies of one or more than one nutrients. Anemia can be classified based on:

Cell size (MCV) which is done as part of the complete blood count:

- Macrocytic (large) MCV   100 + fL (femtoliters)
- Normocytic (normal) MCV   80-99 fL
- Microcytic (small) MCV   <80 fL

Based on hemoglobin content (MCH):
- Hypochromic (pale color)
- Normochromic (normal color).

Iron deficiency anemia is characterized by the production of small (microcytic) erythrocytes and represents the endpoint of a long period of iron deprivation. It is stage IV of iron deficiency, when all iron stores are depleted. In the preceding three stages, although iron stores are depleted, there is no dysfunction. Several tests can be used to assess iron status, but each has its limitations:

- Total iron-binding capacity (TIBC)—capacity of transferrin to bind iron
- Transferrin—globulin that binds/transports Fe
- Percent saturation of transferrin (calculated by dividing serum iron by the TIBC)
- TIBC increases in iron deficiency
- As stored iron falls, saturation of transferrin decreases
- Serum iron: Poor indicator, highly variable day-to-day and during the day
- Ferritin—most sensitive—chief storage form of iron; directly proportional to iron stored in cells
- Zinc protoporphyrin/heme (ZPP/H) ratio—protoporphyrin binds iron to form heme or zinc to form zinc protoporphyrin. In the presence of iron deficiency, ratio will rise (iron deficiency defined as ratio >1:12,000) but is not affected by hematocrit or other causes of anemia, specific to iron deficiency.
- **Megaloblastic anemias:** This is a form of anemia characterized by the presence of large, immature, and abnormal red blood cell progenitors in the bone marrow and 95% of cases are attributable to folic acid or vitamin B_{12} deficiency.
- Folate deficiency also causes anemia. Folate stores are depleted after 2-4 months on deficient diet. Folate deficiency results in megaloblastic anemia, low leukocytes, and platelets.
- To differentiate anemia due to folate deficiency from that caused by vitamin B_{12} deficiency, it is necessary to measure serum B_{12} and serum folate, although RBC folate is more reflective of body stores. Anemia caused by the deficiency of vitamin B_{12}, is referred as 'Pernicious anemia', in which there is destruction of perietal cells in the stomach that produces intrinsic factor that support absorption of vitamin B_{12}.
- High formiminoglutamic acid (FIGLU) in the urine is also diagnostic criteria for megaloblastic anemia or liver disease.

The stages of folate deficiency are as follows:
- Stage I—early negative folate balance (serum depletion)
- Stage II—negative folate balance (cell depletion)
- Stage III—damaged folate metabolism with folate-deficient erythropoiesis
- Stage IV—clinical folate deficiency anemia.

Many nutritional indices are altered in PEM and other nutrient deficiency disorders are measured in body fluids.

PROTEIN STATUS

Protein is the major nutrient upon which body structure and function is based. Unlike fat and carbohydrate, it is not stored in a non-functional form in the body. Gain or loss of protein represents an equivalent gain or loss of function. Hence protein nutriture can be very crucial. Although protein status can be assessed by anthropometric, biochemical, clinical and dietary data, each of them has some limitations. Being objective and quantitative, biochemical indices are better indicators which may facilitatetreatment for improving protein status.

Some of the biochemical assessment of protein status is done by evaluation of somatic protein and visceral protein status. Somatic protein is found within skeletal muscle (75%) and visceral protein within the organs or viscera of the body (liver, kidneys, pancreas, heart and so on), the erythrocytes (red blood cells), and the granulocytes and lymphocytes (white blood cells), as well as in the serum proteins. The somatic and visceral pools are metabolically active forms of protein (known as body cell mass), which can be drawn on, when necessary, to meet various bodily needs. Protein status in children can be used to assess muscle development or growth retardation. It is important to assess protein in critical stages such as Protein-Energy Malnutrition (PEM), infection, burns, trauma,children who fail to thrive, persons with cancer and acquired immune deficiency syndrome (AIDS), ambulatory patients and juvenile rheumatoid arthritis.

Unlike carbohydrate and fat, protein cannot be stored in any non-functional form. Insufficiency of protein in the body may lead to catabolism of tissue and organs and impair body functions. Visceral protein can be accessed through serum protein. There are 4 important serum proteins that are often measured to assess protein status: (1) Albumin, (2) Prealbumin, (3) Transferrin and (4) Retinol Binding protein (RBP) as shown in Table 13.10A.

There are many acute phase proteins such as CRP and ORM which are useful during inflammation and protein like IGF-1 are valuable to assess growth during pregnancy, pre-puberty, anorexia, obesity and pituitary functions. Table 13.10B gives indications of such protein markers.

Indicators used to assess protein status: Several proteins are used as biochemical indices of protein status. These proteins are indicators of acute phase response and disease activity. They are used because inflammation affects body composition, in particular, muscle mass and function. When there is inflammation, cytokines are released and they induce catabolism of muscle. Albumin levels decrease with inflammation. Therefore, although malnutrition results in lower protein levels, inflammation also reduces the levels of proteins like albumin. Besides nutritional status, other factors can modify their concentrations such as hydration status, hepatopathies, infection, and inflammation. Therefore, it is advisable that these should not be used exclusively for nutritional diagnosis. Most of these proteins are synthesized in the liver; hence, a decreased concentration may be an indicator of PEM. The proteins generally measured are as follows and they differ in their half-lives. The normal range for each cut-off levels is given in Table 13.11. Among the various proteins that are used, albumin is the most frequently used for nutritional assessment.

Somatomedin C or insulin-like growth factor is considered as a good parameter to assess the intensity of metabolic response. It is a low molecular weight peptide and mediates the action of growth hormone. The limitation is that it is complex and expensive to determine. Also, its concentration is decreased in acute states of inflammation. Other proteins may be measured but these are not related to the nutritional status. These are protein C, alpha-1 antitrypsin, alpha-1-acid glycoprotein, fibrinogen, and haptoglobin.

The amount of muscle mass can be assessed. In malnutrition, or in hypercatabolic state, there is degradation of skeletal muscle. The indicators that can be used are:

Urinary creatinine: This is a degradation product of creatine that is excreted in urine. Synthesis of creatinine is constant in muscle and reflects muscle catabolism or protein status. It is lowered during starvation, stress, and prolonged periods of immobilization. It helps to determine whether there is nutritional deficiency but by itself is not useful for prognosis or for follow-up with patients. The limitations in using this metabolite as an indicator is that several factors influence interpretation, e.g., age, stress, dietary protein intake, and renal function. Also, a 24-hour collection is required and if incomplete collection is done or if there is oliguria, the interpretation will be incorrect and so will be the diagnosis of whether the person is malnourished or not.

Creatinine height index (CHI): Creatine is metabolized to creatinine at more or less stable rate and reflects the amount of muscle mass. It is a measure of lean muscle mass and can be calculated as:

Table 13.11: Normal cut-off values for different types of serum proteins.

Proteins	Half-life (in days)	Functions	Normal range and cut-off points	Advantages and limitations
Serum albumin	20	A transport protein for several substances, e.g., Ca, Mg, Zn, Se, lipids, free fatty acids, bilirubin, and many drugs	35–50 g/dL—normal >50 g/dL—possible dehydration <35 g/dL—could indicate malnutrition or overhydration or inflammation <25 g/dL—reflects leakage or loss due to burns, or from GI tract/renal, cirrhosis, and malignancy	When there is inflammation, levels of these substances decrease in parallel with decrease in albumin Albumin is a better prognostic indicator than an indicator of nutritional status Since its half-life is 20 days, it is a good indicator of chronic protein malnutrition
Transferrin and serum TIBC	8	An intravascular iron transport protein. It is an acute phase protein that responds acutely to changes in protein status	45–70 µmol/L—normal <45 µmol/L/<200 mg/dL—protein malnutrition >70 mg/dL	Levels are lowered when iron stores increase in pernicious anemia, sepsis, stress, malabsorption, inflammation, and liver disease Levels increase when there is iron deficiency, if person is on estrogen therapy, when person is dehydrated, and during pregnancy Therefore, this is not a sensitive indicator of protein nutritional status
Serum orosomucoid	5	–	0.55–1.05 g/L—normal <0.55 g/L—in malnutrition and due to protein losses >1.05 g/L—inflammation	–
Serum transthyretin/ prealbumin	1–2	Synthesized in liver, partially catabolized in kidney	~0.3 g/L—normal >0.3 g/L—in uremia, dehydration, and alcoholism <0.3 g/L—in fasting, malnutrition, malabsorption, cirrhosis, hepatic failure, overhydration, response to cytokines and hormones, and pregnancy	Responds quickly to nutritional support and rehabilitation but is not sensitive to adapted starvation Thus, it is generally sensitive to nutritional changes but is not a reliable index of nutritional status in diseased state
Insulin Growth Factor -1, IGF-1 or somatomedin C	1 day	–	–	–
Retinol-binding protein (RBP)	0.5	Binding protein for vitamin A	~60 mg/L—normal >60 mg/L—in uremia, alcoholism <60 mg/L—in malnutrition, malabsorption, vitamin A deficiency, cirrhosis, infection, and severe stress	Responds quickly to nutritional support, reflects recent dietary intake but is not sensitive to adapted starvation Can be used to follow-up but is not useful for patients with renal disease

$$\text{CHI (\%)} = \frac{\text{Measured 24-hour urinary creatinine}}{\text{Normal 24-hour urinary creatinine}} \times 100$$

In this, 24-hour urinary creatinine is measured. Ideal creatinine excretion is:
Males: 23 mg creatinine per kg body weight
Females: 18 mg creatinine per kg body weight
A CHI of 60–80% indicates moderate protein deficit and <60% indicates severe protein deficit.

3-methylhistidine: This is also a metabolite of muscle protein catabolism. It is increased when there is hypercatabolism but is decreased in the undernourished. It can be used for nutritional follow-up, and recovery.

Urea excretion: This reflects protein catabolism but the readings are influenced by intravascular volume, increase in nitrogen as well as renal function.

Catabolic index (CI): This helps to assess severity of stress in a patient. It is based on 24-hour urinary excretion of urea and is influenced by endogenous protein catabolism, dietary protein intake, and obligatory urinary urea excretion (UUN). It can be calculated as follows:
CI = UUN (g) – [Dietary nitrogen (g) + 3] × 2 calculated for a 24-hour period
0 = No significant stress; 0–5 = Moderate stress; and >5 = Severe stress

Nitrogen balance: This is noninvasive and can be used to assess metabolic stress. It is useful to follow-up and monitor treatment. However, it is a cumbersome method. Generally, a nitrogen balance between –2 and +2 is aimed for a nutritionally depleted or stressed individual.

Water Soluble Vitamins

Thiamine: Thiamine status can be determined by one of the three tests namely:
1. Erythrocyte transketolase activity
2. Thiamine pyrophosphate
3. Urinary excretion of thiamine before and after thiamine administration, and serum, erythrocyte, or whole blood thiamine levels.

Erythrocyte transketolase activity is a functional test that gives an idea about availability of thiamine, as transketolase is a thiamine-requiring enzyme. Normal values are 0.75–1.30 IU transketolase/Hb. It is a sensitive test that helps to detect deficiency, gives information about tissue reserves of the vitamin, and gives a functional evaluation at cellular level.

Thiamine pyrophosphate: This is a sensitive method for measuring thiamine pyrophosphate in whole blood and erythrocytes, as more than 80% of all thiamine in whole blood are found in erythrocytes. This gives a good idea about the adequacy of body stores as this is depleted from other tissues at the same rate that it is depleted from erythrocytes. It is considered to be a sensitive, specific, and precise method for assessing thiamine status and it is a reliable indicator of total body stores.

Free thiamine can be measured in blood plasma but this does not directly reflect the level in tissues. Rather, tissue thiamine is better reflected by erythrocyte or leukocyte thiamine.

Urinary thiamine levels give an idea about adequacy of the dietary intakes, but do not give information whether the person is deficient or not or to what extent thiamine reserves in the body are depleted. Urinary excretion of thiamine per gram of creatinine has been found to be correlated with thiamine intake. Urinary thiamine levels indicative of marginal deficiency are 90–220 µg/g of creatinine or 133–333 µg/day. Levels indicative of deficiency are <27 µg/g of creatinine or <40 µg/day. For reliable results, it is important to collect a 24-hour urine sample. The acceptable levels and cut-off levels to identify persons at risk are given in Table 13.12.

Folic acid: There are several methods for assessing folate status. The most commonly used is plasma or serum folate. However, these reflect recent dietary intake. RBC folate can be measured and these levels reflect tissue status measuring RBC folate which is costlier and time-consuming. The tests should be performed under fasting conditions, i.e., the person should be fasting for at least 8 hours fast and vitamin B_{12} injection should not have been given before the test.

Normal levels are: Serum folate: 6 mg/dL, RBC folate: 140 ng/mL. However, the reference range of plasma and RBC folate differs with age (Table 13.13).

Deoxyuridine test is done on aspirated bone marrow sample. It is considered to be the most sensitive and functional test to diagnose folate and/or vitamin B_{12} deficiency, but it is expensive and time-consuming. It measures the ability of deoxyuridine to suppress incorporation of thymidine into cultured bone marrow cells.

Table 13.12: Acceptable and cut-off levels of urinary thiamine in different age group.

Urinary thiamine (µg/g creatinine)	Deficient (high risk)	Low (medium risk)	Acceptable (low risk)
1–3 years	<120	120–175	176
4–6 years	<85	85–120	121
7–9 years	<70	70–180	181
10–12 years	<60	60–180	181
13–15 years	<50	50–150	151
Adults	<27	27–65	66
Pregnancy 2nd trimester 3rd trimester	<23 <21	23–54 21–49	55 50

Table 13.13: Normal range of plasma folate and RBC folate in different age groups.

Age groups	Plasma folate	RBC folate
Adults	2–20 ng/mL/4.5–45.3 nmol/L	140–628 ng/mL/317–1,422 nmol/L
Children	5–21 ng/mL/11.3–47.6 nmol/L	>160 ng/mL/>362 nmol/L
Infants	14–51 ng/mL/31.7–115.5 nmol/L	–

Histidine load test: Also called FIGLU/formiminoglutamate (a product of histidine catabolism) excretion test, in this test the patient is given a load of histidine and the resultant urinary excretion of formiminoglutamic acid is measured in urine collected after 6 hours of administered about 2–5 grams of oral histidine. In persons with normal folate status, excretion is about 5–20 mg which increases by 5–10 times in folate deficiency. This test is specific and helps to distinguish folic acid deficiency from vitamin B_{12} in megaloblastic anemia.

Riboflavin: Riboflavin status is generally assessed using the erythrocyte glutathione reductase (EGR) test and the activation coefficient (AC) is used (EGRAC). Glutathione reductase is a FAD-dependent enzyme and the activity coefficient of this enzyme is measured because it reflects tissue saturation and long-term riboflavin status. Activity coefficients are determined with and without addition of FAD in an in vitro assay. A value between 1.2 and 1.4 means riboflavin status is low and when the AC > 1.40, it is indicative of deficiency, whereas a value below 1.2 indicates that riboflavin status is acceptable. The EGRAC is considered to be the "gold standard index". Urinary riboflavin can also be measured. Precautions need to be taken such as protecting urine from light. Interpretive criteria for the urinary excretion of riboflavin are <27 µg/g creatinine for deficient and 27–79 µg/g creatinine for low status. If serum riboflavin is measured, the reference range is 4–24 µg/dL or 106–638 nmol/L of plasma or serum. If urinary riboflavin excretion is <19 µg/g creatinine (without recent riboflavin intake) or <40 µg per day, it can be interpreted that the person has riboflavin deficiency.

Niacin: A 24-hour urinary excretion of N1-methylnicotinamide (NMN) 0.8 mg/day (<5.8 mcmol/day) suggests niacin deficiency. It is thought to be the most reliable measure of intake and body status. A confirmatory test is, if serum tryptophan levels are below the normal reference range, associated with the consumption of a diet low in tryptophan. A ratio of less than 1 mg of metabolites per gram of creatinine is indicative of niacin deficiency.

Photosensitivity test is also done wherein skin is exposed to minimal erythema doses of UV light. Photosensitivity reactions include erythema (redness on the skin), swelling and blistering on exposed parts of the body as well as pruritic (itching), burning, or tingling sensations. A therapeutic trial can be done giving niacin for 5 days, and if the photosensitivity is due to niacin deficiency, there will be an improvement in the cutaneous symptoms within 48 hours of treatment. Also, in niacin deficiency, there are characteristic ECG changes that are normalized with niacin therapy.

Vitamin B_6: Vitamin B_6 status can be measured by direct and indirect methods. Direct methods include measurement of plasma pyridoxal phosphate (PLP) concentrations or measuring urinary levels of 4-pyridoxic acid which is the major inactive metabolite of vitamin B_6. The excretion of 4-pyridoxic acid reflects the body pool. The levels in females are lower than in males. The major limitation is that levels are reduced in riboflavin deficiency. Adequate values are 128–680 nmol/nmol of creatinine or >3.0 µmol/day. Pyridoxal phosphate is the primary active pyridoxal form and is used as the primary index of whole-body pyridoxal levels. However, it is advisable to measure albumin levels as well because PLP levels are dependent on albumin levels so PLP levels can be falsely interpreted as low. Plasma PLP level above 30 nmol/L indicates adequacy.

Indirect methods are tryptophan load test and methionine load test. Also, erythrocyte transaminase can be measured. In the tryptophan load test, a 2-gram load of tryptophan is given and urinary xanthurenic acid (a metabolite) is measured. If urinary xanthurenic acid is <65 µmol/day, it indicates adequacy. The methionine load test primarily reflects vitamin B_6 levels in liver. A 3-gram load of methionine is given and cystathionine is measured in urine. Person is said to have adequate status if the cystathionine excretion is <350 µmol/day.

Erythrocyte transaminases: This entails measurement of erythrocyte alanine aminotransferase (ALT or SGPT) and aspartic acid aminotransferase transaminase activity and/or stimulation indirect indices of vitamin B_6 status. These are long-term indicators of functional pyridoxine status because the lifespan of RBCs is 120 days. Activities of the respective transaminases are measured in vitro in the presence and absence of excess PLP and percent stimulation is calculated. The limitations of this indicator are that index decreases with age and values are falsely low in case of chronic alcoholism. Also, in hemolytic anemia, the lifespan of RBCs is reduced.

Vitamin C

Increase in vitamin C intake increases the plasma ascorbate concentration (PAC). normal range is >50 micromol/L and between 10–50 micromol/L is deficiency. A seum concentration of less than 11.4 micrdomol/L is defined as vitamin D deficiency. A level of less than 0.2 mg/dL has been found to be consistent with scurvy. At 70–80 micromol/L, there is a plateau which is due to decreased absorption rate and increased rate of excretion that is often affected by smoking, age, gender and infection.

Ascorbic acid concentration of WBC is a better indicator than serum ascorbic acid. Plasma vitamin C relfects recent intake whereas levels in leukocytes is reflective of tissue stores and influence on immune function and is less affected by acute dietary changes. A leukocyte vitamin C level of 0 mg/dL is indicative of latent scurvy, 0–7 mg/dL is indicative of deficiency and a level greater than is considered to be adeuate.

Vitamin B_{12}: This B-vitamin is closely related in its function to folic acid. B_{12} status can be assessed in various ways that are listed in Table 13.14.

Assessment of Fat-soluble Vitamins

Vitamin A: Vitamin A status can be assessed by clinical, biological, functional, and histological tests that include xerophthalmia, night blindness, conjunctival impression cytology, and dark adaptometry. The International Vitamin A Consultative Group has recommended night blindness

Table 13.14: Laboratory tests for vitamin B_{12}, micronutrients.

Micronutrients	Tests used	Merits	Demerits/limitations	Normal levels
Vitamin B_{12}	Serum cobalamin	Simple, can be done with limited resources, and sensitivity is good	Reflects recent intakes Serum levels altered by levels of binding proteins, illness, use of oral contraceptives, folate status, and pregnancy Elevated levels in alcoholic liver disease and renal disease	200 pg/mL
	Serum holo-transcobalamin	It is the transport protein in blood and believed to represent the metabolically active fraction Changes in concentrations appear to respond sooner during depletion leading to deficiency It is less likely to be influenced by pregnancy or renal function, has better predictive value than other tests	Levels may be affected by liver disease, macrophage activation, and autoantibodies Relatively expensive	–
	Methylmalonic acid	Measured in urine and serum Simple and reliable indicator	May generate false positives in patients with renal disease, or those with poor renal function Levels can be elevated by intestinal microbial overgrowth Expensive	Serum: Normal value—0.04–0.27 µmol/L Critical value—>0.37 µmol/L Urine: <=2 mg MMA/g creatine or < =3.6 mg MMA/mmol creatine Higher values are regarded as critical
	Schilling test	Helps to determine whether there are defects in absorption of orally administered vitamin Reliable to test adequacy of vitamin B12 absorption Quite sensitive, specific, and accurate Can help confirm diagnosis of pernicious anemia	There can be local reaction to the injection Lightheadedness and nausea may occur	Stage 1: Oral dose of radioactive vitamin B_{12} + injected vitamin B_{12} after 1 hour. If stage I is abnormal, stage II may be done 3–7 days later Stage II: Radioactive vitamin B_{12} along + intrinsic factor Stage II can tell whether low vitamin B_{12} levels are caused by gastric problems that prevent it from producing intrinsic factor Stage III: Antibiotics for 2 weeks. It can tell whether abnormal bacterial growth has caused the low vitamin B_{12} levels Stage IV: This test determines whether low vitamin B_{12} levels are caused by problems with the pancreas

during pregnancy and dark adaptometry testing for population assessment.

Eye signs like xerophthalmia can be used but this is detected when vitamin A depletion has occurred and does not really detect subclinical vitamin A deficiency. Conjunctival impression cytology has been used in field surveys because it does not require expensive equipment but in dry regions, there are difficulties. A small circle of filter paper is quickly touched to the eye surface with the help of a pumping device that holds the paper in position. The filter paper is then put into a fixative solution, followed by staining in order to differentiate goblet cells from endothelial cells. Based on the number of goblet cells (by microscopic examination), eye is considered either normal or abnormal. This test has been found to correlate well with biochemical tests.

Biochemical tests include measuring concentrations of serum retinol and/or breast milk retinol, relative dose response (RDR) and modified relative dose response (MRDR) tests, and deuterated retinol dilution assay.

As such, serum retinol concentrations are generally used in population studies to identify persons at risk of vitamin A deficiency. The drawback is that blood samples are required. Also, in healthy persons, serum retinol is homeostatically controlled and the levels begin to decline only when the liver stores are very low. Retinol-binding protein is an acute phase protein and hence, retinol levels decrease during infection. Status of other nutrients particularly that of iron has a negative effect on serum retinol concentrations as iron deficiency can decrease mobilization of vitamin A from liver stores. Breast milk concentrations can also be measured for population studies and have the advantage of being noninvasive and easier to collect; do not need to be processed much. It is considered that if lactating women in a community have marginal vitamin A status, it is likely that the children are at risk of vitamin A depletion. Serum retinol ≤0.70 µmol/L is indicative of deficiency.

The RDR and MRDR are sensitive indicators of vitamin A status but neither give information about what are the vitamin A reserves in the body nor do they help to differentiate between adequate levels of vitamin A and levels associated with toxicity. The MRDR is probably a better means of determining body reserves of vitamin A.

Other methods that have been developed include dried blood spot retinol determinations, retinol-binding protein concentrations, ratio of retinol-binding protein to transthyretin (this is a static measure, it helps to interpret whether serum retinol concentration is lowered due to infection), and isotope dilution assay using 13C-retinyl acetate and gas chromatography-combustion isotope ratio mass spectrometry (GCC-IRMS) and retinoyl β-glucuronide hydrolysis test. The isotope ratio test has been validated against liver stores.

Vitamin D: The preferred method according to current guidelines is to estimate circulating (after level 25-OHD) in serum. It should be measured using a reliable assay. It has a fairly long half-life of 2–3 weeks. The level of this metabolite has been found to be significantly associated with biochemical, functional, and clinical indices such as PTH levels, bone mineral density, neuromuscular function, and risk of fractures. However, the strength of these associations has been found to vary across different populations. Also, persons who have low levels of vitamin D (25 OHD) can have normal PTH levels. Current guidelines do not recommend measuring $1,25(OH)_2D3$ in order to evaluate vitamin D status. This is because in vitamin D-deficient individuals, secondary hyperparathyroidism can develop due to which expression of 1α-hydroxylase by kidneys is induced. Therefore, even if a person is deficient, $1,25(OH)_2D3$ levels can be normal or even elevated. Also, the half-life of this compound is only 4 hours, besides which there is no internationally accepted reference method or reference material.

Because of the limitation of 25-hydroxy vitamin D, measurement of bioavailable vitamin D has been suggested. However, clinical studies and validation need to be done before it can be accepted as a marker. It has also been suggested that $24,25(OH)_2D3$, a metabolite of vitamin D can be used. Also, calculating the vitamin D metabolite ratio (VMR) may improve assessment. It is the ratio between serum 1,25 (OH) 2 D3 and 25 (OH) D. Vitamin D level of ≥20 ng/mL used to be considered adequate for good bone health, a level below 20 ng/mL was considered as indicative of vitamin D deficiency. Later, it has been suggested that 30–40 ng/mL for children can be considered normal.

Vitamin E: Generally, serum tocopherol is technically easy and simple to measure that is used as an indicator. Some precautions are that the person should have been fasting for 12 hours and should not have consumed alcohol 24 hours prior to the test. The serum samples should be protected from light and the serum needs to be analyzed within 7 days of collection if the specimen is refrigerated or within 28 days if the samples were frozen. The reference range for adults is 5.7–19.9 mg/L. Besides this, the ratio of alpha-tocopherol:total cholesterol ratio is used, as it helps to prevent the overestimation of vitamin E deficiency. The mean ratio of alpha-tocopherol:total cholesterol for adults >18 years of age is 5.1 μmol/mmol. One can also express the ratio of alpha-tocopherol to sum of cholesterol and triglycerides, for which the adult reference interval of lipid ratio is 1.4–5.7 mg/g.

However, other confirmatory tests may be required and it is relatively expensive. Since platelets contain significant concentration of alpha-tocopherol, the platelet tocopherol content appears to be a promising marker of vitamin E status. If one needs an idea about body stores of vitamin E, then tissue tocopherol has to be measured, specifically adipose tissue or liver biopsy samples are needed. However, the limitations are that it cannot be done for large populations. Buccal mucosa has been investigated as alternative, wherein biopsy samples are obtained since by gentle scraping, of cells from buccal mucosa are obtained. The cells adhering to the spatula are suspended in isotonic saline after washing and then analyzed. Results are expressed as μmol of vitamin E/g of protein. However, the usefulness of this test still needs to be established.

A functional indicator of vitamin E status is the erythrocyte hemolysis test. This is based on the antioxidant properties of vitamin E and measures the ability of red blood cells to resist oxidative damage. It requires a small blood sample, is easy to perform but it lacks specificity, and changes in the status of other nutrients can also influence the rate of erythrocyte hemolysis. Also, freshly prepared samples of erythrocytes must be used, making it an impractical method for field studies.

Vitamin K: Circulating phylloquinone levels are generally measured. However, there are challenges in its measurement because its concentrations are 50–25,000 times lower than those of other fat-soluble vitamins. Several conditions affect phylloquinone levels namely dietary intake (concentrations peak 6–10 hours postprandially), possibly the meal pattern, and race/ethnicity. Therefore, phylloquinone should be measured in fasting state and should be corrected for triglycerides as it is transported on triglyceride-rich lipoproteins in circulation, with smaller fractions carried on HDL and LDL cholesterol. Currently, there is no established threshold of plasma/serum phylloquinone to determine either adequacy or deficiency. However, in controlled feeding studies when the adequate intake was met, the circulating phylloquinone levels were approximately 1.0 nM.

Clinically, deficiency can be detected by assessing prothrombin time. However, this test is nonspecific and its sensitivity for measuring K status is low. Also, it does not reflect dietary intakes in healthy adults.

Undercarboxylated prothrombin or proteins induced by deficiency or absence of vitamin K, known as PIVKA-II can be measured in blood as this reflects depletion of vitamin K and/or warfarin use. Osteocalcin is a K-dependent protein that can be detected in serum and is used as a biomarker of bone formation. Undercarboxylated osteocalcin levels increase when there is dietary vitamin K depletion, and decrease when the person is given a vitamin K supplement. It is thought to be a more sensitive indicator than is PIVKA-II and reflects vitamin K better. Another K-dependent protein, matrix Gla protein (MGP), is being studied but further studies are needed. Urinary markers can also be measured. Gamma-carboxyglutamic acid (GLA) can be measured because it is an indicator of the turnover of all vitamin K-dependent proteins. Urinary GLA generally (but not invariably) decreases, when K intake decreases.

Minerals

Iron: Hemoglobin (Hb) is the most widely used screening test for anemia. The normal range for men is 13.5–17.5 g/dL and 12.0–15.5 g/dL for women. The advantages are that there is no need for the person to have fasted, and the test is simple, inexpensive, and rapid. Its major limitation is that anemia is not caused only by iron deficiency and the norms differ by age, sex, pregnancy, altitude, and smoking. Its specificity and sensitivity are low.

Bone marrow iron is a useful indicator of body iron stores. Bone marrow fluid is aspirated and the sample is usually collected from the posterior iliac crest. Microscopic examination of stained bone marrow cells is done. The limitation is that it is not only expensive but it is traumatic and invasive.

Reticulocyte hemoglobin concentration can be measured in whole blood samples. It is an indicator of Hb concentration in new RBCs. Reticulocytes mature for 1–3 days within the bone marrow and circulate for 1–2 days before becoming mature erythrocytes. The reticulocyte Hb concentration gives an indirect measure of the functional iron that is available for new red blood cell production during the preceding three to four days, i.e., it represents the new RBCs that are about 18–36 hours old and so are only recently affected by deficiency. Its major limitation is that it requires expensive equipment in order to obtain reliable results.

Serum or plasma iron: Normal levels are 60–170 µg/dL. It is an indicator of iron bound to transferrin in blood. The person is required to be fasting for about 12 hours before blood is drawn for the measurement. It is advisable to collect samples in the morning because iron levels are highest at this time. Its limitation is that it exhibits diurnal variation after meals. Serum iron levels are low in chronic disease, hence this is not a specific indicator.

Total iron-binding capacity: This is assayed in serum or plasma samples. This is indicative of the total capacity of circulating transferrin bound to iron, the normal range being 240–450 µg/dL. The person needs to be fasting for 8 hours before blood is drawn. One major limitation of this assay is that there is considerable overlap between normal values and values in iron deficiency. This test is not widely used presently as serum ferritin is preferred as an indicator.

Transferrin saturation: This is measured in serum or plasma. It is calculated as: Serum iron divided by total iron-binding capacity. Normal levels are: 15–50% in males and 12–45% in females, with saturation of less than 15% being indicative of iron deficiency. It is widely used but serum ferritin is preferred. It is a sensitive test that helps to detect early hemochromatosis. Its limitation is that the levels are affected by intake of food, alcohol, and some drugs.

Erythrocyte protoporphyrin and zinc protoporphyrin: This is an indicator of restricted iron supply to developing red blood cells and the measurement can be done with whole blood as well as dried blood spots. Zinc protoporphyrin is present in small amounts in RBCs. Most of the protoporphyrin in RBCs combines with iron to form heme and when there is iron deficiency, instead of iron, zinc combines with protoporphyrin to form heme. Thus, in iron deficiency, zinc protoporphyrin levels increase in blood. Assessment of iron status can be done by one of two methods: free erythrocyte porphyrin and zinc porphyrin to heme ratio. For 1–5-year-old children, it is a better indicator than hemoglobin but in adults, its sensitivity and specificity is similar to hemoglobin. The reference range is 0–35 µg/dL.

Serum ferritin: Levels of serum ferritin are directly proportional to iron stores and generally ferritin levels in serum/plasma are assayed. The advantage is that no special preparation is required. Serum ferritin level below 15 ng/mL indicates deficiency. Measurement of serum ferritin along with measurement of soluble transferrin receptors is considered to be the best approach for assessment of iron status. Its limitation is that it is an acute phase protein and so during inflammation or in subclinical infection, ferritin levels are increased.

Soluble transferrin receptors (sTfRs): Transferrin receptors are used by cells to acquire iron for their physiological requirements. When there is iron deficiency, the concentration of surface transferrin receptors increase, particularly on the erythroid precursors on bone marrow, in an attempt to acquire iron. Transferrin receptors are present in serum (circulation) and they reflect the total body concentration of transferrin receptors. Normally, the main source is erythroid precursors but early in iron deficiency, the concentration in serum begins to rise with onset of iron-deficient erythropoiesis. Thus, as iron deficiency progresses and becomes more severe, the levels rise. The ratio of sTfR/ferritin is useful especially in population studies of iron deficiency. It also helps to distinguish between anemia of chronic inflammation and anemia due to iron deficiency. Reference values are 1.8–4.6 mg/L.

Calcium status: Calcium is essential for bone and tooth formation, muscle contraction, blood clotting, and cell membrane integrity. Several methods are used to assess calcium nutritional status such as calcium balance study, serum calcium or radiological examination. None of these are suitable for screening large groups or at population level to determine magnitude of calcium deficiency in a population. Calcium metabolic balance is considered to be the most effective method for assessing calcium status but it has limitations in terms of time, cost and is laborious. Serum calcium is generally measured, it indicates functioning of parathyroid hormone which regulates the calcium levels in the blood. Normally serum calcium values are maintained within a fairly narrow range from 8.5 to 10.5 mg/dL. Values may vary among laboratories as much as 0.5 mg/dL. A low value indicates poor dietary intake of calcium and high value indicates hyperactive parathyroid hormone. When serum levels are high, more calcium is available to be excreted through the urine. It can be high during the day and low in the evening. Urinary calcium levels are more responsive to changes in dietary calcium intake than are serum levels. A diet rich in protein and phosphate can also alter calcium output. Hypocalciuria may also result from renal failure or when the kidneys' ability to reabsorb calcium is impaired. Ratio of calcium to creatinine calculated from 2-hour fasting urine samples is a good indicator of calcium status but requires further study. Radiological changes or bone changes are not a good indicator as they reflect only severe calcium deficiency, and do not provide a diagnosis of calcium deficiency during the early stages of deficiency.

Zinc status: Generally serum or plasma zinc is measured because it reflects dietary intake, responds to zinc supplementation. However, serum zinc is better used for groups or population studies rather than to assess individual status. In population studies, serum zinc will provide information about the magnitude of zinc deficiency and about the magnitude of risk of zinc deficiency. Serum zinc levels are influenced by recent food intake, time of day, age, gender and presence/absence of infection or inflammation. Since zinc is involved in many metabolic processes, including protein synthesis, wound healing, immune function, and tissue growth and maintenance, its deficiency is considered a potential public health issue for which further study is needed. Normal range is 70-125 µg/dL and level below 30 µg/dL indicates severe deficiency whereas 160 µg/dL is associated with toxicity of zinc.

Magnesium status: Magnesium plays a role in regulating the calcium and potassium levels in your body. Generally, serum magnesium is used and normal values ranges from 1.7-2.5 mg/dL or 0.7–1 mmol/L, serum levels can change by dietary magnesium intake, albumin levels, renal excretion and the amount absorbed by the intestines as well as supplementation. However, serum is the best indicator as serum levels can mask deficiency as short-term fluctuations will occur in response to dietary intake. Magnesium excretion (urinary level) is influenced by dietary intake, medication, hormones such as parathyroid hormone, calcitonin, glucagon, gender, age (young women retain magnesium better than do young men), oral contraceptive use, body mass index. Diuretics and some chemotherapeutic agents can cause abnormally high magnesium excretion. In persons who are on long-term diuretic management and diabetics, renal magnesium wasting occurs. Therefore urine levels should not be considered as a good indicator. Magnesium levels in RBC or monocytes have higher magnesium content than does serum/plasma and is considered to be a better indicator. However, there is insufficient information to establish this is a reliable and robust indicator. Another method is intravenous magnesium loading followed by estimation of magnesium in a 24-hour urine sample. Here the percentage retention of the administered dose is estimation. However, this test is expensive, and is impractical for use in clinical settings although it may be used in research studies.

Copper status: There is no reliable biomarker of copper status. Serum copper is measured but is not considered to be a very sensitive indicator because more than 90% of serum copper is carried as part of ceruloplasmin and ceruloplasmin levels are elevated in many inflammatory conditions. Elevated serum copper may reflect the inflammation that accompanies atherosclerosis.

There are many tests done especially hospitalized settings to confirm the pathogenesis of any diseases. These are not direct indication of nutrient deficiency but indicative, e.g., alkaline phosphatase.

CLINICAL ASSESSMENT

Clinical signs and symptoms are assessed by observing different parts of the body externally. Physical examination is an essential feature of nutritional assessment. It is the simplest and most practical method of assessing nutritional status of both individuals and a group of people. It includes assessment of the person's general condition and clinical examination. A number of physical signs need to be looked for, as they are associated with malnutrition and with deficiencies of vitamins and minerals. However, some are specific whereas the others are not specific. At community level, trained auxiliary health workers can detect signs and refer the person to a physician who will then conduct a more detailed examination. Detecting the relevant signs helps to establish and confirm nutritional diagnosis.

In the general clinical examination, special attention is paid to:

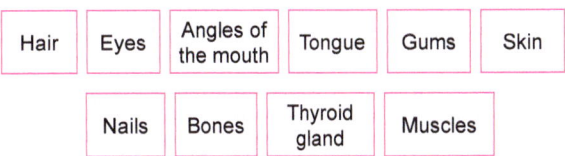

Attention needs to be given to assessment of body fat stores, wasting of muscle mass, edema due to malnutrition or ascites, skin rash, hair thinning, its color and texture and evidence of specific nutritional deficiencies. Detection of relevant signs helps in establishing/confirming nutritional diagnosis. According to the World Health Organization, clinical signs can be put into three groups (Fig. 13.6):

Physical signs need to be recorded as precisely as possible and standard definitions need to be used. Also, it is important to consider that several factors can confound interpretation of signs. For example:
- Excessive exposure to heat or sun, wind, or cold
- Lack of general personal hygiene
- Age of the person. For example, signs of scurvy in a child will present as pain, swollen joints because there is

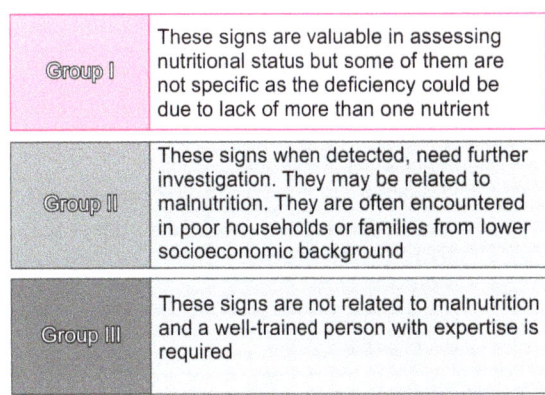

Fig. 13.6: Three groups for assessing clinical signs.

bleeding in the bones. However, in an elderly person, the same nutrient deficiency will appear as small black and blue marks often on the shin bones.

When any clinical sign is detected, it is important to investigate it by conducting biochemical test(s) for confirmation. Example before concluding that pallor is due to anemia, the hemoglobin level needs to be determined for confirmation. Epiphyseal enlargement or costochondral beading needs to be confirmed by X-rays. When thyroid enlargement is seen, laboratory tests are needed to confirm iodine deficiency.

This is an essential feature in most nutrition surveys at community severity. It can be applied to a large group but the disadvantage is that it does not quantify the exact level of nutrient deficiencies as many of the signs are not specific and need to be supported by biochemical tests. Table 13.15 describes the generally used signs of nutritional deficiencies.

Besides deficiency, excess intake has adverse effects, and for some there are signs as listed in the Table 13.16.

Clinical examination has some merits but there are also some limitations (Table 13.17).

Table 13.15: Clinical signs in different organs due to different nutrient deficiencies.

Parts of body	Signs	Attributable to which nutrient deficiency
General appearance	Person appears very thin or wasted, short stature Activity level decreased	Due to inadequate intake of food, lack of sufficient protein
	Edema	Lack of sufficient protein
	Obese	Imbalance between energy intake and energy expenditure
Skin	Pallor	Anemia (iron, folic acid and vitamin B_{12})
	Pigmentation, desquamation	Niacin, protein–energy malnutrition
	Xerosis, follicular hyperkeratosis	Vitamin A
	Petechiae, purpura	Vitamin C
	Bruising	Vitamin C, vitamin K and folic acid
	Symmetrical dermatitis of skin exposed to light, pressure Edema	Niacin
	Scrotal, vulval dermatitis	Riboflavin
	Generalized dermatitis	Zinc, essential fatty acids
	Erythematous rash around mouth and perianal area	Zinc
Hair	Sparse, thin	Zinc, protein, and biotin
	Easy to pull out/easily pluckable, dull, altered texture, and flag sign	Protein deficiency
	Depigmented, normally curly hair lacks curl	–

Contd...

Contd...

Parts of body	Signs	Attributable to which nutrient deficiency
Mouth	Glossitis	Riboflavin, niacin, folic acid, vitamin B_{12}, and protein
	Angular stomatitis	Riboflavin and iron
	Cheilosis	B-complex vitamins
	Leukoplakia	Vitamin A and B-complex (particularly—folic acid, niacin, and vitamin B_{12})
	Sore mouth and tongue	Vitamin B_{12}, vitamin B_6, folic acid, vitamin C, and iron
	Seborrheic dermatitis in nasolabial folds	Riboflavin
	Diffuse pigmentation of facial skin	Protein
Tongue	Glossitis	Niacin, riboflavin, vitamin B_{12}, and folate
Eyes	Night blindness	Vitamin A
	Bitot's spots	Vitamin A
	Corneal xerosis	Vitamin A
	Corneal ulcers, keratomalacia Corneal scars	Vitamin A
	Xerophthalmia	Vitamin A
	Photophobia, blurring	Riboflavin, vitamin A, and zinc
	Retinitis pigmentosa	Vitamin E
	Conjunctival inflammation	Vitamin A
	Small yellowish lumps around eyes (xanthelasma)	Hyperlipidemia
	Tumors (small/large) around joints of hands, legs and skin (xanthomas)	Hyperlipidemia
Nails	Spoon shaped, koilonychia	Anemia (iron deficiency)
Teeth	Caries	Fluoride
	Mottled pitted enamel	Fluoride
	Hypoplastic enamel	Vitamin A, vitamin D
Lower limbs	Edema	Wet beriberi (thiamine deficiency), protein deficiency
	Wrist and foot drop	Dry beriberi (thiamine deficiency)
Bones and joints	Costochondral beading	Vitamin D and vitamin C deficiency
	Craniotabes, frontal bossing and epiphyseal enlargement	Vitamin D
	Bone tenderness	Vitamin C
Muscles	Decreased muscle mass	Insufficient food (protein and calorie inadequacy)
	Tenderness in calves	Thiamine
	Generalized dermatitis	Zinc, essential fatty acids
	Small yellowish lumps around eyes (xanthelasma)	Hyperlipidemia
	Tumors (small/large) around joints of hands, legs and skin (xanthomas)	Hyperlipidemia

Contd...

Table 13.16: Signs of excessive intake of some vitamins.

Vitamins	Signs of excess
Vitamin A	Hepatomegaly, alopecia and headaches
Vitamin B_6	Neuropathy
Pantothenic acid	Diarrhea
Niacin	Vasomotor instability, flushing

Table 13.17: Merits and limitations of clinical examination.

Merits	Limitations
Quick and easy to perform	Clinical signs are manifested at late stage of deficiency Do not enable early detection of nutritional deficiency
Inexpensive	Investigator needs good training
Noninvasive	Signs are sometimes not specific to deficiency of a single nutrient
	Many a times, clinical signs do not correlate with biochemical values or dietary data

DIETARY ASSESSMENT

The purpose of dietary assessment is:
- To identify persons/population groups at risk of becoming malnourished.
- To identify those who are malnourished.
- For intervention purposes:
  - To develop interventions to meet needs of target group
  - To help improve targeting of interventions
  - To measure effectiveness of interventions.
- Trend data to show impact of policy over time.
- As part of nutritional assessment, dietary assessment is used to characterize the dietary patterns of individuals in clinical practice or for research purposes. It is also used to assess exposure to nutrients and nonnutrients and in research studies or in clinical practice, and to study the health effects of dietary patterns, foods, and nutrients. Based on these, dietary guidelines are formulated and issued. Also, nutrition programs are developed for at-risk populations and their impact is monitored.
- Dietary assessment is an important part of nutrition therapy. It is especially relevant to the management of noncommunicable diseases. Measurement of dietary intake is necessary to inform, support, and evaluate interventions. In weight loss regimens, accurate estimation of dietary caloric intake is important for diet planning and counseling as well as assessing effectiveness of the regimens.

However, there are challenges to dietary assessment such as the variability and heterogeneity of cuisines and food choices and the limited knowledge about composition of food for the large number of nutrients and especially of cooked foods in India.

A number of tools are used for dietary assessment:

24-hour recall	Food frequency questionnaire
Food record	Food diary
Food habits questionnaire	24-hour weighment

An ideal method of dietary assessment should be fairly quick, easy to use, inexpensive, and gives precise and accurate estimates of the intakes of foods, nutrients, bioactive substances, additives, and contaminants with minimal error in measurement. Different methods that are used for dietary assessment have been well-explained in a document published by the FAO (2018).

The methods can be used to collect retrospective or prospective information related to diet. Retrospective direct methods include food frequency questionnaire, 24-hour recall, and dietary history. Prospective direct methods include estimated food records, weighed food records, and duplicate meal method. Besides these, a number of innovative methods have been developed such as: personal digital assistant (PDA), image-assisted dietary assessment methods, mobile-based technologies, interactive computer and web-based technologies, and scan and sensor-based technologies (Fig. 13.7).

Generally, 24-hour recall and food frequency questionnaire are used. Similarly, food diary may be used, but each of these has its limitations because it is subjected to considerable bias and error. Thus, none of these can be considered to be "gold standards". One important point is that dietary assessment is based primarily on a person's ability to report consumption. The tool that is used depends on the purpose of assessment in terms of whether one needs/requires information on nutrient intakes, or food patterns or intakes of different food items. Also, it depends whether the information sought is qualitative or quantitative (Table 13.18).

Other problems associated with these methods that are based on self-reporting are that biases result from the presence of social desirability (tendency to avoid social

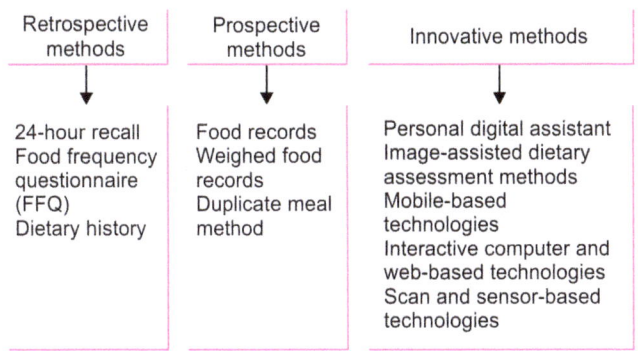

Fig. 13.7: Dietary methods of nutritional assessment.

Table 13.18: Qualitative information versus quantitative information.

Qualitative information	Quantitative information
Can use food group method where foods are grouped according to the nutrients they are good sources of The number of servings from each group may be recorded and compared with the minimum requirement	Amount of energy and other nutrient(s) in each food that is consumed is calculated using food composition tables
Compared to quantitative method is less time-consuming	More time-consuming than the qualitative method

criticism or respond in a manner that is consistent with what is expected norms), either there is some underestimation or overestimation, assumptions are made but food composition tables are not able to give values for each food related to processing and storage losses. Thus, inaccurate measurement of dietary exposure may make it difficult to detect correlations between dietary exposure and disease risk. Besides the limitations of each method, the skill of the person who collects the information is an important factor.

Some of the sources of error in dietary assessment include:
- Type of food consumed (raw, processed, cooked, and preparation practices)
- How much (serving size)
- How often
- Consumed by whom (e.g., young, elderly and immuno-compromised)
- Affected by factors such as:
  - Season
  - Region/culture
  - Wealth/socioeconomic factors/income
  - Age
  - Sex
  - Weight status
  - Education.
- Memory and the ability of the person to recall about episodes of eating and drinking, and general impressions about one's diet
- Desire to reduce the inconvenience of reporting
- Inappropriate for some groups such as children, elderly.

Let us briefly examine each of the methods:

Diet recall (24-hour recall method): As in case of diet record, it allows quantitative assessment of intake and there is less burden on the person whose diet is being assessed. The person does not have to be literate and it is not likely to alter the eating pattern of the person. However, it relies on recall and memory of the person, and if habitual intake has to be captured, recall will have to done on several occasions. A trained interviewer (generally a nutritionist/dietician) asks the person to recall all the foods and beverages consumed in the previous 24 hours. The person who is obtaining the information must have adequate information about cuisines and menu items, cooking methods, preparation practices, including prevalent regional or ethnic foods, and be knowledgeable about foods available in the marketplace. The interview is fairly structured but the interviewer should use probes to help the respondent remember all foods consumed throughout the day and about how foods were prepared. Probing is also useful in recovering many items not originally reported, such as common additions to foods (e.g., butter on toast) and eating occasions that may have not been originally reported (e.g., snacks and beverages). Although it is fairly quick and easy to do, it depends on the memory of the person being interviewed. Also, the previous day's intake may not be representative of usual intakes.

Food diary: Food intake, i.e., types and amounts are recorded by the individual as and when the item (food and/or beverage) is consumed, i.e., at time of consumption. The length of collection period varies from a single up to 7 days. This method is reliable but is burdensome for the person and is difficult to maintain.

Diet history: It is useful for assessing nutritional status, provided the information is collected by a trained interviewer. Details are to be collected about the usual intake, types of food consumed, amount, frequency, and timing of food consumption. It is important to cross-check and verify the information collected.

Diet record: The person himself/herself is required to record all the food and beverages consumed over a 24-hour period which may be extended over three days, usually two weekdays and one weekend day. The individual should be given clear-cut instructions and trained to record his/her food intake. Intake can be measured in terms of household measures or a weighing scale can be provided. One important advantage is that accurate quantitative information is obtained. Alternatively, a portion size guide can be used. This guide could include models and/or pictures, helping to improve the accuracy of estimation, although this places a higher burden on the person who has to record. Recording can be done on paper, or on computer. At the end, the record should be reviewed by a trained person to clarify the entries and to probe for forgotten foods. Diet record cannot be done by children, illiterate persons. In such cases, someone other than the child/illiterate person can be involved for recording. As the number of days of recording intakes is increased, the validity of the information is likely to decrease. Limitations include high burden on the person required to do the food record, can alter the eating behavior of the person, and the person may not complete the day's record of food intake. One advantage is that it can be used for self-monitoring to effect behavior change.

Diet recall using multiple-pass method: The current state-of-the-art 24-hour dietary recall. ntake is reviewed more than once in an effort to retrieve forgotten eating occasions and foods.

It consists of:
- An initial "quick list", in which the respondent reports all the foods and beverages consumed, without interruption from the interviewer.
- A forgotten foods list of nine food categories commonly omitted in 24-hour recall reporting (probe for foods forgotten in step I).
- Time and occasion, in which the time each eating occasion began and what the respondent would call it are reported.
- A detail pass/cycle, in which probing questions ask for more detailed information about the food and the portion size, in addition to review of the eating occasions and times between the eating occasions, and
- Final review, in which any other item not already reported is asked.

A 24-hour recall interview using the multiple-pass approach typically requires between 30 minutes and 45 minutes.

Food Frequency Questionnaire (FFQ)

These are designed to measure habitual intake over a defined period of time. The individual is asked about his/her usual frequency of consumption of different foods for a specific period from a list that is provided. The list will often contain at least 100 foods. The foods included depend on the purpose of using the FFQ information. They can be nonquantitative. For example, a person may be asked whether he/she consumes coffee but no question is asked about the portion size. In many epidemiological studies, FFQs have been used. In quantitative FFQ, how much is consumed will be included. Most FFQ versions ask about portion size. In addition, general questions can be asked about common cooking practices, e.g., type of fat/oil used for cooking. Estimates of intakes are obtained by summing up all the foods based on frequency of consumption, the number of portions, and the serving size (that may be either specified or assumed). However, an FFQ cannot give an accurate estimate of intake of a specified food or nutrient over a specified period of time. Typically, an FFQ should take 30–60 minutes to fill depending on the information that is sought and the number of items in the FFQ.

Modes of administering the FFQ include in-person, other ways that have been used are telephone, email, and nowadays web-based surveys are conducted. The latter are helpful because one can overcome geographical limitations and are less expensive, while larger numbers can be covered.

Limitations of FFQ include recall errors especially when the time between the behavior and the report increases. It may be difficult for the individual to recall frequencies of intakes over a given period of time, e.g., previous weeks/months. Recall is reliable for foods that are rarely eaten but misclassification is very likely for unspecific questions, such as "other vegetables", "other fruits". Precision in quantifying intakes is not possible with a FFQ, more so among children who may not be able to estimate portion size.

Weighed Food Record

This is regarded as the most precise method. The person/subject/respondent is asked to weigh each and every food that he/she eats and record the same, as well as describe the portion size, write the brand name wherever applicable, and write down the details of food preparation. The number of days for which this is done can vary from one single day to as many as seven days. This is essentially used for research purposes and the number of days for which weighment is done depends on the purpose of the research.

The advantages of this method are that it allows assessment of actual or usual intakes but this depends on the number of days for which the diet record is done. It is more accurate than other dietary assessment methods and is said to be the "gold standard" method. There is no reliance on the person's memory, provides the exact portion size consumed, yields information about the food and its preparation, meal patterns, and does not rely on the individual's memory. The specificity of this method is high.

The limitations of this method is that it is both time-consuming and labor-intensive for both the person (investigator) recording and the subject. It requires literacy and numeracy skills if the person himself/herself weighs and records the food intake. Also, the person needs to be motivated especially if the number of days of recording is more. In field situations, a trained field investigator can do the weighing and recording if the information is being collected from an illiterate person or children, elderly, etc. It is possible that the person being studied may alter his/her food intake and meal pattern to reduce the burden. This method is expensive because digital weighing scales are required; staff/investigators need to be well-trained. Also, it is difficult to weigh foods that are eaten away from home as a suitable environment is required for weighing foods (it is a bit cumbersome). Foods that are not eaten frequently may not get captured with this method.

INNOVATIVE METHODOLOGIES FOR DIETARY INTAKE

Traditionally used methods have their limitations in terms of relying on the memory of the person whose diet is being studied and the problem of estimating portion sizes, newer methods have been developed using information and communication technologies. These technologies are aimed to reducing cost of gathering and automatically analyzing the diet (processing dietary information), besides not relying on the person's memory. A big advantage is that with these technologies, personalized feedback and advice can be provided to the individual.

While all of these are attractive, they have limitations in terms of applying such technologies in rural areas, in areas/persons/communities from economically disadvantaged backgrounds, or for persons who have low level of literacy. Hence, most of these technologies presently are more suitable for urban population/more developed regions. Innovative technologies to improve dietary assessment have been classified into four key groups as shown in Figure 13.8.

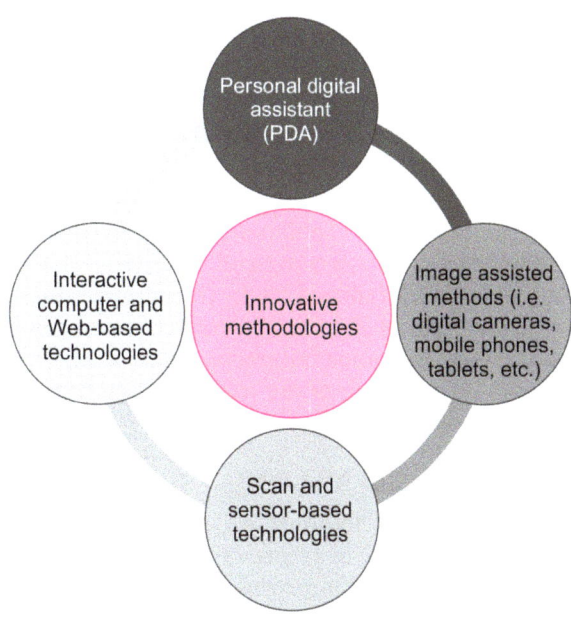

Fig. 13.8: Innovative methodologies for dietary intake.

Personal Digital Assistant (PDA)

This is a handheld computer. It has specially designed dietary software program that is used to register dietary intake. It is useful for self-monitoring. There is a predefined list of food items and the person records his/her intake by selecting the food item consumed. Its merit is that it allows collection of real-time data. The person who intends using this device must be first trained. PDAs currently have a list of approximately 4,000 items. However, the burden on the person is higher as compared to using pen and paper, since the list of foods is very long. PDAs are designed to also help in measuring portion sizes/the amounts of the items consumed with electronic prompts, food photographs, picture books or food models, and household measures. This information is then uploaded and reviewed by dieticians and matched with food composition tables for further nutrient intake analysis.

Image-assisted Dietary Assessment

These are methods that use images of foods for analysis. They could be photographs or videos that have been used to capture food intake when the food is actually eaten. The images are captured using handheld devices/cameras and ideally for each item consumed two sets of images should be taken—one before consumption and one after the person has finished eating so the amount eaten is captured. This helps to make the estimation more accurate and reduces the burden on the person who records. It can be used to complement the traditionally used methods as well as being used by itself as a primary record of food intake. The person who is participating should be given a marker such as a fork/pen/marked table cloth that is placed very near the plate or beneath the container in which he/she eats from, before the images are taken. This helps to improve accuracy of estimating portion size. This can be supplemented by asking the person to write whatever was eaten and to describe whatever cannot be captured from the images, especially if they are not clear. Some people also use a 24-hour recall in order to obtain information about cooking methods, foods that are not visible, and condiments and garnishes used. The photographs/videos can be sent via internet after each meal/snack/eating episode. As with PDA, these are reviewed by a nutritionist who will then estimate the portion size from these images directly or by comparing them with reference portions either on a computer screen or from a printed collection of photographs. Nutrient intakes are then collected using food composition tables or databases on nutrient content of cooked foods. The information can be used with that from 24-hour recall/record in order to identify foods that were consumed but not reported or where there were errors in reporting in the traditional methods, thus reducing memory bias.

Mobile-based Technologies

With greater access to mobiles, this technology has tremendous potential in terms of reducing the burden of recording while also improving accuracy of the record of dietary intakes. With the mobile, i.e., a smartphone or tablet, images/videos are shot of all foods and beverages at every occasion/episode and voice records can also be made. It would be helpful for estimating intakes of children and adolescents, who are attracted to use of technology and are tech-savvy. This technology can be used for short-term dietary assessment. Estimation can be done by the respondent, although, as it is done for the other technologies, a dietician/nutritionist identifies the foods, estimates the portion sizes. Mobile applications have been developed for the purpose of recording food intakes and technologies have been developed to facilitate identifying foods and estimating portion sizes through an automatic analysis of the images of the foods. This is based on digital image segmentation and analysis. The images may be linked directly to food composition databases that allow for calculation of intakes of energy and other nutrients. These technologies are still being studied for their usability. This technology is likely to be useful however, since there is reliance on automated images, underestimation is a possibility if the person does not take photographs before and after consuming every food item/beverage consumed (as this does not allow any retrospective recording of meals), if he/she forgets to photograph a food item or if the quality of the images is poor.

Interactive Computer and Web-based Technologies

This is based on using interactive programs for dietary assessment. The programs are installed on a computer (either a desktop or a portable one) that is connected to the internet. Hence, the term web-based is used. This technology can be used to collect dietary intake information for a short or longer period of time. The traditional method of pen and paper is used but these are introduced into a computer program along with several multimedia attributes such as "colors, food photographs, audio narration, animated guides, graphics and/or touch screens, popup functionalities, and webcams" (FAO, 2018). The person reports his/her food intake for a specific period and this information is interpreted.

Interactive computer based assessment methods have been developed to analyze data gathered using pen and paper and tools such as the FFQ, 24-hour recall, food records, and dietary history. For data collection, participants are asked to report their food intake during a specific period, and this information is added to software that has been developed such that forgotten items can be probed. Food items are coded and once entered into the system, nutrient content of these are calculated based on the multimedia features, adjustable images of portion sizes. One limitation is that the user should be highly literate and have computer skills. Some of these technologies require a nutritionist, and/or high-speed internet access. This may be a problem for people with limited financial resources and access to computers, lack of computer literacy.

Scan and Sensor-based Technologies

Here the person who is recording his/her food intake is required to scan bar codes of purchased food items. This is one of the limitations of this technology because only commercial items that are generally restricted to processed food items and those that have nutrient content printed on the label. This does not place much burden on the respondent and is not likely to alter the person's eating habits much. A sensor-based technology has been developed. This consists of a small electronic device that contains a miniature camera, a microphone, a memory card, and other sensors. The person whose food intake is being monitored is required to wear the device around the neck while eating and the device is supposed to record food intake automatically by collecting visual information in front of the person as he/she eats and/or drinks. This information is stored on the memory card and information is transferred to dieticians' computers as and when it is recorded. It is useful in home settings by use of markers. Outside the home, the device emits small beams that allows for calculating the portion size. The system is linked to a food base so that nutrient intakes can be calculated. In some devices, the number of times the person chews and swallows has been incorporated. This is believed to be a relatively precise way to measure of eating activities that helps to detect and quantify biological activities related to eating food.

These emerging technologies hold great promise but they are still in different stages of development. They need to be validated and often might need modifications and adaptations to make them suitable for use in different populations and countries and different regions within a country.

NUTRITIONAL ASSESSMENT OF HOSPITALIZED PATIENTS

In hospitalized patients, malnutrition is associated with many adverse clinical outcomes. Malnutrition compromises muscle function, respiratory and immune function, which result in poor wound health and poor quality of life. It is likely to increase the duration of hospital stay because it increases postoperative morbidity, is associated with higher cost of treatment, and increased risk of mortality. Depending upon the disease condition of the patient and hospital setting, different types of nutritional assessments are carried out. Generally, malnutrition is based on objective measurements of nutritional status that include:
- Anthropometric—with focus of weight loss or any marked change in any body part
- Body composition
- Biochemical indices
- Dietary intake
- Assessment of oral intake (food and beverage) with a focus on energy intake
- Determination of cell-mediated immunity.

However, each of these has some limitations particularly in hospital settings. For example, body weight readings are inaccurate if there is edema or ascites or if there are fluid derangements. This leads to falsely higher body weight as well as BMI. There are many scores and indicators which can be indicative of malnutrition and associated morbidity and mortality such as nutrition screening, global subjective assessment (GSA), etc. Tests can be used; some are fairly simple and noninvasive whereas others require some biochemical tests to be done:

1. **Malnutrition screening tool:** This is based on weight, percent weight loss, and appetite.
2. **Malnutrition universal screening tool (MUST):** It is based on BMI, percent weight loss, and acute disease effect. However, this has low sensitivity and specificity in oncology patients.
3. **Nutritional risk screening:** It is a simple validated tool. Initially, four questions listed below are to be answered with a simple yes or no.
4. **Prognostic nutritional Index (PNI):** This was designed to indicate risk of a poor outcome after surgery based upon assessment of nutritional status. It was developed by Mullen and coworkers and validated by Dempsey, Buzby, et al. in 1980 in patients undergoing major elective gastrointestinal surgery. It helps to identify patients at risk for postoperative complications.
   PNI = 158 − 16.6 (serum albumin concentration) − 0.78 [triceps skinfold thickness (in mm)] − 0.20 [serum transferrin concentration (in mg/dL)] − 5.8 (delayed hypersensitivity reaction)
   Delayed hypersensitivity reaction is scored as:
   0 = No reaction, 1 = <5 mm induration, and 2 = >5 mm induration
   PNI is categorized as: 50% = High risk, 40–50% = Intermediate risk, and <40% = Low risk
5. **Prognostic hospital index (PHI/HPI):** Prognostic implies the prediction. PHI is a predictor of hospital stay or mortality. This test or assessment is usually carried out in terminally ill or cancer patients. The test was developed by Blackburn, et al. and published in 1981. It is based on serum albumin and skin tests.
   PHI = 0.91 (albumin) − 1.00 (delayed hypersensitivity) − 1.44 (sepsis rating) + 0.98 (diagnosis rating) − 1.09
   Where delayed hypersensitivity reaction is: 0 = Non-reactive, <5 mm induration = 1, and >5 mm induration = 2
   Sepsis rating: Sepsis present = 1 and sepsis absent = 2
   Diagnosis rating: Cancer present = 1 and cancer not present = 2
   An HPI of 0 = 50% probability of survival
   HPI + 1 = 75% survival probability
   HPI − 2 = 10% survival probability
6. **Nutritional risk index (NRI):** This was developed by the Veterans Affairs Total Parenteral Nutrition Cooperative Study Group in 1991. It classifies individuals as either well-nourished or malnourished.
   NRI = 1.519 (serum albumin g/dL) + 41.7 (current weight or usual weight)
   NRI index was first developed to score the severity of postoperative complications using a combination of two simple nutritional indicators: albumin and weight loss.
7. **Instant nutritional assessment** was developed by Seltzer, et al. (1979) and uses two values, namely serum albumin and total lymphocyte count.
8. **Mini nutritional assessment (MNA):** The mini nutritional assessment (MNA) is a simple validated

tool with high sensitivity, specificity, and reliability. It is now well-practiced in clinical settings (in nursing homes or hospitals) to assess nutritional status of elderly persons. It consists of two stages—(1) Screening and (2) Assessment (if patient is at risk). Full MNA consists of 18 questions covering 4 domains focusing on food intake and changes in appetite, weight loss during the last 3 months, mobility, neuropsychological problems/stress, and BMI.

MNA for screening has 6 questions with a total of 14 points. The total possible score for these six questions is 14 (subtotal). Classification by nutritional status is as follows:
12-14 points: Normal nutritional status—no need for complete assessment
8-11 points: At risk of malnutrition—continue assessment
0-7 points: Malnourished

MNA for assessment: It involves 12 questions and 16 points.
The twelve questions focus on whether the person lives independently, whether the person has pressure scores or ulcers, medication, number of meals, markers of protein intake, fluid intake, mode of feeding, self-assessment of nutritional and health status/habits, and two anthropometric measurements, i.e., calf circumference and midarm circumference.
Total points are 30 = Points of MNA for screening (14) + MNA for assessment (16)
Risk of malnutrition is based on the total score as follows:
24-30 points—normal nutritional status
17-23.5 points—at risk of malnutrition
<17 points—malnourished
There is a shorter form of MNA called (MNA-SF) consisting of only 6 questions on food intake/appetite, mobility, weight loss, stress, and psychological distress/acute disease. Recently, calf circumference has been added in case BMI cannot be done. The maximum score is 14. Categorization of patients is as follows:
Normal nutritional status—12-14 points
8-11 points—at risk of malnutrition
≤7 points—malnourished
If the score is less than 11, the patient is at risk of malnutrition and it is recommended that the full MNA can be done.

9. **Subjective global assessment (SGA):** This is a diagnostic tool that identifies risk of complications associated with nutritional status. It is efficient and cost-effective. Its main limitation is that the experience of the observer is important (the clinician's experience and judgment are important to determine whether the patient is well-nourished or severely malnourished) and the tool lacks quantitative criteria.
SGA is a clinical nutritional index involving a standardized questionnaire consisting of dietary intake changes, recent body weight changes, GI symptoms, functional capacity, and physical signs of malnutrition (loss of subcutaneous fat or muscle mass, edema, and ascites), and is the single most useful tool in assessment of malnutrition. It has been validated to assess nutritional status in patients but not with many cancer patients. Initially developed to assess patients for malnutrition, it integrates many traditional parameters in nutritional assessment with current clinical status and functional capacity. The salient information that is required is:
   - Historical information: It consists of weight loss, dietary intake, gastrointestinal symptoms, and functional capacity.
   - Metabolic demands of the underlying disease.
   - Nutrition-related physical examination which includes loss of subcutaneous fat, presence of muscle wasting, edema and ascites (these are important components of SGA).

10. **Patient-generated SGA:** This is an adaptation developed for cancer patients. The advantage is that it is easy to use and inexpensive. It has two sections. In one section, four questions are to be completed by the patient. This includes weight history, presence of nutrition-related symptoms, food intake, and activity or functional level. The second section is completed by the healthcare professional.

11. **Alternative indicators for weight and height:** Calculation of BMI poses problems for patients who are unable to stand, who are critically ill, and are unconscious because it is not possible to measure stature. Also, unless the beds have an inbuilt system of measuring body weight, even weighing the patient poses problems. Body circumferences (abdomen, arm and leg) are used for assessment of nutritional status.

12. **Alternatives for height or stature:** Stature reported by caregivers or family members especially for the aged could be wrong and has often been found to be overestimated. This could lead to errors in calculating the BMI and further classifying the patient by category of nutritional status. One alternative is to measure the skinfold thickness and arm circumference. With these two values, arm muscle area can be calculated. However, in critically ill patients, there may be increased body fluid and arm circumference readings may not be reliable. Recumbent stature, arm span, sternal notch, and knee height may be measured. These are fairly easy to obtain but they may not correctly estimate stature. For example, knee height may be underestimated in relation to real stature.

13. **Study of adductor pollicis muscle (APM):** APM is a fleshy, flat, and triangular fan-like muscle in hand that is connected to thumb. It is used to adduct (move in a direction) the thumb for functioning of thumb and hand in full range. Its measurement can indicate changes in the muscle composition of the whole body, including early changes arising from both malnutrition and recovery of nutritional status. Adductor pollicis muscle thickness (APMT) has been found to be a good prognostic indicator in critically ill patients suffering from either septic or nonseptic complications, and has also been found to be related to the length of hospital stay as well

Table 13.19: Errors due to equipment and technique.

Errors due to equipment	Errors due to technique
Use of incorrect equipment Equipment not calibrated Equipment not installed properly Equipment not maintained properly	Failure to zero the scale before measuring weight Weighing with excess clothing and/or footwear Measuring height with footwear on, feet placed away from the wall, and headpieces or clips, etc. not removed Not using right angle headboard when measuring height Measuring an infant single handedly Not properly extending child when taking length measurements, not positioning child properly/correctly Errors in reading tape or scale Not measuring least count Rounding off measurements

as mortality. This is a simple and sensitive method for hospital settings that can be used to diagnose muscle loss and consequently malnutrition. A large number of hospitalized critical patients are malnourished and have muscle fatigue and loss of contraction force and relaxation rate of APM.

Whatever the indicator used, it is important to avoid errors in measurement by:
- Using correct equipment and checking it for accuracy
- Ensuring use of the correct procedure and following standard procedures
- Ensuring that errors due to use of incorrect equipment and/or technique are avoided (Table 13.19).

NUTRITIONAL ASSESSMENT IN PEDIATRIC POPULATION

Children are the most vulnerable to adverse effects of malnutrition and/or illness, whether it is acute or chronic. Both malnutrition and illness have negative effects on their growth and development. Therefore, growth monitoring is an essential step which can indicate the ups and downs in growth and development of child.

Growth monitoring is important to ensure that children are growing well. This is done by taking serial measurements of weight and height/length (note: mid-upper arm circumference cannot be used for growth monitoring). Besides height and weight, for children under 5 years of age, head circumference can be measured.

Monthly measurements of weight and height as well as BMI are to be plotted on growth charts. The World Health Organization in 2006 made available growth charts developed from data collected from children in different countries. There are separate charts for boys and girls. These charts are based on a Multicentre Growth Reference Study that was undertaken with the specific purpose of generating newer growth reference standards. Data was obtained from healthy infants and children from Brazil, Ghana, India, Norway, Oman, and the United States. The data reflects healthy children who were breastfed and were growing in a nonsmoking environment, which would be favorable for the children to fully achieve their growth potential. It combines longitudinal follow-up measurements from birth until 24 months of postnatal life. In addition, cross-sectional data for children in the age group 0–71 months has been combined. These growth standards are prescriptive, i.e., they inform how children should grow provided that children are nurtured with best health practices. Reference standards are given for length or height for age, weight for age, weight for length or height as well as BMI by age for children up to 60 months of age.

For children above 7–8 years, the charts of the Indian Academy of Pediatrics can be used. However, for preterm/premature infants, different charts need to be used. It is preferable to use intrauterine growth-based charts because the different charts that are available are postnatal growth-based charts. Thus, for such infants, the measurement is plotted based on corrected gestational age for the first 12 months of life and could be extended to 24 or 36 months of age, depending on how the child is growing and the child's size. One of the most widely used growth chart is the Lubchenco growth chart because it is easy to use and gives reference data for weekly age intervals and in percentiles. Another growth chart is the Babson growth chart. In this, the reference values are given for biweekly age intervals from 26 weeks to 40 weeks gestation but instead of percentile, standard deviations are used. In the US, weight charts have been developed. These charts have been developed from large datasets of fetal growth that span the gestational age from 22 weeks to 50 weeks. The charts provide weekly age intervals for weight, length, and head circumference, and percentiles (3rd–97th) are to be used for assessing the nutritional status as well as monitoring the child's growth.

Once the preterm infant becomes 40 weeks of corrected gestational age, the usual growth charts that are used for term infants can be used, as these give the appropriate goal for growth. Charts are available for low birth weight infants who weigh between 1,501 g and 2,500 g [the Infant Health and Development Program (IHDP) charts in the US] and for very low birth weight infants who weigh less than 1,500 g.

Growth velocity: It is the rate of growth or incremental growth (the change in the measurement, for example height or weight) and can be used to detect whether there is a change in the nutritional status of the child. It is also useful to monitor the effectiveness of nutritional/medical nutrition therapy. Standards are available for incremental growth velocity for both sexes for weight, stature, and head circumference from 0 year to 18 years. The time intervals are 1, 3, and 6 months and are presented by percentile, i.e., 3rd–97th or 5th–95th percentiles. In clinical practice, such incremental tables for weight, length, and head circumference can be used for assessment of former premature infants and other children who exhibit growth failure due to other causes. These values for reference growth increments can be given as goals for achieving weight gains daily, weekly, or on monthly basis. Use of these reference standards is also helpful in early detection of growth faltering or whether the child is showing catch-up growth as this method is more sensitive than the normally used growth charts as the latter assess static growth status. Growth charts are also available for assessing height and height velocity in relation to the stage of sexual maturity based on US reference data. Height growth and when height velocity peak is reached is available for early, middle, and late maturers by sex and age at which peak height velocity occurs. These velocity charts for height can be used for those children who are not growing well or who suffer from chronic illness.

Besides these, there are disease-specific charts for children who have any of the following problems: achondroplasia, Brachman de Lange syndrome, cerebral palsy, Down syndrome, Marfan syndrome, myelomeningocele, Noonan syndrome, Prader–Willi syndrome, sickle cell disease, Silver–Russell syndrome, Turner syndrome, and Williams syndrome. The charts cater separately to boys and girls in the age groups of 0–36 months and 2–18 years, respectively. These reference charts can be used alone or along with the other reference growth charts, e.g., the CDC charts. Growth charts are also available for upper arm length, and lower leg length, which are used as alternatives to measurement of stature. The charts of young children below 24 months of age are separate from those for children who are 3 years of age or older.

NUTRITIONAL SCREENING AND ASSESSMENT IN GERIATRIC POPULATION

Nutrition screening is to be treated differently from that of adults because there are several determinants of risk of malnutrition in the elderly that are not encountered in younger adults. BMI alone is not reliable. It is recommended that every elderly person above 65 years of age should be screened once in a year. Tests used should be both sensitive and specific. Those that do not take much time and yet are fairly sensitive and specific are:

a. Mini Nutritional Assessment (MNA)—recommended by ESPEN
b. Malnutrition Universal Screening tool (MUST)—recommended by ESPEN
c. Nutritional risk screening in hospital settings.

There are several other tools used in different countries such as:
- Canadian Nutrition Screening Tool (CNST)
- Australian Nutrition Screening Initiative
- SNAQ—Short Nutritional Assessment Questionnaire
- Malnutrition Risk Screening Tool-Hospital (MRST-H) developed for Malaysian elderly patients
- Geriatric Nutritional Risk Index (GNRI)
- Nutritional Risk Screening (NRS)
- Nutritional Form for the Elderly (NUFFE)

DETERMINE—a mnemonic based on the following: **D**isease, **E**ating poorly, **T**ooth loss/mouth pain, **E**conomic hardship, **R**educed social contact, **M**ultiple medications, **I**nvoluntary weight loss/gain, **N**eeds assistance in self-care, **E**lder age >80 years.

RAPID FIRE

1. What are nutritional screening and nutritional status?
2. What does stand for A, B, C, and D?
3. What is the importance of assessing albumin and prealbumin?
4. Which test is more appropriate to assess lean body mass?
5. What does serum transferrin and ferritin reflect?
6. Name the tests to assess the status of thiamine and niacin.
7. Explain the use of MNA in geriatric population.
8. Define MUST for hospital patients.
9. Suggest two biochemical tests suitable for pediatric population.
10. Which nutrient's deficiencies can easily be identified by observing signs of hair, skin, and eyes?

EXERCISES

1. Identify physical signs of nutritional status in ten persons of different age groups.
2. Try to nutritionally assess and interpret the blood reports of 5 persons.
3. Collect food intake of 5 people using 24-recall method and 5 people's intake using FFQ.
4. Perform MUST and SGA in 2 persons each.
5. Develop a questionnaire to identify the nutritional risk for a person who is obese and diabetic.

SUGGESTED READING

1. Acevedo MG. (2011). Nutrition Assessment: Tools and Techniques. [online] Available from https://www.continuingeducation.com/pdf/rd100_elt-nas-11.pdf. [Last accessed September, 2019].
2. American Society for Parenteral and Robinson D, et al. Enteral Nutrition (ASPEN) Definition of Terms, Style, and Conventions Used in ASPEN Board of Directors–Approved Documents, 2018.
3. Bharadwaj S, Ginoya S, Tandon P, Gohel TD, Guirguis J, Vallabh H, Andrea J J and Hanouneh I. Malnutrition: laboratory markers vs nutritional assessment. Gastroenterol Rep (Oxf). 2016 Nov; 4(4): 272–280.
4. British Association for Parenteral and Enteral Nutrition (BAPEN). (2003). Malnutrition Universal Screening Tool (MUST). [online] Available from http://www.bapen.org.uk/pdfs/must/must_full.pdf. [Last accessed September, 2019].
5. British Association for Parenteral and Enteral Nutrition (BAPEN). (2016). Nutritional Assessment. [online] Available from https://www.bapen.org.uk/nutrition-support/assessment-and-planning/nutritional-assessment. [Last accessed September, 2019].
6. British Dietetics Association (BDA). (2012). Model and Process for Nutrition and Dietetic Practice. [online] Available from https://www.bda.uk.com/publications/professional/model_and_process_for_nutrition_and_dietetic_practice_. [Last accessed September, 2019].
7. Cederholm T, Barazzoni R, Austin P, et al. ESPEN guidelines on definitions and terminology of clinical nutrition. Clin Nutr. 2017;36(3):49-64.
8. Centers for Disease Control and Prevention (CDC). (2017). Clinical Growth Charts. [online] Available from https://www.cdc.gov/growthcharts/clinical_charts.htm. [Last accessed September, 2019].

9. Dradkeh G, Essa MM, Guizani N. Handbook for Nutritional Assessment through Life Cycle. Nutrition and Diet Research Progress. Nova Publisher, 2016.
10. Daradkeh G, Essa MM, Al-Mashaani A, et al. Malnutrition Indicators Which is More Predictive? Nutrition Risk Index (NRI) or Malnutrition Universal Screening Tool (MUST). J Clin Nutr Metab. 2018;2(1):2.
11. Food and Agriculture Organization of the United Nations, Rome, 2018. Dietary Assessment, A resource guide to method selection and application in low resource settings.
12. Food and Agriculture Organization of the United Nations. (2018). Dietary Assessment: A Resource Guide to Method Selection and Application in Low Resource Settings. [online] Available from http://www.fao.org/3/i9940en/I9940EN.pdf. [Last accessed September, 2019].
13. Indian Academy of Pediatrics (IAP). (2019). IAP Growth Charts. [online]. Available from https://www.iapindia.org/iap-growth-charts/. [Last accessed September, 2019].
14. Indian Academy of Pediatrics Growth Charts Committee, Khadilkar V, Yadav S, et al. Revised IAP growth charts for height, weight and body mass index for 5- to 18-year-old Indian Children. Indian Pediatr. 2015;52(1):47-55.
15. Khadilkar V, Khadilkar A. Growth charts: A diagnostic tool. Indian J Endocrinol Metab. 2011. 15(Suppl3): S166–S171.
16. Khadilkar VV, Khadilkar AV. Revised Indian Academy of Pediatrics 2015 growth charts for height, weight and body mass index for 5-18-year-old Indian children. Indian J Endocrinol Metab. 2015;19(2):470-6.
17. Maicá AO, Schweigert ID. Nutritional assessment of severely ill patient. Rev Bras Ter Intensiva. 2008;20(3):286-95.
18. Maqbool A, Olsen IE, Stallings VA. Clinical assessment of nutritional status. In: Duggan C, Watkins JB, Walker WA (Eds). Nutrition in Pediatrics: Basic Science, Clinical Applications, 4th edition. Ontario: BC Decker Inc.; 2008.
19. Meier R, Berner Y, Sobotka L. (2017). Nutritional Assessment and Techniques Module 3.1: Nutritional Screening and Assessment. [online] Available from https://lllnutrition.com/mod_lll/TOPIC3/m31.pdf. [Last accessed September, 2019].
20. Mueller C, Compher C, Ellen DM. ASPEN Clinical Guidelines. Nutrition screening, assessment, and Intervention in Adults. Journal of Parenteral and Enteral Nutrition. 2011;35(1):16-24.
21. National Health and Nutrition Examination Survey III. (1988). Body Measurements (Anthropometry). [online] Available from https://wwwn.cdc.gov/nchs/data/nhanes3/manuals/anthro.pdf. [Last accessed September, 2019].
22. National Institute for Health and Care Excellence (NICE). (2006). Nutrition support for adults: oral nutrition support, enteral tube feeding and parenteral nutrition. [online] Available from https://www.nice.org.uk/guidance/cg32/resources/nutrition-support-for-adults-oral-nutrition-support-enteral-tube-feeding-and-parenteral-nutrition-975383198917. [Last accessed September, 2019].
23. Nestle Nutrition Institute. (2014). Mini Nutritional Assessment. [online] Available from https://www.mna-elderly.com/. [Last accessed September, 2019].
24. Recommended Dietary Allowances, Estimated Average Requirements, A Report of the Expert Group, Indian Council of Medical research, National Institute of Nutrient Requirements for Indians-2020.
25. Rabito EI, Vannucchi GB, Suen VMM, Neto LLC, Marchini JS. Weight and height prediction of immobilized patients. Rev. Nutr. 2006;19(6):655–61.
26. Sauberlich HE. Laboratory Test for the Assessment of Nutritional Status, 2nd edition. CRC, Taylor and Francis group, 1999
27. Secher M, Soto ME, Villars H, et al. The Mini Nutritional Assessment (MNA) after 20 years of research and clinical practice. Rev Clin Gerontol. 2017;17(2):293-310.
28. Seltzer MH, Bastidas JA, Cooper DM, et al. Instant nutritional assessment. JPEN J Parenter Enteral Nutr. 1979;3(3):157-9.
29. Todorovic V, Russell C, Elia M. (2003). THE 'MUST' EXPLANATORY BOOKLET: A Guide to the 'Malnutrition Universal Screening Tool' ('MUST') for Adults. [online] Available from https://www.bapen.org.uk/pdfs/must/must_explan.pdf. [Last accessed September, 2019].
30. Walker HK, Hall WD, Hurst JW. Clinical Methods: The History, Physical, and Laboratory Examinations, 3rd edition. Boston: Butterworths; 1990.
31. World Health Organization (WHO). (1973). Clinical Assessment of Nutritional Status. [online] Available from https://ajph.aphapublications.org/doi/pdf/10.2105/AJPH.63.11_Suppl.18. [Last accessed September, 2019].
32. World Health Organization (WHO). (2006). WHO Child Growth Standards: Length/height-for-age, weight-for-age, weight-for-length, weight-for-height and body mass index-for-age: Methods and development. [online] Available from https://www.who.int/childgrowth/standards/Technical_report.pdf. [Last accessed September, 2019].
33. World Health Organization (WHO). (2013). Guideline: Updates on the Management of Severe Acute Malnutrition in Infants and CHILdrEN. [online] Available from https://apps.who.int/iris/bitstream/handle/10665/95584/9789241506328_eng.pdf?ua=1. [Last accessed September, 2019].
34. World Health Organization (WHO). (2019). Application tools: WHO AnthroPlus software. [online] Available from https://www.who.int/growthref/tools/en/. [Last accessed September, 2019].
35. World Health Organization (WHO). (2019). WHO AnthroPlus v.1.0.4. [online] Available from who-anthroplus.sharewarejunction.com. [Last accessed September, 2019].

CHAPTER 14

Ensuring Food and Nutritional Security: New Technologies

> **KEY CONCERNS**
> - What is food and nutrition security?
> - What are the technologies which can help improve food and nutrition security?
> - What is fortification, biofortification, and genetically modified foods?
> - What is food irradiation?
> - What are the national programs for food and nutrition security?
>
> **KEY CONCEPTS**
> - Concept of food and nutrition security
> - New technologies to ensure food and nutrition security:
>   - Fortification
>   - Biofortification
>   - Supplementation
>   - Irradiation
>   - Biotechnology-genetically modified foods
>   - National programs for food and nutrition security.

INTRODUCTION

Food is essential for survival. Humans obtain the necessary nutrients from food. Hence, food security is a critical issue for all countries and is important for eliminating poverty. Ensuring food and nutrition security is a challenge for India, because of its large population and high levels of undernutrition and poverty. Sustainable development goal (SDG) 2030 and goal no. 2 is zero hunger and achieve food security and improved nutrition and promote sustainable agriculture. Like India, several other countries faced and continue to face problems of food shortages and crisis. Ensuring this sustainable access to nutritious food or nutrition security will require sustainable food production and agricultural practices.

The global food crisis in 1972–74 led to the World Food Summit defining food security in 1974 as *"availability at all times of adequate world food supplies of basic foodstuffs to sustain a steady expansion of food consumption and to offset fluctuations in production and prices."*

However, the most widely accepted definition of food security was adopted at the World Food Summit, Rome, in 1996. As per the United Nations' Committee on World Food Security, food security exists *"when all people, at all times, have physical and economic access to sufficient, safe and nutritious food to meet their dietary needs and food preferences for an active and healthy life."*

> Food security is as a "state in which all the persons obtain a nutritionally adequate, culturally accepted diet all the time through local non-emergency sources."
> **Community on World Food Security (CFS) (2005). Assessment of the world food security situation, Rome**

Food security has four components shown in Figure 14.1:
i. **Food availability**—sources of food supply
ii. **Food access**—purchasing power to buy food

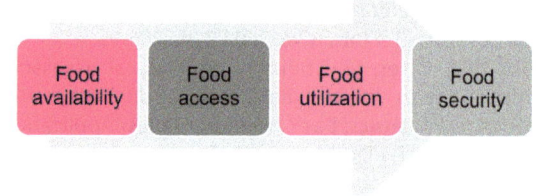

Fig. 14.1: The four components of food security.

iii. **Food utilization**—food preparation, food handling, and storage
iv. **Food security**—food is available throughout the year.

Food security entails physical, social, economical, political and ecological access to balanced diets and safe drinking water, so as to enable every individual to lead a productive and healthy life.

Purchasing power stipulate food security but environmental factors including poor agricultural production, natural calamities and social and political pressures gravely affect the food security.

India ranked 76th in 113 countries assessed by The Global Food Security Index (GFSI) in the year 2018, based on four parameters—affordability, availability and quality and safety. As per the Global Hunger Index, 2018, India was ranked 103rd out of 119 qualifying countries. After the National Food security Act (2013).

Food security is important for its own sake and is instrumental in improving productivity. In any country, the citizens can be healthy, well-nourished only if they have adequate food, and their diets are well balanced, which depends on successful social and economic development. In turn, a nation can develop only when the population is healthy and well nourished. Initially, food security was considered to be important and examined at the regional, national, and global levels and referred shortfalls in supply compared to the requirements for food. However, observations that there are groups or regions or communities who do not have sufficient food even if there is adequate supply at the macrolevel have led to a revision and now include community, household, and even the individual level.

Over half a century, food grain production has increased by leaps and bounds (from 51 million tons in the 1950s to 269 million tons in 2018), making India food sufficient. This is owed to the Green revolution in the late 1960's when India was facing acute food shortage. Production of food grains was focused on wheat and rice being the staple foods for most of us, even today. It helped curb hunger and was a source of income and employment for millions of people. Per capita availability of food grains has increased, to 484g/day in 2018, according to Food and Nutrition Security Analysis (FNSA). It also indicated that population growth and food wastage are big challenges. Despite good economic growth, millions of children, women and others are still malnourished. Engel's law states that rise in income tends to reduce share of income on food as big share of income is spent on non-food items. Expenditure on cereals and cereal products has decreased whereas that on the milk, dairy products, oils and fat has increased. Population has also started recognizing the importance of fruits and vegetables but being perishable in nature, they are wasted more. Changing dietary patterns have led to reduced intakes of energy and protein from cereal products, and energy intake is coming from sugary beverages and processed foods. Such transition has turned out to be unhealthy causing malnourishment, stunted growth, obesity and other associated diseases.

Food and nutrition insecurity have tremendous impact on economic development. Estimates indicate that cost to economic development of undernourishment of children alone is to the tune of billions of dollars. This cost increases even further if the lost productivity and income are taken into account. It is estimated that malnutrition can cost up to one-tenth of a lifetimes' earnings. Food and nutrition security are important for sustainable development.

> **Research Glimpse:** Researchers have proposed five different approaches to food security analysis. These are: (a) food availability; (b) income-based; (c) basic needs; (d) entitlement; and (e) sustainable livelihoods. Having enough food according to the national level is a necessary but not sufficient condition for food security. It is necessary to assess the alternative bundles of commodities such as drinkable water, other goods, or services that directly influence hunger and food security. The researchers have focussed on hunger, undernutrition, or nutritional deprivation rather than "food security" to highlight the need to pay attention to nutritional capability rather than food availability.
>
> *Burchi F, De Muro P. From food availability to nutritional capabilities: Advancing food security analysis. Food Policy. 2016;60:10-9.*

Visualizing the state of Food Security and Nutrition in the World, 2020, Food and Agricultural Organization (FAO), the International Fund for Agricultural Development (IFAD), United Nations Children's Fund (UNICEF), World Food Programme and World Health Organization (WHO) stated that progress towards reaching the target 2.1 of SDG was seemingly off track. COVID-19 pandemic further complexed the situation that may add an additional 83 to 132 million people to the ranks of the undernourished in 2020.

Though India is now self-sufficient in food production and has the capacity to cope with year-to-year fluctuations but unfortunately, our country has not been able to achieve the food security. Millions of households are chronically food insecure. This necessitates change in approach(es) to achieve the second goal among the sustainable development goals (SDG) by 2030 states "By 2030, end hunger and ensure food access by all people, in particular the poor and people in vulnerable situations including infants, to safe, nutritious, and sufficient food all year round." This goal calls for addressing challenges of hunger, food insecurity, and malnutrition in all its forms. However, attainment of this goal is interconnected with the other sustainable development goals.

The common practice was to estimate the number of food insecure households by comparing their calorie intake with required norms. Severity of hunger is indicated by how much is the shortfall or gap between the intakes compared to the pre-determined threshold intake. However, experts argue that energy intake is not enough to measure the food security and nutritional status of the population. This is because non-food factors are also important for food security. It is suggested that the assessment of malnutrition should be based on outcome measures rather than input measures. It has been suggested that outcome measures should include anthropometric measures, clinical signs of malnutrition, biochemical indicators, and physical activity. Outcome indicators are more closely related to health and functional capacity. The South Asia Food and Nutrition Security Initiative (SAFANSI) has a goal of fostering innovative actions that lead to measurable improvements in food and nutrition security such as to set up regulatory standards for fortifying whole, low-fat, and skim milk.

> The Food Insecurity Experience Scale (FIES) is a tool that has been introduced. It is based on direct interviews and measures people's ability to access food.
>
> Another classification is the Integrated Food Security Phase classification that classifies food security crises based on livelihood needs. The classification ranges from food secure to chronically food insecure, to acute food and livelihood crisis, humanitarian emergency to famine/humanitarian catastrophe. Several indicators are used ranging from crude mortality rate, prevalence of malnutrition, food access/availability, dietary diversity, water access/availability, coping strategies, and livelihood assets.

Demand for food will be driven by income and population growth, urbanization, migration, food prices, and income distribution.

There is great amount of interdependence between food security, nutrition, and other aspects that play a crucial role in development. These are inclusive economic growth, population dynamics, decent employment, social protection, energy, water, health, sanitation, natural resource management, and protecting the ecosystems. Also relevant and very important are empowerment of women, addressing gender inequity, as well as rural–urban inequity. Climate change is an important factor that will have an impact on food security.

Food insecurity can be transient or chronic. Transitory or short-term insecurity is usually caused by problems with access or availability such as when there is crop failure, drought, and inflation or during the off season when there is very little or no agricultural production. There are sometimes some unprecedented situations in the locality or country that deprive the people with the assurance of food availability. One such example, at global level is the present COVID-19 pandemic. Short-term insecurity can also occur as a result of illness or unemployment of the person(s) who support(s) the household. In some cases, emergencies that necessitate large amount of expenditure can also result in transitory insecurity. Short-term or transient food insecurity may affect any household. Chronic insecurity refers to insecurity that occurs over a long period of time, with the household/family being unable to meet its food requirements (chronically inadequate diet) and is generally due to lack of purchasing power or poverty. In such communities and households, dietary intakes are generally inadequate. Policy measures taken by governments for the two types of food insecurity are different. For tackling/addressing transient insecurity, the government can have policies such as giving credit to farmers, insurance for crops, try to take measures to stabilize prices in case of inflation, and provide relief in case of problems such as drought by having programs like food for work or some other temporary means of wage earnings all of which would contribute to stabilization of prices and to food consumption by vulnerable groups, i.e., those who are food insecure. Since transient food insecurity cannot be predicted, making plans/programs to tackle it is difficult because the types of interventions required and capacities are different. A household is said to have food security when it is protected or buffered against both transitory and chronic food security.

In case of chronic food insecurity different and multipronged, multisectoral strategies are required involving agriculture, i.e., agricultural production programs, improving the infrastructure, human resource development, endowment of land and non-land assets, etc., to alleviate poverty and improve the standard of living of the poor people. These are long-term mediated interventions. The strategy(ies) should aim at:
- Enhancing the purchasing power of families
- Improving the ability of households to acquire food
- Enabling them to cope with factors that are a threat to food security
- Improving the ability of families to have a level of utilization conducive to good health
- Enabling them to have the ability to cope with factors that interfere with utilization.

Ultimately, households will be food secure when throughout the year, they have access to the quantity and variety of foods that their members require to have good nutritional status and be healthy and active. The food may be produced by the household itself or it can be purchased.

India has instituted several programs that have helped to overcome transient insecurity fairly well. These strategies emphasized achieving self-sufficiency in food grains. India has sizeable buffer stocks, the Public Distribution System (PDS), and the employment programs (Employment Guarantee Scheme/EGS). The Food Corporation of India (FCI) has the responsibility to maintain satisfactory level of operational and buffer stocks of foodgrains to ensure National Food Security. For tackling chronic food insecurity, although poverty reduction is essential, the problems in the food distribution system need to be looked into.

Besides transient and chronic food insecurity, there is also a concept of seasonal food insecurity. Like chronic food insecurity, one can predict seasonal food insecurity, and the sequence of events is known. It often recurs but is of limited duration. This is linked to seasonal fluctuations in several influencing climate, cropping patterns, work opportunities (labor demand), and disease and natural disasters.

> **Research glimpse:** India has been perceived as a development enigma. Recent rates of economic growth have not been matched by similar rates in health and nutritional improvements. To meet the second Sustainable Development Goal (SDG2) of achieving zero hunger by 2030, India faces a substantial challenge in meeting the basic nutritional needs in addition to addressing population, environmental, and dietary pressures. Here the authors have mapped—for the first time—the Indian food system from crop production to household-level availability across three key macronutrients categories of "calories," "digestible protein," and "fat." To better understand the potential of reduced food chain losses and improved crop yields to close future food deficits, scenario analysis was conducted between 2030 and 2050. Under India's current self-sufficiency model, our analysis indicates severe shortfalls in availability of all macronutrients across a large proportion (>60%) of the Indian population. The extent of projected shortfalls continues to grow such that, even in ambitious waste reduction and yield scenarios, enhanced domestic production alone will be inadequate in closing the nutrition supply gap. We suggest that to meet SDG2, India will need to take a combined approach of optimizing domestic production and increasing its participation in global trade.
>
> *Ritchie H, Reay D, Higgins P. Sustainable food security in India—Domestic production and macronutrient availability. PLoS One. 2018;13(3):e0193766.*

Food insecurity can range from mild to moderate to severe as shown in Figure 14.2.

India like many other countries faces and needs to tackle several challenges such as changes in climate and environment and the consequent constraints, degradation of the ecosystems, globalization, and market integration all of which will impact food production, especially small land holders. What is required is a combination of agricultural research, rural education, and adoption of improved technologies, extension and information services for small

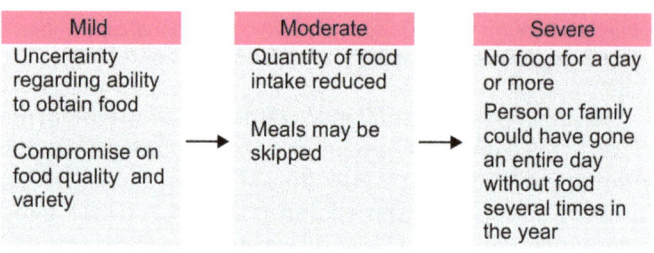

Fig. 14.2: Range of food insecurity.

producers, secure and equitable access to land, water, capital, and importantly infrastructure development.

DIMENSIONS OF FOOD SECURITY

There are four main dimensions of food security:
i. Availability
ii. Access to food
iii. Utilization or absorption (nutrition/nutritional outcomes)
iv. Stability.

These dimensions are explained in Figure 14.3. These four dimensions of food security are interlinked and all of them need to be fulfilled for food security to be realized. Any lacuna or gap in the food supply chain from production to plate affects food security.

Food availability: Food availability implies physical existence of food. It involves availability (in other words supply) of appropriate quality of food in sufficient quantities. Availability will be determined in turn by level of food production, sufficient stocks, and net trade or market and supply chain. It includes domestic food production, i.e., produced locally, food brought in from other regions (national or/and international) including food aid provided by other countries. Availability is influenced by production, food processing, imports and trade, water management on farms, whether there are buffer stocks of food, and import capacity of the country (determined by financial resources to purchase food in international market). During crisis or scarcity, the government may provide food at subsidized prices and even import from other countries in order to ensure availability of food to its people. One time availability of food has no meaning until this availability is sustainable. Adequate food supply must be available at all times to all the people. Buffer stock is a food insurance which is used during seasonal, economic, or climatic crisis.

Access to food: Access involves the physical and economic access to enough food to eat for an active and healthy life. It implies that availability of resources is essential to procure food from the highest level, i.e., government to state to the micro level, i.e., in households and by individuals. Just having an adequate supply of food globally or within a country is not a guarantee for households to have food security. Worldwide, because of this concern, government policies have focused on income generation activities, expenditure avenues, markets, and regulating food prices as the means to achieving food security.

It also indicates that people need to have adequate resources like money to procure or purchase food to satisfy

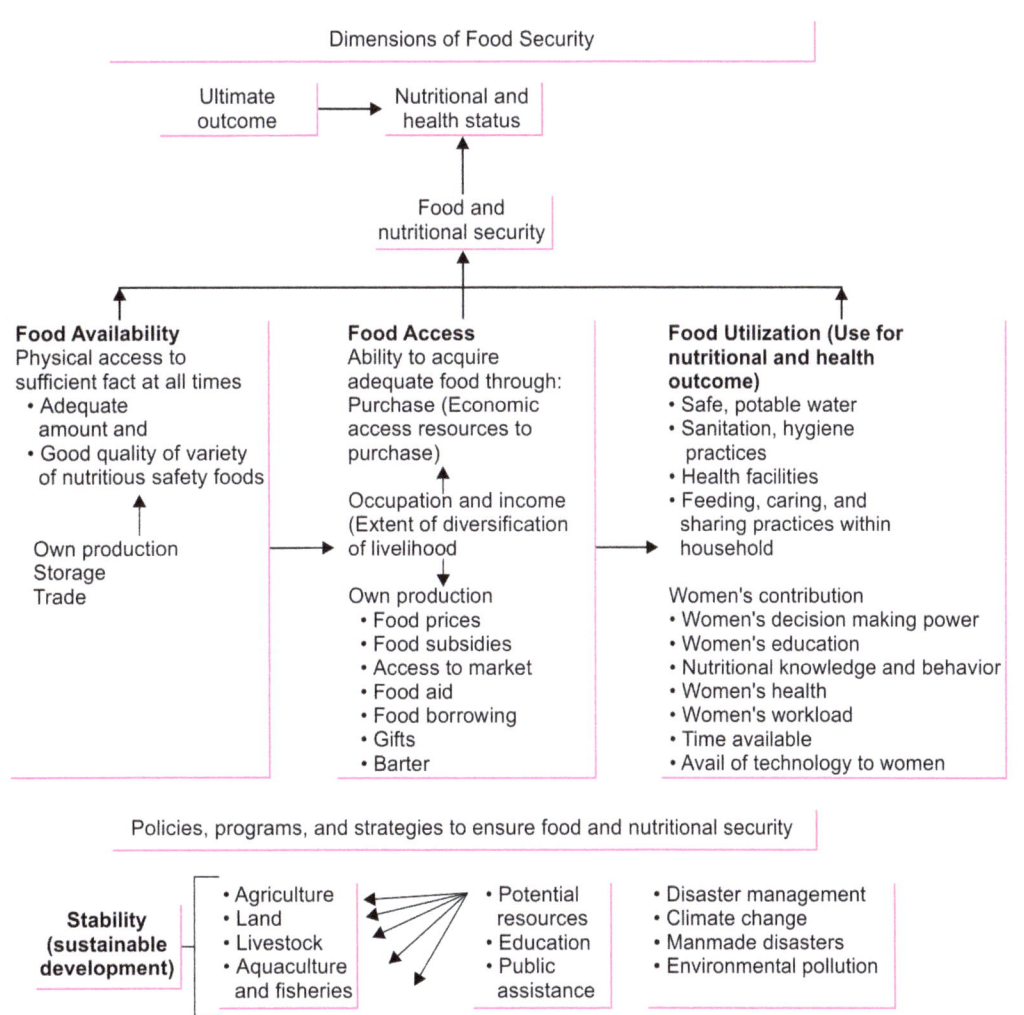

Fig. 14.3: Dimensions of food security.

hunger and fulfill other basic needs. Accessibility to healthy food should be a matter of individual choice but is largely influenced by the legal, political, economic, and social forces. Poverty, purchasing power, level of income, and price fluctuations are determinants of access to food. Although incomes have risen, this has not resulted in improvement in food and nutrient intakes, due to rising food prices. Education and nutrition knowledge influence the purchase of nutritious foods. Expenditure on other pursuits of life may affect access to healthy food. Food can also be available through gifts and donations. Social and development programs also provide access to food. Government programs such as the food for work program (now renamed as National Rural Employment Programme) contribute because people receive food grains as wages instead of money. Schemes like the mid-day meal program also contribute toward food security. But food should also be made affordable. Accessibility to food at household level determines the food consumption, energy intake, nutrient intake, and thus nutritional status. This is influenced by household system of food procurement, livelihoods, family composition, culture, social norms and intra-household food distribution. Climate change, market and transport facilities also govern the regular supply of food.

Utilization of food (Fulfilling food and nutritional needs): At individual level, food must be utilized by the body to fulfill the metabolic and physiological needs for well-being. Utilization implies good health status as an outcome. Not only must the quantity be sufficient but the nutritional quality is important so that nutrient requirements (energy as well as other nutrients) can be fulfilled. Absorption of nutrients and their utilization by the body is important in order to remain active and productive with no nutrient deficiency or diet-related disease(s). Several factors influence utilization including food choices, methods of food preparation, food handling, preparation and storage (that determine food safety and quality), clean water and sanitation and care, and feeding practices. Other concerns are dietary diversity and intra-household food distribution. Therefore, in addition to food, there is a need for basic health and sanitation facilities, along with good education about hygiene and dietary issues. Utilization and nutritional security can be improved by better agricultural biodiversity and nutrition education. Agricultural biodiversity can enhance livelihoods of farmers and decrease poverty in the long run.

Stability for food and nutrition security: All three dimensions (availability, access, and utilization) depend on stability of food supplies and anything that interrupts food supply in terms of availability, access, and/or utilization of that food results in food insecurity. Stability requires appropriate climatic conditions, e.g., rainfall, and good weather for production, good conditions for production such as water supply, pest, and disease management, good economic environment, emergency, and disaster planning and management, e.g., floods and drought mitigation, hurricanes, storms, pest and disease outbreaks, incidents of civil unrest, and political instability. Threats to food security include declining productivity, increasing population, increasing incidence of pockets of poverty, declining income from traditional crops, high dependence on imports, and growing incidence of food-related diseases.

Ensuring food security requires investment in agriculture because it provides livelihoods for 40% of the world's population. It is the largest source of income and employment for poor rural households. In many developing countries, there are small farms that are largely rain fed. These farms are the source of food for up to 80% of the food consumed by populations in developing countries. Food security can be improved by helping the small farmers and their households, by helping them to have more resilient and sustainable farming systems. Lack of electricity is also a constraint.

NUTRITION SECURITY

In India, the need for food security can be traced back to the Bengal famine in 1943 during British rule, when 200,000–300,000 persons perished due to starvation. After several years of Independence, India has been able to overcome the shortages and achieved some self-sufficiency in food. This is attributable to the Green revolution (grain production) in the late 1960s and 1970s and the white revolution (milk production) in the 1970 and 1980s. India produces large amount of milk, fruits, and vegetables; however, these foods are expensive, thus are out of reach for large proportion of the population. Also lack of systems for post-harvest storage results in large losses of fruits and vegetables. In 2010, India was 69th in position on the hunger index. Besides this, large proportion of the population suffers from anemia, iodine deficiency, and vitamin A deficiency and other nutrient deficiencies.

As a concept, food security evolved from the concern that there should be freedom from hunger. Over the years, experts felt that it is essential to include nutrition in food security. Nutrition security evolved in the 1970s from the recognition of multisectoral nutrition planning and the UNICEF conceptual framework. Nutrition security can be defined as "adequate nutritional status in terms of protein, energy, vitamins, and minerals at all times for all members of the household." Thus, nutrition security is more than food security. Nutrition security focuses on adequate nutritional status in terms of protein, energy, vitamins, and minerals for all household members at all times and also adds value to caring and health services and a healthy environment.

Food security ⟶ Nutrition security

The United Nations' Standing Committee on Nutrition has given a definition "Food and nutrition security exists when all people at all times have physical, social, and economic access to food, which is consumed in sufficient quantities and quality to meet their dietary needs and food preferences, and is supported by an environment of adequate sanitation, health services, and care for a healthy and active life."

It is established that food insecurity and malnutrition in all its forms have diverse negative effects on health and well-being. Adverse impacts are on mental and cognitive health and behavioral issues. Food insecurity and malnutrition form a vicious cycle at household or individual level increasing the risk of communicable and non-communicable diseases. There is emerging evidence that there is coexistence of food insecurity and obesity in the same household. As resources for food become scarce, people may choose to eat foods that are sold at lower cost but are also less healthy and more energy dense. Periodic episodes of food insecurity and deprivation have been linked as a possible cause of eating disorders and stress and the related metabolic responses. Mediating factors can be educational level, lifestyle, food environment and habits, and access to clean water, basic sanitation, and quality health services. FAO estimates (2016) indicate that 815 million people in the world—or just over one in nine—are undernourished. The majority of them live in countries struggling with conflict, violence, and fragility. Conflict is often a leading cause of famine and food crises.

The Global Hunger Index (2020) classifies countries on the hunger index as follows:
- Alarming: 35 to 49.9
- Serious: 20 to 34.9
- Moderate: 10 to 19.9
- Low < = 9.9
- India ranks 94th among 132 countries
- India's index in 2000 was 38.9 but has improved in 2020 to 27.2.

Historically, India has made tremendous efforts to improve the food security of the country. The green revolution led to bumper crops and at the macro levels, India manages to have buffer stocks of food grains. India is continuing its efforts to tackle food insecurity and malnutrition in different sections of the society. Also it has the Public Distribution System that provides subsidized food grains through a large network of fair price (ration) shops both in rural and urban areas. The subsidy is provided by the Central government. The PDS is a safety net for the poor since it provides some amount of food grains and oil and protects them against rising prices and inflation to some extent. The scheme has obviously helped considerably since India has not faced large-scale famine and starvation-related deaths in large numbers unlike some African countries. However, there are problems with the PDS and considerable numbers of needy persons/families still do not get the benefit of this safety net. Problems with supply and availability also affect the success of PDS.

> **What are Safety Nets?**
> These are measures that help persons/families to have direct access to food. For this, there are programs which are called social safety net programs. In some countries, financial assistance in the form of income transfers is provided to individuals who are chronically unable to work due to old age or handicaps or for persons who are temporarily out of work/do not have employment due to natural disasters or economic recession. In India, there are such programs like the Employment Guarantee Scheme and Pension Yojana for the Elderly.
> Other programs include feeding programs such as school meals such as the Midday Meal Program in India, food supplementation to preschool children and pregnant and lactating women under ICDS (Integrated Child Development Services), or such as the Public Distribution System (PDS) or subsidized provision of grains to the poor.

Although PDS provides food grains, the issue of hunger especially "hidden hunger," i.e., micronutrient malnutrition is still not completely resolved. This is indicated by results of surveys conducted by National organizations in the country. These organizations have reported a gap between requirements and intakes, indicating that there is still food insecurity. Micronutrient intakes are far from satisfactory and the rates of malnutrition are an indication of the need for policy makers and other professionals including scientists to seriously address the issue of food and nutrition security. The Government of India has set up monitoring systems to obtain information periodically on food and nutrient intakes in different subpopulation of the country. This data is obtained by the National Sample Survey Organization (NSSO) and National Nutrition Monitoring Bureau (NNMB). The NNMB report of 2012 presents findings in terms of food intake and nutrient intakes in terms of percent of recommended dietary allowances fulfilled/met for different age groups. There is a gap between recommended and actual intakes of nutrients; therefore, it is critical that food and security concerns in this country, especially among the vulnerable groups in tribal and rural areas as well as urban slums must be addressed.

Nutrition security has three determinants:
i. Access to food
ii. Care and feeding practices
iii. Sanitation and health.

These are care and feeding, access to food, and water intake. The focus on nutrition adds the aspects of care practices, health services, and a healthy environment, to the definition and concept of food security. Many a times, both food and nutrition security are integrated into a single development goal. This is because it helps to integrate actions better, it facilitates communications, and making decisions as well as taking action in order to eradicate not just hunger but also malnutrition. Also, food and nutrition security reflect the social and economic welfare while they are also determinants of these. They are also linked to structural transformation.

Nutrition security is a broader concept that encompasses food security. FAO in 2010 defined nutrition security as: *"adequate nutritional status in terms of protein, energy, vitamins, and minerals for all household members at all times."*

Food and nutrition security can be explained as *"if adequate food (quantity, quality, safety, sociocultural acceptability) is available and accessible for and satisfactorily utilized by all individuals at all times to live a healthy and happy life."* Since food and nutrition security (FNS) is one of the basic human needs, it is essential that all individuals, at all times, obtain adequate food in quantity, nutritional quality, digestibility, bioavailability, and safety, sociocultural acceptability to live a healthy and active life.

Nutrition security has been defined as "A situation that exists when secure access to an appropriately nutritious diet is coupled with a sanitary environment, adequate health services, and care, in order to ensure a healthy and active life for all household members. Nutrition security differs from food security in that it also considers the aspects of adequate caring practices, health, and hygiene in addition to dietary adequacy" [FAO, IFAD, and WFP, 2015]. Food insecurity exists when people do not have adequate physical, social or economic access to food as defined above. Food security therefore covers availability, access, utilization and stability issues, and because of its focus on the attributes of individuals, food security also embraces their energy, protein and nutrient needs for life, activity, pregnancy, growth and long-term capabilities".

A nutritionally secure person is one who has access to a balanced diet at all times that enables the her/him to lead a healthy and productive life. The nutritional status of each member of a household depends on several conditions and requirements being met: the food available to the household must be shared according to individual needs; the food must be of sufficient variety, quality, and safety; and each family member must have good health status in order to benefit from the food consumed. In order to have good health status, it is essential to have access to safe, potable water, adequate health services, and care. Basic knowledge about nutrition, sanitation, appropriate hygiene practices (environmental, household, personal and food hygiene), food preparation, and storage practices all determine the health and nutritional status of individuals, families, and the community at large. Ensuring nutrition security is a Herculean task not only for the individual but also for the nation. There are many physical, biological, and socioeconomic constraints to attainment of food and nutrition security.

Food and nutrient intakes vary from one day to another and one meal to another. These need to be taken into account when nutrition security is considered. In spite of such large variations in nutrient intakes, the body (under normal healthy conditions) maintains homeostasis and even under conditions of suboptimal intakes, will make an attempt to maintain normal functions to the extent possible. These efforts are made by the body to protect it against long-term, chronic marginal deficits or excessive intakes of one or more nutrients.

Homeostatic mechanisms work in the following ways when dietary intakes are low:
- Use of body stores body stores of energy, vitamins and minerals
- Increased absorption of the nutrient (calcium, iron, zinc, magnesium, copper, and carotene)
- Reduced excretion in urine (sodium and calcium)
- Slowing down of nutrient utilization or turnover (protein).

However, homeostatic mechanisms cannot be taken for granted and too much of a difference or gap between requirements and intakes will ultimately have adverse effects on health whether it is a deficit in intake or excess intake.

Past experiences indicate that meeting the food and nutrition security needs of the world's population is an immense challenge, especially because the amount of arable land available has not increased over the last five decades. In fact, land that can be used for cultivation is being lost to urbanization, construction, desertification, and increasing salinity to the effect that arable land is decreasing.

Added to these woes, is water scarcity and climate change. Climate change is likely to increase the risk of hunger and undernutrition, with the poorest and most vulnerable and marginalized groups being at greater risk. In these households, women and children are likely to be at greater risk. There are several challenges that need to be tackled for ensuring food and nutrition security:
- Increasing population globally and especially in sub-Saharan Africa and South Asia with India being a major contributor to the world population. At the global level, this increase in the population will necessitate 70% increase in total food production
- Poverty not being eradicated
- Depletion of fragile natural resource base
- Urbanization with large proportions living in areas susceptible to floods and landslides
- Nutrition transition and the double burden of malnutrition with the growing incidence of non-communicable, chronic degenerative diseases again more in the developing countries including India
- Climate change and its adverse effects on agricultural production
- Environmental degradation and loss of biodiversity accompanied by reduced food production
- Inflation, rising food prices
- Eroding livelihood systems, lack of support for several agricultural crops, mass migration, and movement of people from rural to urban areas
- Increasing natural and manmade disasters pollution.

What are technolgoy are needed strategies that make use of the advances in science and technology. Integration of agriculture, animal husbandry, and aquaculture is required. Several national and international bodies are working through memberships, associations, and partnerships in different sectors on the issues of food and nutrition security in different countries. Some of the technologies addressed below can help attain food and nutrition security.

TECHNOLOGIES FOR FOOD AND NUTRITION SECURITY

Scientific and technological developments in agriculture, food science, and allied fields have played a tremendous role in improving food production through green and white revolution in the past. However, research and development activities have led to development of new technologies to achieve food and nutrition security such as:
- Value addition
- Supplementation
- Fortification
- Biotechnology
- Genetically modified foods
- Food irradiation.

Value Addition

Value addition is essentially addition of new ingredient or bioactive substance and/or alteration of an ingredient or food process to a commodity/product in order to meet the tastes/

preferences of consumers and enhance the nutritional and health benefits including satiety. Thus, in food products, has a higher degree of quality and/or is likely to be richer value added food products as compared to the original, and may also be safer for consumption. Value addition generally means that the quality of the new product has been upgraded with processing, packaging anti-nutritional factors. Such value-added products generally have the same volume or weight and may be sold for a higher price. The quality of the new product has been upgraded through processing, packaging, or nutritional value was enhanced through enrichment or fortification or reduction of anti-nutritional factors. There are several ways to enhance nutritional quality of the food products as shown in Figure 14.4. However, value addition may be done purely for commercial gain. In the process of value addition, there could be a change in the physical state or form, it may change the economic value by the way it is produced, for example, organic farming or the commodity or product has been segregated to enhance its value. In essence, by value addition, the commodity or product now has greater value. Many consumers today pay attention to nutrition and are willing to pay more for pesticide-free or organic products or nutritious, healthy products as well as those that provide more convenience and are microbiologically safe.

Value-added agriculture means increasing the economic value of a commodity through a particular process, e.g., organically grown fruits and vegetables, regionally branded products, etc. For such products, many consumers are willing to pay a higher price. This can also help in augmenting the income of farmers. Value-added agriculture is an important strategy for agricultural entrepreneurship and rural development.

Many food commodities like pulses, spices, and herbs, lesser known, indigenous fruits and vegetables are nutritious, but are not valued much for a variety of reasons. But most of these foods have great potential in contributing to food and nutrition security.

Modern food processing industry has contributed tremendously to enhancing the availability of shelf-stable foods, but many of these are refined and lack important nutrients. Modern technology and processing have made it possible that foods with limited growing seasons are available year round. The Food and Agricultural Organization declared 2016 as the International Year of Pulses which have been also designated as "nutritious seeds for sustainable future." Government of India declared 2018 as the 'National Year of Millets'. Government of India has led the initiative through the United Nations and has won support from several countries. The Food and Agricultural Organization's Committee on Agriculture has accepted India's proposal and has stated that 2023 will be the 'International Year of Millets'. Both pulses and millets are important nutritionally and can be good for attaining food and nutrition security. Millets require much less water to grow than do rice and wheat and in this era of climate change, cultivating such crops will be invaluable. Both millets and pulses are also functional foods.

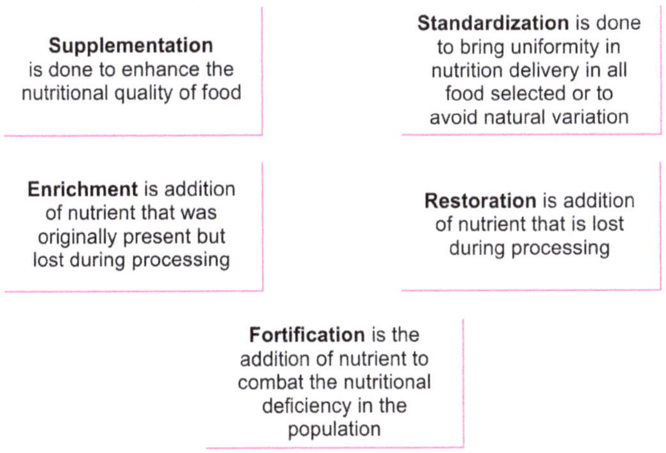

> **Research Glimpse:** Agriculture and industry both play an important role with in food and nutrition security. Agriculture has definitely improved food security but has not been successful in providing nutrition security, but, somewhere lacking in providing nutritional security. Value addition to the existing food crops gives hope to provide nutritional security. Role of food processing industry stand like a pillar for the same. Surplus production of cereals, vegetables, fruits, milk, fish, meat, and poultry is processed and aggressively marketed both inside and outside the country. Value addition coupled with strategic marketing will ensure the perception of consumer thus has shown the potentials of solving the basic problems of food and nutrition security. Value addition coupled with strategic marketing can improve consumer perceptions and has shown potential in solving the basic problems of food and nutrition security.
>
> *Acharya V, Shukla S, Jain S. Agri-produce processing and value addition for nutrition security. International Journal of Applied Home Science. 2017;4(7&8):611-6.*

Restoration: Restoration is the addition of a nutrient to a food in order to restore the original nutrient that might have reduced during processing or storage. Both restoration and enrichment programs usually involve the addition of nutrients that are naturally available or present in the food product.

Standardization is the addition of nutrients to foods to compensate for natural variation, so that a standard level is achieved. Standardization is an important step to ensure a consistent standardized quality of the final food product.

Supplementation

Supplementation "is the supply of nutrients (normally micronutrients) as well as specific bioactive compounds singly or in combination in a quantified dose form. Supplements can take a variety of forms such as tablets, capsules, and pastilles and measured amounts of liquid or small sachets of powder." Provision of iron folate tablets or consuming vitamin mineral or antioxidant in the form of tablet, powders, capsules, and syrups are examples of supplementation. *Supplementation* is the addition of nutrients that are either not normally present or are present in only minute quantities in the food. More than one nutrient may be added, and they may be added in high quantities. Supplementation is a form of providing extra nutrient (s) that is consumed in addition to regular food.

Supplementation is done to enhance the nutritional quality of food

Standardization is done to bring uniformity in nutrition delivery in all food selected or to avoid natural variation

Enrichment is addition of nutrient that was originally present but lost during processing

Restoration is addition of nutrient that is lost during processing

Fortification is the addition of nutrient to combat the nutritional deficiency in the population

Fig. 14.4: Different ways of value addition to food.

Supplementation consists in using specifically designed products to deliver nutrients and other substances to the individual or target group in a unit dose. Each dose or unit or serving is designed to supply a specific quantity of the nutrient(s). The advantage of supplementation is that large numbers of persons can be covered and it is possible to bring about rapid improvement in the nutritional status of the population. It is especially useful for combating deficiencies of vulnerable segments of the population like women in their reproductive years and children. Also in case of micronutrients, the cost and ease of intervention are advantageous. Compared to supplementation, diet-based approaches are relatively slower. The disadvantage is that supplementation does not encourage the population to adopt more healthy eating habits.

In case of nutrients or nutraceuticals, they can be manufactured in different forms such as tablets with or without coatings (needed to mask the unpleasant taste of the active ingredient or to prevent deterioration and act as a barrier to oxygen and moisture), capsules, or liquid supplements.

For some nutrients, the deficiency is a public health problem and there are supplementation programs for combating the problem. For these intensive efficacy and safety studies have been conducted before deciding upon dosages that are recommended by expert groups. In India, the major nutrient deficiencies that are being tackled are PEM, iron, vitamin A, and iodine deficiencies. Zinc and calcium are also important nutrients.

Fortification

Food fortification is one of the most feasible, economical, and achievable nutrition interventions for achieving nutritional security. Food fortification is a means to combat the deficiency of a particular nutrient which is of public health importance. According to the FAO (2003):

"Food fortification means the addition of nutrients at levels higher than those found in the original food."

Evolution of Fortification

One of the earliest reports of food fortification dates back to 4000 BC, when the Persian physician, Melampus, added iron filings to sweet wine to strengthen the sailors' resistance to spears and arrows and to enhance their sexual potency. Fortification is an age old practice initiated in 1833, by the French physician, Boussingault, whose efforts to prevent goiter were successful by adding iodine to salt. Later addition of vitamin D to milk; vitamin A and D to margarine and milk; and addition of B vitamins to cereal products were practised and also accepted by the US FDA in 1965 and governments of several other countries. In India, vanaspati was fortified with vitamin A for a long period of time.

According to the Codex Alimentarius (an international body which defines and prescribes food standards and technologies), fortification is:

"The addition of one or more essential nutrients to a food, whether or not it is normally contained in the food, for the purpose of preventing or correcting a demonstrated deficiency of one or more nutrients in the population or specific population groups."

Fortification differs from enrichment which is *"increasing the level of nutrients present to make the food a "richer" source."*

According to FSSAI (2016), *"fortification means deliberately increasing the content of essential micronutrient in food so as to improve the nutritional quality of food and to provide public health benefit with minimal risk to health."*

Fortification is carried out because deficiencies or potential deficiencies of a specific nutrient exist or are likely to exist in the population. The advantage of fortification is that the nutrient intake of a population can be improved within the context of the indigenous diet and there is little need for the people or consumers to change their dietary behavior and food habits. Also it is cost effective. Conventional foods or ingredients are used to carry the added nutrients. In most cases, it is possible to effectively fortify a food without significantly changing the organoleptic qualities of the food. This is because the amount of micronutrient(s) that is added is very small.

Fortification is usually done at industrial level, but can be done at community or household level by various means. Fortification done for general public is regulated by the government sector. It can be mandatory, e.g., "Universal iodization of salt." Fortification of certain food items like cereals, oil, sugar, and condiments can be mandatory or voluntary depending upon the feasibility or requirement, e.g., bread can be fortified with vitamins and minerals to be served through some feeding programs. The main purpose of fortification is:

- To correct the dietary deficiency of a specific nutrient, e.g., iodine in salt.
- To restore the nutrient lost during food processing, e.g., B-vitamins in breakfast cereals. In this case, the amount of nutrients added is approximately equal to the natural content in the food before processing.
- To improve nutritional quality of a newly manufactured food, e.g., folic acid fortified food
- To add nutrients that may not be present naturally in food
- To ensure that foods manufactured for special purposes have appropriate nutrient content.
- To increase the added nutritional value of a product (commercial view); and to provide certain technological functions in food processing.

Besides this, "functional foods" have been fortified with micronutrients to prevent diseases like osteoporosis, cancer, or heart disease. Similarly, fortified enteral and parenteral feeds are manufactured for hospital patients.

Some terms that are used related to addition of nutrients are as follows:
1. **Fortificant**—the nutrient that is added in the vehicle
2. **Vehicle**—is the food item in which the nutrient (fortificant) is added.

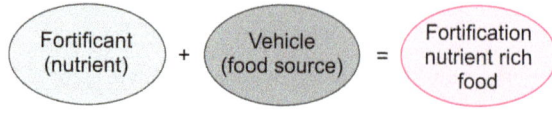

The FAO/WHO Expert Committee on Nutrition has recommended that the following points should be considered when choosing the nutrient for fortification:
- Intake of the nutrient is much below the desirable level among a large number of people, i.e., level of nutrient deficiency prevalent in a given geographical area.
- Food selected should be commonly consumed by the people.
- Addition of the nutrient is not likely to create a nutritional imbalance with other nutrients.
- The nutrient that is added will be stable under customary conditions of storage and processing/cooking that may be done later.
- Additional cost of fortification will not make the fortified food too expensive that it is not within the reach of consumers.
- The compound chosen as a fortificant should have good bioavailability.
- Care should be taken that the fortificant should not cause any undesirable change in color, flavor, or texture of the fortified product.
- Fortificant/nutrient should be mentioned on the label of food.
- The amount of the essential nutrient(s) should be sufficient to correct or prevent the deficiency when the food is consumed in normal amount by the population at risk.
- The nutrient(s) added should be sufficiently stable in the food under customary conditions of packaging, storage, distribution, and use. Some factors should be considered while selecting the nutrient while as shown in Figure 14.5.

Compared with vitamins, iron and iodine are very stable under extreme processing conditions. Vitamin A, on the other hand, is very labile in the processing environment. Vitamin A is both oxygen and temperature sensitive. It has been reported that vitamin A (and also β-carotene) added to foods is sensitive to oxidative damage. In the form of retinol, vitamin A is more labile than its ester form; for this reason, vitamin A esters are usually used for food fortification. The stability of vitamin A is also strongly affected by pH. At a pH of less than 5, vitamin A is susceptible to oxidation. At low pH, vitamin A tends to isomerize from the *trans* to the *cis* configuration, which has a lower vitamin activity. The problem of low pH is encountered especially during juice processing. Fruit juices usually have a low pH (about 3.0). To compensate for low pH, carbonation, which expels oxygen, may be used to stabilize vitamin A. Value-added is defined as the addition of time, place, and/or form utility to a commodity in order to meet the tastes/preferences of consumers.

Methods of fortification: There are different methods of fortification used for different foods:
- Dry mixing—use of premixes at milling stage—for flours
- Coating and spraying after processing—for ready to eat cereals
- Addition at parboiling stage—for milled and processed foods

The most commonly used method is dry mixing. In case of a mixture of vitamins, a premix is added to the flours at the milling stage. Coating and spraying are done for ready-to-eat cereals. More stable vitamins like niacin, riboflavin, vitamin B_6, and vitamin E-acetate are added to formula and more labile vitamins such as vitamin A and thiamin are coated after the processing. Fortification of rice with thiamin is done by soaking parboiled rice with solution of thiamin hydrochloride. Fortification of water-soluble vitamins has been found essential in milled and processed foods because they are usually destroyed in milling.

Vehicle

Selection of food as a vehicle is equally important for food fortification. The factors shown in Figure 14.6 should be considered at the time selecting the vehicle for the fortificant.

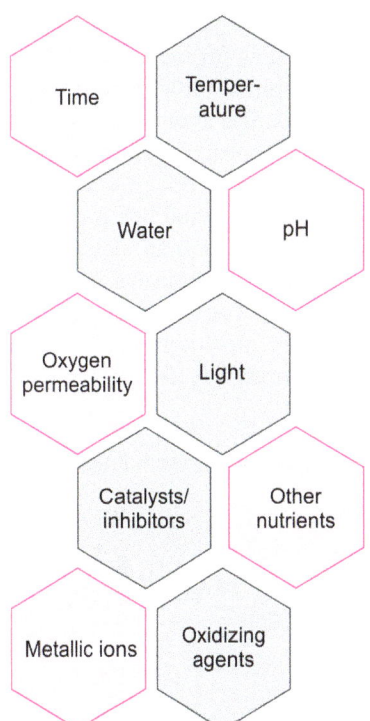

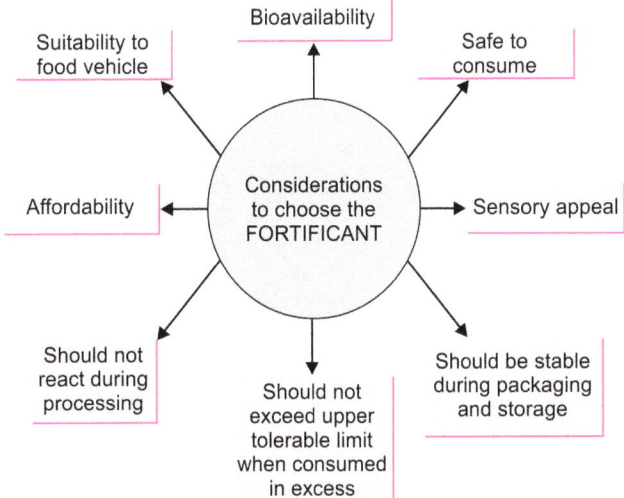

Fig. 14.5: Factors to be considered while selecting a fortificant.

Fig. 14.6: Factors affecting the choice of vehicle.

Selected food (vehicle) should be edible and acceptable by the target population. Cost of fortified foods should not increase much compared to the non-fortified foods. Commonly used foods as vehicles are salt, edible oil, sugar, wheat flour, maize flour, bakery products, and milk products. The range of foods is not very wide because of several limiting factors such as technological and organoleptic restrictions, cost, and consumer expectations. There are several factors that affect the stability of the nutrient: Besides these factors, appearance and stability are important because poor stability or adverse effects of the fortification on the appearance of the food can counteract the benefits of fortification. There may also be interaction between nutrients wherein the fortificant could adversely affect the vitamin content of a food. This may be seen with minerals like iron or zinc.

Deficiency of more than one nutrient may exist, but to fortify foods with every nutrient is not possible for various reasons. There are various chemical compounds which are used as fortificants, e.g., ferrous sulfate for iron fortification. These chemical compounds have different content that determines the possible dose. The fortificant needs to be added in the amount at which the nutrient is bioavailable, stable, and acceptable. It does not also have any adverse effects on the sensory quality of the food or be destroyed or lost during processing, transport, and storage. For some nutrients, fortification of foods is relatively easy as in the case of iodine and for others like iron, it is not easy because there can be changes in color, flavor, and texture of the vehicle. Some of the nutrients that need to be added because their deficiencies are widespread and vehicles used for these are briefly described.

Iodine: Usually, iodide and iodate forms are found suitable for iodine fortification. They are usually added as potassium salts and sometimes calcium and sodium salts. Potassium iodide and potassium iodate are the two major fortificants used for several decades for iodine fortification at the rate 50–150 ppm. Potassium iodide is more stable and more resistant to oxidation and evaporation, but is more expensive. Potassium iodate is therefore preferred for many foods including salt, particularly in hot and humid climates.

Iodates do not require coaddition of stabilizers. Other compounds used in iodization are calcium iodide, calcium iodate, sodium iodide, and sodium iodate. Different salts contain different iodine content as given in Table 14.1. Salt has been chosen for various reasons. Salt is consumed throughout the year by all people, in all geographical regions. Salt iodization technology is easy to implement at a reasonable cost. Iodization does not affect organoleptic quality of foods in which iodized salt is added.

Iron: Iron fortification is very challenging because the selected fortificant compound may or may not be bioavailable and if the bioavailability is good, then it tends to produce undesirable organoleptic effect(s). Over the years, several iron compounds have been used. Table 14.2 lists these compounds with their iron content and possible fortificants. Water-soluble forms are more useful for dry cereal flours, pasta, and milk powders for 1–3 months according to climate. Ferrous sulfate is most commonly used because it is cheap and its bioavailability is high, but it can cause rancidity in food, especially upon prolonged storage.

Table 14.1: Iodine content of different iodine/iodate compounds used as fortificants.

Iodide/Iodate compounds	Iodine content (%)
Calcium iodide	86.5
Calcium iodate	65.0
Potassium iodide	76.5
Potassium iodate	59.5
Sodium iodide	68.0
Sodium iodate	64.0

Table 14.2: Chemical compounds used in iron fortification.

Chemical compound as fortificant	Iron content (%)	Food vehicle
Water-soluble compounds		
Ferrous sulfate.7H_2O	20	Cereal flours, salt, sugar, infant formula, beverages, and dry foods
Ferrous sulfate dried	33	Dry cereal flours, pasta
Ferrous lactate	19	Beverages, infant formula
Ferrous gluconate	12	Cereal, salt, sugar food, infant formula, beverages
Ferrous bisglycinate	20	Fruit juices and soft drinks
Ferric ammonium citrate	18	Cereal, infant formula, beverages
Sodium iron EDTA (sodium ethylenediaminetetraacetic acid)	13	Cereals
Reduced elemental iron by		
Hydrogen (reduced)	96	Wheat flour cookies
Carbon monoxide	96	Cereal flours
Automized iron	97	Cereal flours
Carbonyl iron	99	Cereal flours
Electrolytic iron	97	Breakfast cereals, cereal flours
Poorly water soluble, soluble in dilute acid		
Ferrous fumarate	33	Maize flour, wheat flour
Ferrous succinate	33	Infant cereals
Ferric saccharate	10	Chocolate drink powders
Water insoluble, poorly soluble in dilute acid		
Ferric orthophosphate	29	Rice, infant foods, chocolate foods
Ferric pyrophosphate	25	Extruded rice, salt
Encapsulated forms		
Ferrous sulfate	16	Wheat-based snacks, dairy and soy products, salt, complementary foods
Ferrous fumarate	16	Dry infant formula

Source: WHO/FAO (2006). Guidelines on food fortification with micronutrients/ edited by Lindsay Allen et al. World Health Organization and Food and Agriculture Organization of the United Nations, 2006.

Ferrous sulfate is absorbed like non-heme iron; hence, the presence of ascorbic acid or meat facilitates the absorption of fortified foods. Ferrous fumarate and ferric saccharate are other compounds but they have limitations because they affect the organoleptic properties of the vehicle and may not be suitable in certain medical conditions. Use of elemental iron is governed by the size, shape of iron particle, as well as the composition of meal. Sensory issues can be reduced/handled by encapsulation. Solubility and bioavailability of the iron compound are crucial. However, absorption is also dependent upon the presence of iron inhibitor in the food matrix and prevailing conditions in the gastrointestinal tract. To improve iron availability, addition of ascorbic acid, sodium ethylenediamine tetraacetic acid (sodium EDTA or Na2EDTA) has been found effective. Sodium EDTA is also a food additive and is stable during processing and storage. The removal of phytates by phytase enzyme at industrial level and use of techniques like milling, soaking, germination, and fermentation have shown substantial loss of phytates and increased the bioavailability of iron in the body. Encapsulation needs some coating of stabilizer due to which it mitigates the sensory changes; however, it adds 5–10 times the cost to the product. As per the legislation of the Joint FAO/WHO Expert Committee on Food Additives, use of NaFeEDTA at 0.2 mg Fe/kg body weight per day has been recommended and for high phytate foods like cereals, use of Na2EDTA plus ferrous sulfate rather than NaFeEDTA alone might be a better option.

Vitamin A: Retinol cannot be used in fortification due to its high reactivity to ultraviolet light, oxygen, or air. Retinyl acetate and retinyl palmitate are the major compounds used in food fortification. Vitamin A is a sensitive vitamin and its stability is influenced by pH and metallic ions like iron and copper, hence antioxidants like butylated hydroxyanisole (BHA), butylated hydroxytoluene (BHT), and α-tocopherols (vitamin E) are sometimes used in vitamin A premixes. Dry milk, complementary foods, biscuits, and beverages are successfully fortified with provitamin A or carotene and used commercially or in feeding programs. Oils, margarine, cocoa products, milk products, and margarine are oil-based foods and are generally selected for vitamin A fortification. The use of oil not only facilitates the absorption of the vitamin but also prevents the oxidation of vitamin A during storage. However, sugar, tea, rice, and flour have also been tried out with success. Ambient conditions, storage period, and type of packaging material are important in fortified foods. Different compounds are used in different foods, e.g., oil soluble form of retinyl acetate and retinyl palmitate are used to fortify oil and water-dispersible form of retinyl palmitate is used in sugar.

Vitamin D: Vitamin D2 (ergocalciferol) and D3 (cholecalciferol) are active compounds and are used as fortificants. Both forms are sensitive to oxygen and moisture; hence, they are generally used with an antioxidant (tocopherol) at commercial level. Milk and milk products like dried milk powder, margarine, and vanaspati are usually fortified with vitamin D in India.

Calcium: Calcium salts are used for fortification. Commonly used salts are calcium carbonates, chloride, citrate, gluconate, glycerophosphate, lactate, mono-, di-, and tribasic phosphates, hydroxide, citrate malate, etc. Citrate sometimes gives a tart taste. Calcium fortification is used in infant formula and complementary foods. Low solubility of calcium salts in water is one of the major limitations in their bioavailability. Calcium citrate or calcium malate or the gluconate form are relatively more soluble and are thus used in beverages and juices. Tribasic calcium phosphate or calcium carbonate or calcium lactate is chosen to fortify milk. Stabilizers are used to prevent sedimentation. Calcium salt is selected according to food or vehicle.

Selenium: Selenium is also added to foods particularly in countries like China, where selenium deficiency (Keshan disease) occurs. It is added to milk-based infant foods and sports drinks. Even the soil is fortified with sodium selenate. Selenomethionine has been found to pose certain risks and hence is generally not used for fortification.

Fluoride: Large-scale fortification of water with fluoride is carried out in many parts of the world by using hexa-fluoro-silicate acid (HUSIAC). Salt and milk are also fluoridated in certain parts of the world. Salt fluoridation in Jamaica has been reported to reduce dental decay in children.

Dual Fortification

Addition of two nutrients in one food item is called dual fortification. It means that the fortification is done with more than one nutrient in a single food commodity. Since iodine and iron deficiency coexist in many geographical areas including India, efforts are being made to use fortify salt with these two nutrients. However, this has been a considerable challenge owing to reactivity of the compounds in suitable vehicles. Some success has been achieved with double-fortified salt (DFS) by encapsulation of ferrous fumarate and micronized ground ferric pyrophosphate along with iodized salt. According to Micronutrient Initiative (2014), double-fortified salt is one of the most cost-effective opportunities to overcome iodine deficiency disorders and reduce the prevalence of anemia, thereby improving mental capacity, maternal and infant survival, and human productivity in the target population who is at risk of the deficiencies of these two nutrients.

Government of India is promoting the use of DFS to meet the goal of "Anemia Mukt Bharat." Nutrition International (NI) has developed toolkits and educational materials to create public awareness about the importance of consuming double-fortified salt. Quality control and quality assurance protocols are also essential to scale up the production and distribution of DFS. Dual fortification is being tried for edible oils and sugar in India also. Further evidence indicate that dairy products like whole milk, yoghurt, cheese, yoghurt drinks, dairy-based beverages, milk powder, butter and buttermilk are also good candidates to incorporate essential ingredients like vitamins, minerals, omega-3 fatty acids, probiotics, prebiotics and phytoconstituents to face the challenges of nutrition deficiency and related diseases among all age group of people.

Limitations of fortification

Indiscriminate fortification of foods with protein and other macronutrients as well as micronutrients should be avoided. Fortification of ready to eat foods is also a questionable practice because excessive consumption may lead to obesity and other problems. Fortification of a single ingredient or the whole food product is another big issue of concern. Sugar, vegetable oil, and monosodium glutamate have also been studied for the feasibility to be used as vehicles for the fortification of vitamin A but the efforts have not reached commercial scale as in the case of salt fortification with iodine.

Use of cereals as vehicles is associated two technical constraints, i.e., high levels of phytic acid and extreme sensitivity of unsaturated fat to oxidation during storage due to the presence of highly reactive forms of iron (ferrous sulfate or fumarate). Encapsulation, use of phytase enzyme, or use of microionized form of fortification can reduce the oxidative reaction. Use of fruit juices and drinks for iron fortification poses several problems such as accelerated loss of vitamin C, deterioration of flavor and taste in the presence of thiamine, folic acid, vitamin A, and vitamin C, metallic off-flavors at higher doses, and decolorization of some pigments.

Other Forms of Food Fortification

- **Biofortification**
- **Home fortification**

Biofortification: "Biofortification" or "biological fortification" refers to nutritionally enhanced food crops having improved bioavailability of nutrient(s) to the human population. Staple crops such as rice, maize, cassava, and wheat as well as beans have been biofortified and cultivated using modern biotechnology techniques, conventional plant breeding, and agronomic practices. Biofortified crops that contain higher amounts of essential micronutrients are a feasible and practical approach to cover large proportions of the population. The advantage is that even among poor farmers, benefits of these biofortified crops are reached to the entire family and the excess grain that is sold becomes available through market channels to the general public. Thus, development of these new varieties of crops will help combat nutrient deficiencies. Biofortification is the process of increasing the bioavailable concentrations of essential elements like Fe and Zn in staple food crops through agronomic intervention or genetic selection in order to combat the global problem of malnutrition or hidden hunger.

There are three forms/strategies of biofortification nutritional enhancement:
1. Use of enhanced fertilizers/mineral fertilization, i.e., nutritional enhancement after biofortification
2. Crop breeding through improved plant varieties through conventional breeding
3. Transgenic approaches/nutritional genetic modification.

1. **Biofortification by enhanced fertilizers/mineral fertilization:** Since soil micronutrients influence crop productivity and nutritional quality of food, deficiencies of these nutrients in soil influence the amount present in the diets consumed and can eventually affect nutrition and human health. Use of excess nitrogen, phosphorus, and potassium (NPK) in fertilizer is an old practice to improve crop yield. Agronomic biofortification by spray application on foliage or adding in soil relocates the nutrient availability in the plant. Addition of Zn, Fe, and selenium are considered suitable for this technique (from soil to crop). Soil microorganisms that promote growth may be used, e.g., different species of genera *Bacillus, Pseudomonas, Rhizobium, Azotobacter*. These organisms enhance phytoavailability of minerals or mobility and transfer of nutrients from soil to the edible parts of the plant, thus improving their nutrient content. Some crops are associated with fungi that release organic acids, siderophores, and enzymes that can break down organic compounds and thus increase the mineral concentrations in the crop.

2. **Biofortification by improved plant breeding:** It is usually done on oil producing crops or oil seeds. Plant breeding has immense power to improve nutritional value of foods by increasing vitamins and minerals, antioxidants, fiber, and healthful oils through genetic diversity by which availability of nutrients in food crops can be enhanced. It is one of the more quicker, more reliable yields, and affordable technique. Another breeding strategy for facilitating bioavailability of iron and zinc that are present in cereal grains is to lower the level of phytic acid that is also present in the grains and prevents absorption of zinc and iron.

3. **Transgenic approaches/nutritional genetic modification:** A **transgene** is a gene or genetic material that has been transferred naturally using genetic engineering techniques from one organism to another. There are transgenic plants as well as transgenic animals. Transgenic plants are also called genetically modified plants in which DNA is modified using genetic engineering techniques. Transgenic technique can be applied to those crops when there is limited or very little genetic variation in the nutrient content of different varieties of the same plant, or when a plant does not naturally contain a particular nutrient. The key approach is to identify and characterize gene function followed by utilizing these genes to engineer the metabolism of the plant(s). The purpose of using such technique is not only for plant breeders but can be used to improve the nutritional quality of the food and could be environment-friendly. Also, the amount of time, effort and investment can be quite large. However, the advantages are: (i) once a useful gene has been identified, it can be used for a variety of crops (ii) simultaneously several genes can be inserted that will enhance the micronutrient content in the plant (iii) genetically modify the concentration of the nutrient in different tissue through redistribution (iv) improve the micronutrient availability (v) reduce the antinutrient concentration, thus yielding a crop that has multiple benefits.

With the transgenic approach, levels of vitamins, minerals, selected amino acids and fatty acids have been increased in selected crops. While many plants/crops including cereals, legumes, vegetables, oilseeds, fruits as well as fodder crops are being researched, some crops have been taken to the step of release such as iron rich cassava, golden rice, high lysine maize, high unsaturated fatty acid soybean.

A transgenic gene(s) having desirable and specific characteristic is artificially inserted in the plant. Hence the plant turns into a completely different species. Plants containing transgenes are often called genetically modified or GM crops. Transgenic animal refers to an animal in which deliberate modification of the genome is carried out or a foreign DNA is introduced into the animal, using recombinant DNA technology, and eventually the animal demonstrates the desirable output and behavior.

Genetic engineering could be a tool promising for increasing the bioavailability of iron in staple crops. It has also provided the opportunity to enhance the β-carotene content in orange fleshed sweet potato which was not present in white sweet potato.

However, while reducing the antinutrient content in crops, caution is required because many antinutrients are major plant metabolites with important roles in plant metabolism protecting plants against stress and conferring resistance to crop pests or pathogens. Also, many of these antinutrients like polyphenols are important phytochemicals that have health benefits and protect humans from chronic, non-communicable diseases.

Biofortified crops are developed through joint and collaborative efforts of plant breeders, food scientists, and nutritionists. Several aspects are considered—the concentration of micronutrient in the edible portion of the food crop, the amount of nutrient that can be absorbed after the biofortified food has been processed, especially by traditional methods of processing, genetic variability, soil conditions and climatic zones, cultural factors, and the feasibility of breeding for increased concentrations of several nutrients simultaneously in edible tissues. Yet it is necessary that the yield and other quality characteristics are not affected.

Golden rice is the most popular example of biofortification which is biofortified with β carotene, iron, and zinc. Field trials have assessed its impact on nutritional status on the population at risk, milling, and cooking qualities, and consumer acceptability. Other crops are maize, sweet potato, cassava for iron, and β carotene in India and around the globe. High lysine crops and low phytate maize have shown quite promising results.

The Consultative Group on International Agricultural Research (CGIAR) has been working intensively for years to increase bioavailable Fe and Zn in several staple food crops. Several crops have been targeted such as rice, maize, cassava, sweet potato, beans, pearl millet and wheat, potato, sorghum/jowar, banana/plantain, cowpeas, groundnuts, and lentils. Among these, zinc biofortified rice, wheat, and iron biofortified pearl millet and lentils are products for Asia. For Africa, the products are provitamin A biofortified sweet potato, maize, cassava, plantain, and iron fortified bean, sorghum, and potato. Plant breeding is used as an intervention strategy to address micronutrient malnutrition by breeding/producing staple food crops using efficient lines that make use of untapped resources in the soil with enhanced levels of bioavailable essential minerals and vitamins that will have help to improve the micronutrient status of target populations. Cassava and sweet potato have been chosen to contain high provitamin A carotenoids, while lentil, potato, and sorghum are focused on for increased iron content.

Biofortification is a sustainable, rural-based intervention because it has the inherent advantage of reaching the low income households including remote rural populations who are generally the most nutritionally vulnerable and malnourished. Biofortification costs less than the traditional approach of pharmaceutical supplementation. It has the potential to be fully integrated into the prevailing food chain. Surplus grain grown by small and marginal farmers ultimately will reach urban markets so that biofortified grain over a period of time can also become available to the urban poor. Over a period of time, the benefits can be availed of by several countries as adapted biofortified cultivars become available to farmers in several countries at relatively lower recurrent costs and the germplasm can be shared internationally. Thus, it can complement currently used approaches such as supplementation and industrial fortification which are more expensive and are urban-based.

If biofortification is to be successful, there are important considerations:

- A biofortified crop must be high yielding and profitable to the farmer.
- It should effectively reduce micronutrient malnutrition.
- The biofortified crop must be acceptable to both farmers and consumers in target regions where people are afflicted with micronutrient malnutrition.
- Nutrition education may be required to encourage consumers to preferentially choose and consume the new varieties, and
- How to optimally conserve/retain the nutrient in the biofortified food.

Laboratory Laurel: Fermented milk can contribute to enhance the availability of folate using folate producing probiotics as an aid in fortification. In milk fermentation, some bacteria are folate utilizers thereby decreasing the amount of folate; however, some are folate producers. Hence, judicial selection of a suitable starter culture can increase the dietary folate content. In this regard, some lactic acid bacteria (LAB) such as *Streptococcus thermophilus, Lactococcus lactis,* and *Lactobacillus plantarum* have been reported to produce folate. This study is carried to see the efficacy of a probiotic *L. lactis* CM28 by 16S rRNA strain in folate fortification of skim milk, optimization of its bioavailability, and assess the stability of the produced folate on refrigerated storage. Optimization resulted in a fourfold increase in the extracellular folate (61.02 μg/L) and after deconjugation the total folate detected was 129.53 μg/L. The effect of refrigerated storage on the viability of *L. lactis,* pH, titratable acidity (TA) in terms of percentage lactic acid, and finally on the stability of folate was determined. Only a slight variation in pH and acidity was observed during folate fermentation. During storage, about 90% of the produced folate was retained in an active state.

Jayakumar BD, Nampoothiri KM. Folate fortification of skim milk by a probiotic **Lactococcus lactis CM28 and evaluation of its stability in fermented milk on cold storage.** *J Food Sci Technol.* 2015;52(6): 3513-9.

Home fortification or sprinkles: It is an innovative and simple after innovative method of fortification to nutritionally enrich the meals of the vulnerable population especially young children and others. Single-dose packets containing micronutrient powders (MNP) or multiple vitamins and minerals in powder form are provided. The powder can be sprinkled onto any semi-solid food fed to young children by the mother or on any other food that is consumed at point-of-use. Essentially the sprinkles can be used by any one for a family or an individual.

Ferrous sulfate, fumarate, and electrolytic iron are being used in different food matrices. Packaging and storage conditions have been found to be compatible for long shelf life. Dr Zlotkin and his associates in 2003 developed the single dose sachet containing the nutrient in powder form and it was called "Sprinkles" because it can be sprinkled over the food or mixed into the food. These Sprinkles are encapsulated in a thin soy lipid coating which prevents change in color, taste, and flavor of fortified food. This approach can also be effectively used in hospital kitchens for sick children as well as in public health programs. It is also referred to as Home fortification. Oral iron drops were also used for home fortification but the compliance was poor due to unpleasant and metallic after taste and some abdominal discomfort.

Food to food fortification: Fortification is concerned with addition of nutrient(s) to daily diet and usually carried out at industry level. There are many highly nutrient-dense food ingredients which are now not very difficult to access, e.g., soy isolate, whey protein, nuts, seeds, and many functional foods. When these functional foods are incorporated in food preparation of daily use, it is considered as "food to food fortification". Consumers today are becoming health conscious and use health foods or herbal ingredient to treat a wide variety of aliments. It is talked or written about in different media. Food to food fortification can be done in various ways such as addition of berries and/or dried fruits to breakfast cereals, addition of lemon grass, ginger, tulsi to tea for their health benefits, addition of leafy vegetables like moringa (drumstick leaves) into a variety of preparations, grated vegetables to khichri fruits and/or nuts porridge, addition of sprouted pulses and/or groundnuts to poha, upma and use of flax seeds in dry chutney powders are some examples. Such practices are carried out at home and health centres.

Laboratory Laurel: A study was carried out to develop and characterize omega-3 *dahi* (Indian yoghurt) through fortification of microencapsulated flaxseed oil powder (MFOP). Four different formulations were developed @ 0, 1, 2, and 3% levels and the level of addition was optimized on the basis of sensory scores. *Dahi* fortified at 2% level was observed comparable to control. The samples were tested for titratable acidity, syneresis, firmness, stickiness, oxidative stability (peroxide value), α-linolenic acid (ALA, ω-3) content, and sensory attributes during a storage period of 15 days. MFOP fortified *dahi* showed significantly higher acidity after 12 days of storage. However, peroxide value remained well below (~0.41) the maximum permissible limit (5 mEq peroxides/kg oil) prescribed by the Codex Alimentarius Commission. Gas-liquid chromatography (GLC) profile indicated ~21 % decrease in ALA content in fortified *dahi* after 15 days of storage. Overall, it can be concluded that flaxseed oil microcapsules incorporated in *dahi* could be a potential vehicle for delivery of omega-3 fatty acids.

Goyal A, Sharma V, Sihag MK, et al. Fortification of *dahi (Indian yoghurt)* with omega-3 fatty acids using microencapsulated flaxseed oil microcapsules. J Food Sci Technol. 2016;53(5):2422-33.

Biotechnology

Biotechnology is defined in various ways. Biotechnology is the use of technology in biological science. It has been defined as "any technological application that uses biological systems, living organisms, or derivatives thereof, to make or modify products for specific use." Biotechnology uses biological systems and living organisms or components of organisms to either make or modify products or processes for specific purposes. It utilizes the sciences of biology, chemistry, physics, engineering, computers, and information technology to develop tools and products that will be useful to humans, e.g., use of living organisms to enhance crops, fuels, medical treatments, etc. It also be defined as any technique that uses live organisms in order to make or modify a product or to improve plants/animals or to engineer microorganisms for a specific purpose. Live organisms used could be bacteria/viruses/fungi/yeast/plant cells/animal cells. This could be done through genetic engineering, enzyme and protein engineering, plant tissue culture/animal tissue culture, use of biosensors, bioprocess, and fermentation technology.

With its tremendous scope, modern biotechnology has the potential to meet the tremendous challenges faced in agricultural production to meet the food and nutrient needs of an increasing global population. It is estimated that by 2050 the world population may be about 9 million and food production will need to increase by several times more due to unprecedented natural disastrous episodes like COVID-19, floods, fires etc.

Application of biotechnology in food production is challenging and simultaneously creating the opportunities to enhance the production of different food crops. It is a tool that can help in sustainable development of agriculture, fisheries, forestry, and food industry. If it is properly integrated and used with other techniques, it can contribute in real terms to food security of the increasing needs of a growing world population. Application of biotechnology could contribute to food security by minimizing losses in the food chain as well as reducing waste and harnessing food waste by conversion into useful substances such as biofuels, improve food quality and safety. It could also help to reduce environmental pollution and by increasing food availability and marketability. Food is also processed in order to improve its quality and safety.

Several genetic engineering techniques are used in plant breeding to increase the uptake of a nutrient from soil. Similarly, it is possible to enhance the bioavailability of mineral(s) by either increasing the levels of chelating agents or reducing agents, enzymes, transporter proteins in roots, etc. For example, several genes that can increase the bioavailability of iron and zinc have been identified in plants. For example, Golden Rice 1 contains the PSY (phytoene synthase) gene from daffodil and the CRTI (Phytoene desaturase) gene from the bacterium *Erwinia uredovora*. Replacing PSY with genes from maize and rice can increase the level of β-carotene 23 times in Golden Rice 2.

Biotechnology was initiated in the 1970s with advances in molecular biology and development of DNA-based technology called "recombinant DNA technology." It involves the insertion of desired gene into another chromosome of another living cell. The newly designed gene has inherently different characteristics which may or may not resemble the original genes. It involves the modification/manipulation and transformation in genes, enzymes, and other organic compounds using the organisms. *Bacillus thuringiensis* (Bt) was the first soil bacterium which was used to produce a protein that is toxic to many insects and is thus helpful in protecting the crop.

According to the Codex Alimentarius Commission, biotechnology is, "the application of (i) *in vitro* nucleic acid techniques, including recombinant DNA and the direct injection of nucleic acid into cells or organelles and (ii) the fusion of cells beyond the taxonomic family that overcomes natural physiological reproductive or recombination barriers and is not a technique used in traditional breeding and selection."

Biotechnology offers the techniques to identify select and modify the DNA sequence for specific genetic trait which can be transferred in the recipient plant where those traits are expressed. Development of specific trait is not otherwise possible with traditional breeding practices in agriculture. Over the years, there has been about 20% increase in the use of bio-tech crops (WHO, 2005). Between 1996 and 2017, globally the acreage under biotech crops has increased 100-fold. Increasing the crop yield, improving the nutrient composition of crop, and developing any trait which facilitates processing characteristics and reduces storage losses can be achieved with biotechnology. Modern biotechnology can be applied to plant crops, livestock (dairy products, meat), and fish to produce end products with desirable nutrient composition and certain other traits. Novel traits can be introduced in the food in order to enhance the human health.

Biotechnology has several benefits:
- Increased crop yields through making crops more resistant to insects, pests, tolerance to herbicides
- Slower ripening, and better tasting foods
- Increasing productivity per unit area of land
- Improve food safety by methods that can detect disease causing viruses and bacteria in foods
- Developing new varieties of crops with better color, texture, higher nutrient content
  - Vitamin A-rice containing high level of beta carotene
  - High-iron rice contains the iron carrier protein, ferritin that increases iron storage in rice and absorption in the digestive tract
  - Improved protein content in vegetables like cassava, plantain, and potato
- Developing foods with more favorable nutrient profiles, e.g., higher protein, lower fat, altered fatty acid profile, e.g., less saturated fatty acids and higher amount of monounsaturated fatty acids
  - Altered starch—increased starch content of potato to reduce oil absorption
  - Altered fatty acid composition—high oleic acid in sunflower and soy
- Making foods less allergenic or toxic
  - Peanuts that are less allergenic
  - Reduced cyanide level in cassava
- Developing functional foods for health
  - Increased antioxidant content—increase in lycopene and lutein in tomatoes and isoflavones in soy
- Reducing food spoilage
- Developing foods with extended shelf life.

Examples of foods that have been improved by biotechnology include potatoes with more favorable amino acid content and soybeans with higher amount of oleic acid so that the oil is more suitable for frying in terms of stability, garlic with higher amounts of the compound allicin so that the cholesterol-lowering properties of garlic are enhanced. Other foods that have been improved are peanuts with improved protein profile and tomatoes with higher lycopene content. Modern biotechnology is not only concerned with crop productivity but its uses are also extended to reduce food spoilage; develop new food products of edible nature and extend their shelf life. Microbial culture has also been found useful in production of cheese and other dairy products for a wide range of flavors, colors, and textures. Enzymes are added to flour to improve bread quality. Golden rice, modified food ingredients, dietetic foods, food supplements, medicines, and vaccines are examples of outcome of biotechnology.

Besides helping to improve food and nutrition security, biotechnology can be used to trace the origin of foodstuffs and their authenticity using genetic markers, e.g., genetic tagging of grapevine varieties. A considerable amount of research and development is occurring in the field of human health for development of drugs, vaccines, diagnostic probes, etc.

In food manufacture, biotechnology has been used for centuries in making traditional foods like curds, sauerkraut, fermented sausage, and a variety of other fermented foods. Microbial culture has been used in production of cheese and other dairy products for wide range of flavor, color, and texture.

Chymosin, an enzyme is now used instead of rennet in cheese production. Previously, rennet was obtained from calves' stomachs. Biotechnology has not only eliminated the need to use rennet from calves but it is also of better quality and purity. Besides helping to change plant production, biotechnology can bring important changes in livestock production. In both plant and livestock production, biotechnology has a role in all steps of production, from agrochemical inputs and breeding to final food processing. In fact, work on application of biotechnology in animal production has been comparatively more rapid than in plant biotechnology. Biotechnology can be applied to animal reproduction, selection, breeding, animal health, development of animal feeds, and improved nutrition, improving growth and production of livestock. With reference to reproduction, techniques include embryo transfer, in vitro fertilization, and cloning and sex determination of embryos. All of these are relevant to breeding programs. For example, the cost of importing frozen embryos will definitely be less than importing live animals.

> **Current use of Biotechnology**
> - GM foods
> - Probiotics and Prebiotics
> - Food additives
> - High Fructose corn syrups using enzymes
> - Foods using organisms
> - Biopesticides

> **In the present day scenario, biotechnology is used for manufacturing:**
> - Foods consisting of or containing living/viable organisms.
> - Foods derived from or containing ingredients derived from GMOs, e.g., flour, food protein products, or oil from GM soybeans.
> - Foods containing single ingredients or additives produced by GM microorganisms (GMMs), e.g., colors, vitamins, and essential amino acids that can be used as dietary supplements.
> - Foods containing ingredients processed by enzymes produced through GMMs, e.g., high-fructose corn syrup produced from starch, using the enzyme glucose isomerase (product of a GMM).
> - Rapid production and multiplication of cultivars
> - Production of cultivars that are free of viruses and/or pathogenic agents
> - Rapid adaptation and selecting cultivars that can resist specific stress factors like water resistance, high salinity, or acid in soil
> - Makes seed material available throughout the year rather than in particular seasons
> - Makes it possible to produce species that are difficult to reproduce or grow slowly
> - Tissue culture is relatively inexpensive and is very useful in developing countries for improving local varieties. This has been applied to crops such as banana and potato.

Biotechnology holds immense promise for developing new methods and tests for diagnosis, e.g., use of monoclonal antibodies, development of vaccines to prevent viral and bacterial diseases. This holds promise not only for animals but also for humans. In fact, the first commercially produced genetically engineered product was human insulin. In 1982, biotechnology was used to develop human insulin for diabetes treatment. Prior to this development, insulin was obtained from the pancreas of cows and pigs. The synthetic human insulin has several advantages, including fewer insulin antibodies, less insulin allergy, more rapid absorption, earlier peak, and shorter duration time than the animal insulin.

Biotechnology will help to develop new varieties and multiply disease-free seeds and seeds that are better adapted to specific environments. It can be used to identify bacterial strains specifically suitable for a given crop and particular soil and multiply them on large scale. Nitrogen fixing bacteria can be inoculated into soil. This will help to reduce the use of fertilizer and the associated costs.

Use of biological pesticides could help reduce the use of chemicals. Scientists are exploring the possibility of using fungi with insecticidal effects. Yield can be increased by improving the flowering capacity, increasing photosynthesis, or the uptake of nutrients. Increased production may lead to lower prices and would be beneficial. Cloning plants may help to reduce the labor involved in harvesting because the plants have more uniform characteristics, grow at the same speed, and mature at the same time.

Genetically Modified Foods (GM Foods)

Genetically modified foods are "Food and food ingredients composed of or containing genetically modified organisms (GMO) obtained through modern biotechnology." GMOs are the organisms in which the DNA has been altered in a way that does not occur naturally. It may contain a specific genetic trait which is also may not present in the original organism. The technology used for this purpose is also called "recombinant DNA technology" or "genetic engineering." This technology is used to create genetically modified plants that are then used to cultivate GM crops. GM foods can also be obtained by rearranging the genes already present.

Calgene, the founder of biotech foods designed a tomato that may be grown red and transported as such without spoilage. Conventionally, tomatoes were plucked green, ripened red during storage, and suffered huge losses during transport. The tomato developed by Calgene had a gene added in order to prevent the breakdown of cell walls as the fruit ripened. Thus, the tomatoes remained firm even after long periods of transportation and storage. However, this was withdrawn in 1997 because of public concern and special transportation equipment was needed.

> Genetically modified organism (GMO) are those organism whose genome has been modified using recombinant genetic technology in the laboratory to produce precise and desired physiological traits in a biological product.
>
> Usually inclusion of genes are used from unrelated species. These are also referred as transgenes and organism as trans organism.
>
> Recombinant genetic technology involves the insertion of one or more individual genes from an organism of one species into the DNA of another. It is being used now in agriculture, medicine, research, and environmental management.

The first GM crop was raised in America was maize (corn). It was modified by introducing *Bacillus thuringiensis* (Bt) which can kill corn borer and the corn was called "Bt maize." In addition, this crop survived with one round of pesticide application only, while conventional maize needed six. In 1996, Bt cotton was introduced using the same bacterium. Later other GM crops were developed—soybean, potato, rice, and some fruits and vegetables. Rice and maize have shown promising results to raise the nutrition quality of grains.

Genetically modified crops were initially developed to improve crop protection by increasing the resistance to plant diseases caused by insects or viruses or plants that have better tolerance to herbicides. This ultimately helps the farmer to obtain higher yields because the plants do not have to compete for the soil nutrients with weeds.

Resistance to insects is achieved by inserting the gene that codes for a toxin produced by the organism *Bacillus thuringiensis* (Bt). While this toxin acts against insects, it is safe for human consumption. Insertion of a gene from certain selected disease causing viruses gives the plants resistance to those viruses. For herbicide tolerance, genes from certain bacteria give resistance to herbicides. This helps to decrease the amount of weed killers used. Corn and cotton that have the gene from this organism are known as "Bt corn" and "Bt cotton," respectively. Examples of GM crops are pest resistant

crops, delayed ripening tomatoes, virus resistant squash, herbicide tolerant crops, etc.
- Farm animals (such as pigs, cows, and chickens) are genetically modified for faster growth rates, leaner muscle-to-fat ratios, better resistance to disease, or ability to produce higher levels of omega-3s in the meats.
- Plants are modified to yield higher protein or nutrient levels or to produce healthier oils containing "functional food" components such as omega-3 fatty acids.
- Genetically modified cows can produce milk that contains higher levels of bioactive milk proteins or human blood clotting components or a human breast milk component.
- Biochemical compositional variation between buffalo and cow milk has been revealed in favor of buffalo milk being richer source in nutrient, lower cholesterol content and encouraging heart-health in humans; A1 as well as A2 milks are superior over milch species. Sprayed dried colostrum developed from buffalo milk.
- Low acrylamide potatoes that produce less of the amino acid asparagine which is responsible for formation of acrylamide, a carcinogen. Such potatoes resist bruising and browning when cut and also produce relatively healthier french fries.

Genetic modification is a precise and efficient means of achieving benefits of crop improvement. Over the past 10000 years, agricultural methods evolved and farmers used their observations and knowledge to improve crop production. Farmers rely on plant breeding to add desired traits or eliminate an undesired one. Plants having desirable traits are selected for many generations. The corn or wheat available today is very unlike the corn or wheat as they were when humans first started cultivating crops. The problem is that it takes several growing seasons to produce a plant that expresses the desired trait. In this manner, farmers have produced drought-resistant crops, crops resistant to insects and pests, high yielding crops, or crops with stronger stalks that can withstand the strength of strong wind. In this respect, GM has an advantage because scientists first identify the gene that confers the special desired trait in a plant and the trait can be transferred exactly or precisely. GM technology takes less time than the traditional methods adopted by farmers.

Genetically-modified (GM) crops are of two types: agronomic/input and nutritional/output. With agronomic modifications, the aim is to improve plant growth. All GM crops in production so far are of this type. The most common GM food crops are herbicide-resistant soybeans and pest-resistant maize. But with global warming and water scarcity looming large on the horizon, researchers are focusing on drought and salinity-resistant varieties of many crops. In the market, several GM foods are available such as corn having insect resistance and herbicide tolerance, soybean, oilseed, chicory having herbicide tolerance, squash with virus resistance, and potato with insect resistance and herbicide tolerance.

When GM crops reached the European market, there were protests against genetically modified foods in relation to its safety issues. The issue escalated at global level and Codex Alimentarius Codex (CAC) set up the international standards on GM food through FAO and WHO. In India, the regulatory framework was initiated in 1989 in response to research and development of biotechnology being taken up in this country. All matters related to GM foods are under the Ministry of Environment, Forests, and Climate Change. Guidelines for genetically engineered plants were issued in 2008. For regulation, the Ministry has a statutory body—Genetic Engineering Appraisal Committee (GEAC). The Department of Biotechnology under the Ministry of Science and Technology is the nodal department for promoting biotechnology programs. It also provides support for biosafety regulations. The Food Safety and Standards Authority of India is responsible for regulating genetically engineered foods.

There are several debatable risks of GM crops such as environmental hazards. Some groups argue that genetically modified foods may cause unintended harm to other organisms and reduce the effectiveness of pesticides; as insects become resistant to Bt or other crops, there may be production of "superweeds" through cross breeding of herbicide tolerant crops. They also anticipate human health risks in terms of allergenicity by creating a new allergen or cause allergic reactions in unknown individuals or other unknown reactions. There are also economic concerns, i.e., the lengthy and expensive process of bringing GM crops from lab to land and market, plants may be viable for only one season, and farmers would need to buy seeds every year that is expensive. Intellectual property rights are a concern in terms of impact on farmers.

India is actively involved in development and use of GM crops and research and development of GM foods. Bt cotton has helped to increase cotton productivity and India is now a cotton exporting country. Among food crops, research is focused on GM rice, cabbage, mustard, and brinjal. Bt cotton cultivation would indirectly affect food availability by influencing the amount of cotton available for extraction of cotton seed oil. There are many processed foods such as oil used as cooking medium or ready-to-eat snacks such as chips or breakfast cereal made from GM crops such as soybean, corn, cottonseed, tomato, and potato.

Organic Foods

Environmental contamination and pollution have adverse effects on food quality and pose health risks. Thus, pesticides and insectides have help to reduced crop losses caused by insects and pests. With this and use of fertilizers, grain production has increased and helped to meet grain requirements. However the quality and safety of such grains from health point of view has always been a big question in the minds of consumer. People are looking its solution in organic foods. Food from different sources is organic then what is extra in food.

The word 'organic' implies to all that is grown over the earth and preferably living too and contains carbon and nitrogen. The importance of 'organic food' lies in the use of any laboratory developed and chemical or synthetic fertilizer/pesticide/hormones during food production. The crops cultivated using only natural fertilizers is said to be 'organic crop' and the food produced from such crops is called 'organic food. It is the most natural form of food, full of natural constituents providing health benefits. The only difference may be in the nitrate content. Nitrate is a naturally occurring form of nitrogen found in the air, soil, water, and food (particularly in vegetables) and also within the human body. It is formed from fertilizers, decaying plants, manure, and other organic residues. It is also used as a food additive. Usually, it is non-toxic but excessive consumption is a threat to human health.

It may be to reorient the people and market who are concerned with healthy and safe food. People do not use fertilizers in cultivation of organic foods. The people who are poor people or growing kitchen gardens are also growing organic foods by definition. In cities and metropolises, organic foods are available at a considerably higher cost.

Scientific studies have shown that organically grown fruits and vegetables such as red oranges, apple pulp, tomatoes, strawberries, peaches, pears, and corn contained higher amounts of phenolics, anthocyanins, and carotenoids. This higher content of phytochemicals may be beneficial for health. The higher content in organically grown produce has been attributed to possibly greater activation of the plant defense mechanisms without pesticides, an active soil life where plants and microbes interact better care and handling during production of organic foods. There is a balanced mineral nutrient uptake with excess uptake of easily available nutrients like nitrogen, phosphorus, and potassium being avoided. However, there are studies which report that organic foods may not confer advantage in terms of extra amount of nutrients including antioxidants compared to conventionally grown vegetables and fruits that may be treated with insecticides/pesticides.

Reasons for use of chemical substances were to increase the food production for the growing population and to improve the food security. On the other hand, organic fertilizer and pesticide may not sufficiently protect the enough grains from insect pests for prolonged duration. Rising trend of degenerative diseases was linked with the use of chemical fertilizers to some extent. Organic foodstuffs are produced according to specified standards that emphasize the protection of the environment and controlled use of chemicals in crop production and medicines in animal production.

Growing organic food can be healthy for the soil, environment, and humans. Consuming organic food provide satisfaction of eating healthy food and at the same time selling organic food is also getting profitable. In Europe, the food which is cultivated produced and marketed in accordance to legally regulated standards is called organic food. Plant foods need to be produced in natural environment using only natural resources (water and fertilizers) and animal foods need to be obtained without any treatment with hormones or antibiotics.

Safety of organic food is important because these can easily be attacked by insects, pests, and certain microorganisms. Storage of such food under desired temperature and relative humidity is equally important. FSSAI in 2017 has released the logo of Organic food (jaivik bharat) to indicate authentic organic food if printed on packet.

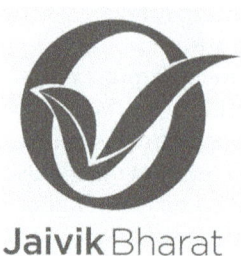

Food Irradiation

Food irradiation is a technology for disinfecting, sterilizing, and preserving food by exposing the it to gamma rays from highly radioactive material such as Cobalt 60 or Cesium 137. It is one of the ways to safeguard food and increase its availability to achieve food and nutrition security. It can be used for a wide variety of food commodities like fruits, potatoes, onions, spices, herbs, and certain ready to eat foods. It is one of the most effective treatments to preserve quality of many foods by destroying the growth of microorganisms and increasing the shelf life of foods. Food irradiation has been found suitable for foods like fruits, potatoes, onions, spices, herbs, and certain ready to eat foods but not for milk and milk products. FSSAI in 2017 has released the logo of Organic food (javik bharat) to indicate authentic organic food if printed on packet.

What is Radiation and Irradiation?

Radiation is the form of intense energy emitted from sources like light, heat, sound, or radioactive substances; it travels through space and penetrates various materials. The nature of radiation energy is defined and measured in terms of wavelength. This energy dislodges the electrons from atoms and molecules and converts into electrically charged particles called ions. The radiation which can produce ions is called ionizing radiation. Ionizing radiation is produced by unstable atoms (in which one electron is missing) and carries excess of energy and/or mass. Radiation can also be non-ionizing as in the case of light, radio, and microwaves.

Radiation: Unstable atoms emit high energy and this emission is referred as radiation and these unstable atoms are said to be radioactive. Atoms that have unstable nuclei emit excess energy or mass in order to reach stability. Radiation is the energy that can be transferred from one entity to other across empty space using radioactive waves namely alpha (α), beta (β), or gamma (γ) rays. Usually, gamma (γ) rays are used in food irradiation, because they are neutral and pure form of energy in contrast to alpha (α) and beta (β). These waves are electromagnetic in nature having shorter wavelength, weak ionizing power, and high penetrative power with high velocity. Most important is that it does not make food or anything in the surroundings radioactive. Gamma radiation is one type of the radiation used for food irradiation.

Irradiation: The process by which any living tissue is exposed to radiation is called irradiation.

Food moves on a conveyor belt through a chamber and receives the desired dose of radiation. Radiation treatment is usually of very short duration (from seconds to a few minutes only). There are three methods of food irradiation, namely, electron beam irradiation, gamma radiation, and X-ray irradiation. Each method is different in terms of time of exposure, penetration power, and safety concerns.

During radiation, electromagnetic waves (energy) strike the electrically charged particles of food called ions and thus it is referred as "ionizing radiation." Energy is absorbed which ionize (s) or excite (s) the biological molecules/food and brings chemical changes in food at molecular level. Water molecule is most affected which instantly influence(s) the water present in the food and alters the food constituents. Radiation also affects the protein molecule, color pigments, and texture of food. Most affected is the DNA of insects, making the food insect free and safe to eat. The impact of irradiation is dose dependent. Higher dose is needed for bacteria because they have less DNA. Radiation delays ripening of fruits and prevents insect infestation in food grains and inhibits sprouting of potatoes, onions, etc.

Functions of Food Irradiation

Food irradiation is also referred to as cold pasteurization or electronic pasteurization. Irradiation uses energy from ionizing radiation while in pasteurization, heat is used; however, both are used to kill pathogenic bacteria in food. It does not significantly increase the temperature or change the physical or sensory characteristics of most foods. It reduces the food losses in various ways, thereby increases the food supply, and significantly contributes to food and nutrition security. Some of them are as follows:

- Great reduction in pathogenic bacteria like *Salmonella*
- Reduction in the food-borne illnesses
- Check on the growth of fungi and certain viruses
- Reduction in insect infestation
- Reduction in food spoilage—leading to increased food supply
- Increased opportunity for trade of food products
- Better quality assurance
- Preserve nutritional quality due to short exposure
- Delay fruit ripening and increase shelf life
- Inhibit sprouting and increase commercial value
- Replace the use of chemicals used to inhibit sprouting
- Replace the use of chemical fumigants for disinfestations in grains, fruits, and vegetables
- To facilitate the shipment and trade as irradiation improve the quality of food by reducing infestation and enhancing shelf life
- Useful for storage in godowns and warehouses
- Color and freshness
- Maintain nutritional quality
- It can be applied to packaged food.

It requires a source of radiant energy and specially constructed containers or compartments to confine the beams, so the personnel will not be exposed. The entire process requires careful handling, tracking, and disposal. An irradiated apple, for example, will still be crisp and juicy. Fresh or frozen meat can be irradiated without cooking. It is an energy-efficient food preservation method that has several advantages over traditional canning. The resulting products are closer to the fresh state in texture, flavor, and color without using additional liquid and there is no loss of natural juices. Food can be irradiated after being packaged or frozen. Effect of irradiation on commonly consumed is shown in Table 14.3.

Dose is of utmost importance which varies from food to food depending on its size of the food or the properties of the food. Dose of radiation is measured in gray (Gy) usually between 0.05 g and 7.0 g. One gray (Gy) dose of radiation is equal to 1 joule of energy absorbed per kg of food material. In radiation processing of foods, the doses are generally measured in kGy (1000 Gy).

Department of Atomic Energy Board of Radiation and Isotope Technology, Mumbai (2014) has suggested different levels of doses for different purposes. Low dose applications (<1 kGy) is used to inhibit sprouting in tubers and bulbs, delay in ripening of fruits and insect disinfestation of cereals, legumes and their products. Medium dose applications (1–10 kGy) is given to increase shelf life improvement of meat, fish, fruits and vegetables, elimination of pathogens in various foods and hygienization of spices (6.0–14.0 kGy). High dose applications (>10 kGy) are recommended for sterilization of packaged food and hospital diets (5.0–25.0 kGy).

Effect of Food Radiation on Food Quality

Effect of radiation depends upon many factors such as dose of irradiation, type of food, and type of packaging, processing technique before and after irradiation, and storage conditions and period. Irradiation does not cause more damage when compared to other methods of food processing. This method is therefore also called a "cold" process because it does not raise the temperature of the food product. Impact of food irradiation on nutritional attributes is shown in Figure 14.7.

Water plays a key role in radiation. Water reacts with various food components and nutrients and forms radiolytic products and water-soluble compounds are affected.

Table 14.3: Foods for irradiation.

Foods for irradiation	Dose (kGy)	Effect of irradiation
Grain, pulses	0.25–1.0	Controls insect infestation
Fruits like bananas, mangos, papayas, guavas, other non-citrus fruits	0.25–0.75	Delays ripening and increase shelf life
Spices (whole and powders)	10.0	Hygienization to reduce microbial load, preserves flavor
Onions, carrots, potatoes, garlic, ginger	0.03–0.15	Inhibits sprouting
Meat, poultry, seafoods	3.0–7.0	Destroys pathogenic organisms, i.e., *Salmonella*, *Campylobacter*, and *Trichinae*
Meat, poultry, seafoods	1.5–3.0	Reduces spoilage organisms and improves shelf life under refrigeration

Source: Udipi and Ghugre (2010) Food Irradiation, Agrotech Publishing Academy, Udaipur. pp 42-43.

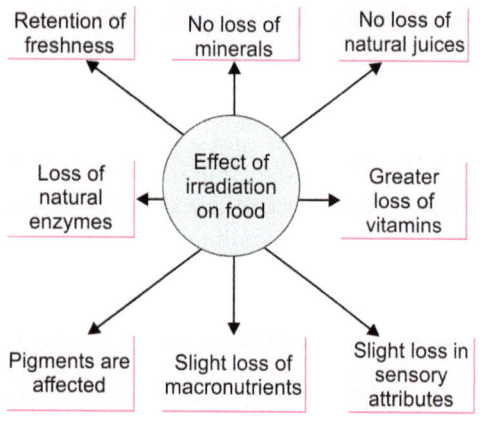

Fig. 14.7: Effects of irradiation on food.

However, the presence of carbohydrates and protein reduces formation of radiolytic products. Therefore, radiation under controlled condition results in negligible losses of macronutrient and vitamin losses are more, although some vitamins are affected. Vitamin B_1, vitamin C, and vitamin A are more sensitive while riboflavin, niacin, and vitamin D are relatively stable. Thiamine in liquid form shows more loss (about 50%) than in dry food (5%). Since dairy products are rich in vitamin A, irradiation is not suited for dairy foods.

Pigments may get affected. Minerals are unaffected. It further depends on storage condition of irradiated food products. Losses are reduced if the food is packaged, sealed and then irradiated. Losses are minimized in frozen foods, and in packaged foods packed in inert nitrogen or if plastic film laminated with aluminum foil is used as packaging material.

Food is irradiated to provide the same benefits as when it is processed by heat, refrigeration, freezing, or treated with chemicals to destroy insects, fungi, or bacteria that cause food to spoil or cause human disease and to make it possible to keep food longer and in better condition in warehouses and homes. Irradiated foods are wholesome and nutritious. All known methods of food processing and even storing food at room temperature for a few hours after harvesting can lower the content of some nutrients, such as vitamins.

Regulations Related to Food Irradiation

It is important to have regulatory bodies at national and international levels. The US FDA has given approval to irradiate certain food products and WHO has also played a role in approving after careful consideration of intensive scientific studies on safety, quality, and health issues. In India, The Department of Atomic Energy (DAE) and The Atomic Energy Regulatory Board (AERB) are regulatory bodies which issue certificates and give approval. The Food and Agriculture Organization (FAO), World Health Organization (WHO), and International Atomic Energy Agency (IAEA) and the Codex Alimentarius Commission have given approval to about 40 food items for food irradiation. Atomic Energy (Radiation Processing of Food and Allied Products) Rules, 2012 look after the aspects related to food irradiation in India. Bhabha Atomic Research Center (BARC) is engaged in research on food irradiation to extend shelf life and to reduce postharvest losses of agriculture commodities. It is also important to put the logo of Rudra symbol with license number to be shown on the packet.

NATIONAL PROGRAMS TO ENSURE FOOD AND NUTRITION SECURITY

The Government of India has numerous programs that are aimed at improving food and nutrition security of its citizens. Some of the important programs with wide coverage are listed herein:

Public Distribution System (PDS): This system evolved as a means to manage food scarcity by distributing food grains at affordable prices, i.e., subsidized rates. Today, it is one of the major food distribution network of the Government of India to avail essential commodities to poor and needy people in the country. It functions through the Department of Food and Public Distribution (DFPD) under Ministry of Consumer Affairs, Food and Public Distribution and operates via Food Corporation of India (FCI). The food grains and other commodities are distributed at Fair price shop or ration shops at subsidized rates. Each household has been provided a ration card. The services of food distribution of PDS are extended under various schemes like Pradhan Mantri Garib Kalyan Yojna and other states' projects during pandemic of COVID-19 in 2020. Also, the State Government is responsible for supervising the functioning of the large and widespread network of the fair shops within each state. In some states, additional items of mass consumption are also distributed through the PDS outlets such as edible oil, iodized salt, and spices to the ration card hold holders.

Besides PDS, Department also allocates grains to midday meal scheme, welfare institutions, and hostels. Additional allocation is made during festivals and natural calamities and other emergency circumstances.

> Public distribution System (PDS) had played a pivotal role in providing food security to considerable proportion of the country's population. To reach poorer sections of society, this programme was redesigned as Targeted Public Distribution System (TPDS) for BPL and APL (below and above poverty line). Since there were several loop holes in the system, Indian Government has undertaken many reforms through National Food Security Act (NFSA, 2013), National Nutrition Strategy (NNS, 2017) and National Nutrition Mission (NNM 2018-2020) and Anemia Mukt Bharat. The main aim of NNM is to reduce undernutrition and low birth weight, stunting, and anemia. These reforms purport to address the inequalities related to age, gender, disability, income as well as to accelerate the pace to achieve SDG2 by 2030.

Targeted Public Distribution System (TPDS): In 1997, TPDS was introduced in order to reach the really needy and for better targeting of such families. TPDS has focused on people in hilly and inaccessible areas, and to target the poor [BPL (below the poverty line)] families to provide food security. Like PDS, TPDS is jointly implemented by the State and Central Governments. States were required to formulate and implement the program for identification of poor for delivery of food grains and its distribution at the Fair Price Shops (FPS) regulated under TDPS Control Order and PDS Control Order rules. Grains are disbursed to BPL families and APL (above poverty line) families.

Antyodya Anna Yojana (AAY): AAY was started with the aim of reducing hunger among the poorest segments of the BPL population. The BPL families are identified and issued Antyodya Ration Card. Beneficiaries in AAY scheme include: (i) landless agricultural laborers, (ii) marginal farmers, (iii) rural artisans/craftsmen such as potters and tanners, (iv) slum dwellers, (v) persons earning their livelihood on a daily basis in the informal sector such as porters, rickshaw pullers, and cobblers, (vi) destitute, and (vii) households headed by widows or terminally ill. They are also entitled to receive 35 kg food grains/month/BPL family. Subsidized rates in AAY (2019) are @ ₹ 3/- for rice and ₹ 2/- for wheat and ₹ 1/- for coarse grains. 5 kg of each foodgrain is provided per month and sugar @ Rs 13.5 per kg to AAY cardholders. The government specifies the rates and the amount to be provided.

Mid Day Meal Scheme (MDMS): Mid Day Meal Scheme is a school meal program of Government of India. It was started in 1995. MDMS is covered by National Food Security Act, 2013. It is meant for the primary and school children between 6 and 11 years studying in government, government-aided, and some local schools. Its aim is to raise the nutritional status of the children. The program also aim to "encourage poor children belonging to disadvantaged children to attend school more regularly, and help them concentrate on classroom activities". Another objective is to "provide nutritional support to children of primary stage in drought-affected areas". The food is meant to serve as a supplement to the children's daily intake and not to substitute home meals/food. In this scheme, each child gets cooked food supplying 300 kcal and 12 grams protein to children enrolled in class one to five for 200 days.

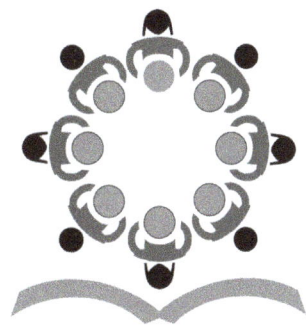

मध्याह्न भोजन योजना
Mid Day Meal Scheme

The nutritional guidelines for the minimum amount of food and calorie content per child per day are given in Table 14.4.

National Food Security Mission: It is a safety net program implemented by the Central Government. The objective is to increase the production of wheat by 8 million tons, rice by 10 million tons, and pulses by 2 million tons so as to ensure food security of the country by the end of the Eleventh Plan (2011–12).

Table 14.4: Entitlement norm per child per day under MDM.

Items	Primary (class one to five)	Secondary (class six to eight)
Calories	450	700
Protein (in gram)	12	20
Rice/wheat (in gram)	100	150
Dal (in gram)	20	30
Vegetables (in gram)	50	75
Oil and fat (in gram)	5	7.5

In case of micronutrients (vitamin A, iron, and folate) tablets and deworming medicines, the students are entitled to receive the amount provided for in the school health program of the National Rural Health Mission.

National Food Security Act (NFSA), 2013: The basic concept of food security globally is to ensure that all people, at all times, should get access to the basic food for an active and healthy life and is characterized by availability, access, utilization, and stability of food. Though the Indian Constitution does not have any explicit provision regarding right to food, the fundamental right to life enshrined in Article 21 of the Constitution may be interpreted to include right to live with human dignity, which may include the right to food and other basic necessities.

Though the issue of food security at the household level was being addressed by the Government from long through the Public Distribution System and the Targeted Public Distribution System, but the enactment of the National Food Security Act (NFSA) 2013 on July 5, 2013 marks a paradigm shift in the approach to food security from welfare to rights based approach. The Act legally entitles up to 75% of the rural population and 50% of the urban population to receive subsidized food grains under Targeted Public Distribution System. About two-thirds of the population therefore is covered under the Act to receive highly subsidized food grains. As a step toward women empowerment, the eldest woman of the household of age 18 years or above is mandated to be the head of the household for the purpose of issuing of ration cards under the Act. The Act is being implemented in all the States/UTs, and on an all India basis.

One of the guiding principles of the Act is its life cycle approach wherein special provisions have been made for pregnant women and lactating mothers and children in the age group of 6 months to 14 years, by entitling them to receive nutritious meal free of cost through a widespread network of Integrated Child Development Services (ICDS) centers, called Anganwadi Centers under ICDS scheme and also through schools under Mid-Day Meal (MDM) scheme. Higher nutritional norms have been prescribed for malnourished children up to 6 years of age. Pregnant women and lactating mothers are further entitled to receive cash maternity benefit of not less than ₹ 6000 to partly compensate for the wage loss during the period of pregnancy and also to supplement nutrition.

In case of non-supply of the entitled quantities of food grains or meals to entitled persons under NFSA, such persons shall be entitled to receive such food security allowance from the concerned State Government to be paid to each person, within such time and manner as may be prescribed by the Central Government. These provisions are governed through Food Security Allowance Rules, 2015.

The National Food Security Act of 2013 provides for reforms. The Direct Benefit Transfer (DBT) Program is viewed as an alternative to the Public Distribution System, "for provisioning of food entitlements". The scheme is linked to Aadhaar and the Government makes payments directly into the Aadhaar linked bank accounts of the beneficiaries/citizens who are below the poverty line. With this money, the beneficiaries can purchase food from the open market. This has been mooted as a means to prevent pilferage, remove malpractices in the existing system, and to bring in transparency. The DBT experiment also "i) reduce the need for huge physical movement of food grains (ii) provide greater autonomy to beneficiaries to choose their consumption basket (iii) enhance dietary diversity (iv) reduce leakages (v) facilitate better targeting. The DBT was started in 2016 in two Union territories, Puducherry and Chandigarh.

Integrated Child Development Services (ICDS): Ministry of Women and Child Development has developed a welfare program for development and protection of children (0-6 years). Integrated Child Development Services (ICDS) scheme is one flagship program of Government of India and it is one of the world's largest and unique programs for early childhood care and development. The ICDS was launched in 1975 with 4981 Anganwadi centers (AWCs) in 33 blocks. Gradually, there were 600,000 AWCs in 5,652 blocks.

It is a symbol of country's commitment toward children and women including adolescent girls, and responds through preschool education on one hand and breaking the cycle of vicious cycles of malnutrition, morbidity, reduced leaning capacity, and mortality on the other. Beneficiaries are children (0-6 years), pregnant women, and lactating mothers.

In 2016-17, the Government restructured and renamed the scheme as umbrella ICDS and included sub-schemes under it. There are several sub-schemes under the Umbrella ICDS besides the core ICDS. These include scheme for adolescent girls (SABLA), child protective services, National Crechè Scheme, National Nutrition Mission, Pradhan Mantri Matru Vandana Yojana and Scheme for welfare of working children in need of care and protection. The Anganwadi services constitute the largest component of services of the Ministry of Women and Child Development.

Objectives of the ICDS scheme are:
- To improve the nutritional and health status of the age group 0–6 years
- To lay the foundation for proper psychological, physical, and social development of the child
- To reduce the incidence of mortality, morbidity, malnutrition, and school dropout
- To achieve effective coordination of policy and implementation among the various departments to promote child development
- To enhance the capability of the mother to look after the normal health and nutritional needs of the child through proper nutrition and health education.

Different services are given in different age groups which are mentioned in Table 14.5.

Activities Key Services of ICDS

Supplementary Nutrition

One of the main component is the supplementary nutrition programme (SNP) wherein hot cooked meals are supplied to preschool children (3-6 years old) and a Take Home Ration (THR) is provided to children aged 6 months to 3 years, adolescent girls as well as pregnant and lactating mothers. SNP is planned and functioning to bridge the gap between recommended dietary allowances (RDA) and average daily intake. It has given 300 days in a year. The type of food varies from state to state. Hot meal cooked at aganwadi center is distributed to the beneficiaries according to the prescribed menu. Food includes preparations with pulses, cereals, oil, vegetables and sugar. Nutritional norms for this supplementary food is given in Table 14.6.

Table 14.5: ICDS services to different beneficiaries.

<3 years	3–6 years	Pregnant women	Lactating mothers	Adolescent girls
Supplementary nutrition	Supplementary nutrition	Supplementary nutrition	Supplementary nutrition	Supplementary nutrition
Health check up	Health check up	Health check up	Health check up	Health and nutrition education
Immunization	Immunization	Immunization	Health and nutrition education	Iron-folic acid (IFA) tablets
Referral services	Referral services	Referral services		
	Non-formal education	Iron-folic acid (IFA) tablets		
		Health and nutrition education		

Table 14.6: Nutrient norms and permissible cost for beneficiaries.

Beneficiaries	Permissible cost (Rs)	Calories	Protein (g)
6 months - 6 years children (severely malnourished)	12.00	800	20–25
6 months - 6 years children (normal)	8.00	500	12–25
Pregnant and lactating women	9.50	600	18–20
Adolescent girls	9.50	600	18–20

1. **Nutrition and health education:** It also uses IEC (information, education and communication) for nutrition and health education in a non-formal way. Intensive innovative media campaign and IEC on key issues such as:
   - Increased rest during pregnancy—especially in the last trimester
   - Appropriate newborn care
   - Promotion of early and exclusive breastfeeding for the first six months of life
   - Initiation of appropriate complementary feeding on completion of six months of age (micronutrient supplementation) along with breast milk
   - Personal hygiene and hand-washing before feeding/after defecation
   - Delayed pregnancies, better birth spacing, and adequate maternal care during pregnancy
   - Prevention of sexually transmitted diseases (STDs) and reproductive tract infections (to prevent low birth weights)
   - Personal hygiene, environmental sanitation
   - Iron-folate supplementation during pregnancy to prevent low birth weights
   - Bi-annual vitamin A supplementation for all children 1–5 years of age
   - Twice-annual de-worming for all (including school children, adolescent girls, and adults).
2. **Health check up:** Growth promotion and counseling (on pre-pregnancy care, early and exclusive breastfeeding, appropriate complementary feeding, and infant and young child nutrition) by AWWs (*weighing scales for all categories, growth charts or cards, IEC materials, etc.*). To strengthen the growth monitoring and promotion component, the project design will pay adequate attention on counseling skills and quality of training of the AWWs; provide AWWs with enough information, skills, and motivation to refer sick children and weak newborns to health facilities; allow enough time in the AWWs schedule to provide the counseling and outreach services. At Primary Health Centre (PHC) staff records the body weight, arrange for immunization and deworming and provide treatment of diarrhea, fever using simple medicines or local remedies.
3. **Referral services:** It implies that sick children and weak newborns to health facilities (*Referral slips/cards, transport vouchers for mothers of sick children, etc.*). Convergence is with the National Rural Health Mission (NRHM). It is provided to the children in the age group of 0–6 years, pregnant, nursing mothers who are at risk. In sickness, they are referred to dispensaries, PHC, general hospital, or nutrition rehabilitation centers.
4. **Immunization:** Six vaccine preventable diseases—poliomyelitis, diphtheria, pertussis, tetanus, tuberculosis and measles are arranged for pregnant women and infants on a selected day. To protect the mother and the children from future illness.

Rajiv Gandhi Scheme for Empowerment of Adolescent Girls: It is also known as "Sabla." Rajiv Gandhi Scheme for Empowerment of Adolescent Girls (RGSEAG)-SABLA introduced in 2011. The objective is to facilitate, educate and empower the girls (11-18 years) to enable them to be self-reliant for self-development, through improved nutrition. Awareness creation about hygiene, good health, sexual and reproduction related issues, is done through formal and non-formal education. It is also for improving the nutritional status and health status.

Kishori Shakti Yojana (KSY): It was proposed by The Ministry of Women and Child Development, Government of India, in the year 2000 and implemented using the infrastructure of ICDS. Under the Nutritional Programme for Adolescent Girls (NPAG) for undernourished adolescent girls (weighing less than 35 kg) and under which 6 kg of free food grain is given to per beneficiary per month.

Annapoorna Scheme: This scheme was initiated in 2002. Under this scheme, 10 kg food grains per month are provided free of cost to the beneficiaries. These beneficiaries are the people who have not been covered under National Old Age Pension Scheme (NOAPS) and they are given "Entitlement card" for issuing the grains.

> **Community Food Banks**
> MS Swaminathan Research Foundation (MSSRF), Chennai, has established a Community Food Security System in 1988. The Community Food bank would be supervised by the society or council chosen by the gram sabha. The Food bank will be managed by the stakeholder council, with different operations assigned to different self-help group. One bank will be set up for every village or cluster of villages with a population ranging from 2000 to 5000. It will be implemented with honesty, political neutrality, and fairness, absence of discrimination based on religion, caste, class, gender, and political belief. It is focused to empower tribal and rural communities for sustainable agricultural and rural development with the use of modern science.

Swarna Jayanti Gram Swarozgar Yojna: It is a merger of several government schemes. It is a kind of self-employment scheme which supports poor self-help groups for training, credit, technology, infrastructure, and marketing. This scheme can indirectly contribute to food security by increasing the purchasing power of households. It strives to provide an environment to encourage urban poor women for self employment.

Sampurna Gramin Rozgar Yojna: Started in 2001, under this scheme, food grains are distributed to the laborers as a part of wages at the BPL rates. National Food for Work Program also works under this yojna, 5 kg food grains are given per man day and in exceptional cases 25 wages is given as cash.

Mahatma Gandhi National Rural Employment Guarantee Program (MGNREGA): This program is an Indian job guarantee scheme which provides a legal guarantee for one hundred days of employment in every financial year to adult members of any rural household willing to do public-work related unskilled manual work at the statutory minimum wages set by the government. It varies in states and hikes with policy changes.

National Rural Health Mission (NRHM): It is run by Ministry of Health with the objective to provide effective healthcare to rural population throughout the country with special focus on 18 states, which have weak public health indicators.

National Urban Health Mission (NUHM): Its objective to extend primary health care services to cities having population above 100,000, particularly to slum dwellers by the senior health professionals using appropriate technology. Provision of health insurance is also made.

Rajiv Gandhi Drinking Water Mission: It promotes a proposed action plan to provide safe drinking water to uncovered habitations.

Total Sanitation Campaign: It covers the improvement in toilet facilities in rural and slum areas. It is well recognized that hygiene has tremendous impact on nutrition. There is also a concept of environmental enteropathy and leaky gut that ultimately increase risk of malnutrition

Rashtriya Krishi Vikas Yojana: It aims to achieve 4% annual growth in agriculture and allied sector in the tenth plan and sponsored by the Central and state government.

National Horticulture Mission: It promotes holistic growth of the horticulture sector covering fruits, vegetables, root and tuber crops, spices, cashew, and cocoa. It is implemented in all states except the North Eastern States, Himachal Pradesh, Jammu and Kashmir, and Uttaranchal for certain reasons.

National Food Security Mission (NFSM) was launched in October 2007. It is regulated by the Ministry of Agriculture and Farmers Welfare and Department of Agriculture, Cooperation, and Farmers Welfare, and operational guidelines are revised from time to time. In 12th plan, the Mission had achieved the targeted and additional production of rice, wheat, and pulses. With overwhelming success, it has been decided to continue the program to 2019–20. Now it will have eight components, viz., (i) NFSM-Rice; (ii) NFSM-Wheat; (iii) NFSM-Pulses; (iv) NFSM-Coarse Cereals (Maize, Barley), (v) NFSM-Sub Mission on Nutri Cereals; (vi) NFSM-Commercial Crops; (vii) NFSM Oilseeds and Oilpalm and (viii) NFSM-Seed Village Program. These Operational Guidelines are for NFSM-Food grains, Commercial Crops, Oilseeds and Oilpalm, Seed Village Program, and Sub Mission on Nutri-cereals.

Rashtriya Poshan Abhiyan or National Nutrition Mission: It is popularly known as Poshan Abhiyan or NNM. It is a PM's overarching scheme for holistic nutrition. It was launched in 2018 and implemented by Ministry of Women and Child Development (MWCD) and along with other ministries. It is also announced to celebrate National Nutrition Month every year in the month of September with a specific theme to work upon to strengthen the nutrition benefits to the people of the country. The key nutrition strategies and interventions are:

- IYCF (Infant and young child feeding)
- Food and nutrition
- Immunization
- Institutional delivery
- WASH (Water, Sanitation, and Hygiene)
- De-worming

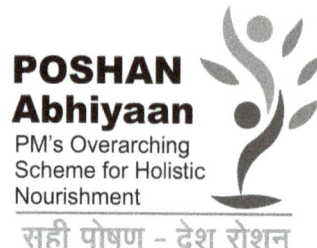

- ORS-Zinc
- Food fortification
- Dietary diversification
- Adolescent nutrition
- Maternal health and nutrition
- ECD (Early childhood development)/ECCE (Early childhood care and education), Convergence
- ICT-RTM (Information and communication technology enabled real-time monitoring)
- Capacity building.

These services and interventions will be monitored by Swasth Bharat Preraks deployed across the country. Under Poshan Abhiyan National Council on Nutrition (NCN) was set which was headed by vice-chair person of NITI (National Institution for Transforming India) Aayog. This is to provide policy direction to address the nutrition challenges in the country and review the programs.

RAPID FIRE

1. Define food security?
2. What are the components of food security?
3. What do you mean by nutrition security?
4. Name nutrients which are used for food fortification.
5. What do you mean by vehicle and name some?
6. Why fortification is a popular to increase nutrition value of food?
7. What is the difference between organic food and GM food?
8. What the national programs which can combat nutritional deficiencies?
9. Suggest two objectives of National Nutrition Mission.
10. How much energy and protein is recommended for target group from ICDS?
11. What is the current status of PDS in your area?
12. What is Anemia Mukta Bharat?
13. How can you contribute to improve nutrition security in your family?
14. Name one to two ministries which are functioning to improve nutritional status of the country.
15. What do you understand by Anganwadi?

EXERCISE

1. Discuss the technologies which can support the food and nutrition security of our country.
2. Find out the fortified food items available in your area and write about its health benefits.
3. Make a ppt role of food irradiation and biotechnological techniques in improving the nutrition security?

4. Visit any Anganwadi and find out the ICDS services being given to whom? What are challenges faced by the centers and what are benefits received by the beneficiaries.

SUGGESTED READING

1. Agarwal A, Alphonso R. Pulses towards nutrition security in India. Res Reach J Home Sci. 2017;16(1):1-10.
2. A Position Paper Indian National Science Academy, Science for Equity Empowerment and Development (SEED) Division, Department of Science and Technology (DST) Symposium on 'Nutrition Security for India–Issues and Way Forward' on August 3–4, 2009 and subsequent discussion with the experts.
3. Balani S. Functioning of the Public Distribution System. An Analytical Report. 2013.
4. Capuano V. Food fortification in India: An overview of how attitudes to food fortification are changing and how they are impacting the legislative landscape, A Leatherhead Food Research white paper 51. 2017.
5. Desjardins E. Nutritional Value of Organic Food: What do we know? Growing up "Organic Conference" Toronto; 2007.
6. FAO, IFAD, UNICEF, WFP, WHO. The State of Food Security and Nutrition in the World 2020. Transforming food systems for affordable healthy diets. Rome, 2020. FAO.https://doi.org/10.40⁶0/ca9692en
7. FAO. PART III: Fortificants: physical characteristics, selection and use with specific food vehicles; 2003.
8. FAO. Technical Consultation of Food Fortification Technogy and quality control, Rome, Italy; 1995.
9. FAO/IFAD/WFP. The State of Food Insecurity in the World 2015- Meeting the 2015 international hunger targets: taking stock of uneven progress, Rome, FAO. 2015.
10. FAO/WHO. Symposium on Nutrition Security for India, Issues and Way Forward- Nutrition Strategies. 3-4, August, 2009, Indian National Science Academy, Rome.
11. FAO 2009: World Food Summit on Food Security. Rome, 16–18 November 2009. Declaration of the World Summit on Food Security. [online] Available from http://www.fda.gov/Food/DietarySupplements/ucm109764.htm. [Last Accessed August, 2019].
12. Fedoroff NV, Battisti DS, Beachy RN, et al. Radically rethinking agriculture for the 21st century. Science. 2010;327(5967):833-4.
13. Food and Agriculture Organization of the United Nations Rome. The state of food security and nutrition in the world building resilience for peace and food security. 2017.
14. Food and Nutrition, Security Analysis, Ministry of Statistics and Programme Implementation and The World Food Programme. India, 2019
15. Food and Nutrition Bulletin. 1998;19(2):100.
16. Government of India NITI Aayog. Evaluation Study on Role of Public Distribution System in Shaping Household and Nutritional Security India. New Delhi: Development Monitoring and Evaluation Office; 2016.
17. Govt. of India. Poshan Abiyan. [online] Available from https://www.india.gov.in/spotlight/poshan-abhiyaan-pms-overarching-scheme-holistic-nourishment. [Last Accessed Auguts, 2019].
18. Hsieh PYH, Ofori JA. Innovations in food technology for health. Asia Pacific J Clin Nutrit. 2007;16(Suppl):65-73.
19. http://www.fao.org/elearning/course/fa/en/pdf/p-01_rg_concept.pdf
20. https://igsss.org/wp-content/uploads/2020/04/Write-up-on-Central-and-state-Govt-Schemes-to-combat-COVID-19-in-India-3.pdf
21. https://www.ilo.org/global/topics/dw4sd/WCMS_568944/lang--en/index.htm.
22. Hubera M, Rembiałkowskab ED, Srednickab S, et al. Organic Food and Impact on Human health: Assessing the status quo and prospects of research NJAS-Wageningen. J Life Sci. 2011;58:103.
23. Hwalla N, Sibelle El Labban and Rachel A. Bahn. Nutrition security is an integral component of food security. Journal Frontiers in Life Science, Focus Issue: Food & Agriculture. 2016;9:3.
24. ICDS. Integrated Child Development Scheme (ICDS), Manual for District Level Functionaries. 2017.
25. ICGFI. Facts about Food Irradiation from International Consultative Group of Food Irradiation, Radiation Processing for Food Preservation and Food Technology, Division of BARC; 1999.
26. Kennert K. Environment, natural resources and food. Achieving food and nutrition security. Actions to meet the global challenge. A Training course reader. In: Went. Internationale Weiterbildung und Entwicklung g GmbH, Capacity Building International, Germany; 2005.
27. Kulshrestha K. Horticultural Crops Value Addition For Nutritional Security. Int J Res–Granthaalayah. 2018;6(10):110-20.
28. Kumar S, Palve A, Joshi C, Srivastava RK, Rukhsar. Crop biofortification for iron (Fe), zinc (Zn) and vitamin A with transgenic approaches. Heliyon. 2019;5(6):e01914.
29. Kunwar R and Sharma V. THE NATIONAL FOOD SECURITY ACT (NFSA) IN INDIA: A REVIEW. Indian Journal of Agriculture, Allied Sciences: A Refereed Research Journal. 2017; 3(4).
30. Micronutrient Initiative. Double fortified salt - feeding the body and the brain. [online] Available from https://www.nutritionintl.org/content/user_files/2014/07/MI-DFS_Brochure-rev3.pdf. [Last Accessed Auguts, 2019].
31. Mishra S, Singh RB. Physiological and Biochemical Significance of Genetically Modified Foods: An Overview. Open Nutraceuticals J. 2013;6:18-26.
32. NITI Aayog – Nourishing India - National nutrition strategy, Government of India. [online] Available from https://niti.gov.in/content/nutrition-strategy-booklet. [Last Accessed Auguts, 2019].
33. Nutritional International. (2019). Governments in India scaling up use of double-fortified salt. [online] Available from https://www.nutritionintl.org/2019/02/governments-in-india-scaling-up-use-of-double-fortified-salt/. [Last Accessed Auguts, 2019].
34. Pant S, Chinwan D. Food fortification and enrichment. Int J Basic Appl Biol. 2014;2(3):166-9.
35. Popkins BM. The dynamics of the Dietary transition in the developing world. In: Caballerao B, Popkins BM (Eds). The Nutrition Transition-Diet and Disease in the Developing World. Amsterdam: Academic Press an Imprint of Elsevier Science; 2002. pp. 111-20.
36. Radhakrishna R, Reddy KV. Food security and nutrition: Vision 2020. [Available from planningcommission.nic.in/reports/genrep/bkpap2020/16_bg2020]. New Delhi: Planning Commission.
37. Rao BS. Food fortification – Principles and applications. In: Bamji MS, Krishnaswamy K, Brahmam GNV (Eds). Text book of Human Nutrition. Oxford: Oxford & Ibh Publishing Co. Pvt Ltd.; 2009.
38. Ritu G, Gupta A. Fortification of Foods with Vitamin D in India. Nutrients. 2014;6(9):3601-23.
39. Sahu KC, Macwan A, Edwin G. COVID-19 Pandemic: Relief Packages Announced by Government: A Brief Summary. April, 2020.
40. Sikka P, Sethi RK. Milk derivatives and their biological activities. Pashudhan. 2006;32(9):1–4.
41. Swaminathan MS. Mission 2007: A nutrition Secure India, Paper presentation at Silver Jubilee Symposium (Nov 2004) Towards National Nutrition Security. 2004.
42. Udipi SA, Ghugre P. Food Irradiation. Agrotech Publishing Academy. 2010.

43. United Nations. Report of the World Food Conference, Rome 5-16 November 1974. New York; 1975.
44. United Nations Standing Committee on Nutrition. Climate change and nutrition security. Message to UNFCCC negotiators. 2010.
45. United Nations System Standing Committee on Nutrition. UNSSCN Nutrition: Nutrition in a Digital World. 2020, Issue 45.
46. US Food and Drug Administration. Center for Food Safety and Applied Nutrition. Overview of Dietary Supplements. 2001.
47. Verma C, Nanda S, Singh RK, et al. A review on impacts of genetically modified food on human health. Open Nutraceuticals J. 2011;4:3-11.
48. Warner K. Chemistry of frying oils. In: Akoh CC, Min DB (Eds). Food Lipids – Chemistry, Nutrition and Biotechnology, 3rd edition. London: CRC Press/Taylor & Francis Group; 2008. pp. 189-200.
49. Weiss J, Takhistov P, McClements, DJ. Functional Materials in Food Nanotechnology. J Food Sci. 2006;71(9):R107-16.
50. Zimmermann MB, Hurrell RF. Improving iron, zinc and vitamin A nutrition through plant biotechnology. Curr Opin Biotechnol. 2002;13:142-5.

15

CHAPTER

New Horizons in Nutrition

KEY CONCERNS
- What are functional foods, probiotics, and dietary supplements?
- How do nutritional requirements for sports people differ from normal persons?
- How are dietary requirements fulfilled for astronauts and for persons living at high altitude?
- What are nutrigenomics and nanotechnology?

KEY CONCEPTS
- Functional foods
- Prebiotics and probiotics
- Dietary supplements
- Sports nutrition
- Nutrition in space travel and high altitude
- Nutrigenomics
- Nanotechnology.

INTRODUCTION

Food is one of the most precious commodities that man has. It has conferred power on those who have certain commodities and puts those who do not at tremendous disadvantage. With the help of science and technology, man has come a long way starting with food production, storage, processing, and how it is served to different people to suit their requirements ranging from promoting good health in general, improving performance, and giving the winning edge to sportspersons to those who go on voyages whether to the Himalayas or to the moon. Man has survived newer and harsher environments by making physiological, psychological, and metabolic adaptations. Hence, man's nutrient needs have also changed depending on whether a person is a marathon runner, swimmer, mountaineer or astronaut.

Nutrition has gone beyond the study of nutrients to the study of bioactive compounds/biodynamic principles in foods opening a new area, i.e., functional foods and nutraceuticals, probiotics, and prebiotics. Bioactive compounds are being intensively investigated for their benefits in preventing many degenerative diseases and promoting good health.

In our quest for healthy and long lives and technological comforts, scientists have developed several new approaches, strategies, and technologies. Nanotechnology is one such promising area for use in food safety, nutrition, food processing and medical science. The human genome project has challenged nutritionists to delve into the relationship between nutrition, food, and genomics.

This chapter touches upon new horizons focusing on nutritional needs of different people working for highly specific goals. Causes and effects of environments and means to adjust in specific environments through food have been discussed.

FUNCTIONAL FOODS

Scientific evidence in the 21st century has given ample support to the age-old statement *"Let food be thy medicine and medicine be thy food"* professed by Hippocrates, as early as 400 BC. Even before Hippocrates, ancient systems of medicine, i.e., Ayurveda, Siddha, Unani in India; Chinese, Egyptian, and several others had been using special foods including herbs, spices, nuts, grains, etc. for promoting health as well as the treatment of various ailments in varying doses and forms.

Practically, all foods are functional as they provide taste, satiety, and nutritive value. However, some foods provide additional health benefits beyond the normal nutritional advantages and such foods are categorized as **functional foods**. In media and marketing ventures, functional foods are often advertised as "superfoods".

Conventional foods	Functional foods
• Taste • Satiety • Nutrition	• Taste • Satiety • Nutrition • Health benefits

Functional foods include whole foods, fortified, enriched foods that have a potentially beneficial effect when consumed in sufficient amounts, confer health benefits. For examples, milk, turmeric, fenugreek, cloves, chillies, *amla*, garlic, apple, soy, and barley among many others. Functionality of foods is attributed to the presence of bioactive ingredients. Innumerable number of bioactive compounds are present in nature. Some of them are phytochemicals, zoochemicals, botanicals, vitamins and minerals, probiotics, phytosterols, bioactive peptides, n-3 fatty acids, etc. These bioactive compounds differ in their source, chemical structure and food behavior. With advancement in science and technology, many bioactive ingredients can now be synthesized commercially.

The concept of functional foods first emerged in Japan in 1980s and was implemented by the Japanese Ministry of Education, Science and Culture in 1984 for addressing the health problems of the aging population. This concept was hailed in many parts of the world, possibly because of increasing prevalence of chronic, noncommunicable diseases, and the high cost of medical care and hospitalization. In different regions of the world, various concepts and terms were advocated. Other terms used are "pharma foods", "health foods", "vita foods", or "designer foods or novel foods". Different countries have conceptualized functional foods in various ways and used different terminologies.

NUTRACEUTICALS

The term "nutraceutical" was coined by Stephen DeFelice in 1989 and is derived from "nutrition" and "pharmaceutics". The term nutraceutical is derived from "nutrition" and "pharmaceutics." The term includes herbal products, dietary supplements (nutrients), and pharmaceutical preparations to aid nutritional as well as medicinal effects on the body.

In the US, "nutraceutical" products are regulated as drugs, food ingredients, and dietary supplements. According to European Nutraceutical Association (ENA, 2016), 'Nutritional products that provide health and medical benefits, including the prevention and treatment of disease'. United Nations Food and Agricultural Organization (FAO) and the World Health Organization (WHO) in the Codex Alimentarius (FAO/WHO 1992) set the guidelines that support production and marketing of foodstuffs and their derivatives. Many countries use these guidelines, which define health claims in terms of—(i) nutrient function; (ii) enhanced health benefits and (iii) reduction of health risks.

In India, the FSSAI regulates health supplements and nutraceuticals through the Food and Safety Standards Act, 2006 and the regulations framed thereunder. India has notified the Food Safety and Standards (health supplements, nutraceuticals, food for special dietary use, food for special medical purpose, functional food, and novel food) Regulations, 2016 in the Gazette of India on 23rd December, 2016. They are scrutinized from time-to-time for various aspects.

Nutraceuticals are specifically designed to provide functional and health benefits from ingredients and technologies, not limited to nutrients alone. They can be presented to consumers as granules, tablets, capsules, liquids, gels, etc., they generally have defined usage levels, and their taste and sensory properties are not highly relevant. Consumers would need guidance for usage from health professionals. In general, nutraceuticals are active molecules derived from plant or animal sources with specific health benefits.

From Conventional to Functional Food

Different amounts of bioactive compounds are effective in different situations and sometimes too much of a bioactive compound in a food can be toxic. Hence, the level of consumable amount must be tested for safety.

Conventional food	Functional food	Nutraceuticals
Food we eat daily basis, e.g. rice, wheat, pulses, fruits, vegetables, etc. These foods provide nutritional benefits for normal body functioning	Food or food ingredients containing bioactive compounds in efficacious dose provide health benefits, e.g. oats, ragi, apple, pomegranate, ginger, garlic, turmeric, saffron, clove, cinnamon, herbs and spices, walnuts, flaxseeds, egg, and meat	Nutritive or bioactive compound(s) found in food, manufactured in the form of pills, powders, syrups, capsules, tablets, etc. For example, curcumin, piperine, omega-3 fatty acid, folic acid, CoQ10, DHA, betaine, glucosamine, alpha-lipoic acid, zinc, calcium, etc.

Japan: In 1991, the Japanese Ministry of Health and Welfare laid down a policy for food manufacturers to label specific foods that were claimed to have health benefit(s), with the term "Food for Specific Health Use" or FOSHU. Japan does not use the term nutraceutical or functional food but uses FOSHU (food for specific health use) even today. For a food to be labeled as FOSHU, it should fulfill the following criteria:
- It should be a food, not capsules, pills/powder containing naturally occurring food components.
- They should be consumed as part of the normal daily diet.
- They should have a defined function in the human body such as:
  - Improving immune function(s)
  - Preventing specific disease(s)
  - Supporting recovery from specific disease
  - Controlling physical and psychic complaints
  - Slowing down the aging process.

China: China uses the term "health foods", i.e., "foods with specific health functions that are suitable for consumption by specific groups of people and that have the effect of regulating human body functions without treating diseases".

Canada: Both terms, functional foods and nutraceuticals are used. Functional food is similar in appearance to conventional foods and consumed as a part of a usual diet and has been demonstrated to have physiological benefits and/or reduce the risk of chronic disease beyond its basic nutritional function, e.g., oats, wheat (insoluble/soluble fiber), modified oil (high oleic acid, low saturated fats), soya, buckwheat, flaxseed, lentil, chickpea, peas, and beans, the effects being attributable to the constituent bioactive principle. Nutraceuticals are products isolated or purified from foods that are generally sold in medicinal form, such as powders, pills, and capsules. A nutraceutical is demonstrated to have a physiological benefit or provides protection against chronic disease.

USA: US regulations 'focuses on safety aspects and acknowledges the term nutraceutical and applies a different set of regulations to them than those of conventional foods and drugs. As per the Dietary Supplement Health and Education Act established in 1994 (DSHEA), it is the manufacturer's responsibility to ensure that a nutraceutical is safe before it is marketed'.

Research glimpse: Authors from the Functional Food Center, USA have discussed and introduced various definitions and discourses about functional foods around the globe. They have also introduced a new definition of "functional foods" developed in a panel discussion in an International Conference in 2014, which was jointly organized by USDA and ARS, i.e., *"natural or processed foods that contains known or unknown biologically-active compounds, which, in defined, effective nontoxic amounts, provide a clinically proven and documented health benefit for the prevention, management, or treatment of chronic disease"*. They have tried to explain the use of each word for marketing these foods.

Martirosyan DM, Singh J. A new definition of functional food by FFC: What makes a new definition unique? Funct Foods Health Dis. 2015;5(6):209-23.

Europe: Instead of the term "nutraceutical", the term "food supplement" is used. The European Commission has defined functional food as "a food that can be regarded as functional if it is satisfactorily demonstrated to affect beneficially one or more target functions in the body, beyond adequate nutritional effect, in a way that is relevant, either an improved state of health and well-being and/or reduction of risk of disease. Functional foods must remain foods and must demonstrate their effects in amounts that can normally be expected to be consumed in the diet; they are not pills or capsules, but part of a normal food pattern". A functional food can be a natural food to which a component has been added or its components have been modified or bioavailability of nutrient modified.

India: In India, several terms like functional foods or nutraceuticals are used for foods that have special dietary uses. Functional food is defined by the Food Safety and Standards Authority of India (FSSAI, 2006) as "processed food which is similar in appearance to conventional food and consumed as a part of normal diet and is demonstrated to have normal physiological benefits beyond basic nutritional functions". Functional foods contain bioactive compounds which may provide health benefits and may reduce the risk of chronic diseases. Functional food should have the sensory properties, i.e., taste, flavor, etc. of normal foods.

Conventional foods can be made into functional foods using one or more of the following approaches (Table 15.1):
- Addition of the bioactive principle to a food
- Replacement of a component that can adversely affect health if it is in excess
- Elimination of a component that can have negative effect(s) on health.

At household level, a food preparation which is made from several selected foods containing active ingredients can become functional. Simple addition of fruits and vegetables, nuts, herbs, and spices in adequate amounts will provide sufficient health benefits beyond normal nutrition. However, bioefficacy of functional foods depends upon some factors shown in the box. These factors influence the type and/or amount of bioactive compound(s).

Factors affecting bioefficacy of functional foods:
- Plant variety
- Stage of maturity at the time of harvest
- Environmental factors
- Processing methods
- Storage conditions

Role of Functional Foods

Functional foods have beneficial effects through one or more of the following properties/effects:
- Possess high antioxidant capacity
- Act as anti-inflammatory agents
- Possess antibacterial and/or antiviral activity
- Help in regulation of basal metabolism
- Slow down aging process
- Improve immune functions

Table 15.1: Approaches to convert conventional foods into functional foods.

Addition	Replacing	Elimination
Phytochemicals	Component which if in excess can be harmful, e.g., gum arabic	Deleterious component inherently present and may cause allergic reaction, e.g., trypsin inhibitor from soybean
Bioactive compounds and peptides	–	–
Dietary fiber	–	–
ω-3 PUFA	–	–
Probiotics	–	–
Household level		
Grains like oats, ragi	Gluten with gluten-free cereals like rice	Reduction of phytates by soaking and fermentation
Legumes like soy	Dehusked pulses with whole pulses	Oxalates with germination and fermenting
Vegetables like green leafy vegetables	Potatoes with sweet potato Fried vegetables with steamed vegetables	Bland taste with seasoning
Fruits—apple, plum, papaya, pomegranate, pineapple, kiwi, and watermelon	Apple with guava Lemon with amla	Peel to remove skin and make softer to eat Cook/preserve/stew some to change taste
Spices like turmeric, black pepper, cinnamon, bay leaves, clove, and cardamom	Cinnamon with fennel	Chillies to reduce pungency
Herbs like mint, rosemary, basil, etc.	Mint with coriander, curry leaves	Reduce quantity as they are very dense in bioactive compounds

- Increase bioavailability of nutrients
- Speed-up the recovery from any disease
- Regulate intestinal transit
- Prevent occurrence of some specific diseases like CVD by having hypolipidemic, hypoglycemic, and hypotensive effects
- Have estrogenic effects
- Promote growth of favorable gut flora and improve gut health
- Have antimutagenic or anticarcinogenic effect.

Bioactive Compounds

Numerous bioactive compounds confer health benefits and many of these have been included in a variety of natural or manufactured products to offer consumers functional foods and nutraceuticals. Some of the major groups of bioactive compounds are shown in Figure 15.1.

Phytochemicals

Phytochemicals are chemical compounds inherently present in plant kingdom. They are mostly secondary metabolites, synthesized by the plants as chemical defense against pathogens and predators. The kind and amount of different phytochemicals are influenced by the plant genetics, cultivar, soil composition and growing conditions, maturity state, and postharvest conditions.

They are abundantly found in nature, notably in fruits and vegetables, cereal grains, leaves, fruits, seeds, herbs and spices and some man-made drinks. They are high molecular weight polymers each having distinct chemical structure, having diverse properties. They impart color, eye appeal or attraction, taste, aroma, and flavor to the food that they are present in. Bioactive compounds influence certain physiological processes in the body and thereby exert health

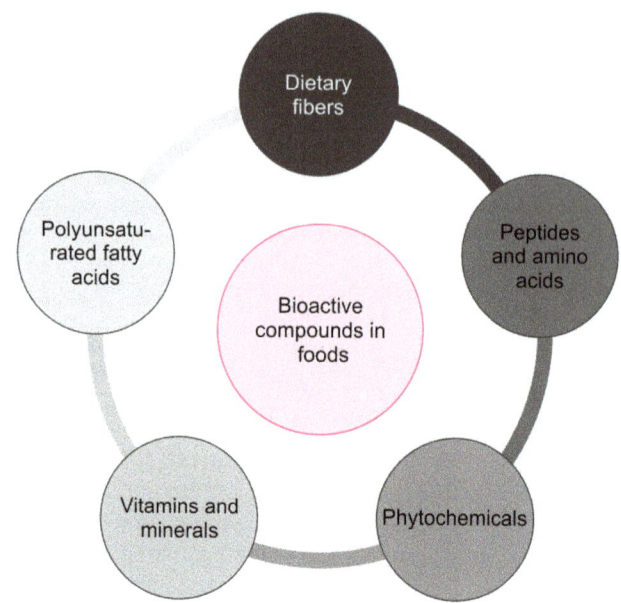

Fig. 15.1: Major groups of bioactive compounds.

benefits. Most of them exhibit high antioxidant capacity or ability to scavenge free radicals thus prevent pathogenesis and/or progression of many chronic diseases like cancer and CVDs and delay aging.

Many phytochemicals were considered to be toxic or antinutrients because they either prevent absorption of certain nutrients or reduced bioaccessibility or bioavailability of certain nutrients. Now there are ample evidence that they have many beneficial effects on health. More than 30,000 phytochemicals have been perhaps identified and about 5–10,000 are present in the foods that are commonly included in the human diet. Classification of phytochemicals are shown in Figure 15.2.

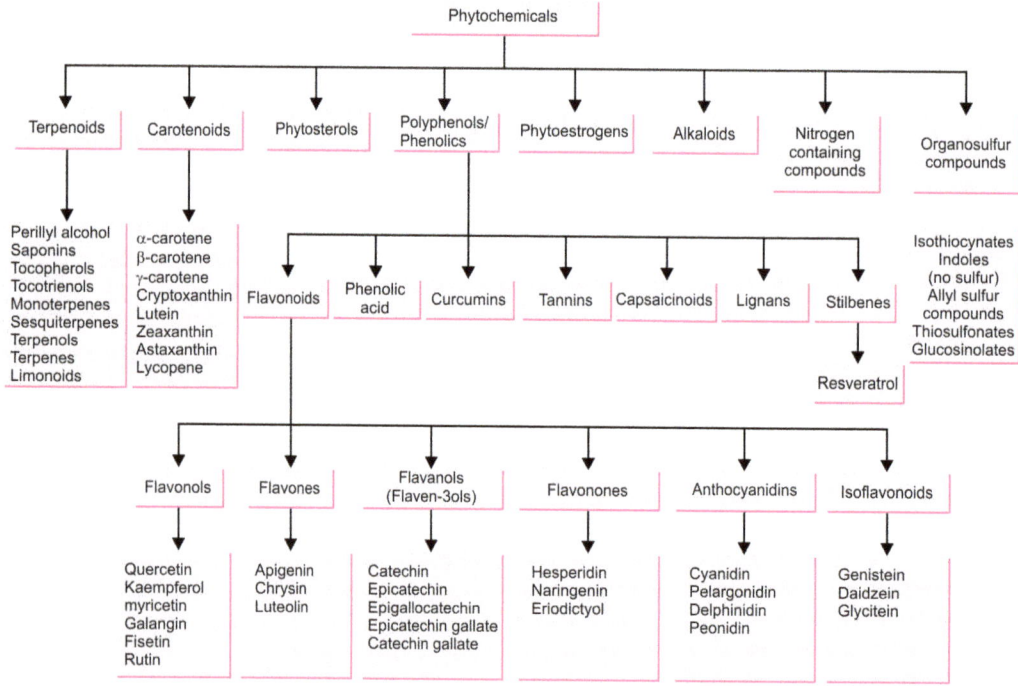

Fig. 15.2: Classification of phytochemicals.

Terpenoids: Terpenoids are diverse organic compounds, in which the primary subunit is isoprene. These compounds are, therefore, also referred to as isoprenoids. Isoprene is a basically a five-carbon, hydrocarbon that can condense with other isoprene molecules to form a wide range of compounds, that have numerous physiological roles in the human body. One example is limonene that imparts typical flavor and fragrance to citrus fruits. It is responsible for the bitterness that is sometimes found in orange juice. Terpenoids are found in a variety of plants and include different compounds such as terpenes, chlorophyll, saponins, tocopherols, tocotrienols, and monoterpenes and sesquiterpenes. Each of these has different chemical structures and biological functions. and shift terpene to limonoids little inside as it is within terpenoids group terpenoids carotenoids, etc. are subheadings of phytochemicals.

Terpenes: Terpenes are compounds of very low molecular weight and are thus are volatile in nature. They are responsible for the aroma, flavor of most essential oils and foods. Many of the terpenes such as monoterpenes, sesquiterpenes. Herbs and spices including their extracts, infusions, tincture and essential oils are rich sources of monoterpenes like limonene, pinene, myrcene, linalool, etc. and each terpene has distinct in its aroma, taste and medical benefits. They have antiseptic properties and also show stimulating and protective effects. Essential oils are potent antioxidants, free radical scavengers, and metal chelators, as well as having antinociceptive, neuroprotective, anticonvulsant, and anti-inflammatory properties. Hence, they are effective in several inflammatory diseases. Essential oils are used by respiratory, olfactory (inhalation), and integumentary systems (skin, hair, and nails). The antioxidant capacity as measured by ORAC (Oxygen Radical Absorbance Capacity) of essential oils is several times higher than raw food. Avoid comparing the ORAC value because weight of raw food consumed is in grams and volume of essential oils is in drops or mL (and that is not consumed internally). Sesquiterpenes have been shown to support cell-to-cell communication in the brain. Perillyl alcohol is found in the essential oils of lavender, lemongrass, sage, and peppermint etc and used in cleaning agents and also in certain medical applications.

Saponins: Saponins are a diverse group of compounds found in legumes like chickpea, soybean, and peanuts as well as in herbs and spices like fenugreek, nutmeg, sage, and thyme. They impart a bitter taste and often affect nutrient absorption. They have been found to reduce cholesterol and have beneficial effects on some cancers. Saponins also have anti-inflammatory, immunomodulatory, and antiallergic properties.

Limonoids: Limonoids are triterpenoids found in citrus fruits and other plants of Cucurbitaceae, Rutaceae, and Meliaceae (neem, mahogany) families. Bitter principle of citrus juice is largely due to the limonoids. Grapefruits and oranges have higher concentration of limonoids than other citrus fruits. They demonstrate significant antioxidant properties and inhibitory action against proliferation of tumor cells.

Carotenoids: Carotenoids are a family of more than 600 fat-soluble compounds. Main sources of carotenoids are yellow-, orange-, and red-colored fruits and vegetables. They are synthesized *de novo* by plants and microorganisms but not by humans, thus they need to be obtained from dietary sources. Some carotenoids like α-carotene, β-carotene, and β-cryptoxanthin show vitamin A activity. Different carotenoids have different biological functions. Carotenoids are also associated with cellular protection, regulation of cell growth, cell differentiation, and apoptosis. Carotenoids can be divided into two groups on the basis of molecular structures, as shown in the Figure 15.3.

Being lipid soluble, accessibility of carotenoids may be limited during food processing and digestion. Food processing has a marked effect on their bioavailability and this difference can be as much as 70% between raw carrot and carrot juice. The relative bioavailability of β-carotene from vegetables compared with purified β-carotene may range 3–6% for green leafy vegetables, 19–34% for carrots, and 22–24% for broccoli. Red, orange, and yellow fruits and vegetables predominantly contain α- and β-carotene and lycopene and green leafy vegetables contain mainly lutein and zeaxanthin. There are many types of carotenoids that are commonly found in food and useful for the body are shown in Figure 15.3 and Table 15.2.

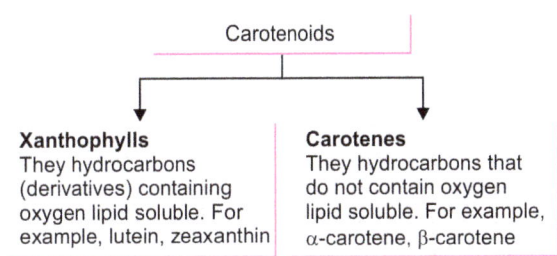

Fig. 15.3: Two groups of carotenoids.

Table 15.2: Different carotenoids—their physiological functions and foods sources.

Carotenoids	Food sources	Physiological effects
Yellow carotenoids Lutein Zeaxanthin	Lutein—spinach and parsley Zeaxanthin—corn, avocado, and egg yolk	Powerful antioxidant for eye—prevent age-related macular degeneration Work in association with LDL and HDL and helps in terminating chain reaction of free radicals
Orange carotenoids α-carotene β-carotene γ-carotene	Carrot Sweet potato Pumpkin Papaya Mango Apricot	↓ LDL-C LDL-C oxidation ↑ Antioxidant effect Better skin protection against UV light
Red carotenoids Lycopene (plant tissue) Astaxanthin (skin of seafoods)	Tomato Watermelon Grapefruit Pink guava Color of the skin coat of crab, salmon, and shrimp	Reduces damage to DNA and proteins Strong antioxidant against singlet oxygen (similar to vitamin E)

Carotenes: Variety of carotenes such as α-carotene, β-carotene and α- and β-cryptoxanthin, lutein, luteolin, and lycopene are carotenoids found in citrus species (grapefruit, oranges, lemon, tangerine, and mandarin). Some carotenoids like α-carotene, β-carotene, and β-cryptoxanthin show vitamin A activity, although the most biologically active is β-carotene. Carotenes, particularly β-carotene, provide photoprotection from bright sunlight to the eyes. They can reduce LDL cholesterol levels and are powerful antioxidants which reduce damage to DNA and proteins. They stimulate expression of genes directly involved in regulation of cell communication processes and may have antitumor activity. They are best absorbed when consumed with some fat.

Lutein and zeaxanthin are naturally occurring yellow pigments. They are xanthophylls belonging to the carotenoid family. Structurally, both are similar. They are found in higher concentrations in the macula of the eye and play a significant role in prevention of macular degeneration, glaucoma, and cataracts which are usually age-related eye diseases. Lutein and zeaxanthin protect the eye by filtration of harmful light (blue light filters). They act as antioxidants and provide protection from oxidative stress caused by cigarette smoke and sunlight. They are also associated with a decreased risk of cartilage defects. They are commonly found in foods such as egg yolk, yellow bell pepper, and pumpkin, yellow color underneath the chlorophyll in green leafy vegetables like spinach, peas, and broccoli.

Lycopene: Lycopene has become popular in recent years as a potent free radical quencher. Its antioxidant activity against singlet oxygen is 47 and 100 times greater than that of β-carotene and vitamin E, respectively. Lycopene is also a potent neuroprotective, antiproliferative, anticancer, and anti-inflammatory, a cognition enhancer and hypocholesterolemic agent. Lycopene is tightly bound to macromolecules within the food matrix, so that its bioavailability from food is relatively poor. However, cooking or processing lycopene-rich foods like tomatoes can liberate lycopene from complexes and enhance its bioavailability. Since lycopene is highly lipophilic, consumption with lipids increase its bioavailability. The red color of tomato has been ascribed to lycopene. Tomato is one of the best sources; lycopene content of tomato varies between 0.9–4.2 mg/100 g depending upon the variety. Tomato sauce and ketchup are concentrated sources of lycopene (33–68 mg/100 g) compared to unprocessed tomatoes. Tomato paste has more lycopene than fresh tomato. It is also present in apricots, guavas, watermelons, papayas, pink grapefruit, and rosehips.

Polyphenols: They are the largest family of phytochemicals, widely distributed in the plant kingdom. The different types of phenolic compounds are shown in Figure 15.2.

They are generally found in fruits and vegetables. They are abundantly available in the human diet and have been linked to many health benefits. Due to their presence, fruits and vegetables are highly valued for health promotion and health protection. They are potent antioxidants, complementing the antioxidant activity of vitamins and enzymes and provide defense mechanisms against oxidative stress and lipid peroxidation caused by reactive oxygen species (ROS). Polyphenols do not act individually and may regenerate antioxidant vitamins. Also, they may induce antioxidant enzymes such as glutathione peroxidase, catalase, and superoxide dismutase. These enzymes are important for defense against ROS such as hydroperoxides, hydrogen peroxide, and superoxide anions. Other beneficial effects include protection against CVD, diabetes, cancer, etc. Polyphenols have the potential to inhibit key enzymes that are responsible for the digestion of dietary carbohydrates (α-amylase and α-glucosidase) and thus modify the postprandial glycemic response.

Polyphenols are a collective term for several subgroups of phenolic compounds. They have been found to exert tremendous health benefits to human beings. Polyphenols differ in their chemical structures and physicochemical properties that significantly affect their stability, bioavailability, and physiological functions related to human health. Their availability varies greatly with the type of compound, type of food and part(s) of the plant as well as the type of food processing. Polyphenols are classified as nonflavonoids and flavonoids based on source of origin, biological function, and chemical structure. Functionality of the compound depends not only on the chemical structure of the compound but also its interaction with other compounds, environmental exposure, cooking, and processing methods and storage. This is because they are easily oxidized when exposed to heat, light, and oxygen. Amount of phenolic compounds is also influenced by the sanitizing methods such as the use of sodium hypochlorite and ozonization and sanitation time.

Phenolic Acids: Phenolic acids are nonflavonoid polyphenols consisting of two main groups: hydroxybenzoic acid and hydrocinnamic acid. Important derivatives of hydroxybenzoic acids are gallic acid and ellagic acid which are found in raspberries, cranberries, pomegranates, and in some nuts. Other phenolic acids include benzoic acid, cinnamic acid, hydroxycinnamic acid, coumaric acid, and ferulic acid. Derivatives of hydrocinnamic acid are caffeic acid, quinic acid, and together form chlorogenic acid that is high in coffee beans; foods like pineapple, cinnamon, apple, maize, peanuts, wheat, rye, barley, and oats.

Coumarin has vanilla-like flavor and is found in plants like cinnamon, cherries, strawberries, licorice, etc. It has blood-thinning, fungicidal, and antitumor activities. Coumarin can be toxic when used at high doses for a long period and should not be taken with anticoagulants. Phenolic acids can occur in free and bound forms. Generally, fruits and vegetables contain free phenolic acids whereas bran or hull of grains and seeds contain bound form. Bound phenolic acids need to be released by subjecting them to hydrolysis by acid/alkali/enzymes. Possible health effects include reducing DNA damage and decreased risk of colon and esophageal cancer by food sources such as berries, peanuts, and wheat. Several phenolic acids containing foods have antioxidant, antimicrobial, anti-inflammatory, antithrombosis, and anticancer activities.

Flavonoids: Flavonoids comprise more than 5,000 individual compounds. Many of them are present in the form of glycosides, i.e., bound to a sugar moiety. The structure and the presence or absence of the sugar influences the biological activities of different flavonoids. They are nonnutritive compounds of plants and belong to a subclass of polyphenols. Flavonoids are well-known for scavenging free radicals, i.e., high antioxidant capacity, thus acting as antioxidants and play anti-inflammatory role. They can also modulate the cell signaling and gene expression. Figure 15.2 gives the classification based on their chemical nature.

Though flavonoids are widely distributed in the plant kingdom, their bioavailability is a great concern. Consuming one to two extra servings every day may significantly reduce the risk of diseases. However, proper combination of foods tends to improve the absorption in the body, e.g., naringenin from oranges is better absorbed with cooked tomato paste and grapefruit juice. Excessive consumption of flavonoids needs to be avoided in pregnancy.

Flavonols are found in fruits, vegetables, and tea while isoflavonols are present in leguminous plants such as soy. One of the flavonols, quercetin is a very potent antioxidant and has anti-inflammatory property. It is found to increase energy expenditure (thermogenesis) and fat oxidation and reduces circulatory inflammatory markers and is helpful in relieving allergy symptoms. It is abundantly present in apple skin, red onions, buckwheat, red grapes, and green tea. Other efficacious flavonols are rutin, hesperidin, and naringin which are slightly bitter in taste and are mainly found in peels of citrus fruits. Rutin is found in asparagus, buckwheat (seeds and flower), amaranth leaves, figs, grapes, and citrus fruits that are helpful in strengthening the capillary wall. Quercetin and rutin protect the body from radiation-induced free radicals. Rutin possesses antimicrobial, antifungal, and antiallergic properties, and is used in many pharmacological formulations for diabetes, hypertension, and neurodegenerative diseases associated with oxidative stress and cognitive deficits.

Hesperidin is present in oranges and other citrus fruits, helps to regenerate vitamin C, and slows proliferation of cancer cells and replication of some viruses. Naringin is present in grapefruit and gives its characteristic bitter taste. It has a role in controlling LDL cholesterol and protects against alcohol-induced stomach ulcers as well as protects against radiation-induced DNA damage. A food may contain more than one type of flavonoid compound and exerts multiple health benefits that are summarized in Table 15.3.

Table 15.3: Different flavonoids and their food sources and physiological effects.

Flavonoids	Food sources	Physiological effects
Flavonols	Licorice roots, dill weed, onion, berries, ginger, tea, fennel leaves, kale, okra, pepper, parsley, saffron, radish, broccoli, chia seeds, olives, and buckwheat	↑ Antioxidant effect ↑ HDL ↓ TC and LDL-C oxidation ↓ Platelet aggregation
Quercetin	Onion, apple skin, grapes, berries, cherries, broccoli, and citrus fruits	↓ Inflammation ↓ Oxidative stress ↓ Metabolic disorders
Kaempferol	Tea, broccoli, apples, strawberries, and beans	↓ Cancer cell growth Cardioprotective and neuroprotective
Rutin	Buckwheat, apples, onions, citrus fruits, figs and green tea	↓ Neuroinflammation Blocks inflammatory enzymes and useful in Alzheimer disease (AD) and arthritis
Flavones	Oranges, sorghum, oregano, peppermint, celery, saffron, celery seed, and pepper	Protection against UV radiation Antihistaminic Antispasmodic Helps in delivering oxygen
Apigenin	Parsley, onions, oranges, beer, chamomile tea, and wheat sprouts	Antispasmodic Prevents malignancies
Luteolin	Thyme fresh, celery, green peppers, and chamomile tea	Anti-inflammatory, cardioprotective
Flavonols (Flavan-3-ols)	Apple skin, banana, red wine, tea (black, green, white), black grapes, peaches, plums, broad bean, and pecan nut	↓ TC and LDL-C oxidation ↓ Platelet aggregation ↓ BP ↑ Insulin sensitivity ↑ Flow-mediated dilatation
Catechin	Green tea, apple, dark chocolates, blue berries, red wine, cherries, and guava	Inflammatory bowel disease (IBD) Activates glutathione peroxidases (GPOs) and glutathione (GSH)
Epicatechin	Tea, apple, and cocoa	↓ Risk of cancer, diabetes, osteoporosis, and cardiovascular and neurodegenerative diseases
Epicatechin-3-gallate	Tea (green, black, white, and oolong), raw strawberry	Anti-inflammatory, anticancer, anticollagenase, and antifibrosis effects
Flavanones	Orange, grapefruit, lemon, and mint	Anti-inflammatory, antiallergenic

Contd...

Contd...

Flavonoids	Food sources	Physiological effects
Hesperidin	Oranges, lime, grapefruit, and peppermint	↑ Microvascular endothelial function—reduces diastolic blood pressure ↑ Production of nitric oxide
Naringenin	Grapefruit, lime, mandarin, and tangerine	↓ Intestinal disorders including IBD ↓ Intestinal inflammation
Eriodictyol	Lemon, peppermint, oregano, and thyme	↓ Lipid peroxidation Anti-inflammatory
Anthocyanidins	Berries, currants, grapes, cherries, plum, red cabbage, eggplant, red onion, raddish, pistachio nuts, black and red beans, and sweet potato	Improve visual and neurological health
Anthocyanins	Red-purple color flowers, berries, blackcurrant, and purple-colored fruits and vegetables	Antidiabetic, anticancer, anti-inflammatory, antimicrobial, and antiobesity effects ↓ Cardiovascular diseases (CVDs)
Pelargonidin	Berries, pomegranate, and plum	Improves immune functions and endothelial functions Anti-inflammatory
Isoflavonoids Genistein, and glycitein	Soya bean and soy products Present in small amounts in other pulses	↑ Cognition ↓ Risk reduction of certain cancers, cardiovascular and skin diseases, osteoporosis and obesity, as well as menopausal symptoms
Phenolic acids	Wine, coffee, potatoes, olives, citrus, and grains	↓ Hypertension Role in growth, reproduction, and defense against environmental stress and microorganisms
Gallic acid	Wine, tea, apple, flaxseed, and corn	Useful in gastrointestinal, neuropsychological, metabolic, and cardiovascular disorders Prevents rancidity in oils and fats
p-coumaric acid	Barley, wheat, corn, and oats	Anticancer, antimicrobial, antivirus, anti-inflammatory, antiplatelet aggregation, anxiolytic, antipyretic, analgesic, and antiarthritis
Ferulic acid	Wheat, brown rice, corn, oats, parsley, and spinach	Protective role in keratinocytes, fibroblasts, collagen, elastin inhibits melanogenesis thus used in cosmetic applications
Hydroxycinnamic acid	Cinnamon	Photoprotective, anti-inflammatory ↓ Hypercholesterolemia and hyperglycemia
Stilbenes	Grapes, peanuts, and berries	Anti-inflammatory Anticancerous
Resveratrol	Grapes, peanuts, and berries	Anti-inflammatory Anticancerous Cardioprotective
Lignans		
Phytoestrogens—lignans	Sesame seeds, flaxseeds	Source of omega-3, cardioprotective, neuroprotective, and good for bones
Sesamin, sesamolin, and sesamol	Sesame seeds, linseed (flaxseeds)	↓ Oxidative stress Chemoprotective
Tannins	Wine, tea, barley, buckwheat, sorghum, cacao, nuts, cinnamon, apples, avocado, apricot, herbal tea, and bitternut	Anticarcinogenic and antimutagenic and antimicrobial

Capsaicinoids: Some polyphenols contain amides. Two groups that have been shown to have significance for human health are capsaicinoids in chillies and avenanthramides in oats. Capsaicinoids such as capsaicin confer the pungency to chillies, and have antioxidant and anti-inflammatory properties. Both capsaicinoids and avenanthramides have also been shown to reduce LDL oxidation.

Curcuminoids: Turmeric is highly valued due to the presence of curcumin that imparts yellow color to turmeric and confers therapeutic properties to this spice. It contains a mixture of curcumin, demethoxycurcumin (DMC) and bisdemethoxycurcumin (BDMC). It functions as an antioxidant but in higher concentration can also have prooxidant properties. It has protective effect against certain cancers. It also has anti-inflammatory, hypoglycemic, and antidepressant activities; thus, it may be useful in diabetes, atherosclerosis, arthritis, and some neurological disorders.

Tannins: Tannins are generally associated with tea and known to inhibit iron absorption. It is also present in *amla* in good amount. It protects vitamin C. Hence, vitamin C from amla and lemon is not lost even when exposed to heat. Besides tea, tannins are present in the outer layers of grains, legumes, and some fruits like grapefruit, lime, and lemon. Tannins give astringent taste because they combine with protein in the saliva. Tannin along with vitamin C helps to strengthen collagen and prevents urinary tract infection. Cranberries and pomegranates are helpful in these conditions. Tannins are known to inhibit lipid peroxidation and lipoxygenases *in vitro*, and are able to scavenge radicals such as hydroxyl, superoxide, and peroxyl, which are known to be important in cellular prooxidant state.

Lignans: Lignans belongs to phytoestrogen group of phytochemicals. Along with isoflavonoids, it shows estrogenic behavior. It is present in flaxseed, pumpkin seed, and sunflower seeds.

Stilbenes: Stilbenes are produced in plants in response to injury or infection. Only dietary source of stilbene compound is resveratrol. The *French paradox* refers to the French being protected from cardiovascular diseases by red wine despite their consuming good amounts of foods containing saturated fatty acids. Red wine is a good source of resveratrol, with other sources being some varieties of grapes, mulberries, cranberries, and peanuts, pistachios. Resveratrol prevents low-density lipoprotein (LDL) oxidation and may have beneficial effects on osteoclasts and osteoblasts. It has shown anticancer, antiaging, cardioprotective, anti-inflammatory, and neuroprotective effects.

Probiotics

The ever-growing quest to find out the reasons for good health and freedom from diseases in olden days has always given birth to new approaches within traditional systems of food processing and consumption. Use of yogurt has been found to improve the intestinal flora in the large intestine, thereby improving digestion and gut health. There are roughly 100 trillion viable bacteria consisting of more than 500 species including *Bifidobacteria*, *Lactobacillus*, and *Enterococcus* species.

In 1908, Prof Metchnikoff observed that lifespan of people who consume fermented foods is longer. In 1915, Newman used *Lactobacillus* for treating cystitis (infection of the bladder). In 1965, the term "probiotic" was coined by Lilly and Stillwell.

Probiotics are defined as "live microorganisms which when administered in adequate amounts confer heath benefits on the host". They can be used in food and also in nonfood preparations. They are postulated to exert a wide range of health benefits such as restoration and maintenance of healthy gut microflora, lowering cholesterol, management of lactose intolerance, inflammatory bowel disease, malabsorption syndrome, and diarrhea. They may be helpful in urogenital and vaginal infections, protection against colon cancer, antihypertensive effects, and antiallergy. The viable number of organisms in food with added probiotic ingredients shall be $\geq 10^8$ CFU/g.

When intestinal flora is in balance, it is known as "eubiosis" and when there is imbalance, it is called "dysbiosis". In dysbiosis, there is growth of pathogenic bacteria causing several pathological conditions and inflammatory diseases like inflammatory bowel disease (IBD) or ulcerative colitis. Deficiency of hydrochloric acid in stomach can also cause dysbiosis. It can also be caused by high sugar and fried food, use of antibiotics, use of radiation, bacterial and parasitic infection, yeast such as *Candida*, environment pollutants, stress, and age. In absence of sufficient HCl, protein is not digested and some bacteria are not destroyed and reach the large intestine.

Bifidus factor from mother's milk contributes to the growth of *Bifidobacteria* in the intestine of newborns. *Bifidobacteria* carries immune-boosting properties and inhibits the growth of *Rotavirus* responsible for infantile diarrhea. The bacteria also help in digestion of milk. Cesarean babies and bottle-fed babies have less chances of developing enough *Bifidobacteria*.

Probiotic yoghurt, ice cream, cheddar cheese, and sour cream are now commercially available which can help to restore the intestinal flora. Nutritive value of such products may not change but with probiotic inclusion, therapeutic effect multiplies. Such products can also be consumed by lactose-intolerant people.

> **Research Glimpse:** *Saccharomyces cerevisiae*, a yeast has been used in food fermentation for making bread, etc. since ages. *Saccharomyces cerevisiae var. boulardii* has shown probiotic effect and health benefits. It works through: (1) hydrolysis of phytate, (2) folate biofortification, (3) as fructo-oligosaccharides, (4) detoxification of mycotoxins, and (5) antioxidative properties. It shows anti-inflammatory effect and improves immune response. By folate fortification, it reduces the risk of NTD. Nutritionally, it improves the bioavailability of minerals like iron, calcium, and zinc.
>
> *Moslehi-Jenabian S, Pedersen LL, Jespersen L. Beneficial effects of probiotic and food borne yeasts on human health. Nutrients. 2010;2(4):449-73.*

Prebiotics: Prebiotics are indigestible carbohydrates that promote the growth of bacteria like *Bifidobacteria* and other spp. Oligosaccharides, inulin, resistant starch, gums, and mucilages are prebiotic materials. These substances are not digested in the small intestine and are fermented by the microflora in the large intestine.

In 2010, the International Scientific Association for Probiotics and Prebiotics (ISAPP) has redefined the definition focusing on the functionality of prebiotics: "a selectively fermented ingredient that results in specific changes in the composition and/or activity of the gastrointestinal microbiota, thus conferring benefit(s) upon host health". It modulates the composition of gut microbiome and its activity and thereby confers physiological health. Gut flora has demonstrated tremendous impact on health of the person. In the past, it has been observed that breastfed infants are healthier than formula-fed babies owing to the composition of microbial species in the gut.

By modifying the ecology of the gut, prebiotics tend to reduce the pH and control the growth of pathogenic bacteria. Their fermentation results in production of short-chain fatty acids (SCFAs) like acetate, butyrate, and propionate. SCFAs are absorbed through the epithelial wall of the intestine and reach the liver via the portal vein. Acetate and propionate are metabolized in liver and contribute to energy in muscles and other peripheral tissues. Propionate also helps in reducing cholesterol level. Butyrate is associated with sodium and water retention as well as cell growth and differentiation. Production of SCFA is largely dependent on the energy intake and the kind of dietary fiber in the diet. Prebiotics also helps in absorption of calcium, magnesium, and iron which otherwise was bound by the dietary fiber.

Some organic acids like citric acid, malic acid, capric and valeric acid found in many plant products including honey, are also found to have positive effect on the gut flora and provide health benefits.

Synbiotics: A synbiotic is a mixture of probiotics and prebiotic that benefits the host.

> **Research glimpse:** Scientific and regulatory definitions of prebiotics differ greatly, although health benefits of these compounds are uniformly agreed upon to be due to their fermentability by gut microbiota. Scientific evidence suggests that 8 categories of compounds exhibit health benefits related to their metabolism by colonic taxa. Health benefits of prebiotic dietary fibers are: (1) Increase in *Bifidobacteria* and *Lactobacilli*, (2) Production of beneficial metabolites, (3) Increase in calcium absorption, (4) Decrease in protein fermentation, (5) Decrease in pathogenic bacteria populations, (6) Decrease in allergy risk, (7) Effect on gut, and (8) Improved immune system defense barrier permeability.
>
> Prebiotic dietary fibers are specific, microbiota-shaping compounds that function as a carbon source for growth of beneficial taxa, thus delivering a specific or selective change that confers the host health related to its metabolism.
>
> *Carlson JL, Erickson JM, Lloyd BB, et al. Health Effects and Sources of Prebiotic Dietary Fiber. Curr Dev Nutr. 2018;2(3):nzy005.*

The Indian consumer is exposed to "nutritious" and "healthy foods" through advertisements. These foods are labeled as: health or nutritional supplements, food supplements, and dietary supplements. The definitions for each of these as per the Food Safety and Standards Authority of India (2010) are as follows:

Health Supplements
"Foods which are specially processed or formulated to satisfy particular dietary requirements which exist because of a particular physical or physiological condition or specific diseases and disorders and which are presented as such wherein the composition of these foodstuffs must differ significantly from the composition of ordinary foods of comparable nature".

Food Supplements
A food supplement is a product that will perform a physiological role beyond the provision of simple nutritive requirement. It may be a food or part of food containing health-promoting ingredient from plants, animals, or microbes, minerals and/or vitamins, and probiotics or prebiotics. The purpose of food supplement is to supplement the normal diet with beneficial physiological/nutritional effect. These products may be either in the form of conventional food or conventional form such as capsule, powder, soft gel, gel cap, tablet, or liquid.

Dietary Supplements
Various definitions have been given by different countries. In 1994, the "Dietary Supplement Health and Education Act (DSHEA)" in the USA defined a dietary supplement as "a product (other than tobacco) taken by mouth that is intended to supplement the diet which bears or contains one or more of the following dietary ingredients: a vitamin, a mineral, a herb or other botanical, an amino acid, a dietary substance for use by man to supplement the diet by increasing the total daily intake, or a concentrate, metabolite, constituent, extract, or combinations of these ingredients. It is intended for ingestion in pill, capsule, tablet, or liquid form and is not represented for use as a conventional food or as the sole item of a meal or diet and is labeled as a dietary supplement".

The Indian definition [**Food Safety Standards Association of India (FSSAI, 2010)**] is "the term dietary supplement means a product (other than tobacco) intended to supplement the diet that bears or contains one or more of the following dietary ingredients: (A) a vitamin, (B) a mineral, (C) a herb or other botanical, (D) an amino acid, (E) a dietary substance for use by man to supplement the diet by increasing the total dietary intake, or (F) a concentrate, metabolite, constituent, extract, or a combination of any ingredient described in clause (A), (B), (C), (D), (E), or (F).

Dietary supplements are further defined as products that are labeled as dietary supplements and are not represented for use as a conventional food or as a sole item of a meal or the diet. Supplements can be marketed for ingestion in a variety of doses, forms including capsules, powder, soft gel, gel cap, tablet, liquid or, indeed, any other form so long as they are not represented as conventional foods or as sole items of a meal or of the diet".

This implies that dietary supplements are ingredients intended to supplement the diet but they are not an integral part of the regular meal. They may provide therapeutic support to boost health and energy. The consumer should be able to understand, differentiate, and make informed choices without involvement of health professionals. People usually self-prescribe these and some people may consider them as a convenient means and good replacements for deficient diet and improve health. These supplements are sometimes incorporated in food preparations like biscuits, sports drink, beverages, and dietetic foods. They are easily and commercially available and can be purchased without prescription under different brand names. They usually carry a health claim on the bottle or brochure.

Use of dietary supplements is an age old practice. Certain herbs and many botanical products have been used. Traditional healthcare practitioners from different countries like China, Germany, and India used several herbal preparations like ginseng, *shilajit*, and *Ginkgo biloba* for various health conditions. Vitamins and minerals are often prescribed for children, women, and patients. Dietary supplements are often used for the following reasons:

1. To improve the nutritional quality of the diet
2. To reduce the deficiency of a particular nutrient
3. To improve the utilization of another nutrient
4. To improve the energy level and stamina
5. To improve sports performance
6. To reduce the risk of several diseases
7. To have preventive or curing effect for certain diseases and disorders
8. To gain extra health benefits.

Side effects of dietary supplements: Some individuals tend to ignore the value of normal healthy diet and replace the meal with supplements. They use them indiscriminately, as an easy and cost-effective way to treat or cure the disease.

Use of protein supplements is common among athletes and many others. It is not really required to build muscles because muscular workout is needed to build the muscles and excess protein intake may be harmful. Protein intake from dietary supplements instead of food sources are not advisable for all women of childbearing age, pregnant and lactating mothers, infants, children, adolescents, and elders. Some supplements may contain unusual combinations or very high amounts of some amino acids. Indiscriminate use of protein supplements may increase the load on the kidney and increase risk of problem such as osteoporosis. Excessive dose of calcium supplements may increase the risk of hypercalcemia, calcification of soft tissues, and impaired kidney functions.

Today market is flooded with herbal supplements with tall claims about cures for various diseases. The consumer must be aware that many of them do not have any scientific evidence. Some popular ones are *Echinacea* which is used to improve immunity and reduce the episodes of cold and asthma but it is also found to aggravate arthritis. Ginseng is considered to be a heart stimulant but it can lead to headaches and palpitation. Many of such herbs are very rich in minerals and phytochemicals which require specific dose needs to be taken under abled guidance professional. Some of the supplements and their medical use are given in Table 15.4. There can be many more supplements and one supplement may provide more than one benefits. Indiscriminate use can be injurious to health.

Table 15.4: Some dietary or nutritional supplements and their claims.

Dietary or nutritional supplements	Used for and/or claims
Echinacea	To improve immunity and promote wound healing
Ginseng	To improve resistance to stress
Brahmi	To improve memory and nervous system functions
Tryptophan, valerian	Sleeping aid
Kava kava	Relaxant
St John's wort	Antidepressant
Licorice	Good for throat
Shilajit	Good for cold and cough
Bee pollen	Improves athlete performance and has antioxidant activity
Aloe vera	Heals digestive disorders as well as in skin and hair
Spirulina	Source of vitamin B_{12}
Alfalfa	It has alkaline effect so neutralizes acidity
Flaxseed oil	Rich in omega-3 essential fatty acids
Green tea	Contains high percentage of polyphenols and acts as antioxidant
Wheat grass	High chlorophyll detoxify the systems and protects cell functions
Acidophilus milk	Improves digestion

Cautions in use of dietary supplements:
- They should be used only when required and under guidance
- They should not be used in place of a meal
- Read the label and available literature before use for usage, dose, and storage
- Storage conditions may affect the potency.

SPORTS NUTRITION

Sports nutrition focuses on the type, amount and timing of each nutrient to be given to the sports persons for their peak performances. Doing some exercises for fitness for shorter duration may not increase the nutritional demand in the body. People sometimes take them unnecessarily and face health hazards. Hence, it is necessary to understand different types of exercises and changes occurring during exercises also. Sports and exercise are beneficial in several ways including improvement in aerobic power, enhanced oxygen uptake, improving blood lipid profiles, better glucose tolerance and enhanced self-assurance, and physical well-being, all of which contribute to better quality of life. Sports and physical fitness are characterized by numerous biochemical and physiological changes in the body affecting the body composition, body secretions, cellular functions, and metabolic reactions. There are many types of activities which are shown in Figure 15.4.

Physical activity: Any bodily movement done by contraction and expansion of the skeletal muscles that involves energy expenditure is called physical activity.

Exercise: Exercise is a subset of physical activities that is planned and structured and involves repetitive movement to improve or maintain physical fitness.

Physical fitness: Physical fitness is a set of attributes which an individual can attain in order to perform and sustain physical activity with ease and agility.

Games: It is a structured form of play usually played for recreational purpose, e.g., ludo, kho-kho, *gilli danda*, video games, etc.

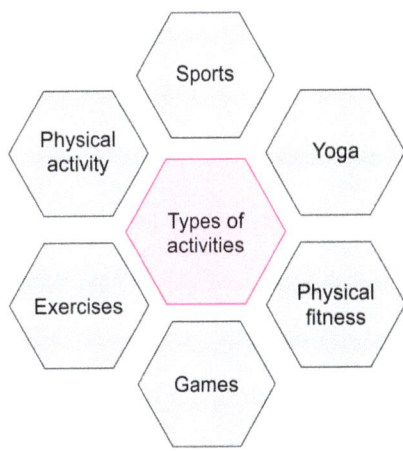

Fig. 15.4: Different types of activities.

Sports: It is an intensive physical activity that involves casual or organized competitive games that require physical fitness and skill to play. It is competitive for the player (sportsperson) and recreational for the viewers, but many people play sports for recreation purposes as well. There is a wide range of sports played at local, national, and international levels such as cricket, weightlifting, tennis, table tennis, badminton, hockey, baseball, football, soccer, polo, kabaddi, swimming, etc. Each type of sports requires training to develop the specific characteristics that are required to do well in the sports activity. Some require muscular strength, some require agility and flexibility, and some require endurance and speed. In order to perform well, nutrition plays a very important role, besides undertaking intensive training. Sports are divided into four main categories based on the skills required. Different sports are mentioned in Table 15.5.

Yoga: Yoga is a holistic way of achieving physical, mental, and spiritual health. It is combinations of activities that involves, breath control, mental focus and physical posture. It enhances the muscle strength, flexibility, respiration, circulation in the body as well as increases the mental focus and agility.

Table 15.5: Different type of sports.

Sports	Tool or technique used	Examples
Adventure sports	Sports specific gadgets	Kayaking, bobsleigh, canoeing, surfing, cross-country skiing, and rafting
Aquatic sports	Water body (river or sea like)	Snorkeling, swimming, bodyboarding, diving, synchronized swimming, rowing, and scuba diving
Strength and agility sports	Sports specific gadgets	Aerobics, aikido, artistic gymnastics, baton twirling, boxing, discus throw, fencing, figure skating, judo, karate, kickboxing, long jump, pole vault, wrestling, etc.
Ball sports	Sports specific tools	Baseball, basketball, handball, dodgeball, tennis, badminton, golf, hockey, ice hockey, soccer, squash, table tennis, etc.
Extreme sports	Sports specific gadget	Base jumping, abseiling, gliding, parachuting, skydiving, paragliding, etc.
Mountain sports	Hills and suitable gadget	Climbing, cross-country cycling, hiking, and mountaineering
Motorized sports	Sports specific vehicle	Drifting, formula racing, and kart racing
Mind sports	Attention and critical thinking Specific tools, e.g., chess board and pawns for chess	Chess, bridge, mahjong
Sports with animals	Specific animal like horse	Polo, horseback riding

Types of Exercise

Different types of exercises are shown in Figure 15.5.

Isometric exercises: Muscle tension is increased by contraction of the muscle without moving the knees or hips, tightening the thigh and leg muscles. It is usually carried out in rehabilitation centers, for strengthening muscles without any special equipment and with little chance of injury.

Isotonic exercises: These are movements of muscles along with movement of a joint or increasing their length, e.g., bending and stretching of arms, legs and back, chin-ups, push-ups, and sit-ups. It is also done with dumb-bells and frequently used in weight training to increase the resistance force. Such exercises improve the circulation and condition the heart.

Isokinetic exercises: Isokinetic exercise involves use of machines to control range and speed of motion. It combines both isometrics and weight training, e.g., bicycle set at 90 revolutions/min.

Strength-building exercises: These include isometric, isotonic, and isokinetic exercises. They are used for improving muscle strength and mass, bone strength, and the body's metabolism, e.g., carrying baby or baggage. It requires balance in walking.

Aerobic exercises: Also known as cardio exercise, because they help in cardiovascular conditioning. Aerobic exercise

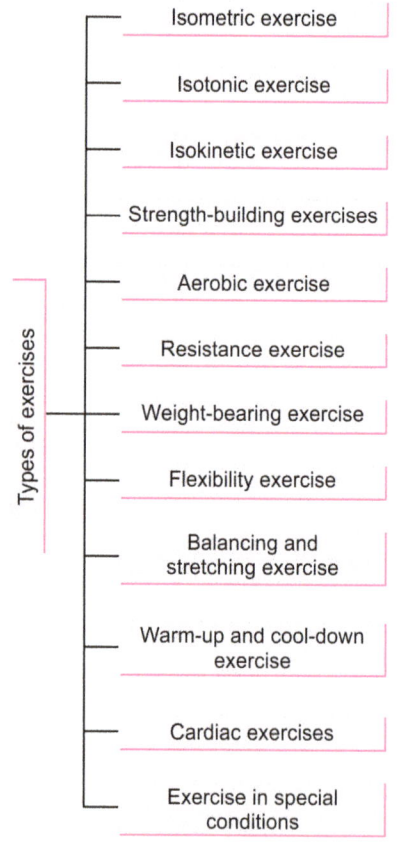

Fig. 15.5: Different types of exercises.

stimulates/speeds up the heart rate and breathing rate that increase in a way that can be sustained for the exercise session and thus improves heart and lung fitness. Some exercises involve repetitive movements with slow intensity. Aerobic means with oxygen whereas anaerobic ("without oxygen"). If aerobic exercise is performed at a high level of intensity, they can become anaerobic, e.g., sprinting or lifting a heavy weight. Examples of aerobic exercises are cardio machines, spinning, running, swimming, walking, jogging, rope skipping, hiking, aerobics classes, dancing, cross-country skiing, kickboxing, bicycling, and aerobic dance and other types. It involves large muscles moved in a rhythmic manner for sustained periods and increased uptake of oxygen. They are performed at relatively high speed in controlled manner while maintaining the balance of the body. They also aid in strengthening muscles used for the exercises. Aerobic exercises tend to utilize more calories and are often prescribed in weight loss programs. They can be performed for longer duration with practice and training.

Resistance exercises: They involve movement of muscle groups against resistance or applied force or weight or gravity. It is done to improve the muscle mass and muscle strength. It also increases focus and reduces the risk of injuries. It requires perseverance, patience, and practice. It is good for reducing visceral fat as it increases the oxygen consumption. Many persons find them difficult in the beginning, particularly elders and obese whose body fat is high or muscle mass is low. These are performed in gyms also using tools, equipments and techniques.

Weight-bearing exercises: They involve movement of muscle groups against resistance or applied force or weight or gravity. They are done to enhance bone mass, strengthen and condition the body. They are suggested to postmenopusal women and in cases of osteoporosis. It should be done slowly and gradually. Jerky or enthusiastic weightlifting can be injurious. In gyms, machines help in use of certain group of muscles. These exercises are used to above. They can be performed in bouts, for a very short period of time, because they are very difficult to sustain for long due to anaerobic conditions of the body, e.g., lifting weights.

Flexibility exercises: Flexibility exercises refer to activities designed to preserve or extend range of motion around a joint. Examples can be rotating or flexing extremities. Yoga and Sukshma Vyayama is good for improving flexibility. Others include dancing, e.g., Zumba, pilates, tai chi.

Balance exercises: Balance exercises involve posture which extends the arms and legs in different angles with support while centering the centre core of the body. It need tremendous focus to avoid fall. As a result it enhances the harmony, relaxation, focus and flexibility in the body. Dancing, yoga, gentle stretching, and tai chi are good examples.

Warm-up and cool-down exercises: Warm-up exercises involve simple bending and extending the different joints of the body for loosening the body parts and prepare it for further movements. It is done for 10–15 minutes. Similarly before finishing the final round of exercises, body is cooled down by slowing down the body movements. It helps to recover fast.

Cardiac exercises: The body movements are done in a way that raise the heartbeats such as brisk walk, jumping, cycling, etc. These are undertaken to improve the efficiency of their oxygen use, increase fitness level, and reduce and prevent cardiac disorders and diseases. Endurance and aerobic exercises may be used at lower intensity and speed. If they are to be done at high intensity and greater speed, these should be done only under supervision and guidance.

Exercise in special conditions: Age is important for selection of exercise. Children and teenagers can perform and sustain exercise or physical activities for longer duration (60 minutes) whereas adults and elders may be able to perform for 30 minutes on average, according to their level of physical fitness. For pregnant women, 30 minutes of moderate physical activity everyday are recommended. In case of people with asthma, high blood pressure, diabetes, osteoporosis, and obesity, the exercise regimen should be followed after consultation with the doctor. Warm-ups and simple walking can be done.

Levels of Physical Activity

There are three levels of physical activity that are classified on the basis of intensity:

Light: These activities generally entail energy expenditure of less than 3.5 kcal/min or less than 3.0 Metabolic equivalent (METS). These include casual walking, bicycling at a speed <5 km/h, stretching, sitting, light weight training, leisurely sports like playing catch, floating, boating, fishing, golf using a cart, lighthouse work, as well as occupations that require extended periods of sitting.

Moderate: These are activities for which the energy cost is 3.5–7 calories/min or 3.0–6.0 METS. This includes walking briskly (about 3–4.5 miles/h), hiking, roller skating at a leisurely pace, low impact aerobics, aqua aerobics, light calisthenics, gymnastics, climbing, gardening/yard work, dancing, bicycling (5–9 miles/h), and weight training (a general light workout), yogasanas, jumping on a trampoline, boxing, competitive tennis, volleyball, badminton, diving, canoeing, housework that involves intense scrubbing/cleaning, recreational swimming, golf-carrying clubs, shoveling snow, carrying a child weighing more than 50 pounds, and occupations that require extended amount of time standing or walking.

Vigorous: These activities have an energy cost of more than 7 calories/min or >6 METS. Examples are running/jogging (5 miles/h), bicycling (more than 10 miles/h), swimming (freestyle laps), aerobics, brisk walking (>4.5 miles/h), weightlifting (vigorous effort), wheeling a wheelchair, mountain climbing, backpacking, fast pace in-line skating, high impact aerobics, vigorous calisthenics, karate, judo, tae kwon do, jujitsu, jumping rope, circuit weight training, vigorous dancing, most aerobic machines like stair climber, elliptical competitive sports and heavy yard work, such as digging, cutting wood, synchronized swimming, treading water, downhill skiing, and occupations that require heavy lifting or rapid movement.

> "If physical activity does not increase the heart rate, it is not intense enough to be counted in the category of "45 minutes of exercise a day". Activities that do not increase the heart rate include walking at a casual pace, grocery shopping, and doing light household chores".
>
> *Dietary guidelines for Indians—A Manual. National Institute of Nutrition: Hyderabad; 2010. p. 58.*

Worldwide different expert groups and organizations have recommended the duration of physical activity which may be used in health and in certain disease conditions. The recommendations of the WHO (2020) are:

Adults

1. Adults in the age group of 18–64 years should do 150 to 300 minutes of moderate intensity aerobic physical activity or 75 to 150 minutes of vigorous intensity aerobic physical activity throughout the week. Alternatively, they can undertake a combination of both.
2. Aerobic activity should be done in bouts, each for about 10 minutes.
3. If additional health benefits are desired, moderate intensity aerobic physical activity should be increased more than 300 min/week or 150 min/week of vigorous intensity physical activity or an equivalent combination of both types of physical activities.
4. At least 2 days in a week, adults should undertake muscle-strengthening activities that involve major muscle groups. These activities should be done at moderate intensity and should involve all major muscle groups.

Children and Adolescents

Recommendations are also made for children and young persons in the age group of 5–17 years. They should undertake physical activity that includes play, games, sports, transportation, recreation, physical education, or planned exercises, in the context of family, school, and community activities. In order to improve cardiorespiratory and muscular fitness, bone health, cardiovascular and metabolic health biomarkers, and reduced symptoms of anxiety and depression, the following are recommended:

1. Children and young people should do at least 60 minutes of moderate-to-vigorous-intensity physical activities daily.
2. Physical activities done for more than 60 minutes daily will provide additional health benefits.
3. Most of daily physical activity should be aerobic. Vigorous-intensity activities should be incorporated, to strengthen muscle and bone, at least 3 times/days per week.

Recommendations for children are given by age group. It is recommended that vigorous-intensity activity should be included in children's routine at least three times/day in a week, that muscle and bone-strengthening, i.e., weight-bearing activities should be performed at least thrice in a week and as is recommended for adults, the amount and intensity should be gradually increased over a period of time.

Age groups	Recommendations for physical activity
3–5 years	Should be physically active and have all possible opportunities to move throughout the day
6–17 years	At least 60 minutes of moderate-to-vigorous-intensity physical exercise daily, most of which should be aerobic

Older Individuals

Also, recommendations have been made for adults who are 65 years of age and older. For these persons, "physical activity includes recreational or leisure-time physical activities, transportation (e.g., walking or cycling), occupational (if the person is still engaged in work any kind of profession), household chores, play, games, sports, or planned exercises, in the context of daily, family, and community activities. In order to improve cardiorespiratory and muscular fitness, bone and functional health, and reduce the risk of non-communicable diseases (NCDs), depression, and cognitive decline, the following are recommended".

If the elders are healthy enough and have good muscle mass they can continue to do the similar exercises recommended for adults. If an individual has poor mobility, the activity should be done at least three times in a week but it should be such that it will enhance balance and prevent falls. On two days a week at least, muscle-strengthening activities that involve major muscle groups should be done. If their health condition does not permit undertaking the recommended activities, they should be as physically active as is possible within the constraints of their physical condition. Older adults are recommended to do at least 150–300 minutes moderate intensity aerobic physical activity and at least 75–150 minutes of vigorous aerobic physical activity throughout the week (WHO, 2020).

Various intensity of exercise recommendations have been proposed American Heart Association (AHA) for different age groups and health conditions. With training and practice intensity and duration of exercise can be increased. If they are healthy enough and have good muscle mass they can continue to do the similar exercises recommended for adults.

Recommendations have been made by several countries including the UK, Canada, and Australia. The NIH, UK encourages physical activity for babies and toddlers in addition to other age groups.

Benefits of Physical Activity

- Helps to maintain body weight and desired body composition
- Helps to reduce body fat and increases lean body mass
- Helps to gain muscle mass, muscle strength, and improve stamina and flexibility in body movements
- Helps to build strong bones, muscles, and strengthen joints
- Reduces the risk of chronic diseases such as type-2 diabetes, high blood pressure, heart disease, osteoporosis, arthritis, and some cancers
- Increases level of HDL (good cholesterol)
- Improves mood, sense of well-being and self-esteem, and wards off depression.

Physiological Changes during Exercise

A sportsperson is expected to be physically fit. Physical fitness includes strength (the ability of the muscle to work against resistance), muscular endurance (the ability of the muscle to contract repeatedly without becoming exhausted during a given period of time), joint flexibility (the capacity that the joints have to move through a full range of motion and recover without injury), cardiovascular endurance (ability of the cardiovascular and respiratory system to sustain efforts over a given period of time), and desirable body composition, speed, agility, and balance. Besides these characteristics, the sportsperson must have resistance to fatigue syndrome, resistance to infection as well as recover as early as possible in case of injuries. Sportspersons are expected to perform well in various environments.

Physical fitness can be improved by training to use different sets of muscles for sustained periods of time. It not only improves skills but also alters physiology which is different in both aerobic and anaerobic conditions. Physiological changes brought about by exercise are:

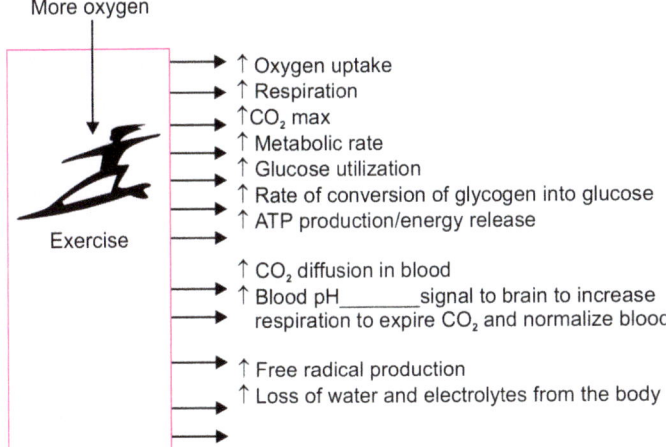

Significant changes are described herein:

Body composition: The proportion of lean body mass (LBM) and fat mass (percent body fat) are critical in many sports events, e.g., low % body fat is desirable for swimmers (6–14%) whereas it can be a little higher (18–24%) for basketball players. There are gender differences in body composition. Men have less body fat (15–17%) than women (25–27%). LBM is equally important. Loss of LBM is detrimental and adversely affects speed, mobility, strength, and alertness.

Aerobic capacity: Aerobic capacity of the individual indicates the ability of the person to sustain high-intensity exercises like endurance or cardio exercises. It is measured as VO_2 max. It is the level of maximal potential of the individual when breathing reaches to the point of exhaustion. At this point/stage, metabolically, there is a shift from aerobic to anaerobic state. VO_2 max is measured as maximal uptake of oxygen volume. It is measured as milliliters of oxygen used in one min/kg body weight. VO_2 max (>60) indicates that there is improvement in circulation and cardiac function and reduces risk of heart disease. It determines the performance capacity of the individual and varies widely from individual to individual and from one type of sport to another. Training and practice can improve the VO_2 max.

Glycogen stores: Under normal conditions, liver can store about 50–75 g glycogen and muscles store 300–400 g glycogen. Sports performed for longer duration require more glycogen in the muscles which can be increased by carbohydrate loading technique to 600 g, because glycogen can easily converted to glucose to produce ATP during the event. A carbohydrate-loading diet can increase glycogen storage in muscle by as much as 100 percent of the normal amount. It is important to begin exercise and sports with ample glycogen stores to improve performance, and restoring stores is equally important for complete recovery as well as to maintain one's capacity for exercise that will be done subsequently.

> **Glycogen stores in the body**
> **Under normal conditions**
> Muscles—300–400g (=1,200–1,600 kcal)
> Liver—80–90 g (=320–360 kcal)
> **Carbohydrate loading**
> Muscles—600 g (=2,400 kcal)

Water and electrolyte balance: Exercise induces sweating due to which there is loss of water and electrolytes. Hence, dehydration can occur during exercise and sports and reduces the stamina. Water and electrolytes need to be replenished to prevent dehydration and its consequences.

Timing of ingestion of nutrients: Timing of ingestion of nutrients influences the response of the body to both nutrients and adaption to exercise. Daily ingestion of high-CHO meals (~65% CHO) is recommended to maintain muscle glycogen. Increased ingestion rates are employed (~70% CHO) in the 5-7 days leading up to the competition/event, as a means of maximizing muscle and liver glycogen stores and in order to sustain blood glucose during exercise.

ATP production: ATP production increases with increased oxygen uptake. At the same time, ATP is utilized by the body for energy utilized for performing the sports activity and for the normal body processes. Normally, ATP is produced in mitochondria of muscle cells and requires oxygen. However, the muscle cells need to work in absence of oxygen. In endurance or resistance activities which are of short duration (10-20 seconds) as in weightlifting and shot-put, muscles utilize another high-energy phosphate compound creatine phosphate (CP) which can be used to resynthesize ATP. Under anaerobic conditions, pyruvate is converted to lactic acid which is eventually used for ATP production.

Energy expenditure: Energy expenditure is proportional to the intensity of exercise. Intensity means the rate of exertion during exercise, that can be measured by VO_2 max (oxygen consumption) and heart rate. As the intensity of aerobic exercise increases, energy expenditure also increases during and after exercise, e.g., in cardiovascular exercises like running on a treadmill, running on plain surface will be less intense than running on hill (inclined position) although, it may be at the same speed. Resistance training also requires more calories because of intensity. Lifting more weight uses more calories in shorter duration than lifting lighter weight for longer duration. Well-trained persons with practice may expend fewer calories because their oxygen uptake is faster, thereby their breathing and heart rate also increase and their repair of muscles is also faster.

Excessive production of free radicals: Increase in oxygen uptake followed by ATP production will naturally release more free radicals resulting in oxidative damage of the cell membranes and cause oxidative stress. Adequate supply of antioxidants during exercise may lessen the adverse effect of free radicals. Otherwise, free radicals can play havoc on fluidity and integrity of cell membrane, cellular activities, and eventually adversely affects the body functioning.

Different Types of Stress

Stress can ruin the performance of an athlete/sportsperson and the right kind of stress could enhance your performance. The announcement of the sports event can motivate the person. A person can have "eustress" which is a good form of stress because it is associated with a feeling of fulfillment, and some athletes feel good about it because they are challenged to perform better. The other type of stress is "distress" that is primarily anxiety, nervousness, worry, and apprehension that is caused by a feeling or perceived inability to meet the demands of the sport. An individual undergoes following types of stresses:

Physical stress: Sports involve use of the body in various dimensions that will take toll on the muscles and bones. Naturally after some time, depending upon the body's capacity, a person does get tired or fatigued. Optimal nutrition and rest can help the person to recover in a fairly short time quickly. The fatigue for longer duration may result in muscular tension and stiffness in different muscle groups that interferes with flexibility, agility and mental and motor actions during the game. There is risk of injuries that might need therapies also. Physical stress implies a low energy level, anxiety, breathlessness, headaches, gastric disturbances, and tight muscles, high or low blood pressure, etc. It can also be caused by trauma (injury, infection, and surgery), overexertion, and environmental pollution (heavy metals, radiations, pesticides, noise, inadequate light, and electromagnetic field). Hormonal imbalances, malnutrition, food allergies, unhealthy eating habits, and other poor lifestyle habits including sleeping and training schedule cause physical stress. Stress relieving techniques can reduce stress.

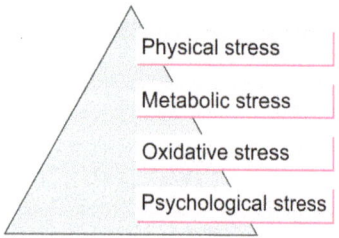

Metabolic stress: Inadequacy or imbalance in the supply of any substrate (energy, nitrogen, vitamins, minerals, water, and electrolytes) required for metabolism can hamper the functioning of metabolic pathways, thereby bringing changes in the rate of metabolic activities, BMR. Imbalance or alterations in BMR and metabolic demand is called **metabolic stress**. This can be for shorter duration and can be compensated by supplying adequate substrates in time. During exercise and sports, the metabolic demands and metabolic stress increase. Poor dietary habits, lack of physical activity, lifestyle factors, negative attitude, smoking, alcohol consumption, pollutants, accumulation of metabolic waste. Environmental changes also influence the metabolic demands of the body and thus cause metabolic stress.

Metabolic stress alters glucose uptake by the muscles and other tissues and adjusts the secretion of insulin and other hormones. Supply of adequate energy through carbohydrates and fat is important. Sometimes there is synthesis of amino acids that occurs from ingested dietary protein/amino acids or by catabolism of body protein. Hence, dietary protein must contain adequate and digestible amounts of nutritionally indispensable amino acids as well as conditionally amino acids and other sources of nitrogen for protein synthesis. Maintenance of body fluid composition and proper hydration can be ensured with adequate intake of water and electrolytes.

Metabolic stress also brings about changes in the biochemical environment within cells and can affect the cell signaling mechanisms as well as immune response. Consequently metabolism may slow down, causing problems like difficulty in weight loss, moodiness, poor concentration, sleep disturbances, reduced energy level, lethargy, and rise in blood glucose level. Low BMR reduces the intention of exercise and training for desired duration and adversely affects the performance in sports events. Chronic metabolic stress leads to lower BMR, elevation of insulin, cortisol, and lower levels of other hormones. These changes can in turn result in accumulation of visceral fat which increases risk of systemic inflammation and oxidative stress. Metabolic stress also causes anabolic and catabolic imbalances characterized by aging of cells that affect their normal physiological functioning. Elevated levels of cortisol, blood glucose, insulin, and low androgen and growth hormone levels lead to oxidative stress.

Oxidative stress: Oxygen is an essential element for living organisms. Oxygen uptake increases during sports activities. During oxidative reactions, there is production of highly reactive oxygen molecules within the mitochondria.

Generation of reactive oxygen species (ROS) or free radicals is an outcome of aerobic metabolism. Different types of ROS include superoxide anion, hydrogen peroxide, hydroxyl radicals, and singlet oxygen. They can react with almost all cellular components, lipids, carbohydrates, proteins, and nucleic acids including DNA and can cause oxidation in them resulting in formation of numerous harmful products like advanced glycation end products (AGEs) or lead to lipid peroxidation. When ROS tends to oxidize DNA or break the DNA strand, it can critically affect cell function and can also result in mutation.

The imbalance between production of ROS or FR and body's ability to detoxify them or supply of antioxidants is called **oxidative stress** (OS). Oxidative stress can be either transient or chronic, but it disturbs cellular metabolism and regulation in terms of: (i) cell signaling, (ii) defense against infections, (iii) modification of molecules, and (iv) damage to cellular constituents.

There is enough physical stress in sports and the intensity and duration of exercise influences the magnitude of oxidative stress. Antioxidant defenses of skeletal muscles are poor.

During OS, there is reduced level of glutathione and glutathione peroxidase. High-fat and high-carbohydrate diet cause more production of ROS. OS exerts major influence on cell aging and tissue damage particularly of brain and cardiac cells. With prolonged duration and intensity of exercise, age, and poor diet, free radical generation accelerates due to lipid peroxidation and impaired antioxidant activity in the cell membrane. Oxidative stress is greatly influenced by psychological factors and lifestyle.

Under normal conditions, cells are well-equipped with the antioxidant defense system to deal with FR in the form of glutathione and enzymes like catalase and superoxide dismutase (SOD) as well as of antioxidants obtained from dietary sources in the form of vitamins E, C, carotenoids, flavonoids, etc. Consumption of foods having high antioxidant activity helps in removing the excess ROS, detoxifying the system, and maintaining homeostasis. There are numerous vegetables fruits, herbs, spices and essential oils which have high antioxidant capacity (in terms of ORAC or Oxygen Radical Absorbance Capacity) values. These foods should not be over consumed rather under supervision of trained health professionals. Other methods of relaxation, avoidance of high fat, high-sugar diet, and refined foods are also useful.

Psychological stress: It has been established that free radicals affect cognitive functions, mood and focus, and the ability to perform different activities including daily activities. Elevated oxidative stress induces the release of the catecholamines—epinephrine and norepinephrine and interleukin-2 (IL-2) particularly during mental and physical stress which may often be encountered in competitive sports. Release of norepinephrine may induce DNA damage.

In competitive events, psychological stress increases and when in excess, it affects the performance and increases the vulnerability to sports injury. It reduces concentration and increases anxiety, aggression, and irritability. Oxidative stress further increases psychological stress, which tends to alter the hormonal and immunological response.

Anxiety can be prevented by use of the following techniques: diaphragmatic breathing, relaxation techniques, visualization (the game, opponents), muscle relaxation, and focusing on what can be controlled. Adequate sleep is also important for good performance.

Sports nutrition deals with the role of dietary components in physical fitness and sports. It is the application of the principles of nutrition to sports in relation to physical and physiological changes occurring in the body of a sportsperson or athlete. Fuel and fluids are of paramount importance in their diets. It is well-established that provision of right food and fluids at the right time, in the right amounts can help sportspersons to perform at their best. Inappropriate dietary intake can adversely influence performance, reduce chances of winning the game, and have serious effects on health. Nutrient needs differ during training, competition, and rest days that require special meal planning for pre-event, during, and postexercise sessions.

Nutritional requirements of a sportsperson also differ from nonsports persons because of their body composition and physiology. Hence, nutritionally adequate diet in athletes and sports persons is essential for:
- Providing fuel for energy
- Providing adequate protein to build and maintain muscles mass and repair tissues
- Replenishing body fluids
- Providing dietary antioxidants
- Enhancing muscle strength
- Improving endurance
- Achievement of peak performance
- Preventing of injury and fatigue
- Promoting speedy recovery after game or injury
- Improving immunity and capability to resist infection.

Energy and Nutritional Needs of Sportspersons

Like every other activity, sports activities also require energy and other nutrients. Sports differ in type and intensity, amount of energy expenditure hence, the calorie requirement will also be different. The International Life Sciences Institute-India, National Institute of Nutrition and Sports Authority of India jointly developed guidelines in 2007 for nutrition and hydration to achieve excellence in sports. According to these guidelines, sports and games have been classified as per the energy expenditure which is shown in Table 15.6A. Table 15.6B clearly indicates that energy requirements for each group are based on body weight and per kg/day. The percent contribution of each of the three macronutrients to total energy intake is also recommended. Table 15.7 extends the nutritional guidelines along with level of fitness and duration of sports activity.

Table 15.6A: Classification of sports and games based on energy expenditure.

Categories	Events
Group-I	Power events of higher-weight category (80 kg and above)—weightlifting, boxing, wrestling, judo, and throwing events
Group-II	Endurance events—marathon, long-distance running, and walking road cycling, rowing, and middle- and long-distance swimming
Group-III	Team events, athletics, and power events of middle-weight category (65 kg)—hockey, football, volleyball, basketball, tennis, sprints, jumpers, boxing, wrestling, weightlifting, judo, and swimming
Group-IV	Events of light-weight category—gymnastics, table tennis, yachting, boxing, wrestling, weightlifting, and judo
Group-V	Skill games—shooting, archery

Source: International Life Sciences Institute-India, National Institute of Nutrition, Sports Authority of India. (2007). Nutrition and Hydration Guidelines for Excellence in Sports Performance.

Table 15.6B: Average body weight and energy expenditure levels assumed and allowance suggested.

Event categories	Body weight (kg)	Energy allowance		Calories ratio CHO:PROT:FAT		
		kcal/kg/day	kcal/day			
Group-I	85	70	6,000	55	15	30
Group-II	65	80	5,200	60	15	25*
Group-III	65	70	4,500	60	15	25
				64	15	21*
Group-IV	60	60	3,600	65	15	20
Group-V	60	50	3,600	55	15	30

* = means glycogen loading

Source: International Life Sciences Institute-India, National Institute of Nutrition, Sports Authority of India. (2007). Nutrition and Hydration Guidelines for Excellence in Sports Performance.

Table 15.7: Energy and nutrient requirements for fitness and different levels of sports.

Level of activity	Suggested for body weight	Duration of activity	Energy requirement	Carbohydrates	Proteins	Fat
General fitness	50–80 kg	30–40 min/ 3 times/week	1,800–2,400 kcal or 25–35 kcal/kg/day	45–55% of total calories or 3–5g/kg/day	15–20% of total calories Or 0.8-1.0 g/kg/day	25–35% of total calories or 0.5–1.5 g/kg/day
Athlete intense training	50–70 kg	2–3 h/day for 5–6 times/week	2,000–7,000 kcal or 40–70 kcal/kg/day	5–8 g/kg/day or 250–1,200 g/day for 50–150 kg person	1.2–2.0 g/kg/day Or 60–300 g for 50–150 kg person	20–35% of total calories
High volume (training)	50–70 kg	3–6 h/day 1–2 workout for 5–6 days/week	More than 600–1,200 kcal during training	8–10 g/kg/day or 400–1,500 g/day for 50–150 kg person	1.7–2.2 g/kg/day Or 85–330 g for 50–150 kg person	50% of total calories

Source: Kerksick CM, Wilborn CD, Roberts MD, et al. ISSN exercise and sports nutrition review update: research and recommendations. J Int Soc Sports Nutr. 2018;15(1):38.

Insufficient energy intake during training may lead to loss of muscle mass (fat-free mass), increased resting heart rate, and psychological issues like apathy, heightened stress, and other adverse outcomes. It can also result in loss of quality sleep, incomplete recovery, and hormonal fluctuations. Negative energy balance is a debatable particularly in aesthetic sports and females with eating disorders. Adequate intake of carbohydrates, protein, and fat is necessary to optimize the training and performance.

Gastric discomfort, travel and training schedules, nonavailability of nutrient dense foods, and changes in timings of meal intake are some factors that can influence nutrient intakes. On average, 4-6 meals a day + snacks are sufficient to meet the demand. Snacks can be bars, sports drink are conveniently used by athletes to maintain the energy levels.

Role of Carbohydrate in Sports

Carbohydrate is the major source of energy (fuel) for the working muscles. Carbohydrates are crucial before, during, and after intense and high-volume bouts of training and event because the rapidity with which a carbohydrate is digested and raises blood sugar, has an impact on exercise intensity and duration. Optimal carbohydrate intake plays an important role to replenish the lost muscle and liver glycogen. Glycogen in liver and muscle is the source of energy during exercise particularly during prolonged bouts of moderate-to-high-intensity exercise. Carbohydrate availability from liver and muscle glycogen is a critical determinant. Restoring endogenous glycogen stores is a crucial factor determining recovery especially for effective endurance performance. Provision of constant supply of glucose to the exercising muscle and brain even during prolonged exercise.

Normally carbohydrates come from starches from grains and fruits and also from engineered sports products. However, carbohydrates also come from refined sugars but this sugar should only be reserved for the situations of quick glycogen synthesis at accelerated rate. When rapid glycogen resynthesis is required, the experts indicated that consuming approximately 0.5–0.6 g/kg of rapidly absorbed carbohydrate is advised. Approximately 300g of carbohydrates are required by an athlete for intake of 2000 kcal/day. Menu must include unrefined wholesome complex carbohydrates until specified. Then >0.8 g carbohydrate/kg/h or 1.2 g/kg/h for first 4 hours is required for recovery. It relates to timing or concomitant ingestion of other macronutrients and nonnutrients (caffeine) and carbohydrate type (glycemic index) is important. In the hours immediately postexercise, it is important to consume carbohydrate in order to speed glycogen synthesis.

Liver can store only 80-90 g of glycogen whereas muscles can store 300-400 g of glycogen. Rest of the ingested carbohydrate (glucose) is converted into fat and stored in adipose tissue. Since fat cannot directly be converted into glucose like glycogen, therefore fat is not a good source of energy for exercising muscles. Glycogen stores determine the stamina and performance in sports and depleted stores result in fatigue and poor performance. There is a technique which is used, during competition of sports events, to increase glycogen store. This is known as "glycogen loading" or "carbohydrate loading".

Carbohydrate Loading

Carbohydrate loading is a process used by athletes who participate in endurance exercise or sports to delay the onset of fatigue by increasing the body glycogen stores (in muscles). Endurance athletes include those who participate in long distance events that last 90 minutes or more, i.e., marathon runners, cyclists, swimmers, and others. Carbohydrate loading is not required for shorter athletic activities, such as recreational biking or swimming, weightlifting, and 5- or 10-mile (8- or 16-kilometer) runs.

> **Carbohydrate loading** is a method of boosting glycogen level in the body prior to competition. It enables the body to draw maximum fuel during competition.
> It is important to remember that everyone who is involved in sports need not go on a carbohydrate-loading diet.

This strategy was developed by a Swedish scientist, Gunvar Ahlborg (1967). In this process, muscles are first depleted of glycogen, and then loaded with carbohydrates in order to increase the accumulation of carbohydrates (glycogen) in muscles. During this period, the athlete also reduces the scale of activity. During bouts of endurance exercise, fatigue generally coincides with low muscle glycogen content. By simply eating some carbohydrates during exercise and having glucose available in the blood is not enough to sustain exercise for an extended period of time. This has led researchers to believe that it may be necessary to load one's body with glucose prior to prolonged exercise. Carbohydrate loading (>6 g/kg/day) prior to participation in an endurance exercise competition has been shown to help delay the onset of fatigue by approximately 20% during endurance events lasting longer than 90 minutes. Endurance running severely taxes carbohydrate stores which, unlike fat reserves, can be performance limiting because they are comparably small.

Carbohydrate loading is carried out in 2 phases, 6–7 days prior to a competitive event:

Phase I or depletion phase: For the first three days, the athlete consumes less carbohydrate so that it supplies about 50–55% of total calorie intake. The remaining energy should come from protein and fat. Training and exercises are continued at the normal level so as to deplete the body's glycogen stores and prepare for the body to store more glycogen in the next phase of the diet.

Phase II, i.e., loading phase: Three to four days before the event, carbohydrate intake should be increased to supply about 70% of total calorie intake. Simultaneously, there will be a decrease in protein and fat intake. Smaller athletes can consume about 4.5 g of carbohydrate per pound of body weight and those with larger body size can consume about 3.5 g per pound of body weight. After this carbohydrate is digested and metabolized, it is stored in the form of glycogen in muscles. Maximal level of glycogen is generally achieved after 1–3 days after consuming high glycemic, high carbohydrates (600–1,000 g or 8–10 g/kg body weight/day). It is also suggested that carbohydrate is combined with protein and free amino acids to stimulate protein synthesis.

At this time, the exercise is to be reduced so as to not utilize the energy that is being stored and on the day prior to the event, the athlete is advised to rest completely. An athlete who has diabetes should consult his/her doctor before adopting a carbohydrate-loading diet.

It is required in specific cases and should be done in under supervision only. However, there can be some problems with such a diet:

- **Weight gain:** Much of this weight is extra water, but if it hampers performance, it may be advisable not to consume the extra carbohydrates.
- **Digestive discomfort:** It may be advisable to limit some high-fiber foods for one or two days before your event, especially those that cause bloating and flatulence.
- **Blood sugar changes:** Carbohydrate loading can affect blood sugar levels. It is worthwhile to monitor blood sugar during training or practice sessions. Anyone planning to start on a carbohydrate-loading diet should consult a doctor and dietician.
- **Other side effects** have been experienced by some individuals like muscle stiffness, diarrhea, chest pain, depression, and lethargy.

Recovery phase: When energy is available, muscles also absorb amino acids from the blood which help in protein synthesis in muscles. This also helps in reducing breakdown of muscle protein and speeds up the recovery process. Hence, consumption of carbohydrates and protein together in a ratio of 3:1 or 4:1 is suggested. Prolonged deprivation of carbohydrates can cause ketoacidosis. For utilization of carbohydrates, adequate intakes of vitamin B, iron, and magnesium are also essential. The amount of carbohydrates and the type of carbohydrates are crucial. Oxidation rates of different sources of dietary carbohydrates (exogenous) differ. It is higher in disaccharides and polysaccharides, e.g., sucrose and maltodextrin as compared to monosaccharides like glucose and fructose. However, combination of glucose and sucrose or fructose and maltodextrin has been found to promote oxidation of carbohydrate more than oxidation of other forms of carbohydrate. Hence, such combinations may be beneficial and inclusion of different foods that are sources of these can be chosen in different meals.

Tips for carbohydrates foods for sportsmen	
Add (low-medium glycemic foods)	**Avoid (high glycemic foods)**
• Whole grain cereals—wheat, jowar, ragi, other whole grain millets, brown rice • Pulses—*rajma, mung, urad,* chickpea, pea, *chana,* lentil, soy bean as well as sprouted form • Fruits—banana, apricot, apple, sapota, custard apple, papaya, watermelon, pineapple, sweet lime, pear, peach, etc. • Vegetables—all including green leafy vegetables • Sugar—jaggery, jam, and jelly	• Rice, sugar, honey, chocolates, and Indian sweets • Refined flours and preparations made with them • Junk foods, fried foods like samosa, bhature, chaat, burger, pizza, chips, kachori, farsan etc. • Excess of sugar candy

Besides these, the amount of carbohydrate intake required to be consumed varies for at different timings of sports event, i.e., pre-exercise, during, and postexercise. Carbohydrate intake is often manipulated and different types of carbohydrates may be required at different timings of sports events. There are many factors to be considered for selection of carbohydrate:

Factors to be considered while selecting carbohydrate rich foods
- Intensity and duration of exercise
- Glycogen stores in liver and muscles
- Types of event
- Fatigue
- Timing of ingestion
- Type of carbohydrates
- Amount of energy expenditure
- Season of event, food habits
- Geographical location

Different types of carbohydrates are oxidized at different rates in skeletal muscles due to the involvement of different transporter protein that regulates the carbohydrate uptake. Combination of glucose, sucrose, maltodextrin, and fructose support carbohydrate oxidation. Oxidation rate, carbohydrate type, fasting status, and duration of exercise are crucial. It has been suggested that using glucose and fructose together as a mixture or glucose and sucrose mixtures will replete the liver glycogen at a rate that is faster than if glucose alone is used, although it may not do much for repleting muscle glycogen. Also, this combination does not give much gastric distress when given at a rate ≥1.2 g/kg of body weight per hour.

Role of Protein in Sports

In sports, proteins are not only important for protein synthesis but also training adaptation. Protein is associated with muscle building, repairing, and preventing their damage in sports. It is also essential for the formation of ligaments, tendons, cartilage, bones as well as hormones, enzymes, antibodies, and neurotransmitters. Sports performance and recovery are greatly influenced by the quality of protein and supply of the amino acids at the appropriate time. However, ingestion of protein alone does not build the muscles. Training and exercise are essential because they have an anabolic effect and promote protein synthesis.

When protein is consumed before or after a workout, it induces a significant increase in muscle protein synthesis. Proteins differ in their sources, amino acid composition, and method of processing. These factors influence the availability of amino acids and peptides which may possess biological activity. Alpha-lactalbumin and lactoferrin have high bioavailability. The rate of digestion and/or absorption and metabolic activity of protein are also important considerations.

It is important to consider that each amino acid has a specific metabolic or biochemical role in the body. Deficiency of one can affect the functioning of others. Hence, all the essential amino acids need to be ingested in sufficient amounts through diet. Some of the important amino acids are branched-chain amino acids (leucine, isoleucine, and valine), arginine, glutamine, tyrosine, tryptophan, tyrosine, glycine, and lysine.

Protein requirement for activities of different intensity is given in Table 15.8. According to Indian guidelines (2007), protein intake in grams can be 1–1.5 times the body weight in kgs and should contribute 10–15% of the total calories. The type of sport and total energy intake also influence protein requirements. Protein intake should be considered because it influences physiological factors that influence physical performance. This includes muscle remodeling, glycogen resynthesis, energy production, and maintenance of nonmuscle structural tissues. Athletes need not only ensure adequate protein intakes but they need to pay attention to the protein quality, type, and timing of intake. Two grams/kg of body weight has been recommended for junior athletes to enable development of muscle mass, muscle regeneration, and the additional requirements due to sports activities. The amount of protein will depend not only on the exercise, its mode, and intensity but also the protein quality, and the energy and carbohydrate status of the sportsperson. As far as is possible, the athlete should consume good quality protein. Timing of intake is important in order to obtain the benefit to the greatest extent possible in terms of recovery and gaining lean body mass. Protein should be consumed during the periworkout period within 0–2 hours of the exercise. For achieving better muscle adaptation to training, it is recommended that athletes consume 0.3 g of high quality protein per kilogram of body weight within 0–2 hours after exercise. Subsequently, protein of high quality can be consumed every 3–5 hours. Also, consuming protein before sleeping can help to increase muscle protein synthesis as well as to improve metabolism next morning.

Sportspersons who are undergoing intense training may need to consume more than two times the RDA (1.5–2.0 g/kg/day) in order to maintain the protein balance. It has been noted by the Food and Nutrition Board, USA that the risk of adverse effects from excess protein from food is very low. This may not apply to very high protein intakes from foods and supplements because there is limited scientific evidence regarding the potential adverse effects. At levels of two to three times the RDA (0.8 g/kg/day) in case of adults and 0.85 g/kg/day in adolescents, the risk is not higher for possible side effects such as kidney stones or adverse effects on kidney function, dehydration, or bone health or glucose as well as lipids, creatine, and blood urea nitrogen. However, high intakes of single amino acid preparations hamper the absorption of other amino acids resulting in nitrogen imbalance. It may increase the risk of urinary loss of calcium.

Table 15.8: Protein requirements of sportspersons.

Categories of the sportspersons	RDA for protein
Sedentary adult	0.8 g/kg BW/day
Physically active adult	0.8–1.0 g/kg BW/day
Endurance athlete	1.2–1.4 g/kg BW/day
Strength athlete	1.4–1.8 g/kg BW/day
Adolescent athlete	1.0–2.0 g/kg BW/day
Maximum for adult athlete	2.0 g/kg BW/day

Source: International Life Sciences Institute-India, National Institute of Nutrition, Sports Authority of India. (2007). Nutrition and Hydration Guidelines for Excellence in Sports Performance.

High-protein diet along with low carbohydrates may deter athletic performance. It is important to remember that all essential amino acids are necessary for muscle protein synthesis. Supplements of arginine, glutamine, beta-alanine, and branched-chain amino acids are touted, but there is limited scientific evidence of their improving performance.

> **Protein foods for sportspeople:**
> Egg
> Whey protein
> Soy and soy products
> Milk (casein)
> Low fat dairy products
> Grains
> Nuts nuts and seeds

If the diet provides insufficient amount of protein, it can increase protein catabolism and the sportsperson may have negative nitrogen balance which may slow down the recovery. Over a period of time, this can result in muscle wasting and training intolerance. The timing of protein intake has several benefits like improved recovery and greater gain in fat-free mass or lean body mass. Preexercise intake of essential amino acids or protein increases muscle protein synthesis. Intake of protein to carbohydrate during exercise (both acute and endurance exercise) in a ratio of 3:1 to 4:1 helps to increase endurance performance. After the event (postexercise), a ratio of 1:3 (protein to carbohydrate) will help to stimulate glycogen synthesis. At all three time points, addition of 0.15–0.25 g of protein/kg/day to carbohydrate may help restore muscle glycogen stores. On glycogen depletion, protein is utilized for energy at the end of the workout. Therefore, consumption of both carbohydrate and protein is required for physical activity, maintenance, and repair.

Foods like egg, whey protein, soy and milk (casein), low fat dairy products, grains, nuts, seeds, and beans provide good quality protein. Each source may differ in its amino acid composition and biological value. Judicious selection and combination of foods are helpful. Use of protein powders, supplements, or special amino acid preparations is not always necessary. Many protein foods like red meat, cream cheese are also rich in saturated fats and thus are not a good choice.

> **Research Glimpse:** Sports nutrition products are developed and targeted mainly for athletes to improve their nutrient intake, performance, and muscle growth. The fastest growing consumer groups for these products are recreational sportspersons and lifestyle users. In high-protein diets, more undigested protein-derived constituents end up in the large intestine compared to moderate- or low-protein diets, and hence, more bacterial amino acid metabolism takes place in the colon, having both positive and negative systemic and metabolic effects on the host. BCAA supplementation regulates some brain neurotransmitter production and thus in fatigue development during exercise. Furthermore, due to fast digestion and absorption, whey protein supplements are a popular protein source for athletes. Gut microbiota deserves attention when regarding personalized nutrition.
>
> *Kårlund A, Gómez-Gallego C, Turpeinen AM, et al. Protein Supplements and their Relation with Nutrition, Microbiota Composition and Health: Is More Protein Always Better for Sportspeople? Nutrients. 2019;11(4):E829.*

Whey provides highly soluble protein which is absorbed in a few hours. Whey protein also contains immunoglobulins which promote immunity. It also supports glutathione function which is an antioxidant in the body. Egg white contains soluble, i.e., albumin which is of high biological value and supports protein synthesis. Egg yolk is rich in cholesterol that supports synthesis of testosterone hormone needed for stamina and also contains other nutrients. Soy is a vegetarian source of protein and its isoflavones content has shown positive effect in sports activity particularly in female athletes. Casein is a slow-releasing protein, taking up to several hours to release its amino acids and hence may be suitable for long duration exercise and in recovery phase. It has been observed that if amino acid level is adequate during recovery phase, maximal protein synthesis can be achieved and at the same time recovery period can be shortened. A judicious combination of the protein source is advisable. It is important to remember that total daily intake of not only protein but that of energy as well is crucial in enabling a person to adapt the exercise.

Role of Fat in Sports

Fat provides more than double the calories (9 kcal/g) as compared to carbohydrates (4 kcal/g). However, glucose, but not fat, is the primary fuel for energy during exercise. The body utilizes fat for moderate to slow activities carried out for long duration. Fat is composed of glycerol and fatty acids. Fatty acids undergo β-oxidation in the presence of oxygen to produce energy. Glycerol from fat can be converted into glucose whereas fatty acids cannot. Glycerol can provide energy under anaerobic conditions as well. Also, carbohydrate must be present to avail energy from fat as it is involved in breakdown of fatty acids.

The type of fatty acids from dietary fats play significant role. High-fat diet has been found favorable for prolonged and endurance sports like marathon and skiing. It is also useful during intensive training. One-third (30%) of the total calories in the beginning for first few weeks and more than that (40–45%) at the end of training can be suggested. However, high-fat diet should be avoided at the time of event. Good food choices are skimmed milk, low-fat yogurt, fats from nuts, seeds, vegetable oils (canola, olive, peanut), and avocados.

Consumption of saturated fats within prescribed limit (10–15% of total fat intake) support functioning and synthesis of certain hormones like testosterone which aid muscle building and stamina. Excess intake can increase body fat and cause cardiac problems. Consumption of unsaturated fats particularly essential fatty acids helps in maintaining energy level, prevents inflammation of muscles cells, and speeds up the recovery.

Limiting the fat intake excessively limits the food choices, reduces the absorption of fat-soluble vitamins, and tends to cause deficiency of essential fatty acids.

Role of Vitamins and Minerals in Sports

Role of micronutrients is related to metabolism and utilization of macronutrients enhancing immunity and reducing production of free radicals. Vitamin C, B1, B2, B3 and B6 is associated with energy production, whereas folate and vitamin B_{12} are involved in production of red blood cells, DNA, and protein synthesis thus being important for tissue repair and maintenance. The antioxidant nutrients—such as vitamins A, E, and C; beta-carotene—support prevention of free-radical chain reaction and play a role in protecting the cell membranes from oxidative stress which is high in sports. In absence of antioxidant vitamins, lipid peroxidation may occur which will directly influence the cardiac input and lower down the stamina. Vitamin C is also required for formation of collagen and absorption of iron. Vitamin K controls bleeding in injury. Vitamin D improves utilization of calcium and phosphorus and it is important for bone health and immunity. Consumption of high amount of carbohydrates without vitamins will cause more metabolic stress. Certain vitamins like vitamin B_6, choline, thiamine, zinc are essential for brain function. Iron is crucial for oxygen delivery to muscles for energy production; iron is important for female athletes because they are at high risk of anemia.

Dietary antioxidants: Since intensive exercise involves considerable production of reactive oxygen species (ROS) which increases the requirements of antioxidants. Vitamins A, C, and E and several phytochemicals from dietary sources can mitigate the harmful effects of ROS in the body.

Role of Water and Electrolytes in Sports

Water and fluids intake is absolutely necessary in sports. Constant hydration is required to avoid dehydration, transport the nutrients across the cells and remove waste from there; provide lubrication to joints and maintain body temperature and body structure. Sportsperson, should continue sipping water (not gulping) throughout training and event. Plain drinking water and/or sports drink (which contain some sodium, potassium chloride, and simple sugar) can be used. Fluid intake helps to:

- Transport nutrients and fluids to cells
- Excrete the waste products from the body
- Lubricate the joints and digestive tract for smooth functioning
- Maintain the body temperature
- Maintain acid-base balance
- Reduce metabolic and psychological stress.

Under normal conditions, thirst sensation is not a very good indicator for need for water in the body. Athletes should drink fluids regularly before they get really thirsty. Serious thirst indicates that the body is in a state of dehydration. ILSI-NIN- SAI (2007) have give consequences of different stages of dehydration.

Drinking large volume of water in a dehydrated state can also cause gastric distress. The amount of water needed varies from person to person and from day to day, depending upon the individual's metabolism, environmental conditions, activity level, and hydration status. Fluid requirements are high in heavy exercise and in hot adverse conditions due to loss of body fluids. When the body is dehydrated, blood circulation decreases and the muscles do not receive enough

Table 15.9: Guidelines for fluid intake at different timings of the event.

Timings	Amount	Types of beverage
Before activity 1–2 hours 10–15 minutes	500 mL Up to 600 mL	Plain cold/cool water Plain cold/cool water, diluted fruit juice, and glucose-electrolyte drink
During activity Every 10–15 minutes	150–250 mL	Plain cold water, glucose-electrolyte drink, and diluted fruit juice
After activity Begin immediately	Compensate loss in body weight (in grams) with equal amount of fluid (in mL)	Plain water, mild sweet-tasting beverage

Source: International Life Sciences Institute-India, National Institute of Nutrition, Sports Authority of India. (2007). Nutrition and Hydration Guidelines for Excellence in Sports Performance.

oxygen for maximum performance. Playing in hot weather accelerates the loss of body water, thus more water and electrolytes are needed. It is approximately 1.5–2.0 times more. Sportspersons need to consume 1.0–1.5 times of the body weight. Sweat loss is higher in heavy exercise (may be 1–2 L/h) which depends upon intensity and duration, temperature, humidity, etc. Hence, in hot environments, fluid requirements may increase up to 5–16 L/day.

To maintain fluid balance and hydration, the person must drink 500–600 mL before exercise and 100–150 mL every half an hour during exercise. Following guidelines have been given for fluid replacement in Table 15.9.

Sports drinks can be helpful, especially for events lasting for 60 minutes or longer. They replace loss of water as well as electrolytes much faster. Warmer fluids are suggested in cooler to cold environment. Cool drinks like diluted fruit juice or sports drink are advised in warm–hot weather.

Composition of drink is very important. Presence of carbohydrate and sodium can delay fatigue and promote fluid retention. They are palatable so there are fair chances of increase in fluid intake. Sodium, potassium, and phosphorus should not be overlooked.

Role of Nutrition and Recommendations: Pre-exercise, During, and Postexercise

Sports performance may be influenced by the timing and the composition of meals and foods consumed before, during, and after exercise. Given below are salient features.

Pre-event Meals

This phase is for preparing the body for maximal output. The pre-event meal plan focuses on energy stores, i.e., glycogen stores. High-carbohydrate diet providing 60–70% calories from carbohydrates is advocated. Pre-event meals are usually planned 1–2 hours or 3–4 hours before exercise. If the event is in the morning, dinner can be high in carbohydrate and if the event is in the evening, breakfast and lunch should be high-carbohydrate meals followed by light snacks.

Combination of glucose, fructose, sucrose, and maltodextrin can be used, but large amounts of fructose are not recommended due to the greater likelihood of gastrointestinal problems. Ratio of carbohydrate to protein needs to considered and 4:1 is more acceptable.

Large meal rich in carbohydrate should be consumed 3–4 hours prior to prolonged exercise. If taken 15–60 minutes before the exercise, it can cause hypoglycemia and exert negative influence on performance. However, it may be beneficial in high-intensity exercises. Liquid meal prior to competition may be helpful. Yogurt and banana providing 200–400 kcal food can be taken. Partial replacement may be done effectively with beverages/reconstitutable powders containing maltodextrin.

Foods to be taken 1–2 hours before exercise:
- Liquid meal supplement, milkshake or fruit smoothie, sandwiches, and sports bar
- Breakfast cereals with milk, cereal bars, and fruit flavored yoghurt, fresh fruits
- 500 mL water before 1–2 hours
- 600 mL other fluids before 15–20 minutes
- Emptying of bladder 15 minutes prior to the event is a must.

Foods to be taken 3–4 hours before exercise:
- Indian thali containing dal, *chapatti*, rice, vegetable + curd + fruit (in less quantity)
- Baked beans on toast, sandwich with paneer filling/meat filling
- Fruit salad with yoghurt
- Pasta or rice with low-fat ingredients (e.g., tomato, vegetables, lean meat)
- 1.5–3 L of water above normal intake on the day of event.

During Event

This phase involves constant utilization of energy reserves from the body and loss of body fluids. The loss can be replenished instantly through beverage intake. Carbohydrate ingestion during exercise can delay fatigue and increase exercise time. It can also promote glycogen synthesis and spare breakdown of muscle glycogen. A drink containing 10% carbohydrate could delay hypoglycemia during an event of 2–3 hours like cycling. Sports drink or any other fluid preferably containing simple carbohydrate, e.g., glucose (4–8%) and protein in ratio of 4:1 help to reduce fatigue.

Postevent Requirements

This phase is for rehydration, refueling, and repairing at rest. During this phase, glycogen stores are rebuilt and proteins need to be synthesized. Protein intake with adequate amino acid composition helps in repairing and rebuilding muscle mass and adequate carbohydrate intake will support synthesis of glycogen.

Postexercise (within 30 minutes), the sportsperson should be provided about 8–10 g carbohydrate and 0.2–0.5 g protein or in ratio of 3:1 to promote glycogen synthesis and tissue repair. Further, athletes can consume carbohydrates at 1–1.5 g/kg bodyweight within half an hour to 4 hours after the event (Table 15.10). High-glycemic foods are easily digested and help in reducing the protein catabolism and enhance nitrogen retention which is favorable for muscular activities. Use of antioxidants helps to reduce oxidative stress.

Table 15.10: Postexercise needs for selected nutrients.

Water	To replace fluid lost as sweat and to aid the process of "glycogen fixation"
Electrolytes	To replenish minerals lost in sweat (e.g., sodium, chloride, calcium, magnesium)
Carbohydrate	To replenish muscle glycogen, the body's premium grade fuel for strenuous exercise and also to top up liver glycogen stores, maintain correct blood sugar levels
Protein	To repair and regenerate muscle fibers damaged during exercise, to promote muscle growth and adaptation, and to replenish the amino acid pool within the body

ERGOGENIC AIDS

According to the International Society of Sports Nutrition (2010), an ergogenic aid is any training technique, mechanical device, nutritional practice, pharmacological method, or psychological technique that can improve exercise performance capacity and/or enhance training adaptations. This includes aids that may help prepare an individual to exercise, improve the efficiency of exercise, and/or enhance recovery from exercise. Ergogenic aids may also allow an individual to tolerate heavy training to a greater degree by helping them recover faster or help them stay injury free and/or healthy during intense training.

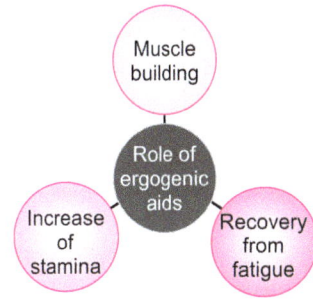

Ergogenic aids can be dietary supplements. Numerous dietary supplements have been studied for use in sports as ergogenic aids. Some of them are branched-chain amino acids, carnitine, creatine, glucosamine, chondroitin sulfate, taurine, bicarbonates, and ginseng. However, various human studies have shown conflicting results; hence, their use is also under consideration.

NUTRITION AT HIGH ALTITUDE

Thousands of people around the globe travel to mountains and hill (high altitude) for tourism, religious purposes, adventure, various sports and country's safety (military and army). Mountaineering and climbing (rock climbing, skiing), and traveling in hills have received attention in recent years for several purposes. It is also important for military and mining operations. Millions of people reside there permanently. Hills are several feet above the sea level (>5,000 ft), where oxygen supply is relatively less, atmospheric pressure is less, and weather is also cold. The human body gets acclimatized in few days or weeks to high altitude by making certain physiological changes such as increasing breathing depth and rate in low oxygen atmosphere. High altitude is a hypoxic environment which alters the cardiorespiratory system. Nutritional and physiological requirements are different. In low oxygen environment, concentrations of many substrates in the blood may vary. It may cause fatigue, headache, and alteration in appetite which may take 2-3 weeks to restore normalcy.

At high altitude, the physiology of persons may be altered which affects body composition and body functions in the following ways:
- Breathing becomes fast because of hyperventilation of lungs that is due to low oxygen pressure in air
- Hypoxia (poor availability of oxygen in body tissues)
- Sore muscles due to low pH of muscles
- Increase in BMR, increase in energy expenditure thus increasing the energy requirement
- Loss of muscle mass as well as loss of fat mass resulting in wrinkled skin
- Loss of body water because of increased respiration in cold dry air having low vapor pressure.
- Loss of body weight due to high metabolic rate at high altitude
- Body uses more of carbohydrates as fuel rather than fat because to be used as fuel, fat needs more oxygen, and in low oxygen atmosphere, carbohydrates are good source of fuel for the body.

At approx 2100 m/7000 feet above sea level, oxyhemoglobin saturation begins to decrease rapidly. There are three altitude regions that reflect the lower amount of oxygen in the atmosphere, namely:
- High altitude   = 1,500–3,500 meters (4,900–11,500 ft)
- Very high altitude = 3,500–5,500 meters (11,500–18,000 ft)
- Extreme altitude = above 5,500 meters (18,000 ft)

Chronic oxygen deprivation at high altitudes (above 5,000 m) results in many physiological changes, loss of body mass, body fat and protein stores. Reduced oxygen pressure and hypoxia as well as cold tend to reduce the maximal oxygen consumption (VO_2 max), which dramatically reduces the work efficiency and performance. Person tries to breathe in more air per minute (hyperventilation). There can be low arterial pressure of oxygen, which stimulates the chemoreceptors of the heart and respiratory center of the brain signaling for increased rate of breathing through which delivery of oxygen is improved.

Such kind of responses may be visible at low altitudes (1,500–5,000 m) in some individuals in the form of acute mountain sickness (AMS). Common symptoms of AMS are headache, nausea, vomiting, lethargy, and anorexia. Usually, these symptoms vanish when the journey is over or in a day or two after rest (simple remedy like chewing of ginger can be effective). Due to hyperventilation together with dry environment, there is risk of severe dehydration too. In addition, there is decreased thirst and increased diuresis. Chronic mountain sickness (CMS) occurs after prolonged stay at high altitude which leads to polycythemia (more number of red blood cells and low plasma volume) and hypoxemia. Some of the common problems faced by people ascending high altitude are loss of appetite, fatigue, breathlessness, insomnia, abdominal pain, constipation, nausea, and blisters in hands and feet. Longer stay at high altitudes may cause water and salt retention. Hence, food and salt needs are reduced.

During prolonged stay, plasma volume may decrease and oxygen carrying capacity is expanded by the secretion of erythropoietin (EPO) which stimulates the production of RBC. A significant reduction in the concentration of ferritin in the blood at altitudes above 2,000 m was observed. Low levels of ferritin and iron in the blood can impair the increase in hemoglobin concentration in athletes exposed to hypoxia. However, there is a limit to the body's ability to adapt. Altitude above 8000 m/26000 ft is referred to as death zone, because it is believed that the human body does not have the capacity to adapt or acclimatize.

Altered physiology at high altitude tends to alter the nutritional requirements and nutrient utilization. There can be increased requirement of energy (carbohydrate, fat, and protein), vitamin (vitamin E), and minerals (iron).

Energy: Climbing requires energy which is drawn from the muscle as well as utilization of body fat. The extent of utilization of fat and/or muscles depends upon the person's energy intake and energy expenditure. Energy expenditure is largely determined by the intensity and duration of work performed, availability of the nutrients, body stores of energy, and environmental conditions. When body tissues are used for energy, there will be loss of adipose tissues and muscle. Most studies reveal that significant weight loss occurs at altitudes. Though there is increase in BMR in high altitude and there is decreased supply of oxygen to the body that is often accompanied by both weight loss and lean mass loss. Energy requirement can be increased by 275–300 kcal/d, since expenditure is high. Depending upon the energy cost of different activities, the increase in energy cost of activities can vary from 7–25%. Mountain climbers should consume high-energy diet (may be more than 4,000 kcal/day) of which 60–70% of the calories are from carbohydrate, 20–25% from fat, and 15–20% from protein. Thus, energy is mainly obtained from carbohydrates.

Carbohydrates: Continual supply of sugar is beneficial at high altitude (HA). It can easily refuel the body. It helps in maintaining blood sugar level and glucose supply to the brain, replaces muscle glycogen, and prevents catabolism of protein for energy. Carbohydrate is beneficial because its respiratory quotient is 1.0 and can keep pace with the energy metabolism. On the other hand, if fat is exclusively taken then RQ is 0.7. High-carbohydrate diet increases the glucose metabolism.

Accessibility to food on hills may be limited, hence simple energy foods can be carried such as confectionary and bakery items. Hot beverages may be consumed if available. Simple carbohydrates are digested fast and the person may feel hungry soon, hence intake of complex carbohydrates is needed. Fruits are a better choice since they are good sources of energy, micronutrients, and phytochemicals. Low-carbohydrate intake can lead to low energy, confusion, lack of coordination, and disorientation. As per suggestions by Nutrition Foundation of India (1999), up to 750 g carbohydrates can be given for 4800 kcal diet at above 9000–12000 feet height.

Fat: At altitude >4,500 m, fat intake needs to be restricted especially above 6,300 m because at high altitude there is hypoxia, decreased respiratory capacity which tend to alter the rate of fat oxidation. However, butter, cream, nuts, and seeds are good sources for obtaining essential fatty acids.

Protein: Significant loss of muscle mass is observed at higher altitude which may increase the protein requirement. However, loss of muscle mass is largely attributed to loss of total body weight and fat mass and negative energy balance. Positive or negative nitrogen balance can be seen in high altitude depending upon the food intake in initial stay. Prolonged stay by the people who are living at high altitude for some duration in high hills may find difficulty to regain muscle mass. Intensive mountaineering sports may increase the protein requirement. Weight loss at altitude is frequently observed. Overall digestibility of protein is not significantly impaired up to 5,000 m. Adequate intake of calories will protect muscle catabolism and decrease in lean body mass. Supplements of branched-chain amino acids (leucine, isoleucine, and valine) have been found by some researchers to prevent loss of muscle at high altitude.

Water and electrolytes: There can be loss of total body water. People with AMS can have fluid shifts from intracellular to the extracellular compartment or from the extracellular to the intracellular compartment by 1 L.

Vitamins and minerals: There is not much scientific evidence regarding increase in the vitamin requirements for people living at high altitudes and in cold climate. Increase in vitamin B1, B2, B3, vitamin C, iron and calcium has supported the utilization of macronutrients and improved the performance. However, increased intake of vitamin E (tocopherol) has shown improvement in rheological characteristics of the blood and in limiting the lipid peroxidation. Increased need for iron and zinc has been postulated but it is not necessary to increase the requirement because there is increased absorption. Adequate intake of iron is essential. Use of foods containing vitamins C, E, and other antioxidants can reduce the oxidative stress and prevent cell damage caused by oxidative stress.

Dietary intake is greatly influenced by the climatic region. At high altitude, it is rather difficult to have wide variety of foods because few plants flourish and fish, poultry, and livestock are also difficult to raise. Provision of sweet and salt taste foods were found more acceptable rather bitter and sour. However, local plant foods including herbs and spices should be added in the diet for better acclimatization.

> **Laboratory Laurel:** Defence Institute of Physiology and Allied Sciences (DIPAS) has evaluated the energy requirements using standard methods such as oxygen consumption and latest techniques (doubly labeled water and accelerometry-based activity monitoring devices). The ratio scale for different categories like for armed forces at altitude and chilly cold environment was found to be in the range of 3,600–5,000 kcal with adequate intakes of other nutrients. For soldiers particularly those who consume MRE (Meal Ready-to-Eat), DIPAS found that there is no need of extra vitamin supplements. However, development of certain nutraceutical products has shown promising results.
>
> *DRDO. Environmental, Physiological and Human Factor. Res Bull Def Res Develop Org. 2011;19(6):6.*

Altitude exposure leads to considerable weight loss possibly due to lower food intake caused by loss of appetite, by hypoxia, nonavailability of familiar food, lack of comfort, negative energy balance partly due to increased basal metabolic rate, and/or high levels of activity vis-à-vis lower food intake. Other causes of weight loss are: loss of body water due to increased insensible loss through increased ventilation at high altitudes in mountainous/hilly regions, decreased fluid intake, and/or changes in fluid metabolism. Absorption of nutrients may also be affected and there can be loss of muscle mass due to lack of physical exercise and/or direct effects of hypoxia on protein synthesis. Initially, the weight loss is largely attributable to fluid loss and later due to loss of fat mass and muscle wasting. Up to altitudes around 5,000 m weight loss from fat and muscle may be avoided by adequate food intake consumed in a comfortable environment. Evidence suggests that in populations who are residing at high altitude circulating levels of high density cholesterol are higher. Higher total cholesterol has also been observed and has been attributed to erythropoiesis that occurs due to acclimatization.

NUTRITION IN SPACE

With scientific advancement, man has undertaken space travel. Nutrition is of paramount importance in maintaining the good health and optimal performance of astronauts during space flights. Astronauts tend to lose weight during flight and there is loss of bones as well as muscle. In micro gravity there is high level of oxidative damage. During space flights, astronauts undergo some physiological changes; hence, providing nutritious, appetizing high quality food products with long shelf-life is very crucial. Space foods include the products which were created and processed for consumption by "astronauts" in space satellites.

In addition to being nutritious and shelf-stable, space foods need to be designed in a way that they are easy to hold and consume in the weightless environment of the manned spacecraft and also to store for the next mealtime safely in a limited space available in the spacecraft. Various food processing and packaging technologies are used in preparation of space food.

Waste management is of paramount importance. Waste includes leftover food or biological human excreta. It is collected in special systems and germicides are used to kill bacteria that cause decay and odor.

Looking back in history, during space travel, explorers always had to face the problem of how to carry enough food for their space journey. Adequate storage space and food carried during the journey being edible throughout the voyage were major challenges. Space food systems evolved as the US space programs were developed. How space food was designed over a period of time through various voyages is briefly discussed in this section.

Mercury (1959–1963)

In the early mercury project, due to a short duration flight, complete meals were not used. The physiology of chewing, drinking, and swallowing solid and liquid food in a microgravity environment was tested. The astronauts carried bite-sized cubes, freeze-dried foods, and semi-liquids in an aluminum toothpaste-type tubes. However, they found it unappetizing, and experienced many difficulties in rehydrating the foods. Eating food from tube was also not appreciated much.

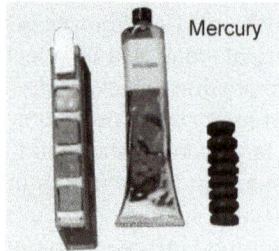

Gemini (1965–1966)

Mercury experiences were taken into consideration. Hence, tubes were discontinued. Gelatin coatings were used and process of rehydration was also simplified. Varieties of foods were made available and included grape and orange drinks, cinnamon toasted bread cubes, fruit cocktail, chocolate cubes, turkey bites, apple sauce, cream of chicken soup, shrimp cocktail, beef stew, chicken and rice, and turkey and gravy.

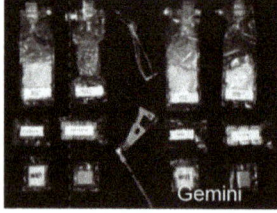

Apollo (1975)

Improvements in food design were continued and in Apollo, rehydratable food was encased in a pressure-type plastic zipper which was convenient to scoop out with a spoon and consumed. Bowls and spoons were introduced. For rehydration, water was injected into the package through the nozzle of a water gun.

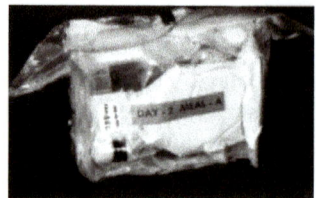

Skylab

Skylab provided a dining experience unlike any other space flight. The Skylab laboratory included a freezer, refrigerator, warming trays, and a table. The arrangement was sufficient for three astronauts for approximately 112 days. Rehydratable beverages were packed in collapsible accordion-like beverage dispensers. All other foods were packaged in aluminum cans of various sizes or rehydratable packages. Menus included processed food as well as ice cream.

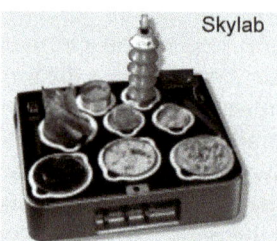

Apollo-Soyuz

During the Apollo-Soyuz test project, similar meals were provided as on the Apollo and Skylab flights. It consisted of Russian meals packaged in metal cans and aluminum tubes. Their spacecraft also had a small heating unit on board.

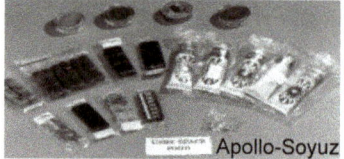

Space Shuttle

For space shuttle program, earth-like feeding approach was designed. Food varieties were expanded to 74 different kinds of food and 20 kinds of beverages. On the shuttle, food was prepared at a galley installed in the orbiter's mid-deck. This modular unit contained a water dispenser and an oven. A meal tray was used as a dinner plate. The tray was attached to the astronauts lap by a strap or could be attached to the wall. Eating utensils consisted of a knife, a fork, a spoon, and a pair of scissors to open the food packages.

Type of Space Food

Designing food for the space flights has always been an immense challenge. The food is required to be nutritious, should result in minimal changes in physiology of the crew, sustain them during the long voyage, be appetizing, and workable in the zero-gravity environment. Packaging is very important. Menus are sorted by space dieticians. Food is prepared with all the necessary and stringent processing conditions. Color codes and bar codes are usually used for each crew member. Each meal tray is labeled with all instructions for content and the method of rehydration. Then food trays are racked, locked, and shipped 10–14 days prior to the launch of the shuttle. Different types of foods used in space are given in Table 15.11. Certain foods are not allowed in space craft. For example, bread, cookies, salt and pepper, alcohol, soda or carbonated beverages, fish, chips, ice-creams. Some of them may leave crumb and that can float around and get stuck in the sensitive instruments there while others may distract the astronauts or fish failed due to poor shelf life.

Table 15.11: Different types of food and their properties.

Different types of foods	Different properties of space food
Freeze-dried or rehydratable food	Moisture is removed from the food during packaging food materials like soups, casseroles, scrambled eggs, and breakfast cereals. Usually, foods are pitted, peeled, and cut into small pieces and cooked before freeze drying. These fruits and vegetables are washed by spray of water. Some quickly scalded or blanched vegetables like peas and corn are used before freezing. These foods are easy to store and transport. They regain shape when soaked in water then ready to eat
Thermostabilized food	Thermostabilized foods are processed at high heat to destroy microorganisms so that they can be stored at room temperature. Fruits and tuna fish are thermostabilized in cans. Puddings are packaged in plastic cups. These foods are preferred as they are less time-consuming and easy to cook because they only need to be warmed (reheated) before eating
Intermediate moisture food	Intermediate moisture foods are preserved by taking some water out of the product while leaving enough in, to maintain the soft texture. Hence, they can be eaten without any preparation. They include dried peaches, pears, apricots, and beef jerky
Natural form of food	These foods are ready to eat and are packaged in flexible pouches. Examples include nuts, granola bars
Irradiated food	Irradiated foods are cooked and packaged in flexible foil pouches and sterilized by ionizing radiation so they can be kept at room temperature. Beef steak and smoked turkey are the only irradiated products being used at this time. Fruits and vegetables are also included
Frozen food	Precooked and frozen foods are quickly frozen to prevent formation of large ice crystals. This process maintains the original texture of the food and its "fresh" taste. They include quiches, casseroles, and chicken pot pie
Fresh food	Fresh foods like apple, banana, etc. are just sanitized and packed in plastic bags before loading in shuttle. These need to be consumed within 2–3 days
Refrigerated food	These foods require cold or cool temperatures to prevent spoilage. Examples include cream cheese and sour cream

Effect of Space Voyage on Nutritional Status of Astronauts

Spacecraft and its environment bring many significant changes in the physiology of the astronauts. This is largely attributed to the microgravity environment. Also, the astronauts are exposed to a much higher level of radiation than humans on Earth. Exposure to weightlessness or microgravity and radiation in the spacecraft affects almost every system in the body, including the bones, muscles, heart and blood vessels, and nerves.

In the first few days, space travelers may feel nauseated (known as space motion sickness). Other body changes include changes in the vestibular receptors of the ears due to lack of the gravity vector, creating confusion.

Metabolic, psychological, and oxidative stresses are common. Important physiological changes occur in—body fluids, blood mass, muscles and bone, immune system, digestion, psychological changes.

Body fluids: Body fluids are redistributed after the launch. There is less fluids in legs and hypotension that is soon reversed on return from space. Motion sickness in space flights is often experienced. Unique puffy appearance of the face is also seen.

Blood: There may be reduction of about 10% in the blood volume. It may be because plasma/body fluid is decreased as well as reduction in red blood cells. This may be a possible adaptation for the duration of the space flight and becomes normal on return.

> **Laboratory Laurel:** "Space anemia" is a term that reflects the loss of erythrocytes and hemoglobin. It is observed that hemolysis occurs due to change in the rheology of erythrocytes in that microgravity environment. Composition of cell membranes may also be influenced by external factors such as hypothermia, hypoxia, or variation in gravitational strength. Change in fatty acid composition of the cell membrane may increase fragility. There may be splitting of water in space environment by solar radiation or low wavelength electromagnetic radiations (such as gamma rays) that may increase generation of hydroxyl radicals. These tend to initiate chain reactions leading to lipid peroxidation. Use of antioxidants may mitigate the oxidative effects. However, further experiments are needed to integrate the dietary approach to reduce oxidative stress and space anemia.
>
> *Rizzo AM, Corsetto PA, Montorfano G, et al. Effects of long-term space flight on erythrocytes and oxidative stress of rodents. PLoS One. 2012;7(3):e32361.*

Muscles and bones: There is gradual loss of muscle mass and strength. Muscle loss or muscle atrophy brings structural changes in muscle, i.e., reduction in the size of muscle fibers. Persons might find difficulty in maintaining upright postures due to nongravitational environment. The loss can be 20–30% depending upon the duration of flight. Poor nutrition and stress may accelerate the loss. In flight, protein degradation increases and protein synthesis decreases by 20–50%. On return to gravitational environment, astronauts frequently complain of muscle soreness and tightness in the calf muscles and hamstrings. However, there is full recovery in 1–2 months postflight. Microgravity also induces bone loss. Other factors which accelerate bone loss are low level of light or no sunlight, low levels of parathyroid hormone, and vitamin D. Studies show that there is much higher loss of calcium through urine and calcium absorption is also reduced during flight. This leads to loss of bone density (1–2%). During spaceflights, bone resorption increases significantly, and formation either remains unchanged or decreases slightly. There can also be respiratory acidosis, causing pH imbalance and bone loss.

Psychological changes: Stress may develop due to isolation from their regular environment in the world. However, astronauts are well-trained for expeditionary behavior skills.

Immune dysregulation: Cell-mediated immunity is impaired which normalizes in a week or two after return to earth. Circulating levels of glucocorticoids and catecholamines increase and in turn may mediate the changes in the immune system.

Nutritional Requirements of Astronauts

Nutritional requirements of astronauts are greatly influenced by the physiological changes that occur during spaceflight. Space-nutrition specialists need to consider individual nutritional requirements as well as the cultural food preferences of astronauts. There is also a need for ensuring that there is adequate clean air, drinkable water, and effective waste collection systems.

Important nutrients for astronauts are:
- **Calcium**: Absorption is very low even with calcium supplements.
- **Sodium**: Space diet is often high in sodium.
- **Vitamin D**: Absence of sunlight causes its deficiency and affects bone. It needs to be provided by dietary sources or supplements.
- **Iron**: RBCs are adversely affected releasing the iron when newly formed RBCs are released in circulation under weightless environment leading to the increase in iron availability. Iron overload is observed; therefore, overdose of iron is not advisable.
- **Russian and American** astronauts are assumed to require about 3,600 and 3,200 kcal, respectively and the calorie distribution is about 17% from protein, 32% from fat, and 51% from carbohydrates.
- **Water**: Food consists of mainly vegetables and fruits, meat, and fish which are dehydrated to remove 70% water in order to reduce the bulk and weight. It is packaged in a way which can easily be rehydrated with hot water and can be eaten in breakfast, lunch, tea, and dinner.
  Water is generated in electrical fuel system by combining hydrogen and oxygen. It is purer than municipal water, only it is bland in taste due to lack of dissolved solids. It is stored in command module which is compartmentalized to store cold water (10°C) and hot water (80°C).
- **Antioxidants:** Since oxidative stress is higher in space, there is need for special formulation to combat this stress and development of ROS. Reactive oxygen species (ROS) will be formed by ionizing radiation due to exposure to solar and galactic radiation. Lipid peroxidation can be caused by those oxidants and thus alter cellular membranes. Proteins can be made dysfunctional and mutations in DNA can occur. In space antioxidants like vitamin A and vitamin C (ascorbic acid) and vitamin E (tocopherols) are destroyed. The required antioxidants in space are vitamin A and beta-carotene, vitamin C (ascorbic acid), and vitamin E (tocopherols) as well as several phytochemicals.

NANOTECHNOLOGY

Nanotechnology has revolutionized not only the food and agriculture industry, but several other industries as well such as oil and gas, consumer goods, aerospace, chemical, construction, and electronics among others. Nanotechnology has potential applications in food processing, food packaging, food monitoring, production of functional foods, and development of desired foods products by modifying the color, flavor, or nutritional properties. Food safety and extended shelf-life of food products are the need of hour as food gets spoiled due to moisture, oxygen, heat, light, and microorganisms. Nanotechnology can provide solutions for reducing food spoilage and food wastage and eventually help to improve food security and reduce hunger and malnutrition. Nanotechnology is being studied in a number of scientific fields such as biotechnology, molecular biology, and its study has revolutionized the science of food and nutrition and expanded its horizons. It has a role in diverse sectors like agriculture, environment, communication technology, and health. Pharma and packaging industry have already taken numerous initiatives to use nanotechnology in a variety of ways.

Nanotechnology may be defined as the technology that is used to create functional materials or devices or systems by manipulating at nanoscale (nanoscale is one billionth fractions of a meter). One nanometer (nm) is one thousandth of a micrometer (μm), one millionth of millimeter (mm), and one billionth of a meter (m). The expression nanoscale is used to refer to objects with dimensions in the order 1–100 nm. There are numerous substances such as cell components and biomolecules—hormones, DNA nutrients like amino acids, sugars, fatty acids, and phytochemicals that are nanomolecules. Nanoparticles have a large surface area, which typically results in greater chemical activity, biological activity, and catalytic behavior compared to large particles of the same chemical composition.

At nanoscale, novel properties and functions occur. Thus, nanotechnology has opened the gates and offers tremendous possibilities to create materials and devices which can be used for diagnostic and screening purposes in the field of nutrition and medical science. It helps to examine the biological processes occurring in the body as well as deliver many valuable components, food additives, fortificants, dietary supplements, etc. that were difficult to deliver previously, e.g., titanium dioxide with a particle size smaller than 100 nm is widely used as a food additive and antimicrobial agent for food packaging and storage containers. Silver nanoparticles are also used for these purposes. Delivery of such molecules may be achieved by association colloids, biopolymeric nanoparticles, and nanoemulsions. It is being investigated in dairy industry also. Nanoparticles possess unique structural, chemical, mechanical, magnetic, electrical, and biological properties. Because of their small size, nanoparticles can be used to deliver drugs to target tissues more precisely in controlled manner.

Nanotechnology implies the fabrication, characterization, and manipulation in the properties of the matter to the nanosize, thereby atoms and molecules of the matter can be developed into wide variety of products of food and health importance and also modulate their delivery system. Nanotechnology may prove a boon to mankind and is considered one of the major breakthroughs in medical science, food science, and several other fields like aerospace, microelectronics. It is being utilized in nutrition research to obtain accurate information regarding the location of a nutrient or bioactive substances in cells or tissues. It is envisaged that use of nanotechnology will enable scientists to understand interaction between nutrients and biomolecules within tissues to assess bioavailability of nutrients and to assess nutritional status.

In nutrition science, nanotechnology has proven its role in the development of dietetic foods and delivery of the nutrients and phytochemicals to the body where natural forms of food or drug cannot be consumed. Several diagnostic tools can identify the target point of disease generation and help in the treatment of the same. Some of the uses in relation to food science and nutrition have been shown here.

Potential Uses of Nanotechnology

Nanotechnology has potential applications in all aspects of food sectors including food processing, food packaging, food monitoring, production of functional foods, development of foods capable of modifying their color, flavor, or nutritional properties according to a person's dietary needs as well as production of stronger flavorings, colorings, and nutritional food additives. Nanoparticles are added to many foods to improve flow properties, color, and stability during processing, or to increase shelf-life. Nanoformulations are being developed to improve bioavailability, protect active ingredients against biodegradation, or to reduce side effects. Uses are as follows:

- Improves uptake of nutrients which are low in bioavailability or poorly absorbed
- Improves the delivery system through nanoemulsion and polymer micelle formation
- Improves nutritional status, hydration, and immune system in the body
- Investigate and monitor the cellular and molecular functions
- Monitor dysregulation/altered biological processes and systems in diseases
- Supply oxygen to organs that have inadequate oxygen
- Helps in reducing the health problems
- Development of functional foods and nutraceuticals
- Sensoceuticals to enhance the flavors, color, and aroma
- Nano-food packaging which increases shelf-stability and shelf-life of the foods
- Nanocoatings to protect food from pathogenic organisms
- Use in food packaging to contain additional nutrients
- Increases stability and sensory quality of food products
- Microencapsulation of bioactive compounds
- Nanocapsules in cooking oil may improve the use of plant sterols
- Nanosensors to detect pathogenic bacteria
- Gene therapy and tissue engineering.

Nanoemulsions consist of small droplets (1–100 nm—maximum 500 nm) that appear to be transparent or translucent with a bluish tint. They are generally used to increase the bioavailability of phytochemicals which are entrapped in the nanoemulsions; otherwise they pose functional problems due to their instability and poor water solubility. Nanoemulsion stability implies a high interfacial tension and nanoemulsions are stabilized by protein/polysaccharide complexes to attain controlled release of phytochemicals like green tea polyphenols and curcumin. It also enhances the bioavailability of the encapsulated phytochemicals.

Nanocoatings and sensoceuticals enhance the flavors and aromas in food and have been found to be helpful in deriving pleasure of eating by individual with taste and smell impairment. Nano-food packaging is used in designing functional foods. Hence, it affects the accessibility of food which leaves impact on nutritional status. Nanoscale edible coatings as thin as 5 nm wide, invisible to the human eye, are being developed to be used on meats, cheese, fruits, vegetables, confectionery, bakery goods, and fast foods.

> **Laboratory Laurel:** In 2011, it was again suggested that nanostructured oxides and phosphates of Fe and atomically mixed Fe/Zn are more promising for food fortification and other nutritional applications over existing ferrous sulfate ($FeSO_4$), NaFeEDTA, and electrolytic iron. Because new product shows high solubility at neutral pH and better sensory appeal and at gastric pH, soft agglomerates of micron size break up and rapidly dissolve in surrounding area thus increasing the bioavailability. No Fe compound was later detected in submucosa suggesting the complete utilization of iron.
>
> *Zimmermann MB, Hilty FM. Nanocompounds of iron and zinc: their potential in nutrition. Nanoscale. 2011;3(6):2390-8.*

Nanosensor: A nanosensor consists of an electronic data processing part and a sensing layer or part which can translate a signal such as light or the presence of an organic substance or gas into an electronic signal. The electrodes or the active layer can be structured at the nanometer scale. Nanosensors can help in detection of pathogenic bacteria, insects or fungus within the grain or storage bins or food containers enable the diagnosis of spoiled food easily. Consequently, humans can be saved from infectious diseases. It can also help to eliminate the toxin or dead cells at molecular level from the body. A single nanosensor can rapidly and accurately detect the presence of any number of insects, different bacteria and pathogens including fungi. The sprays containing nanoparticles may react with bacteria or insects and illuminate them. Hence, use of nanosensors can be a very useful tool for safety and prevention of food spoilage in the food chain. Packaging equipped with nanosensors is also designed to track either the internal or external conditions of food products, pellets, and containers throughout the food supply chain. It can also be applied in food analysis to pinpoint the toxin produced by the microorganism even at low level. Food poisoning episodes can be prevented.

Microencapsulation: Silicon-based nanoparticles offer a light weight, more heat resistant, and stronger covering for foods which require vacuum covering to stay fresh. Microencapsulation can enhance the bioavailability of vital food components. Nanomolecules can travel through the bloodstream, cross the blood–brain barrier, and nourish the various parts of the body. Similarly, medicines in nanosize particles can enter the body and reach the defective target cellular constituent. Hence, there is a great hope in medical science for drug delivery particularly in cancer therapy. Microencapsulation promotes delivery of nutrients and phytochemicals and enhances their absorption at the target sites. It has a potential to change the ways the food is processed, packaged, transported, and delivered to consumers.

Nanoencapsulated active ingredients like vitamins and fatty acids are used in the production of functional foods such as soft drinks, ice cream, chocolate, and chips that are marketed as healthy foods by reducing fat, carbohydrate, or calorie content or by increasing protein, fiber, or vitamin contents. Encapsulated materials are available commercially for use in processing and preservations of beverages, meat, cheese, and other foods. Nanoencapsulation is a promising technology that can be used to deliver nutrients by fortifying foods such as dairy products, cereals, breads and beverages with vitamins, minerals, omega-3 fatty acids, probiotics, bioactive peptides, antioxidants, and plant sterols. Other active ingredients, preservatives, and enzymes are also added to foods in microscale capsules. Many developed countries are using this technology to enrich their products.

Being such a young technology that has only recently come to be considered for application in food industry, knowledge gaps still exist. Most of the toxicology research carried out so far has been in the occupational sector of nanotechnology, where workers are exposed to nanoparticles for short periods of time and the path of intake is more likely inhalation or absorption (through the skin), then ingestion/oral intake, which was pointed out in both the meetings. Biodegradability of nanoparticles is another risk that needs to be taken care of.

There is concern that nanoparticles may be more toxic because they are more reactive and more mobile. They may produce greater oxidative stress as a consequence of generation of free radicals which in turn will have adverse health consequences. Also, enhanced bioavailability of specific nutrients and food additives delivered using nanotechnology needs further investigations.

"The US-FDA stated that if the chemicals have already been approved for commercial use in large particle form, nanoparticles of these chemicals do not legally require any additional authorization or trigger new safety testing. Also, food ingredients that are classified as "generally recognized as safe" (GRAS) do not require any premarket authorization from the FDA. The GRAS system also fails to differentiate between substances in larger particle or nanoparticle form".

NUTRIGENOMICS AND NUTRIGENETICS

"Nutrigenetics and nutrigenomics include the study of genetic variations and their effects on dietary response and the role of nutrients and bioactive compounds in foods in gene expression respectively". Nutrigenetics studies the relationships among genes, diet, and health outcomes. Nutrigenomics, a related but distinct field, that includes the study of how genes and nutrients interact at the molecular level, in order to provide a molecular understanding of how common chemicals in the diet affect health by altering gene expression and the structure of an individual's genome. It studies the possible interaction of different foods with specific genes to increase the risk of common chronic diseases such as type 2 diabetes, obesity, heart disease, stroke and certain cancers.

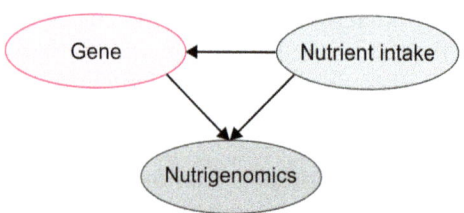

- Nutrigenetics term was used first time by Dr R.O Brennan in 1975 in his book Nutrigenetics.
- Nutrigenomics is a branch of genetic research of how foods affect our genes and how, in return, genetic variations affect the way we react to nutrients in foods.
- Nutrigenetics encompasses the study of individual differences at the genetic level that influences individual responses to diet.

Interaction of gene and dietary components can bring subtle changes in human health. Three factors are recognized as important in the science of nutrigenetics and nutrigenomics. (i) There is considerable diversity among different ethnic groups and individuals in the inherited genome. This affects the metabolism, nutrient availability, etc. (ii) There are considerable inter-individual differences in food choices, food and nutrient availability and these are largely dependent and shaped by one's culture, religion, financial status, taste and preferences, value systems as well as geographic location. (iii) Nutritional status and excess or lack of a nutrient(s) have an effect on gene expression and genome stability, and ultimately result in phenotypes that increase risk of disease particularly NCDs during the various life stages. This gene-diet interaction can play a role in onset of disease, incidence and severity of disease, and by dietary interventions, pathogenesis and progression of disease can perhaps be reduced. Study of nutrigenomics can help in development of personalized nutrition based on their genotype because the genotype and phenotype of every individual is different.

Nutrigenomics employs the gene technologies to unravel the interaction between nutritional pathways and gene expression or influence of dietary intake on health and disease depending upon the genotypes. This includes how individual nutrients influence gene stability and regulate gene expression and transcription as well as genetic mutations may affect nutrient metabolism, utilization, and risk of various diseases. It also opens the gates for treatment of diseases even like cancer. In nutrigenomics, the aim is to gain understanding about relationship between health and disease during the life span in the context of changing physiological states and needs such as growth, pregnancy, and aging.

With the success of the Human Genome Project, numerous genes have been identified and the role of different nutrients on genes has been elucidated and how genes also influence the nutrient absorption, metabolism, excretion, taste perception, and degree of satiation. Scientists envisage that nutrigenomics will be useful in routine clinical practice to prevent and cure degenerative diseases as well as reduce the need for drug and medicines.

Some Terms used to understand Nutrigenomics

Genome: Entire set of genes in the DNA embedded in the chromosomes of a given organism is called genome.

Human genome: It is a blueprint of 30,000 different protein which serves as a base for different structural components in the body, hormones, enzymes, etc.

Genomics: It is the study of the entire human genome and involves studying the actions of single genes as well as the interactions of multiple genes with each other and with the environment.

Genotype: An individual or cell with a specific genetic makeup is referred as genotype.

Phenotype: Genetic expression of a physical property in an individual.

Inheritance: It means inheriting some specific genes from individual parent or both the parents. Some genes are dominant and some are recessed. Actual trait of dominant gene determines the phenotype, e.g., one parent has blue eye and another has brown eye. The child may have blue eye due to the dominant gene. Most genes contain the information needed to make functional molecules called proteins.

Transcription: It is the process of making an RNA copy of a gene sequence. The copy is called messenger RNA (mRNA). During the process of transcription, the information stored in DNA is transferred to RNA (ribonucleic acid) in the cell nucleus.

Translation: It is assembly of polypeptide chain that is based on the sequence of mRNA. It is the process of translating the sequence of mRNA molecule during protein synthesis to a sequence of amino acids to make up the polypeptide chain. In the genetic code, in the mRNA, the sequence of base pairs (groups of three bases) encode for specific amino acids.

Polymorphism: DNA sequence of specific gene that varies among individuals.

Single nucleotide polymorphism (SNP): It relates to exchange of one nucleotide with another.

Gene expression: Together, transcription and translation are known as gene expression. Gene expression is the process by which cell converts genetic code in mRNA and protein. It translates the specific from encoded DNA into a protein in RNA during production of mRNA. Expression is regulated by many variables like dietary components.

Metabolomics: It involves identification of molecular interactions between the different molecules produced by metabolism of various nutrients and bioactive compounds and processes through which genome-encoded proteins are expressed.

It has been observed that deficiency of nutrients like folate, zinc, vitamin B6, vitamin B12, and riboflavin may cause mutation or breakage or weakening of DNA strands. Different nutrients have different effects on DNA (Table 15.12).

The *MTHFR* gene provides instructions for synthesis of the enzyme methylenetetrahydrofolate reductase. This enzyme plays a role in processing amino acids. Methylenetetrahydrofolate reductase plays an important role in folate metabolism and maintenance of homocysteine level in the blood. *MTHFR* gene can be modified depending on the amount of two essential nutrients: folate, which is the substrate for *MTHFR*, and riboflavin, a cofactor of *MTHFR*. Deficiency of these nutrients can affect *MTHFR* gene expression and thereby folate level.

There is clear evidence that glucose, fatty acids, amino acids, iron, and vitamins regulate gene expression. Omega-3 fatty acids affect transcription factor responsible for lipid metabolism. Gene expression of n-3 is associated with inflammation, lipid metabolism, and energy utilization. Protein quantity and quality influences the expression of a number of genes. In rat model, low-protein diets were found to alter expression of many genes, including those involved in insulin biosynthesis, secretion, and cellular remodeling.

Folate is also related to DNA methylation. DNA methyltransferase enzyme catalyzes one carbon transfer from S-adenosyl methionine (SAM) to a specific site of DNA. SAM metabolizes various nutrients such as folic acid, vitamin B_6, B_{12}, and methionine. Deficiency of these nutrients

Table 15.12: Nutrients involved in gene stability.

For DNA functionality	Nutrients involved
Gene expression	β-carotene
Increase in genome stability	Higher intake of vitamin E, retinol, folic acid, nicotinic acid, calcium, zinc, selenium, and epigallocatechin-3-gallate
Decrease in genome stability	Higher intake of riboflavin, pantothenic acid, and biotin
DNA damage	Deficiency of folate, zinc, vitamin B6, and vitamin B12
DNA weakening	Deficiency of folate and other methyl donor
DNA oxidation	Excess iron, inadequacy of vitamin A, C, E, selenium, and carotenoids
Inhibition of DNA repair	Niacin

Source: Schmelz EM, Wang MD, Merill AH. Genomics, proteomics, metabolomics and system biology approaches to nutrition. In: Bowman BA, Russell RM (Eds). Present Knowledge in Nutrition, 9th edition. Washington: International Life Sciences Institute; 2006. p. 8.

adversely affects DNA methylation and increases the risk of development of noncommunicable diseases (NCDs). Besides these nutrients, vitamins C and E, selenium, zinc, and niacin bring changes in DNA.

Maternal undernutrition including deficiencies of specific nutrients may alter chromatin structure during critical windows of development. Even this short-term exposure to unbalanced environment/deficiencies can result in long-lasting changes in the gene expression pattern.

Exercise has been found to turn on many genes in skeletal muscle including some genes coding for substances that have an anti-inflammatory effect. Further, in the recovery phase, other genes turned on and it has been observed that gene expression is influenced by age.

Flavonoids interact with major classes of enzymes and influence enzymatic activity and affect cell signaling. They can induce detoxification enzymes like glutathione S-transferase and others. Genes for these enzymes are regulated by antioxidants. Quercetin can modulate the gene expression of proinflammatory cytokines like tumor factor alpha by human peripheral blood mononuclear cells. It is assumed that quercetin has anti-inflammatory effect.

> Nutrigenetics specifically investigates the modifying effects of inheritance (or acquired mutations in the case of cancer) in nutrition-related genes on micronutrient uptake and metabolism as well as dietary effects on health.
>
> The field of nutrigenomics harness multiple disciplines and includes dietary effects on genome stability (DNA damage at the molecular and chromosome level), epigenome alterations (DNA methylation), RNA and micro-RNA expression (transcriptomics), protein expression (proteomics) and metabolite changes (metabolomics), all of which can be studied independently or in an integrated manner to diagnose health status and/or disease trajectory.
>
> *Fenech M, El-Sohemy A, Cahill L, Ferguson LR, French TA, Tai ES, et al. Nutrigenetics and nutrigenomics: Viewpoints on the current status and applications in nutrition research and practice. J Nutrigenet Nutrigenomics. 2011;4(2):69-89.*

It is envisaged that nutrigenomics and nutrigenetics will pave the way toward personalized nutrition. Nutritionists and dietitians would need to recognize that a person's response to diet will be influenced by the genetic background and that diet recommendations may need to be individualized based on a person's genetic makeup.

RAPID FIRE

1. Why certain foods are called functional foods?
2. What do you mean by nutraceuticals?
3. What is the difference between health supplements and dietary supplements?
4. What is the difference between prebiotic and probiotic?
5. List the benefits of prebiotics and probiotics.
6. What are the different categories of sports events and their energy requirement?
7. What physiological changes occur during exercise?
8. What is carbohydrate loading?
9. What is the composition of meals—pregame, during the event, and postgame?
10. List the key points for ensuring good nutrition of person living at high altitude.
11. What are the effects of space voyage on astronauts?
12. What is nanotechnology?
13. List the potential uses of nanotechnology in food and nutrition.
14. What is nutrigenomics?
15. What is the role of different nutrients in gene stability?

EXERCISES

1. Collect information from the market what functional foods, nutraceuticals and dietary supplements are available and for what purpose they are sold.
2. Find 2–3 sports people and find their dietary pattern and discuss as per your understanding.
3. Prepare the presentation on nutragenomics, space foods, food for mountaineer, any one.

SUGGESTED READING

1. Abdel-Salam AM. Functional foods: hopefulness to good health. Am J Food Tech. 2010;5(2):86-99.
2. Al-Dhabi NA, Arasu MV, Park CH, et al. An up-to-date review of rutin and its biological and pharmacological activities. EXCLI J. 2015;14:59-63.
3. Alfadul SM, Elneshwy AA. Use of nanotechnology in food processing, packaging and safety – review. Afr J Food Agricult Nutr Develop. 2010;10(6):2721-39.
4. Anand David AV, Arulmoli R, Parasuraman S. Overviews of biological importance of quercetin: A bioactive flavonoid. Pharmacogn Rev. 2016;10(20):84-9.
5. Arvanitoyannis IS, Van Houwelingen-Koukaliaroglou M. Functional foods: a survey of health claims, pros and cons, and current legislation. Crit Rev Food Sci Nutr. 2005;45(5):385-404.
6. Bakonyi T, Radak Z. High altitude and free radicals. J Sports Sci Med. 2004;3(2):64-9.
7. Beheshtipour H, Mortazavian AM, Mohammadi R, et al. Supplementation of Spirulina platensis and Chlorella vulgaris Algae into Probiotic Fermented Milks. Comprehen Rev Food Sci Food Safety. 2013;12(2):144-54.
8. Bhaskarachary K. Traditional Foods, Functional Foods and Nutraceuticals. Proc Indian Nat Sci Acad. 2016;82(5):565-77.
9. Bhinde G, Mandalika S. Nutritional Guidelines for Sports persons. Jaypee Health Science Publishers. New Delhi, 2018.
10. Chen AY, Chen YC. A review of the dietary flavonoid, kaempferol on human health and cancer chemoprevention. Food Chem. 2013;138(4):2099-107.
11. Ghosh D, Bagchi D, Konishi T (Eds). Clinical Aspects of Functional Foods and Nutraceuticals.
12. Das S, Santani DD, Dhalla NS. Experimental evidence for the cardioprotective effects of red wine. Exp Clin Cardiol. 2007;12(1):5-10.
13. Douglas GL, Zwart SR, Smith SM. Space food for thought: Challenges and considerations for food and nutrition on exploration missions. J Nutr. 2020; 150 (9):2242–44.
14. Food Safety and Standards Authority of India (FSSAI). (2010). Panel on Functional foods, Nutraceuticals, Dietetic Products and Other similar products. [online] Available from https://fssai.gov.in/cms/Panel-on-Functional-foods-Nutraceuticals-Dietetic-Products-and-Other-similar-products-f-s.php. [Last accessed September, 2019].

15. Ganeshpurkar A, Saluja AK. The Pharmacological Potential of Rutin. Saudi Pharm J. 2017;25(2):149-64.
16. Gurung RB, Pandey RP, Sohng JK. Natural sources. In: Stacks NM (Ed). Apigenin and Naringenin: Natural Sources, Pharmacology and Role in Cancer Prevention. United States: Nova Science Publishers; 2015.
17. Hasler CM. Functional foods: benefits, concerns and challenges-a position paper American Council on Science and Health. J Nutr. 2002;132(12):3772-81.
18. Health Canada, Therapeutic Products Programme and the Food Directorate from the Health Protection Branch. (1998). Nutraceuticals/Functional Foods and Health Claims on Foods. [online] Available from https://www.canada.ca/content/dam/hc-sc/migration/hc-sc/fn-an/alt_formats/hpfb-dgpsa/pdf/label-etiquet/nutra-funct_foods-nutra-fonct_aliment-eng.pdf. [Last accessed September, 2019].
19. http://www.fssai.gov.in/portals/0/pdf/food-act.pdf.
20. https://www.academia.edu/11921202/WHO_child_growth_standards_and_the_identification_of_severe_acute_malnutrition_in_infants_and_children.
21. https://www.cdc.gov/nccdphp/dnpa/physical/pdf/PA_Intensity_table_2_1.pdf
22. Institute of Medicine (US) Committee on Military Nutrition Research, Marriott BM, Carlson SJ. Nutritional Needs in Cold and in High-Altitude Environments: Applications for Military Personnel in Field Operations. Washington: National Academies Press; 1996.
23. International Food Information Council (IFIC). (2002). Functional Foods Attitudinal Research. Washington: International Food Information Council; 2002.
24. International Food Information Council (IFIC). The consumer view on functional foods: yesterday and today. Food Insight. 2002.
25. Jiang N, Doseff AI, Grotewold E. Flavones: From biosynthesis to health benefits. Plants (Basel). 2016;5(2):E27.
26. Kahkeshani N, Farzaei F, Fotouhi M, et al. Pharmacological effects of gallic acid in health and diseases: A mechanistic review. Iran J Basic Med Sci. 2019;22(3):225-37.
27. Kaput J, Perlina A, Hatipoglu B, et al. Nutrigenomics: concepts and applications to pharmacogenomics and clinical medicine. Pharmacogenomics. 2007;8(4):369-90.
28. Kayser B. Nutrition and high altitude exposure. Int J Sports Med. 1992;13 (Suppl) 1:S129-32.
29. Kerksick CM, Arent S, Schoenfeld BJ, et al. International society of sports nutrition position stand: nutrient timing. J Int Soc Sports Nutr. 2017;14:33.
30. Kerksick CM, Wilborn CD, Roberts MD, et al. ISSN exercise and sports nutrition review update: research and recommendations. J Int Soc Sports Nutr. 2018;15(1):38.
31. Khoo HE, Azlan A, Tang ST, et al. Anthocyanidins and anthocyanins: colored pigments as food, pharmaceutical ingredients, and the potential health benefits. Food Nutr Res. 2017;61(1):1361779.
32. Kumari M, Jain S. Tannins: An antinutrient with positive effect to manage diabetes. Res J Recent Sci. 2012;1(12):70-3.
33. Kumar S, Kumar D. Designer milk and role of gene manipulation in producing low fat and high protein milk. Trends Biosci. 2015;8(6):1568-75.
34. Michalczyk M, Czuba M, Zydek G, et al. Dietary recommendations for cyclists during altitude training. Nutrients. 2016;8(6):E377.
35. Minatel IO, Borges CV, Ferreira MI, et al. Phenolic compounds: functional properties, impact of processing and bioavailability. In: Soto-Hernandez M, Palma-Tenango M, Garcia-Mateos M (Eds). Phenolic Compounds: Biological Activity. New Delhi: InTech; 2017.
36. Misra A, Nigam P, Hills AP, et al. Consensus physical activity guidelines for asian Indians, Diabetes Technol Ther. 2012;14(1):83-98.
37. Murray B, Rosenbloom C. Fundamentals of glycogen metabolism for coaches and athletes. Nutrition Reviews. 2018;76(4):243-59.
38. Nasri H, Baradaran A, Shirzad H, et al. New concepts in nutraceuticals as alternative for pharmaceuticals. Int J Prev Med. 2014;5(12):1487-99.
39. National Aeronautics and Space Administration (NASA). (1999). Space Food and Nutrition: An Educator's Guide with Activities in Science and Mathematics. [online] Available from https://www.nasa.gov/pdf/143163main_Space.Food.and.Nutrition.pdf. [Last accessed September, 2019].
40. Niyati A, Devla MN, Acharya SR, et al. Dietary supplements: A legal status in India and in foreign countries. Int J Pharma Pharmaceut Sci. 2011;3(3 Suppl):7-12.
41. Ou S, Kwok KC. Ferulic acid: pharmaceutical functions, preparation and applications in foods. J Sci Food Agricult. 2004;84(11):1261-9.
42. Ozcan T, Akpinar-Bayizit A, Yilmaz-Ersan L, et al. Phenolics in Human Health. Int J Chem Engineer Appl. 2014;5(5):393-6.
43. Palafox-Carlos H, Ayala-Zavala JF, González-Aguilar GA. The role of dietary fiber in the bioaccessibility and bioavailability of fruit and vegetable antioxidants. J Food Sci. 2011;76(1):R6-15.
44. Pereira DM, Valentão P, Pereira JA, et al. Phenolics: From Chemistry to Biology. Molecules. 2009;14(6):2202-11.
45. Position of the American Dietetic Association: functional foods. J Am Diet Assoc. 1999;99(10):1278-85.
46. Position of the American Dietetic Association: phytochemicals and functional foods. J Am Diet Assoc. 1995;95(4):493-6.
47. Prakash D, Gupta KR. The antioxidant phytochemicals of nutraceutical importance. Open Nutraceut J. 2009;2(1):20-35.
48. Ray KS, Subbulakshmi G, Subhadra M. Methodologies for Fitness Assessment. New Delhi: Ane Books Pvt. Ltd.; 2010.
49. Reddy VS, Palika R, Ismail A, et al. Nutrigenomics: Opportunities and Challenges for Public Health Nutrition. Indian J Med Res, 2018;148:632-41.
50. Rizza S, Muniyappa R, Iantorno M, et al. Citrus polyphenol hesperidin stimulates production of nitric oxide in endothelial cells while improving endothelial function and reducing inflammatory markers in patients with metabolic syndrome. J Clin Endocrinol Metab. 2011;96(5):E782-92.
51. Safety assessment and potential health benefits of food components based on selected scientific criteria. ILSI North America Technical Committee on Food Components for Health Promotion. Crit Rev Food Sci Nutr. 1999;39(3):203-316.
52. Saibabu V, Fatima Z, Khan LA, et al. Therapeutic potential of dietary phenolic acids. Adv Pharmacol Sci. 2015;2015:823539.
53. Santini A, Cammarata SM, Capone G, Lanaro A, Gian Carlo Tenore GC, Pani L, Novellino E. Nutraceuticals: opening the debate for a regulatory framework. Br J Clin Pharmacol. 2018 84(4): 659–72.
54. Shafiee MN. Space food technology: Production and recent developments. Int J Adv Res Technol. 2017;6(2):120-9.
55. Shahidi F, Ambigaipalan P. Phenolics and polyphenolics in foods, beverages and spices: Antioxidant activity and health effects – A review. J Funct Foods. 2015;18:820-97.
56. Shipp J, El-Sayed M, Abdel-Aal. Food applications and physiological effects of anthocyanins as functional food ingredients. Open Food Sci J. 2010;4:7-22.
57. Simon-Schnass IM. Nutrition at high altitude. J Nutr. 1992;122(3 Suppl):778-81.
58. Singh SN, Sridharan K, Selvamurthy W. Nutrition in High Altitudes. Bull Nutr Foundation India. 1999;20(3):1-3.
59. Srinivas PR, Philbert M, Tania QV, et al. Application of nanotechnology in food and dairy processing: an overview. Pak J Food Sci. 2012;22(1):23-31.
60. Srinivas PR, Philbert M, Vu TQ, et al. Nanotechnology research: Applications in nutritional sciences. J Nutr. 2010;140(1):119-24.

61. Subbulakshmi G, Subhadra M. Functional Foods and Nutrition. New Delhi: Astral International Pvt. Ltd.; 2014.
62. Tamang JP, Shin DH, Jung SJ, et al. Functional properties of microorganisms in fermented foods. Front Microbiol. 2016;7:578.
63. Tsao R. Chemistry and biochemistry of dietary polyphenols. Nutrients. 2010;2(12):1231-46.
64. United States Department of Agriculture (USDA). (2007). USDA Database for the Flavonoid Content of Selected Foods, Release 3.1 (December 2013). [online] Available from https://www.ars.usda.gov/northeast-area/beltsville-md-bhnrc/beltsville-human-nutrition-research-center/nutrient-data-laboratory/docs/usda-database-for-the-flavonoid-content-of-selected-foods-release-31-december-2013/. [Last accessed September, 2019].
65. USDA Foreign Agricultural Service. (2018). New FSSAI Directives for Certain Ingredients under Functional Foods. [online] Available from https://gain.fas.usda.gov/Recent%20GAIN%20Publications/New%20FSSAI%20Directives%20for%20Certain%20Ingredients%20under%20Functional%20Foods_New%20Delhi_India_9-12-2018.pdf. [Last accessed September, 2019].
66. Vauzour D, Rodriguez-Mateos A, Corona G, et al. Polyphenols and human health: prevention of disease and mechanisms of action. Nutrients. 2010;2(11):1106-31.
67. Williams D, Kuipers A, Mukai C, et al. Acclimation during space flight: effects on human physiology. CMAJ. 2009;180(13):1317-23.
68. World Health Organization (WHO), Food and Agriculture Organization of the United Nations (FAO UN). (2006). Probiotics in food: Health and nutritional properties and guidelines for evaluation. [online] Available from http://www.fao.org/3/a-a0512e.pdf. [Last accessed September, 2019].

16 CHAPTER

Nutrition and Health Significance of Food Ingredients

> **KEY CONCERNS AND KEY CONCEPTS**
> What is the nutritional significance of individual food items in the food groups:
> - Cereal, millets, and their products
> - Pulses and oils seeds
> - Milk and milk products
> - Meat, fish, poultry, and egg
> - Fruits and vegetables
> - Fats and oils
> - Sugars and sweeteners
> - Spices and condiments
> - Herbs–fresh and dried
> - Tea, coffee, and cocoa

INTRODUCTION

For centuries, India has had a system of food beliefs related to health and diseases as well as for different life stages of the life cycle. This is evident in scriptures such as Bhagvad Gita. Ayurveda which is around 5000 years old considers food (*ahar*) as one of the pillars for being healthy. Foods were considered to have specific properties/attributes and in most Indian communities, numerous ingredients are an integral part of their diets, some ingredients that are seasonal are preserved, and many recommended for specific uses. The Charaka Samhita states:

> "*Tat cha nityam prayunjeet svasthyam yen anuvartate. Ajaatanam vikaranam anuttpattikaram cha yat.*"(*Charaka Samhita: Sutra Sthana: 5*) "The diet which besides providing the basic nutrition to the body, helps to maintain the healthy state of the body, and prevents the occurrence of diseases should be consumed." "At different stages of life, the constitution of the human body changes and it requires modulating one's eating habits to sustain normal physiological functions, health, and well-being." In Ayurveda, food is characterized by the action on the individual. Food can alter moods and food is believed to have an effect on psychological dispositions; there is a subtle link between disease manifestation and six psychological states—lust, anger, greed, desire, attachment, and ego.

Traditionally, Indian foods were classified into three main categories (Table 16.1). Cooked vegetables, milk, fresh fruits, and honey were considered *Satvika foods* meant for the truly wise persons. Foods meat, liquor, garlic, spicy, and sour foods were classified as *Tamasika foods* that bring out undesirable qualities of human behavior and the foods that give enough energy and vigor to carry out daily work were categorized as *Rajsik foods*.

A similar classification is mentioned in the Bhagvad Gita. Ayurveda recommends consumption of seasonal foods.

Table 16.1: Satvic, Rajasic and Tamasic foods.

Sattva (contented state)	Light food—balances doshas, brings mental harmony, evokes conscious awareness	Fresh vegetables, rice, milk, butter, honey, fruits, nuts in right quantity
Rajas (excited state)	Rich food—stimulates fantasy, jealousy, ego, to some extent needed in modest amount	Garlic, coffee, wine, fried, too spicy, too hot
Tamas (lethargic disposition/ dull/sluggish)	Impure and stale or unhealthy food Enhances emotions like greed, ignorance, and laziness	Frozen foods, peanuts, certain root vegetables, leftover food, meats that need more energy to digest

Season played and still plays a big role because various foods grow/are produced in different seasons. In the Rig Veda, about 67 medicinal plants were described and in the Atharva Veda, 293 such plants were described. The Charaka and Sushruta Samhitas are texts dealing with healing and longevity. The Ashtanga Hridaya besides dealing with medicine contains dietetics as an integral component and in Ayurveda, diet and herbal preparations are an integral part of the practice in order to restore harmony or balance. Thus, food is viewed as medicine. It could be used as a primary mode of treatment, a precursor for specific treatment, in preparation of rasayanas, as an adjuvant to other treatment, for specific disease conditions, besides giving guidelines for physiological conditions.

It is evident that since the evolution of man, a wide variety of ingredients are being used. In traditional systems of medicine and in each culture, various foods have been ascribed properties associated with health. Each food ingredient inherently contains various types of chemical components in the form of nutrients, phytochemicals, essential oils, flavor compounds, pigments, and enzymes. By virtue of these valuable components, different food ingredients not only provide essential nutrients, impart color, flavor, texture, and variety to diets but also have medicinal value, making them valuable for disease prevention and health promotion.

This chapter deals with the nutritional and health significance of foods commonly consumed in various forms. Foods have been categorized on the basis of the similarity in their biological nature and nutritional benefits:

1. Cereal, millets, and their products
2. Pulses and legumes
3. Vegetables and fruits
4. Nuts
5. Milk and milk products
6. Egg, seafood, fish, and meat
7. Fats and oils
8. Sugars and sweeteners
9. Spices and condiments
10. Herbs—fresh and dried
11. Tea, coffee, and cocoa

CEREALS, MILLETS, AND THEIR PRODUCTS

Cereals belong to the family of cereal grasses. The word "cereal" is derived from "Ceres," the goddess of harvest and agriculture. Cultivation of cereals began around 10,000 BC. Wheat, rice, maize, rye, oats, and barley are cultivated and consumed throughout the world in various forms. Most of them are part of staple diets. Some cereals or their parts are also used in animal feed, ethanol production, and in various other non-food industries. Besides these, there are some pseudocereals or lesser known cereals like amaranth and buckwheat which are used in some parts of the world. With advances in agro-biotechnology and DNA-recombinant technology, it is possible to enrich the grain itself with selected nutrients. Golden rice is one example which contains higher amount of vitamin A, iron and zinc. High lysine wheat and maize varieties are also cultivated.

In general, cereals and millets are rich in carbohydrate, low in fat, and good sources of protein, vitamins, minerals, and fiber. Cereals are low in lysine, threonine, and tryptophan and high in methionine; hence, protein quality of cereals is considered to be poor, which is basically due to the high concentration of the storage protein prolamine that has low lysine content. Prolamine content is higher in maize and sorghum but very low in oats and rice. Hence, biological value of oats and rice protein is relatively high. Plant breeders have developed varieties with better amino acid profile of cereal proteins.

Consumption of cereals/millets with pulses complements the amino acid composition of both. Nutrient composition of the different cereals varies considerably and is influenced by cultivar, agro-climatic conditions, milling, extraction, storage conditions, and food preparation methods. According to the National Nutrition Monitoring Bureau (NNMB) report (2012) based on cereal consumption, average consumption of cereals and millets in Indian households is 375 g/day/person (ranging from 286 g in Gujarat and 430–434 g in Odisha and Uttar Pradesh). Consumption of millets ranged from 46 g (Madhya Pradesh) to 153 g (Gujarat).

Cereals and millets need to be processed before consumption because these are hard seeds. Different methods are used to make them edible and these procedures have remarkable impact on nutritional quality as well as their effects on health. Cooking further influence the palatability, digestibility, and satiety. Excessive milling increases losses of vitamins, minerals, and important phytoconstituents with health benefits including fiber. Therefore, national and international health organizations and expert groups advocate the consumption of whole grain foods as they are protective against the development of several degenerative (non-communicable) diseases like diabetes, obesity, heart diseases, and certain cancers. They are good sources of calcium, iron, and zinc but the presence of phytates limits the bioavailability of these minerals. Certain cereals/millets contain considerable amount of phytate that binds calcium, iron, and zinc and reduces their bioavailability. However, traditional domestic processing techniques like soaking, germination, fermentation, and puffing reduce the phytate content, thus enhancing the availability of minerals.

Grain Structure

Structurally, cereal grain is a monocotyledon signifying one endosperm. The grain can be divided into three major parts—bran, endosperm, and germ. For example, in wheat, endosperm constitutes 80–85%, bran 13–17%, and the germ a small fraction 2–3%. In between the endosperm and bran, is a layer called aleurone layer which protects the grain.

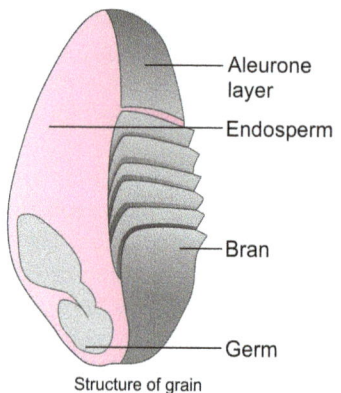

Structure of grain

Bran is separated from the starchy endosperm during the first stage of milling. Edible portion of bran is largely composed of dietary fiber consisting of cellulose, hemicelluloses, and lignin (also *see* Chapter 2). Endosperm is primarily a store house of starch and some vitamins like pantothenic acid. Some amount of protein and fat is also present. The aleurone layer is important in terms of its nutritional composition and health benefits. It is rich in protein, B vitamins like niacin, thiamine, and pentosans. It also contains enzymes which play role in germination. Wheat germ is separate entity and wheat germ oil is the richest source of vitamin E. Amino acid composition of wheat germ promotes growth. However, it is most susceptible to milling rate. Higher extraction rate chips off the aleurone layer with consequent loss of nutritional quality of grain. The nutritional benefits and health significance of individual cereals which are commonly

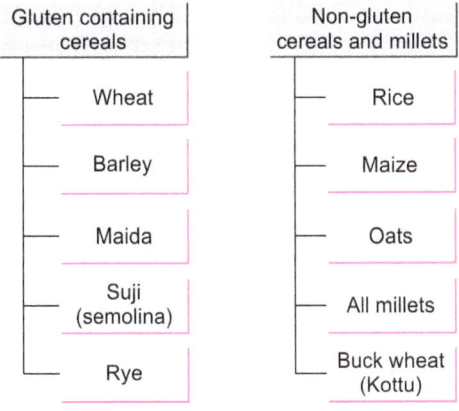

Fig. 16.1: Gluten and non-gluten cereals.

consumed in India are as follows. Some cereals contain gluten (a protein to which some people are found allergic to) whereas other grains including millets do not contain gluten; these are shown in Figure 16.1.

Wheat (Triticum aestivum)

Wheat is a staple grain, primarily consumed in the form of *chapatti*, *paratha*, *puri*, and bread. It is also used in making certain snacks. Commonly used wheat products are wheat flour, *dalia*, *suji* (*rawa*), and *maida*. Pasta, noodles, and vermicelli are other commonly used products. Wheat endosperm also contains pigments like carotene and xanthophylls due to which pasta looks yellowish in color. Lutein another important carotenoid, with high antioxidant activity, is present in the bran and germ fractions of wheat. Lutein, along with zeaxanthin, is important for health of skin and eyes in humans. Fiber and several antioxidants present in different part of the wheat grain are useful in improving the insulin sensitivity and reduce risk of metabolic syndrome and certain cancers (breast cancer).

Wheat is considered to be nutritious and health promoting. Satiety value of wheat is higher than other foods. It provides significant amount of calories, protein, carbohydrates, B vitamins, trace elements, and dietary fiber. Refining does not have significant effect on protein and carbohydrate content on dry weight basis but drastically reduces the in vitamins content and some trace elements. Refined wheat flour (*maida*) less vitamins and minerals than whole wheat flour as they are lost during refining.

There are two types of wheat, "hard wheat" and "soft wheat." Both differ in nutrient composition and rheological properties. These properties depend on the structures and interactions of the grain storage proteins, namely gliadin and glutenin which together form "gluten" a protein that determines the quality of wheat. Gluten develops during dough making, with formation small case. Formation of gluten makes the dough stretchable that can entrap air. Hence, gluten is important in *chapatti* or bread making.

Hard wheat like durum wheat contains 10–18% protein and more gluten that make the dough stretch more. This property is necessary and is used in bread and pasta making but undesirable for biscuits, cakes, and muffins. Therefore, soft wheat containing 8–11% protein is used in biscuits and cakes. Wheat is used in a wide range of processed food products by industry. However, gluten may be a problem in certain pathological conditions like celiac disease, in which the person has gluten intolerance or is gluten-sensitive. Hence, a gluten-free diet is recommended in celiac disease; however, it is not advisable for persons who are healthy and do not have celiac disease.

Different types of wheat products are processed and/or manufactured. Table 16.2 indicates their uses,

Table 16.2: Wheat products, their common food preparations, nutritional, and health significance.

Wheat and wheat products	Uses	Nutritional and health significance
Wheat	Germinated, puffed	Good source of energy, protein, fiber, thiamine, vitamin E, low fat content, supplies considerable proportion of dietary zinc and iron
Wheat flour	*Chapatti*, *puri*, *naan*, bread, or *laddoo*	Staple food gives satiety and contains nutrients mentioned above. Sieving can reduce dietary fiber and vitamins and minerals
Broken or cracked wheat (*Dalia*)	Porridge—sweet without milk, Lapsi salted with or without vegetables	Contain more amount of nutrients than other wheat products, hence more nutritious as part of the germ, bran and parts of aleurone layer are retained
Semolina (*Suji* or *rawa*)	*Halwa* (*sheera*), *upma*, *laddoo*, other snacks	Usually roasted before use. Provides energy and protein but lesser amount of vitamins and fiber than wheat. Easy to digest and easy to cook
Vermicelli	Extruded form made from flour—used in upma, kheer, etc.	Provides energy and some protein, good digestibility, and easy to cook
Refined flour or *maida*	White bread, biscuits, cakes, etc., *samosa*, *kachori*, fried snacks like *mathri*, *bhatura*, etc.	Provides starch, some protein but little vitamins, minerals, and fiber. Over consumption is linked to constipation, obesity, diabetes, etc.
Bulgur wheat	Commonly used in Turkish, Middle East, and Mediterranean dishes like soups, breads	It is parboiled, dried, and the bran is partially removed. It looks like cracked wheat. It is more digestible and high in fiber and has a nutty flavor
Pasta/Spaghetti Macaroni	Available in different shapes and sizes. Boiled before use; various dishes are made	Usually made from durum wheat contain good quality protein. Some nutrient addition is done since the preparations contain egg, meat, cheese, or vegetable puree like spinach, tomato, etc.
Noodles	Boiled and seasoned noodles/instant noodles	Usually made with *maida* or soft wheat. High in calories (saturated fats) and sodium and some food additives and low in fiber and micronutrients. Advised to avoid or eat in limited amount and frequency

nutritional value, and health significance processed and/or manufactured.

Rice (Oryza sativa)

Today rice is a staple food for more than half of the world's population, particularly in Asia. There are innumerable varieties of rice cultivated in different parts of the world. Asian rice is most widely known and it is estimated that there are about 40,000 varieties. There are wide variation in different varieties owing to agroclimatic and genetic conditions and substantially in terms of amylose and amylopectin content. Unpolished rice contains important nutrients. People are used to consuming white rice that is milled and polished to improve its acceptability but during polishing, the B vitamins are lost. Basmati rice is highly valued for its fragrance, cooking and nutritional quality. Similarly, in Maharashtra, there is a rice called "ambe mohar" which has a typical fragrance. Golden rice is genetically modified to increase β-carotene in rice grain itself. Brown rice is relatively richer in several nutrients than polished rice. Black rice popular in North eastern region is rich in anthocyanin and sweet and nutty in flavour. Parboiled rice has better nutritive value than white, milled, polished rice. Further, water-soluble vitamins are also lost during several washings and cooking, particularly when excess water is thrown out in order to reduce the starch. Protein quality of rice is good because of its amino acid composition. Polished rice does not contain much iron but rice flakes and puffed rice contain more iron. Rice is easy to digest and used in most digestive disorders. Many people perceive satiety after consuming rice. Rice contains less magnesium, zinc, copper, and manganese than wheat but unlike wheat it does not contain any gluten. Amino acid score and NPU of rice is higher than wheat hence it is easily digested, thereby raises blood sugar levels faster than wheat. Some long grain varieties do elevate the blood glucose level owing to their high amylose content. However, few rice varieties have been found to have low glycemic index (<60). At the same time, white rice, especially, is considered a culprit for raising the blood sugar level. It is not the rice but the glycemic index of the food. In case of rice, it is the ratio of amylose and amylopectin that determines the GI and outcome of rice consumption. Rice cultivars containing high amount of amylose has low GI and does not raise the blood sugar level. However, all varieties do not have a high GI, and the GI of different varieties has been found to range from around 40 to about 90. During cooking rice, starch undergoes gelatinization. When cooled, starch is retrograded and contributes to the resistant starch content (Table 16.3).

Brown rice: Brown rice is unmilled rice containing the seed coat and germ and only the inedible hull is removed from the paddy. It has a higher content of nutritional components, particularly dietary fiber, phytic acid, vitamins E and B, and γ-aminobutyric acid (GABA), phytochemicals, than ordinary milled rice. These biofunctional components exist mainly in the germ and bran layers, most of which are removed by polishing or milling. However, brown rice takes longer to cook and cooked brown rice is harder to chew than white rice. It has a nutty flavor and is susceptible to rancidity. Brown rice is available as germinated and non-germinated form. Germinated brown rice has a better texture, better palatability and contain high amount of GABA. This kind of rice shows good glycemic control.

Table 16.3: Rice forms and their nutritional and health significance.

Rice products	Uses	Health significance
Paddy	Rice bran is used to extract rice bran oil (RBO)	Rice grain is enclosed in a thick rough inedible casing. Rice is harvested in this form that is called paddy. Husk is removed to various degrees and husk is used in industries including oil industry to get RBO.
Brown rice	Rice preparations	Only husk of the paddy is removed and grain has brown streaks. It contains the germ, endosperm and the fibrous bran. Thus it takes more time to cook. It provides similar energy but higher amount of fiber, vitamins, minerals, phytochemicals as compared to white rice.
Milled rice (polished white rice)	Rice preparations like *pulav*, *biryani*, *kheer*, *khichri*, etc.	Milling rice includes polishing. During milling the husk, bran and even germ is removed depending upon the degree of polishing which results in significant loss of fiber and all other nutrients.
Parboiled rice	*Pulav* and *biryani*	Parboiling involves 3 steps namely soaking, steaming and drying in which paddy is soaked for several hours, then partially boiled before drying. It is followed by removing the husk. This rice has better nutritional profile, as parboiling drives the nutrients, especially thiamine, from the bran to the endosperm and starch gets gelatinized hence it is harder in texture.
Rice flakes	*Poha* or *chivda* and various dishes made with poha	Rice flakes are popularly called *poha*. Process of making *poha* consists of soaking for 4–6 hours, after which the paddy is pressed and roasted, which makes it more digestible, nutritious as nutrients are transferred from husk to the grain.
Puffed rice	Used in many preparations, e.g., *namkeen*, *laddoo*, *bhel*, *jhalmuri*	It is also called *laiya*, *kurmura*, *murmura*, etc. The process of puffing the rice makes it nutritious but its volume is high hence consumed less hence good for dieters and its powder is also used in complementary and some therapeutic foods.
Rice flour	Foods for infants and other dishes including chapati and making noodles	Gluten-free, hence used in many gluten-free preparation as filler and making it more crispier.

Red rice: In some parts of India and Sri Lanka, some varieties of red rice are cultivated and consumed. Traditional red varieties contain higher levels of protein with well-balanced amino acids and higher contents of fat, fiber, and vitamin E (tocopherols and tocotrienols) than the new-improved ones. Wide variation is observed in their antioxidant capacity, major phenolics, and nutritional parameters. Proanthocyanidins are the major pigment detected only in the traditional red varieties but not in the new varieties.

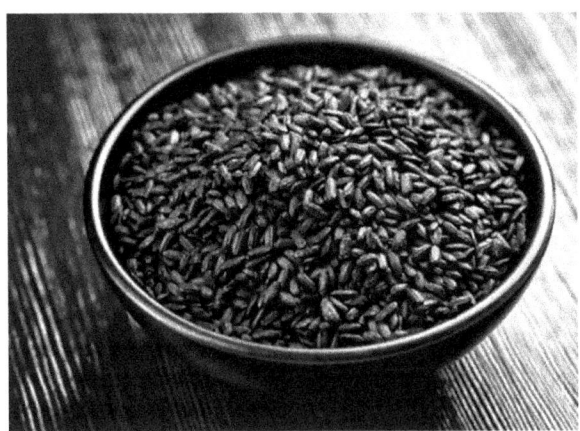

Black rice: Black (purple) rice is becoming popular and it is also belongs to *Oryza sativa L*. It has good nutrition value, and phytochemical properties. Black rice is cultivated in some parts of India and contains a high amount of anthocyanins that give this rice good antioxidant properties. This rice was considered to be medicinal rice or longevity rice. It has been found to be have cardioprotective effects.

Maize/Corn (Zea Mays)

Maize is a staple food in many developing countries. The term maize is derived from Spanish term *maiz*. The word "maize" is generally used in agriculture and scientific citations whereas the word 'corn' is used for the same grain in countries like USA. However, there is considerable difference in the properties of maize flour and corn flour. Maize contains varying amount of nutrients while corn flour is so processed that it is mainly starch. There are numerous varieties of corn. Sugar-rich varieties are called sweet corn and are often consumed as vegetables. Baby corn is also used in some cuisines.

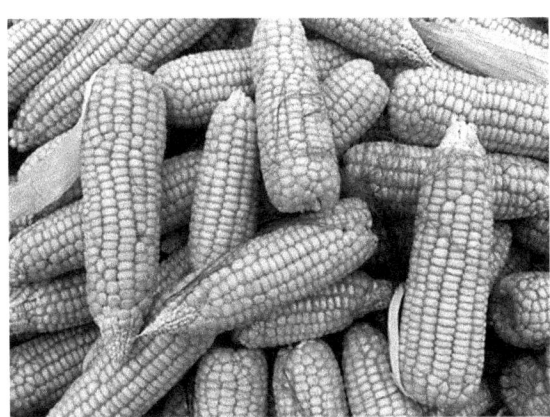

Some maize varieties are yellow and some are white or cream. Nowadays purple and black maize cobs can also been seen in some geographical area. Since pigments have demonstrated different health benefits. For example, yellow corn is rich in carotenoids (α and β carotenes, xanthophylls, cryptoxanthin) and total phenolic compounds and antioxidant capacity, vitamins, starch, and dietary fiber and low in fat as compared to white or cream varieties. Due to its composition, corn is useful in heart disease, high cholesterol, and hypertension. It is also a useful ingredient in gluten-free diets as it does not contain gluten. High-carotenoid genotype contains more amounts of total phenolics, ferulic acid, and antioxidant activity as compared to white corn. Cooking with lime is called nixtalization. Corn is also frequently used in extrusion processing. Nixtallization and extrusion retain more phytochemicals particularly ferulic acid which is good anti-aging compound.

However, the protein quality and niacin content of maize are significantly low. People living on maize diets showed signs of pellagra and kwashiorkor. High leucine content in the grain is found to adversely affect the niacin metabolism which may result in symptoms of pellagra. Nixtallization process tends to release the niacin and tryptophan, making these compounds more bioavailable. The protein quality of maize is poor because the protein present in maize—zein contains lower amounts of lysine and tryptophan compared to other grains. Thus, diets based solely on maize are not suitable for growth of children. However, treatment of maize with alkali can enhance the availability of niacin. High protein maize (HPM) varieties have been developed for better nutritional quality. On the other hand, being gluten-free, corn/maize is suitable for patients with celiac disease.

> **Nixtamalization:** It is a traditional process used in Mexico and Central America for centuries. Dried maize seeds are soaked and cooked in alkaline water usually lime water before dehulling the grains. The term refers to removal of the pericarp of any grain using an alkaline process. This process tends to increase bioavailability of niacin, iron, and zinc, increase the calcium content, and also reduce the mycotoxin. The grain is more easily ground. At industrial level, enzymes are used for nixtamalization.

Different forms of maize or corn are used as food and may vary in their starch content. Hence, different varieties of corn are used for different purposes. Besides being a good source of carbohydrate, maize provides fiber.

Maize flour: Dried seeds of maize are milled into the flour. "Makke di roti" is a popular dish eaten with "sarson ka saag" in northern India. Maize/corn can be ground to fine, medium, or coarse and also referred as corn meal. Corn meal is used to make corn bread in some countries whereas corn flour is used as a thickener in preparations like stew, sauces, etc.

Corn flour: During its manufacture, only endosperm/starch is retained while fiber, germ and nutrients are removed. It is an ingredient generally used as a thickening agent in soups and curries; for coating cutlets and kebabs; bulk agent in desserts and Indian sweets; and in confectionary, chewing gums, and bakery. It is also used in non-food industries like textile, paper, powders, adhesives and medical use.

Corn syrup: Corn is treated with acid and enzymes to make corn syrup. It is used as a sweetener in cakes, cookies, and candy to keep them moist. It is usually composed of dextrin, dextrose, and other carbohydrates. Another form of corn syrup is High Fructose Corn Syrup (HFCS) which contains relatively more amount of fructose and is relatively lower in cost. It is used worldwide in food and beverages. The reason for using HFCS instead of plain sugar is attributed to it high sweetness (>70%), easy transportation, and storage. Commercial soft drinks, ice-creams, jams, and jellies usually contain HFCS. However, consumption of high fructose corn syrup has been found to increase the risk of obesity, particularly central obesity, elevated circulating triglyceride levels, diabetes, and heart disease.

Corn oil: Corn oil is obtained from maize kernels. It contains considerable amount of PUFA (both n-6 and n-3) including essential fatty acids, phytosterols, and tocopherols. Hence, it provides several health benefits. It is a good choice for salad oil as well as for cooking and frying.

Popcorn: It is essentially popped kernels of maize made by passing through steam under high pressure and heat. Soon the endosperm bursts and the kernel is "popped." The volume of popcorn is large; it is light in weight, cheap, and a popular snack. Popcorn is high in dietary fiber, low in fat and calories, and contains no sugar (unless it is caramel popcorn) and very little sodium (until salted). Hence, it is good for weight watchers and people with dietary restrictions. Addition of salt, butter, spices, caramel, etc., may make popcorn more tasty and desirable, but the additions are not very good for health. Popcorn is used for many non-food purposes like decorative strings and as packaging material.

Cornflakes: The first commercial cereal food was invented by WL Kellogg in the 1860s, while searching for a digestible bread substitute for a patient in a sanatorium in America. Incidentally, the person forgot to switch off the boiling cereal. Rather than throwing the lot, he rolled the overcooked grain, dried them, and found to his surprise that each grain is converted into a flake. This serendipitous discovery led to the development of a new product called "Cornflakes", a well known product use it as a **Breakfast cereal**. It is a ready-to-use product usually marketed in packaged form. It is sometimes fortified with vitamins and minerals and different flavors like chocolate. Cornflakes are crisp in texture and usually consumed after addition of milk or fruit juice and considered as a full meal for breakfast. The fried form is also used in snacks. Cornflakes have been found to have a high glycemic index. New researches indicate that consumption of cornflakes may be linked to obesity and cardiovascular function.

Oats (Avena sativa)

Oats are usually cultivated in countries like England and Scotland but not much in tropical countries. Due to its benefits in many chronic diseases, it is being used in different parts of the world including India. Oats are processed like other grains and different types of processed oats are commercially available. Steel cut oats are made by crushing the oat grain (also called oat groats) into pieces. Oat flakes are made by flattening the oats between two rotating rollers. Oat groats are the whole grains composed of endosperm and the germ. Oatmeal is made from whole or steel-cut groats with two rotating roller oat groats from which hull is removed. Rolled oats are prepared by light steaming of oat groats followed by rolling through the roller mill, where they are flattened to various thicknesses. Quick cooking oats are made by rolling the flakes very thin and/or steaming them longer so that it cooks faster. Instant oats are also precooked as quick cooking oats, but it may be finer and also contain additional ingredients for extra flavour and texture. Oat flour is the whole grain flour.

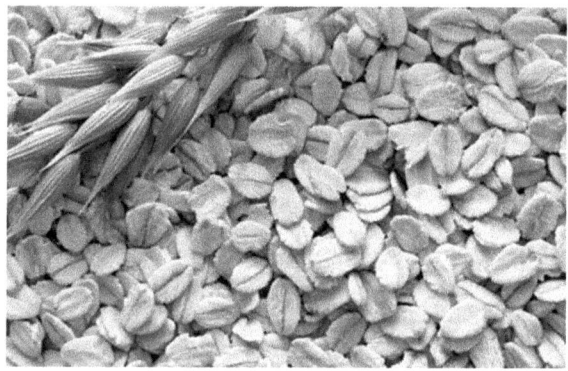

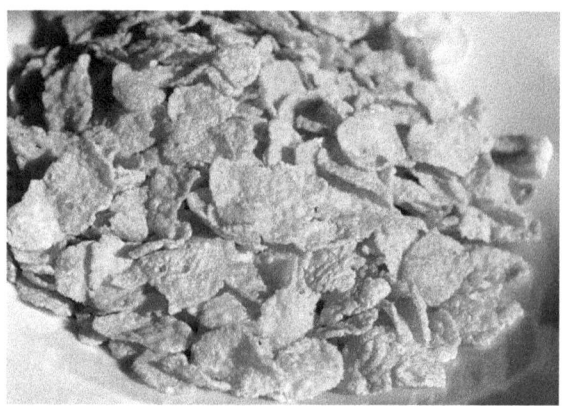

Oats are richer in protein and fat compared to other grains. It is highly valued for its content of soluble fiber (β glucan) which helps to reduce LDL cholesterol in blood. About 3 g of β glucan is required for the beneficial effect. The soluble fiber in oats reduces glycemic index of foods into which it is incorporated in sufficient amounts and can improve postprandial glycemic and insulinemic responses. It is a good source of selenium, avenanthramides, tocotrienols, and tocopherols all being antioxidants which protect against oxidative stress. Avenanthramides are polyphenols that have been shown to have anti-inflammatory, anti-proliferative, and anti-itching properties. Thus, oats exhibit a protective role against coronary heart disease, colon cancer, and skin irritation. It is gluten-free and well suited for people who cannot tolerate gluten, e.g., celiac disease. Oats are also a good source of magnesium. They are used as a breakfast cereal, in porridge, cookies, and cakes and in many dietetic food products. Oats' consumption has been advised in cardiovascular disease, diabetes, certain cancers, obesity, poor immune system, bowel health, and during menopause.

Barley (Hordeum vulgare)

Barley is an age old food grain which has been written about in Ayurveda. It was the first staple food of Aryans and is mentioned in the *Rigveda*. It is comparable to oats in terms of nutritional and health benefits like cholesterol-reducing and blood sugar control properties due to the presence of β-glucan, a soluble fiber. Some studies have shown it to be useful in weight management. The fiber in barley is present in the whole grain rather than just in the outer layer as in case of other cereals. It is rich in thiamine, riboflavin, and niacin. It is also rich in selenium and tocotrienols and thus has antioxidant capacity. It is low in fat, easy to digest, and useful during illness. Pearl barley (seed) is generally used in the form of porridge. Barley water is often given in urinary and kidney problems. Gripe water given to infants is made from barley. It is also used in malted form, popularly used in food supplements and infant food. Malting is also done in breweries and distilleries. Malting is a treatment in which barley grain is steeped in water and allowed to germinate for 4–6 days. During germination, dormant enzymes are activated and convert the starch into maltose. Making the malted grain malted grain more digestible. Malted barley contains more amount enzymes (amylase) and simple sugars, thus it is more easily digested and may be suitable for infants and invalids. However, malted barley has more gluten content than the original barley so it needs to be avoided in gluten-free diets.

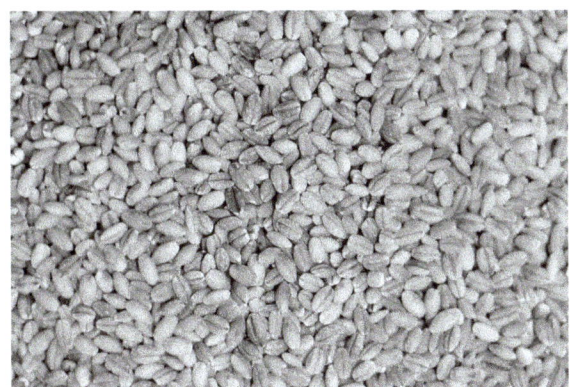

LESSER KNOWN CEREALS OR PSEUDO-CEREALS

Some seeds are like cereals and categorized as pseudo-cereals because of similarities in cultivation and usage. They have good nutritional value and have been found effective in treatment of several diseases. These include buck wheat, rye, and amaranth. One pseudocereal that has become popular is quinoa. Triticale is a hybrid of wheat and rye.

Buck Wheat (Kottu) (Fagopyrum esculentum)

It is also known as "kottu" and is used as the main ingredient in foods consumed during religious fasts in some parts of India. Worldwide it is used to make noodles, pasta, pancakes, confectionaries, and other products. It is generally ground into flour and used. The flour can be white or brownish. It has gained popularity owing to its nutritional and health benefits. It is gluten free and contains soluble fiber, minerals (zinc, copper, manganese, magnesium, selenium, potassium, sodium, calcium), and B vitamins (thiamine, riboflavin, and niacin). The biological value of buckwheat protein is high but digestibility of its protein is low. It is good for reducing cholesterol, constipation, and obesity. Some people have allergic reaction which may be triggered by low molecular weight proteins like legumin present in buckwheat.

Rye (Secale cereale)

It is not grown in our country but rye bread in popular in European counties. Rye grains are like wheat in shape but longer, more slender and the color varies from yellowish brown to grayish green. Its protein content (approx 15%) is higher than that of other cereals. It contains manganese, tryptophan, dietary fiber, and selenium. It is a good source of magnesium. Lignan (a non-starch polysaccharide) content is high. This is considered to provide protection against breast cancer among menopausal women and many other diseases. Rye bread has a lower glycemic index than bread made from refined white flour (*maida*). Sometimes caramel is added to wheat flour and may be labeled as rye bread but this is not the true rye bread. Rye also contains other beneficial components like fructans, arabinoxylan (similar to β-glucans), plant sterols, and saponins. Rye appears to have good satiating properties and hence may be useful for weight loss and weight control.

Triticale

It is a cereal grain made by man, a hybrid of wheat and rye first developed in laboratory in Germany and Scotland. Later due to its high yield and good nutrition it was considered for growing commercially in other countries as well. Flour is dark in color and used in bread making. This cereal is also used to make noodles, soft wheat type products, and for malting. Its composition is close to that of wheat but it has a higher free sugar content and it provides good amino acid balance with high lysine. Thiamine, niacin, and iron content are much higher than in other cereals.

Amaranth Seed (L. amaranthus)

In India, Amaranth seeds which are tiny like mustard seeds, are frequently used during religious fasts in the form of *laddoo* or *chikki*. Its flour is also used along with other flours. Since it is gluten-free, difficult to knead alone to make a dough like we use for *chapatis*. It contains 62% carbohydrate which is lower than in other cereals and the pseudocereal quinoa. It contains much higher amount of protein than other cereals and is similar to that of quinoa. This cereal is exceptionally high in lysine thus the protein quality is good. It is also rich in vitamins and minerals like calcium, iron and selenium, and several antioxidants and fiber. Thus, it can be used in prevention of malnutrition and many inflammatory diseases.

Quinoa (*Chenopodium quinoa*)

Botanically, this pseudocereal is related to spinach. It was first cultivated more than 4000 years ago by the Incas who considered it to be "the mother of all grains." It is a staple food in South America. Its protein content is 14–18% which is higher than in other cereals. It provides 69 g or carbohydrate, approximately 6 g of fat and 399 kcal per 100 g. Its lysine content is almost two times more than in rice and wheat. It has very low niacin content compared to other cereals but contains more tocopherols. it is also a good source of calcium (like amaranth) and iron but contains anti-nutrients like saponins and phytate. Recently it is considered as highly nutritious super food. May be its richness in many nutrients such as carbohydrates, insoluble dietary fiber, protein, thiamine, riboflavin, biotin, folates, tocopherols, calcium, iron, selenium and zinc as compared to other commonly consumed cereals. Perhaps this is the only cereal like grain which contain high amount of alpha linoleic acid (204 mg) and total unsaturated polyunsaturated fatty acid (2406 mg). Quinoa is consumed like *daliya*, in salads after soaking and steaming and prescribed in weight management. Also it is gluten-free.

Millets

Millets are one of the oldest foods known to man. Millets are small seeded grains cultivated in semiarid zones, where water resources are limited. They are used as food and animal fodder. Millets are resistant to insect and bird attacks and can be stored easily. These are hard cereals and sometimes hard to digest too. Therefore, skill is needed to develop food products of mass choice. Common millets are sorghum (*Jowar* or *cholam*), pearl millet (*Bajra*), and finger millet (*ragi* or *nachni*). There are some other lesser known millets such as proso millet, fox tail millet, and kodo millet. Along with maize, millets are referred as "coarse grains" and consumed by poorer sections of society and more in rural than urban areas. However, they are gaining popularity for their health benefits.

They are good sources of energy, protein, vitamins like thiamine, riboflavin, and niacin and vitamin E and minerals like iron, magnesium, and potassium. They also contain fiber which often binds minerals. Presence of phenolic substances in millets reduces mineral availability but gives them an advantage because polyphenols have health benefits. Sorghum contains a bitter compound called "durrin." Pearl millet contains a goitrogen. Roasting improves the flavor; kneading dough with warm water or mixing with glutinous flour improves bread quality.

Common domestic processes like soaking, germination, or malting can enhance nutritional quality of millets. Millets are useful for gluten-free diets. Certain experiments have shown that millets may be high glycemic food. Ragi is a good source of calcium and hence can be used for infant food as well as dietetic food. Main preparations from millets are *rotis*/*bhakri*. Beside this *jowar* is puffed, *bajra* is used to make *khichri* and *ragi* is used to make *kheer* or *sheera* for children.

Jowar/Cholam or Sorghum (*Sorghum vulgare*)

It is an ancient grain and now being popularized as functional food or health food. It is rich in protein, niacin, iron, and dietary fiber. Total protein content is at par with wheat, but its protein quality is poor due to its high leucine and tannin content, hence addition of legume flour improves its nutritional quality. Its starch content is similar to wheat but, the lower α-amylase (40–50%) and amylolytic (10%) activity affects its rheological properties. Sorghum is used to bake bread (especially in gluten-free bread) porridge, tortillas, gruel, steam-cooked products, alcoholic, non-alcoholic beverages, and so on. Sorghum contains a wide range of phytochemicals such as tannins, phenolic acids, anthocyanins, phytosterols, and policosanols. It has shown high potential in reducing the risk of certain types of cancers, CVD, and obesity compared to other cereals. Being gluten-free, it is considered for celiac disease (CD).

Bajra or Pearl Millet (*Pennisetum glaucum*)

In some parts of the country, bajra is included in regular diet. It is very high in dietary fiber, iron, and zinc and hence it is helpful in controlling anemia, constipation, diabetes, and CVD. It is being considered for fine quality brewing and many other diversified uses. Like other millets, pearl millet has low tannin but high saponin content. Amino acid profile is also comparable with other grains and it is high in lysine, methionine, and threonine. It is rich in B vitamins and minerals like P, K, Mg, Cu, Fe, Zn, and Mn. Wet pearls have characteristic odor and flavor.

Ragi or Finger Millet (*Eleusine coracana*)

Ragi is also known as *Nachni* in Western India and also used as a staple. It is used for pregnant women, lactating mothers, as well as children. In India, it is used to make complementary food for infants. Its protein, vitamin, and mineral content is close to wheat and other grains but it exceeds in calcium content than others. The presence of trace elements like manganese, phosphorus, iron, copper, chromium, magnesium, molybdenum, zinc, and selenium makes ragi a wonder grain. It is believed to have good laxative effect and used for people with liver disease, high-blood pressure, obesity, and osteoporosis. It is used as flour with which a wide variety of dishes are prepared.

READY-TO-USE CEREAL PRODUCTS

In the 1960s, the trend of Meal-Ready to Eat (MRE) was initiated by the armed forces, because there was a requirement for rations in individual packs that are easy to transport and store. These may have long shelf life of up to 3 years. Gradually, food products were developed with characteristics like just heat and eat; they are called "**Ready-To-Eat (RTE)**"and "**Ready-To-Use (RUF)**." Bread, cookies, desserts, beverages, and many others are examples of RTE foods. Such products became popular across the world due to their convenience in use, taste, and cost effectiveness. There seems to be no limit for such foods in the market. Market is flooded with such products; hence, individual mention will be beyond the coverage of this book. Also, dry mixes, frozen foods, partially cooked, and shelf stable foods are available. These products require minimal cooking to obtain good quality food and snack. RTE is very handy for persons who do not have time to cook or who do not know cooking. A large variety of RTE food products are available and they can be categorized as follows:

Ready-To-Cook (RTC)/Ready-To-Use Mixes

The raw ingredients used in these are dried; powdered or small pieces can be cooked using very simple cooking procedures, e.g., instant mixes like cake mixes, pasta products like noodles, macaroni, vermicelli, etc. Rice, *pulao*, or *biryani* mixes, dosa mix, idli mix, upma mix, gulab jamun mix and wide variety are also available. An unlimited number of ready to eat snacks have always been made across the country. Many of these are traditional. To these are added extruded snacks. These are dry powders/mixes containing the ingredients in dehydrated or frozen form. The mix generally provides the same texture, taste, and appearance of the preparation as when it is made with fresh ingredients, e.g., *upma*, *idli*, *dosa*, *pulao*, cake mixes, etc. These are available in packed form with directions for use on label. Such mixes save considerable time which is otherwise used in procurement of all raw materials, preprocessing, and cooking. People who are not well versed with cooking can read the instructions on the label and cook some of these preparations. Some of them are cost effective, whereas others are expensive, depending on the cost of ingredients and cost of manufacturing and marketing. Nutrition facts labels on most products provide some information. Brand value and interaction with the users provide better information and feedback.

Ready-To-Eat (RTE) and Ready-To-Serve (RTS) Foods

These foods do not require any further cooking. They have been cooked and are kept as fresh as possible and edible using a variety of processing, preserving, and packaging methods. They can be eaten without any elaborate procedure after opening the packet or tin, e.g., baked beans, sweet corn, tinned soups, precooked sausages, chicken products, curries, etc. Infant foods, biscuits, and some breakfast cereals are also examples of RTE foods. They can be used anytime and are a good option for travelers. Now fresh foods like *idli* are also available but they have a short shelf life. Some frozen foods are also available.

Processed and packaged breakfast cereals are usually available in ready-to-eat or ready-to-cook form, e.g., corn flakes, *muesli*, and oat porridge. They can be consumed as cold or warm generally with milk, curd, or fruit juice and sometimes as a snack. Fruits like banana, apple, strawberry, mango, and nuts like almonds and raisins are often added. Nutrient composition may vary among products and brands depending upon the ingredients used. Breakfast cereals usually supply good amount of energy and other nutrients. They are generally low in fat and high in dietary fiber and also in carbohydrates. Addition of milk, fruit juice, or other ingredients enhances their nutritional value. Muesli consists of uncooked rolled oats, or a mixture of different types of roasted uncooked grains, dried fruits, and nuts. Different combinations are made with different types of cereals. Muesli is comparatively rich in energy, starch, protein, fiber, and other nutrients. Sugar content is higher than oatmeal as it contains sugar or honey coating on the grains and other items in muesli.

PULSES, LEGUMES, BEANS, AND PEAS

Pulses are dried seeds belonging to the family called "Leguminosae." Legume is a generic name that is often used interchangeably with the word pulses. Codex Alimentarius Commission of FAO/WHO Food Standard program (2007) has clarified the difference between pulses and legumes, on the basis of fat content. Pulses are dry seeds of leguminous plants which are distinguished from leguminous oil seeds due to low oil content. Leguminous oil seeds include soybean and peanut and the crops which are harvested green are used as vegetables (green beans, peas, and sprouts). Commonly cultivated and consumed pulses in India include mungbean (green gram), chickpea (Bengal gram), urd bean (black gram), lentil (masur), pigeon pea (arhar), cowpea, horse gram, Lupins and bambara beans, peas, dry beans, dry broad beans, cow pea, chickpea, pigeon pea, lentil, bambara beans, vetches, lupins, and minor pulses.

In 2016, FAO declared pulses as "nutritious seeds for sustainable future" and the year as "International Year of Pulses" (IYP) to increase public awareness about nutritional benefits of pulses. Pulses are powerhouses of protein, energy, dietary fiber, a number of micronutrients, and bioactive compounds from plant sources. The Indian Institute of Pulses Research, Kanpur, referred pulses as "Health Food" or "Nutri-Rich Food." India has a commonly used variety of pulses, many of which are grown and consumed locally, in different parts of India.

Pulses are dicotyledenous in nature; hence, they can be used whole or decorticated/dehusked (called as *dal*). It includes all forms of beans and peas, dried, powdered, canned, and cooked. Only whole pulses are sprouted because they carry the germ portion but dehulled pulses or *dals* are devoid of germ, and so cannot be sprouted. Pulses are one of the basic components of Indian cuisine or Indian vegetarian *thali* as *dal bhat*, or *dal roti*. Some of the pulses form one of the ingredients in several popular snack items like idli, dosa, besansev, dhokla, cheela, pakodas, and sweets like laddoo and burfi.

Pulses are known for their high protein content. They are good sources of lysine and branch chain amino acids but they are deficient in methionine. Hence, they can be used by all age groups including children, sports activities, and diabetics. If their protein quality is improved by complementation, they can be used to reduce PEM. They are low in fat, and have no cholesterol. On the other hand, they are rich in dietary fiber, folate, and other vitamins and minerals like iron, calcium, zinc, and magnesium. They are slowly digested and hence have a low glycemic index. Pulses confer satiety and may should be retained help in weight loss regimes.

Presence of omega-3 (ALNA) and other unsaturated fatty acids, phytosterols, isoflavones, and lignans further could help to reduce the risk of many non-communicable diseases. High concentrations of polyphenols are found in seed coat as compared to cotyledons, e.g., more flavonoids were reported in the seed coat of lentils.

Pulses are also found to contain anti-nutritional factors. Anti-nutritional factors (ANF's) are usually the secondary metabolites that are naturally present in plants that constitute the plants' defense mechanism or their own protection from predatory animals and insects. On the one hand, while these ANFs have been found to exhibit certain inhibitory actions, on the other hand, these have shown several health benefits. Some of the ANFs are tannins, phytic acid, oligosaccharides, protease inhibitors etc. and some of these are described in Table 16.4 along with the simple ways to remove them. Oligosaccharides cause flatulence and gastric distention. Phytates tend to chelate multivalent metal ions (especially Fe, Ca and Zn) there by reduce their absorption but also exert some protective health effects.

Kidney bean/*Rajmah*, black gram/*urad*, and Bengal gram/*kala channa* are very good sources of omega-3 fatty acids particularly for people who abstain from fish consumption. *Kala channa* has been reported to be helpful in controlling

Table 16.4: Anti-nutritional factors in pulses.

Anti-nutritional factors	Food sources	Inhibitory function	Household ways to remove/reduce them	Health effects
Trypsin inhibitor	Soybean (trypsin inhibitor), white beans, chickpeas, navy bean, black gram, cowpea, peanuts	Inhibits the activity of trypsin enzyme which digests protein in stomach. It results in growth retardation deplete sulphur amino acids	Autoclaving or pressure cooking at 120°C for 30 minutes	Possess anti-carcinogenic and anti-inflammatory activity
Lathyrogens	*Kesari dal*	It is a neurotoxin named BOAO (β-N-oxalyl L αβ-diamino propionic acid). Disrupts the collagen	Soaking in water for 12 hours followed by steaming for 20–30 minutes or soak for 1 hour leach out the water and sundry. New varieties may be devoid of this toxin	It cripples and paralyzes the lower legs usually in man
DOPA	Fava beans	DOPA (dihydroxyl phenylalanine) and two other glycosides affect metabolism of glutathione in RBC	Boiling and germination can reduce it	May cause allergic reactions
Hemagglutinins/lectins	Field bean, horse gram	Interferes with digestion of proteins and absorption of certain minerals	Soaking and boiling	May influence blood glucose response, affect insulin homeostasis, and may be anti-carcinogenic. It may release histamine and cause allergy or inflammation and may also lead to auto-immune diseases in some people
Cyanogenic glycosides	All legumes except in lima beans usually within safe limit (10–20 mg/100 g)	Inhibit functioning of β-glucosidase may cause cyanide poisoning	Heat treatment	Can serve as biopesticides, may have anti-cancer role
Saponins	Soybeans	Causes nausea and vomiting	Soaking and remove foam during pulse cooking	Shown to have hypoglycemic effect, reduce blood cholesterol concentrations, enhance immune response, and may inhibit growth of cancer cells. Also possess antioxidant capacity
Goitrogens	Soybeans	Interfere with thyroid functions	Dehulling, pressure cooking	May disrupt production of thyroid hormones and cause hypothyroidism.
Tannins	Seed coat of most legumes like peas, beans, and cereals	Slow down the starch digestion	Dehusking, soaking, steaming, boiling	Have antioxidant effects, inhibit proliferation of microorganisms, may protect animals against parasitic infections
Alpha amylase inhibitors	Legume like kidney, beans, lupins some	Inhibits amylase activity and prevent utilization of bean starch by the body	Soaking. Use of salt/alkaline may increase the amount of antinutrient leaching and also loss of desirable nutrient like soluble protein and vitamins	May help to decrease postprandial glucose hyperglycemia and insulin levels, thus may decrease energy intakes. Useful in obesity and diabetes

blood sugar. *Urad* contains a mucilaginous kind of slimy substance, composed of arabinose, rhammanose, and galacturonic acid which make the pulse preparation a little slimy due to which it is suitable for fermented food products like "*idli*," *dosa*, and "*vada*." These pulses are considered nourishing but are more difficult to digest compared to *moong* and other pulses. Cowpeas/*lobia*/*rongi*/*chowli* is a good source of iron and folic acid; peas and *kabuli channa* is rich in zinc. Pea protein is gaining importance because of its good amino acid composition and being non-allergic. Lentil/*masur* provides protein, iron, thiamine, and meager amount of fat and is easy to cook and digest. Moth bean contains high amount of iron, thiamine, and fiber but has poor digestibility because its seed coat contains a toxic compound which needs to be removed by soaking and germinating the seeds before use. It contains alpha linoleic acid, calcium, iron, magnesium, potassium and B vitamins.

Green gram/*mung* is a pulse, highly valued for its good digestibility, palatability, and cooking quality. It is a good source of protein and iron. It can easily be germinated in 1-2 days. The germinated seeds also contain vitamin C and enhanced bioavailbility of minerals like iron, zinc and calcium. It does not cause flatulence and gastric discomfort like other whole pulses and is useful in illness. It is grown in winter months and often contains hard seeds that are not viable and hard to cook. Prolonged storage naturally removes the hardness that can also be removed by soaking *dal* in hot water (80°C) for 20 minutes.

Pulses like *channa*, *moong*, *urad*, and *masoor* are converted into two types of *dals*, i.e., with husk and without husk. Color of whole and dehusked pulse may be different, green gram is yellow inside, black *urad* is white, and brown *channa* is golden yellow. They are equally good in nutritional value on dry weight basis except for loss of some nutrients and dietary fiber. *Dals* are relatively easier to cook and digest than the whole pulse. Pulse seed coats are rich in insoluble fibres and polyphenols such as flavonol glycosides, anthocyanins and tannins which are responsible for the seed coat color. These specialized phytochemicals are being explored for designing of nutraceuticals.

Red gram is popularly known as "*arhar dal*" in northern part of India and "*tuar dal*" in western and southern parts of India. It is relished very much in dehusked forms. Whole dried seeds contain a toxic compound in the seed coat. Fresh seeds are used as vegetables in certain states.

Kesari dal: There is another dal called *kesari dal* (*Lathyrus sativus*) that is similar in appearance to *tuar dal* and frequently consumed in Madhya Pradesh and Maharashtra. Consumption of *kesari dal* is responsible for causing lathyrism (nerve disease causing paralysis of lower limbs, usually in males). It is due to the presence of a toxic compound known as BOAA (β-N-oxalyl-L-α, β di-aminopropionic acid) in *kesari dal*. Soaking and prolonged autoclaving may minimize it.

Cluster bean (guar gum) is valuable owing to the presence of soluble fiber. Fiber from guar gum is helpful in control of blood sugar level. It is consumed fresh and dried both as vegetable. Its viscosity is exploited for manufacturing of adhesives and thickeners in non-food industries.

Soybean (*Glycine max*): Soybean is very popular in food industry, oil industry, and now valued for its health benefits. Although it belongs to the *Leguminosae* family, it is considered more as an oil seed rather than a pulse owing to its high fat content and high protein. Its biological value is almost similar that of egg. It also contains phytoestrogens such as isoflavones and other bioactive molecules like phenolic acids, phytosterols, saponins, and tannins. Isoflavones like genistein and daidzein tend to reduce menopausal symptoms in some women. These have also been found to have protective effects in other degenerative diseases also.

Soybean is difficult to cook and digest. It has a beany flavor that is often found unacceptable. Soy allergy is also found in many people. It contains several anti-nutritive factors like protease inhibitors, trypsin inhibitors, goitrogens, and hemagglutinins/lectins.

High production, low cost, health benefits, nutritional richness, and technical advantages have made soybean a favorite legume in food industry, many cuisines, and many cultures and countries. However, more recently, the American Heart Association (AHA) has observed certain conflicting results with the role of isoflavones in menopause and cancer prevention. Regular consumption of soy may restrict the absorption of most minerals due to the presence of high amount of phytates in soybean as compared to other pulses.

In Asia, fermented soy products like miso, natto, and soy sauce are traditionally used. In India, soy flour (whole or defatted) is used in some households and baking industries to enrich bread. Addition of soy flour to several products has become a regular feature for its functional advantage due to the presence of lecithin. Soy milk is available in different flavors. When enriched with calcium and vitamins, it is considered a milk replacement for infants and children who are lactose intolerant or who have cow's milk allergy. Other products are soy curd and soy cheese which is also called "Tofu." Some of the soy products are tempeh and miso.

Tempeh is an Indonesian food made by fermenting the cooked and dehulled soyabean which is inoculated with *Rhizopus* spp and kept for 1-3 days at 30°C. It has been observed that soy from GM crop does not give good quality tempeh. During fermentation, fat and thiamine decrease with corresponding increase in vitamins B_2, B_3, and fiber. Tempeh can also be made with wheat and cassava which are also rich in vitamin B_{12}. It has meat-like taste and peanut butter-like consistency.

Miso is another fermented soy product which originated in Japan. Washed rice is steamed, cooled, and inoculated with *Aspergillus oryzae* then incubated for 50 hours at 27°C. The resultant product is referred to as "koji." Next soaked soybean is crushed, mixed with "koji" and inoculated with *Sacchromyces rouxxi*, and fermented for 2 months at 35°C. It is then blended and mashed again and kept for one week at room temperature. During this process, it becomes rich in B vitamins like B_2 and B_{12}, with a protein content that ranges from 10 to 12%.

Soy sauce is one of the most popular flavoring agents in Japan and China. Soaked and cooked soybeans are mixed with roasted, charred, and milled wheat. *Aspergillus oryzae* are grown in this mixture for 2 days at 25-30°C. The mixture is stirred in 1.5 volumes of salt solution and fermented for 3 years or in certain cases, one month only. It is filtered under pressure, heated, pasteurized, and bottled. The energy and protein content is six times less than soybean and fat is only 1.5%. However, salt and mineral content is very high.

Soy concentrate and soy isolate: Soy concentrate is prepared from defatted soy flakes and contains 72% protein. It also retains dietary fiber from soybean. Soy isolate contains about 90% protein. It is considered a good choice of protein supplements among vegetarian sportspersons indulged in intense training and the method employed may retain isoflavones.

Full fat soy flour is used for fortifying cereals/millets/pulses at 10-15% level in the preparation of traditional recipes. It is available in sealed polythene bags and hermetically sealed metal containers. The shelf life is about one month at normal retail shelf temperatures.

Medium fat soy flour is used for fortification with other cereals/millets/pulses at 10-15% level in the preparation of traditional recipes. In chickpea flour and papad, it can be added up to 20 and 40%, respectively. The keeping quality is about six months at normal retail shelf temperatures and has to be used within a month after opening the packet. It contains protein 45% (min) and fat 7% (max).

Defatted soy flour is also a common ingredient in blended food aid products and can also be fortified with various micronutrients. It contains 50% protein and 1.5% fat.

Soy protein isolate is made from defatted soy meal and is used as an ingredient in high protein foods including dairy foods, nutritional supplements, meat systems, infant formulas, nutritional beverages, cream soups, sauces, and snacks. It is also a good source of protein in milk replacers. Due to high protein content, it is highly suited for those people who have high protein needs due to growth (children), famine (acute needs), and chronic diseases (HIV/AIDS/tuberculosis).

Texturized soy protein is made wholly from either defatted soy meal flakes or soy protein concentrates. It is widely used as an ingredient in ground meat for patties, sausages, and meatloaf. It is commercially available as soy chunks in different sizes and frequently used by vegetarian population in the diet. It contains 50% protein (min) and fat 3% (max).

Soy milk (plain/flavored) is ready to drink and applicable to all sections of people suffering from lactose intolerance (infants/youth/old/pregnant, etc.). The soymilk may consist of pure water, soybean extract, sugar, and salt. It has 3-4% protein, 1.5-2.0% fat, and 8-10% carbohydrates. Flavored soymilk may consist of pure water, soybean extract, sugar, salt, flavors, and permitted food colors. Plain soy milk is packed in 200/500 mL polythene bags/glass bottles/tetra packs. The soy milk has shelf life of six months when packaged in tetra packs.

VEGETABLES

Vegetables are plant food materials, grown seasonally across the globe. They may be cultivated or collected when they grow wild in certain seasons. The types of vegetables and varieties vary widely from region to region. Vegetables add variety, color, texture, flavor, and appeal to the meal and contribute to heath in myriad ways. They are obtained from different parts of the plant, e.g., potato is a tuber and carrot is a root. Cauliflower is a flower and cabbage is a leaf. All vegetables have some or the other health benefits. Many are considered functional foods also, e.g., garlic, ginger, tomato.

Usually locally cultivated, seasonal vegetables are consumed. With advancement in agriculture, postharvest, and transport systems, they are also available and consumed off season. However, it is traditionally said that the off-season vegetables should be avoided. Nutritional and health benefits are maximum when in season. Vegetables form a part of main meals and are consumed with or without spices and condiments; in many forms like raw, boiled, seasoned, fried, baked, canned, dehydrated, and fermented.

Vegetables in general are perishable, although some roots and tubers can be stored for longer periods. Green leafy vegetables are most perishable owing to 90% moisture content. Hence, they need to be procured and consumed as soon as possible. In some parts of the country, vegetables are dehydrated and used. Frozen vegetables are also now available in the market for ready use. Texture and color are important in selection, cooking, consumption, and storage of vegetables. Color or pigments contain health protective components. For example, yellow orange colored vegetables are good sources of carotenoids. Beta carotene is a source of vitamin A and it along with other carotenoids exerts several health benefits.

Vegetables in general are low in energy, protein and fat but relatively high in fiber, certain vitamins and minerals, and phytochemicals like carotenoids, flavonoids, and other compounds. Their nutritional composition differs considerably depending on the cultivar, plant genetics, agricultural factors, storage, handling, processing, packaging, and the method of processing and preparation. They are broadly categorized into 3 categories: (1) Roots and tubers, (2) Green leafy vegetables and (3) Other vegetables.

Roots and Tubers

Roots and tubers generally are grown beneath the soil and are cultivated once or twice a year. They can be stored for months in proper storage conditions. They are mostly rich in starch. Example, onion and garlic are not rich in starch. They also contain several nutrients and phytochemicals due to which they are health promoting and protective. They are relatively cheap depending upon the variety and geographical location. Carrots, radish, turnip, and beet root are roots; potatoes, sweet potato, and yams are tubers. This group also includes onion and garlic although onion is a bulb and garlic is a stem.

Potatoes (*Solanum tuberosum*): Potato is very popular because of its comparatively low cost, taste, and because it can be mixed with a wide variety of other food ingredients.

It is relished by most people of all age groups. It provides 14.8% carbohydrate, 1.54% protein and 0.23% fat, respectively and is a good source of the amino acid lysine. It is a good source of potassium but like other potassium containing foods, it may need to be consumed in small amounts in potassium - restricted diets. Often diabetics are advised not to eat potatoes. However, the American Diabetes Association (ADA) recommends that starchy vegetables like potato can be included as part of a healthful diet. Although the glycemic index of potato is high, the method of cooking and presence of other ingredients also play a significant role, e.g., potatoes when fried, they supply even more energy, can increase content of trans fat, and so would not be healthy, but a small amount could be consumed with high fiber foods that may lower the GI value. Cooking and consuming yellow fleshed potato with skin add health value due to the presence of zeaxanthin. Potato is eaten boiled, deep fried, baked, and used in curries, salads, and snack items like potato chips. Fried potatoes/French fries contain several times more calories than boiled or steamed preparations. Evidence shows that there is formation of acrylamide (a toxic/carcinogenic compound) during prolonged frying of potato at high temperature (>250°F). Potato starch is of high value not only for food industry but for paper and textile industry too. Green potato or potatoes with sprouts contain a toxic compound known as solanin. Hence, it is advisable to avoid consuming them; it may cause hallucination, confusion, and some gastrointestinal disorder.

Sweet potato (*Ipomoea batatas*): Sweet potato is different from potato because it belongs to a different genus. It has white, red, orange, or purple skin and is either white or yellow inside. Each type differs in composition. It is consumed boiled or baked with or without seasoning. Some people use it to make *halwa*, *kheer*, or *chips*. Sweet potato is a good source of β carotene. Its bioaccessibility is better when cooked with some amount of fat. Orange-fleshed sweet potato contains more amounts of carotenoids and can be a good vehicle for combating vitamin A deficiency. Purple sweet potato is rich in anthocyanin and exhibits antioxidant activity. The sweet word may be misleading for diabetics. Researchers suggest that it might be due to the presence of the special protein called arabinogalactan. Sweet potatoes contain more fiber than potatoes and have a lower GI than potatoes. Besides presence of carotenoids in sweet potato, method of cooking determines the glycemic index. Roasted and baked sweet potato has higher GI as compared to boiled and steamed due to formation of resistance starch during boiling and baking destroy it.

Yam (yam elephant, Suran, or zimikand) (*Amorphophallus paeoniifolius*): It is very rich in starch, dietary fiber, B vitamins and carotenes and generally used in curries, but it is sticky and irritating to tongue and throat. Care needs to be taken while cutting by smearing hands with oil. Some acidifying agent such as lemon juice and tamarind pulp may be used to overcome the irritating effect or it may be fried. The tuber contains relatively high levels of total phenolics and tannins.

Tapioca or Cassava: This tuber is common in some Asian and African countries and is used in some parts of India. Tapioca contains a bitter and toxic compound known as "cyanogens." It is boiled, mashed, grated, or roasted. "Garri" is a popular tapioca product in Nigeria. Cassava is also used to make chips. It is being used by traditional medical systems for many ailments.

Arrowroot: Arrowroot is a tropical herb with starchy rhizome. It produces very fine quality of starch and is used popularly in all foods for mixing and coating without affecting the taste of the product like puddings. It is also used to give bulk in the diets of invalids.

Beet root (*Beta vulgaris*): Beet is a red purple root. Its color is due to the presence of pigments called betalains. Betalains are water soluble. Hence, beet is used as natural dye/food color. At household level, also its juice is used to provide red color to *pulav*, *puri*, and *halwa*. Betalains have been shown to have antioxidant, anti-inflammatory properties and perhaps inhibit tumor growth. Beet is also used for sugar production at industry level. It is rich in pectin and hemicelluloses that are used in many non-food industries. Its juice has been reported to enhance vigor and reduce anemia. The combination of carrot, beet, and lemon has been found to be acceptable. It is generally eaten raw or cooked in salad, sandwiches, or juice along with other vegetables.

Carrot (*Daucus carota*): Carrot is one of the most popular red or orange color vegetables, sweet in taste, and relished by people of all age groups. It contains abundance of α, γ, and β carotene which are potentially beneficially for eye sight, immune system, and vitality. Raw carrot has moderate GI, although carrot juice has high GI which is an important consideration for diabetics. It is consumed in cooked form in a wide variety of vegetable preparations, the popular being "gajar ka halwa," carrot cake, pickles, kanji, and salad.

Colocasia (*arbi*) (*Colocasia esculenta*): It is a good source of starch and the granules of this starch are finer than cereal starch. Thus, it is more digestible and suitable for special feeding. It also contains some amount of protein, folate, potassium, and phenolic compounds. Energy value of potato and colocasia is similar (97 kcal). It is slimy in nature; hence, while cooking some souring/acidic agent like tamarind or *amchur* (dehydrated raw mango powder) needs to be included in the preparation. It is eaten as a vegetable in some parts of India and is commonly used during religious fasts. Its flour is also prepared and used in making extruded products.

Radish (*Raphanus sativus*): Radish is a root vegetable similar to turnip in texture and belongs to the mustard family. It is usually white and pink. White radish is long, shaped like a carrot, whereas pink radish looks like a small turnip or beet. It has a lingering, highly pungent, and sulfurous odor and acrid, sharp flavor. It is eaten as such, sliced, grated in salads, and used as stuffing in *parathas* and in pickle. It has a negligible amount of protein, sodium, and fat and may be useful in diabetes, obesity, hypertension and kidney problems. It is a low GI food and has an alkalizing effect. In rat model, it has been found to have anti-inflammatory properties.

Turnip (*Brassica rapa glabra*): Turnip is also a root vegetable belonging to the *Brassica* family. It is shaped like beet and is pinkish white in color. Its taste and flavor are fairly similar to radish. It adds variety, volume, and fiber to the diet. Like other vegetables of *Brassica* family, turnip also contains goitrogens. Turnips contain phytochemicals that may be protective against cancer.

Onion (*Allium cepa*): Onion is of the most popular ingredients in almost all cuisines across the globe. Several varieties of onion are available—white, and purple, big and small. Its use is sometimes culturally prohibited in some Hindu and Jain families. It is generally not used as a vegetable but in salads, pickles, sauces, seasoning, and gravies. Its strong odor, pungent taste, and flavor are due to sulfur-containing compounds. Onions and other allium vegetables contain thiosulfinates, sulfides, and sulfoxides, which are odoriferous sulfur compounds responsible for the strong odor and flavor. Cutting onion is a tear-producing activity and that is due to the presence of lacrimatory compound, propyl disulfide. Its sulfur-containing amino acids help to manage cholesterol. Onion is not as potent as garlic since the sulfur compounds in onion are only about one-quarter the level found in garlic. Raw onion is considered to beat the heat in hot summer. Onion is effective against many bacteria including *Bacillus subtilis, Salmonella,* and *E. coli*. It may also have cancer preventive effects.

Garlic (*Allium Sativum*): Garlic has an exceptionally strong flavor which is either liked or rejected. It is a popular ingredient like onion in seasoning, chutney, pickles, sauces, and gravies. Immature garlic with green stalks is used in some special preparations. Some communities and households shun the use of garlic due to traditional beliefs or due to its strong lingering odor. Garlic is valued for its therapeutic properties. It is antiseptic, antibacterial, antihypertensive, and antithrombotic and helps to lower total blood cholesterol and LDL and raises HDL cholesterol.

Green Leafy Vegetables

Mint, coriander, onion stalks, and other green leafy vegetables (GLV) like spinach, fenugreek, amaranth, lettuce, and shepu are green in color because they contain the pigment—chlorophyll. Chlorophyll is associated with some health benefits such as—anti-aging, treatment for acne, may be helpful in treating anemia, may serve as a deodorant, and help in wound healing. Vegetables are also rich in carotenoids although their yellowish color is camouflaged under the green color of chlorophyll. Darker colored vegetables contain more amounts of carotenoids. There can be large difference in the content of total carotenoids and β carotene. Total carotenoids include other carotenoids like alpha carotene, cryptoxanthin, xanthophylls, lutein, and zeaxanthin. GLVs are considered to be the powerhouse of nutrients except for fat and carbohydrates. It indicates that although spinach is considered a good source of iron, there are many other leaves which contain more iron such as fenugreek leaves, moringa (drumstick) leaves, and parsley. However, phytates and oxalates in GLV like *bathua*, and amaranth tend to inhibit mineral absorption. Oxalates are likely to bind with calcium and precipitate forming renal stones/calculi. GLVs are rich in vitamin K and some of them provide omega-3 fatty acids which is good for vegetarians. They are also good sources of dietary fiber. GLVs have a high water content, thus they are highly perishable. Perusal of Table 16.5 reveals the wide variation in the nutritive values of different types of GLVs. The data is obtained from IFCT (2017).

Besides carotenoids, GLVs are also rich in various flavonoids and phenolic acids. Hence, they extend health benefits by reducing the risk of several chronic diseases. Total dietary fiber and insoluble dietary fiber are very high in curry leaves. Processing has no effect on dietary fiber and some of the bioflavonoids. However, water-soluble compounds are lost during washing and cooking. Vitamin A is also lost significantly while sun drying and deep frying.

Amaranth (*Amaranthus cruentus, chowli ka saag*): There are many *Amaranthus* species and since ancient times it is considered a natural protector against chronic aliments. Its anti-cancerous, anti-viral, hepatoprotective, neuroprotecive, cardioprotective, and antidiabetic properties are currently in the limelight. Plethora of phytochemicals include alkaloids, flavonoids, glycosides, phenolic acids, steroids, saponins, amino acids, vitamins, minerals, terpenoids, lipids, betaine,

Table 16.5: Important nutrients in commonly consumed green leafy vegetables.

Name	Protein (g)	β Carotene (µg)	Omega-3 (mg)	Riboflavin (mg)	Folic Acid (µg)	Vitamin C (mg)	Calcium (mg)	Iron (mg)	Oxalate (mg)	Magnesium (mg)
Amaranth	3.9	8457	214	0.27	70.3	83.5	245	4.36	823	177
Bathua	2.5	1075	169	0.51	42.5	41.0	211	2.66	1077	48
Fenugreek	3.7	9245	362	0.22	75.3	58.3	274	5.69	34	63
Drum stick	6.4	1754	446	0.45	42.9	108	314	4.56	120	97
Lettuce	1.5	1285	134	0.09	30.7	11.9	56	2.73	364	43
Radish	2.2	2591	203	0.13	53.1	65.7	234	3.82	53	58
Colocasia	3.4	5758	335	0.07	159	40.7	216	3.41	701	59
Spinach	2.1	2605	220	0.10	142	30.2	82	2.95	592	87
Mustard	3.5	2619	240	0.18	110	60.3	191	2.84	2	52
Parsley	5.6	2710	255	0.10	197	133	288	5.51	128	49

catechins, tannins, and carotenoids which make its extract a promising neutraceutical material.

Amaranth leaves are red and green in color and both are commonly consumed. They are rich in carotenoids, folates, and vitamin C. They have a high oxalate content that prevents absorption of minerals. The seeds of amaranth are rich in protein, contain good amount of lysine, calcium, and unsaturated fatty acids and have the potential to be used for managing malnutrition. It is used as gluten-free flour.

Bathua (*Chenopodium album*): It is a fairly good source of iron, magnesium, vitamin A (carotenoids) and vitamin C. It contains good amount of essential amino acids like lysine, methionine, leucine and isoleucine. It contains good amount of polyphenols thus exhibit free radical scavenging capacity or antioxidant properties. The plant has been traditionally used as a blood purifier, diuretic, sedative, hepatoprotective, antiscorbutic laxative, and as an anthelmintic against roundworm and hookworm.

Spinach (*Spinacia oleracea*): Spinach is popularly considered a good source of dietary fiber, iron, folic acid, and β carotene and lutein. It also contains numerous bioactive compunds due to which it showed anti-inflammatory, anticancer, hypoglycemic, and lipid-lowering effects. Carotenoids are protective for many diseases including neurogenerative diseases. It also contains good amounts of oxalates, hence when eaten with calcium rich foods; the oxalate reduces the bioavailability of calcium. It is a natural laxative owing to its fiber content.

Fenugreek leaves (Methi) (*Trigonellafoenum graecum*): Nutritionally among GLV, it is exceptionally rich in protein, calcium, β carotene, fiber, vitamins C, riboflavin, carotene, dietary fiber and wide range of flavonoids, and polyphenolic compounds. Hence Methi leaves has shown hepatoprotective, antiulcer and hypoglycemic effects. It is used almost all over India. Both tender and mature leaves are used. Fenugreek leaves contain saponins known as graecunins. Its consumption are good for diabetic and anemic persons as well as by breast-feeding mothers.

Mustard leaves (*Brassica campestris*): It is an excellent source of β carotene, vitamin C, and iron like methi leaves and it also contains some amount of protein. "*Makke di roti* and *sarson da saag*" is a traditional meal of north India. They are a good source of fiber, riboflavin, niacin, pantothenic acid, folic acid, vitamin C and β carotene, vitamins B_6, K, E, and minerals like calcium, manganese, and iron. Its phytate content inhibits absorption of calcium, magnesium, and iron. It also contains glucosinolates that are metabolized in the body into indoles and isothiocyanates. In animals, these have been found to inactivate carcinogens, and have anti-viral, anti-bacterial, and anti-inflammatory properties. Mustard leaves have been shown to lower cholesterol. Mustard leaves contain oxalate and hence should be restricted in diets of persons with renal stones. Also, persons who are prescribed anticoagulants like warfarin need to be vigilant because these greens have a high vitamin K content that could alter the coagulation time.

Coriander leaves (*Coriandrum sativum*): It is a very popular and fragrant garnish used for numerous preparations in India and other countries. It has been used since prehistoric times and was used by physicians. It is also used in chutneys and sometimes in seasoning but is not used to make vegetable preparations like other GLVs. In Maharashtra, it is used to make a snack "kothimbir/coriander wadi." Coriander leaves have been used since prehistoric times and by many including Greek physicians. Leaves are excellent source of vitamin C and also good source of thiamine, zinc, and dietary fiber. It is known for its antioxidant, anti-diabetic, anti-inflammatory, anti-anxiety, antimicrobial activity, hepatoprotective and diuretic activity. It is a cooling herb and also exhibits hormone balancing effect. It is contains a wide range of bioflavonoids and polyphenols due to which it exhibits pharmacological action against LDL oxidation.

Mint (*Mentha arvensis*): Like coriander, it is also not used for vegetable preparations but has much wider range of usage in preparations like *chutney*, *jal-jeera*, garnish, as an additive. Dried mint is also used. It has a stronger flavor. It is cool and gives freshness and is thus useful in hot summer. "Pudina hara" is a commercial over the counter (OTC) preparation, the capsules of which contain mint extract. Menthol is an active component which is used in its crystalline form. It is present in the essential oil of mint. Nutritionally mint leaves provide folic acid, iron, and protein. Mint is traditionally used as a carminative, anti-spasmodic and prevents/relieves chest congestion from cough and cold when used its vapor.

Curry leaves (*Murraya koenigii*): They are popular as a seasoning ingredient for many south Indian preparations. It is rich in calcium, β carotene, and protein. It has been reported to be useful for controlling blood sugar level because it contains an inhibitor of the enzyme alpha amylase. It has antioxidant property, antiulcer activity, and antimicrobial activity. Flavonoids present in leaves show a wide range of biological activities. The antioxidant properties are capable of scavenging free superoxide radicals, thus providing antiaging benefits as well as reducing the risk of cancer. Its leaves are also found to prevent hair fall and premature greying.

Drumstick leaves (*Moringa oleifera*): It is an excellent source of vitamin C and β carotene, protein, and fiber and is consumed like other GLVs. Its high nutritional content exhibits high promise to combat vitamin A deficiency and malnutrition. It contains phytosterols, alkaloids, flavonoids like anthocyanins, proanthocyanidins, and cinnamates, quercetin, and chlorogenic acid. It has been found to have anti-hyperglycemic activity and play a role in reducing dyslipidemia, has anti-oxidant, and anti-inflammatory properties.

Lettuce (*Lactuca sativa*): Lettuce as the Hindi name suggests ("salad patta") is used in salad only. It may not be used as good source of vitamins and minerals but its high content of water makes lettuce worth adding in salad. There are different varieties of lettuce available in market. It is a very low calorie food and can be included in weight management.

Shepu (Sowa or dill) (*Peucedanum graveolens*): Shepu or dill is primarily a medicinal herb and very strong in flavor. It is usually consumed in combination with other vegetables. It has been used during lactation. It is rich in iron, choline, flavonoids, and monoterpenes (volatile compound due to which dill has typical fragrance). It is said to have effect on cancer and obesity. It is often used in many ayurvedic preparations meant for vata aliments (swelling in joints).

Radish leaves (*Paphanus sativus*): Radish leaves are a very rich source of riboflavin, calcium, and fiber. They are relished in some parts of India as a vegetable.

Cabbage (*Brassica oleracea*): Cabbage may not look like other GLVs but it is categorized as a leafy vegetable. It is very low in calories and a good source of vitamin C. It is good for people on low calorie diets. However, it contains goitrogens. Its juice has been reported to useful in peptic ulcer as it contains an anti-ulcerative U factor. It is eaten raw, steamed; shredded or whole leaves are used. It contains sulfur compounds. Over cooking and pressure cooking may spoil the flavor of cabbage.

Cauliflower leaves (*Brassica oleracea*): Normally they are not consumed by people, rather they are thrown or used as animal feed. But nutritionally they are extraordinarily rich in iron and high in fiber. It can easily be incorporated in other foods to enhance the nutritional quality of food particularly iron content. However, if pesticide has been used to reduce worms in the cauliflower, it is advisable not to use the leaves.

Colocasia leaves (*Colocasia esculenta*): There are two varieties, black and green. Black variety is nutritionally rich but causes severe irritation in throat that can be prevented by use of tamarind. Green variety is also rich in thiamine, riboflavin, iron, and β carotene (*see* Table 16.5). They are big in size and used to make "patra" (Gujarati name) or "alu wadi" (in Maharashtra) or "patora" (north India). Some people use it for vegetable preparation. It can be used to enhance the nutritive value of food.

Onion stalks (*Allium cepa*): Onion stalks is also called as spring onion, green onion, and scallion and frequently being used in Chinese cuisines. It is very rich in iron and zinc. Its medicinal qualities lie in its sulfur compounds like onion, although their content is lower than that in the bulb.

Cowpea leaves (chawli saag) (*Vigna unguiculata*): They are good sources of fiber, iron, calcium, magnesium, potassium, sodium, fat, β carotene, vitamin C, and folate. It is mainly used as cooked vegetable. The leaves have a low glycemic index and contain antioxidants. The leaves contain higher amounts of amino acids (leucine, lysine, methionine, cysteine, phenylalanine, valine, tryptophan, and histidine) than the seeds.

Bengal gram leaves (chana ka saag) (*Cicer arietinum*): Cooked as a vegetable, they are a good source of fiber, iron, protein, calcium, zinc, manganese, copper, and boron as well as vitamins C and B_6. Strength and endurance have been reported in people eating chana saag. It may be suggested for people indulged in heavy duty work including sports persons.

Beet greens (*Beta vulgaris*): Beet greens (the young leafy tops of beetroot) are a good source of iron, calcium, copper, manganese, β carotene, thiamine, riboflavin, and vitamin K besides being a good source of fiber. It does not contain much fat. Its high potassium content aids to reduce high blood pressure. It also provides some folate. It has good antioxidant properties due to the pigments (lutein, zeaxanthin, and beta-carotene) present in beet leaves.

Turnip leaves (*Brassica rapa*): Good source of riboflavin, iron, phosphorus, magnesium, and calcium but contains insignificant amount of protein and fat and some amount of β carotene and vitamin K. The leaves contain high amount of nitrate. Nitrate has beneficial effects on cardiovascular system. It is helpful in reducing anemia and osteoporosis. It has high oxalates also and thus limits the absorption of certain nutrients.

Betel leaves (Paan) (*Piper betle*): This is not used for cooking but served and chewed after meal filling with or areca nut, other aromatic ingredients, and folded. It has a strong, pungent, and aromatic flavor and is used as a mouth freshener. Sometimes silver foil is also used to cover it. It improves digestion. It contains iron, magnesium, and calcium, can be added with other GLVs of choice, and the juice can be extracted with or without water. Lemon juice, salt, or sugar can be added as per taste to treat anemia. The presence of compound like chavicol in betel oil, chavicol, phenol, eugenol, terpene, and campene are responsible for its medicinal properties (due to the antioxidant properties). The dried leaf powder has been shown to reduce blood glucose levels. The leaves are also helpful in modifying lipid levels and have anti-mutagenic, anti-proliferative, and antibacterial properties. *Note:* When consumed with tobacco and betel nut, the risk of oral cancer increases.

Celery (*Apium graveolens*): It belongs to the carrot family that includes parsnips, and parsley is similar to coriander leaves and again not common in our country. It is a good source of iron, vitamin C, and β carotene as well as vitamin K, folate, potassium, and fiber, but low in calories. The leaves resemble coriander leaves but are much larger. It is usually used in soups for weight loss and detoxification. It is said to lower inflammation, reduce blood pressure (attributable probably to celery seeds), and prevent age-related vision loss. It is a good source of phenolics. A molecule apigenin present in celery is being studied for its anticancer properties as well as for stimulating neurogenesis.

Amaranth leaves (*A. dubius*): There are several varieties of it such as *A. hypochondriacus*, *A. caudatus*, and *A. cruentusetc* in red and green varieties. They are a good source of iron, vitamin C, and beta carotene; antioxidants like lutein, zeaxanthin. They also provide vitamin K, folate, B_6, riboflavin, thiamine, niacin, and potassium. They are a better source of manganese, magnesium, copper than spinach.

Parsley (*Portulaca oleracea*): Also known as *luni bhaji* in Hindi or Ghol in Marathi, it has soft, succulent, triangular dark green leaves that are an excellent source of omega-3 fatty acids, providing about 255 mg of alpha linolenic acid. It is native to Mediterranean region of southern Europe and western Asia. Now people have started using it at other places also. There are varieties with differences in leaf size, thickness, leaf arrangement, and pigment distribution. The leaves are mucilaginous, thick, and are slightly sour and salty to taste. Both leaves and stem are edible. It is rich in dietary fiber. It is an excellent source of beta carotene, vitamin C, riboflavin, niacin, pyridoxine, folic acid, iron, magnesium, calcium, potassium, and manganese. Purslane also contains betalain alkaloid pigments (reddish betacyanins and yellow beta xanthins). These have potent anti-oxidant and anti-mutagenic properties.

Other Vegetables

Other vegetables include several gourd vegetables, different fresh beans, peas, vegetables of brassica family. Vegetables belonging to *Brassica* family are referred to as cruciferous vegetables. They are good sources of phytochemicals that provide protection from chronic degenerative diseases. There are many exotic vegetables used in different parts of the world and now available and consumed in some societies of India. These are asparagus, bok choy, brussels sprouts, purple cabbage, Romaine lettuce, etc. They are also exploited for their taste, texture, flavor and health significance.

Cauliflower (*Brassica oleracca var. Botrytis*): Cauliflower is a white flowered vegetable, belonging to the *Brassica* family. It is quite popular and is widely used in vegetable preparations, *pulao*, *pakoras* (*cutlets*), *pickles*, and salad. It contains isothiocynates, sulfur compounds that give a typical taste to the vegetable and also produce flatulence if eaten in excess. It is low in fat and sodium but is a good source of vitamin C and choline. Its white, creamish color is due to presence of a pigment called anthoxanthines which become yellowish in presence of alkali. White color of potato and rice is also due to this pigment. Being a part of the *Brassica* family, it may contain phytochemicals like glucosinolates and S-methyl cysteine sulfoxide. Glucosinolates are said to have goitrogenic effect and S-methyl cysteine sulfoxide has been shown to possess anti-carcinogenic properties. Cauliflower intake is restricted in conditions like gout because its purine content may increase the uric acid level in the blood.

Broccoli (*Brassica oleracea italica*): Broccoli is a newer addition to the Indian market and is known as green cauliflower locally. It is a member of the Brassica family. It is an excellent dietary source of phytochemicals like glucosinolates, phenolics and other antioxidants. It is rich in vitamins (C, K_1, etc.) and minerals (Ca, Mg, Na, K, Fe, Zn, etc.). Though glucosinolates are goitrogenic, but have a protective role in certain cancers and skin diseases.

Banana flower/banana blossom (*Musa paradisica*): It is also known as banana heart and is a drop-shaped purple/maroon colored flower that hangs at the end of a cluster of bananas. Generally consumed in southern and western parts of India and in West Bengal as a vegetable. Only tender flowers that are creamish in color are used and extra caution is required when it is cleaned, as the outer flowers are inedible. The flowers contain substantial amounts of phenolic compounds. The extract of banana flower has been shown to contain several phytochemicals, namely, alkaloids, glycosides, steroids, saponins, tannins, flavonoids, and terpenoids. Banana flower is traditionally used in many illnesses like diarrhea and dysentery and may also play a role in diabetes. It is believed to reduce PMS (premenstrual syndrome). Nutritionally, it is a good source of potassium, magnesium, calcium, phosphorus, fiber, and vitamin E.

Peas (fresh green) (*Pisum sativum var Arvense*): Peas belongs to the leguminous family. Fresh peas are used as vegetable. Dried peas are also used, although there is a vast difference in their nutritional composition. Snow pea is another delicacy; its pods are consumed. Fresh green peas are a favorite among persons of all ages because of the color, taste, and flavor. Frozen and canned peas are easily available and used in vegetables, pulav, snacks, soups, and filling. New researches indicate that pea protein may replace soy protein because it is of high quality and nonallergic. It is comparable with whey protein which is used in synthesis of muscle protein after resistance exercise.

Beans: Beans belongs to vegetables group of leguminous family. Fresh pods of many legumes are harvested, cooked, and consumed for their taste and flavor as vegetables. They are easy to grow in kitchen gardens as creepers which can rise on any side of the house or tree. Wide variety of fresh beans are consumed throughout the world such as french beans (*Phaseolus vulgaris*), field beans (*Dolichos lablab*), cluster beans or *Guar ki Phalli* (*Cyamopsis tetragonoloba*), and double beans or *Papri* (*Faba vulgaris*). They are good sources of protein and fiber. They tend to produce flatulence due to the presence of sugars of raffinose family and high fiber. Cluster beans are very rich in soluble fiber and galactomannans that are helpful for diabetes and lowering cholesterol in many pharmaceutical and non-food industries.

Cucumber (*Cucumis sativa*): Cucumber is cool, refreshing, high in water content, low calories, and useful in acidity and weight loss diet regimens. It is generally eaten raw as a salad or in raitas. In the Western world, it is preserved in vinegar to make pickles. It also contains glycolic, salicylic, and lactic acids. Its extract has been found to help in healing corneal burns in an experimental model. The presence of silica in the peel of cucumber supports bone health and is also found to be effective in skin care and detoxification.

Tomato (*Lycopersicon esculentum*): It is a good source of vitamin C and carotene particularly lycopene, which has health benefits. Availability of lycopene is better in cooked tomato than raw. Lycopene is several times a more potent antioxidant than β carotene and α tocopherol. Evidence showed its protective role in certain cancer including prostate cancer as it reduces the harmful effects caused by DNA damage. It is used in a wide variety of preparations like salads, soups, ketchup, sauces, and as an ingredient in gravies of various curries, and pickles, juice, chutney. It is also available in puree, powder, and sun-dried form.

Pumpkin (*Cucurbita moschata*): It is large in size having very hard skin. Thus, it can be stored for long duration without cutting. It is yellow and cream or even orange in color and relatively cheap and relatively safe to consume. It is used in vegetable preparations, in soups, sauces, juice, and gravies and as filler in pies. Pumpkin is a good source of potassium, β carotene, fiber, and may be useful in diabetes and cancer. Its seeds are getting popular owing to its high content of essential amino acids such as tryptophan and good amount of minerals (magnesium, zinc, copper, selenium, and calcium but are low in sodium), PUFA, sterols, squalene, and tocopherols. Some studies suggest that pumpkin seed oil may be useful in treating benign prostatic hyperplasia and urinary disorders.

Brinjal (Eggplant) (*Solanum melongena*): There are many sizes and shapes, the skin color varying from blackish purple to white and green. Some varieties are bicolored or striped. Its nutritional contribution is less than leafy vegetables or carrots but add variety and bulk to the diet. Large rounds brinjals are roasted/boiled to make "bharta." It is a good source of fiber, potassium, and B_6. The anthocyanins may be good for heart health due to the presence of chlorogenic acid which has antioxidant and anti-inflammatory function and reduces LDL. Brinjal also contains a compound called nasunin that may improve blood flow to the brain. It is useful to include this vegetable in low calorie regimes. It can safely be used by diabetic patients.

Lady's finger (or okra/*bhindi*) (*Abelmoschus esculentus*): It is one of the most relished and easy-to-cook vegetables. It is rich in many nutrients, including carotene, B_6, folic acid, iron, magnesium, and calcium and soluble fiber like gums, pectin, and mucilages. It is a good source of fiber and in rat model has been shown to reduce blood glucose and normalize the lipid profile. It contains antioxidants and flavonoids and exhibits hepatoprotective effects. Its soluble fiber content, help in managing blood glucose levels.

Bottle gourd (white gourd/lauki/dudhi/ghia) (*Lagenaria siceraria*): It is considered to be "cool" and good for most people since it is easily digested. Some people advice its use during illness. It is considered to have diuretic properties and thus useful to detoxify the system. Juice is considered to be good for diarrhea, peptic ulcer, acidity, and flatulence.

A protein, langenin, isolated from seeds, has been reported to have antitumor, antiviral, antiproliferative, and anti-HIV properties. Juice of fresh fruits significantly decreases the serum cholesterol, triglyceride levels by inhibition of lipoprotein lipase, and lecithin-cholesterol acyltransferase activity making triglycerides available for uptake and metabolism by tissues. It is a low calorie vegetable and used to make vegetables as well as *halwa* and *burfi*.

Ridge gourd (*Torai*) (*Luffa acutangula*): There are two types of torai, one with ridges and one without ridges. It is a low calorie vegetable and low in fat. It is a good source of dietary fiber, vitamin C, riboflavin, zinc, thiamine, iron, magnesium, and manganese. It is good to eat in weight loss regime particularly in summers for its cooling properties. The seed are rich in glycolipids, phospholipids, and protein.

Ash gourd (Petha) (*Benincasa hispida*): It is whitish or light green and has high moisture content. Its juice is considered to be beneficial for peptic ulcer, acidity, and flatulence and "cooling." It is highly alkaline and is thus useful in acidity. It increases urine output and washes out the waste products from the body, due to its diuretic action. Shelled seeds promote tissue growth. When taken with coconut milk, they expel worms from the intestine. In Northern India it is consumed as *pethe ki mithai* rather than a vegetable. This sweets uses only ash gourd and sugar but zero fat. In South, it is used more in vegetable preparations like "Avial" and other preparations.

Bitter gourd (Karela) (*Momordica charantia*): It is also called bitter melon, bitter apple and many other names in different communities. It comes in different sizes and shapes. Small variety is called uchhe. The main reason for bitterness is the presence of antioxidants, phenols, flavonoids, terpenes, glucosinolates and anthraquinones. The triterpenoid in bitter gourd exhibits not only bitterness but also an anti-diabetic effect. Further they are being used in traditional medicines for infection, malaria, hypertension, wound healing and even in certain cancers.

Parwar (pointed gourd or patol) (*Benincasa hispida*): Its skin is a little hard and waxy so the name and it can stay fresh for a longer time than other vegetables. In Ayurveda, it is considered to be a blood purifier, improves appetite, digestion and useful in constipation, weight, cholesterol and diabetes management. It is used as cooked vegetable. Parwar sweet with khoa filling is a delicacy of north India.

Round gourd (Tinda) (*Citrullus vulgaris var. Fistulosus*): It is light green, round in shape, and used in similar way as bottle gourd and parwar. It is also cool and a low calorie vegetable. Ayurveda uses this vegetable for reducing pitta conditions.

Scarlet gourd (Kundru): It is a small, soft, parwar like look and used in a similar way. It has been found to help in controlling high fever, biliousness, and blood sugar.

Capsicum (shimlamirch/bell pepper) (*Capsicum annuum*): It is available in three bright colors—green, red, and yellow and the color difference is due to the type of carotenoids present in them. Green contains more chlorophyll; yellow contains lutein, and zeaxanthin and red pepper is rich in astaxanthin and lycopene. These capsicums are light in weight and mild in pungency and widely used in many cuisines. Green capsicum (giant chilli) is a very rich source of vitamin C and thiamine and several polyphenols showing antioxidant property. It is said to increase the body metabolism by reducing adipose tissue and helps to burn calories more effectively.

Lotus stem (kamalkakri): Lotus flower blooms on lotus stem that is hollow inside. Lotus stem is consumed as vegetable and considered rich in nutrients. Fresh kamal kakdi is relished in Kashmiri cuisine and many vegetable recipe forms like kofta by several communities. Dry lotus stem contains exceptionally high amount of iron and is a good source calcium.

Asparagus (*Asparagus officinalis*): Asparagus is rich in folic acid, fiber, and vitamins A, B, C, and K and trace elements (fluoride, manganese). It is considered to be very effective in detoxification of liver as well as lungs. It is eaten steamed especially with hollandaise sauce. It is not a common vegetable in India, but is available in select stores. It contains polyphenols and has been found to possess anti-hyperlipidemic and antioxidant properties.

Mushroom (Khumbhi): There are many varieties like button, shitake, oyester, etc., and some wild types can be toxic, so care is needed during selection. It is used raw, fried, dried, and used in soups, on pizzas and even cooked as a vegetable. It contains good amount of copper, iodine, manganese, and selenium. It helps in strengthening the immune system and lowering cholesterol and body weight.

FRUITS

Botanically fruits are the seed bearing structures formed from the ovary after flowering. They are generally fleshy and are highly valued for their distinctive flavor, taste, freshness, juiciness, color, texture, and nutrition. They are used in every state from wellness to illness. The goodness of fruits is attributed to the presence of numerous phytochemicals out/other bioactive compounds. Fruits are consumed by all age groups and in all sections of society. Most fruits are usually consumed raw with or without peel. Some are eaten whole with skin like apple, pear, cherries, and berries; some are peeled, like banana, oranges, mango, and litchi. They do not require cooking until preserved and processed for making products like dried fruit, jams, nectar, squashes, juices, etc. They are perishable and sensitive to postharvest treatments.

Fruits are classified as:
- Pomes, e.g., apple, pear
- Stone fruits, e.g., peach, plum, cherry
- Berries, e.g., strawberry, cape gooseberry, raspberry
- Tropical and subtropical fruits, e.g., pineapple, banana, dates, avocado
- Hard shelled fruits, e.g., bael.

Pomes

Pomes belong to the rose (*Rosaceae*) family which is characterized by waxy layer on the fruit peel and small seeds in the core of the fruit. The fruit peel is rich in flavonoids and hence consumed. These fruits, on cutting, turn brown due to the presence of presence of PPO (polyphenol oxidase) enzyme in them. The fruits also contain several organic acids in which malic acid is the major acid that helps in removing uric acid and thus pome fruits are useful in gout and arthritis. They have a low glycemic index. They are useful in several chronic diseases like diabetes, CVD, and obesity.

Apple (*Malus sylvestris*): "An apple a day keeps the doctor away" is an age old saying and it works even today. There is a large variety of apples, each having distinct size, color, and flavor. Apple contains abundance of health-protecting components in each part of the fruit. Apple is rich in polyphenols such as quercetin, catechin, phloridzin, chlorogenic acid. Apple peel contains significant amount of quercetin glycosides (flavonol) and chlorogenic acid. Thus, it is advisable to eat apple with the skin. Apple catechins may be more bioavailable than those present in tea. Apple consumption may be protective against cancer and asthma. It is high in fiber (soluble fiber), low in glycemic index, and low in fat which makes apple more useful in diabetes, obesity, and CVD. Apple also helps in removing the uric acid due to the presence of malic acid, quinic acid, citric acid, and pyruvic acid thus, apples are good in gout and arthritis. of gout and arthritis. The trace elements like selenium, chromium, boron, and molybdenum in apple keep the circulatory, musculoskeletal, and nervous systems healthy. Apple is consumed whole, cut, and used to prepare juice, jelly, jam, pies, dried apple pieces, apple cider, brandy, and vinegar.

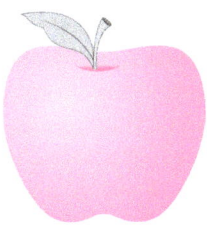

Pear (*Prunus persica*): Pear is relatively similar to apple in its health protective properties. It is a natural source of sorbitol (a sugar alcohol); xylose, arabinose, and mucilages (non-starch polysaccharides); and malic, citric, and oxalic acid (organic acids). Thus, pear is useful in obesity, diabetes, gout, and constipation. It is eaten raw, stewed, and canned.

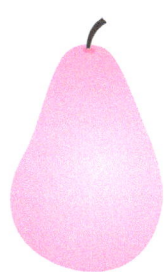

Tropical Fruits

Watermelon (*Tarbooj*) (*Citrullus vulgaris*): Watermelon is large in size, green from outside, and with bright red pulp inside containing black seeds. It is consumed raw in the form of fruit pieces or fruit juice. It contains large amount of water, hence it is very cooling in summer and helps to quench thirst. It is reputed to be beneficial for acidity and other digestive disturbances. It is also useful in anemia. Its red color is due to the presence of lycopene and lutein, the carotenoids; however, it does not contain β carotene. It is low in calories and also low in glycemic load. Being sweet in taste, it can be consumed in controlled quantity by obese and diabetic people. Its low potassium content makes it good fruit in contrast to muskmelon or potato.

Watermelon seeds are frequently used in many forms—raw, roasted, or ground or its oil. These are rich in protein and fat and are exceptionally rich in an amino acid, arginine and linoleic acid.

Muskmelon (*Kharbooja* or cantaloupe) (*Cucumis melo*): It is available in many sizes and color (white to yellow) and is somewhat similar to water melon. It is also cooling, refreshing, and is useful in conditions like acidity, constipation, urinary tract infection, heat stroke, and heart disease. The fruit has been found to have anti-oxidant and anti-inflammatory properties. In contrast to watermelon, muskmelon is high in potassium and thiamine and good for hypertensive people and weight watchers but not for patients with renal problems. Its seeds are also consumed roasted and ground. They are rich in protein and unsaturated fatty acids. They have been found to have good antioxidant potential. The raw fruit is used in pickles in Japan and has been found to have antimutagenic properties.

Sapota (*Chikoo or sapodilla*) (*Achras sapota*): It is brown in color having light brown, brownish yellow to reddish brown pulp, the texture varying from gritty to smooth. Sapota is a good source of energy, potassium, and fiber. It also contains antioxidant polyphenols and tannins. Its high fiber content makes it a good laxative and is useful in constipation. It has a high glycemic index but low glycemic load. It can be consumed by diabetic persons in limited amount. It is used as fresh fruit, is processed into candy, and used in ice cream.

Banana (*Ripe*) (*Musa paradisiaca*): Many varieties are available in India such as green, "elaichi" (small yellow bananas), red, and large yellow bananas from Kerala. People grow plantain tree in their gardens and have a regular supply of fruit. It is available round the year, is comparatively cheap, and can be consumed by all. It is useful to feed infants and sick persons. It is eaten fresh, mashed for infants, and used to make milkshakes, smoothies, ice cream, and jams. "Halwa" is also prepared from the large yellow bananas in South India. Raw banana is also used as a vegetable. It is good for heart and blood and effective in ulcer and diabetes. Banana contains alkaloids, flavonoids, glycosides, saponins, steroids, tannins, and xanthoproteins. It demonstrates antibacterial activity.

It is an excellent source of vitamin B_6 and potassium. It gives instant satiety and energy. Starch from banana is important. Ripe banana contains simple sugars and is easy to digest whereas raw banana contains resistant starch which delays gastric emptying and thus it is found useful in cholesterol management. It is good for enhancing mood as it contains good amount of tryptophan which can be converted into a relaxing neurotransmitter called serotonin and vitamin B_6 helps in this conversion. High potassium content of banana helps in electrolyte balance. It is also used for constipation. It tends to reduce excretion of calcium and thus strengthen bones and formation of kidney stones.

Custard Apple (*sharifa or seetaphal*) (*Annona cherimola, A. Reticulata*): It is rich in dietary fiber, vitamins (vitamin C, vitamin B_6, and carotenoids), and minerals (iron, magnesium, and copper). It is cool, alkaline, so it is useful for acidity. It is useful for good digestion, anemia, and relaxation of muscles. It is eaten as such in the ripe form and is used to make milkshakes, ice cream, and is added to shrikhand. The seeds, like those of other *Annona* species, are crushed and used as insecticide. The seeds contain several alkaloids.

Guava (*Psidium guajava*): Guava is a popular fruit available in winter and rainy season and can easily be grown in kitchen gardens. Nutritionally it is known for its high content of vitamin C and dietary fiber particularly pectin. Pink guava is considered more nutritious due to the presence of lycopene. Guava is considered to be a laxative. It contains a number of major pharmacologically active ingredients such as flavonoids, guayavolic acid, guavanoic acid, guajadial, guajaverin, and other active principles. With vitamin C, these ingredients give it antioxidant properties. It is eaten as such and used in the preparation of jelly, guava nectar, cheese (a sweet), and toffee. The plant is reported to possess several therapeutic properties such as antidiarrheal, antimicrobial, hepatoprotective, anti-plasmodial, antispasmodic, cardioactive, anti-diabetic, anti-inflammatory, anti-nociceptive (reduces sensitivity to painful stimuli), and anti-tussive (effective against cough) activities.

Papaya (*Carica papaya*): Papaya is a well-known tropical fruit, cultivated and consumed throughout the years. It is known for its β carotene content, lycopene and vitamin C. It helps to digest protein but it is not suited in celiac disease. It is also consumed as juice, and in smoothies. It is also dehydrated. Raw papaya is used as a vegetable, is candied, and also added in meat to hasten the tenderization because it contains the proteolytic enzyme papain.

Pomegranate (*Punica granatum*): Pomegranate contains red juicy pearls or seeds that are consumed. It is a good source of riboflavin, vitamin C, iron, potassium, and copper. It is high in sugar but due to its high content of anthocyanin and ellagic acid (both are polyphenols and antioxidants); it is used in diabetes too and in small amount to prevent cardiovascular disease. Juice drunk in small amount helps in convalescent period. It also has fiber (2.8 mg). Pomegranate juice protects against oxidative stress. The fruit and the juice contain lignans—isolariciresinol, medioresinol, matairesinol, pinoresinol, secoisolariciresinol, and syringaresinol. The seeds have been reported to contain estrogenic compounds. The pericarp of pomegranate has been traditionally used for treatment of diarrhea. In a rat model, the dehydrated skin reduced blood glucose and lipid levels and raised HDL and hemoglobin.

Bael Fruit (*Aegle marmelos*): It is rich in potassium, contains very little sodium and is also rich in thiamine. It is fibrous with good amount of mucilages, thus it is good for dysentery as well as constipation. However, excess can also cause these symptoms. It is cool and a relatively cheap option in summer season. It contains tannins and pectin. Its pulp is used for direct consumption or bael *sharbet* is also consumed in summer season. The fruit has been observed to possess several properties—analgesic, anti-hyperlipidemic, anti-diabetic, and anti-cancer. The pulp contains marmelosin, psoralen, and other polyphenolic compounds. Psoralen increases tolerance of skin to sunlight and marmelosin is useful as a laxative and a diuretic. The fruit contains coumarins and β-sitosterol. Seeds of bael fruit have antifungal property and the fruit may be useful in gastric ulcer and chronic fatigue syndrome found to be useful in gastric ulcer.

Figs (*Ficus carica*): Both fresh and dried forms are used. Fig has good amount of dietary fiber, both insoluble and soluble fibers are in which make the fruit good for bowel health. It is frequently added to ice creams. Figs contain oxalates, polyphenols and have several health benefits including antioxidant, anti-viral, anti-helminthic, hypoglycemic, and hypotriglyceridemic. In animal models, it has been observed to have hepatoprotective properties.

Pineapple (*Ananas comosus*): It has a typical tough and waxy rind. It is a good source of vitamin C, thiamine, riboflavin, and iron. It is eaten fresh, made into juice, squash, canned, and made into jam, or dehydrated. The presence of organic acids and enzymes makes the fruit and its juice is useful in conditions such as gout, arthritis, and dyspepsia. However, drinking large quantity of pineapple juice can lead to stomach upset. Bromelin, a proteolytic enzyme is present in pineapple which curdles milk or curds/yoghurt when mixed with them, thus it is suggested to stew the pineapple first. Bromelin helps in denaturation and digestion of protein. It has beneficial biological properties—antioxidant and anti-inflammatory. It is a good source of polyphenols.

Avocado (*Persea* spp): Avocado is an exceptional fruit (also known as alligator pear or butter fruit), which is not at all sweet but is very rich in fat (10–20%), having a substantial percentage of MUFA. Fat from avocado is found to decrease triglycerides and LDL cholesterol and increase HDL in the blood. It is a good source of fiber, potassium, magnesium, vitamin E, K, B6, riboflavin, niacin, pantothenic acid, and folate. It is not sweet like other fruits but is used fresh usually to make guacamole sauce, bread spread, and sandwich filling. Its oil is also used in cosmetics owing to its high humectant and nourishing nature. Its lutein and zeaxanthin content are effective for preventing macular degeneration of eyes. It is also a source of β carotene and omega-3 fatty acids. It also contains beta-sitosterol and other plant sterols that help to maintain healthy cholesterol levels. Avocados also contain substances that have anti-microbial activity, especially *E. coli*.

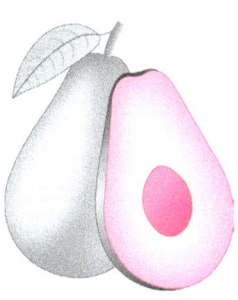

Berries

Berries have low fat and energy content, and are good sources of fiber and micronutrients like folic acid, selenium, carotenoids including lutein. They contain polyphenols especially flavonoids—anthocyanidins and ellagitannins. Anthocyanin is a pigment found in red, purple, and blue-colored fruits, vegetables, and flowers. It also provides health benefits. Flavonoids protect the body from free radicals and oxidative stress. Thus, berries may be cardioprotective and reduce the risk of acute myocardial infarction.

Raspberries (*Rubus idaeus*): They are rich in vitamin C, carotene, and anthocyanins. They are rich in pigments and contain many polyphenols (anthocyanidins) and organic acids like malic acid. Anthocyanidins possess antioxidative and antimicrobial properties and play an important role in visual and neurological health as well as provide protection against various non-communicable diseases including cancer. The fruit is valued for its antioxidant and anti-inflammatory properties. It is useful in many health conditions like gout, eczema, and indigestion. It is highly valued for its sweet flavor which is used in jams, custard, ice creams, and other desserts.

Strawberries (*Fragaria* spp): Its bright red color, shape, size, memorable aroma, and flavor attract everyone. It contains more than 200 flavor compounds. It is valuable for its vitamin C, iron, and fiber content. Also, it is a rich source of phenolic compounds like ellagic acid. It has good antioxidant capacity and is beneficial in reducing total and LDL cholesterol. It is also found to reduce an inflammatory marker, CRP (C-reactive protein), and therefore may be protective against inflammatory diseases, pain, and cancer. Strawberry products include jam, nectar, yogurt, and ice cream as well as milkshakes. A topping or garnish with red strawberry adds visual appeal to any preparation.

Cape gooseberries (rasbhari) (*Physalis peruviana*): It is a good source of carotene, thiamine, and vitamin C, minerals, and tannins. It has antioxidant and anti-inflammatory properties and may have a preventive role in several diseases like cancer and cardiovascular disease.

Blue berries (*Vaccinium corymbosum*): They are a good source of vitamin C, bioflavonoids, and glycosides. Hence, these berries possess high antioxidant capacity reflected in a high Oxygen Radical Absorbance Capacity (ORAC) value, a unit to report antioxidant capacity. It is valued for fighting infection, thus its soup is found to be a good remedy for diarrhea. Most of the health benefits are attributed to the anthocyanins that give the typical color. It has been shown that they reduce total and LDL cholesterol, triglycerides, abdominal fat, and hence the risk of heart disease as well as improving fasting glucose and insulin sensitivity. This is attributable to its antioxidant property and probably to a compound present called pterostilbene. A compound in blueberries has been found to prevent bacteria from adhering to the cells that line the walls of the urinary tract and thus may protect against urinary tract infection. It is consumed as fresh ripe fruit and in jams, juice, and ice creams. In studies with rat models, these berries slowed the age-related loss in mental capacity.

Cranberries (*Vaccinium macrocarpon, V.*): Cranberry juice has been popular for treating urinary tract infection (UTI) in folklore for ages. It is alkaline in nature and provides a shield between epithelial cells and bacteria thereby having anti-infective properties. It may be due to the presence of many nutrients and phytochemicals. The proanthocyanidins have also been reported to prevent dental plaque formation. In some people, regular cranberry juice consumption for months can kill the *H. pylori* bacteria, which can cause stomach cancer and ulcers. It may also be useful for increasing HDL and decreasing LDL.

Kiwi Fruit (*Actinidia sinensis*): Kiwi is a recent addition in Indian fruit market. It is considered to be a rich and nutrient-dense fruit as it contains good amount of vitamin C, E, folate, vitamin B_6, and minerals like manganese, magnesium, iron, and zinc. It has been reported to contain omega-3 fatty acid which is rare in fruits. It is a good source of carotenoids and phenolics and contains calcium oxalate, chlorophyll, as well as papain, a proteolytic enzyme. It is not usually mixed with milk. It is consumed raw, and is frequently used in desserts. Kiwi fruit may have immunoprotective properties. It contains pectin which functions as a prebiotic and may be beneficial for gut health.

Citrus Fruits

Among fruits, citrus fruits are highly valued for their content of vitamin C and bioflavonoids. They are also rich in water-soluble vitamins, minerals—phosphorus, potassium, magnesium, copper, sugars, and non-starch polysaccharides, and a variety of phytochemicals such as monoterpenes, limonoids (triterpenes), flavanoids, carotenoids, and hydroxycinnamic acid. Naringin, naringenin, nobelitin, narirutin, and hesperidin are the most important flavonoids thus far isolated from citrus fruits. These phytochemicals show anti-carcinogenic mechanisms attributable to their antioxidant capabilities; their effects on cell differentiation, and increased activity of the enzymes that detoxify carcinogens, and blocking of nitrosamines. In addition, citrus fruits do not contain fat or much sodium and being a plant food, no cholesterol. Some citrus juices become bitter after being refrigerated overnight. This is because they contain limonoids that are generally present in the peel. These compounds also give the fruits their characteristic aroma.

Lime (*Citrus aurantiifolia*): Its juice contains more reducing sugars, citric acid and malic acid. It is helpful in maintaining fluid and electrolyte balance. Being acidic, it leaves alkaline ash, thus it is found to be useful in treating nausea. Drinking diluted lime juice enhances freshness and reduces anxiety, lethargy, and depressive mood.

Lemon (*Citrus Limon*): Since ages lemon has been found to cure scurvy among sailors, has been used as an antidote to poison by Romans, and is popularly used to combat common cold though it is still folklore. It is a good source of folic acid, potassium and vitamin C. Regular use may delay aging, fat accumulation, and treat colitis. Its juice is sprinkled over salad, cooked vegetables, chats, and chutneys. Squash and pickles are also commercially manufactured. Its rind contains pectin, hemicelluloses and phenolic compounds and is thus considered as functional food and used in nutraceuticals. Lemon peel is also expressed to obtain essential oil that contains a wide range of terpene compounds and exhibit antifungal, antiseptic, and antioxidative properties.

Sweet Lime (*Citrus sinensis*): Sweet lime is also called mosambi. It is rich in vitamin C and a good source of potassium. It enhances immunity and helps to resist infections and aids healing in motion sickness and weight loss. Its juice is a commonly relished drink for its freshness and is also used in indigestion.

Orange (*Citrus aurantium*): It is rich source of carotenes and vitamin C. Its fatty acid composition and amino acid composition and folate make orange worth eating on regular basis in any form. Its peel also has many pigments having bioflavonoids and pectin; thus peel is also added in many food preparations in spite of its bitter taste, e.g., in marmalade. Bitter taste comes from the compound limonene present in the white pith just below the skin. It also causes cloudiness in juice, so care is needed to remove it. The phytochemical present includes flavonoids like hesperidins and naringenin, carotenoids. Naringenin is largely present in the albedo (inner layer) and pith and have potential to improve endothelial function and thus cardiovascular health. Naringenin has anti-inflammatory and antioxidant properties and also exhibits anti-cancer effects.

Tangerine (Kinnow) (*Citrus reticulata*): It is similar to orange but grown in different agro climatic conditions, so it may vary in chemical composition. Orange color of tangerine is due to carotene and xanthophylls. It is also a good source of flavonoids. It has high content of potassium which is useful for maintaining blood pressure but is not advisable for patients with renal disease. It is also good for people with liver damage. It contains oxalic acid.

Grape fruit (Chakotra) (*Citrus x paradisi*): It is a very large sized fruit. It is either pink or white from inside. Pink grapefruit (the flesh) contains lycopene. It is good for detoxification of liver and is considered good for weight loss too, and lowering cholesterol lowering blood cholesterol. The bitter principle in skin of the fruit is naringin. It has more terpenes and other flavor components which makes it different from other citrus fruits and seeds. Grapefruit and other citrus fruits and seeds of grapefruits interact with certain drugs and thus reduce their effect. The peel is candied and is a good source of pectin. It is used in nutraceuticals and and has antifungal action agent.

Mandarin (*Citrus reticulata*): It is slightly different from orange (tightly skinned). It contains pectin, vitamin C, and bioflavonoids particularly hesperidin. The essential oil of mandarin is used certain food products like ice creams and squashes. It has relaxing and stimulating properties at the same time, thus it may be useful for anxiety and depression. Its essential oil is frequently used in cosmetics.

Drupes or Stone Fruits

Drupes are succulent fruits with the seed enclosed in an inner stony layer of the fruit wall. The skin is usually thin and the seed is also known as "pit." Examples of drupes are cherries, olives, mango, and peach.

Apricot (*Prunus armeniaca*): The color ranges from creamish to greenish white to orange and orange red. Fresh and dried are both eaten as such. The fruit is frozen and used in manufacture of jelly, jam, juice, nectar, and extruded products. Among stone fruits, it has a higher carbohydrate content, contains some fiber, minerals like potassium, magnesium, iron, calcium, selenium, and vitamins C, K, E, riboflavin, thiamine, niacin, beta-carotene, folic acid, B_6, and pantothenic acid. It contains malic acid and other organic acids. It has good free radical scavenging activity. Apricot seed oil is good for skin nourishment. It has been reported that daily consumption of Japanese apricots inhibited gastric mucosal inflammation and chronic gastritis progression caused by *H. pylori* infection. In animal models, it was found to reduce hepatic steatosis.

Jackfruit (*Artocarpus heterophyllus*): Jackfruit belongs to the *Moraceae* family to which fig, mulberry, and breadfruit also belong. It is the national fruit of Sri Lanka and Bangladesh and the state fruit of both Kerala and Tamil Nadu. In India, both raw and ripe jackfruits including the seeds are consumed. It is the largest tree-borne fruit. It is a multiple fruit containing hundreds to thousands of individual flowers. The fleshy petals of the fruit are eaten. Jackfruit is a good source of carotenoids, volatile acids, sterols, tannins, compounds like morin, dihydromorin, cynomacurin, artocarpin, isoartocarpin, cyloartocarpin, artocarpesin, oxydihydroartocarpesin, artocarpetin, norartocarpetin, cycloartinone, and artocarpanone. Artocarpesin has been found to reduce obesity-associated inflammation; artocarpin has been found to alter cell morphology and induce apoptosis in a breast cancer cell line. Jackfruit inhibits alpha-amylase activity.

Breadfruit (*Artocar pusaltilis*): It is closely related to jackfruit. It is a very high-yielding food plant and in a single season, the plant can produce up to 200 fruits that are approximately the same size as grapefruits. It is high in moisture and contains very little protein and fat. It is a rich source of prenylated polyphenols—geranylated flavones and has good superoxide anion-scavenging activity that are anti-inflammatory and inhibit reactive oxygen species (ROS) generation. The seeds contain chitin-binding lectins. A compound present in the fruit, frutackin, promoted hemagglutination and growth inhibition against fungi *Fusarium moniliforme* and *Saccharomyces cerevisiaein vitro*; pathogenic organisms like *S. aureus*, *P. aeruginosa*, *S. mutans*, and *E. faecalis*.

Mango (*Mangifera indica*): Mangoes are rich in various carotenoids such as β carotene; leucoxanthin, violaxanthin, with considerable difference among the varieties. Numerous varieties are available in India. Carotenes are more in Alphonso followed by Langra and Fazli. Mango is good for managing vitamin A deficiency symptoms and improves vitality and strength. It has considerable amount of vitamin C, thiamine, riboflavin, and niacin and many organic acids like malic acid, sugars and minerals like magnesium. Its typical flavor is due to the presence of esters, alcohols, and lactones. Raw (green) mango is used to make pickles and "panna" a drink made in summer. Its dry powder is called *amchur* or raw mango powder and frequently used for its sourness in many cuisines. The pulp of ripe fruit is highly relished as such used in the preparation like milkshakes, ice cream, barfi, aamras, aampapad, etc. Canned slices of pulp and juice are also available. Polyphenolics from mango have been found to have anticancer properties due to the presence of gallotannins. Mangiferin a flavonoid is present in leaves and has strong antioxidant capacity. Mango has a number of pharmacological actions and possible health benefits. The compounds present in the fruit, peel, stalks, leaves, bark, kernel, and stone/seed make this fruit valuable because they confer the following properties: antioxidant: iron-chelating property, antiviral, anticancer, antidiabetic, antiaging, immunomodulatory, hepatoprotective and analgesic effects, modulation of glucose metabolism, reduces cholesterol, triglycerides and free fatty acids, have cardioprotective effects, and may prevent cell proliferation.

Sweet Cherry (*Prunus avium*): Its bright red color and round, small size attract everyone and make it suitable for toppings on ice cream and other desserts. It is a powerhouse of phytonutrients and organic acids and contains many carotenoids. As a result, regular use can control the pain and crippling that occurs in gout. It is used fresh, canned, in jam, preserves, and candied. Cherries have a high content of antioxidants (anthocyanin, quercetin, and hydroxycinnamates), potassium, vitamin C, and melatonin. It has several potential preventive health benefits related to cancer, cardiovascular disease, diabetes, inflammatory diseases, and Alzheimer's disease. They also elicit a low glycemic response.

Peach (*Prunus persica*): It is a good source of vitamin C and dietary fiber, potassium, xylose, sorbitol, and many types of carotenoids like xanthophylls, zeaxanthin, beta cryptoxanthin, and lutein. It has good antioxidant capacity and therefore may provide protection against chronic diseases. It is fresh, canned, used in jam, juice, stewed, and in pieces. In a rat model, peach and nectarine intake was found to protect DNA from damage.

Litchi (*Nephelium litchi*): White flesh of litchi is rich in vitamin C, some minerals, and polyphenols including bioflavonoids giving it good antioxidant capacity. It is good for digestion being astringent and diuretic. It is consumed fresh or in the form of squash. It is not they are a medium glycemic index fruit.

Loquat (*Eriobotrya japonica*): It contains wide variety of carotenoids and antioxidants. It is also a good source of potassium. It is believed to be good for eyes, cognitive functions, dental health and also preventive for cancer.

Plum (*Prunus domestica*): It contains many types of sugars and sugar alcohols. Anthocyanin content is high along with catechin, rutin, chlorogenic acid, and caffeic acid. It is a source of the amino acids, glutamine and threonine. Plums are good for diabetes, heart diseases, and cancer. Fresh, dried (prunes) jam, brandy. Seeds should not be consumed as they contain hydrogen cyanide (HCN) which is not only bitter but toxic too. Dried plums or prunes may be beneficial for bone health. In an experiment with postmenopausal women, a group was asked to consume dried plums and was given calcium and vitamin D supplements. Prune group had significantly higher bone mineral density in the ulna and spine, than the group given dried apples and the calcium vitamin D supplements.

Phalsa (*Grewia asiatica*): It is dark purple in color and of pea size with seeds in the center. Its anthocyanin and β carotene contents are high. It is good for eyes and blood disorders and is reputed to be "cooling" for the body and quenches thirst. It contains good amount of oxalic acid. Its sharbat is a popular drink in summer in northern part of India or it is eaten raw. It is an effective antioxidant. In an experimental mouse model, the fruit extract was found to be protective against radiation-induced peroxidation in the cerebrum.

Jamun (Jumbo fruit) (*Syzygium cumini*): It is also known as malabar plum, java plum, black plum, or Indian blackberry. The most commonly found variety is generally oblong and has a deep purple to bluish color. The pulp of the fruit is gray to pink in color, and has a relatively large seed. Another variety is seedless ranging in color from purple to white in color. It is rich in polyphenols. The glycoside in the seed, jamboline, shows antidiabetic properties and the jambolan compound present in its fruit is said to mimic the action of sulfonylurea and biguanides that are used for medical treatment of type 2 diabetes mellitus. The pulp of the fruit also has an antioxidant effect. It has low potassium content. The fruit is also known to have anticancer and antihyperlipidemic roles. The fruit has also been known to have antibacterial activity against some Gram positive and Gram negative bacterial strains including *Bacillus cereus* and *Salmonella paratyphii*. It is eaten fresh, and the extract of fruit and seed is available in capsule, tablet forms.

Ber (Zizyphus) (*Ziziphus jujuba*): It is rich in vitamin C and other nutrients including polyphenols which makes it useful for health. It has a high content of flavonoids—quercetin, kaempferol, and phloretin derivatives. It is usually eaten raw. It is used traditionally as a tonic, an aphrodisiac and anxiolytic (reduces anxiety). It is reputed to have anticancer, antifungal, antibacterial, antiulcer, anti-inflammatory, hypotensive, cardiotonic, antioxidant, immunostimulant, and wound healing properties.

Grapes (*Vitis viifera*): Grapes are a rich source of polyphenolics, for which grapes are highly valued in disease prevention. Resveratrol that is present in some grape varieties and red wine is one of the most potent antioxidants and has a significant role in prevention of heart disease and cholesterol management. Grapes are green and purple (called blue variety). Blue variety contains more amount of resveratrol and flavans called catechin. The fruit is eaten fresh, as juice, jelly, wine, and, in dried form. Red wine and purple grape juices have been reported to enhance platelet and endothelial production of nitric oxide and improve endothelial function and protect against LDL oxidation. Due to this, red wine is considered to provide protection against cardiovascular disease. In Ayurveda, grapes are considered to be cool and nourishing fruit and prescribed in gastritis, fever, urinary problem, etc. Dried forms are also called "draksha or raisins" and are very useful treating digestive disorders and hangovers or dullness.

Dried Fruits

Raisins: Raisins are dried grapes. They are sweet in nature, a concentrated source of energy, vitamins, and trace elements, like iron, manganese, boron, copper, and zinc. They are packed with polyphenolics having as antioxidant and anti-inflammatory properties with beneficial health effects. It helps in preventing anemia and delaying aging, several degenerative diseases including diabetes, CVD, macular degeneration and bone loss.

Black currants (Munnka) (*Ribes nigrum*): It is a good source of iron which is similar to charoli (piyal seeds) spinach. It is low in fat. It is found good for constipation. It is used fresh as well as in muffins and cakes. Black currants are a rich source of anthocyanins, proanthocyanidins, quercetin, myricetin, phenolic acids, and isorhamnetin. Its vitamin C and bioactive phenolics give black currants high antioxidant activity. Thus, they may confer multiple health benefits including the inhibition of development of certain cancers, cardiovascular, and inflammation related diseases. They were found to provide neuroprotection against oxidative stress.

Dates (*Phoenix dactylifera*): Dried dates are rich in iron and carbohydrates and also contain some amounts of protein. They can be used as a nutritious sugar substitute. Both fresh and dried dates contain good amount of insoluble fiber. Dates contain fluorine which protects against dental caries. They also contain selenium. Some date varieties have been found to have a low glycemic index. Dates possess antioxidant and anti-mutagenic activity due to the presence of compounds with free-radical-scavenging activity.

Nuts

Nuts are seeds or fruits of different plants. They are one-seeded fruits with a hard pericarp or ripened ovary wall. They are good sources of protein, fat, vitamin E, fiber, plant sterols, essential fatty acids, vitamins, minerals, and a wide variety of phytochemicals. By virtue of these vital components, they are highly valued for their medicinal properties. Commonly consumed nuts are almonds, cashewnut, pistachios, walnut, and hazel nuts that are consumed raw, roasted, sliced, fried, powdered, or in paste form as an ingredient of some sweet or savory preparation, as snacks or as garnishing. A small amount of nuts may provide considerable health benefits like building stamina, boosting immunity, improving memory, reducing weight and aging process, and regulating blood cholesterol and diabetes. However, excessive consumption of these may increase weight due to the high energy and fat content. Nuts are usually not consumed in large quantity hence they are not major contributors of energy and protein. It is best to avoid sugar or chocolate coated and salted nuts. However, they are nutrient dense food items and significantly improve the quality of diet.

Almonds (*Prunus dulcis*): Since ages, almonds have been valued for improving memory and cognitive functions and control satiety. It is still a valid reason to continue to add in the daily diet. Almonds are consumed raw, roasted, soaked with or without skin; halved or slivered. Its paste form is added to gravies and milkshakes. Soaking and removing skin facilitates better absorption of nutrients and removes the toxic components naturally present in the skin only. They are frequently used in Indian sweets and as a garnish for barfis, chocolates, marzipan, etc. Nutritionally, they are rich in fat and protein, B vitamins, and minerals. They contain good amount of chromium, iron, and alpha linoleic acid but does not provide carotenes or vitamin C. Almonds also contain oxalates, hence those who have oxalate renal stones need to be cautious in their consumption. Play a role in lowering down the cholesterol that may be due to the presence of unsaturated fats and also in weight management. It has been suggested the chewing almonds for more than 30–40 times may affect the release of appetite suppressing hormones and thus suppress hunger. It is also used for cosmetic purposes. Bitter almond contains a toxic substance called amygdalin and should not be eaten.

Cashewnut (*Anacardium occidentale*): They are one of the most relished nuts; eaten raw, roasted, used in gravies and in sweets like kajukatli. Immature cashewnut is also eaten. It is very rich in zinc, magnesium, thiamine, and also contain chromium, selenium, and copper which may be beneficial in diabetes, dyslipidemia, protection of heart, and oxidative stress by supporting functioning of antioxidant enzymes like SOD. Roasting cashewnuts at 130°C for 30 minutes may increase availability of the phenolic compounds and flavonoids present.

Pumpkin seed (*Cucurbita moschata*): Pleasing green colored seeds, they are a rich source of protein, fat, phosphorus, and iron, zinc, calcium, magnesium, potassium, and other nutrients such as tocopherols, PUFAs, fiber, as well as sterols and squalene. The seeds are also a good source of tryptophan. They are consumed roasted as a snack or mixed with salad, shakes, and savories. The seeds are a good source of phytochemicals having antioxidant and anti-inflammatory properties.

Pistachios (*Pistacia vera*): Pista as it is known in India is very rich in thiamine, and riboflavin. It is used raw, roasted, plain, and salted. Its green color enhances the visual appeal of sweets and ice cream. They have been found to improve the lipid profile but also decreased HDL levels. Pistachios have a highest levels of potassium, γ-tocopherol, vitamin K, phytosterols, xanthophyll carotenoids, certain minerals (Cu, Fe and Mg), vitamin B_6, and thiamine. It possesses high antioxidant and anti-inflammatory potential.

Walnut (*Juglans regia*): It is said that the shape of the walnut resembles the shape of the brain, thus it is beneficial for the brain development and its functioning. Secret of this notion lies in the presence of high amounts of omega-3 fatty acids (alpha linolenic acid); tocopherol and boron. Walnuts are endowed with antioxidant and anti-inflammatory bioactivity and it has been reported to have potential role in inhibition of initiation and progression of several cardiovascular and neurodegenerative diseases. Walnuts are found to be protective for cardiac health and prevent cancer (prostrate) that may be attributable to flavonoids like ellagic acid. Walnuts contain more phenolic compounds including ellagic acid and melatonin than other nuts. Walnuts have been shown to reduce total and LDL cholesterol but not triglycerides or HDL cholesterol. They are also good sources of arginine, folate, fiber, and tannins. Walnuts when consumed in prescribed limit helps to reduce weight because the nut provides satiety and fullness.

Hazelnuts (*Corylus spp*): Hazelnuts are also associated with CVD prevention owing to their monounsaturated fatty acids (MUFA) content that protect low-density lipoproteins (LDL) against oxidation and increase HDL. They are rich in various bioactive substances such as tocopherol, phytosterols, B vitamin, iron, potassium, selenium, and the amino acid arginine and exert their respective benefits.

Pecans (*Carya illinoensis*): Pecan nuts have high fat content and are also a good source of dietary fiber, vitamin E, copper, and magnesium as well as antioxidant phytochemicals. They have a low glycemic index. They have been found to lower LDL cholesterol and bring favorable changes in serum insulin and insulin sensitivity.

Sesame seeds (til) (gingelly seed) (*Sesamum indicum*): Til or sesame seeds can be white or black. It is an excellent source of protein, calcium, zinc, and thiamine. It contains oxalates in high amount. Hence, it should be used in limited amounts with caution by persons susceptible to oxalate renal stones. It is generally roasted before use. It is used to make laddoo, chikki, gajak, and used as garnish for some preparations and ingredients in dry chutney as well as tahini, a popular paste used in humus. Certain communities prefer its oil in various cuisines as well as in body message for daily use while others do not due its odor. It is considered good for bone health owing to its high calcium content. Seasamol and sesamolin are major components which have a cholesterol lowering effect and also have antihypertensive action. It also increases HDL and lowers LDL levels. It contains polyphenols including lignans. It also contains cephalin, a phospholipid that has been reported to have hemostatic activity. It is mildly laxative, and may also have antibacterial activity against *Staphylococcus, Streptococcus,* and some common fungi. The oil has wide medical and pharmaceutical applications. Black sesame seeds have antiaging properties also.

Garden cress seeds or chandrashoor (*halim/aliv/chandrashoor*) (*Lepidium sativum*): Traditionally it is considered to be excellent for lactating mothers, as a galactogogue. It is a good source of protein, iron, and fat, dietary fiber and linolenic acid. It is used to make laddoo or porridge. It has been found to be useful for healing fractures in an animal model. Hence, seeds are also recommended in inflammation, muscular pain, and rheumatism.

Groundnuts/peanuts (*Arachis hypogea*): It is popular, cheap, and easily accessible to everyone. It is also considered an oilseed because edible oil is extracted and used. It is an excellent source of niacin, thiamine, folic acid, protein, and fat. Refined vegetable groundnut oil contains 21% MUFA and 10% PUFA. Peanuts are rather inexpensive nuts. It is rich in polyphenols particularly p-coumaric acid and resveratrol, thus it has been considered as antiaging agent. It also provides protection against cancer and radiation exposure. Roasted, boiled, seasoned, groundnut is an ingredient of many dishes, garnish in salads in some parts of Maharashtra. A handful of peanuts have been reported to play a beneficial role in weight management by providing satiety. Boiled peanuts have been found to be healthier than fried or roasted ones due to the presence of phytochemicals like isoflavones (biochanin and genistein) and transresveratrol.

Chilgoza/Pine nuts (*Pinus geradiana*): Also called neoza in India, it is generally used raw in winters. It contains half the amount of thiamine than cashewnut but more than double the amount of niacin than charoli and the same amount of iron. It is rich in manganese and like other nuts it is a good source of protein, and packed with several compounds having antioxidant capacity and thereby effective for treatment of various health disorders. It has low carbohydrate content, but is a good source of magnesium, potassium, and phosphorus. It also contains iron, zinc, calcium, manganese, and copper. Almost half of the fat is linoleic acid and approximately one-third is oleic acid.

Piyal seed (Charoli/chironji) (*Buchanania latifolia*): It is a small seed, generally used in sweets for garnishing, and is relatively cheap compared to other nuts. Like other nuts, it is also high in fat, protein, and thiamine, riboflavin, iron, and magnesium. Besides these, it contains comparatively very high amount of arginine and leucine.

Coconut dry (*Cocos nucifera*): It is also called copra. Various sizes of shavings are available and used in different food preparations like *halwa*, *kheer*, *chivra*, etc. It is rich in fat that is saturated but due to the presence of high proportion of lauric acid, it is said to be heart friendly and also provide numerous health benefits. It also contains a good amount of protein and iron, hence useful for pregnant and lactating mothers; coconut oil is obtained from dry coconut. The oil is relished in south Indian cuisine.

Sunflower seed (*Helianthus annuus*): This seed is one of the most important oilseed crops. It has high antioxidant capacity. Besides being rich in fat, protein, and iron, the seeds are rich in choline, tocopherol, and phenolics compounds, making them good inhibitors of lipid oxidation, which is beneficial in terms of preventing cardiovascular diseases.

Flax seed (*Linum usitatissimum*): Flax was used by Hippocrates and treasured throughout the Roman Empire as a health food for its healing properties. Now it has been rediscovered as a health food owing to its tremendous health benefits. It is exceptionally rich in ω-3 fatty acid, i.e., alpha linolenic acid (a very good source of omega-3 fatty acid for vegetarians), protein, and fiber in the form of lignan. Its viscous fiber is also beneficial. It is commercially available in the form of seeds and oil. It enhances immunity and brain cognitive function and is also good for bowel and bone health. Since ω-3 fatty acid is sensitive and easily destroyed, the oil should be well protected from heat and exposure to air. The seeds are slightly roasted, ground, and can be used in curd, milk, and a variety of products without affecting the taste and flavor.

Brazil nut (*Bertholletia excels*): Brazil nut is the richest source of selenium and also contains good amounts of healthy fat, tocopherols, squalene, protein, and minerals. It also extends antioxidant and anti-inflammatory effect due to which it reduces the oxidative stress and its associated diseases.

Macdamia nut (*Macadamia integrifolia*): Macdamia nut is extremely rich in fat but a good balance of unsaturated fatty acids but has a good balance of obesity and CVD. It is less susceptible to oxidation and more stable in cooking. Its oil is similar to olive oil in composition and helps to balance the omega-6 and omega-3 composition. It is also very rich in vitamin E, phytosterols, and polyphenols. Macadamia oil (MO) is a versatile fat widely used in the pharmaceutical and cosmetic purposes.

MILK AND MILK PRODUCTS

Milk is nearly a complete food in itself for infants, providing necessary nutrients in adequate amounts (except iron and vitamin C) to sustain life. Infants survive only on milk (preferably human milk). Milk is obtained from different female mammals, e.g., cow, buffalo, goat, sheep, and camel. However, commonly consumed milk comes from cows and buffaloes.

Raw milk or pasteurized milk has a mild but characteristic taste due to the presence of around 400 aroma compounds. Milk is highly perishable and cannot be stored for long. Milk is pasteurized at low temperatures (68°C for 30 minutes) to avoid spoilage by undesirable microorganisms, to destroy pathogenic (disease-causing) microorganisms, and to extend its storability/shelf life. Pasteurized milk does not have a cooked flavor. In order to extend the shelf life, various heat treatment techniques are generally applied such as pasteurization, ultraheat and short time (UHT), sterilization and drying, etc. Milk may also be homogenized, i.e., the size of the fat globules in milk is reduced further so that the fat does not separate out. Composition of milk obtained from different species is typical, which makes it very useful in making a wide variety of milk products that may be useful in many health conditions.

Nutrient composition of milk and dairy products is highly influenced by the type of feed or feeding practices used for the cattle (cows, etc.). Cows grazing on free pasture (grass fed) produce milk with higher amount of omega-3, CLA, vitamin E, and carotenes as compared to those who are fed other food. Milk is a good source of protein, fat, calcium, and several other nutrients. Besides calcium, other minerals present in milk are sulfur, magnesium, manganese, iodine, zinc, etc. It is also rich in riboflavin, vitamin B_{12}, vitamin A, and vitamin K. Milk does not contain niacin but contains the amino acid tryptophan which can be converted into niacin. It is a very poor source of iron and vitamin C. The major sugar in milk is lactose consisting of galactose and glucose. No other food contains galactose or lactose in free form. It helps in growth and development and also aids calcium absorption. Milk contains small amounts of glucose and other sugars. Lactose is easily converted into lactic acid in the presence of lactobacillus many oligosacchrides or lower pH. This is the basis for making curd and other fermented milk products.

The major protein in milk is casein which is present as calcium caseinate. When any acidic substance is added to milk, it curdles. Casein is the protein that coagulates and is the solid part which is separated and called paneer. Other proteins present in milk are lactoglobulin, lactoalbumin, and lactoferrin which remain in the whey (liquid fraction) when milk curdles. These proteins are highly nutritious and provide immunological benefits. Whey water is used during illness. Milk proteins have a high biological value as they contain all essential amino acids to promote growth.

Most of the milk fat is triglycerides, with smaller amounts of phospholipids, sterols, free fatty acids, etc. Milk characteristically contains short chain fatty acids like butyric acid and caproic acid which are also present in butter and responsible for distinct flavor. Milk fat is very finely distributed as small globules (diameter 0.1–10 μm) in the aqueous/liquid phase. Milk fat primarily consists of fat droplets or globules which are surrounded by a thin membrane for stabilization of fat globules in the milk serum. Nutrient composition of both globule and membrane is different. The fat globules contain triglycerides, diglycerides, fatty acids, sterols, carotenoids, fat soluble vitamins, and the membrane consists of phospholipids, lipoproteins, glycerides, cerebrosides, proteins, enzymes, metals, and water. On heating milk in an open container, protein coagulates and fat rises to the surface, being lighter (having lower specific gravity) than water, due to this milk fall over the edge of the vessel while boiling. This coagulated layer contains fat and protein and forms a thick layer on the surface of the milk. It is called "skin" which is also referred as "malai." Formation of skin holds the steam and does not allow much of it to escape. Raw milk also forms cream layer on top of the milk on standing at low temperature. This cream layer can be separated out.

The fat content of milk from different animal varies considerably (with source of milk) and processing also influences fat content. Buffalo's milk has a much higher fat content than cow's milk. Milk fat can also be altered by various processing methods. In the dairy industry, the cream may be separated to remove fat and the fat content of the milk can be standardized. Fat is removed to different extents to produce full fat/whole, standardized, toned, low fat, and skimmed milk. Milk is generally marketed with the fat content being specified. According to FSSAI (2019) double toned, toned full cream milk has minimum of 1.5, 3.0 and 6.0% fat respectively. Skim milk has not more that 0.5% fat. It is adjusted with total solids in the milk. Skimmed milk is devoid of fat and often used in low fat diets. Thus, protein content of skimmed milk is higher particularly in skimmed milk powder per unit weight compared to whole milk or whole milk powder. Due to the higher protein content, it is used for malnourished persons, in food aid and feeding programs, as well as in pathological conditions. Removal of fat delays spoilage of skimmed milk.

Milk contains different types of proteins predominantly casein (solid) and whey protein (milk serum). Casein has mainly four fractions, due to which different milk products like cheese and yogurt or curd can be prepared and their quality is also affected. Whey protein fractions exhibit immunological and other health benefits. Absorption of calcium and lactose from milk is also linked to casein and whey protein, respectively.

Milk often becomes brown or gets scorched on the sides or bottom of the pan. This is due to a chemical reaction that occurs whenever sugar and protein are heated together. The reaction is known as "Maillard reaction." It is also responsible for cooked or caramel type flavor in the milk.

There is a large variety of liquid milk available in the market ranging from cow's milk, buffalo's milk, skimmed milk, double toned milk, toned, whole milk, flavored milk, and fortified milk. Among milk products, paneer, curds, or yoghurt, many types of cheese, khoa, milk powders, ice cream, lassi, and condensed milk are easily available and consumed. Besides these, a wide range of sweets are manufactured with milk or khoa or paneer such as rosogolla, gulab jamun, rasmalai, basundi, rabri, etc. Nutritional and health significance of various milk products are given in Table 16.6.

Table 16.6: Uses and nutritional and health significance of milk products.

Milk products	Uses	Nutritional and health significance
Evaporated milk	Used as replacement for milk in food industry	A concentrated source of protein, calcium, and fat so good for malnourished children. It is unsweetened condensed milk reduced from 2.5 parts of whole milk to 1 part and the finished product is packed in tin containers. It has a cooked flavor but not caramelized. Easy to store and transport.
Condensed milk	Used as an ingredient to make tea, sweets like gajar halwa, coconut laddoo, bread spread, cakes, or to replace milk and sugar	It is also evaporated but to higher concentration and 30–40% sucrose is added to it. It contains 31% milk solids, 9% fat, and 60% sugar. Concentrated form if used without dilution can be harmful. Can cause dental caries, obesity. Useful in treating protein energy malnutrition for community nutrition programs. Easy to store and transport.
Skimmed milk (liquid)	Drinking fat-free milk and other uses where fat needs to be restricted	Comparatively high in protein and calcium but not fat. It contains 0.5% fat only and lesser amounts of fat-soluble vitamins and cholesterol. Good for liver disorders, obesity. It is better avoided by growing children in order to relatively low in other essential nutrients.
Skimmed milk powder	Used to make fat-free original milk and nutrient dense food products.	Very high in protein and calcium and low in fat. It is widely used as a good source of protein for management of malnutrition or high protein diet. Needs extra care during storage. Sometimes stabilizers are added to lengthen shelf life.
Whole milk powder	Useful in scarcity of fresh milk and adds creaminess and nutrient density of food preparations	Concentrated source of protein, calcium, and carbohydrates can be used to fortify other food products to make nutrient dense. Easy to store. Ideally temperature should be <25°C and relative humidity should be <65%. Avoid rancidity and maillard reaction.

Contd...

Contd...

Milk products	Uses	Nutritional and health significance
Instant dairy whitener	Tea/coffee, milkshakes	Source of protein and calcium easy to mix in hot and cold beverages, easily digestible. Other ingredients are also used to mimic the qualities of the milk. Plant oils are used in production of dairy whiteners.
Khoa (Mawa)	Used to make Indian sweets and sometimes used in fillings of snack or as an ingredient of gravy	Concentrated source of protein, calcium, and fat. Should be consumed in limits even by healthy people, e.g., occasionally in festive season.
Curd	Curd, lassi, raita, chakka (hung curd), a sweet called "shrikhand"	Source of protein, calcium, vitamin B_{12}, magnesium and important fatty acids. Fresh and sweet (without sugar) impart several health benefits through improving gut microbiome using variety of bacteria evolved while making curd.
Yoghurt	Available as plain yoghurt or with fruit in which fruit or fruit puree is added	Yogurt is similar to Indian curd, the fine line difference is in the method of preparation and bacterial strains in its culture. Both provide health benefits like improving digestion, immunity, bone health, cooling in summer.
Acidophilus milk	Used as such, as a probiotic	Milk is fermented with *Lactobacillus acidophilus*. It helps in balancing the gut flora, thus used for digestive disorder and yeast infection. It can also be used by lactose intolerant individuals.
Paneer	Used as ingredient in filling of many snack items, spreads, fried to add in gravy, vegetable preparations; used in some sweets, e.g., rosogolla	Concentrated source of protein, calcium, and carbohydrates. An addition to other products enriches them.
Whey water	Used as drink and sometimes in curries and to make new batch of paneer	Whey proteins constitute 14 to 24% of the total proteins. Whey is rich in proteins like lactalbumin, lactoglobulin, lactoferrins, lactoperoxidase, catalase, phosphatases, and riboflavin. Good in illness and convalescence because of its immune enhancing proteins. Lactoferrins are commercially are used in antibacterial medicines both for animals and humans.
Whey protein concentrate	Used as a powder usually by sports persons or as a supplement to enrich the protein in other foods	Concentrated source of protein which is easily digested and strengthens the muscles, improves stamina and vitality. It tended to reduce total cholesterol and LDL cholesterol as well as fasting insulin levels.

Cheese

Cheese is one of the most ancient forms of manufactured food. It is thought that cheese-making may go as far back as 10,000 BC, when sheep and goats were first domesticated in the Middle East and early herdsmen used to consume milk. Due to contaminating bacteria, milk has a short shelf life, especially in warm climates. Therefore, it might have happened that sour milk naturally separated into curds and whey, the solid curd provided an edible and nourishing food. The basic reason for purposely processing milk into cheese is to preserve a perishable food and to convert it into a stable and storable product. It also expands the variety of food because it is astonishingly high in palatability, versatility in culinary world.

Milk has mainly two phases, i.e., liquid phase is whey and the solid phase is coagulum, constituting about 20–25 g/100 g. Coagulum is converted into cheese that can be strained, molded, salted, fermented, and/or ripened for more or less time. Protein and lactose are drained in whey. Digestibility of protein from cheese is very high (95%). Various peptides have been identified from variety of cheeses which have health benefits. It also contains fat-soluble vitamins. Some vitamins are also synthesized during ripening of cheese such as folate and vitamin B_{12}. Calcium in cheese is also absorbed and is bioavailable.

A very wide range of varieties are prepared using different starter cultures and techniques to ripen the cheese. In India, paneer is used which is basically unripened coagulum and often made at household level. Some cheeses are hard and some soft. Commonly used varieties of cheese are Cheddar, Cottage, Mozzarella, Parmesan, Roquefort, Swiss, Brick, Camembert, Ricotta, etc. Each variety has a distinct texture, flavor, and color that largely depend on the duration of ripening and environmental conditions. In ripened cheese, edible bacterial or fungal culture is added and kept for maturation till desired flavor and textures are obtained. European and western cuisines include cheese in a large variety of preparations besides consuming it as such. Even in India, cheese is a popular product, frequently used in sandwich fillings, toppings, and mixed with other ingredients to make a variety of snacks, sauces, desserts, spreads, dips, and salads. It is eaten with fruits or crackers, with macaroni, and in soufflés. It is convenient to use but not economical.

Cheese is a rich source of bioavailable calcium, protein, carbohydrates, bioactive peptides, amino acids, fat, fatty acids, vitamins, and minerals. Fresh cheese has lower amount of fat and higher amount of lactose than semi-hard and hard cheeses that have been ripened. Ripened cheese has no lactose but its fat content is higher. Chewing a piece of cheese after a sugary food brings plaque pH rapidly back to neutrality. However, it contains high amount of sodium, and should be restricted for persons who are advised sodium restriction, e.g., those with renal problems and hypertension.

Cheese is a good source of conjugated linoleic acid (CLA). Conjugated linolenic acid and sphingolipids present in cheese may have anticarcinogenic properties, although their content varies widely with the type of cheese. Soft cheese contains more than hard cheese varieties. Hard cheeses have much higher protein and fat than soft cheeses. Fresh cheese has lactose whereas soft and hard cheeses do not. Thus, hard cheese can be used in lactose free diets. There is evidence to suggest that two bioactive tripeptides, VPP and IPP, found in sour milk fermented with *Lactobacillus helveticus*, lower blood pressure. These peptides were also detected in specific cheese varieties in significant quantities. The high calcium content in cheese is well known to contribute to the formation and maintenance of strong bones and teeth, also has a positive effect on blood pressure, and helps in losing weight in combination with low-energy diets.

EGGS

Eggs have been used as food since times immemorial. Egg is one of nature's perfect protein foods. Egg from hen is commonly consumed throughout the world. Eggs of other birds may also be consumed, e.g., ducks, quail, geese, seagulls, etc. However, if the word "eggs" is used without specifying the source, it may be assumed that it refers to chicken/hen's eggs. Eggs are soft or hard-boiled, scrambled, fried, dried, powdered, or frozen and used in a wide variety of food preparations like bakery products, etc. Eggs are also used as an emulsifier in gelling or thickening agent in custard and as leavening agent in cakes. For example—when an egg is beaten, the protein of the egg forms a thin film around air, forming bubbles. Incorporating this air provides the leavening to the cake, giving the cake, its fluffy and spongy texture.

Egg is an important source of nourishment at affordable price. A medium egg weighs approximately 40-50 g and provides 67 kcal and 6.6 g protein. It contains relatively no carbohydrate, no fiber, and no vitamin C. Its fat is present in egg yolk which is mainly saturated fat. Egg yolk also contains cholesterol. Egg white does not have any fat content. It has been observed that feed of the hen influences the nutrient composition of egg. If the hen is given food rich in omega 3 fatty acids, it is reflected in the lipid content of the egg. Eggs also contain a large number of active lipid components, such as unsaturated fatty acids, phospholipids, choline, and carotenoids. Dietary phospholipids are important in controlling the cholesterol metabolism, HDL functions, and inflammation.

There has been lot of debate to consume egg or not, to avoid dietary cholesterol. There are many confounding factors such as genes, hormones, other dietary components, lifestyle, and the nutritional status of the subjects which determine the pathogenesis of CVD. After scrutiny of several researches eventually US Dietary Guidelines Advisory Committee (DGAC) eliminated this restriction from the latest version of dietary guideline in 2015.

Egg protein is one of the best high quality proteins because it contains all the essential amino acids and is considered a "reference protein" to compare protein quality of other foods. The biological value (BV) of egg is 100. Egg protein has a potential for antioxidant capacity due to which it plays a role in protection from degenerative diseases. The egg albumin which is present in egg white is pure soluble protein. Eggs are easily digested. Beside its high quality protein, it contains appreciable amount of vitamins particularly riboflavin, pantothenic acid, folic acid, vitamins B_{12}, A, D, and E. Among minerals, egg contains iodine, phosphorus, zinc, selenium, calcium, and iron. Egg offers numerous health benefits—like presence of choline that boost brain functions particularly in fetal and neonatal stage; selenium curbs damages from free radicals and aids in prevention of heart diseases; high sulfur content promotes healthy hair and nails and high phosphorus supports bone health.

Structurally, egg is divided in three main parts each having distinct features and functions: (1) egg shell, (2) egg white, and (3) egg yolk.

Egg shell: It is white or brown in color, rigid, and brittle in appearance but the shell is porous. The brown color is due to hen's species and does not reflect the nutritional content of the egg. The shell is made up of calcium carbonate, magnesium carbonate and phosphate, mucopolysaccharides, and other organic matter. It protects the egg from microbial spoilage by restricting penetration by microorganisms. Being porous, it is permeable to gases.

Egg white: It contains a variety of proteins and some of them are glycoproteins. Main egg white protein is albumin. The albumin is present in three layers which vary in thickness. The outermost layer near the shell is thin, and then there is a thick layer of white and another thin layer near the yolk. As the egg ages, the albumin/the white gradually becomes thinner in consistency. Other proteins are conalbumin, ovomucoid, ovomucin, avidin, lysozyme, and other proteins. Ovomucin is responsible for foaming of egg white. Ovalbumin is denatured rapidly. All proteins have biological activities and protect the egg. Egg white does not contain fat, so it is very useful in cases when high quality protein diet is advised.

Egg yolk: Egg yolk is the cream or yellow round portion in the center. Yolk is held in the center with chalazae (invisible) passing through egg white. The yellow color of egg yolk is due to the presence of carotenoids like lutein, zeaxanthin, and cryptoxanthin, which are useful in delaying macular degeneration of eyes and cataract caused by aging. Lecithin a phospholipid is naturally present in egg and helps to emulsify fat. It is also a component of cell membrane.

Egg can be separated into its white and yolk which can be dried and powdered for further use. Egg is used in a wide variety of processed foods like bakery products, noodles, pastries, mayonnaise, salad dressings, soup powders, ice creams among others.

FISH AND SEAFOODS

Fish is found in abundance in ponds, lakes, rivers, and sea. It is a prime food for populations residing in coastal regions. Fish has excellent nutritional value, providing high quality and easily digestible protein and a wide variety of vitamins and minerals, including vitamins A and D, phosphorus, magnesium, selenium, and iodine in marine fish. Fish oils in fatty fish are the richest source of omega 3 fatty acid that is vital for brain development in infants and maintains cardiac and bone health in adults. Thus, fish fulfills a very important role in human nutrition. Fish may also be categorized according to the environment in which it lives: fresh fish like carp and salmon and sea fish such as sardines, catfish, and mackerel.

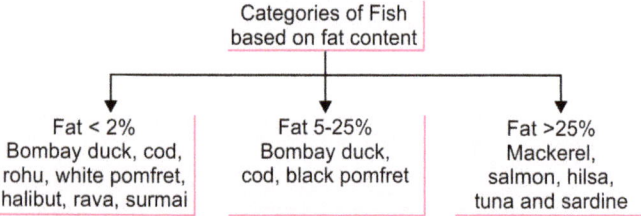

Fish can be classified into two—(1) Fin fish and (2) shell fish.

Fin Fish: Fin fish have a bony skeleton and they are found in fresh water and salt water and are easy to catch. They can further be divided into three categories as per their fat content. Fat content varies among different species and includes lecithin, free cholesterol, triglycerides, waxes, and free fatty acids. Fish also contains inositol and phosphotidylethalomaine. Most of the lipids are digestible but most of it is unsaturated fatty acids, that increase susceptibility for rancidity easily and there is deterioration of flavor. Fish liver contains extraordinarily large amounts of vitamins A and D. Though, fish liver is rarely eaten, but instead used to extract fish liver oil. Tuna and halibut contain more of vitamin A while mackerel, salmon, and sardine contain more of vitamin D. Flesh of salmon is reported to have good amount of pantothenic acid. Fish supplies good amount of minerals and is a good natural source of iodine and fluorine. Muscle protein is similar to that of mammals which is easy to digest.

Shell Fish: They are devoid of vertebral column and fins but have a hard covering on their body, called "shell." Shellfish are again categorized into two. They are considered as sea food. Shell fish contain more of thiamine and riboflavin and vitamin B_{12}. They contain more minerals than fin fish particularly calcium, magnesium, iron, and iodine.

1. **Crustaceans:** These have a shell and a segmented body, e.g., lobster, crab, prawn, and shrimp.
2. **Mollusks:** These have a soft unsegmented body covered by a calcified shell, e.g., oyster, mussels, clams, and scallops.

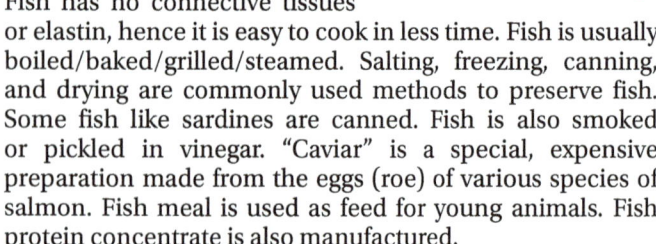

Fish has no connective tissues or elastin, hence it is easy to cook in less time. Fish is usually boiled/baked/grilled/steamed. Salting, freezing, canning, and drying are commonly used methods to preserve fish. Some fish like sardines are canned. Fish is also smoked or pickled in vinegar. "Caviar" is a special, expensive preparation made from the eggs (roe) of various species of salmon. Fish meal is used as feed for young animals. Fish protein concentrate is also manufactured.

> Consumption of one to two servings of fatty fish per week lowers the risk of CHD and sudden death. Fish oil capsules are also a good source of n-3 PUFAs. On the other hand, there is growing concern over the potential harmful effects of mercury, dioxins, and polychlorinated biphenyls (PCBs) present in some fish species. Water source in which fish are farmed also determines content of these toxins.

Cod liver oil is obtained from the liver of cod fish (Gadidae). It contains high concentrations of eicosapentaenoic acid (EPA) and docosahexaenoic acid (DHA) and also contains Vitamin A and D. It is often prescribed for prevention of rickets and improves cognitive functions in children. While fish oils from other fish contain EPA and DHA, they are not good sources of vitamin A and D. Fish oil is obtained from fatty fish like salmon, herring and cod liver oil comes from Atlantic or Pacific cod and delivered in the form of capsule. They are consumed as a accessible and effective source of omega-3 for reducing the inflammatory conditions in the body.

Fish spoils within 2–3 days even in a refrigerator, as it contains 70–80% water and unsaturated fatty acids. It is easily attacked by microbes. Glycogen level in muscles of fish is high, that is easily converted into lactic acid resulting in a decrease in pH. During spoilage, a compound known as trimethyl amine (TMO) is formed that gives an obnoxious stale fishy smell.

The Food and Agriculture Organization (FAO, 2010) has accepted seafood as an essential food for humans owing to the abundant presence of high-quality proteins, n-3 polyunsaturated fatty acids (PUFAs), and other nutrients, such as minerals, trace elements, and vitamins. Consumption of seafoods has also increased in recent years. Seafood is regarded as a support to maintain and protect health from CVD and other chronic diseases. In addition, n-3 PUFAs have been shown to play a beneficial role in body weight and satiety regulation, reducing inflammation and thus could help in inflammatory diseases like rheumatoid arthritis. Consumption of fish and/or EPA/DHA may protect against the development of Alzheimer's disease. Sea foods are rich sources of different forms of dietary phospholipids thereby they are good in improving blood lipid profile and brain functions. Further sea foods are also demonstrate high amino acid score and digestibility. Lobster is rich in the amino acid, taurine. Some sea foods are being exploited in cosmetic and pharmaceutical industries using their collagen, gelatin, oily substances and many proteins.

MEAT AND POULTRY

Animal foods have been used to satisfy hunger since evolution of mankind and even today, they are used extensively for human consumption. Meat refers to those parts of animals that are used as food and include muscles, connective tissues, and organs of warm-blooded and four legged animals like cattle, sheep, pig, goat, horse, camel, and mule. Meat flavor and quality are largely dependent upon the type of animal, species, age, and part of the body. There are different names for different kinds of meat used for consumption:

Mutton: Flesh of sheep of both sexes age above 12 months of age. Flesh of younger sheep or lambs is known as lamb meat. Lamb meat has milder flavor and taste than mutton.

Yearling mutton: Carcass of young sheep aged between 12 and 20 months.

Mature mutton: Flesh of sheep whose age is 20 months at the time of slaughter.

Beef: Meat of cattle over 1 year old.
Pork: Meat of pig or swine between ages of 3 and 12 months.
Veal: Meat of calves usually slaughtered after 1 month up to 14 weeks of age.
Organ meat: Liver, kidney, heart, thymus, pancreas, and brain.
Red meat: Meat which has higher amount of fat and cholesterol.
Lean meat: Meat from which fat layer has been removed.
Sausages: Made of minced and ground meat and are enclosed in casings (intestine).

Meat contains good quality protein, high amount of fat (mostly saturated fat), heme iron that is more bioavailable than is not in iron from plant sources (non-heme iron), and B vitamins such as thiamine, riboflavin, and niacin and zinc. Carbohydrates in meat are glycogen and glucose. It does not contain fiber and vitamin C. Calcium in meat comes from bones. Meat protein comes from muscles and collagen. Muscle protein is of two types—myosin and actin. Collagen is a soluble protein which during moist heat cooking is converted into gelatin. Connective tissues also contain mucopolysaccharides. Muscles are surrounded with fat layers. This is called marbling which plays a significant role in flavor. Fat composition varies as per diet of the animal, genetic background, age, and amount of exercise before slaughter. Fat increases the water holding capacity, thus contributes to the juiciness of meat. Fat is rich in saturated fatty acids and cholesterol content. However, lean meat contains more unsaturated fatty acids and high percentage of phospholipids. Pork tends to have higher fat content than other meat.

Meat contains two pigments, namely, hemoglobin and myoglobin. Hemoglobin is a red pigment present in the red blood cells and myoglobin that is present in muscle, provides purplish color; however, it changes with availability of the oxygen. On slaughter, it is exposed to oxygen and forms a pigment called oxymyoglobin which is bright red in color. When oxygen supply stops, it becomes purple. On exposure to air, it is again bright red which is often fixed with use of nitrites; otherwise, myoglobin is soon converted into another pigment known as metmyoglobin which is brownish gray in color.

The amount of myoglobin in red and white meat varies considerably. Immediately after slaughter, the muscle is soft, limp, and dry. But a few hours after death, the carcass becomes rigid. The process of stiffening of the muscle is called "Rigor mortis." The onset of rigor mortis occurs in beef muscle within 10-24 hours, in pork within 4-18 hours, and in chicken within 2-4 hours after slaughter. Meat is aged or ripened at low temperature to make meat tender. Tenderness is further enhanced by mincing; use of proteolytic enzymes such as papain from green papaya, ficin from fig, and bromelain from pineapple; use of salts such as sodium chloride, sodium bicarbonate, calcium chloride, magnesium chloride, and acids like lime or vinegar. Meat is often marinated with spices to increase flavor and improve the texture of meat. Smoking is another method used to improve flavor. Cooking methods used are roasting, broiling, pan broiling, frying, braising, stewing, and pressure cooking.

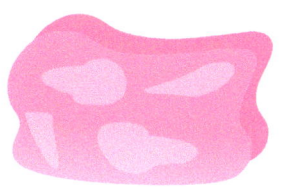

Poultry refers to all domesticated birds that are bred for consumption. Chicken, ducks, geese, turkey, and pigeons are used as meat. Common terms used are broilers (8–10 weeks old when bones are soft), rooster (3-5 months old), stag (male chicken), and cock (>10 months old). Poultry meat has a high protein content 18-22 g % depending upon the body part of the bird used. Similarly, the fat content and other nutrients will depend on the body part. Poultry meat contains more of unsaturated fatty acids and is a good source of B vitamins and minerals. Light colored meat is rich in niacin whereas dark colored meat is a good source of riboflavin. It also does not contain any fiber or vitamin C.

Meat is processed using mechanical, chemical, or enzymatic processes essentially to extend shelf life and to manufacture a variety of meat products including canned meat, ham, a variety of sausages, bacon, cold cuts, meat pastes, and meat extracts which are used in soup powders and sauce powders. Processes used include cooking, curing, smoking, freezing, etc. Shelf life of meat can be increased to a considerable extent by freezing. Drying is an ancient method often used in combination with salting, curing, and smoking. Salting of meat is done by addition of salt or by immersing the meat in 15-20% brine. In some preparations, sugar or spices may be added. Processed meat contains additional salts, phosphates, nitrate or nitrite, and hydrocolloids. Nitrite is added to arrest microbial growth (particularly of *Clostridium botulism*) and preserve the color of the meat. However, use of nitrite is a health concern. It can combine with amines (breakdown product of proteins) in the stomach and form nitrosamines which is carcinogenic in nature. Some processors add ascorbic acid or its salt like sodium ascorbate to retain the color.

Meat Analogs: Meat analogs are meat like substances made from plants. They are vegan meats or mock meat. Analog means they are structurally similar but vary in composition. They are being acceptable in the market as an cheaper alternative to high protein meat products. the concern over the diseases in animals and many environmental issues can also be taken care with such food forms such as fillings in burgers, tacos patties etc. Food scientists are working to develop taste and flavour similar to meat.

SUGARS AND SWEETENERS

In nature, a wide variety of sugars are available. However, only a few of these are used as sweeteners. Sucrose is the principal sugar used all over the world. Other sugars that are used include glucose, invert sugar which contains a mixture of glucose and fructose, maltose, lactose, and fructose. Some of these are derived from carbohydrate, e.g., starch. Some sugars and sugar alcohols are also used in industry (food and pharmaceutical) such as sorbitol, xylitol, mannitol, maltitol, lactulose, and lactitol. Those of economic importance are sucrose, glucose, fructose, lactose, high fructose corn syrup (HFCS), invert sugar, mannitol, sorbitol, xylitol, glucose syrup, and maltose syrup. Use in foods and food manufacture/processing essentially depends on the relative sweetness of sugar (Table 16.7). Sugar, jaggery (gur), and honey are forms of sugar which are used on daily basis. Sugar provides empty calories. Sugar is used to sweeten tea, coffee, cocoa, and beverages. Used in manufacture of sweets and confectionery, jams, jelly and squashes, candied fruit, bakery products, biscuits, and decorations like icing. Jaggery has been used as sweetening agent since ages and nutritionally is better than white sugar as it contains minerals and some phenolic compounds. Maple syrup is another sweetening agents which is being used now in India also. It is dark in color and rich in mineral and several compounds showing antioxidant and anti-inflammatory effects.

FATS AND OILS

Since ancient times, fats and oils have been used in every household for a wide variety of purposes like seasoning, sautéing, shallow frying, deep-frying, smearing, garnishing, salad dressing, and pickle making. Oils are also valued for cosmetic and religious purposes. However, today in general, people have started believing that fat should be totally avoided in the diet for a healthy heart. This is a myth, because fat is not consumed just for taste but also for health. All biological membranes in the body including nerves contain different types of lipids, i.e., phospholipids, glycolipids, and sterols. Thus, the body always needs some amount of fat, in order to perform several important functions such as providing energy, protecting the organs, providing insulation, providing the building blocks for steroid hormones, aiding in absorption of fat-soluble vitamins, and other biological functions. However, there is no doubt that excessive amount of fat consumption and lack of exercise is responsible for many physiological disorders and degenerative diseases.

Fats and oils are generally used for cooking and are exposed to thermal oxidation at high temperatures during preparation of various food items. Repeated use of cooking oils accelerates the oxidation. Results of studies indicate that oxidation has deleterious effects such as generation of cytotoxic compounds, loss of carotenoids, phenolics, and vitamins thus reducing the overall antioxidant properties of the oils which have adverse effects on health. Hence, cooking oils should not be overheated and the same oil should neither be repeatedly used for frying, nor for seasoning, sautéing or shortening.

The fatty acid composition of individual fat varies considerably. The composition of animal fat is largely affected by the kind and breed of animal and what the animal was fed (the composition of the feed). Animal fats include beef fat, sheep tallow, and lard (hog fat). Composition of lard is affected by the feed of the animal whereas beef

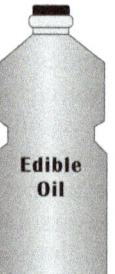
Edible Oil

Table 16.7: Different types of sugars and their nutritional and health significance.

Food item	Nutritional and health significance
Sugar	It contains only calories and no other nutrient. It adds energy value to the diet. Excessive consumption can cause dental caries, obesity, diabetes, and rise in triglyceride levels in blood, lethargy, and depression.
	Present in a variety of foods such as sugar cane, sugar beet, sweet corn, palm sap, fruits, and onion. Generally made from cane sugar or beet sugar. Other sources are dates, palm sap, maple, and sorghum.
Jaggery	It is obtained from cane sugar, date, and palm sap. In addition to carbohydrates, unrefined jaggery contains many minerals. Date and palm jaggery contains more iron.
Honey	It is obtained from honeybee combs. Flower honey is sweet, highly aromatic, and can vary in color. Flavor and color are influenced by the kinds of flowers/plant from which the nectar is obtained.
	It contains 80% sugars (fructose and glucose and small amounts of disaccharides and oligosaccharides). It also contains some amino acids, enzymes, and fatty acids. In addition, it contains many vitamins and minerals like chromium. Among other valuable components are furfural, and hydroxyl methyl furfural which act as antimicrobial agents. Natural honey contains caproic acid and valeric acid which are short chain fatty acids. Honey also contains several phytochemicals which confer medicinal value to honey as has been mentioned in various texts of ancient medicines like Ayurveda. These play a role in inhibiting the growth of unhealthy microorganisms and yeast. Honey also protects the gut environment from toxic effects.
Dextrin	Dextrin is a product developed after partial hydrolysis of starch. It is slightly gummy in texture and sweet in taste. It is used in fermentation of sugars at industrial level.
High fructose corn syrup (HFCS)	HFCS contains varying amounts of fructose (42–90%) with the remainder being glucose. There are different types of HFSC varying in fructose content, e.g., HFSC 55 that contains 55% fructose is commonly used in soft drinks. Being liquid in nature, it is easy to blend and also provides less kcals (3 kcal/g). Depending upon the cost of corn production, it is a cheaper source of sweetener. It can be used by persons with sucrase deficiency. It has the same effect on blood glucose as sugar and not recommended as an alternative sweetener, hence it should be avoided by persons who have insulin resistance, diabetes and high uric acid. Fructose is broken down into purines. It increases the oxidative stress in the body.
Fructose	Metabolized by liver and does not require insulin for entry into liver cells. It also provides 4 kcal/g.
	In well-controlled diabetics, does not affect blood glucose much but in patients with severe insulin deficiency, blood glucose rises. It can cause osmotic diarrhea, if consumption is more than 75 g/day. Fructose intake from fruits, vegetables and honey should not be considered as harmful because fruits also contain several other phytochemicals, fiber and other nutrients. Total fructose is also not very high in fruits (due to their high moisture content) unless they are consumed in large amounts. Fructose is a constituent of white sugar and HFCS which is present in many processed foods and beverages. Thus if such processed foods are consumed in large quantity, it has adverse implications for health.
Molasses	Produced after cane sugar or beet sugar processing. Contains a mixture of sucrose (approx 60%) and other components. Used in food production or for production of acids like citric acid or in production of amino acids, baker's yeast, production of ethanol, glycerol, acetone, rum.

fat is not. Other animal fats are marine (fish) oils obtained from sea mammals like whales, seals, and fish like herring. Sheep tallow is harder than beef tallow and because it has an unpleasant odor, it is generally not used as edible fat. Beef fat when heated to 30–34°C gives two fractions—oleomargarine which is liquid and oleostearin that is solid. Oleomargarine is soft; the consistency is similar to melted butter and is used in margarine and for bakery products. Oleostearin has a higher melting point and is used to manufacture shortenings (fat used in bakery industry). Poor quality tallow is used more as a raw material for non-food products.

Across the world, almost all the oils used in food preparations are of plant origin. Some oils are obtained from fruit pulp such as olive oil and palm oil. The others are obtained from a variety of seeds, e.g., groundnut oil, mustard oil, seasame oil. Oil seeds are rich in oil which can be extracted for manufacturing vegetable oils. Fats and oils are not only used for cooking but also for soap making, in cosmetics, and for pharmaceutical purposes. Edible oils are necessary for health but are harmful in excess or if the oil has got oxidized but is still consumed.

Butter and ghee are obtained from cow's and buffalo's milk. Coconut, corn, cottonseed, peanut (groundnut), safflower, soybean, sunflower seed, sesame, mustard, flaxseed, and rape seed oils are obtained from their respective oil seeds and categorized as vegetable oils. Oil is also extracted from some nuts such as almond, grape seed, and walnut and these oils are used for medicinal and cosmetic purposes.

Butter: Butter is made from cream separated out from whole milk by fermentation and agitation. It is made from either sour cream or non-soured, sweet cream. It is a water-in-oil emulsion and lighter in weight or less dense than the protein and water in cream. Hence, it separates out from the rest and rises to the surface. 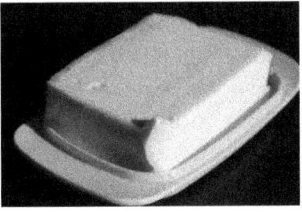 Butter contains less fat compared to other fats because it contains some moisture whereas the others do not. It contains about 80% fat, some amount of protein, non-fat solids, and about 16% water. Therefore, calorie value of butter is lesser than other fats (7 kcal/g). It has short chain fatty acids like butyric acid which makes butter easy to digest. Butyric acid plays an important role in the gastrointestinal tract. Animal studies show that it is immunomodulatory, improved smooth muscle contractility, and regulated neurotransmission, may be useful in diarrhea, have a protective effect in inflammatory response of the gut, probably through maintaining symbiosis (gut microflora) and homeostasis in the human body. Yellowish color of butter depends on the carotene content of the milk; or it can be added artificially by using annatto dye. Salt is often used in commercial butter. The buttery flavor is due to the compound, diacetyl. It has a low smoke point and hence is not good for seasoning and frying. Butter that is sold in the market contains added antioxidants to extend shelf life and some permitted color. Otherwise, butter has a short shelf life because it contains moisture and is susceptible to hydrolytic rancidity. It is used as bread spread and added to cake batter and soups, etc. In India, traditionally butter and buttermilk are made at the same time. The cream or malai is churned with water. Butter floats on the surface. When butter is heated, it is called ghee.

Ghee: It can be obtained from butter of both cow and buffalo's milk. Ghee is manufactured at household and commercial level. Cow's ghee has religious significance among Hindus and is valued in Ayurveda for its health giving properties. Its yellowish color indicates the presence of carotene pigments. Ghee is relished for its flavor that includes carbonyls, lactones, and free fatty acids and is greatly influenced by the fermentation of the cream or butter and the heating processes. It contains conjugated linoleic acid (CLA) which has been found to be useful for weight loss and may be helpful for heart health. Buffalo's ghee lacks vitamin A but the yield is higher than cow's ghee since the fat content of buffalo's milk is more than cow's milk. Ghee is used for seasoning and as an ingredient in many sweet preparations like laddoos. However, overheating ghee may produce oxidation products that are harmful.

Cream: Cream is separated either by centrifugation or by holding the raw milk at refrigeration temperatures (cream being lighter it rises to the surface). It contains protein as well as fat and has more water content than butter. It also contains fat-soluble vitamins. It has a short shelf life unless treated appropriately. Nowadays, it is available in Tetrapak containers and this cream can be stored for longer periods. It is an essential ingredient in some of the desserts, like ice cream and cakes. To enrich gravies and soups, cream is also mixed in or used as a garnish.

Margarine: Margarine is a fat, basically prepared with beef or mutton fat but, if there is objection to the use of animal fat, then it is manufactured using soybean, cottonseed, coconut, or palm oil by partial hydrogenation. It used to contain good amount of trans fats but regulations are now in place, FSSAI as well as at international level, upper limits have been set for trans fats content. As a result, bakery fats or margarine generally tend to contain negligible amounts or the amount is within the prescribed limit of trans fats. Owing to its physical properties, it is still being used in several commercial food products, especially in bakery products. Nowadays, low calorie margarine is also manufactured which contains more amount of water; thereby energy value is reduced per gram. Butter and margarine are very similar in terms of spreadability, plasticity, and melting point. It contains 80% fat, 16% water, and other milk solids. Color, salt, flavors (diacetyl), emulsifiers (lecithin), preservatives (sorbic acid), and antioxidants are often added. The flavor and preservatives are also used to prolong shelf life. Margarine is often fortified with vitamin A, D, and E. However, it has softer creamy texture and better spreadability as compared to butter. In some countries, it is used as a butter substitute. Such margarine contains small amount of skimmed milk or skimmed milk powder and color, salt. In some cases, it may be enriched to contain about 30%

linoleic acid. It is a good option as a shortening agent in bakery products. It seems to be a good medium to enrich with desirable nutrients and reduce the risk of diseases.

Lard: Lard is the fatty tissue of hog/swine. Lard is prepared by rendering method. It is used in bakery products to give them plasticity and creamy texture. Quality of lard depends on the location of fatty tissue in the animal body and method of heating. The best quality is obtained from "belly trimmings," i.e., abdominal fat. It can be bleached, deodorized, and emulsified. It melts at lower temperatures and does not have a very long shelf life. It is mainly used in bakery products as a shortening agent. However, it contains about 47% MUFA, 41% SFA, and 11% PUFA with a small amount of n-3 fatty acid. If the pigs were raised on pasture, the lard may also contain vitamins D and K_2.

Vegetable oils: They are used as crude oil and refined oil. Crude oil extracts contain phospholipids, pigments, gums, and free fatty acids as well as several antioxidants like tocopherols, oryzanol, carotenes, tocotrienols, and phytosterols. Sometimes undesirable products like soaps, hydroperoxides, etc., are also present which give undesirable odor. Therefore, industrially edible oils are refined and deodorized. But in this process, many of the important health giving compounds are lost because the seeds are crushed and heated to very high temperatures (up to 270°C in a steam bath) for deodorization and to start the oil extraction process. The high temperatures can result in loss of antioxidants like tocopherols and sterols, produce free radicals and TFA, and polymeric components, which are potentially atherogenic and mutagenic. Refined oils are more susceptible to get rancid due to the presence of unsaturated fatty acids and require antioxidants. Therefore, nowadays many people are opting for physically refined cold pressed oils rather than chemically refined oils. For physical refining, crude oils obtained from oil-bearing seeds are processed in a way that maximum nutritional quality is maintained, while eliminating the undesirable material. Cooking particularly deep frying with refined oils with high PUFA can degrade them easily to toxic components like free radicals, transfats, malondialdehyde (MDA), etc., which are potentially mutagenic and atherogenic. Traditional cooking oils like mustard, sesame, and coconut were discarded in favor of other high n-6 containing oils. However, research indicates that the traditionally used oils have health benefits more than the n-6 containing oils. The properties of different oils are briefly described.

Coconut oil: India is the largest producer of coconut oil. Its saturated fatty acid composition includes 45% lauric acid and 18% myristic acid. Due to the presence of lauric acid, it is considered as a medium chain triglyceride (MCT). Lauric acid and monolaurin (a substance derived from lauric acid) can destroy pathogens including bacteria, viruses, and fungi. It is found useful in the managing many health

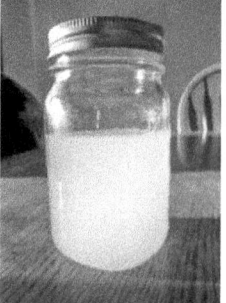

states including improving HDL cholesterol, hypothyroid, Alzheimer's disease, obesity, skin allergies, hair fall etc. Like any other oil it should be used in limited amounts. It is useful in diseases where fat absorption is impaired. Typical sweetness and flavor are due to the presence of delta lactone. The oil is cool and used for burns. Use of coconut oil for cooking is limited to southern parts of India where it is grown. It is popularly used as hair oil.

Corn oil: Corn oil contains more amounts of PUFA as compared to MUFA providing additional health benefits, compared to coconut oil. It is suitable for frying because of high smoke point. It is good as a shortening agent and fat replacements like margarine. It is considered to lower cholesterol and is also useful for skin health.

Cottonseed oil: As the name suggests that the cottonseed oil is obtained from the extraction of cotton seed plant. Hull of the seed is used for lint and fiber to make cotton cloth. Since seeds are rich i, oil and protein hence used for oil extraction. Its oil is very rich in polyunsaturated fatty acids particularly linoleic acid which is good for heart. The cotton seed contain a phenolic compound, i.e., gossypol which to toxic to animal feeding that is removed during refining process then oil is safe to consume.

Palm kernel oil: Palm is a fruit native to Malaysia and Indonesia. Palm oil was also used traditionally in some parts of Africa. Palm fruit is covered by skin with oil bearing fibrous pulp. Palm fruit contains a hard shell like that of coconut; inside which is the palm kernel. Oil from the outer skin is referred as palm oil and oil from kernel is called palm kernel oil. Oils from this fruit are unique as it high in saturated fatty acids whereas all other seed oils contain mostly unsaturated fatty acids. Palm kernel oil is rich in unsaturated fatty acids and in addition it contains stearin due to which it may be solid in nature. Palmolein is manufactured which contains 47% saturated fatty acids, 41% oleic acid (MUFA), linoleic acid, and linolenic acid an (n-3) fatty acid.

Palm oil: It contains about 50% saturated (mainly palmitic acid) and 50% unsaturated fatty acids (mainly oleic and linoleic acid). It contains very high amount of β carotene. It also contains μ carotene and lycopene as well as tocopherol and tocotrienols. Dark red color of the oil indicates higher amount of carotene. However, repeated heating reduces the β carotene content. It is a good replacement for transfats. Many brands contain a blend of palm oil with other vegetable oils like soybean and canola oil.

Olive oil: Olive oil is extracted from the pulp of olive fruits. Its yield is only around 20% which explains its high cost. But it is highly valued for its health benefits due to the high MUFA content (76%), tocopherol, phytosterol (β sitosterol), and phytoestrogen. It has been found to be useful in reducing pain and reducing cholesterol. Its squalene content protects retina. It is also used for cosmetic purposes in skin and hair care products.

Olive oil can be categorized as Virgin oil and Extra Virgin oil. When remaining pulp after first extraction is steeped in hot water to gain extra yield of oil, it is called Virgin oil. When olive oil is extracted using cold press method, the chances of oxidation of unsaturated fatty acids are reduced and the oil contains maximum phytochemicals and other valuable components and this oil is called Extra Virgin oil. Virgin olive oil contains comparatively lesser amount of phytochemicals; however, MUFA content is not lost.

Peanut oil (Groundnut): Groundnut seeds yield approximately 40-50% oil which contains 52% MUFA and 26% PUFA and the remaining are SFA. Its content of oleic acid and tocopherol, phytosterol, resvertol, and squalene make groundnut oil effective for cardiovascular health and prevention of cancer. However, refined groundnut has negligible amounts of these beneficial compounds. Its high smoking point is good for frying and it is one of the most popular oils used by Indians.

Canola oil: Canola spp. *B. napus* is commonly known as rapeseed. Rapeseed was identified in 2000 BC as a high-erucic acid crop, containing >40% erucic acid in the oil. Canadian scientists developed low erucic variety of rapeseed and Canada registered the word "canola" to describe a new oilseed, which was low in erucic acid and low in glucosinolates. Later, it has been used as edible oil and USFDA granted it GRAS status. During refining, these compounds are removed. High content of MUFA, some amount of omega 3 fatty acid, tocopherol, and phytosterol make it worthwhile to be used for health purposes. Positive effects of MUFAs compared with SFAs have been reported on regulation of plasma lipids and lipoproteins, susceptibility of low-density lipoprotein (LDL) oxidation, and insulin sensitivity.

Sesame oil: Oil from sesame(gingelly) seeds contains MUFA and PUFA having 1% linolenic acid (omega 3) and lecithin (fat emulsifying agent). Though its use in cooking is limited in some regions, people use it for therapeutic massage of infants, to relieve aches and pain and help in wound healing. In Ayurveda, sesame oil has been given value to pacify vata and pitta generating diseases and soothe and nourish the skin and muscles.

Safflower oil: It contains PUFA and is used as an edible oil or is used in oil blends. It is used in making spreads as well as in skin care products.

Soyabean oil: Soy bean oil is popular. Its health benefits are due to high PUFA (60%) and omega-3 content. It has a high smoke point and hence is useful for deep frying.

Sunflower oil: It is light, slightly sweet, and cheaper than other edible oils and thus is most used. It contains PUFA, tocopherol and tocopherol and some phytochemicals. At high temperature, it is easily decomposed. It is good for use in blended oils. High oleic sunflower oil is also commercially available now.

Rapeseed oil: Although it contains a good amount of omega-3 fatty acids, it also contains a toxic compound known as erucic acid. For human consumption, use of refined rapeseed oil is recommended. Scientists have developed rapeseed with low erucic acid content to overcome the problem or low erucic varieties like canola should be used.

Mustard oil: Mustard oil is frequently used in many parts of the country. For some it is highly palatable but is not liked by some because of its sharp nutty flavor due to the presence of isothiocyanate which is released when the oil is heated. Mustard oil also contains erucic acid which has adverse effects on heart. During refining, erucic acid is removed while the health benefits of MUFA and omega 3 are retained. Mustard oil also contains certain phenolic compounds which act as natural antioxidants. Mustard oil has long shelf life.

Mustard oil is often subjected to adulteration with argemone oil which contains neurotoxins responsible for dropsy (edema or fluid accumulation). In 1998, an epidemic of dropsy was recorded and the entire stock of oil was seized by government authorities.

Rice bran oil (RBO): RBO is extracted from rice bran which yields approximately 25% oil. It is rich in tocopherol (80 mg), tocotrienols, phytosterols, and γ oryzanol, all exhibiting antioxidant properties and many health benefits. RBO also contains MUFA. It is a little brownish in color due to methyl fumarate and has a typical flavor due to the presence of squalene.

Flaxseed oil: Flaxseed oil is also known as linseed oil or "alsi" in Hindi. It contains high amount of alpha linolenic acid (50%), lignan, and γ tocopherol. ALA is better absorbed in small intestine. The oil helps to produce anti-inflammatory prostaglandins; hence, it is useful in arthritis and other inflammatory conditions. It also improves immune system and reduces the risk of atherosclerosis. Flax seed oil is comparable to fish oil in its fatty acid composition. Therefore, flaxseed oil is a good option for vegetarians. High ALA content makes the oil sensitive to oxidation or rancidity with exposure to heat, air, and light. The oil is not used for cooking rather by adding in curd, salad even cooked food. It usually does not alter the taste and provide numerous health benefits.

Vanaspati: Soy bean, cottonseed, or palm oil and other oils are often used to make vanaspati by hydrogenation. Thus, it is also called hydrogenated fat. During the process, oil is converted into solid fat that behaves like saturated fats. Purpose of hydrogenation is to get a type of fat that resembles ghee in consistency, at an economical price. Chemical properties and configuration of vegetable oils are changed. Vanaspati is a solid fat having transfats which have adverse health effects. It is used both at household as well as industrial level. It is also fortified with vitamin D. It has a long shelf life.

Oil blends: Mixing or blending of two or more vegetable oils is done to improve the fatty acid composition, e.g., blend of rice bran and safflower oils. Each oil has its own fatty acid composition and properties. Each of the individual oils may not have the fatty acid profile desired from the health perspective; hence, two or more oils are blended in different proportions by different companies. Combination of oil blends needs technological adaptation.

Exotic oils: The quest for exotic foods and food ingredients has led to numerous cuisines becoming popular around the globe for palatability and health resonance. In this journey olive oil caught the focus for its role for healthy heart. Now other exotic oils are on the way such as the oils obtained from avocado, walnut, macadamia, hemp seed, *Camellia*, flax seed, hazelnut, grape seed, pistachio, almond etc. Such oils are usually used in the areas where these foods are cultivated. Macadamia oil has a very high lipid content (> 70%) and more appropriate n-6: n-3 ratio and that is reported to reduce insulin resistance and inflammatory diseases. Avocado oil contains high MUFA phytosterols, vitamins and various antioxidants. Some studies suggest its role in the improvement in postprandial insulin and glucose levels and showing anti-inflammatory effects. Walnut oil has been found to raise the HDL and reduce the LDL- cholesterol and other beneficial effects. Hemp seeds oil contains several antioxidant compounds and have good heat stability and can withstand the high temperatures in cooking. New technological advancements have brought out oil sprays to reduce the consumption of fats and oils. Since these exotic oils are very expensive hence research on them is limited and they are nor commonly used cooking oils.

SPICES, HERBS, AND CONDIMENTS

Spices

Spice is an aromatic plant part used in very small amounts in food preparations for seasoning, taste, flavor, aroma, color, and texture. A wide variety of spices are available for all types of cuisines around the world. They are used as whole, crushed, and powdered. They can be used fresh and/or dried. Different combinations of spices are used in seasonings, curries, and sauces to deliver distinct aroma and flavor to the dish. In addition to their culinary use, they provide medicinal benefits as well. Many of the spices inherently possess antiviral, antibacterial, antifungal, anti-inflammatory, carminative, diuretic properties which are mainly due to the presence of essential oils and phytochemicals. The nutrient content of these spices varies but because they are used in small amount, their nutritional contribution may be negligible but the essential oils and phytochemicals present in them demonstrate myriad health benefits.

Some spices are said to be "hot" in nature such as black pepper, nutmeg, cinnamon, ginger, clove, and some are said to be "cool" like fennel seeds, cumin, and coriander seed. Being anti-bacterial and antifungal, some spices can be used to prevent food infections and digestive disorders. Most microorganisms proliferate in a hot and humid environment. Spices often tend to check their growth and prevent food spoilage. Some spices can irritate the epithelial lining of the stomach whereas some can enhance the secretion of digestive juices and thus help in digestion. There are several household remedies for which spices and/or condiments are used. Flatulence, nausea, and acidity are problems often solved by consumption of some spices like fennel, *ajwain*, black pepper. Tea is recommended for chills. Some spices are also used for cosmetic purposes. Since spices are expensive, they need to be preserved well. They should cautiously be protected from adulteration with harmful dyes and other substances. Discussion on adulteration is not within the scope of this book. Health significance of different spices is summarized in Table 16.8.

Table 16.8: Health significance of different spices.

Spice name	Health significance
All spice (Jamaican Pepper)	Not used much in India but in Jamaica and Guatemala. Has characteristic flavors of clove, nutmeg, cinnamon, and black pepper. Used in the treatment of bruises, sore muscles, respiratory congestion, and tooth ache
Aniseed (choti saunf)	Carminative, useful in dyspepsia, indigestion, it is mucolytic, so good in cough. Believed to promote menstruation and milk secretion during lactation, possibly has antidiabetic, hypolipidemic, and antioxidant activities may become bitter in humid atmosphere
Asafoetida (hing)	It is a gum resin exuded from rhizome of Ferula plant. Has very strong flavor. It exhibits carminative (relieve flatulence), relaxant, neuroprotective, digestive, antioxidant, and antispasmodic, hypotensive properties
Bay leaf (Tejpatta)	Antimicrobial and antibacterial; hypoglycemic, and also improves the lipid profile and possess antioxidant activity and anti-inflammatory
Black pepper	Provides distinct flavor and pungency; analgesic, antipyretic, antimicrobial, anti-inflammatory, antioxidant, insecticidal, increases shelf life, its key component, piperine improves the cognitive brain functioning, enhances drug bioavailability, and improves gastrointestinal functionality
Bishop's seed (ajwain/omum)	Rich source of calcium, selenium, zinc and iron carminative. It has a very bitter pungent, strong flavor. It is antiseptic, antibacterial, anti-inflammatory and its key component thymol is blood purifier and chest congestion
Caraway (shahi jeera)	Ayurveda uses it for balancing vatakapha. It improves digestion and reduces pain due to indigestion. Essential oil of caraway is used to control vertigo
Green cardamom (hari or choti elaichi)	Queen of aroma in Indian foods, rich in choline so good for depression and memory booster. It contains chemicals that might treat intestinal spasms, destroys some bacteria, and may help in immunity
Black cardamom (kali or badi elaichi)	Possess anti-inflammatory properties, good for sore throat, nausea, reduce bad breath. Used to balance tridosha as per Ayurveda
Chillies (red dried)	Rich in iron, thiamine, riboflavin, niacin; contain a component called "capsaicin" which produces burning sensation in mouth. Capsaicin helps in weight loss. Pungency sensation reaches to the brain and blocks the sensation of pain thus useful in reducing pain and also nasal congestion. Helps to increase the secretion of saliva and gastric juice, hence may increase appetite but in excess irritates the stomach, it tends to increase the immunity and metabolism

Contd...

Contd...

Spice name	Health significance
Cinnamon	Reduces blood sugar. It contains cinnamaldehyde, eugenol, cinnamic acid, and cinnamate. It has got good anti-inflammatory, anti-oxidant, anti-ulcer, anti-microbial, anti-diabetic, memory enhancer, and many other properties. Reduces cold, cough, and asthma
Clove	Very high value for antioxidant capacity, good for throat and intestinal infection. It helps in digestion and relieves pain. Clove oil is popularly used for tooth ache and rheumatic pains. It is rich in eugenol and gallic acid. It can withstand high processing temperature
Coriander seeds	Rich in calcium, fiber, and choline; helps in constipation. Boost memory and reduce depression, urinary tract infection and improve thyroid activity
Cumin seeds	Rich in calcium, good for digestive disorder. It works as stimulant, antispasmodic, carminative and antimicrobial, anti-inflammatory, analgesic, antioxidant, anticancer, antidiabetic
Dill (Suwa)	Good for digestion; carminative, stomachic, and diuretic and reputed to be a galactogogue (the substance that increases the milk secretion in lactating mothers)
Fennel (badi saunf)	Sweet and appetizing, flavorful, digestive, diuretic, antibacterial, antifungal, antioxidant, hepatoprotective, believed to be a galactogogue, ingredient of gripe water, reduce colic pain in infants
Fenugreek seeds	Rich in protein and fiber hence useful in nutraceutical ingredient; galactogogue; gel like texture in soaked seed has hypoglycemic effect which is attributed to the presence of an active compound trigonella—protect from oxidative damage, anti-hyperlipidic and used in weight management and also pain management
Ginger (dried/sounth)	Used as anti-inflammatory agent, it contains gingerol, shagoal, and zingerone and many volatile compounds which give ginger pungent strong aroma and flavor. It has been used in tooth aches, nausea, gingitivitis, and joint pains
Kokum	Cooling agent. Being sour, it often replaces tamarind. Kokum butter from seeds of the fruit is also used. It is rich in hydroxycitric acid
Mace (javitri)	Used for diarrhea, nausea, stomach cramps, gas; it is useful in treating insomnia. Excess can lead to hallucination
Mango dried powder (amchur)	Good source of iron useful to combat indigestion and constipation. excess can be harmful in vata dosha or joint pain
Mustard (rai)	Rich in niacin, protein, fat. Mustard seeds can be black and yellow. Its oil is frequently used in many cuisines. Its pungency is due to organic isothiocyanates. Besides using as edible oil, it is frequently used for hair oil and base to prepare herbal oil for joint pain. It has strong anti-inflammatory properties
Niger seed (ram til or kala til)	It is a concentrated source of energy, protein, oil (contain more of linoleic acid), and iron and also phytosterols. Its oil has been found to play role in many degenerative diseases including arthritis, it may promote weight gain in weak persons
Nigella seeds (kalonji)	It is widely used in the treatment of various diseases like respiratory problems, rheumatism and skin disorders, etc. as its seeds demonstrate anti-inflammatory, spasmolytic, bronchodilator, gastroprotective, hepatoprotective, renal protective and antioxidant properties. It is an active component thymoquinone and other compounds of high biological efficacy besides rich in protein, selenium and phytosterols
Nutmeg (Jaiphal)	Nutmeg is an oval seed and mace is the red cover on this seed. Induces sleep. It is rich in myristicin and elemicin because of which excessive consumption can cause hallucination and constipation. Useful in inflammation in sprains
Pepper (black/white)	White pepper is lesser mature hence milder than black pepper. Both are the same fruits. White pepper helps in improving brain functions, black pepper is used in fever, cold, cough and build up the immunity
Pepper long/pipali	Mucolytic, used in cough. It is often used in Ayurveda for common aliments of respiratory and digestive tracts
Pomegranate seeds (anardana) (dried form)	It has been found to contain several types of lignans in varying quantities, and many other polyphenolic compounds due to which they can be used for prevention of many chronic diseases
Poppy seeds (khuskhus)	It is a good source of protein, fat, and minerals like calcium, iron, magnesium, zinc, copper, etc. Since opium is also obtained from poppy seeds, due to its narcotic effect, excess use is not advisable in domestic food preparations
Saffron (Kesar/zafran)	The stigma of flower is used as commercial saffron. Its rich dark orange color is due to the presence of carotenoids including α and β carotene. Saffron exhibits its chemopreventive effects by the modulation of lipid peroxidation, antioxidants, and detoxification due to the presence of carotenoids. It is useful for vitality and vigor and for cosmetic effect
Turmeric (haldi)	Rich in iron, niacin; anti-inflammatory agent in muscular injuries. Contains curcumin that has tremendous health benefits and essential for enhancing immunity
Tamarind	Used as acidifying or souring agent, use of tamarind is considered to give freedom from food infection because of highly acidic nature

Herbs

Any specific parts of plants—berries, flowers, roots, and fruits, highly valued for their flavor, aroma, and medicinal properties are called herb. Most herbs are leafy parts of the plant. They are used both in fresh and in dried forms. Dried herbs need to be stored in air tight bottles or bags away from heat, light, and insects. Herbs are skillfully used in culinary art as well as in cosmetic and pharmaceutical formulations preparations. Some herbs like holy basil (tulsi) are used in religious practices and also for immunity enhancing and other medicinal properties. Herbs are power packed with nutrients and phytochemicals. They are usually added at the end of cooking or as garnishes thereby adding visual appeal and top note flavors to the dish. They are being used in seasoning of *pulav, biryani*, ingredient of *garam masala*, stews, relishes, etc. They can easily replace salt and sugar and are thus useful in dietetic foods. They inherently possess antiviral, antibacterial, antifungal, anti-inflammatory, carminative, and diuretic properties. Therefore, they are used in many household remedies. Excessive use may have side effects. Some people are allergic to specific herbs. Most of the herbs have legacies of folklores that signify their value. The medicinal properties of various herbs are used in Ayurveda and Unani systems and many of these properties have been investigated by pharmacologists. Hence, only a few are given in Table 16.9.

Besides being marketed whole, spices are coarsely or finely ground. Generally, grinding reduces shelf life of the powders, results in loss of aroma and pharmocogical effect. Crushed spices and powders also absorb aromas from other sources in the environment where they are stored. Hence they should be stored in a cool, dry place to minimize spoilage and loss of aroma. Individual spice powders and blends are available such as jal jeera powder, garam masala, chat masala, tea masala, etc. In food industry, spice extracts and oleoresins are increasingly being used because they are easier to handle than spice powders and generally do not contain large number of microorganisms, in contrast to spice powders.

Condiments

Condiment is a single substance or mixture of substances that is added to the food preparation or consumed singly to add flavour, taste and pleasure in the meal. They are used to complement foods such as salad dressing, seasoning, vinegar, mustard, and salt and pepper corns. Chutneys, sauces, and pickles are not considered condiments (Table 16.10).

Table 16.9: Nutritional and health significance of some commonly used herbs.

Herb	Nutritional and health significance
Basil leaves	Antimicrobial, antibacterial used for variety of digestive and respiratory disorders. Relieves mental fatigue and improves concentration. Use basil leaves to repel flying insects. Prolonged use of raw leaves by chewing can erode tooth enamel due to the presence of high content of methyl chavicol. Its leaf extract has been found to be hypoglycemic
Bay leaves	Good for indigestion and flatulence, decoction used as gargle for sore throat, antiseptic
Coriander leaves	Good source of vitamin C, improves iron absorption from food, carminative
Chamomile dried flowers	Powerful analgesic, and anti-inflammatory; calming properties—useful for insomnia; antioxidant and antimicrobial, cholesterol lowering in animals useful in improving liver function and bile flow; skin infection
Dill (sowa) leaves	Good source of folic acid, used during lactation; very good for women, health problems like painful or irregular menstruation
Fennel (badi saunf)	Sweet flavor, used during lactation, carminative
Lemon grass	Possesses anti-inflammatory, antifungal, stimulant, antispasmodic, carminative properties. Good for digestive system, removes lethargy, and relieves body pain
Marjoram leaves (fresh and dried)	Bactericidal effect; useful in abdominal pain, distention; rheumatism; essential oil when mixed with almond oil can be applied externally for relaxation and high blood pressure
Mint leaves (fresh and dried)	Fresh and cool due to menthol content, carminative, useful in diarrhea, vomiting, nausea, and helpful in expelling worms; analgesic and anti-inflammatory
Oregano (fresh and dried)	Analgesic and anti-inflammatory; useful in respiratory system problems; good to reduce bloated feeling upon over consumption of food
Parsley	Rich in iron, calcium, zinc, vitamins A, B, C, and also contain boron and good amount of chlorophyll which is good for bones and brain. Useful in improving liver function and bile flow; diuretic and laxative and dyspepsia. It also helpful in minimizing the onion and garlic odor
Rosemary (fresh and dried)	Highly antioxidant, useful in gout, promote perspiration and bile flow, good for digestive system, and nervous system, stimulant; good for hair growth. It is used as natural form of antioxidant in various foods and oils
Sage	Useful for management of excessive perspiration, fatigue. Useful for health problems like painful or irregular menstruation and menopausal symptoms
Thyme	Potent antiseptic; good for intestinal infection and parasites, improves immunity, good in bronchitis, cold and cough; good in case of rheumatism and arthritis. Its active ingredient is thymol

Table 16.10: Nutritional and health significance and uses of different condiments.

Condiments	Nutritional and health significance
Pepper corns	Used in digestive disorders. Excessive use can irritate stomach and intestine
Vinegar	Rich in minerals. Quality and use depends on its original ingredient; used in diluted form as gargle for sore throat; disinfectant and helps to increase the flavor of other herbs and spices which are placed or preserved in vinegar. Used in digestive disorders. Excessive use can irritate stomach and intestine
Mustard	Causes sensation of heat in stomach and stimulates digestion
Salt	It is sodium chloride. Human body requires sodium and chloride both of which are electrolytes. Excessive intake is detrimental to health. Sodium restriction is usually recommended for controlling hypertension and for patients with kidney disease
Rock salt	Also known as halite. It is also sodium chloride.
Salt substitutes	Since sodium is restricted in several diseases. It also contain other trace elements. it is high in fluoride so need to be avoided in areas having fluorosis. however It often alters the taste and used in many beverages and chaat masalas. Salt substitutes are suggested. These contain potassium, magnesium, or calcium salts of glutamic acid, lactic acid, hydrochloric, tartaric or citric acids, potassium sulfate. These should also be used with caution, e.g., potassium is also restricted in renal failure
Iodized salt	This is common salt or sodium chloride fortified with sodium, potassium, or calcium iodide in order to prevent iodine deficiency, i.e., goiter, a disease of the thyroid gland

Popular Brewed Beverages

Tea (*Camellia sinensis*, leaves): Tea is the most popular beverage consumed in almost every nook and corner of the world. Based on the distinct manufacturing processes, tea can be classified into three main types, namely, green tea, oolong tea, and black tea. Green tea is non-fermented tea while black tea generally refers to the fermented one. Oolong tea is the partially fermented product. In green tea, green tea catechins (GTC) remain relatively unchanged compared with the fresh tea leaves, whereas in black tea, they are oxidized and polymerized to the "pigments" called theaflavins (TF) and thearubigins (TR) during fermentation. In contrast, oolong tea contains a mixture of GTC, TF, and TR. It is known that both green tea and black tea water extracts can reduce serum total cholesterol (TC) and triacylglycerols (TG) in both humans and animals. In addition, many studies have demonstrated that dietary green tea and black tea have strong free-radical scavenging activity both *in vitro* and *in vivo*. Now white tea is also relished and advocated for its high antioxidant compounds.

There are different ways in which tea is processed. Tea has its origins in China but Darjeeling tea and Assam tea are famous all over the world. Tea is basically a hot beverage but iced tea is now becoming popular. Green tea is being popularized in India as a functional food owing to its high antioxidant capacity. Variety of flavors and tea from different origins are available. Green tea gives a beverage which is very light, clear, and slightly bitter in taste. The Chinese and Japanese add to its aroma by incorporating rose, rosehip, marigold, aprajita or jasmine flowers and orange or lemon peel.

Tea is prepared in different ways all over the world and varies hence widely in color, taste, and aroma. Despite being every one's choice, the recipe for the method of preparation is a highly individual choice. Some people drink green or black tea just for its aroma. Some people drink black tea with lemon, and others add milk and sugar to the decoction. In some parts of India, ginger, mint, lemon grass, cardamom, or a mixture of spices called tea masala in addition to tea leaves, are added along with milk and sugar.

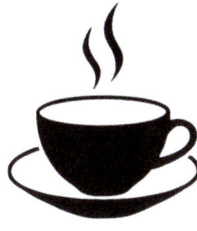

Tea contains tannins which gives it the astringent taste. Bitterness of tea is generally ascribed to the combination of catechins, saponins, caffeine, and amino acids. Depending on molecular weight, catechins can be bitter or astringent, whereas saponins are often described as acrid. Color of tea comes from the component called theaflavin (yellow) and thearubigins (red color). The nutrient content of tea decoction is negligible. However, the tannin in tea reduces the bioavailability of iron and other minerals when tea is consumed with other foods. Therefore, it is advisable not to consume tea with iron rich foods. Vitamin C is not destroyed by tannin and vitamin C enhances the absorption of iron. Lemon tea seems to have relatively less effect on bioavailability. The stimulating effect of tea can be attributed to its caffeine and theobromine content.

High consumption of tea is said to cause acidity. On consumption of tea with milk, tannin forms complex with milk protein which is further broken down in the stomach and can cause acidity. On the other hand, tea lowers the risk of adverse effect of cholesterol on heart. It also provides protection against bacterial attack. In many diseases, weak tea is permitted but in case of dyspepsia or many digestive disorders, it is better to avoid tea.

Coffee: Coffee is obtained from beans of a plant. Coffee beans are the seeds of crimson fruits from which the outer pericarp is completely removed. The seeds may be raw or roasted, whole, or ground. Generally, coffee beans are roasted and ground into powder.

The aroma of coffee powder is not stable since the aroma compounds are volatile and rapidly lost. Like tea, coffee is also popular worldwide and used for taste, aroma, and stimulation. Coffee extract is made by boiling the coffee in water for 10 minutes and then filtering or by steeping a bag filled with ground coffee in hot water, or by the filtration-percolation method. Coffee products are made like instant coffee and decaffeinated coffee.

Caffeine is the main component responsible for the stimulating effect of coffee. Excessive consumption (four to seven cups of coffee a day) has affects the nervous system causing irritability, restlessness, sleep disturbances, rapid pulse rate, and frequent urination. It may raise the basal metabolic rate. Coffee contains antioxidants that may give some protection against heart disease and development of diabetes but it also increases homocysteine levels that increase risk of heart disease. Decaffeinated coffee does not have these benefits. It also contains two substances that raise cholesterol levels—kahweol and cafestol. Decaffeinated coffee also raises blood cholesterol. Coffee products are used not only for preparation of coffee beverages but also as flavorings for desserts, cakes, cookies, and ice cream.

Cocoa: The cacao tree originated in South America and was known in Mexico and Central America more than 1000 years ago. Linnaeus called this tree "theobroma" meaning "Food of the God." From cacao beans, a beverage was prepared followed by cocoa butter and the ever popular chocolate. Unlike tea and coffee, cocoa as a beverage is neither an aqueous extract nor a clear brew, rather it is a suspension. Cocoa contains stimulating alkaloids especially theobromine and to a smaller extent caffeine. Cocoa contains flavonoids that have good antioxidant capacity, lower blood pressure, improve blood flow to brain and heart, and have anti-aggregatory effect on platelets. When cocoa is processed into chocolate products, it goes through several steps such as fermentation, alkalizing, and roasting to reduce strong pungent taste of natural cocoa. This results in loss of flavanols. Most commercial chocolates are highly processed.

Cocoa products contain substantial amounts of fat, carbohydrates, and protein. Cocoa butter is made up of equal amounts of oleic, stearic, and palmitic acids. Cacao beans contain approximately 50% fat; hence, cocoa butter is a very significant ingredient. Cocoa powder is produced by removing the cocoa butter, most of which is used in chocolate manufacture. Cocoa powders are available according to the extent of defatting. Cocoa powder is used in manufacture of cakes, fillings, icings, pudding powders, ice cream, and cocoa/chocolate beverages. Other products made from cocoa include chocolate syrup, etc. Varieties of chocolate in different forms from fancy balls and bars to blooms and borders with chocolate syrups hold the breath of all age groups on all occasions. A wide range of chocolate varieties are available throughout the globe.

Recent researches have shown that Cocoa and chocolate are rich in antioxidants and help in lowering cholesterol and high blood pressure. The component called "theobromine" is responsible for its mood elevating effect. Chocolate is essentially composed of cocoa powder, sugar, milk solid (in milk chocolate), and suspended crystalline matrix of cocoa butter (one-third of total fat used) as it is more stable to oxidation.

RAPID FIRE

1. What are the most valuable components found in cereals and pulses other than nutrients?
2. What is importance of Breakfast Cereals?
3. What is nutritional importance of whole pulse?
4. Name some green leafy vegetables which are rich in iron and folic acid.
5. Name some fruits which carry some antioxidant activity and help in prevention of chronic disease.
6. Name some nuts and oils with high omega-3 fatty acids and what is its importance.
7. What are advantages of having liquid milk over fermented milk products?
8. Name some spices which can provide good amount of iron, fiber, and B-vitamins.
9. Differentiate fresh and dried herbs in terms of health contribution.
10. Why are tea and coffee popular all over the world?

EXERCISE

1. Collect the information on different types of fruits, vegetables, herbs, and spices in your community/area and write their nutritional and health benefits.
2. Discuss the role of any five cereals and millets which is commonly consumed in your area and which other foods can be added to improve their nutritional quality.
3. Discuss the health contribution of any 20 foods ingredients which you have consumed in last 24 hours.

SUGGESTED READING

1. Abdullaev FI, Espinosa-Aguirre JJ. Biomedical properties of saffron and its potential use in cancer therapy and chemoprevention trials. Can Detect Prevent. 2004;28:426-32.
2. Afify AE-MMR, El-Beltagi HS, Abd El-Salam SM, et al. Bioavailability of iron, zinc, phytate and phytase activity during soaking and germination of white sorghum varieties. PLoS One. 2011;6(10):e25512.
3. Agarwal S, Rao AV. Tomato lycopene and its role in human health and chronic diseases. CMAJ. 2000;163(6):739-44.
4. Agrawal P, Rai V, Singh RB. Randomized placebo controlled Single blind trial of holy basil leaves in patients with non-insulin requiring diabetes mellitus. International Journal of Clinical Pharmacology and Therapeutics. 1996;34(9):406-9.
5. Al-Snafi AE. The pharmacological activities of *Cuminum cyminum*: A review. IOSR J Pharma. 2016;6(2):46-65.
6. Amalraj A, Gopi S. Biological activities and medicinal properties of Asafoetida: a review. J Tradit Complement Med. 2017;7(3):347-59.
7. Amon AS, Soro RY, Koffi PKB, et al. Biochemical characteristics of flours from ivorian taro (Colocasia Esculenta, Cv Yatan) corm as affected by boiling time. Adv J Food Sci Technol. 2011;3(6):424-35.
8. Anandh MA, Lakshmanan V, Anjaneyulu ASR. Designers meat product. Indian Food Industry. 2003;22(4):40-5.
9. Anderson JW, Major AW. Pulses and lipaemia, short- and long-term effect: Potential in the prevention of cardiovascular disease. Br J Nutri. 2002;88(Suppl. 3):S263-71.
10. Anjum FM, Nadeem M, Khan MI, et al. Nutritional and therapeutic potential of sunflower seeds: a review. Br Food J. 2012;114(4):544-52.
11. Ayyanar M, Subhash-Babu P. Syzygium cumini (L.) Skeels: A review of its phytochemical constituents and traditional uses. Asian Pac J Trop Biomed. 2012;2(3):240-6.
12. Bailey A, Ortiz L, Radecka H. The book of Ingredients. London: Mermaid Books; 1980.
13. Balamurugan R, Chandragunasekaran AS, Chellappan G, Rajaram K, Ramamoorthi G, Balakrishnan SR. Probiotic potential of lactic acid bacteria present in home made curd in southern India. Indian J Med Res. 2014;140(3):345–55.
14. Bernard D. Food Commodities. London: Willium Helnemann Ltd.; 1978.
15. Berrios JD, Morales BP, Cámara BM, et al. Carbohydrate composition of raw and extruded pulse flours. Food Res Int. 2010;43:531-6.
16. Bhowmik D, Kumar KPS, Paswan S, et al. Tomato-A natural medicine and its health benefits. J Pharmacogn Phytochemistr. 2012;1(1):33-44.
17. Bisht VK, Negi JS, Bhandari AK, et al. Amomum subulatum Roxb: Traditional, phytochemical and biological activities—An overview. African J Agricult Res. 2011;6(24):5386-90.
18. Bocarsly ME, Powell ES, Avena NM, et al. High-fructose corn syrup causes characteristics of obesity in rats: Increased body weight, body fat and triglyceride levels. Pharmacol Biochemistr Behav. 2010;97(1):101-6.
19. Bonzanini F, Bruni R, Palla G, et al. Identification and distribution of lignans in Punicagranatum L. fruit endocarp, pulp, seeds, wood knots and commercial juices by GC–MS. Food Chemistr. 2009;117:745-9.
20. Brogren M, Savage GP. Bioavailability of soluble oxalate from spinach eaten with and without milk products. Asia Pacific J Clin Nutr. 2003;12(2):219-24.
21. Bullo M, Falgarrona J, Hernandez-Alonso P, Salas-Salvado J. Nutrition attributes and health effects of pistachio nuts. Br J Nutr. 2015;113(Suppl 2):S79-93.
22. Cassady BA, Hollis JH, Fulford AD, et al. "Mastication of almonds: effects of lipid bioaccessibility, appetite, and hormone response." Am J Clinl Nutr. 2009;89:794-800.
23. Cazzola R, Garziano MP, Loreggian L, et al. First insights of macadamia nut oil as dietary fat. Potential Health Benefits Agro Food Industry Hi Tech. 2018;29(6):18-20.
24. Chandrashekhar SH, Taklikar S. Impact of Niger seeds supplementation on hemoglobin level of women with anemia. Int J Med Sci Pub Health. 2016;5(8):1721-3.

25. Chawla PC. CSIRí's Breakthrough in Baby Food in Progress, Promise and Prospects. 2010;60(13):146-8.
26. Chizoba EF. A Comprehensive Review on Coriander and its Medicinal properties. Int J Sci Res Rev. 2015;4(2):28-50.
27. Christa K, Soral-Śmietana M. Buckwheat grains and buckwheat products – nutritional and prophylactic value of their components – a review. Czech J Food Sci. 2008;26:153-62.
28. Chukwumah Y, Walker L, Vogler B, et al. Changes in the phytochemical composition and profile of raw, boiled, and roasted peanuts. J Agricul Food Chemistr. 2007;55:9266-73.
29. Coulibaly A, Kouakou B, Chen J. Phytic acid in cereal grains: structure, healthy or harmful ways to reduce phytic acid in cereal grains and their effects on nutritional quality. Am J Plant Nutr Fertil Technol. 2011;1:1-22.
30. Craig SA. Betaine in Human Nutrition. Am J Clin Nutr. 2004;80(3):539-49.
31. Dhandevi PEM, JEEWON R. Fruit and Vegetable Intake: Benefits and Progress of Nutrition Education Interventions. Narrative Review Article. Iran J Public Health. 2015;44(10):1309-21.
32. Doke S, Guha M. Garden cress (Lepidium sativum L) seed - an important medicinal source: a review. J Nat Prod Plant Resour. 2014;4(1):69-80.
33. Economos C, Clay WD. Nutritional and health benefits of citrus fruits. FAO, Food Nutrition, and Agriculture, 1999.
34. Enyiukwu DN, Amadioha AC, Ononuju CC. Nutritional significance of cowpea leaves for human consumption. Greener Trend Food Sci Nutr. 2018;1(1):1-10.
35. Eun-Kyung Choi EK, Myoung-Hwan K, Soo-Hyun P, et al. Eriobotrya japonica improves cognitive function in healthy adolescents: a 12-week, randomized double-blind, placebo-controlled clinical trial. Int J Pharmacol. 2016;12(4):370-8.
36. Fabraini G, Lintas C. Protein and enzymes composition of drum wheat. In: Durum Wheat – Chemistry and Technology. St. Paul Minnesota, USA Feillet: American Association of Cereal Chemist, Inc.; 1988. pp. 93-120.
37. Falade AO, Oboh G, Okoh AI. Potential health implications of the consumption of thermally-oxidized cooking oils – a review. Pol J Food Nutr Sci. 2017;67(2):95-105.
38. Fard MA, Shojaii A. Review of pharmacological properties and chemical constituents of Pimpinella anisum. ISRN Pharm. 2012;2012:510-795.
39. Fatima T, Showkat U, Hussain SZ. Nutritional and health benefits of walnuts. J Pharmacogn Phytochemistr. 2018;7(2):1269-71.
40. Gandhi AP. Review article: Quality of soybean and its food products. Int Food Res J. 2009;16:11-9.
41. Goldberg I. Functional Foods: Designer Foods, Pharmafoods, Nutraceuticals. New York: Chapman; 2008.
42. Gopalan C, Shatri BVR. Nutritive value of Indian foods. Hyderabad: National Institute of Nutrition Indian Council Of Medical Research; 2004.
43. Halton TL, Willett WC, Liu S, et al. Potato and French fry consumption and risk of type 2 diabetes in women. Am J Clin Nutr. 2006;83(2):284-90.
44. Hosomi R, Yoshida M, Fukunaga K. Seafood consumption and components for health. Glob J Health Sci. 2012;4(3):72-86.
45. https://www.foodsafetymantra.com/2019/03/fssai-categorization-of-milk-products-and-their-standards
46. Ideda S, Tomura K, Ymashita Y, et al. Nutritional profile of minerals in buckwheat and its products. Rome: Proceedings of th 8th ISB; 2001. pp. 485-8.
47. Jelen P. Introduction to Food Processing. Virginia: Reston Publishig Company, Inc A Prentice Hall company; 1985.
48. Jnnalgadda SS, Harnack L, Liu RH, et al. Health benefits associated with whole grains –Summary of American Society for Nutrition 2010 Satellite Symposium. J Nutr. 2011;141:1011S-22S.
49. Jonathan WW (Jr), Zscheile FP, Brunson AM. The Carotenoids of Yellow Corn Grain (reprinted from the Journal of the American Chemical Society, 64, 2603 (I9~2)). [Contribution from the purdue university agricultural experiment station and the bureau of plant industry, USDA].
50. Jones JM. Breakfast cereals and how they are made. In Fast RB, Caldwell EF (Eds). Cereal Nutrition. St. Paul Minnesota: American Association of Cereal Chemist, Inc.; 2000. pp. 411-37.
51. Jones JM. Cereal Nutrition in Breakfast Cereals and how they are made. In: Robert BF, Elwood F (Eds). Minnesota: Caldwell from American association of Cereal Chemist); 2003.
52. Kahlon TS, Chapman MH, Smith GE. In vitro binding of bile acids by okra, beets, asparagus, eggplant, turnips, green beans, carrots, and cauliflower. Food Chemistr. 2007;103:676-80.
53. Kalinova J, Dadakova E. Rutin and total quercetin content in amaranth (Amaranthus spp.). Plant Food Hum Nutr. 2009;64(1):68-74.
54. Kanchan R, Tiwari A, Chakroborthy S. Stevia: Herb with a lot of potential. Beverage and Food World. 2009;36(1):42-44.
55. Kaviarasan S, Vijayalakshmi K, Anuradha CV. Polyphenol-rich extract of fenugreek seeds protect erythrocytes from oxidative damage. Plant Food Hum Nutr. 2004;59(4):143-7.
56. Khoo HE, Azlan A, Tang ST, et al. Anthocyanidins and anthocyanins: colored pigments as food, pharmaceutical ingredients, and the potential health benefits. Food Nutr Res. 2017;61(1):1361-779.
57. Kristensen M, Jensen MG, Aarestrup J, et al. Flaxseed dietary fibers lower cholesterol and increase fecal fat excretion, but magnitude of effect depends on food type. Nutr Metabol. 2012;9:8.
58. Kuang H, Yang F, Zhang Y, et al. The impact of egg nutrient composition and its consumption on cholesterol homeostasis. Cholesterol. 2018;6303810.
59. Kulamarva AG, Sosle VR, Vijaya Raghavan GS. Nutritional and rheological properties of sorghum. Int J Food Propert. 2009;12(1):55-69.
60. Kumar P, Yadava RK, Gollen B, et al. Nutritional contents and medicinal properties of wheat: a review. Life Sci Med Res. 2011;2011:1-10.
61. Kushwaha S. Nutritional composition of drumstick (Moringa Oleifera). Int J Res. 2015;2(5):688-91.
62. Lin L, Allemekinders H, Dansby A, et al. Evidence of health benefits of canola oil. Nutr Rev. 2013;71(6): 370-85.
63. Lokeshwar BL, Zhang L. Medicinal properties of the Jamaican pepper plant Pimentadioica and Allspice. Curr Drug Targets. 2012;13(14):1900–6.
64. Machado de Souza RG, Raquel Machado Schincaglia RM, Pimentel GD, et al. Nuts and human health outcomes: a systematic review. Nutrients. 2017;9(12):1311.
65. Mahmood A, Ngah N, Omar MN. Phytochemicals Constituent and Antioxidant Activities in Musa x Paradisiaca Flower. Eur J Sci Res. 2011;66(2):311-8.
66. Malik S. Pearl millet-nutritional value and medicinal uses! IJARIIE. 2015;1(3):414-8.
67. Manay NS, Shadaksharaswamy M. Food - Facts and Principles. New Delhi: New Age International; 2008. pp. 131-382.
68. Manchanda SC. Selecting healthy edible oil in the Indian context. Ind Heart J. 2016;68(4):447-9.
69. McChesney, Monica J. Relationship between high-fructose corn syrup, uric acid, and metabolic syndrome. Journal of Pediatric Surgical Nursing. 2016-5(4):88.
70. McCrory MA, Hamaker BR, Lovejoy JC, et al. Pulse consumption, satiety and weight management. Adv Nutr. 2010;1:17-30.
71. Mergoum M, Gomez-MacPHerson H. Triticale improvement and production. FAO Plant Production and Protection Paper No 179.

72. Meydani M. Potential health benefits of avenanthramides of oats. Nutr Rev. 2009;67(12):731-5.
73. Moreno DA, Carvajal M, López-Berenguer C, et al. Chemical and biological characterisation of nutraceutical compounds of broccoli. J Pharmaceut Biomed Anal. 2006;41:1508-22.
74. Muller HG. An Introduction to tropical Food Science. Cambridge, New York: Cambridge University Press; 1988.
75. Nambiar VP, Parnami GS, Mammen D. Impact of antioxidants from drumstick leaves on the lipid profile of hyperlipidemics. Journal of Herbal Medicine and Toxicology. 2010;4(1):165–72.
76. Nambiar VS, Daniel M, Guinl P. Characterization of polyphenols from coriander Leaves (coriandrum sativum), red amaranthus (*A paniculatus*) and green amaranthus (*A frumentaceus*) using paper chromatography: and their health implications. J Herb Med Toxicol. 2010;4(1):173-7.
77. Olas B. Honey and its phenolic compounds as an effective natural medicine for cardiovascular diseases in humans? Nutrients. 2020;12(2):283.
78. Oplinger ES, Oelke EA, Brinkman MA, et al. Buckwheat. Alternative Field Crops Manual Univ of Wisconsin. 1989.
79. Ozaki S, Okit N, Suzuki S, et al. Structural characterization and hypoglycemic effects of arabinogalactan- protein from the tuberous cortex of the white-skinned sweet potato *(Ipomoea batatas L.)*. J Agricul Food Chemistr. 2010;58(22):11593-9.
80. Pandian S, Sivasankar C, Muthuramalingam P, et al. An amazing nutritional value in wonderful finger millet makes this "The Most Lovable Food Crop" to the World. Sci J Food Sci Nutr. 2017;3(2):34-6.
81. Petera K, Gandh P. Rediscovering the therapeutic potential of Amaranthus species: A review. Egyptian J Basic Appl Sci. 2017;4:196-205.
82. Peter KV. Handbook of Herbs and Spices. New York: Woodhead Publishing Limited/CRC Press; 2002.
83. Poonia A, Upadhayay A. *Chenopodium album* Linn: review of nutritive value and biological properties. J Food Sci Technol. 2015;52(7):3977-85.
84. Poulose SM, Marshall G. Miller Barbara Shukitt-Hale. Role of walnuts in maintaining brain health with age. J Nutr. 2014;144(4):561S-6S.
85. Pratiwi R, Purwestri YA. Black rice as a functional food in Indonesia. Funct Food Heal Dis. 2018;7(3):182-94.
86. Rafiqa S, Kaula R, Sofia SA, et al. Citrus peel as a source of functional ingredient: a review. J Saudi Soc Agricul Sc. 2018;17:351-8.
87. Ramulu P, Rao PU. Total, insoluble and soluble dietary fiber contents of Indian fruits. J Food Composit Anal. 2003;16:677-85.
88. Richard DM. The energetics of nut consumption. Asia Pac J Clin Nutr. 2008;17(S1):337-9.
89. Richardson DP, Ansell J, Drummond LN. The nutritional and health attribute of kiwifruit: a review. Eur J Nutr. 2018;57(8):2659-76.
90. Sarkar P, Kumar L, Dhumal C, et al. Traditional and ayurvedic foods of Indian origin. J Ethn Food. 2015;2(3):97-109.
91. Shahidi F, Ambigaipalan P. Phenolics and polyphenolics in foods, beverages and spices: Antioxidant activity and health effects – A review. J Funct Food. 2015;18:820-97.
92. Singh B, Jatinder Pal Singh JP, Shevkani K, Singh N, Kaur A. Bioactive constituents in pulses and their health benefits, J Food Sci Technol. 2017;54(4):858-70.
93. Subbulakshmi G, Udipi SA. Food Processing and Preservation. New Delhi: New Age International Publishers; 2007.
94. Upadhyay A, Karn SK. Brown rice: Nutritional composition and health benefits. J Food Sci Technol Nepal. 2018;10:48-54.
95. Vangalapati M, Satya SN, Prakash, SDV, et al. A review on pharmacological activities and clinical effects of cinnamon species. Res J Pharmaceut Biol Chem Sci. 2012;3(1):653.
96. Joshi VK, Kumar S. Meat analogues: Plant based alternatives to meat products - A review. Intl J Food Ferment Technol. 015;5(2):107-19.
97. Walther B, Schmid A, Siebier R, et al. Cheese in nutrition and health. Dairy Sci. Technol. 2008;88(2008):389-405.
98. Yadav M, Jain S, Tomar R, et al. Medicinal and biological potential of pumpkin: an updated review. Nutr Res Rev. 2010;23:184-90.
99. Yang J. Brazil nuts and associated health benefits: A review. LWT Food Sci Technol. 2009;42:1573-80.
100. Yousuf B, Gul K, Wani AA, et al. Health benefits of anthocyanins and their encapsulation for potential use in food systems: a review. Crit Rev Food Sci Nutr. 2016;56(13):2223-30.
101. Šramková Z, Gregová E, Šturdík E. Chemical composition and nutritional quality of wheat grain. Acta Chimica Slovaca. 2009;2(1):115-38.

CHAPTER 17

Nutritional Implications of Food Processing and Packaging

> **KEY CONCERNS**
> - What are the different types of food processing at different levels?
> - Which chemical reactions occurring during processing?
> - How do processing and packaging influence nutritional value?
> - Do different reactions or end products have an impact on health?
>
> **KEY CONCEPTS**
> - Methods of food processing
> - Benefits of food processing
> - Chemical reactions occurring during processing
> - Packaging materials–their merits and demerits

INTRODUCTION

Since prehistoric times, attempts have been made to prevent food spoilage and increase food accessibility as safeguards against food scarcity. Food preservation methods have evolved as science and technology progressed and today a variety of methods are used to improve the shelf life of foods. The tremendous advances in food science and food technology have stretched the possibilities of food preservation and development of food products beyond imagination with almost exponential growth in development in food industry and delivery of high-quality, varied, and shelf-stable food products consumers. Food processing is often confused with food preservation. Some of the procedures used may be similar, but the two concepts are different. Food preservation aims to reduce food spoilage thereby preventing occurrence of food-borne diseases and extend shelf life. Whereas food processing focuses on processing of raw food ingredients to varied extents in order to convert them into edible food products. It also deals with food packaging and storage systems. Advances in food processing techniques not only limit the growth of harmful microorganisms but they also ensure product safety, quality, and retain nutrients as far as is possible. Many of these are also sustainable, environment-friendly processes, e.g., sun drying.

Food processing and food packaging are multioperational and multifaceted activities. Food processing involves the conversion of farm produce or raw food into edible food products and food packaging entails the protection of food from outside influences and extends shelf life. Edible food is expected to comply with physiological needs, cost, social, cultural, and religious norms with regard to food. It is well established that certain foods such as fruits, vegetables, herbs, and spices are associated with reducing the risk of chronic degenerative diseases. Processing, packaging, and storage tend to alter their health-promoting properties and also bring about certain changes in organoleptic and nutritional characteristics of the food. These changes are inevitable due to external and internal factors listed in Table 17.1.

Food processing has numerous benefits which are given in Figure 17.1. However, processing techniques tends to modify the functional properties of the food and can greatly influence the nutritional quality and stability of food. Therefore, judicious selection of processing method(s) along with sufficient precautionary measures is necessary to retain maximum nutritional and bioactive components intact and the functional properties within the foods or food products.

Food processing brings about various changes in the food in terms of color, texture, functionality, nutritive value, and

Table 17.1: External and internal factors involved in changes during food processing.

External factors	Internal factors
- Oxygen or air - Heat (temperature) - Light - Microorganisms and insects - Relative humidity - pH or acidity - Use of chemicals or gas in processing or holding - Cooking/processing methods - Cooking utensils, such as size and volume of cooking vessel, lid or foil covering food during cooking - Knives, saucepans, frying pans - Cooking/processing time - Cooking/processing temperature - Final internal temperature - Surface to volume ratio - Type of food tissue and texture of food surface - Amount food cooked - Amount of liquid added - Amount fat added - Type of fat added. Food cooked with or without bones. Time passed between the termination of cooking and consumption - Enzymes - Sulfite and chlorine - Inhibitors and interactions	- Physical nature of the food itself - Chemical properties of the food - Nutritional composition of food - Moisture content/water activity - Enzymes present in food - Stage of maturity - Kind of pretreatment

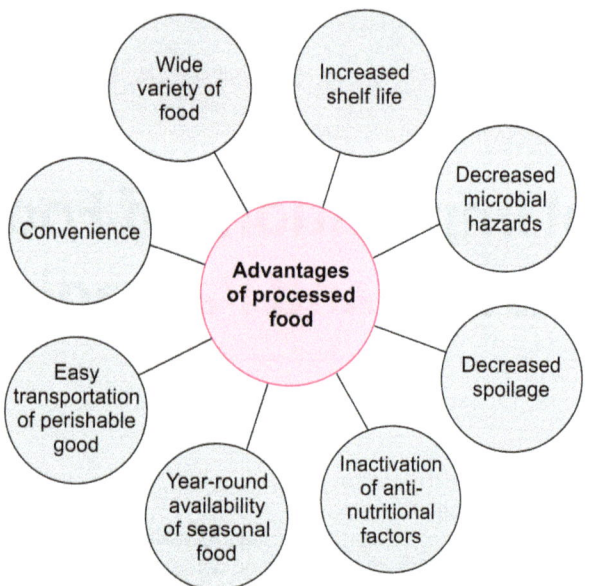

Fig. 17.1: Advantages of processing foods.

formation of new compounds. Some changes are desirable and some are undesirable. Some of these changes are given in Table 17.2.

These changes may occur from farm to kitchen, production harvesting. Physical changes modify appearance, color, texture and consistence and chemical changes influence the sensory, nutritional, and health properties/aspects of the food. Food processing technologies may alter, the bioaccessibility of a specific compound by denaturation or other changes in the structure. Some of the changes may even result in the formation toxic, mutagenic, carcinogenic, and teratogenic compounds.

BROWNING

Browning can be frequently observed on many food items like apple, banana, potato, and brinjal when they are bruised or cut or processed. This may be due to chemical reactions occurring when exposed surface of food comes in contact with air, water, heat, and enzymes during processing and storage of food. Browning affects the flavor, texture, and nutritional aspects. Sometimes the phenomenon of browning is used purposefully while making cakes, meat, coffee, and gulab jamuns, etc. In many other cases, browning can spoil the food to make it unacceptable and unhealthy. This could be a major cause of financial loss to food growers and suppliers.

> **Biochemical changes occurring during food processing**
> - Browning
>   – Enzymatic browning
>   – Nonenzymatic browning
>   - Maillard reaction
>   - Caramelization
> - Gelatinization
> - Dextrinization
> - Denaturation
> - Coagulation
> - Gelation
> - Gel formation
> - Rancidity.

With the impact of many external and internal factors, the process of browning may result in production of chemicals like melanoidin and advanced glycation end-products

Table 17.2: Physicochemical changes in food products during food processing.

Desirable Changes	Criteria	Undesirable Changes
Roasting: Browning of coffee beans Baking: Browning of cake Frying: Browning of Gulab Jamun	Color	Burning of food product Browning of peeled apple, potato Dull green color of GLV on heating
Release of flavor compounds on frying, baking, roasting, simmering	Flavor	Off-flavor and off smell in rancid food Acridity during frying Bitterness on cooking with lemon
Paste on grinding Soft texture on pressure cooking Crispy chips/papad on frying, roasting	Texture	Hardness in meat or protein foods with over heating Leakage of water on thawing Ropiness in over fermentation
Milling grain into flour facilitates dough kneading Peeling, chopping makes food easy to cook Fermenting batter helps in making soft idli or crisp dosa Cooking makes the food easy to chew and digest	Functionality	Uncooked or burnt food is a waste and inedible Cooking in acidic make food hard and difficult to chew Making spongy and soft cake is difficult if baking is not done properly Dosa or pancake gets stick to cooking pan when batter is not fermented or beaten properly
Germination synthesizes vitamin C and improve bioavailability of minerals like zinc, iron, calcium Soaking pulses removes antinutritional factors Simmering retains more nutrients and flavor compounds in the gravy	Nutritive value	Use of soda for softening of pulses reduce thiamine content Frequent washing and boiling leach out B vitamins Heating reduces vitamin C Deep frying reduces vitamin A and B vitamins
Development of aromatic and hetrocyclic compounds, aldehydes, release pleasing aroma and flavor, e.g., benzaldehyde in almonds, citral from lemons	Development of new compounds	Deep frying for long on polymerization of oil release many AGE products which are carcinogenic Development of acrylamides

(AGEs). While melanoidin has been studied to exhibit anticancer and antioxidant properties, advanced glycation end-products have been known to be carcinogenic. Thus, it is a major area of concern and needs careful study to take corrective measures. There are two different physico-chemical reactions involved in browning of foods which are as follows:

1. Enzymatic browning
2. Nonenzymatic browning.

Enzymatic Browning

Enzymatic browning is an oxidative reaction that occurs in fruits and vegetables like apple, potato, banana or brinjal, when they are exposed to oxygen or air during peeling, cutting bruising and soon become brown in color. Soon a chemical process begins in which phenolic compounds are oxidized by polyphenol oxidase (PPO) enzyme present in food itself and eventually a black-brown phenolic compounds called "melanin" is formed on the cut surface. PPO is present in the plastids of plant cells and the phenolics are found in vacuoles. In an intact fruit or vegetable, the two are physically/spatially apart but when the tissue is damaged, they are now in enough proximity for the reaction to occur.

Different polyphenolic compounds are present in different fruits and vegetables hence, the rate and extent of browning also differ. PPO plays a natural defense mechanism in the plants against microorganisms and insects attack. Enzymatic browning is undesirable for food processers and food growers, as this browning badly affects the organoleptic properties of fresh fruits and vegetables, thus often cause substantial economic losses to them. Nutritionally phenolic content and vitamin C are significantly reduced their myriad health benefits such as reduced risk of CVD and certain cancers. Melanin being antimicrobial, antibacterial, and antioxidant prevents further damage to the plant tissue. However, enzymatic browning is exploited for fermentation of tea leaves, coffee beans and darkening of raisins, dates, and prunes.

When enzymatic browning occurs in produce, the cut/bruised fruits/vegetables lose their appeal, taste, and flavor; hence, it is better to prevent browning. Use of sugar blocks, the oxygen supply, and use of acid medium inhibits enzyme action. Browning can be prevented at household and industrial levels by:

- Cutting or peel fruits and vegetables just before use
- Dipping in water, acid or sugar solution
- Blanching preferably steam blanching
- Refrigeration
- Dehydration
- Irradiation
- High pressure treatment
- Use of super critical carbon dioxide
- Use of inhibitors such as sulfur compounds, ascorbic acid, and antioxidants.

Blanching destroys the PPO enzyme by denaturing it (due to heat) thus prevent browning; however, it causes loss of vitamin C. Other methods can be used as well; the choice of method may vary with the type of food, variety, usage, storage period, transport system and facility available.

Nonenzymatic Browning

As the name suggests nonenzymatic browning does not involve any enzyme. Nonenzymatic browning is also of two types: (1) Maillard Reaction (MR) and (2) Caramelization.

Maillard Reaction (MR)

The Maillard reaction (named after the French chemist Louis Camille Maillard who discovered this in 1912), does not involve any enzyme. The products of this reaction are known as Maillard reaction products (MRPs) and/or advanced glycation end-products (AGEs) depending on duration of treatment and food compounds involved. At high temperature amino acids and reducing sugars react with each other and the products of this reaction give a range of color and impart flavor and aroma in the food. At various stages in the process, different compounds are formed. MR is accelerated in conditions like high relative humidity, high temperature, high pH (alkaline), high protein content, and low water content maximum at water activity (AW) 0.6–0.7.

MR occurs only in reducing sugars. Pentoses (xylose, ribose, and arabinose) are more reactive than hexoses (glucose, fructose, and galactose). Sugar alcohols or polyols (sorbitol, xylitol) do not participate in Maillard reaction. Xylose and arginine produce more browning. Sometimes oxidized lipids may also participate in this reaction. MR occurs in almost all foods during heating or storage. At various stages in the process, different compounds are formed. Thus, MRs bring significant changes in food color, organoleptic properties, protein functionality, and protein digestibility. This reaction is therefore also used in food industry, e.g., browning in roasted, baked, and fried foods. MR reaction is an inevitable reaction in certain food products, hence some undesirable browning mostly occurs during storage due to various factors that need to be managed.

Maillard reaction also takes place in living organisms. Among the MRPs, melanoidins that are highly colored are said to have beneficial effects on health as an antioxidant, and antibiotic effects. Heterocyclic compounds that are formed exhibit antioxidant capacity. Melanoidin can be formed even if a product is kept at low temperature for prolonged period. However, when exposed to high temperature (>180°C), acrylamide is produced. Also, acrylamide is neurotoxic and is a carcinogen.

In the reaction, lysine is converted to carboxymethyl lysine and carboxyethyl lysine (CEL). Ne-Carboxymethyl lysine and carboxyethyl lysine have been implicated to have a role in increasing risk of diabetes and cardiovascular diseases. Because MR modifies lysine, its availability is reduced. MR also causes losses of tryptophan, histidine, and arginine. In addition, it lowers the digestibility of protein, although the digestibility of carbohydrate and its availability is not affected much.

Cooking at high temperature may generate MRPs which can be good or bad for health. Extrusion, microwave, and infrared heating tend to generate acrylamides. Time and temperature critically influence the formation of MRPs. Pasteurization and ultra-high temperature (UHT) of milk often lead to the formation of MRPs because milk is rich in protein and sugar. Studies show that various compounds such as MRPs, acrylamide, furosine, hydroxymethylfurfural (HMF), pyrrole, pyrazine, furan, imidazole, and many heterocyclic compounds are formed, which exude distinct flavor but many of them are classified as possible human carcinogens, e.g., furan in excess can cause adverse reactions in eyes, skin, and lung. Pyrolysates play important role in the development and progression of diabetes and age-related degenerative diseases. Most undesirable changes occur during boiling, broiling, frying, and baking at high temperature for prolonged periods.

Foods rich in lysine and ribose form a very dark brown color and strong flavor, e.g., whey protein, egg wash, cheese topping are used for browning. Cysteine, sulfur-containing amino acid in meat tends to form heterocyclic compounds which are responsible for meat flavor. Since different foods have different amino acid composition hence flavor compounds formed are also different.

In advanced stages of MR as stated above also "Advanced glycation end-products" (AGEs) are formed. AGEs are formed both in foods during processing as well as under normal physiologic conditions of human body. The process of formation of AGEs is called glycation. Glycation tends to alter the structure and functional properties of proteins influencing cellular metabolism. Glycation is one of the major reasons for the complications in diabetes such as retinopathy, nephropathy, neuropathy, cardiomyopathyand many inflammatory diseases like rheumatoid arthritis and also aging. During long-standing hyperglycemia or diabetes, glucose forms complex with plasma proteins through glycation resulting in excessive production of AGEs in different tissues and organs of the human body. Its formation in vivo contributes to the progress of degenerative diseases associated with inflammatory conditions and complications in diabetes. High blood glucose forms a complex with plasma protein through a process of glycation. Blood test of HbA1c among diabetic patients indicates glycation reaction in the body.

> Acrylamide is a naturally occurring compound in foods and is also formed during Maillard reaction. Potato chips or French fries are found to contain acrylamide. This compound is usually formed with the reaction of asparagine and reducing sugar at temperature above 120 °C. Large dose of acrylamide consumption can damage mucous membrane and cause birth defects, inflammation and some chronic diseases. Asparagine in potato and cereals and fat seem to be the main culprits in development of acrylamide. Soaking peeled potatoes in acidic solution 10-15 minutes before frying or use of herb-like rosemary may mitigate the formation of acrylamide.

Caramelization

Caramelization is an oxidative process of sugar degradation in the presence of heat which results in a product that has typically nutty or burnt sugar flavor and brown color and is called caramel. Caramelization occurs in three steps, at 160–180°C when a high concentration of carbohydrate is heated. However, the temperature depends on the sugar that is used. Fructose caramelizes at 110°C, galactose, glucose and sucrose at 160°C, whereas maltose caramelizes at 180°C.

When sugar (sucrose) is heated first it breaks down into fructose, and glucose. This is known as inversion of sucrose. The next step is condensation wherein the sugars lose water and react with each other, forming difructose-anhydride. Further, dehydration occurs. And the aldoses isomerize to ketoses. Also, low molecular compounds like organic acids, aldehydes, and ketones are formed. Some of them are volatile and contribute to characteristic flavor. The amount of these intermediate products depends on the pH, water activity, redox potential, and food structure. The molecules then fragment which then polymerize and produce the characteristic caramel color and browned sugar flavor associated with the process. The three main products from sucrose caramelization are the dehydration products caramelan and two polymers, carmelen and caramelin. The thermal processing can be controlled to obtain desirable properties. Excess cooking of sugar, leads to the caramel having bitter taste and lacking sweetness.

The kind of caramel depends upon the type of sugar present in food, e.g., caramel produced from table sugar produces different caramel product as compared to caramel produced from cocoa beans or coffee so resulting in different flavor. Caramelization is used in food industries for sugar candies and Indian sweets. The commonly formed flavor compounds are:

Although both caramelization and MR result in formation of brown pigments, the flavors generated by each are different. Also, caramelization occurs at a higher temperature (160–180°C) than MR (100–140°C). Another difference is MR involves not only sugar molecules but protein and/or lipid whereas, in caramelization only sugar is used.

> *Diacetyl:* This is formed during in the initial stages of caramelization and contributes a buttery or butterscotch flavor.
> *Hydroxymethylfurfural (HMF):* It has a sweet aroma and flavor, whereas other furans have a nutty flavor. HMF is also considered toxic at higher level. It is developed during thermal treatment, smoking, addition of nuts like raisins in bread and prolonged storage of dry food products (milk powder) at high temperature (above 37°C).
> *Maltol:* This has toasty flavor and aroma of freshly baked bread.
> *Esters and lactones:* These compounds have a sweet flavor. Lactone is associated with creamy butter like flavor in dairy products.

Gelatinization

Gelatinization is an irreversible physicochemical process of converting starch into a viscous paste-like form when starch is heated with water. Starch is not soluble in cold water (it forms a suspension) but when it is heated in water, it brings structural changes, the intermolecular bonds are broken down and the hydroxyl hydrogen and oxygen can engage more water, and starch granules swell. The process of gelatinization usually begins at 60–70°C, the starch granules begin to absorb water and swell. At 80°C, the starch particles absorb about five times their volume of water, until they burst open. Gelatinization is complete when the temperature reaches 100°C. One sign of gelatinization is that the starch that was originally opaque now becomes translucent. This can easily be demonstrated with rice starch or arrowroot starch or sago starch. If the starch to water ratio is high enough, it forms a paste.

For different starches gelatinization commences at different temperatures, occurs at a different rate and is influenced by the proportion of amylose and amylopectin as well as the amount of water used. Completion of gelatinization process is indicated by translucency of the starch. Also, the gelatinization process is influenced by cooking temperature that is called "Gelatinization temperature," e.g., cereal starch gelatinizes at much higher temperature (95–100°C). If starch is cooked for a longer duration, the molecules disintegrate and the starch loses its functionality. On letting the paste/mixture is left to stand undisturbed and cooled, the molecules bond and form a three dimensional network, resulting in a semi-rigid structure called gel, taking the shape of the container. The process is called **gelation**. A gel does not flow.

Starch consists of amylose and amylopectin. Amylose is linear polymer of glucose linked with alpha 1-4 linkage and hydrogen bonding and amylopectin is a branched chain in which branches are linked with alpha 1-6 linkage. Hence, amylose being linear chain forms gel that is viscous and translucent whereas amylopectin (waxy starch) having branched chain does not form gel and forms a clear paste. As it cools amylose forms solid gel and if amylopectin is high it remain in liquid form and called sol. These properties (called rheological properties) can be modified and used in various applications by food industry in various food products.

The amylose content has physiological significance as it determines the glycemic index (GI) e.g., long grain rice has low glycemic response due to high amylose content. Short grain sticky rice have relatively high GI. Thus, all rice varieties and cultivars are not the same. GI factors may be avoided. A higher amylose concentration retards gelatinization process. Starch in peas and corn that contains more amylose gelatinizes at 120°C. High amylose foods also contain resistant starch and/or dietary fiber that influence gelatinization and have implications for management of diabetes mellitus or weight management.

Gelatinization improves the digestibility of starch. It increases the availability of starch for digestion by amylolytic enzymes. Starch granules are not completely dissolved during food processing, thus food is in a dispersed state in which starch granules and/or granular remnants constitute the dispersed phase. The degree of gelatinization determines the rate of digestibility of the particular starch. Consequently even food processes, which result in a low degree of gelatinization (e.g., steaming and flaking of cereals), produce postprandial blood glucose and insulin increment similar to that with completely gelatinized foods. It is widely used throughout the world in making a vast variety of foods ranging from rice, bread, pasta, kheer, and pudding. Various factors influence gelatinization including the type of starch, size of starch granules, temperature, amount of liquid, stirring, presence of acid, fat, and protein. Starches from different sources gelatinize at different temperatures, e.g., wheat gelatinizes at a higher temperature and tapioca at lower temperature because the latter has more amylopectin. Addition of acid in the form of lime juice or vinegar hydrolyzes/breaks down the starch molecules and so reduces viscosity making the paste thinner and addition of fat and protein delays the process. Sugar delays gelatinization because it competes with the starch for water so less water is available for gelatinization, decreases viscosity and increases gelatinization temperature. The more sugar added, the longer the delay, with disaccharides having a stronger effect than monosaccharides. Acid (>4.0 pH) weakens the ability of starch to thicken resulting in a thin paste. Addition of acid after gelatinization helps to stabilize the gel. Stirring in early stages helps to prevent lump formation and gives uniform consistency and if continued it results in thin, slippery starch paste.

When gelatinized starch is cooled for a prolonged period of time, especially if starch-based foods are exposed to freeze-thaw cycles, the polysaccharides (amylose and amylopectin) in the gelatinized starch recrystallize or reassociate, this process is known as **retrogradation**. Retrogradation is one of the causes for staling of bakery products like bread or cake. The product becomes less moist and the firmness of the crumb increases. It also becomes less crisp and less sticky and there is change in flavor and aroma. Retrogradation also occurs in many snack products and breakfast cereals. Retrogradation reduces starch digestibility and has an impact on the development of resistant starch and GI value of carbohydrate foods.

Many factors influence starch retrogradation, such as storage temperature, the composition of the food including water content, sugar, lipids, salts, use of antistaling enzymes. For example, staling of bread is most rapid at 0–4°C. Amylose undergoes retrogradation more readily as it is a smaller and unbranched molecule. Therefore, in starch-based foods that are likely to be exposed to freeze-thaw cycles, waxy starch with low amylose content can be used to reduce the level of retrogradation.

Dextrinization

When starch is exposed to dry heat, it is partially broken down into dextrin that has a brown color and typical or distinct flavour, e.g., toasted bread or *chapatti*. Particularly, amylopectin is broken down into dextrin that does not form paste as is seen with gelatinization. In gelatinization the starch molecule absorbs water and swells whereas in dextrinization, the food loses moisture and the starch is degraded. Due to this, food with considerable dextrin content cannot be used much for thickening and imparting viscosity to a product. The color of toast, biscuits and cakes is due to dextrinization. Also, products can become more crisp in texture. Dextrinization improves digestibility of starch.

Denaturation

Denaturation is the process of unfolding of the complex, well defined, folded structure of a protein. It occurs under the influence of heat, acid, alkali or enzyme. It facilitates digestion of protein food in the stomach, where the enzyme pepsin and acidic medium support digestion. Achlorhydria (low acid in stomach) hinders the digestion of protein. Further, proteolytic enzymes in the small intestines complete digestion of protein foods. Denaturation is influenced by temperature, pH; hence cooking at high temperature and presence of acid toughens the protein and reduces the bioavailability of the amino acids particularly lysine. It is also influenced by mechanical pressure, e.g., whisking an egg. Denaturation thus brings about changes in texture, flavor and color that vary from food to food, e.g., marinating meat where acid partially tenderizes the meat before cooking. Denaturation also results in loss of shape of the protein and irreversible loss of function. However, it enhances the digestibility of dietary protein. Sensitivity of protein to heat depends on the nature of the protein, its concentration, pH, amount of moisture, ions present. Denaturation of different proteins is influenced by temperature, pH and mechanical pressure. Different types of protein are composed of different amino acids, thus they are denatured differently and digested differently. Sometimes denaturation has a detrimental effect on protein as it inactivates the enzymes that are also protein in nature. Overheating toughens the protein food and adversely affects the bioavailability of the amino acids particularly lysine. It also brings changes in texture, flavor and color that vary from food to food.

Denaturation decreases solubility, alters water binding capacity, loss of biological capacity, increased susceptibility to attack by proteases or proteolytic enzymes. Functional properties of egg proteins are denaturation, coagulation, gelation, foaming that are extensively used in cookery.

Coagulation

Coagulation is an irreversible process of random rearrangement (aggregation) of denatured proteins into a soft semisolid mass. It occurs at 60–75°C in egg white and can vary from protein to protein, e.g., omelet is a mixture of coagulated egg proteins and paneer is coagulated casein. Protein gets separated from other nutrients. Heat application for a long time causes changes in protein structure and entraps the liquid which helps in the formation of a gel. Coagulation is observed in boiled egg and many other products. Coagulation is influenced by temperature, time, acidic medium, dilution, sugar, salt, and fat. Sugar and dilution raise the coagulation temperature. Acidity and salt speed up coagulation. For example when egg white is heated to 60–75°C, it becomes opaque and firm.

Gelation

Gelation is the irreversible formation of three-dimensional network of denatured protein in orderly manner in which water is entrapped. It generally occurs when protein is still in solution and has not precipitated out. The end product is a firm structure called gel. Calcium and sulphydryl groups give extra strength to the protein gel but excess amount of both inhibit the gel formation. Egg custard and curds are examples of gelation.

Gel Formation

Gel is a soft solid viscoelastic product. It is a commonly used process in food preparations or foods, e.g., yogurt, jellies, etc. Gel formation process occurs under certain optimal conditions such as temperature, presence of ions, pH and the concentration of gelling agents. In food gels polysaccharides and proteins behave as gelling agents. Surface active compounds like lecithin is also used for gel formation, e.g., gelatin gels.

Rancidity

Rancidity is chemical decomposition of oil, fats, and lipids. When fats or lipids are exposed to atmospheric oxygen or heat/light/moisture/bacterial or fungal contamination, certain physicochemical changes occur in the natural properties of the fat leading to the development of characteristic unpalatable/unpleasant odor or taste or abnormal color particularly when it stored for a long period of time. This process can occur in raw foodstuffs, refined or used edible oils, including snack foods cooked in such oil. There are three types of rancidity:
1. Hydrolytic rancidity—involve water
2. Oxidative rancidity—involve air/oxygen
3. Ketonic/microbial rancidity—involve microbes.

Hydrolytic Rancidity

It implies the hydrolysis or breakdown of fats in presence of water, a catalyst or by the action of the enzyme lipase. Free fatty acids and glycerol are liberated from the triglyceride. It generally occurs when fats are exposed to high temperature and moisture. Butter is susceptible to hydrolytic rancidity because it contains moisture. The unpleasant odor associated with hydrolytic rancidity is due to the free and volatile short chain fatty acids. Some microorganisms possess lipase enzyme that catalyze hydrolytic rancidity in which ketones and other hydrolytic products are present.

Oxidative Rancidity

This rancidity occurs due to oxidation of fat or oil wherein oxygen is added at the unsaturated double bond of unsaturated fatty acid of oil, i.e., lipid peroxidation occurs. This reaction is catalyzed by exposure to oxygen, light, ultraviolet light, heavy metals and/or heat producing peroxide derivatives. Oxidative rancidity occurs in three stages: Initiation, propagation, and termination (Fig. 17.2). In the first stage, when the oil is exposed to light or metal ions and/or heat, highly reactive free radicals are formed. This is followed by the second stage—propagation wherein a chain reaction is started and new reactive radicals are formed as shown in Figure 17.2. In the termination stage, two radicals combine and neutralize each other, forming stable oxidation products. These products are responsible for the typical rancid odor of oxidized fats/oils/foods.

Pigments like chlorophyll and some carotenoids accelerate auto-oxidation of fats in the presence of light. The reaction occurs as soon as fats, oils and any fatty foods come into contact with air. These derivatives on decomposition yield

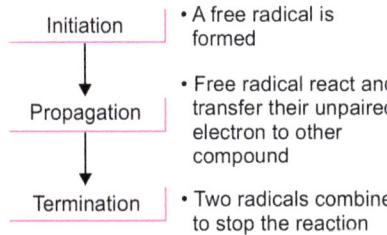

Fig. 17.2: Stages of oxidative rancidity.

peroxides, aldehydes, ketones and dicarboxylic acids that are toxic and have offensive odor. Saturated fats resist rancidity more than unsaturated fats that have unsaturated double bonds.

Lipid peroxidation: Lipid peroxidation means that oxygen reacts with unsaturated fatty acids in a fat or oil, forming free radicals or reactive oxygen species (ROS), initiating a chain reaction. It is an autocatalytic process that includes initiation, propagation and termination and can be a cyclic process. It occurs in any lipid containing a double bond, i.e., PUFA and cholesterol. Oxidation of fat is higher in PUFA during heating, contact with air (oxygen) and contact with metals like iron. Presence of antioxidant(s) can terminate the free radical chain reaction.

Lipid oxidation leads to formation of aldehydes and ketones that further interact with sugars or proteins and form a wide range of compounds which impart flavor to the food particularly in the fried food. Some of the products are of concerns related to health. These are hydroperoxides, malondialdehyde, 4-hydroxynonenal, and advanced glyoxidation end products (AGE). The nature and proportion of these products can vary widely in foods and depend on the composition of the food as well as numerous environmental factors.

Lipid oxidation results in deterioration of quality of food by producing off-flavor and loss of nutrients like vitamins A, D, E, K, carotenoids, and essential fatty acids when oil is exposed to heat and air like during frying and storage. Lipid oxidation severely compromises the quality of some foods and limits the shelf-life of foods due to development of oxidized or off-flavor as a result of rancidity. In oils, colored compounds are formed, resulting in a change in the color of the oil. The food product cooked thereafter possesses burnt, smoky, fishy, rubbery, and acrid characteristics. The color change is mainly due to nonenzymatic browning that occurs due to the reaction between the sugars and amino groups present in the food that is fried. This is particularly seen in foods containing protein foods, especially whey protein. Color change and formation of color compound(s) indicate the degradation of the oil and indicates the deterioration in the nutritional and sensory qualities of both the food being fried and the frying oil.

All foods that contain lipids are susceptible to oxidation but those foods that are dehydrated, subjected to high temperatures or cooked and subsequently stored, e.g., dehydrated eggs, cheeses and meats, foods fried in frying oils, and cooked (uncured) meats, are more susceptible. Cooking, grinding, mixing, exposure to air are important factors. Use of antioxidants and appropriate packaging materials that do not allow entry of air into the package or vacuum or modified atmosphere packaging (use of gases like nitrogen or carbon dioxide) for processed food products, can retard oxidation. Some products are volatile and get evaporated, so they are not very harmful, in contrast to the nonvolatile products that are formed.

Oxidation of oils/fats produces lipid peroxides which are unstable and further degrades with formation of secondary oxidation products such as malondialdehyde (MDA). Toxic compounds that are carcinogenic, e.g., hydroperoxides damage the DNA. Coronary artery disease (CAD) may be in part caused by the consumption of lipid oxidation products. Lipid peroxidation is found to play a major role in pathogenesis of atherosclerosis, may be in oxidizing the LDL cholesterol and also neurodegenerative diseases. At high temperatures, interaction with food molecules like protein and lipids in meat tends to produce other compounds like advanced glycoxidation end products (AGEs) and advanced lipid end products (ALEs) which are linked to aging and cellular damage.

The process of lipid oxidation (LP) can be delayed or mitigated by:
- Avoiding exposure of the fats/oils/fatty foods to light, oxygen, high temperature, bacteria or fungi
- Proper storage of oil—keeping them in closed containers in a cool, dark, and dry place
- Checking the temperature while cooking can help to protect the food and oil.
- Avoid frequent and reheating of the oil
- Avoid heating of butter at high temperature
- Avoid leaving crumbs or pieces of food in the oil after frying, strain the oil before storage
- Use of various natural and synthetic antioxidants.
- Some vegetables, spices and herbs like in traditional food preparations have been found to inhibit the lipid peroxidation. Use of garlic, paprika, tejpattta is common. Rosemary extract has been investigated to prevent spoilage of oil.
- Pasteurization of foods like milk to inactivate the enzyme lipase.

Ketonic/Microbial Rancidity

This is due to contamination of the fats/oils or fatty foods with fungi like *Aspergillus niger*. The chemical structures in the fat are hydrolyzed by the lipases produced by the contaminating microorganisms. Due to the microbial action, ketones, fatty aldehydes, short chain fatty acids, and fatty alcohols are formed. This rancidity is accelerated by the presence of moisture.

NUTRITION ASPECTS OF DIFFERENT METHODS OF FOOD PROCESSING

Several factors influence the nutritional content of food products. These include genetic makeup of the plant or animal, the soil in which plants were grown, feed given to the animal, use of fertilizers, maturity at harvest, packaging, storage conditions, method of processing/cooking and storage methods, and conditions after processing.

Besides making food safe, edible, palatable, digestible and nutritious, food Processing benefits, include removal of antinutrients and toxins, improvement of flavor, easing marketing and distribution tasks, availability of many seasonal foods around the year, enabling transportation of delicate perishable foods across long distances, preservation of food, and rendering foodstuffs shelf stable said above the word safe. Concentration of the nutrient that was originally present affects nutrient concentrations of the food after processing. Losses depend on the nutrient and exposure to different environments/treatments. Nutrients losses may occur by different means as shown in Figure 17.3.

During food processing, one or more chemical reactions may occur simultaneously. This is largely attributable to the composition of the food, other ingredients added and the method of cooking. The effect of food processing depends on the stability and sensitivity of various nutrients to the different conditions to which the food(s) is exposed such as light, temperature, air/oxygen, metals.

Varied methods of food pre-preparations and cooking are employed in a wide range of food preparations/food products. Selection of processing method(s) is largely based on the nature of the final product, availability of raw material, available tools and equipment as well as time, and skills needed to cook the food. In some foods only one method may be used but in general, a combination of methods is generally employed. Cooking usually involves some thermal, i.e., heat treatment that can be moist or dry heat. Concentrations of important constituents are altered by various processing methods such as milling, fermentation, germination, and thermal processing. The time and temperature of processing, product composition, and storage are all factors that substantially impact the nutritional quality of foods. Germination, fermentation, and malting have been used successfully for ages and they enhance the nutritional quality of food.

Cleaning, cutting and chopping is generally required for preparation of most recipes; and is referred to as primary processing. Primary processing is generally a manual and nonthermal process but on large scale, in food industry this is often done mechanically and/or chemically, sometimes cutting and chopping can be done by equipment under controlled conditions. Selection of appropriate the processing method is important in order to maintain maximal nutrition in the food product. Some methods like boiling, steaming, etc. are commonly used at both household and industry levels, but methods like irradiation require special setup and equipment.

Advances in technology, transport and communication has brought drastic changes in food processing. Both thermal and nonthermal techniques are frequently used in food processing. Thermal methods involve moist and dry heat methods of cooking while nonthermal include primary processing, germination and fermentation, along with newer methods.

The type of processing and the method used actually determines the extent of physicochemical changes. These changes either enhance or degrade the safety, sensory, and nutritional qualities of the food product. It can also accelerate or delay the food process of spoilage and nutritional losses. There are mainly three types of processing commonly used in food processing before raw food is utilized for human consumption as shown in Figure 17.4.

Primary processing is the conversion of raw food items into edible usable or consumable food ingredients, many of which need to be cooked or consumed later. It involves pre-preparation steps like cleaning, soaking, peeling, cutting, grating, sizing, and milling, etc. Most of these operations are usually done manually; however, sometimes machines like potato peeler, slicers, cutters, etc. that save time and labor are

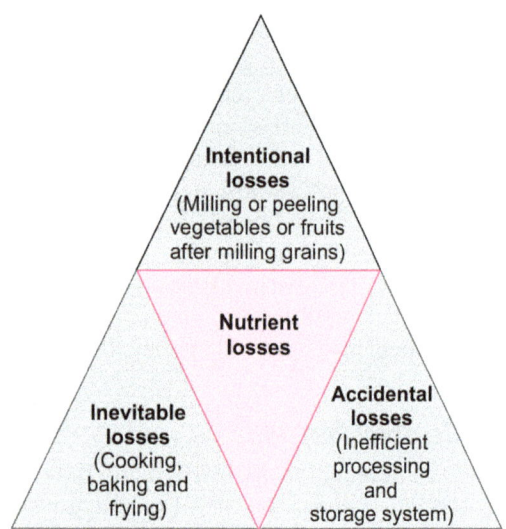

Fig. 17.3: Different means of nutrient losses.

Primary processing
- Conversion of raw food material into usable/edible food ingredient
- Done before cooking
- Examples: Cleaning, sorting, cutting, peeling, chopping, grating, slicing, mashing, grinding, etc.

Secondary processing
- Conversion of raw ingredients into cooked food items
- Actual cooking process
- Boiling, steaming, sauteing, roasting, baking, grilling, pressure cooking, etc.

Tertiary processing
- Final presentation of food
- Food is ready for consumption
- Use to produce commercial food products

Fig. 17.4: Different stages of food processing.

also used to perform these tasks. Primary processing usually does not include any heat treatment or cooking.

Secondary processing is the actual cooking process that involves transformation of primary processed food ingredients into the edible/consumable food products. It includes cooking methods like boiling, steaming, roasting, baking, etc. It enhances palatability, digestibility and bioavailability of certain nutrients and other health promoting compounds and at the same time heat treatment used in processing robs some essential nutrients.

Tertiary processing involves final presentation of food ready for consumption. It helps to maintain quality characteristics of the food, and extend shelf life for future consumption.

Primary Processing

Cleaning, Washing, and Soaking

Cleaning is the first and preliminary step of cooking, food processing and also food consumption. It ensures food safety and freedom from harmful microorganisms and thus helps to delay spoilage. It can be carried out manually, mechanically or chemically with or without water, in accordance with the nature of food. Cleaning can be dry or wet. The type of method used has nutritional and health implications. Cleaning for long duration and/or use of abrasive material can strip some vitamins and other components of health importance.

Washing removes dirt, debris, pesticides, and microorganisms. Prolonged or frequent washing with water tends to leach out some water-soluble compounds to varying extent such as vitamins, some phenolic compounds, and pigments including chlorophyll.

Soaking may or may not be necessary in all food preparations. However, soaking is a prerequisite step in parboiling, germination, and fermentation. Soaking whole pulses like rajmah, etc. is commonly done to reduce cooking time. It also reduces antinutritional factors to some extent and improves the bioavailability of nutrients such as minerals (iron, zinc, and calcium). Soaking of rice and cut vegetables for short duration is often practiced to hydrate the food and help retain the texture. However, soaking for long period leaches out the water soluble vitamins and water soluble pigments and other compounds.

Peeling, Chopping, and Cutting

Cutting, chopping and peeling of fruits and vegetables is common. During this, the cut surface is exposed to air and depending upon the type of food and the size of the cut pieces, enzymatic browning occurs in some fruits and vegetables, e.g., it occurs intensively in apple and potato but not in papaya and cauliflower. The cut or peeled surface is also at risk of microbial contamination resulting in food spoilage and loss of nutritional quality. Surface area of cut surface also determines the extent of nutrient loss. Smaller size pieces have more surface area than larger pieces. Hence, cutting fruits and vegetables into bigger pieces reduces the surface area exposed to air and helps to reduce losses of vitamins that are easily oxidized, especially vitamin C and folate. Dipping the cut pieces in mild acid like lemon solution may reduce browning.

Peel is a protective covering of food and protects the nutrients and antioxidants. Peeling exposes the flesh of the fruit/vegetable to air or oxygen that then reacts with antioxidant vitamins such as vitamin C, E and A and some phenolics compounds hence they are lost. Also, cutting raises the respiration rate which increases the breakdown of sugars into carbon dioxide leading to drastic changes in appearance, taste and texture of the cut food. In order to keep cut food for a longer duration, it is generally kept at refrigeration temperature, as low temperature reduces the respiration rate. However, not all nutrients are lost. For example, protein, fat and many compounds including B complex vitamins are not lost after peeling and cutting.

The knife used in peeling and cutting also play a role in nutrient loss or nutrient retention. Using a sharp knife, for cutting vegetables or fruit, does not bruise the produce as much as a dull blade will. As a result, there is less leakage of calcium and potassium and less production of off-odors. Also, a clean knife should be used in order to ensure that bacteria or mold is not introduced, which will lead to spoilage.

Peeling is not always necessary for certain fruits like apple, banana, grapes, pear, but it is essential for fruits like watermelon, orange, pineapple, papaya, and pomegranate. Peeling entails removal of the skin or peel of the fruit or vegetables. Discarding the peel of fruits results in loss of many nutrients and phytochemicals, e.g., quercitin from skin of the apple. Fruit/vegetable skin possesses dietary fiber, minerals and numerous phytochemicals that have antiviral, antibacterial, and cardioprotective properties as given above. Hence, unnecessary removal of a thick layer while peeling should be avoided to protect health benefits of food.

Milling

Milling of cereals involves removing the hull from the harvested mature grains usually cereals like wheat, rice, millets and convert the grain into edible form. It is mechanical separation of the endosperm from the germ, seed coat, and pericarp. Rice milling involves obtaining the edible rice kernel from paddy. Harvested grains contain an external/top layer, i.e., husk and bran; below which is the aleurone layer. Some parts of each layer are removed by milling of dehusked grains. The extent of delayering determines the extent of loss. Wheat milling includes production of whole wheat flour, semolina (suji), and refined flour (maida). These layers contain good amounts of soluble and insoluble fiber, niacin, vitamin B_6, vitamin E, potassium, magnesium, calcium, iron and zinc and many phytochemicals. Removal of aleurone layer causes maximum nutritional loss of these nutrients. The extent of milling grain or the proportion of whole grain that is ultimately converted to flour is referred to as extraction rate, i.e., the percentage of flour or a product like semolina obtained from a given quantity of grain. Extraction rates vary depending on the type of flour produced. Since many of the nutrients are found in the germ and bran, flours with a higher extraction rate have a higher nutritional value. In general, the higher the extraction rate less is the removal of bran, aleurone layer, and germ. Higher extraction rate generally retains more of the micronutrients present in the grain. At 100% extraction rate, i.e., in whole wheat flour, maximum nutrients are retained as the aleurone layer and germ are conserved, whereas at 65–70% extraction rate, refined flour is obtained and there is considerable loss of nutrients because most of the B vitamins, iron, and calcium are concentrated in the aleurone layer. Commercial milling results in loss of 58% of thiamine, 58–65% of riboflavin, and 85% of the vitamin B6 from whole wheat.

Milling of rice is an abrasive process that involves removal of husk of paddy, (hulling) polishing of endosperm to get white rice and removal of broken kernel and paddy husk or hull. Hulling is done either by hand or rolling/grinding the rice grains between stones. However, on large scale this is done in mills by automated processes. During hulling 80–90% of the kernel hulls are removed. Rice bran is not used as an edible source of dietary fiber and vitamins but it is used for making rice bran oil.

The bran is rich in fiber, minerals (magnesium, potassium, and zinc), ferulic acid, phytic acid and other nutrients including GABA, hence brown rice is more nutritious however they take longer to cook. The brown rice is further processed to remove the outer bran layers from the grain. Removal of all bran layers gives white polished rice that may be coated with glucose to increase luster. Rice milling or polishing drastically affects the nutrient composition of rice. Highly polished rice is devoid of some nutrients. Milled rice is easy to cook more palatability but is mainly starch, has a high glycemic index.

Milling does not affect adversely the carbohydrate, fat, and protein. However, flours cannot be stored for longer time otherwise they get rancid fast which is attributed to the presence of active lipase and lipoxygenase. These enzymes decompose fat and release free fatty acid thereby flours get rancid and impart bitter taste to the product. Stability of flours is increased by keeping them at low temperature and low humidity. Inert gases are also used but they may increase the cost.

> **Laboratory Laurel:** In some cases premilling treatments are given to ease the milling process but it tends to alter the nutritional composition and in vitro availability. In the present study pearl millet or bajra grains were given four treatments, i.e., acid treatment (2 hours, 12 hours, 18 hours, and 24 hours), dry heat treatment (30 minutes, 60 minutes, 90 minutes, and 120 minutes), blanching treatment (30 seconds, 60 seconds, and 90 seconds) and malting. In-vitro iron availability was assessed. Raw pearl millet contains 11.93 mg iron/100 g. Total iron content was reduced in all the treatments. However, in vitro iron availability improved after all four treatments. Acid treatments significantly reduced iron and longer duration further reduced the iron. It is because iron is present in pericarp of the grain and that is leached out during acid treatment. Maximum in vitro iron availability was noted in 120 minutes dry heat treatment followed by 90 seconds blanching treatment. However, longer dry heat treatment makes the grains darker having cooked flavor. Researcher concluded that 90 second blanching treatment is suitable for product development because of high in vitro iron and low free fatty acid content without diminishing its color.
>
> *Bhati D, Bhatnagar V, Acharya V. Effect of pre-milling processing techniques on pearl millet grains with special reference to in vitro iron availability Asian J Dairy Food Res. 2016;35(1):76-80.*

Parboiling

Parboiling is a process of steeping the paddy in water for a few days followed by heat treatment. During this process, nutrients like iron and thiamine are transported from bran to the rice kernel and starch is gelatinized, e.g., during making of poha or flattened rice and parboiled rice. Therefore parboiled rice is yellowish in color, and grains are separated during cooking. Starch is pregelatinized making parboiled rice more digestible and nutritious. The rice is also less sticky. Lipase is inactivated during parboiling hence parboiled rice does not become rancid quickly. This method is also used in making malt from millet like barley.

Secondary Processing

This consists of methods that are used to convert primary processed foods into other foods. During this a food can be mixed with other foods and ingredients. Often, the physical form of the food also changes considerable. Examples of secondary processing methods are juicing, stewing, canning, kneading, cooking, and drying. These methods are either used to make ready to use or ready to eat foods, i.e., to create a final edible product. Various food processing methods are used to cook the food which are shown in Figure 17.5.

Moist Heat Methods

Moist heat methods of cooking involve heating the food by conduction and convection with direct or indirect inclusion of water, any liquid, or steam. It includes boiling, steaming, pressure cooking, simmering, stewing, poaching, blanching, pasteurization, sterilization, and canning. All these methods eliminate pathogens to varying degrees, thus rendering the food safe for consumption. Cooking results in changes in color, texture, taste, flavor and nutritive value, and storability of food (*see* Table 17.2). Considerable loss of ascorbic acid occurs because it is easily oxidized, especially in aqueous solutions and the losses are enhanced by high temperatures, relative humidity and physical damage. Moist heat prevents formation of maillard reaction products, thus boiling, steaming, simmering, poaching are rather more healthy options for cooking. Choice of cooking methods are governed the type of food and desired cooked product. Differences in temperature in different moist heat cooking methods and their impact on nutritional, sensory, and microbiological attributes of cooked foods are given in Table 17.3.

Boiling is the most popular method of cooking wherein foods are immersed and cooked in boiling water. Boiling results in loss of valuable nutrients. The longer the food is immersed in water, greater is the loss. Hence, it is advisable to cook food in less water in the shortest possible time for maximum retention of nutrients. Boiling is used to soften the food, but it also brings changes in color and flavor also, e.g., purple-colored cabbage loses its anthocyanin content when it is boiled, so it looks unappealing and dull along with loss of health benefits of anthocyanin. Boiled food often tastes bland.

Boiling is also associated with losses of folate, B vitamins and vitamin C and reduction of minerals like potassium,

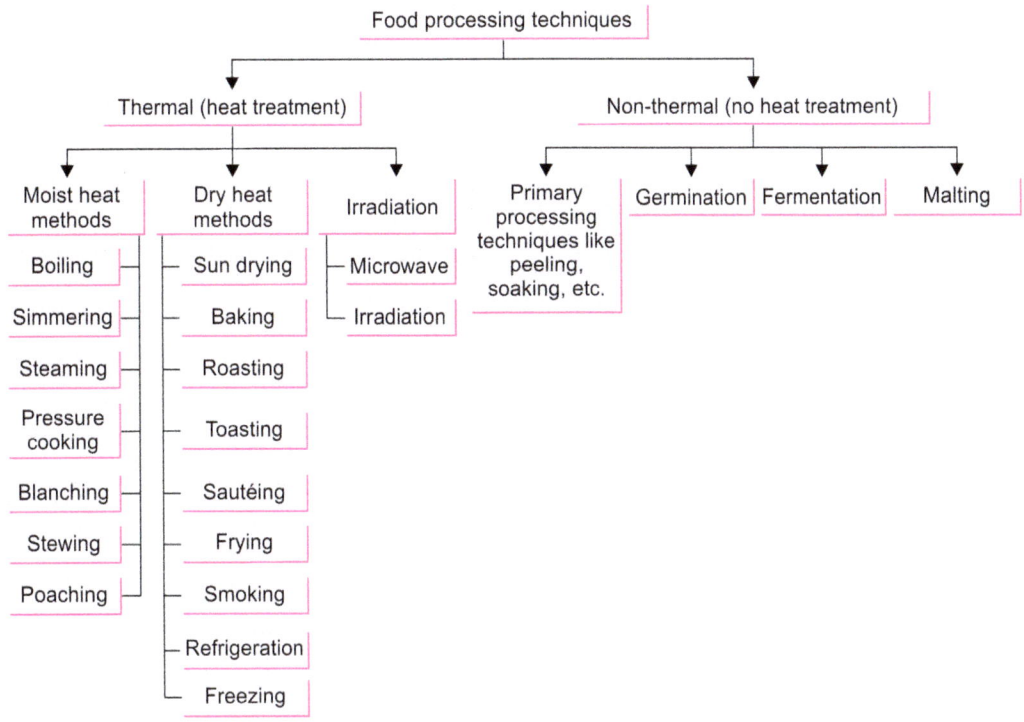

Fig. 17.5: Different techniques of food processing.

Table 17.3: Possible impact on nutrient in moist heat cooking methods.

Moist heat cooking Methods	Temperature used	Possible impact on nutrient
Boiling	100°C/212°F	Loss of folate, vitamin C, and some minerals like potassium and pigments like anthocyanin Preservation of antioxidant activity and carotenoids. Gelatinization of starch and denaturation of protein make the food digestible Leaching out of soluble nutrients, e.g., B-complex vitamins if boiling water is discarded
Steaming	121°C/249.8°F	One of the best methods to retain maximum nutrients Minimal loss of proteins and sugar, folates, vitamin C, chlorophyll, carotenoids, and many phenolic compounds
Pressure cooking	121°C	Nutrients, color and flavor are well preserved. Development of sulfur flavor in cauliflower, cabbage, capsicum due to release of sulfur compounds Destruction of antinutritional factors Loss of fiber, cellulose, hemicelluloses and polyphenolic compounds
Simmering	85–93°C (185–200°F)	Nutrients are retained in the gravy that is also consumed
Stewing	55–60°C for meat and 80–95°C for vegetables	Nutrients are retained maximum as they are transferred in the cooking water which is also consumed
Poaching	82°C/180°F	Slow heating preserves nutrients
Blanching	100°C	Inactivates enzymes to stop further ripening which may otherwise cause losses of nutrients. Vitamin C is lost
Pasteurization • Low Temperature Long Time (LTLT) • High Temperature Short Time (HTST) • Ultra heat treatment (UHT)	• 63°C for 30 minutes and rapidly cooled at 10°C • 72°C held for 15 seconds only • 135°C held for 1–2 seconds	Eliminates spoilage bacteria and enzymes and extends shelf life. Nutrients are not lost as in other processes Drastic alteration in temperature and cooking time may lead to nutrient loss and development of cooked flavour in raw food (milk)

phosphorus, magnesium, sulfur, zinc, and iron due to leaching. However, losses are higher in shredded, cubed or cut potato but boiling potato whole especially prevents these losses. In potassium-restricted diets, e.g., kidney dialysis, potato is peeled, cut and boiled, and cooking water is discarded to reduce its potassium content.

Losses of vitamins occur due to heat, oxidation and leaching. Aflatoxin is also lost to some extent although the losses may be more when the excess water is discarded or the product is pressure cooked instead of being boiled. Pigments like chlorophyll may also be lost.

Boiling has its advantages such as starch gets gelatinized, thus increasing the digestibility of starch. Also, protein is denatured making the boiled food more digestible. However, some amount of starch and free amino acids can leach into the water or react with each other in the Maillard reaction. There is no loss of dietary fiber. It also increases the bioavailability of minerals and total antioxidant capacity of foods. The water in which food is boiled should be preserved for further use in soups, gravies, etc. as it contains good amount of nutrients leached out from food during boiling. Losses can be reduced by using just the amount of water required so that all the water is absorbed and covering the container.

Steaming: Food is exposed to steam generated by water vapor from the steamer which is a closed container. There is a sharp rise in temperature, thus it helps to cook the food faster and keeps it moist. It limits overcooking and burning (121°C) retains more nutrients. Steaming is considered one of the best methods of cooking as far as nutrient retention is concerned. There is minimal loss of soluble proteins and sugar, folates, vitamin C, chlorophyll, carotenoids (β carotene, lutein, zeaxanthin and cryptoxanthin) and many phenolic compounds such as glucosinolates as compared to other cooking methods. Vegetables should not be overcooked by steaming in order to retain nutrients and better flavor.

Pressure cooking involves cooking under pressure. It is considered a convenient way of cooking because it takes less time to cook most of the foods. In household level cookers, 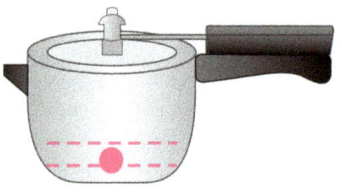 the pressure is about 5 psi due to build-up of steam along with 121°C temperature. Temperature rises with increase in pressure. Heat penetrates the food evenly thus food cooks uniformly. Nutrients, color and flavor are well preserved in pressure cooking. However, flavor of cabbage, capsicum or strong flavored vegetables is often spoiled due to release of sulfur compounds so should not be pressure cooked. Some antinutritional factors like lectins are also destroyed in pressure cooking, which is advantageous. Pressure cooking significantly decreases the fiber, cellulose, and hemicelluloses and also polyphenolic compounds except lignin. It also increases starch digestibility. Soaking beans in a salt solution, discarding the solution and cooking with fresh water is the best way to improve the nutritional quality of beans.

Simmering means to cook slowly at a temperature (85–96°C) lower than boiling temperature, and preferably using well-fitting lid. Simmering is useful for better mixing, thickening and developing the flavor of foods and is suitable for preparation of gravies and sauces. Nutrients and other compounds are leached out and remain in the gravy. If simmering is done in an open pan for prolonged duration, the nutrient loss is higher.

Stewing involves cooking on low flame of uniformly cut pieces of food (usually fruits or meat) completely submerged/immersed in liquid or water, with or without whole spices till softens. The food is consumed whole along with liquid to have maximum flavour and nourishment. Preparations like stews are nourishing and healthy and advocated for people on low fat diet.

Poaching is a delicate method of cooking for egg and fish. The food is submerged gently into plain hot water and is cooked slowly at temperature (93–95 °C), for a fairly short period of time. Protein of food gets coagulated and most of the nutrients are retained.

Blanching is primarily a pretreatment/operation applied to vegetables or fruits prior to freezing, canning, or drying, although fruits are generally not blanched. Traditionally, blanching was done by first immersing the food into boiling water for a short time varying from seconds to a few minutes (depending on the fruit/vegetable), then immersing it in cold water and then removing it. Instead of immersing in cold water, cold dry air may be blown over the product so that evaporative cooling occurs. Besides, hot water, blanching is nowadays done using steam or microwave and hot gas blanching. Blanching is done to inactivate enzymes; modify texture; preserve color, flavor, and nutritional value; as well as remove trapped air. Inactivation of enzymes like polyphenol oxidase also prevents browning. Blanching enhances the drying rates and makes removal of peel/skin and dicing the produce easier. Blanching also reduces the microbial load and pesticide residues/toxic constituents and helps to retain the color and flavor of the vegetables although vitamin C is lost.

Dry Heat Methods

Dry heat methods are those in which heat is conducted by hot air, hot metal, radiation or hot fat/oil as the medium of cooking, without use of additional moisture/water. Commonly used methods are roasting, baking, grilling, drying, dehydration, etc. Food is exposed to high heat, i.e., 148.8°C (300°F) or more. The heat source is generally placed either from below or above the food and brings the temperature of food to much higher level than does moist heat. Heated air can come from an open or closed area and with or without presence of a liquid medium. Food cooks in its own moisture when the food surface is exposed to hot environment resulting in rise in the temperature of the food surface to more than 100°C. It tends to evaporate the moisture from the food and food becomes dry and crispy. In case of products like cakes/bread the outer surface becomes brown (due to nonenzymatic browning) and crisp. The process prolongs the shelf life due to the reduced moisture content and reduces spoilage of the food product. High heat and loss of water tend to reduce the heat labile and water-soluble components of food. Losses of some volatile and heat labile components due to heat and water loss occur. However, there is remarkable improvement in palatability of food, digestibility, and bioavailability of some nutrients.

In cereal foods and meat foods or any foods containing sugars and protein cooked by dry heat cooking methods like roasting and grilling, the possibility of Maillard Reaction and formation of advanced glycation-products (AGEs), acrylamides, and heterocyclic amines which are carcinogenic in nature, is quite high. On the other hand, when these methods are employed at low temperature for a longer duration, they numerous volatile flavor compounds are formed. Volatile organic compounds are organic molecules that include esters, alcohols, aldehydes, ketones, phenols, terpenes, etc. Food containing fats and fatty acids may often develop (rancidity) off-flavor and change color when undergo dry heat methods.

Puffing

Puffing and Popping: Puffing and popping are age-old processing techniques in countries like ours and have been widely as a cheap and simple method of food preparation and to develop ready-to eat-foods. During popping, grains are exposed to very high temperature (240–270°C) for very short time (5–10 seconds) usually under pressure. There is sudden expansion of the endosperm and internal moisture creates the vapor pressure inside the grain which explodes making the grain volume increase several times in volume. At the same time volatile flavor compounds are released imparting a delicious aroma and flavor to the grain.

Puffing and popping is usually done with hot air, hot sand, frying in hot oil, microwave and gun puffing. Kernel properties like shape, size density, moisture content and thickness of the seed coat determine whether grain will be popped, puffed or parched. Popping is done for soft grains having high moisture content (>12%), e.g., corn is well suited for popping.

Popping occurs at about 177°C, which is equivalent to a pressure of 135 psi inside the kernel. In puffing, there is sudden release of super-heated vapor and the grains are cooked from inside, expanding the endosperm. Also, water vapors escape through the microspores of the grain rupturing the pericarp with great force.

Grains like rice, wheat, amaranth or some millets do not contain required moisture (12% for popping) rather they have low moisture, hence they are puffed to get dry, voluminous, and crispy products. Though there are many factors which affect the process and outcome of puffing; however, low moisture content and high amylose content in cereal grains limits the popping capacity hence they are puffed.

Puffed rice, popcorn and puffed wheat, puffed amaranth (Chowli or ramdana), and millets are common examples of puffing. Various factors as shown in Figure 17.6 influence popping qualities of cereals such as season, varietal difference, grain characters, i.e., bran content, bran thickness, kernel size, shape and density, moisture content, type of endosperm, method of popping, microspore size, popping temperature, e.g., large kernels generally give lower popping volume than small kernels, because they contain a high percentage of soft endosperm. There is considerable increase in size of the grain, e.g., 8–16-fold for wheat and 6–8-fold for rice grains. Puffed grains become voluminous and light in weight. Type of starch is also important, e.g., rice with high amylose content is not suitable for puffing because it gives a lower puffing index than rice with medium amylose content. Puffed grains get sterilized (seed microflora is destroyed) at such high temperature. So puffing makes the grains safe to consume. Moisture content is reduced, thus shelf life is increased. There is gelatinization of starch and degradation of dietary fibers, thus the digestibility of starch is much improved. Puffing alters the morphology and composition of grain. It increases the water holding capacity of the grain and the flours made from puffed grains. Puffing reduces the phytate content and improves of iron bioavailability to some extent.

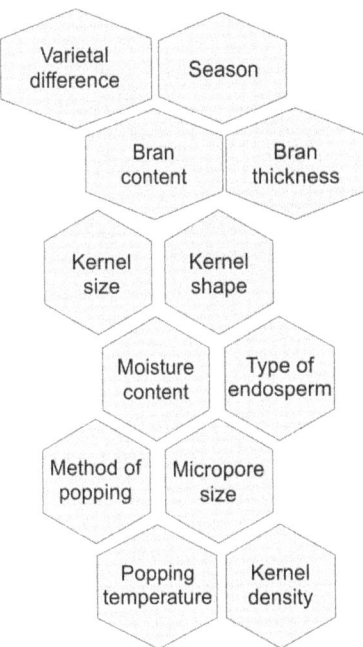

Fig. 17.6: Factors affecting puffing and popping.

Puffed rice has a high glycemic index, thus it can raise the levels of insulin and blood glucose level considerably. However, there are novel processes to make puffed rice with three times more protein and eight times more dietary fiber than commercial puffed rice with better taste and crunch.

Laboratory Laurel: Supercritical fluid technology is a novel technology to develop new food products using low temperature and high expansion, in contrast (to extrusion (SCFC) technology in order to develop puffed grains. In the concerned experiment puffed rice is fortified with protein, dietary fiber and micronutrients and evaluated the end product for nutritional and textural qualities. This technique could retain nutrients better particularly which were used for fortification, e.g., 55–58% retention of vitamin A, 64–76% vitamin C, and 98.6% for all amino acids including lysine. Hence, fortified puffed rice contained 8% dietary fiber, 21.5% protein and iron, zinc, vitamin A and C, and found suitable for breakfast cereal, snack food and school lunch programs, and market place.

Paraman I, Wagner ME, Rizvi SSH. Micronutrient and protein-fortified whole grain puffed rice made by supercritical fluid extrusion. J Agric Food Chem. 2012;60(44):11188-94.

Toasting

Toasting is a process of dry heating and browning the semi-cooked or cooked food by exposing to radiant heat. During toasting, starch is partially broken down into dextrin due to dextrinization that imparts a slightly sweet taste and improves digestibility of the carbohydrate. Food also becomes crisp due to evaporation of water. Browning occurs due to Maillard reaction and caramelization. Roasting or toasting and parching legumes are practiced largely in India and Africa.

Roasting

Roasting is a very popular method of dry heat cooking in an open or controlled manner. It is popular in many parts of the world. There are many ways of roasting, i.e., hot iron vessel (tawa or griddle or karai), sand, microwave, oven, grill, etc.

The whole husked or unhusked grain is exposed to high heat either directly by placing the whole grains and grams. A little water is first sprinkled on the grain, with or without salt. Generally, the grain is mixed with sand, the ratio being 1:4 on a volume: volume basis. The pulse–sand mixture is kept in an open pan on the fire, and the sand generally reaches a temperature of 240°C and roasted. Changes occurring during roasting as shown in Figure 17.7 improves the flavor and texture of the grain.

Research Glimpse: People consume varying amounts of acrylamide mainly through the diet. Acrylamide develops during cooking at high temperature (more than 120°C). It is formed more during frying or baking and not during boiling or microwaving. Temperature and time are crucial in formation of acrylamide. It generally develops in starchy foods such as potato chips (French fries), cereal and bakery products and that is attributed to with high carbohydrate, free asparagine, reducing sugars, pH, water content, ammonium bicarbonate, and high concentration of competing amino acids in them. It is found in low levels in as meat and fish. Unfortunately acrylamide intake may increase the risks of kidney and breast cancer. Though no permissible limit has been set worldwide for acrylamide consumption in diet till date but its daily intake has been estimated to be about 0.85 μg per kg body weight, normal conditions. Its dietary intake differs from country to country. Addition of antioxidants influences the Maillard reaction, which results in acrylamide formation. Rosemary extracts, bamboo leaves and green tea extract could effectively reduce acrylamide presence in different heated foods.

Krishnakumar T, Visvanathan R. Acrylamide in food products: A review. J Food Process Technol. 2014;5:344.

Roasting pulses denatures the protein and hence improves digestibility. Although some amount of amino acids is lost, but biological value of proteins improves. Thiamine and riboflavin are also lost to some extent. Roasting also significantly reduces antinutritional factors like phytic acid, phenols, and saponins and enhances nutritional quality and digestibility. During roasting several compounds that exert antioxidant capacity are formed. Different foods release different compounds. For example, during roasting of coffee bean, structural changes occur that result in the formation of melanoidins by Maillard and caramelization reactions. Formation of melanoidins coincides with the loss of some of chlorogenic acid found in coffee beans. Polyphenolic compounds such as *chlorogenic acid, resveratrol* are potent antioxidants found in roasted coffee and peanut. These compounds provide protection against many chronic diseases and delay hunger. However, roasting for longer duration and high temperature results in a loss of phenolic compounds, but this loss is compensated by formation of MR compound called melanoidin which is also a potent antioxidant. Hence, antioxidant capacity is not lost. When foods that contain fat are exposed to heat during roasting, rancidity is accelerated. Free fatty acids are released and exposure to air increases the susceptibility of roasted foods to rancidity. Chopped or roasted nuts spoil faster due to oxidative rancidity. Nuts contain more of unsaturated fatty acids. During storage nuts are exposed to air resulting in oxidation thereby rancidity. Hence nuts should be stored in air-tight jars and at low temperature.

Laboratory Laurels: The concentrations of B vitamins, carotenoids, and tocopherols in nuts differ in different varieties and are influenced by roasting. Thiamine, riboflavin, pyridoxine, lutein, zeaxanthin, β-carotene and α-/γ-tocopherol were determined in raw and roasted nuts using HPLC. Pistachios were rich in lutein/zeaxanthin and contained highest β-carotene levels among nuts. Almonds and hazelnuts were abundant in α-tocopherol (>4-fold the RDI for tocopherol equivalents) while pistachios and walnuts were rich in γ-tocopherol. Roasted almonds and walnuts showed lower levels of thiamine, carotenoids, and tocopherols. It is concluded that reduction in micronutrient content by roasting varies from nut to nut.

Stuetz W, Schlormann W, Glei M. B-vitamins, carotenoids and α-/γ-tocopherol in raw and roasted nuts. Food Chem. 2017;15(221): 222-7.

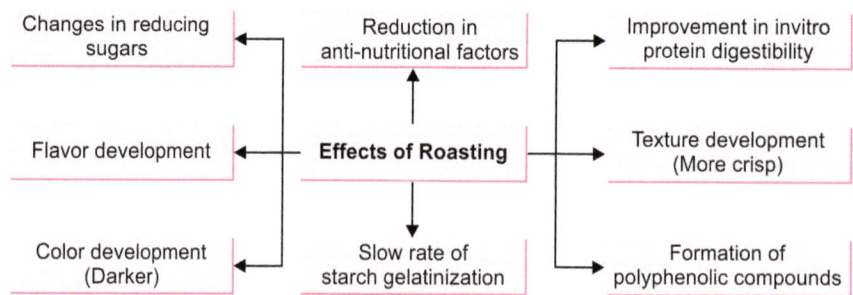

Fig. 17.7: Changes in food during roasting.

> **Laboratory Laurel:** This study was to determined the effect of thermal processing on tocopherols and carotenoids in tomatoes. Sliced tomatoes were heated in an oven at 100, 130, and 160°C for 5, 10, and 20 minutes, and then freeze-dried. These samples were analyzed for average concentrations of total lycopene, lutein, β-carotene, α-tocopherol, and γ-tocopherol and compared with fresh tomatoes. A significant increase was observed in tomatoes baked at 160°C for 20 minutes to the tune of 75% lycopene, 81% β-carotene, and 32% α-tocopherol. Heating induced isomerization of different isomers of lycopene. However, β-carotene was less influenced by heat treatment for isomerization. It suggested that thermal processes might break down cell walls and enhance the release of carotenoids and tocopherols from the matrix, as well as increase isomerization of lycopene and β-carotene.
>
> *Hwang ES, Stacewicz SM, Bowen PE. Effects of heat treatment on the carotenoid and tocopherol composition of tomato. J Food Sci. 2012;77(10):C1109-14.*

Grilling and Broiling: Grilled food is highly relished for its flavor all over the world. In grilling, the food is exposed to direct dry heat from below or above. In broiling, food is exposed to heat from above only. Food is generally placed on the grid or grate or a tava. Heat is transferred via thermal radiation. Heating source used is coal, gas or electric current. Barbecuing is a form of grilling and often done with lid closed over the food. In broiling, food is placed in an open pan and heat is transferred by thermal convection from above. These methods are generally used in cooking meat and meat products. The time required for cooking depends on the thickness of meat, the fat content and personal preferences for color, flavor and texture including the extent to which the meat is cooked. Grilling chars the external surface to some extent and the surface of the food cook quickly. Heat from the open fire tends to seal the outer surface of the food which supports release of flavor compounds, cooks the food using its own moisture and prevents the loss of vital compounds from the food. Hence it imparts a distinctive appearance and improves the flavor because browning occurs due to Maillard reaction.

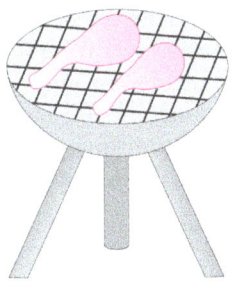

High heat (>260°C) is used in broiling and barbecuing in order to obtain the typical flavor. High temperature may tend to form heterocyclic amines, benzopyrenes, and polycyclic aromatic hydrocarbon (PAH) compounds that are responsible for the typical flavor, tenderness, and juiciness in meat. Unfortunately these compounds are known to cause DNA mutation and certain cancers. During grilling when fat from meat drips onto hot coal of the grill, the smoke increases formation of PAH thereby increases the risk of cancer. It is advisable to select leaner cuts of meat; marinate before grilling, grill at lower temperature and avoid overcooking. Figure 17.8 shows the differences among three methods of dry heat cooking.

- Formation of heterocyclic amines (HCAs), benzopyrenes, polycyclic aromatic hydrocarbon (PAH) provide typical flavor, tenderness and juiciness in meat (also causes DNA mutation and certain cancers)
- Destruction of anti-nutritional factors and bacteria

Grilling	Broiling	Barbecuing
• Intense high heat from **BELOW** • Charring and caramelizing • Preheating is necessary • Fat drips over	• Intense high heat from **ABOVE** • Charring and caramelization • Preheating is necessary • Fat drip into the pan below	• Form of grilling • Cooking in hot air with closed lid

Fig. 17.8: Difference among three high temperature cooking.

Smoking

Curing and smoking meat are age-old methods of food preservation. Intensive meat smoking is a combination of two effects, drying the meat by reducing its moisture content through hot air and the condensation of smoke particles on the meat surface together with their penetration into the inner layers of the product. Both have preservative effects and prolong the shelf-life of the product. Thickness of the meat parts is important. When the thickness is 3–15 cm, uniform drying does not occur. Faulty drying and smoking have a negative influence on rehydration capacity.

In smoking, meat is exposed directly to smoke that may be generated by a number of methods. Wood is generally used to generate smoke because wood smoke produces large number of flavor compounds like carbonyls (aldehydes and ketones), organic acids, phenols, organic bases, alcohols, hydrocarbons, and polycyclic aromatic compounds and gases like carbon monoxide, carbon dioxide, oxygen, and nitrogen.

Wood contains cellulose, hemicellulose, and lignin. Thermal decomposition of cellulose gives anhydroglucose, carbonyl-containing compounds, and furans. Hemicellulose undergoes decomposition similarly yielding acetic acid and carbon dioxide. The carbonyl-containing compounds give a sweet or burnt-sweet aroma. Also, the carbonyl-containing compounds interact with the proteins in the food and contribute to changes in the texture. Due to Maillard reaction and the products resulting from it, the color becomes golden-brown or brown.

Pyrolysis of lignin yields different types of phenolic compounds. The phenolic compounds contribute to the flavor of smoke. Thus, a mixture of compounds is obtained that impart the flavor and aroma but also have antioxidant and antibacterial properties. Development of polyphenolic compounds adds value to nutritional quality of smoked food, e.g., carbonyls improve the bioavailability of the protein in meat.

Smoking develops typical flavor in foods like meat. Some of these compounds are fungistatic and prevent the growth of molds. The kind of wood, method of heat transfer, humidity and circulation within the smoke room, influence the development of flavor. Intensive or prolonged smoking may increase the shelf life of the product but has unfavorable impact on the flavor since the concentrated compounds give the food an unpleasant tarry flavor. Also shelf life of smoked products stored at high temperatures is not likely to be long.

Oxidative changes in fat and destruction of vitamins also occur due to heat. Production of AGE products and nitrosamines are common in smoked meat products and both of them are very toxic and carcinogenic and have been established to be responsible for several inflammatory and chronic diseases. One of the concerns of smoking is that PAH are formed. In liquid smoke, these PAH may be removed and the intensity of flavor and color in the refined liquid smoke may be adjusted.

Baking: Food is cooked by convection using dry hot air in a closed airtight chamber (oven or tandoor). It is primarily used for the preparation of bread, cakes, pastries and pies, tarts, cookies, biscuits and many other vegetable and meat dishes.

Baking is of two types:
1. *Dry baking*: When baking, steam is formed from the water present in the food; this steam with the dry heat of the oven cooks the food, e.g., cakes, pastry, baked jacket potatoes.
2. *Steam baking*: When baking certain foods, e.g., bread, the oven humidity is increased by placing a bowl of water or injection of steam into the oven, thus increasing the water content of the food and so improving the eating quality. Humidity is an important criterion in cooking. High humidity in oven enhances moistness, volume, sponginess, good crust, glaze and color to the final product.

In a convection oven, the heat transfer is enhanced by the use of a fan. The fan creates forced convection within the oven, which not only heats the food faster but also encourages even distribution of heat. Food is cooked by the steam generated within it. Water evaporates bringing the hard or crisp texture. Crust formation and browning in baking due to relatively high temperature >140–220°C is due to the Maillard Reaction. Starch molecules dextrinize and sugar caramelizes which also impart color and flavor. Protein is denatured. Since baking is done in a closed environment, there is better retention of vitamins and minerals. However, nutrients that are heat sensitive like vitamin C will be lost, the extent varying with the duration of baking. Baked potatoes are found to be more nutritious than boiled and fried ones. Baking tends to enhance the antioxidant properties.

Microwave Cooking

Microwave cooking has become very popular because of the convenience, good quality product, and low maintenance. It takes less time to heat or cook the food and keep things word-clean. Some people also find it to be cost effective other than the initial cost of microwave oven. Microwave is commonly used to heat foods as well.

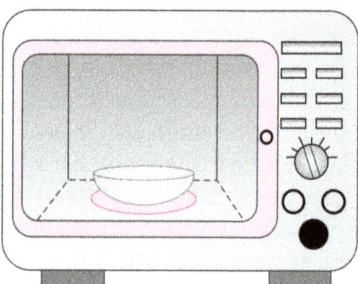

Microwaves are high-frequency electromagnetic waves of radiant energy similar to the electromagnetic radiation of light or radio waves with only difference in wave length. The wave length of microwaves is between 1,000 MHz and 300,000 MHz. Microwave ovens use high-power radio waves to cook food evenly. In microwave ovens, only 2450 MHz microwaves are used where they are absorbed by the water or other polar molecules and vibrate at intensely high speed that helps in heating or cooking the food, by raising the temperature of food above boiling point. In microwave ovens, microwaves originate from a Magnetron tube fitted inside the microwave oven that converts electric energy into microwave energy. According to the WHO, microwave energy can be absorbed by the water, fluid, and body tissues. It produces heat in exposed tissues particularly the organs with poor blood supply and temperature control. Long exposure can be rather damaging.

Cooking with microwaves differs radically from conventional cooking methods because the heat is generated inside the food rather than being transferred to the exterior of the food by conduction, convection or radiation. Microwaves are electromagnetic waves originating from a magnetron. A Magnetron is a vacuum tube that converts electric energy into microwave energy. Microwaves have longer wavelengths than infrared rays or visible light. Microwaves pass through glass and plastic, and are absorbed by any object that contains water. All foods contain varying degrees of moisture, no matter how dry they appear. How food is cooked in microwave is shown in Figure 17.9.

Microwave-oven energy is also more penetrating than heat that emanates from an oven or stove or gas range. It immediately reaches molecules about an inch or so below the surface. Heating the product in a thin layer provides uniform cooking while heating in thick layer may leave the food uneven and uncooked. Thick layer may cause for growth of microorganisms which may spoil the food.

Microwave cooking varies with the composition of food particularly the water content. Fat, protein fiber, etc.

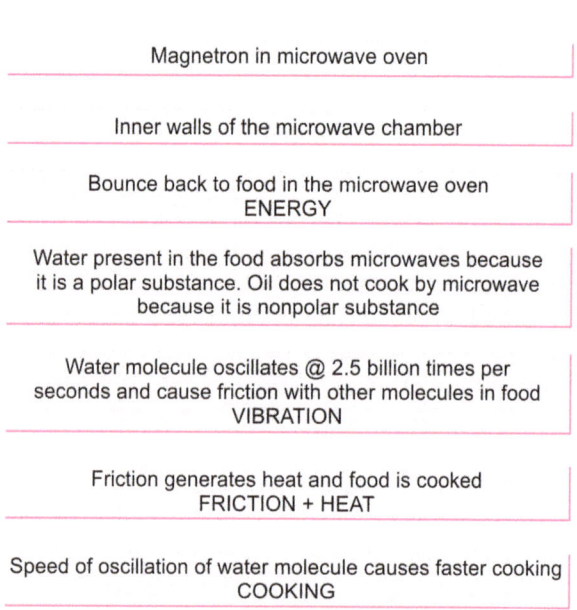

Fig. 17.9: Cooking process in microwave oven.

may delay the cooking as they are nonpolar substances. Microwaves are also been used for drying, pasteurization, sterilization, blanching, roasting, popping, and baking as well as for heating, cooking, tempering, and thawing. These methods are used singly or in combination. Cooking does not stop when the microwave is turned off. It continues to cook as the heat on the outside travels to the middle of the food by conduction. This additional cooking must be taken into account especially in large thick solid foods. This period of time is called the standing or resting time.

Although cooking with microwave is faster than conventional methods of cooking; protein foods do not become brown when cooked in a microwave. From the perspective of nutrient content, food cooked in microwave contains similar nutrients as cooked in conventional ovens and sometimes the loss is less. Nutrients loss is minimal possibly due to shorter exposure of heat to the food. There is reduced oxidation; hence the nutrients like vitamin A and E are less likely to be destroyed. Loss of water-soluble compounds like vitamin C occurs, the extent of loss being similar to other methods of heating. Effect on polyphenols and carotenoids is likely to be less, although retention of different compounds varies with the food. It is also safe because the microwave heat penetrates deeper into the food and for shorter duration as compared to conventional ovens. However, significant loss of amino acids, trypsin inhibitor and inactivation of vitamin B_{12} has been reported. The loss of flavonoids is not evident and it can be assessed by retention of color in the food. Capsicum remains green and tomato still looks red.

Microwaves are electromagnetic waves that are exploited in wide range of frequencies (i.e., 300 MHz to 300 GHz) in households, industry, communications and medical pursuits. In 2011, the International Agency for Research on Cancer (IARC) prophesied that microwave radiation might have carcinogenic effects. Without ignoring its beneficial effects, some negative incidence of these waves attracted the attention of public and researchers. During microwave heating enormous amount of energy enters into the food molecules and that may be sufficient to break protein molecules concomitantly forming different and sometimes unfamiliar new molecules. Microwave radiation affects the oxidative state of the liver, kidney and hemoglobin macromolecule. Harsh effects may be observed in terms of accumulation of lipids, induction of lipid peroxidation of cell membranes and appearance of degenerative processes. The liver biomarker enzymes viz alkaline phosphatase (ALP), alanine aminotransferase (ALT) and aspartate aminotransferase (AST) have been found to be significantly changed under the effect of 50 Hz magnetic field. There are reports of a significant increase in disorders in the digestive system associated with eating foods heated in microwave ovens, as well as a significant decrease (60% to 90%) in the nutritional quality of food. These research trends suggest that microwaves should be used with caution.

When heating small amounts of food, it is advisable to place a glass of water in the oven in order to absorb the excess energy so that there will be no damage to the microwave generator.

There are some limitations to microwave cooking. The waves are emitted downward from the top of the microwave oven cavity. They bounce off the metal sides of the cavity and hit the food from different angles but do not strike the food evenly. Although the microwave has a rotating turntable that moves the food, yet there are still problems with uneven heating. Also, microwave energy penetrates to a depth of about 25 mm. Thus, food does not get heated evenly and therefore there may be "hot" spots and "cold" spots. In the "cold" spots, microorganisms are likely to multiply and may cause food borne illnesses. Stuffed poultry should not be cooked in the microwave oven, because it is difficult to reach the desired temperature to kill the microorganisms present. The outer edges of the food get hot while the center remains cool. Microwave ovens cannot be used for sterilizing baby bottles etc. Salt added at the beginning of cooking toughens protein food especially meat.

Use of plastic containers not designed for microwave use may introduce potentially harmful chemicals into food. Chemicals in plastic containers and plastic wrap can migrate into food with which it comes into contact during microwave heating. Polyvinyl chloride is a resin that helps make plastic wraps stretchy and clingy. This compound can seep into food during microwave cooking, especially if the food is high in fat. Polyvinyl chloride (PVC) containers are made flexible using phthalates and Bisphenol-A (BPA) which poses threat to health.

Use of unspecialized plastic or foam containers or use of containers of "take-away" or "use and throw" types should not be used for microwaving. It should be melt or get warped during microwaving, but harmful chemicals from these materials can enter the food.

Frying

Fat is used as a medium of cooking in frying. The quantity of fat used in cooking determines the type of frying namely, sautéing, shallow frying and deep frying. Depending upon the amount of fat used and absorbed by the food, energy content, i.e., kcal and density of the food is also increased. Retention or loss of other nutrients depends upon many other factors like temperature, type of oil, food composition, etc. Nutritional aspects of oil degradation in frying are associated with lipid peroxidation.

Sauteing and stir-frying use minimum amount of fat to partially cook the food in open air at higher temperature for a very short period of time. It is done to reduce the rawness and improve flavor and add little crispness. Since food is exposed to heat and air for short period of time; it retains maximum freshness, (color) and nutrients and polyphenolic compounds of the food. Browning may or may not occur depending upon the amount of oil used, temperature, duration of the process and the type of food.

Shallow frying includes use of some oil to cook the food like paratha, tikki usually on a flat hot surface of griddle or tava. It imparts good amount of crispness, color and flavor. Browning is the result of MR. prolonged exposure may form AGE products. Black residues or soot on the food may be harmful. Cooking with oil having low smoke point could be harmful such as using butter or extra virgin oil. Cooking beyond smoke point may initiate decomposition of oil resulting in formation of cancer causing compounds. Increase in energy value of food corresponds to the amount of oil used in preparation. It enhances the absorption of fat-soluble vitamins. It reduces the loss of other components by coating of the oil over the food. Duration of contact of food with the heat source affects the nutritional quality.

Deep frying: Food is cooked by immersing it into hot oil (about 160–180°C). During frying the heat gets transferred from oil to the food due to which water quickly gets evaporated and steam builds up the pressure altering the microstructure of the food. Hence porosity of food increases. The size and number of pores and the space between the pores (tortuosity) determines the oil absorption and thereby the taste, flavor, lightness, puffiness, crispiness and calorie content. There is loss of moisture during high heat of frying. It leads to formation of more porous material resulting in high absorption of oil in making French fries; further, oil viscosity increases that result in thicker adherence of oil layer to the food.

Fat also decomposes, yielding several volatile and non-volatile compounds. Certain volatile compounds like aldehydes generated are different in oils stored at ambient temperature or on exposure of high heat. Some of these compounds imparts typical flavor but some are harmful to health. Fats may undergo hydrolysis, oxidation and polymerization depending upon the type of oil, food composition, temperature, and duration of frying. Hydrolysis occurs by interaction of water, oil, and heat. It results in breakdown of triglyceride into fatty acids and glycerol. Glycerol evaporates at more than 150°C and reduces the stability of the oil. During oxidation, free radicals, hydroperoxides and other compounds are formed. Prolonged heating at high temperature (>190°C) hydroperoxides are converted into aldehydes and ketones. Some aldehydes impart characteristic flavor to the fried food and some may also contribute to off-odor. Certain hydroperoxides are harmful and carcinogenic. Polymerization indicates the deterioration of oil resulting from formation of polymers increasing the viscosity and darkening of the oil. There is formation of acrolein that tends to irritates mucous membrane and causes abdominal discomforts, lung and eye irritation, at low levels of exposure.

Small amounts of acrolein can be present in fried foods, cooking oils, and roasted coffee. Acrolein can enter into a variety of foods and even water supply if it has been used as an aquatic herbicide in irrigation canals.

Deep frying is crucial in terms of desirable taste, flavor, color, and texture of the fried food. The food is usually coated with a batter that helps in protecting the surface of the food from intense heat, prevents excessive moisture loss, and modifies the rapid penetration of heat into the food. Absorption of fat varies from food to food depending upon the food composition. Foods rich in sugar, starch or moisture/water absorb more oil as compared to foods containing protein like pulses. Cooking time depends on the quantity of food, its size and shape, water content, ratio of fat to food, the type of oil has its own nutritional implications owing to their fatty acid composition. At temperatures above the smoke point and with lower temperatures the food will absorb more oil than it would have at the right temperature and become greasy.

Use of high temperature reduces the water activity and helps in destruction of microorganisms, thus improving the safety of foods. Reactions occurring during frying are shown in Figure 17.10. Starch gets gelatinized and sugar dextrinized. Frying does not have much adverse impact on the protein or mineral content of fried food. However, the dietary fiber content of potatoes is increased after frying due to the formation of resistant starch. There may be changes in the structure and behavior of heat labile nutrients such as tocopherols (oxidation of fat soluble vitamins like vitamin E), essential amino acids, and fatty acids and loss of water-soluble compounds due to water evaporation from the food during deep-fat frying. Although some unsaturated fatty acids and antioxidant vitamins are lost due to oxidation, fried foods is generally a good source of vitamin E. There is moderate loss of antioxidants. The high temperature and short transit time of the frying process cause less loss of heat labile vitamins than other types of cooking. For example, vitamin C concentrations of French-fried potatoes are as high as in raw potatoes, and thiamine is well retained in fried potato products as well as in fried pork meat. It is inevitable that fried foods have increased energy density, since some fat is absorbed by the food during frying. However, this also results in highly palatable foods with a high nutritional content.

Frying and fried food have always been of high concern for the industry as well as health professionals. Water is released during frying. This enhances heat transfer but may cause deterioration of oil. In commercial operations, continuous use of the same batch of oil leads to more degeneration and production of aldehydes. These aldehydes are volatile and the person cooking these is exposed to them and would inhale

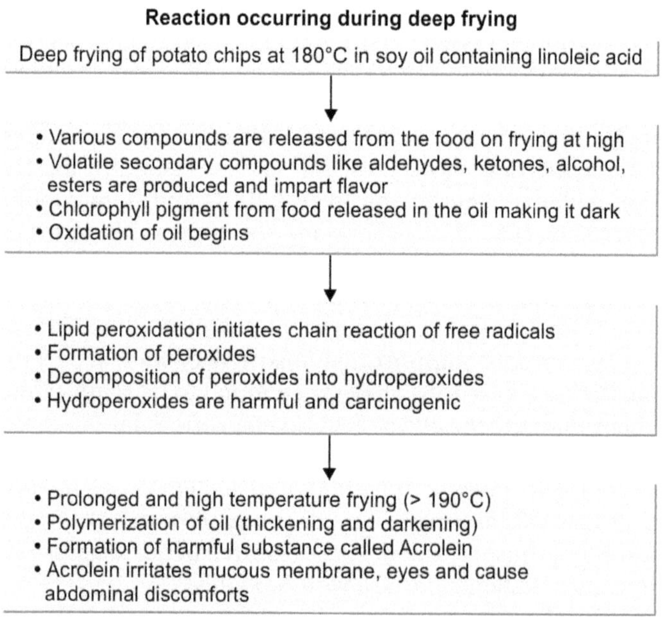

Reaction occurring during deep frying

Deep frying of potato chips at 180°C in soy oil containing linoleic acid

↓

- Various compounds are released from the food on frying at high
- Volatile secondary compounds like aldehydes, ketones, alcohol, esters are produced and impart flavor
- Chlorophyll pigment from food released in the oil making it dark
- Oxidation of oil begins

↓

- Lipid peroxidation initiates chain reaction of free radicals
- Formation of peroxides
- Decomposition of peroxides into hydroperoxides
- Hydroperoxides are harmful and carcinogenic

↓

- Prolonged and high temperature frying (> 190°C)
- Polymerization of oil (thickening and darkening)
- Formation of harmful substance called Acrolein
- Acrolein irritates mucous membrane, eyes and cause abdominal discomforts

Fig. 17.10: Physico-chemical changes during deep frying.

them. Thus even without eating the food, it puts persons who work in such establishments at risk even if they have not eaten the food.

Fatty acid composition of oil used in frying affects the extent of lipid peroxidation and its consequences, e.g., use of soy and rape seed oil contain more unsaturated fatty acids which accelerates the oxidation of oil and formation of trans fats. The amount of trans fats formed depends on the frying conditions, frying materials. TFA formation is not desirable as its consumption increases the risk for cardiovascular diseases.

Butter is also not suitable because of its low melting point and presence of short chain fatty acid. It burns easily. Hydrogenated fat like vanaspati is well suited due to lower degree of unsaturation, but it is not advisable due to the presence of transfats.

Oxidation of fats is reduced by the use of antioxidants. Commercial oils are fortified with them but after constant use they lose their capacity. Wide range these compounds such as BHT, TBQR, and lecithin are used. Natural form of antioxidant, rosemary extract and, ginger oleoresin are being investigated with promising results. They also reduce loss of tocopherol. Besides use of commercial antioxidants, spices used in food preparation prevent spoilage of fat such as ginger, garlic, chili, bay leaf, etc.

Consumption of oxidized oil is very detrimental to health. It may also oxidize the LDL and thus is a high risk for heart diseases, etc. Biological effects of ingestion of frying oil can result in oxidative stress, impaired glucose tolerance and altered thyroid and lipid functions and gene expression in the body.

Drying and Dehydration

Drying and dehydration both entail removal of water/moisture from the food. But both are different in application and outcome. Food is dried using nonconventional energy sources like sun and wind while dehydration uses artificial source of energy. In commercial operations, dehydration is done under controlled conditions, i.e., temperature, humidity, and air flow. Various designs of chambers and many dehydrators are commercially available for the purpose. Drying is economical but dehydration yields better quality product. Generally dehydration removes 80–90% of the moisture in foods.

Effects of dehydration
- No significant loss of carbohydrate, protein, and dietary fiber
- Increase calorie content
- Loss of vitamin thiamine, riboflavin, pyridoxine, ascorbic acid due to heat
- Loss of tocopherol
- Increased utilization of fat-soluble vitamins
- Increased antioxidant activity of antioxidants compounds
- Negligible antinutritional components,
- Kills microorganisms so relatively safe.

Drying: Usually when drying is done by simple methods like placing the food under the sun (Sun drying) at home, foods are dried under uncontrolled conditions such as under the sun or shade, e.g., papads are sun dried under the sun whereas green leaves and herbs are usually dried in shade.

Dehydrated foods take less space as they are reduced in volume, lighter in weight and easy to transport. Liquid can be converted into powder form, e.g., milk powder. This may reduce the cost of packaging, storage, and transportation. Since it removes moisture from the food, it reduces the chances of food spoilage by microorganisms (bacteria and yeasts, molds). It also slows down enzymatic action that may spoil foods and makes food safe for consumption. Seasonal surplus can be well utilized to provide food security during times of scarcity. Drying can convert the raw food into a new food. On dry weight basis, the nutrient content is very high in some food products, e.g., liquid milk contains approximately 4 g% of protein whereas milk powder contains about 25 g% protein. Similarly, the carbohydrate and fat contents are higher in the dried/dehydrated product than in the original food. There is also denaturation of proteins.

In grains, vegetables and fruits, removal of water tends to change the cellular structure of the food, altering its shape, size, color texture, and mouth feel. Although other nutrients are also concentrated, exposure to heat and air/oxygen as well as light leads to loss of vitamins like ascorbic acid, thiamine and beta-carotene, folic acid, and riboflavin with water-soluble nutrients and other compounds being lost to a greater extent. Similarly, oxidation of essential fatty acids occurs. Dehydration may adversely affect the functionality of amino acids like lysine, threonine and methionine. Enzymatic and nonenzymatic browning may occur resulting in discoloration. Rehydration is possible in some foods but may not match the original counterparts in terms of their original form and quality characteristics. This is particularly seen in dehydrated fruits and vegetables. Improper drying can increase the risk of food spoilage.

It also influences the nutritional quality of food. Rancidity may occur because the lipase and lipoxygenase are active even at low temperature. Off odor may occur due to accumulation of volatile compounds and oxidation of unsaturated fats, particularly in dairy products. Dehydration is done in several ways:

- **Hot air bed drying** wherein solid foods are placed on perforated trays and hot air is blown through the tray under carefully controlled conditions regulating the time and temperature.
- **Drum drying:** In this, food is sprayed onto heated drums or rollers and the dried powder is scraped off.
- **Spray-drying** is used for liquid foods, such as milk. The finely sprayed food is blown into a hot air chamber, where it dries as granules and drops to the bottom for collection.

Loss of nutrients also depends upon the extent of cutting and chopping the food, drying temperature, duration of drying, drying equipment, exposure to air and light, and storage conditions.

Milk powder is made by either spray drying or drum drying. Thiamine and riboflavin and vitamin C losses are higher in drum drying while niacin and pyridoxine losses are more in spray drying. Vitamin D content is reduced which is often compensated for by fortification of dried milk powder.

Vitamin A is retained in drum drying, however, substantial loss is observed in dry skim milk powder due to oxidation.

Dehydration is also associated with discoloration and browning which can make a product unacceptable. It causes loss of pigments like chlorophyll and other compounds having antioxidant capacity. Drying of meat at high temperature reduces its biological value and vitamin content. Smoking and curing enhance palatability and stability of meat. To retain color, nitrate or nitrites are used, but heating converts these into nitrosamines that is an intense irritant to the gastric lining and is carcinogenic in nature. It is suggested that sodium nitrate is not carcinogenic and the other options used by industry are sodium ascorbate, erythorbic acid, and sodium erythorbate.

Freeze drying is another method used wherein sublimation is used to remove moisture, i.e., solid ice in the food maintained at freezing temperature is directly converted into vapors without transition through the liquid state. During freeze drying, food is frozen and then placed in the freeze dryer, the dryer is sealed and a vacuum is created and maintained. Sublimation of water is accelerated under vacuum. Application of heat from radiant heaters within the shelves of the freeze drier provides the energy required for sublimation to occur. The amount of heat applied to the food is carefully controlled to maximize the rate of drying without causing transition of water from the solid to the liquid phase. One of the important advantages of freeze drying is that foods retain their original shape and can be rehydrated almost completely. Chemical changes that occur with other methods of drying do not occur with freeze drying.

Freeze drying is done for high value foods and mixtures of foods including seasonings as in ready-to-eat or ready-to-cook foods. It is an expensive commercial method. Many fruit powders, curd powder, etc. are manufactured by freeze drying. It retains maximum nutritional quality. Off flavor may develop in vegetables if they are not blanched or improperly blanched because enzymatic activity continues.

Packaging and storage after dehydration is very important and nutrient loss can be reduced by storing food at low temperature or in conditions where oxygen is low. Pasteurization and homogenization can prevent freeze burn in milk foods. Deterioration of fish is prevented by vacuum packaging, wrapping it in plastic film or using a protective coating. Starch undergoes retrogradation making food denser and squeezing of its water makes the product a rubbery gel. Therefore modified cellulose, alginates, and gums are used in frozen starch foods.

Freezing

Freezing is subjecting varied types of cooked and uncooked foods to low temperatures below −18°C. Primarily, freezing is used to prolong the shelf life and preserves the quality characteristics of foods. There is maximum retention of freshness, color, and certain nutrients except for losses associated with pretreatment like blanching. Freezing itself does not destroy any nutrients. Fruits in general are not blanched prior to freezing owing to their delicate nature and inherent acidity. Frozen food should be stored at 0°C or less in the freezer. Although frozen food can be stored for about a year or longer, prolonged storage tends to deteriorate the quality of food products. Freezing slows the movement of molecules, enzymatic activities and kills most bacteria, yeasts, and molds. Thus, microorganisms that cause food spoilage or food borne illnesses do not grow and the food is safe. Parasites are also destroyed by sub-zero freezing temperatures. Color changes can occur in frozen foods. Meat for example may turn brown due to lack of oxygen, freez burn (grayish brown leathery spots caused by air coming in contact with the surface of food) or prolonged storage. Products like cream, fat-laden foods or mayonnaise should not be frozen.

Before use of frozen food, thawing is essential. Thawing is the process of melting the ice crystals which are formed during freezing of food. Food contains varying amount of moisture/water which forms the ice crystals formed in the plant tissues.

Water makes up approximately 80–90% of the weight of most fruits and vegetables. This water and other chemical substances are held within the fairly rigid cell walls which give them the structure, and texture. When fruits and vegetables are frozen, the water contained in the plant cells freezes and expands. During thawing, ice crystals cause the cell walls to rupture followed by melting of ice into water that leaks out. Loss of moisture might cause redistribution of chemical composition within the food. There is disruption of cell components causing release of chemically reactive components that changes the texture of the product. This results in drastic alterations in physical, chemical properties of food, e.g., when frozen tomatoes are thawed, they become mushy and watery and lose their shape and firmness. There is significant loss (20–50%) of vitamin C in frozen fruits and vegetables stored for 1 year at −18 to −20°C. Frequent freeze-thaw-freeze cycles result in more mechanical damage, denaturation of protein and loss of water holding capacity as well as loss of nutrients so such practices should be avoided. Foods containing high moisture content like spinach pose greater threat to nutritional quality as compared to foods having low moisture content or water activity such as pea. Protein and minerals are not generally affected by freezing.

> **Laboratory Laurel:** In this study, effect of freeze–thaw cycles on the nutritional quality of selected Nigerian soups was investigated. Soups (*Ila, Ewedu, Ogbono,* and *Kuka*) were prepared using standard recipes; packaged in plastic and aluminum containers; frozen in laboratory scale chest freezer at −20°C, and thawed with microwave oven, hot water (100°C), and at ambient condition for four cycles of 5-day interval. After each cycle, chemical compositions of the samples were determined for moisture, protein, fat, crude fiber, ash, and carbohydrate using AOAC methods. Samples packaged in plastic containers and thawed in microwave oven had highest moisture content retention when compared with the freshly prepared soup. Reduction in fat content indicated an increase in lipid oxidation. Losses in crude fiber were observed in all soups owing to enzyme-induced degradation. Though soups are good sources of vitamins and minerals but freeze-thaw cycle causes deterioration in their nutritional quality. Microwave-thawed plastic soups showed minimum nutritional losses and freeze-thaw cycle should not be extended beyond the third cycle to avoid deterioration.
>
> *Raji AO, Akinoso R, Raji MO. Effect of freeze–thaw cycles on the nutritional quality of some selected Nigerian soups. Food Sci Nutr. 2015;4(2):163-80.*

Frequent freezing-thawing-freezing cycles must be avoided, as there can be loss of water-soluble vitamins and increased risk of lipid peroxidation and discolouration. There is serious threat with meat as ice crystals forms in between the muscle fibers and damage the microstructure of the meat. Losses are higher in spinach and broccoli as both have larger surface area and high moisture content to leach out as compared to peas. Rapid thawing is beneficial. Cooking without thawing may prevent thawing losses but it increases cooking time. Also, once the food is thawed the microorganisms begin to multiply and will grow at the same rate that they do in fresh food. Thus, thawed food must be heated and cooked well as quickly as possible is done for any other perishable food. These losses can be prevented or minimized by steam blanching followed by cooling that does not involve direct immersion of water. Microwave blanching shows lesser degree of losses. Fats in meat can become rancid during storage. Vitamin C loss upto 50% has been observed during prolonged storage of vegetables. Some spices and seasonings change during freezer storage. Pepper, cloves, garlic and synthetic vanilla tend to become strong and bitter, and onion change flavor during freezing, salt loses flavor and has a tendency to increase rancidity of any item containing fat.

Food Irradiation

Like microwave, irradiation also employs radiant energy. Irradiation is also called cold pasteurization. Food irradiation is basically used for preservation of food. It destroys the microorganisms, inactivates the enzymes in foods but can damage some of the food constituents, hence the dosage of radiation is very crucial. It is not a method of cooking that can be used at household level. It does not significantly increase the temperature or change the physical or sensory characteristics of most foods. Food irradiation is usually done for fruits and vegetables at low doses; for potatoes to prevent sprouting, to poultry, pork and ground beef, herbs and spices to reduce the microbial load. An irradiated apple may remain crispy and juicy. Fresh or frozen meat can be irradiated without cooking. Irradiated foods are wholesome and nutritious. Its merits compared to other methods are:

- It can help ensure food safety and improve food security.
- It does not produce ice crystals like in deep freezing hence the texture is not affected
- It does not leave any harmful residues like chemical treatment
- It can be used to treat even the packaged foods.

Food irradiation is primarily used to disinfect the food by reducing the bacteria and insects and thus increase the shelf life. The rays used have good penetrating power so they can inactivate the microorganisms and enzymes not only on the food surface but at deeper level. Sometimes it can alter the chemical structure of the organic and biochemical compounds at molecular level particularly when given in high doses. Penetration of ionizing radiation depends upon the nature of food and the characteristics of the rays. It also reduces sprouting. Dosage of radiation determines the outcome of the product. Irradiation can alter macronutrients and vitamin contents but will not affect the mineral content. Nutritional quality of irradiated foods depends on the dose and the source, temperature, moisture content and presence or absence of oxygen. Generally doses upto 1 kGy do not result in significant losses. Amino acids, vitamins, and sugars are more susceptible to chemical changes such as hydrolysis and oxidative degeneration of carbohydrate, denaturation of proteins and auto-oxidation and polymerization of lipids.

Radiation at higher doses (50 kGy) has adverse effects on nutrients, pigments, flavors, enzymes and so on. But at lower doses (10 kGy) most vitamins are saved, however, vitamin C and thiamine and fat-soluble vitamins are most sensitive. Thus, food containing $\propto$ tocopherol (oils and dairy products) are not irradiated and it can also develop off-flavor in them. Loss of vitamin C has not been observed in onion and garlic at lower dose (0.15 kGy) that is used for inhibition of sprouting. While many organisms are destroyed, spores of *Clostridium botulism* are quite resistant to irradiation.

> **Laboratory Laurel:** Ber (*Ziziphus mauritiana*) is a seasonal and underutilized fruit of India. Ber fruits are highly nutritious, rich in ascorbic acid, vitamin B, many minerals and several phenolics having antioxidant power. Its storage life is short thus requiring postharvest management. Ber fruits were procured from local market and subjected to irradiation treatments at dose of 0.25 kGy for 15 minutes, 0.50 kGy for 30 minutes, and 0.75 kGy for 45 minutes, and 1.00 kGy for 60 minutes at room temperature 32–35 °C in gamma irradiation unit ANGRAU, Rajendra Nagar, Hyderabad. After irradiation, of Ber fruits were used to antioxidant analysis for Scavenging DPPH radical activity, reducing power assay, super oxide anion radical activity, TBARS, total phenolic content, and total flavonoid content. Gamma irradiation treatment up to 1.0 kGy elevated the scavenging DPPH radical activity (9%), super oxide anion radical activity (26%) and total flavonoid content (208%) compared to fresh Ber fruit and reduced the phenolics content. Conclusively 0.25 to 0.5kGy is better dose to retain the natural antioxidant in fruit.
> *Kavitha C, Kuna A, Supraja T, et al. Effect of gamma irradiation on antioxidant properties of ber (Ziziphus mauritiana) fruit. J Food Sci Technol. 2015;52(5):3123-8.*

International Atomic Energy Agency (IAEA) has released new guidelines to improve food irradiation practices worldwide in partnership with FAO/WHO. Irradiation up to an average dose of 10 kGy causes negligible nutritional and pathological and environmental loss. Irradiation in plastic containers can increase the risk of development of off-odors owing to volatile compound.

Fermentation

Fermentation is the process in which healthy living microorganisms utilize carbohydrates (sugars) and produce acid and CO_2 that provides leavening to the products. This brings about changes in texture, volume, taste and flavor and nutritive value, and digestibility of the final product. It is an ancient method of food preservation and is used to prepare several food products in varied cuisines of the world. In many parts of India, particularly the North Eastern states have a rich heritage of fermented foods and beverages using local food crops and other biological resources. Fermentation technology has been established as an independent branch of science. Its contribution is large in human nutrition and culinary art. It not only enhances the bioavailability of nutrients but also supports synthesis of B vitamins such as thiamine, riboflavin, niacin, and biotin and reduces antinutritional factors and, toxic products. Fermentation takes time depending upon the product but the time required for cooking is generally less.

Fermentation is essentially of two types: (1) **lactic acid fermentation** and (2) **ethanolic fermentation**. Grains, vegetables, pulses, milk are used singly or in combination in fermentation to make a wide variety of food preparations. Fermentation involves use of specific species of microorganisms, e.g., lactobacilli used in curd making. Different microorganisms and their strains are used and by varying the temperature, duration as well as substrate, hundreds of products that vary in taste and texture are made. Bacterial or yeast fermentations are more common in India, while fungal fermentation is more widely practiced in the far East. Fungi bring about saccharification and proteolysis of the starting materials, bacteria cause acidification and leavening while yeast ferment the sugar to produce alcohol and esters which impart typical desirable flavors to the products. Specific species are used to obtain desirable products and during fermentation various physicochemical changes occur. These changes include synthesis of enzymes and other compounds, liquefaction and acidification as well as breakdown and reduction of some compounds. Fermentation provides numerous benefits as shown in Figure 17.11.

Some of the Fermented Products

Some of fermented products used in different communities are given in Table 17.4.

During fermentation some undesirable products are also formed, e.g., putrefaction which is controlled by addition of salt. It is necessary to carefully control quality of raw materials and the entire process to prevent contamination by pathogenic organisms like *Clostridium botulinum* and spoilage. Since fermented foods are widely accepted, this processing technique can easily be used for value addition to enhance the nutritive value. Certain leaves like of basil, curry, drumstick can be added to food during fermentation, e.g., addition of curry leaves have increased the protein content of kulcha, bhature and wadis and reduced the phytic acid.

Many a times other ingredients are used in fermented food products, e.g., salt draws the water and sugar from the food and prevents growth of undesirable bacteria, besides providing flavor. Amount of acid, salt, sugar, and oxygen can be controlled and their concentrations influence the product outcome. Excess of any one ingredient can adversely affect the final product.

Germination

Germination is the process of sprouting, which may further grow into a new plant, signifying the viability of the seed. Whole seeds of some cereals, whole pulses, nuts, spices are usually germinated for human consumption. The process requires moist conditions. Seeds are generally soaked for 8 to 12 hours, the water is decanted and the seeds are allowed to sprout that takes 1–3 days or longer. During germination, the nutrients stored in the seed are made available for the embryo and growing seedling, several enzymes are activated to make nutrients available to the growing plant. Phytochemicals may be synthesized to protect the seedling. All of these changes are also beneficial to man. The flavor of sprouted and cooked legumes is better than that of the raw legumes. Sprouted pulses can be eaten raw or steamed. Sprouted pulses tend to contain higher amount of thiamine and ascorbic acid, higher protein and starch digestibility and

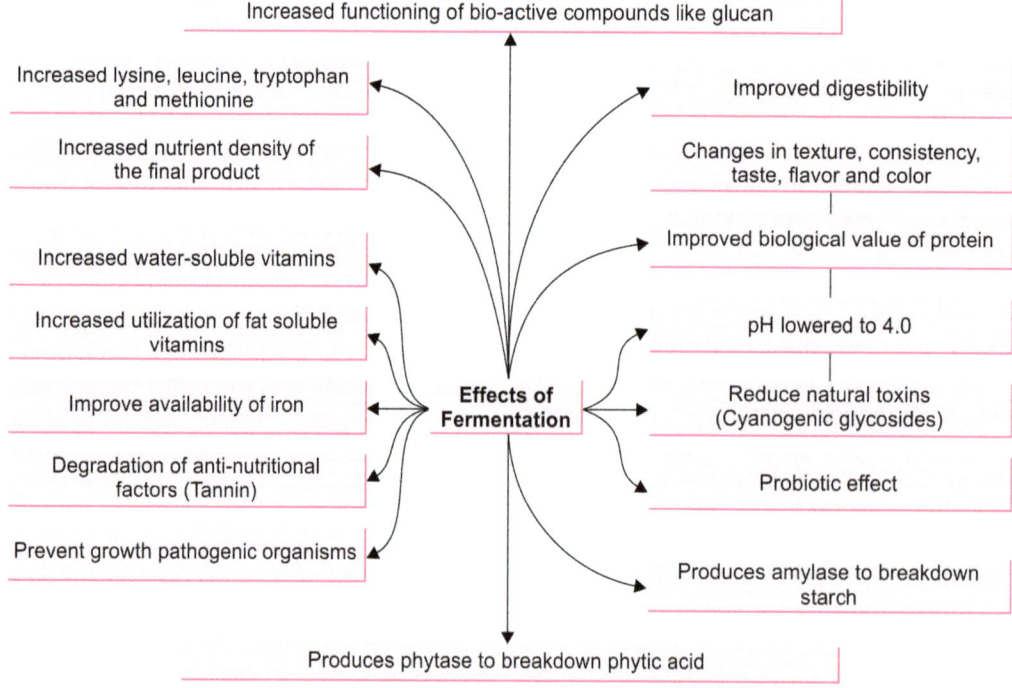

Fig. 17.11: Effects of fermentation in food and its utilization in the body.

Table 17.4: Fermented foods of India.

Food product	Raw ingredients	Impact on nutritional quality
Fermented milk products		
Curd	Boiled milk + starter	Prebiotic effect due to more lactic acid and more free amino acid
Cultured butter milk	Skim milk with lactic acid and aroma producing microorganisms	High protein, lactose, calcium, potassium, zinc, and B vitamins including vitamin B_{12}
Acidophilus milk	Whole or skim milk + *L. acidophilus*	Reduce gas forming organisms in intestines
Butter	Milk cream or malai fermented with curd starter	Better yield of butter which some B vitamins and minerals. Desi ghee prepared from this has high yield (98%) and has long shelf life without refrigeration
Fermented Cereal products		
Appam	Rice + Toddy	Synthesis of B vitamins
Bhatura, Kulcha, Naan	Refined wheat flour + previous batch of dough as starter or curd	Improved availability of Fe, Zn, Ca and Mg due to reduction in phytate
Jalebi	Refined wheat flour + previous batch of batter as starter or curd	Rich in sugar, fat thus in calories
Fermented legume products		
Wari, Bhallae, Vada, Papad	Black gram (urad)	Significant rise in thiamin, riboflavin and cyanocobalamin. Soluble nitrogen and free amino acids are increased. High level of amylase helps to assimilate starch
Fermented cereal-legume products		
Idli, dosa	Rice + urad dal in different combinations	Improve digestibility of protein digestibility and increase availability of essential amino acids, choline, thiamin, riboflavin, folic acid, cyanocobalamin and ascorbic acid
Dhokla	Rice and urad dal + curd or Bengal gram dal	
Fermented vegetable products		
Pickles	Variety of vegetables like carrot, turnip, mango	Salting and low pH aid gastric secretion. Antimicrobial effect is obtained from spices. Too much can be irritating
Meat and fish products		
Tungtap	Fermented fish product of Meghalaya	Increased amounts of vitamins, higher protein solubility, and improved amino acid patterns

bioavailable iron, even after cooking. Germination is less effective in reducing trypsin inhibitor, hemagglutinin activity, tannins and saponins but more effective in reducing phytic acid, stachyose, and raffinose. Cooking germinated grains reduced lysine, total aromatic, and sulfur-containing amino acids although the grains have been found to contain more of these than the FAO/WHO reference amino acid pattern and greater retention of all minerals and B vitamins. The significant changes are shown in Figure 17.12.

Reduced storage substances: Total starch may be less because it is degraded into smaller compounds by amylase, the activity of which is stimulated.

Enhanced activity of enzymes: Hydration and germination induce enzymatic activity. Amylase degrades starch making the food more digestible. Amylose may be degraded more than amylopectin. Oligosaccharides are practically degraded and thus reduce the flatus production by pulses. Invertase, protease, and lipase activities are also increased.

Increased availability of lysine: Lysine is the limiting amino acid in cereals. Lysine and tryptophan are synthesized during germination thus improving the amino acid content.

Synthesis of vitamin C: Synthesis of vitamin C occurs during germination.

Reduction of antinutritional factors: Germination aids in removal of antinutritional factors like phytates, oxalates, and trypsin inhibitor and tannins. Phytic acid binds the minerals like iron and reduces their bioavailability. Phytic acid is degraded by the enzyme phytase that is activated during germination.

Increased bioavailability of minerals: Bioavailability of minerals like iron, zinc and calcium is improved due to reduction in various antinutritional factors like phytate, tannins.

Improved digestibility: Besides breaking down starch, oligosaccharides like stachyose and raffinose are also broken down. This improves the digestibility and reduces flatus formation that is often a problem with consumption of pulses.

Synthesis of more polyphenols: During germination, there is synthesis of phenylalanine ammonia lyase an enzyme involved in synthesis of polyphenols.

Malting

Malting is a two-step process of converting some cereals into malt. It involves controlled germination followed by controlled drying. After germination, the grain is dried at high temperature or kilned. During this, MR and caramelization occur, giving the grain the typical malted flavor and an attractive brown color.

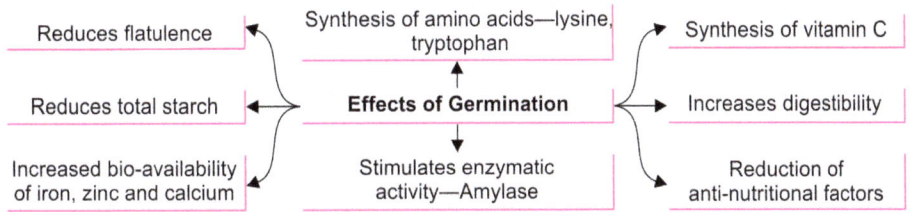

Fig. 17.12: Favorable changes occurring in food during germination.

The amylases degrade starch into maltose and other simpler sugars and proteases degrade protein thereby increasing the bioavailability of nutrients and digestibility. Malting is a common process used for beer manufacture in breweries, to produce malt extract for hot malted beverages, cereal and confectionary flavoring and coloring. All cereals can be malted, but in the brewing industry barley is preferred. For brewing generally the whole kernel is used.

It is also used to prepare amylase-rich foods (ARF) that can be used to make porridges with thinner consistency and make the porridge/gruel more nutrient-dense as more of the powder can be packed in per unit volume. Use of ARF is practiced in the development of complementary foods for infants. Malt is also used in the bakery industry as an enzyme or flavor source and in the breakfast food industry as a flavoring agent. Kibbled malt is used in some baked products for the crunchy texture and nutty taste. Malt extract is a hydrolysate of germinated barley grains. It contains about 90% carbohydrate, but mainly in the form of maltose. it also rich in mainly niacin, magnesium and potassium and some phenolic compounds like ferulic acid, (+)-catechins and (-)-epicatechin. it is good to combat oxidative stress. it is suitable to use in place of refined sugar. Malt syrup is used in some health drinks. The malt syrups contain about 60-65% carbohydrates, 5.5-6.0% protein, 20-25% moisture, and 1.5% ash. Food manufacturers generally utilize malt products such as dried malt extracts, malt syrups, or malt flours. Malted milk shakes and malt vinegar are other products.

Pasteurization

The process of Pasteurization is named after Louis Pasteur who discovered that pathogenic microorganisms were destroyed at temperatures below the boiling point. Pasteurization is basically a high heat treatment to kill pathogens (but does not kill all microorganisms) and protect the food from spoilage for short duration. It limits the formation of undesirable compounds like MR products. One of the main benefits is that the taste and quality of the product remain unaffected. This is the most important process that is applied to milk, worldwide. Pasteurization is now used/carried out for other foods including milk products like cheese, egg, beer, fruit and vegetable juices. The temperature and time are strictly controlled. Uncontrolled temperature may give rise to cooked flavor and browning in milk that is undesirable.

> **Pasteurization for milk**
> - **Normal:** 62.8°C (145°F) for <30 minutes
> - **HTST (high temperature and short time):** 72°C for <16 seconds followed by rapid cooling to 10°C
> - **UHT (ultra-high temperature):** 130°C for 2-3 seconds followed by cooling

Pasteurization has tremendous benefits in terms of microbiological safety and also improves nutritional quality. Some benefits are as follows:
- Destroys many pathogenic bacteria like *Salmonella spp.*
- Delays spoilage or increase shelf life from hours to days
- Inactivates an enzyme called lipase, thus prevents development of off-flavor
- Prevents deterioration of egg or milk and their products.
- Does not affect the fat-soluble vitamins, calcium, phosphorus in milk
- Loss of water soluble vitamins is less than 10%. This extent of loss occurs during normal handling and processing of foods at home.

Sterilization

Sterilization is another high heat treatment to kill pathogens and destroy the spores which otherwise may grow under conducive environment and spoil the food. It includes steaming under high pressure and is frequently used in food preservation including sterilization of storage containers and lids. It is a harsh treatment for food resulting in loss of nutrients and organoleptic qualities. However, it provides sterile food that maintains its shape and color to maximum and has long shelf stability. It is important to balance the benefits of sterilization with the adverse effects on the nutritional and organoleptic qualities. This method is often used to sterilize foods packed in cans or packaged food that are treated at significantly high temperature for a specific/defined time period. Autoclaving or retort sterilization leads to formation of significant amounts of acrylamide, a neurotoxic and carcinogenic product that may occur due to are action between asparagine and reducing sugars. Increase in temperature and/or time contribute to increased loss of thiamine. Vitamin A is also destroyed at high temperature. Now many novel methods are being developed to sterilize foods such as microwave, filtration, ionizing radiation (gamma and electron beam), and gas (ethylene oxide and formaldehyde). Various permutation and combination of temperature and time for different food products need to be studied in order to optimize the quality.

During sterilization, spore-forming microorganisms are killed which are not destroyed in pasteurization. Milk is sterilized in bottles, at 110°C for 30-40 minutes, followed by cooling. Maillard reaction or caramelization often occur resulting in brown color and cooked flavor. Other solid cooked products may also be darkened because of contact with the hot can. Loss of vitamins occurs especially vitamin C and folate. Vegetables, pasta, etc. become softer than desired.

In order to overcome these, high pressure sterilization is applied to some products such as fruit juices, jams, jellies, some meat products, yoghurt. Elevated pressure upto 900 MPa is applied for a short time ranging from a few seconds to minutes, the temperature being 60-90°C. Quality of such products is superior to conventional heat sterilization in terms of flavor, texture, and retention of nutrients. However, the nutrient content depends on the formulation of the product, the packaging system and the amount of pressure used.

Ultra-high temperature (UHT) sterilization is a newer process. Milk for example is heated at 135°C, for 2-5 seconds. Besides milk, other foods that are sterilized by UHT are juices, cream, wine, salad dressings, baby foods, tomato products, fruit and vegetable juices, soups, and stews. UHT does not affect vitamin A and D. These foods have a shelf life of longer than 6 months. Since foods are exposed for a very short time to high temperature effects on sensory qualities and nutrients is much less.

Canning

Nicolas Appert is known as the "Father of Canning" for his innovative approach in improving the food quality to serve the French Military force in the 18th century. Canning is usually done for fresh and perishable solid foods like fruits, vegetables, and meat and fish products. Canned products can safely be stored for several months and are easy to transport.

The canning process involves placing foods in jars/cans or similar containers and heating them to a temperature that destroys microorganisms that cause food to spoil. During the heating process, air is driven out of the container and as it cools a vacuum seal is formed. This vacuum seal prevents air from getting back into the product and thus prevents the entry of contaminating especially pathogenic microorganisms. The advantage is that it gives ready to eat food that remains wholesome and safe for months or even years without addition of preservatives.

Canning prevents the direct contact of food with oxygen; therefore, nutrient losses are significantly reduced. Color and texture of food is also maintained to maximum. However, there are losses of vitamin C due to exposure to heat and leaching out into the liquid in which fruits or vegetables may be placed in the container, although there is not much loss during storage. There is decrease in the polyphenolic compounds due to blanching (which is an essential preliminary step) and canning. UHT application further prevents the losses; however, some nutrient losses are inevitable due to pretreatment which forms a part of canning process. Different foods require different temperature for treatments. Canned food may also develop metallic or cooked flavor depending upon the type of food and other ingredients used in it. Canned food is usually kept either in syrup (sugar solution) or brine (salt solution) due to which canned foods either contain extra sugar or extra sodium and both are harmful for health and cause of many degenerative diseases.

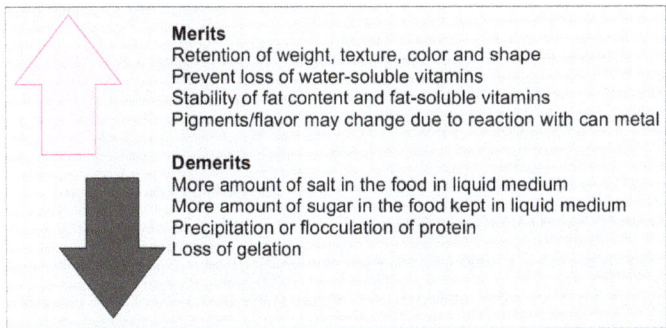

Acidic food like tomato juice is sterilized at slightly lower temperature whereas nonacidic foods like meat are sterilized at temperatures above 100°C usually 121°C. Fat-soluble vitamins like carotenoids and vitamin D remain unchanged; riboflavin and niacin are stable. Acidic medium in the can and sealing prevents loss of vitamin C and thiamin during storage.

Over a period of time, bright green color of chlorophyll may turn olive green, anthocyanin may show some pink shades and lycopene may decolorize, may be due to reaction of tomato with can metal. Hence, canning of tomato product may be done in glass jars. Calcium chloride used in tomato to maintain the shape of the tomato can be considered as an advantage because it may enhance some calcium content in the tomato.

> **Laboratory Laurels:** In this study effect of different cooking methods including blanching, boiling, microwaving and steaming on vitamin content and retention of nutrients in vegetables is evaluated. True retention (TR) values for all vitamins were calculated using the following formula:
>
> $$TR\,(\%) = \frac{\text{Nutrient content per g of cooked food} \times \text{g of food after cooking}}{\text{Nutrient content per g of raw food} \times \text{g of food before cooking}} = 100$$
>
> The retention of vitamin C ranged from 0.0 to 91.1% for all cooked samples. Generally, higher retention of vitamin C was observed after microwaving and lowest after boiling. Different methods have shown retention α-tocopherol and β-carotene, Microwave cooking prevents loss of vitamin K in spinach and chard but accelerates in the crown daisy and mallow. However, the extent of loss or retention depends on vegetables and cooking processes.
>
> *Lee S, Choi Y, Jeong HS, et al. Effect of different cooking methods on the content of vitamins and true retention in selected vegetables. Food Sci Biotechnol. 2018;27(2):333-42.*

Flavor compounds are altered and are affected by liquid medium present in the can. Prolonged storage and high temperature induce changes in starch, fat, and protein. Starch gelatinizes and increases in viscosity. Protein may degrade, flocculate, coagulate or precipitate. Though fats are rather stable during canning, the metal ions of the can, light, moisture, and heat may cause oxidative rancidity. Flavor reversion of PUFA has been observed.

Extrusion

Extrusion technology is used worldwide to produce cereal products including breakfast cereals, pasta, snack foods, etc. The extrusion process uses a combination of high pressure, heat and mechanical force that brings about physical and chemical changes in raw material and produces a new food product in a short time. With extrusion a wide range of food products with varied shapes, texture and sizes can be manufactured from different flours. The grain flour is forced/pushed through a small hole and it is simultaneously subjected to high temperature using a dye that is specially designed to obtain the desired shape. The product expands and has a high volume. The time taken for production is relatively less and because high temperature is used in the extrusion process, it reduces microbial load and inactivates enzymes in the extruded product. Extruded products generally have a low moisture content and water activity. Biochemical changes in extrusion cooking include gelatinization of starch that results in reduction in viscosity of starch, and higher temperatures result in greater reduction in viscosity. Also, there is denaturation of proteins, lipid modification, complexes are formed between starch and lipids, protein and lipids, inactivation of enzymes, formation of volatile flavor compounds and increase in soluble dietary fiber; there by improving digestibility of the extruded products. Extrusion also destroys antinutritional factors and microorganisms and extends the shelf life. However, extruded products tend to alter the glycemic index. Maillard reaction sometimes is induced in these products to enhance palatability and acceptability but its undesirable effects need to be considered in terms of their role in inflammation and degenerative diseases.

NOVEL FOOD PROCESSING TECHNOLOGIES

Conventional heat treatments help to ensure that food is tasty and safe but sometimes undesirable changes take place nutritionally and in the sensorial properties of the foods do occur. They also suffer from some disadvantages such as consuming fossil fuel or electricity and are not environment-friendly. Therefore, new technologies that are more environment friendly in terms of being less polluting, with less emission, being more energy efficient and using less water are used. Nonthermal technologies have been developed to extend shelf life of foods, without exposing them to heat and ensure that the products will retain their fresh-like qualities. Besides these, new thermal technologies like ohmic heating and dielectric heating have been developed. The nonthermal technologies include pulsed electric field or radiofrequency electric field, ultrasound, pulsed light treatment, high-pressure processing, ionizing radiation ultraviolet radiation, dense phase carbon dioxide, high voltage arc discharge, cold plasma, and use of ozone.

Ohmic heating: It is also known as Joule heating, electrical resistance heating, and direct electrical resistance heating. It is a process of passing an electric current (heat) in the food which is evenly and rapidly distributed into the food. It inactivates the microorganisms and some anti-nutritional factors. This novel technology is generally used for fruits and vegetables. After heating, it is important that the food is packed aseptically after it is cooled. It tends to cause less damage to food in comparison conventional methods, thus the food is fresh and product quality is good. Now it is being used in blanching, evaporation, dehydration, fermentation, sterilization, pasteurization, and heating of foods. It also helps to improve extraction, expression, drying, and fermentation, blanching, and peeling. It produces high quality products minimum changes in sensorial and nutritional qualities. It is not suitable for food containing fats and oils.

Magnetic heating: This is based on interaction between an electromagnetic alternating field and the dipoles and ionic charges contained in the food. This enables volumetric heating of the product and has the potential to be used for pasteurization and sterilization of liquid foods, although knowledge of the dielectric properties of the food is required.

Use of ultrasound or ultrasonic: Ultrasound is a non-thermal technology. Supersonic or ultrasonic are sound waves having velocities greater than that of sound, i.e., 20 kHz are used. It results in minimal flavor loss, reduces the time required for processing, saves energy, and gives a product with better quality and improved shelf life. It also inactivates microorganisms. It has applications such as improving the tenderness and juiciness of meat, pasteurization of milk. It inactivates enzymes that are resistant to heat such as polyphenol oxidase as well as other enzymes like lipases, proteases, lipoxygenase.

Use of modified atmosphere: Modified atmosphere packaging (MAP) is used for minimally processed foods like fish, meat, fruits and vegetables; wherein the atmosphere is modified within the package or container by reducing oxygen concentration and/or increasing carbon dioxide concentration. The package or container may be flushed with nitrogen to prevent oxidation or vacuum packaging. A well-known example is vacuum packaging of nuts.

High pressure processing: High-pressure processing (HPP) is a kind of mild preservation of foods and is effective against microorganisms because it results in the rupture of microbial membranes and therefore death of microorganisms. Also, biochemical reactions are regulated by the application of pressure. The pressure applied is generally 200–600 megapascal (MPa) at ambient temperature. At this temperature and pressure, most yeasts and molds are inactivated, as are gram negative organisms although it is not as effective on gram-positive organisms. The advantage of this processing method is that the product retains its fresh-like appearance, does not get crushed or deshaped and the organoleptic characteristics and nutritional quality is not significantly affected. Effect on bioavailability varies from one food to another and can differ between nutrients. However, there is not much nutrient, loss of flavor or color. Protein denaturation occurs although enzymes are not affected much. Gel formation has been seen in soy, meat, fish, and egg albumin. The process can help in tenderizing meat. Change also occurs in starches making the treated product sweeter and more susceptible to amylase activity. However, effects on starchy foods differ with the food.

> An adiabatic process is one where no heat enters or leaves a system. Here we compress a gas is compressed adiabatically inside a bicycle pump. The gas increases its internal energy, so increasing its temperature in accordance with the first law of thermodynamics.

Depending on the food can induce chemical/biochemical reactions thus affecting quality attributes and with very high pressure, enzymatic activity may be lost. Compared to pasteurization, this process increases shelf life two- to three-fold and therefore it can be used for foods that cannot be subjected to thermal pasteurization.

Pulsed electric fields (PEF): It is used to process and preserve liquid and semiliquid nature foods by exposing the food to short bursts/pulses of light. It is more efficient than conventional heat treatments in terms of better retention of flavor, color and nutritional value, improved protein functionality, increased shelf-life and reduced pathogen levels (it is lethal to microorganisms because ultraviolet light is used). Carotenoids and vitamin C were better preserved. Research shows that this method can deactivate peanut allergens.

Cold plasma: This process consists of using an ionized gas, the charged particles of which can rupture the cell membrane of microorganisms and help to inactivate pathogens on the surface of fresh and processed foods. The process can be used to decontaminate raw produce including fruits like apples, mangoes, melons, and cooked meat and cheese. The effect on nutrient content, chemical, and sensory properties of foods and their shelf life is being investigated.

Dense phase carbon dioxide: Dense phase carbon dioxide (CO_2) or supercritical and liquid CO_2 is a form of cold pasteurization method. Under pressure, CO_2 exerts molecular effects on microorganisms and enzymes. It can be used to treat juices and dairy based beverages. In such products, there was no adverse effect on anthocyanins, soluble phenolics, and antioxidant capacity as well as sensory qualities. This process can be used to extract lycopene from tomatoes, caffeine from tea or coffee, flavor and aroma from hops in breweries, fat from animal products, e.g., powdered eggs and freeze-drying of vegetables. Besides this, in the pharmaceutical industry it is used to extract medicinal compounds from herbs.

PACKAGING

Packaging provides a shield between food and surrounding environment in order to protect the food from environmental stressors. Packaging is crucial in retaining the food quality and facilitating the food availability and accessibility. Packaged foods are sometimes considered healthy and more nutritious because they are guarded from external influences and also largely untouched by human hands directly, rather every step of food handling from harvest to packaging is done by special machines. This ensures the quality of food for the consumer. The choice of type of food packaging depends upon the type of food, quantity of food, and whether it is to be refrigerated or not. Nutritional quality of some food can also be preserved by just keeping the food in the refrigerator. At industry level, different methods may be used for packaging.

Packaging is an integral part of harvesting and food processing and is essential for preserving food quality, minimizing food wastage and reducing use of preservatives in food. Packaging serves the important function of protecting the food from dirt and pollutants and against chemical and physical damage, contamination by microorganisms, insect pests, and other contaminants. Purpose of packaging is to preserve the quality of food; product in identification, extend the shelf life and ease the transport and storage. Packaging also helps to protect the form, shape and texture of the food inside, prevent the loss of flavors and odors. It also assists in regulating the water or moisture content of the food to keep it as fresh as possible. It also contains information that will give consumers knowledge about the ingredients used, the shelf life, how to use the product and its composition including the nutritional information. Nowadays packaging has become a source of consumer attraction at the point of sale or acceptance and convenience in use along with maintenance of quality till end use.

Several factors need to be taken into account for selecting the packaging material for different foods. Certain foods like fruits continue to respire and milk contains water and microorganisms can grow very rapidly. There is constant uptake of oxygen by the fruits and evolution of carbon dioxide, ethylene gas, water, and other volatiles. This exchange continues through packaging films. Rate of respiration varies from fruit to fruit. Respiration is also influenced by stage of maturity, membrane permeability, temperature, oxygen, carbon dioxide, partial pressure, ethylene gas concentration, and light. Regulating these factors, respiration rate can be modified and this is done by packaging system. The goal of food packaging is that it should contain the food as cost-effectively as possible, satisfy the requirements of both the industry and consumers, meet government regulations and have as little adverse impact on environment as is possible and protect food from chemical, biological, and physical damage.

Structure of packaging film, thickness, area, temperature, oxygen, carbon dioxide, concentration, all play significant roles in packaging and regulating the quality of foods. Based on scientific principles, new convenient packaging methods and materials are available to the food processors to make best choice of packaging system and maintain the quality of food. Beside quality of food, there are many other factors which consumers look for in the package which are as follows:

- Attractive in color, design, shape and size according to the food product
- Easy to open and close again without any additional tool requirement
- Seal should be temper proof
- Easy to dispense and having resealing features
- Communication to consumers
- Instructions to use and other label requirements should clear, understandable and usable
- Packaging material must be printable or can sustain ink for some label later also
- Packaging material should be compatible with food rather leaving its own odor in food
- Package should be biodegradable or recyclable
- It should be convenient to carry, transport and store
- Retention of fresh like quality of food
- Maximum retention of nutrients and flavor compounds
- Nontoxic particularly ingress of environmental pollutant
- Protect against contamination from microorganisms, insects, rodents, and other animals
- Provide barrier to moisture loss or entry of moisture, and entry of oxygen as well as protection from light and humidity
- Protect from mechanical damage caused by pressure, shock, vibrations and enable the food to sustain impact, abrasion or crushing.

There is a wide variety of packaging materials and packaging systems that are customized according to the food (perishable or nonperishable) or predicted shelf life (days to years) and the type of storage (room to granaries and cold storage). The choice of packaging material should be such that it serves the functions and yet does not adversely affect the nutritional quality of the food product. In order to ensure that the food retains its qualities, packing material need to have certain properties as listed below:

Environmental factors	Important package properties
Mechanical shock	Strength
Oxygen, water vapor	Impermeability (prevent migration in and out of package)
Light	Transparency, opacity and light transmission
Biological agents	Penetrability

Protection of foods from entry of oxygen into the package will help to prevent rancidity, oxidation of essential fatty acids. This is important in high fat foods like potato chips, roasted salted and nuts, and fried snacks and savories. Also, loss of labile vitamins like vitamin C and folate, e.g., in cut fruits and vegetables can be prevented. Similarly, opacity of the packaging material prevents loss of riboflavin.

PACKAGING MATERIALS AND THEIR IMPACT ON NUTRITION AND SAFETY

Traditionally cloth, paper, leaves, wood, glass, and metal were used in food packaging to provide mechanical protection and thereby reduce some nutrient losses. Most of these materials were locally available and inexpensive. However, man has exploited natural resources too extensively and these have now become expensive propositions. Also, with advancement in packaging technology and high demand of packaged food for several reasons, several new materials are now available, such as polystyrene, polythene, tetra packs, microwave friendly packaging, and retort pouches. An important issue today is biodegradability of the packaging material and several environment friendly materials are being developed. Food Safety and Standards of India (FSSAI) have issued new Food Safety and Standards (Packaging) Regulations in, 2018, that are specific to packaging requirements taking health concerns of the consumers.

Different materials are used for different foods and for different purposes. The design and construction of the package significantly influences the shelf life of a food product in terms of maintaining product quality and freshness during distribution and storage. Duration of storage and the mode of transport also determine the selection of packaging material.

Retention of nutrients is largely dependent on the storage conditions like in jute bags. High temperature, high relative humidity and insect infestation, and rodents significantly lower down the nutritional quality of food. Cotton bags are used to retain freshness and prevent moisture loss and thereby preserve many nutrients also.

Paper is relatively strong and safe. It protects food from light, thus it reduces loss of riboflavin, e.g., wrapping green leafy vegetables in brown paper saves their riboflavin content. Parchment paper is used to make tea bags as it reduces the loss of flavor compounds which are also flavonoids in nature and have health benefits. Sulfate paper is stronger, more durable and suitable for foods like sugar, flours and fruits that are packed in this paper. Sulfite paper is lighter, weak and used for lining in confectionary and bakery products. Grease proof paper is also sulfite paper with high gloss, resistant to water, and prevents rancidity in foods containing fats/oils. Wax paper also reduces the loss of moisture and oil from the foods, e.g., used for wrapping bread. White board paper is used in making boxes for biscuits and cakes. When coated from inside with polyvinyl chloride can be used for ice creams.

Tin and aluminum are steady, durable, and tamper-proof packaging material. Metal containers particularly with airtight lids provide barrier to oxygen, moisture and external contamination, e.g., tin cans. They provide barriers to moisture, oxygen and other gases, and volatile aroma and prevent its migration. Internal atmosphere in metal cans is greatly influenced by pH, oxygen, sulfur dioxide and nitrogen present in food. These factors can cause corrosion in tin and spoil the food to the level of toxicity. Pressure is also developed inside the can, leading to bulging or bursting and allows the entry of food poisoning bacteria. Aluminum poisoning has also been observed during heat processing. Inner coating or lamination inside the container prevents these harmful effects. Aluminum foil is suitable for short-term use, to keep food warm; however, it also preserves nutritional as well as sensory qualities of food. Aluminum foil is an integral layer of tetra pack. Steel containers are also used in packaging. In hot weather, metal gets heated and accelerates the chemical reactions within the food, thus speeding up the deterioration. Sometimes insect infestation find conducive atmosphere in metal containers. Since, food cannot be seen from outside and left unchecked for longer duration, huge losses can occur, there is risk of unseen spoilage and if consumed can be injurious to health (food poisoning or food allergy, etc.).

> **Laboratory Laurel:** This study was carried out to determine the risk of leaching of aluminum from aluminum foil in different food solutions. Minced meat was used to prepare six different food solutions using tomato juice, citric acid, apple vinegar, salt, and spices. Three techniques namely weight loss (WL) measurements, Environmental Scanning Electron Microscopy (ESEM), and Inductively Coupled Plasma-Mass Spectrometry (ICP-MS) were used analysis. Use of aluminum foil for cooking contributed significantly increase the daily intake of aluminum through the cooked foods. The amount of leaching was high in acidic solutions, and even higher with the addition of spices. WHO has recommended tolerable daily intake of 1 mg/kg body weight/day for aluminum and in this experiment obtained values were unacceptable. This research paper also indicated that aluminum salts can be absorbed by the gut and get concentrated in various human tissues including bone, parathyroid, and brain. High concentration of aluminum in brain tissues is associated with Alzheimer's disease patients. Researchers advocate that aluminum foil may be used for packing but not for cooking.
>
> *Bassioni G, Mohammed FS, Zubaidy E Al, et al. Risk assessment of using aluminum foil in food preparation. Int J Electrochem Sci. 2012;7:4498-509.*

Glass is an inert material and does not react with food. Food is most safe and can be seen from outside. Therefore any indication of spoilage can be handled and food can be saved much more easily. Sun exposure can be effective in case of pickle making but undesirable for milk. Milk is a rich source of riboflavin and is light sensitive and so gets destroyed in light. Glass is good for sterilization purpose.

Glass is used for liquid food like milk, sauces, drinks, fruit juices, etc. and filling is done aseptically, before sterilization of bottles. Another big disadvantage is breakages and injuries caused by broken glass.

Plastics are polymers of varying chemical composition with various micron sizes (thickness or density). Commonly used plastic polymers are cellophanes, polyethylene, polypropylene (PP), PVC, and polyamide. Plastic contains variety of chemicals, polymers, plasticizers, light absorbers, colorants, and antioxidants. These ingredients are included depending upon the kind of final product required. BPA (Bisphenol A), Pthalates, Di(2-ethylhexyl) adipate (DEHA), perchlorate, styrene are some of the ingredients which are scrutinized world over to leave significant impact on health. These are potential carcinogen and endocrine disruptors. Many of them affect reproductive functions and imbalance hormones. Risk of respiratory diseases, diabetes, and obesity is also increased. Perchlorate inhibits iodine uptake and causes hypothyroidism. Endocrine disrupters are the chemical compounds that alter the normal functioning of the endocrine system of both humans and animals. They can come from environment and manmade chemicals.

There are thermostable films that are meant for microwave and radiation. Depending on the permeability and strength of the polymer used, they provide sufficient barrier to moisture, oxygen, and other environmental hazards except heat. Plastic melts on heating. Poor quality plastic absorbs odors from the surroundings and has its own unpalatable aroma and thus causes heavy loss of food. This can be toxic as well. Oxidation of polymers may result in formation of peroxide, alcohol and carbonyl compounds and excess of them can be health hazardous. Besides heating there is tendency of migration or leaching or microplastic components in to the product (food product, beverage, oil /fat based).

Thermoplastics can easily be shaped and molded into various products such as bottles, jugs, and plastic films; hence they are highly suitable for food packaging. Other advantages include low cost, thermosealability, microwaveability, transparency, light weight among others. Almost all thermoplastics are recyclable. However, there are health safety concerns regarding components used in plastics, e.g., bisphenol A (BPA). Zipper technology is also being used in food packaging of different food material particularly the ready to eat snacks for convenience of the consumers.

Plastic materials are manufactured either as a single film or as a combination with other plastics or bonding plastic to other materials such as paper or aluminum. Such bonded material is called laminates. Paper is also laminated with cellophane, polypropylene or glassine. These laminated coatings provide a gas barrier and thereby limit the respiration rate in fresh produce and preserves aromatic flavor and texture. There are coatings on glassine that are rather more stiff and protective. Tetra packs are made of protective grades of paper, plastic and metal foil and provide maximum protection to food. Tetra pack is good for liquid food in which nutrient loss is minimized. Laminated paper is used to package dried products such as soups, herbs, and spices. There are many other plastic materials that provide a barrier to oxygen and limit the peroxidation of unsaturated fatty acid.

BIO-BASED PACKAGING AND EDIBLE FILMS

Need for attractive, convenient, durable, and safe packaging is an all-time requirement. With issues being raised about harmful effects related to use of plastic material, several bio-based materials are being investigated like polymers extracted from biomass, e.g., polysaccharides, protein and fat-based materials. These are derived from starches from potato, corn, wheat, rice derivatives; cellulose from cotton, wood, other derivatives and gums from guar gum, locust bean, alginate, carrageenan, pectin, chitosan or chitin. Considerable research and pilot studies have been carried out for bio-based packaging material so that they provide protection from water vapor, gases, odors, dust, shock, microorganisms. Some examples of bio-based packaging are wheat gluten film for mushroom, chitosan film for mangoes, starch based laminates for fruits, cut vegetables and, dry products.

Bio-based films are biodegradable and sometimes these are edible too. An edible film is a thin layer formed over the food as a coating or placed on or between food components. These are usually the food-grade proteins and other food-grade additives like plasticizers, surfactants, acid or base, salts or enzymes. Edible film is applied over or between foods by immersion, spraying, or panning. Whey protein and soy protein are commonly used. Edible film provides physical protection and selective barrier to oxygen, carbon dioxide, moisture, aroma, and lipids. It improves the appearance of coated foods, e.g., whey protein isolate-sucrose coatings provided the highest and most stable gloss. Edible films can be used as carriers of active ingredients such as antioxidants, flavors, fortified nutrients, colorants, antimicrobial agents.

TYPES OF FOOD PACKAGING

The main aim of packaging is to preserve the shelf life of the food by providing the appropriate environment and providing a barrier to entry of external gases, moisture, and microorganism from the environment. Oxygen levels inside the pack need to be controlled to delay respiration in perishable foods like fruits and vegetables and to prevent the growth of aerobic microorganisms and insects. However, in oxygen-free environment, anaerobic bacteria may grow and spoil food. Presence of oxygen in a package can accelerate the oxidative reaction and facilitate growth of aerobic bacteria and mold. Since oxidation reduces the nutritive quality of food and produce off-odor, off-flavor, and undesirable color changes. Hence oxygen scavengers are used. Carbon dioxide has some inhibitory action on some bacteria (psychotropic). In liquids, it is converted to carbonic acid and reduces the pH and has an effect on enzymatic activity. The ratio of oxygen to carbon dioxide is very important in packaging. Each food has its specific requirement (depending on its composition) for the gaseous environment within the food package. Controlled atmosphere packaging and modified atmosphere packaging are used for this purpose. Controlled atmosphere packaging controls the amount of oxygen and carbon dioxide levels inside the packaging environment so that the respiration by fruits and vegetables and production of ethylene by them is limited. Consequently, ripening and spoilage is limited. Nitrogen has been found to protect the food during storage. Packaging conditions influence the content of phytonutrients and other non-nutrients. High concentration of phytonutrients could protect fresh cut vegetables and fruits against oxidation. Excess moisture also increases chances of food spoilage. Ingredients like sugar and salt are hygroscopic. Therefore, there is need to used moisture control agents, e.g., silica gel may be packed in sachets to prevent condensation of moisture on the food product. Also, a combination of low temperature with appropriate packaging can help to keep the product fresh and preserve the acceptability of the food product. Certain tropical fruits may lose quality due to chilling injury when they are exposed to 0–10°C.

Vacuum packaging: Air is removed from the package thereby creating a vacuum, after which the package is then hermetically sealed. Air-tight sealing ensures that the oxygen level inside the package is low ensuring that entry of microorganisms as well as growth of existing aerobic bacteria and/or fungi is restricted; enzymatic activity is checked resulting in retention of flavor, color, and nutritional quality of food. Also, volatile components do not evaporate and deterioration of flavor and odor is prevented. Thus, foods like cereals and cereal products, meat products, bakery and fat-rich foods, maintain their freshness and flavor 3–5 times longer and have good shelf life than with conventional storage methods. Other advantages include elimination of freezer burn, moist foods do not get dehydrated and dry foods like sugar will not "cake."

Modified atmosphere packaging (MAP): Modified atmosphere packaging includes one of the following: Either reduction in the proportion of oxygen/total replacement of oxygen/an increase in the proportion of other gases like carbon dioxide or nitrogen. Different ratio of oxygen and carbon dioxide (80% O_2 and 20% CO_2) are filled which vary from food to food. Increase in CO_2 extends the shelf life and at the same time O_2 is reduced and nitrogen is added as filler. Carbon dioxide is bacteriostatic, prevents rancidity and slows down the respiration of products. Chemical agents are also added to retain the color and freshness in the food product. However, this atmosphere may change over a period of time during storage due to respiration of the food and/or the permeability of the packaging material. MAP helps to prevent spoilage by anaerobic bacteria and retain the color better. Content of vitamin C, flavonoids, glucosinolates are influenced by the proportion of gases used particularly O_2 and CO_2.

All three gases, i.e., O_2, CO_2, and N are common and readily available, safe, economical, and are not considered to be chemical additives. However, the optimum level of each gas that is to be used for different food products must be individualized to achieve the best possible results while minimizing the negative effects. For fruit and vegetables, the packaging films need to be permeable that help to achieve the correct atmosphere according to the product's natural respiration.

Active packaging: In this, subsidiary materials or constituents are deliberately included either in or on the packaging material, or in the package headspace to enhance the performance of the packaging and to maintain/extend the shelf life of the product. Sachets and pads may be placed inside the package or incorporated into the packaging material. Nanotechnology has a lot to offer in active packaging. Nanoparticles may be incorporated into the packaging material to impart antimicrobial activities or there may be oxygen and ethylene-scavenging systems. Other applications include oxygen scavengers, carbon dioxide generating systems, flavor and odor absorbers/releasers, antioxidants, humidity control.

Intelligent packaging: It is intended to preserve food better and provide more convenience to consumers by enabling sensing, detection and recording external and internal changes in the food environment. Some of the features can be incorporating indicators for quality and freshness such as temperature indicators, time-temperature integrators, or gas-level control.

Nanopackaging: Nanomaterials are incorporated into the packaging material with enhanced mechanical and thermal properties to ensure better protection of foods from external mechanical, thermal, chemical, or microbiological effects. This would endow packaged foods with an additional level of safety and functionality and increase shelf life of foods. Packaging can release nanoscale antimicrobials, antioxidants, flavors, fragrances or nutraceuticals into the food or beverages to extend its shelf life or to improve its taste or smell. Other functions can be to detect the development of spoilage within the food, deliver flavor compounds, enhance nutrient delivery, antimicrobial compounds, and bioactive compounds into the food.

PACKAGING FOR DIFFERENT TYPES OF FOODS

Different packaging materials are used for different foods, depending on the purpose, e.g., to maximize safety, hygiene, ease in storage and transport and also protect the color, texture, flavor, and nutritive value. The International Conference on Electronics Packaging (ICEP) has recommended some standardized practices with regard to use of plastic and other materials in food. The Bureau of Indian Standards (BIS) given in Table 17.5 depicts the kind of packaging material for specific food.

Cereals and cereal products: Grains are usually kept in jute bags and stacked in ware houses where temperature and relative humidity tend to fluctuate, if not controlled. Alternatively, grains and cereal flours, semolina are packed in high density polythene woven sacks. The chances of rodents, insects or fungi attack may cause huge losses, both in quantity and quality. Poor storage conditions cause lipid peroxidation leading to off flavor and loss of vitamins. Insect infestation increases the uric acid content in the grain which

Table 17.5: Packaging material for specific food.

Product	Packaging material
Pasteurized flavored milk	• Glass bottles LDPE lined cartons • Aseptic cartons
Fermented milk products and dahi	• Glass bottles or any other dahi suitable containers and capped.
Channa, khoa, cheese, chakka shrikhand	• Biaxially oriented polypropylene (BOPP also called OPP) BONF/EVA BONF/IONOMER, BOPP/EVA • Metal cans coated with a suitable lacquer
Burfi	• Paper-board container • Barrier laminates like BOPP/LDPE • Tinplate containers having inner lining of parchment paper • Board carton lined on the inside with fat and moisture proof parchment paper
Ice-cream	• Mild steel tinned • Aluminium or stainless steel nonreturnable containers • Paper-board • Metallic foil • Paper board containers shall be made water-resistant by coating or impregnation with wax or resin. • Sterilized and wrapped spoons to be supplied with small nonreturnable containers
Canned rosogolla	• Open top sterilized sanitary cans • Polystyrene tubs
Vacuum Pan Sugar, Refined • Sugar, Raw Sugar, white sugar • Sugar Used in food Preservation Industry	• Polyethylene coated hessian bags, Polyethylene coated raffia bags and A-twill jute bags
Flours and starches • Maize, Tapioca Arrowroot	• LDPE-coated jute bags • LDPE-coated raffia bags • A-twill jute bags
Cereal grains	• LDPE-coated jute bags • Raffia bags
Corn flakes	• HDPE bags made of 300 gauge HDPE and properly sealed • LDPE-lined cartons
Rolled oats	• Air-tight containers made of tinplate • LDPE-lined cartons
Papad	Pouches made from PET/LDPE and BOPP/LDPE
Bread	• In sliced form, in LDPE coated poster paper or clean waxed paper • Grease-proof paper
Biscuits and confectionary	• Cellulose film waxed paper or foil, Polyethylene, Cello/LDPE, BOPP/LDPE, PET/LDPE, Paper/LDPE, Foil/LDPE
Cakes	• Waxed paper • Grease-proof polyethylene • Glassine/LDPE • Tins
Roasted groundnut kernels	• Flexible food grade pouches • Sealed containers

Contd...

Product	Packaging material
Ready-to-Eat, protein-rich multi-extruded foods	• Moisture-proof paper bags layered, polyethylene lined • Pouches made from BOPP/ LDPE, Glassine/ LDPE • High density polyethylene woven bags having 300 gauge LDPE liner for bulk • 250 gauge high-density polyethylene bags
Whole spices	• Jute, cloth, paper or polyethylene bags • LDPE-coated jute bags or raffia bags (woven polypropylene bags) • Double gunny bags for black pepper, whole • Jute bags with or without moisture-proof lining • Tinplate or wooden cases, lined with polyethylene or waterproof or kraft paper • Jute bags lined with polyethylene
Ground spices	• Paper bags • Bags made of suitable barrier films/laminates, such as PET/LDPE, PET/EVA, BOPP/EVA
Tomato ketchup	• Glass containers, jars • Plastic containers made of PET
Oils	• Tinplate containers • Glass bottles • Rigid plastic containers of HDPE, food grade PVC, PET • Flexible pouches made of plastic film/foil/laminate • Flexible pouches of ionomer and coextruded nylon/ionomer • High molecular HDPE, linear low density polyethylene, nylon-6, ethylene vinyl acetate copolymer, ethylene acrylic acid copolymer, polyester (PET)
Fat	• Flexible packs • Tin containers

(PET; polyethylene terephthalate; PVC, polyvinyl chloride; EVA, ethylene-vinyl acetate; LDPE, low density polyethylene; BOPP, biaxially oriented polypropylene)

is detrimental to health. Loss of food grains directly affects the nutritional status of people. Good quality or lined jute bags and improved condition in storage areas and warehouses are required. Besides these, other packaging material is used in cereals products, e.g., LDEP pouches for pasta and vermicelli.

Milk and milk products: These food products are most sensitive to microorganisms, light, heat and packaging material and their packaging requires careful consideration. Since milk is used on daily basis it should be safe and wholesome throughout the processing, storage and distribution chain until it reaches the consumer. Usually big metal cans are used to transport liquid milk and supplied manually to consumers at earliest as commonly practiced in India. Nowadays plastic pouches usually made of low-density polyethylene (LDPE) films are used. Glass bottles were used previously for retail milk distribution as they were convenient for pasteurization, sealing, and reusable. However, they have been phased out and are avoided presently, because there are higher chances of breaking. Also, the milk is exposed to light that destroys riboflavin. Aseptic packaging is used for UHT milk. Tetra packs that are made up of polyethylene-coated paper-board with aluminum foil laminates are used. Tetra pack reduces the nutrient losses as there are barriers for light, moisture, and oxygen. It also helps to maintain the natural flavor of milk and extend the life. The fortification of milk with vitamin D has also become possible due to use of tetra pack.

Butter is packaged in various materials like mica filled HDPE base plastic; two parchment papers; two aluminized metallized paper and aluminum foil glue laminated to bleached sulfite paper. Butter needs to be protected from oxidation in order to reduce the development of off flavor and vitamin loss. Cardboard or metallic types of packaging materials are used for different types of cheese; wax coating, vegetable parchment, aluminum foil, and laminated foil (9 μm) are used. Paper coated with paraffin or PVC/PVDC copolymer or aluminum foil (15-20 μm) is advisable for cream. However, LDPE or PP is suitable enamel. Vacuum packaging is often used for milk products like milk powder which reduces the oxidation and browning due to Maillard reaction and nutrient losses associated with MR.

Fruits and vegetables: Extensive losses of fruits and vegetables occur to the tune of 40-50% in season, in developing countries due to their inherent perishable nature and due to lack of suitable storage and packaging systems. They continue to respire even after harvesting from the plant, although different produce have different respiration rates, therefore one type of packaging system is not suitable for all or most produce.

Selection of packaging material for fruits is largely based on the respiration rate and ethylene production by the fruits. Ethylene is a natural product of fruits and vegetables that plays an important role in ripening. Ethylene production is reduced in low oxygen and high CO_2 atmosphere. Continued ethylene production soon deteriorates the quality of fruit as it becomes overripe. Physical damage during postharvest handling increases respiration, ethylene production, and loss of water and other valuable components including nutrients.

Fruits are often packed in wooden strip boxes and sometimes cartons or plastic bags depending upon the quantity and the type of fruit to be packed. In most packages, holes are made which are done to release the ethylene gas which normally produces during ripening of fruits. Overproduction of ethylene tends to spoil the fruit, making it inedible. Canning methods used to be preferred for fruits like pineapple and vegetable like peas and mushrooms in which can are used which protects the fiber, folate content better than freezing the fruit.

Plastic polymeric films like LDPE (low density polyethylene) provide a good moisture barrier and oxygen permeability. Tray packs (made with white pigmented LDPE) are used with over wrap heat shrinkable stretch film. Modified atmosphere packaging (MAP) with modified desired gas mixture delays respiration and increases concentration of CO_2 thus protecting the fruit quality. Controlled atmosphere (CA) packaging extends the humidity control and prevents mold growth. Use of xylitol, potassium chloride, and sodium chloride has been tried along with LDEP film for gas exchange. Oxygen concentration affects β carotene and sugar content and CO_2 helps in retention of color, flavor, acidity, enzymatic activity, and vitamin C. Flexi-pouches made up of PET-PP and PVC are frequently used in packaging of fruits and vegetables. Fruit juices are packed in cans, glass bottles, tetra packs. New materials like "lamicon" and "lamipet" having high resistance to gas permeation are also tried. Liquid bags are used for beverages like fruit juices, tea coffee, milk shakes, honey sports drinks, ice creams, yogurt, etc.

Meat, meat products, and fish: Being high in protein and fat, animal foods are more prone to microbial spoilage and rancidity. Oxidation or lack of oxygen convert oxymyoglobin (red color) to reduced myoglobin (brown color) resulting in dull colored meat. Vacuum packaging is more desirable to control oxygen concentration and enzymatic activity and prevent oxidation. Fish is very susceptible to deterioration. Though they are consumed fresh, they may need some amount of packaging and duration. Keeping temperature low and use of MAP has been found to be useful. Similar conditions may be used for sea foods.

Tea-coffee and spices: Since aroma and flavor compounds are volatile substances and for that tea and coffee are highly valued, it is of utmost importance to retain these compounds. Therefore, complete oxygen barrier and vapor control is required in the packaging system. Double bag of cellophane, polyethylene, glassine, polyolefins are used. Vacuum packaging in PET, foil/PVDC/PE is appropriate. They extend shelf life too. Plywood chests with lining of foil or cellulose film are used for large scale transport of tea. Foil laminates and HDEP containers are suggested for spices to protect precious volatile oils. Conventional metal and glass containers are also used at household level.

Beverages: Glass is found optimal for beverages which protect its color, flavor, and other contents to maximum quality. Beverages in glass are appealing, attractive and convenient to use but liable to break if not handled properly. Tetra packs, metal cans, plastics, and PET bottles are also used.

Oil and fats: Fats and oils undergo rancidity in presence of moisture, heat, and air. Therefore, it is necessary to store these in air-tight containers at cool dark places; however, refrigeration is not required. After use, oil must be filtered as residue of previous batch will accelerate the spoilage of fat. Low-density polyethylene is a good, heat sealable and cheaper option, but it has relatively high gas permeability. Thus this packaging material makes oil sensitive to spoilage and there is poor odor resistance. High density versions are better for oils. PVC containers provide good protection from light and air and prevent rancidity. Antioxidants like tocopherol and synthetic ones like BHT, BHA and TBHQ and metal chelators like citric acid and EDTA (ethylenediaminetetracetic acid) are added at the time of manufacturing the oil for prevention of auto-oxidation in fats and oils.

Nuts: Since nuts are precious source of nutrients and are expensive, their packaging is very important. They contain high amount of fat particularly unsaturated fatty acids including omega-3 fatty acids, which are susceptible to rancidity. Hence, extra care is needed for their packaging.

The quantity of nuts and also the size and shape of nuts also determines the choice of packaging material and the type of packaging. In recent years, some nuts like peanuts, walnuts are packaged in shrink wrap plastic films to avoid rancidity. Storing them at low temperature in air-tight containers is also beneficial. Now small and bite-size packaging is also in demand for various reasons. Thin coating of aluminum in the packaging may provide better protection by providing the barrier to oil, gases, moisture, light, odor or aroma of the food product.

RAPID FIRE

1. Describe the effect of peeling potatoes on food quality.
2. What is the role of blanching in freezing and canning?
3. What is the difference between baking and roasting with regard to browning?
4. What are the harmful effects of grilling meat on high fire?
5. What is the difference in denaturation of protein from meat and of pulse?
6. Define Maillard reaction and what is its relationship with AGE products?
7. Define lipid peroxidation and describe its impact on food quality.
8. Why germinated pulses are considered healthful?
9. How tetra packs are more advantageous over common paper cartons?
10. Identify two advantages of each of MAP, CA, and Nanopackaging?

EXERCISE

1. Explain the impact of any four moist heat methods on nutritional quality of food with examples.
2. What is the difference between microwave and irradiation in terms of their principle of function and also their role in preservation of food quality and nutritive value?
3. Select five each of fermented and roasted products used in your area and explain their nutritional contribution after treatment.
4. Choose any ten food preparations and explain their method of cooking and the chemical reaction occurring in them affecting their nutritional quality.
5. Select any ten food packets and try to identify the type of packaging material in them and explain their nutritional advantages and disadvantages.

SUGGESTED READING

1. Agrahar-Murugkar D, Subbulakshmi G. Preparation techniques and nutritive value of fermented foods from the Khasi Tribes of Meghalaya. Ecol Food Nutr. 2006;45(1): 27-38.
2. Arora S, Singh R. Food engineering for biotechnologists In: Marwaha SS, Arora JK. (Eds). Food Processing: Biotechnological Applications. New Delhi: Asia Tech Publishers Inc; 2000. pp. 25-58
3. Barretta DM, Lloydb B. Advanced preservation methods and nutrient retention in fruits and vegetables. J Sci Food Agric. 2012;92:7-22.
4. Bethke PC, Jansky SH. The effects of boiling and leaching on the content of potassium and other minerals in potatoes. J Food Sci. 2008;75(5):80-85.
5. Bettison J. Packaging for fruit products. In: Fruit Processing, Nutrition, Products, and Quality Management. Maryland: An ASPEN Publishers; 2001. pp. 205-22.
6. Choe E. Effects and Mechanism of minor compound in oil on lipid peroxidation. In: Akoh CC, Min DB (Eds). Food Lipids: Chemistry, Nutrition and Biotechnology, 3rd, edition. London: CRC Press, Taylor & Francis group; 2008. pp. 449-67.
7. Davis B. Food Commodities. London: William Helnemann Ltd.; 1978.
8. Del Caro A, Piga A, Vacca V, et al. Changes of flavonoids, vitamin C and antioxidant capacity in minimally processed citrus segments and juices during storage. Food Chemistry. 2004;84:99-105.
9. Dev SL, Chakravati R. Food preservation. In: Marwaha SS, Arora JK (Eds). Food Processing: Biotechnological Applications. New Delhi: Asiatech Publishers Inc; 2000. pp. 79-108.
10. Ecoursesonline. Caramelization and its significance.[online] Available from http://ecoursesonline.iasri.res.in/mod/page/view.php?id=90187. [Last Accessed on September, 2019].
11. FAO (food and Agriculture Organization) 2016; Bio-based food packaging in Sustainable Development Challenges and opportunities to utilize biomass residues from agriculture and forestry; http://www.fao.org/forestry/45849-023667e93ce5f79f4df3c74688c2067cc.pdf; as a feedstock for bio-based food packaging.
12. Fourie PC. Fruit and human nutrition. In: Fruit Processing Nutrition, Products, and Quality Management. Maryland: An ASPEN Publishers; 2001. pp. 37-52.
13. Gazette Notification on Food Safety and Standards (Packaging and Labelling) first amendment Regulations, 2020 relating to Display of Information in food service establishment [Uploaded on : 26-08-2020]
14. Gil MI, Aguayo E, Kader AA. Quality changes and nutrient retention in fresh-cut versus whole fruits during storage. J Agric Food Chem. 2006;54:4284-96.
15. Harris RS, Karmas E. Nutritional Evaluation of Food Processing, 2nd edition. Connecticut: The AVI Publishing Company Inc; 1975.
16. http://icpe.in/icpefoodnpackaging/pdfs/28_national_international.pdf -
17. https://www.fssai.gov.in/upload/notifications/2020/08/5f4611c4eca96Gazette_Notification_Information_Display_Food_26_08_2020.pdf
18. IS : 10106 (Part 2, sec 6) – 1990 Packaging Code : Packaging materials : Flexible laminates, and BIS Plastics for Food Packaging: National And International Standards.
19. Johnson LA. Recovery, refining, converting, and stabilizing edible fats and oils peroxidation. In: Akoh CC, Min DB (Eds). Food Lipids: Chemistry, Nutrition and Biotechnology, 3rd edition. London: CRC Press, Taylor & Francis Group; 2008. pp. 206-35.
20. Jose CF, Tulipani MA, Romandini S, et al. Contribution of honey in nutrition and human health: A review. Mediterr J Nutr Metab. 2009;2:1-9.
21. Majid I, Nayik GA, Dar SM, Nanda V. Novel food packaging technologies: Innovations and future prospective. Journal of the Saudi Society of Agricultural Sciences. 2018. 17 (4): 454-62.
22. Mandal S, Yadav S, Neema RK. Antioxidants: A review. J Chem Pharmaceut Res. 2009;1(1):102-4.
23. Mirajkar M, Menon S. Food Science and Processing Technology, Vol. I. Biochemistry of Food and Nutrition, New Delhi: Kanishka Publishers; 2002.
24. Monteiro CA. Nutrition and health: The issue is not food, nor nutrients, so much as processing. Public Health Nutr. 2008;2:729-31.
25. Moore J, Luther M, Cheng Z, et al. Effects of baking conditions, dough fermentation, and bran particle size on antioxidant properties of whole-wheat pizza crusts. J Agric Food Chem. 2009;57(3):832-9.

26. Navale SA, Swami SB, Thakor NJ. Extrusion cooking technology for foods: A review. J Ready-to-Eat Food. 2015;2(3):66-80.
27. Oliviero T, Capuano E, Cämmerer B, et al. Influence of roasting on the antioxidant activity and HMF formation of a cocoa bean model systems. J Agric Food Chem. 2009;57(1):147-52.
28. Pacholi S, Likhitkar S, D'Souza A. Active packaging in keeping the food fresh: A review. Int J Eng Res Adv Technol. 2017;3(9):19.
29. Pardeshi IL. Convenience foods and its packaging effects on human health: A review. J Ready-to-Eat Food. 2014;1(4):127-32.
30. Parra Cde La, Saldivar SO, Liu RH. Effect of processing on the phytochemical profiles and antioxidant activity of corn for production of Masa, Tortillas, and Tortilla Chips. J Agric Food Chem. 2007;55(10):4177-83.
31. Parveen R, Butt S, Yasin M, et al. Storage and frying behavior of sunflower oil blended with peanut oil. J Food Saf. 2011;13:214-20.
32. Pawara SG, Pardeshib IL, Rajput SG. Convenience foods and its packaging effects on human health: A review. Journal of Ready to Eat Food. Jakraya Publications (P) Ltd. 2014;1(4):127-32.
33. Reid T, Munyanyi M, Mduluza T. Effect of cooking and preservation on nutritional and phytochemical composition of the mushroom Amanita zambiana. Food Sci Nutr. 2017;5(3):538-44.
34. Richardson T, Finley JW. Chemical Changes in Food during Processing. New Delhi, India: CBS Publishers & Distributors. 1997.
35. Robertson GL. Food Packaging, Principles and Practice. New York: Marcel Dekker, Inc.; 1993.
36. Sadowska-Bartosz I, Bartosz G. Prevention of protein glycation by natural compounds. Molecules. 2015;20:3309-34.
37. Soni SK, Arora JK. Indian fermented foods: Biotechnological approaches. In: Marwaha SS, Arora JK (Eds). Food Processing: Biotechnological Applications. New Delhi: Asiatech Publishers Inc; 2000. pp. 143-90.
38. Subbulakshmi G, Udipi SA. Food Processing and Preservation. New Delhi: New Age International Publishers; 2021.
39. Tamanna N, Mahmood N. Food processing and Maillard reaction p'oducts: Effect on human health and nutrition. Int J Food Sci. 2015;2015:6.
40. Tatum V. Effect of processing and storage on fatty acids in edible Oils. In: Chow CK (Ed). Fatty Acids in Foods and Their Health Implications, 2nd edition. New York: Marcel Dekker, Inc.; 2000. pp. 411-23.
41. Toivonen PMA, Stan S. The effect of washing on physicochemical changes in packaged, sliced green peppers. Int J Food Sci Technol. 2004;39:43-51.
42. Udipi SA, Ghugre P. Food Irradiation. Udaipur: Agrotech Publishing Academy; 2010.
43. United States Department of Agriculture, USDA Table of Nutrient Retention Factors, Release 6 (2007). [online] Available from:https://www.ars.usda.gov [Accessed September 2019].
44. Valentino R, D'Esposito V, Ariemma F, et al. Bisphenol A environmental exposure and the detrimental effects on human metabolic health: Is it necessary to revise the risk assessment in vulnerable population? J Endocrinol Invest. 2016;39:259-63.
45. Warner K. Chemistry of frying oils. In: Akoh CC, Min DB (Eds). Food Lipids: Chemistry, Nutrition and Biotechnology, 3rd edition. London: CRC Press, Taylor & Francis Group; 2008. pp. 189-200.
46. World Health Organization (WHO). FAO/WHO consultations on the health implications of acrylamide in foods. Summary report of a meeting held in Geneva. 2002.

APPENDIX 1

Food Sources of Energy (100 g Edible Portion)

Food Codes from IFCT, 2017	Food Name	Carbohydrate (g)	Protein (g)	Fat (g)	Energy (KJ)	Energy (kcal) - calculated
A. Cereals and Millets						
A003	Bajra	61.8	11	5.4	1456	348
A004	Barley	61.3	10.9	1.3	1331	318
A005	Jowar	67.7	10	1.7	1398	334
A006	Maize (dry)	64.8	8.8	3.8	1398	334
A009	Quinoa	53.65	13.1	5.5	1374	328
A010	Ragi	66.8	7.2	1.9	1342	321
A015	Rice (milled)	78.2	7.9	0.52	1491	356
A011	Rice flakes	76.8	7.4	1.1	1480	354
A012	Rice puffed	77.7	7.5	1.6	1514	362
A013	Rice, brown	74.8	9.2	1.6	1480	354
A016	Rice, small	65.6	10.1	3.9	1449	346
A022	Semolina (rawa)	68.4	11.4	0.74	1396	334
A018	Maida (wheat flour, refined)	74.3	10.4	0.76	1472	352
A024	Vermicelli (roasted)	71.4	10.4	0.49	1423	340
A019	Whole wheat flour	64.2	10.6	1.5	1340	320
B. Grain Legumes						
B001	Bengal Gram, Dal	46.7	21.6	5.3	1377	329
B002	Bengal Gram, Whole	39.6	18.8	5.1	1201	287
B003	Black Gram, Dal	51	23.1	1.7	1356	324
B006	Cow Pea, (White)	53.8	21.3	1.14	1340	320
B010	Green Gram, Dal	52.6	23.9	1.4	1363	326
B011	Green Gram, Whole	46.1	22.5	1.14	1229	294
B012	Horse gram whole (kulthi)	57.2	21.7	0.62	1379	330
B013	Lentil, Dal	52.5	24.4	0.75	1349	322
B014	Lentil, whole	48.5	22.5	0.64	1251	299
B017	Peas (dry)	48.9	20.4	1.9	1269	303
B020	Rajmah, red	48.6	19.9	1.8	1252	299
B021	Red Gram, Dal	55.2	21.7	1.6	1384	331
B025	Soybean, white	10.2	37.8	19.4	1579	377
F. Roots and Tubers						
F001	Beet root	6.2	2	0.14	149	36
F002	Carrot, Orange	5.6	1	0.47	139	33
F003	Carrot, Red	6.7	1	0.47	160	38
F004	Colocasia	17.9	3.3	0.17	372	89
F005	Lotus Root	14.7	1.9	0.93	332	79

Food Sources of Energy (100 g Edible Portion)

Food Codes from IFCT, 2017	Food Name	Carbohydrate (g)	Protein (g)	Fat (g)	Energy (KJ)	Energy (kcal) - calculated
F006	Potato, Big	14.9	1.5	0.23	292	70
F007	Potato, Small	12.9	1.4	0.22	255	61
F010	Radish, White	6.6	0.77	0.15	135	32
F011	Radish, Round, Red skin	6.1	0.89	0.16	130	31
F013	Sweet Potato, Brown skin	24.3	1.3	0.26	456	109
F014	Sweet Potato, Pink skin	23.9	1.27	0.33	452	108
F016	Water Chestnut	21.5	0.86	0.37	400	96
F018	Yam, Ordinary	17.7	2.2	0.17	349	83
D. Other Vegetables						
D001	Ash Gourd	0.85	0.79	0.14	73	17
D004	Bitter Gourd	2.8	1.4	0.24	87	21
D007	Bottle Gourd	1.7	0.53	0.13	46	11
D010	Brinjal	3.5	1.8	0.4	114	27
D032	Broad Bean	2.1	3.9	0.15	123	29
D033	Capsicum, Green	1.8	1.1	0.34	68	16
D034	Capsicum, Red	2.1	1.5	0.5	83	20
D035	Capsicum, Yellow	1.9	1.4	1.41	78	19
D036	Cauliflower	2	2.2	0.44	96	23
D037	Celery Stalk	2.3	0.98	0.24	69	16
D039	Cluster Beans	4.9	3.6	0.37	168	40
D042	Corn, Baby corn	11.7	2.7	1.3	306	73
D044	Cucumber, Short	2.8	0.83	0.18	73	17
D046	Drumsticks	3.8	2.6	0.12	123	29
D047	Field Beans, Broad	2.8	3.1	0.64	129	31
D051	Jack Fruit	3.5	2	0.35	110	26
D056	Ladies Finger	3.6	2.1	0.22	115	27
D057	Mango, Green Raw	10.6	0.7	0.1	205	49
D058	Onion, Stalks	3	2.1	0.26	107	26
D059	Papaya, Raw	4.4	0.5	0.23	100	24
D060	Parwar	3.5	1.5	0.3	101	24
D061	Peas, Fresh	11.9	7.3	0.13	340	81
D062	Plantain, Flower	2.2	1.5	0.63	89	21
D063	Plantain, Green	17.6	1.2	0,23	334	80
D065	Pumpkin, Green	4.2	0.87	0.18	103	25
D066	Pumpkin, Orange	4	0.84	0.16	97	23
D068	Ridge Gourd	1.7	0.91	0.14	55	13
D070	Tinda	1.9	1	0.17	58	14
D076	Tomato	2.7	0.9	0.5	82	20
D077	Zucchini, Green	2.3	1.1	0.5	84	20
H. Nuts and Oil Seeds						
H001	Almonds	3	18.4	58.5	2549	609
H005	Cashew Nuts	25.5	18.8	45.2	2438	583
H006	Coconut, Dry	8	7.3	63.3	2611	624
H008	Garden Cress, Seeds	33.7	23.4	23.7	1863	445
H009	Gingelly (Black), Kala Til	10.3	19.2	43.1	2124	508
H011	Gingelly (White), Safed Til	10.8	21.7	43.1	2174	520
H012	Groundnut	17.3	23.7	39.6	2176	520
H014	Flax Seeds (Linseeds)	11	18.6	35.7	1857	444
H015	Niger Seeds	23	18.9	38.6	2144	512
H017	Pine Seed	26.8	12.6	48.8	2486	594

Food Codes from IFCT, 2017	Food Name	Carbohydrate (g)	Protein (g)	Fat (g)	Energy (KJ)	Energy (kcal) - calculated
H018	Pistachio	15.8	23.3	42.5	2257	539
H020	Sunflower Seeds	6.9	23.5	51.9	2453	586
H021	Walnut	10.1	14.9	64.3	2809	671
E. Fruits						
E001	Apple, Big	13.1	0.3	0.6	261	62
E002	Apple, Green	10.7	0.5	0.5	214	51
E005	Apricot, Dried	72.6	3.2	0.7	1321	316
E007	Avocado Fruit	1.8	3	13.9	604	144
E008	Bael Fruit	28.2	2.6	0.6	569	136
E009	Banana Ripe	25	1.3	0.3	463	111
E013	Black Berry	10.6	0.9	0.6	227	54
E014	Cherries, Red	11.9	1.5	0.5	250	60
E015	Currants, Black	9.9	1.5	0.5	227	54
E016	Custard Apple	20.4	1.6	0.7	414	99
E017	Dates, Dry Pale	74.9	2.5	0.35	1340	320
E020	Fig	16.3	2	0.4	341	82
E021	Goose Berry (Amla)	5	0.3	0.2	99	24
E022	Grapes, Seeded, Black	13.2	0.8	0.3	254	61
E023	Grapes, Green, Seeded	12.2	0.8	0.3	235	56
E026	Grapes, Seedless, Green	11.8	0.6	0.3	224	54
E028	Guava, White Flesh	5.1	1.4	0.3	135	32
E029	Guava, Pink Flesh	9.1	2	0.3	195	47
E030	Jack Fruit, Ripe	14	2.7	0.15	302	72
E031	Jambu Fruit, Ripe	12.3	0.8	0.2	235	56
E032	Karonda	2.9	1.2	1.7	141	34
E033	Lemon Juice	7	0.4	0.8	153	37
E034	Sweet Lime, Pulp	5.2	0.8	0.2	114	27
E035	Lichi	11.41	1	0.3	225	54
E042	Mango, Ripe, totapari	12.8	0.4	0.5	248	59
E043	Mangosteen	11.4	0.6	0.2	219	52
E044	Tamarind	13.5	3.6	1.1	342	82
E045	Muskmelon	4.2	0.42	0.35	97	23
E047	Orange	7.9	0.7	0.13	156	37
E049	Papaya, Ripe	4.6	0.4	0,2	100	24
E050	Peach	7.8	0.9	0.4	168	40
E051	Pear	8.1	0.4	0.3	157	38
E052	Phalsa	15.11	1.7	0.1	299	71
E053	Pineapple	9.4	0.5	0.2	180	43
E054	Plum	12.1	0.6	0,4	238	57
E055	Pomegranate	11.6	1.3	0.2	229	55
E057	Raisins, Dried, Black	71.3	2.6	0.3	1279	306
E058	Raisin, Dry, Golden	68.8	2.8	0.4	1241	297
E060	Sapota	13.9	0.9	1.3	307	73
E062	Star Fruit	4.5	0.8	0.4	110	26
E063	Strawberry	3.4	1	0.6	103	25
E064	Tamarind, Pulp	67.4	2.9	0.2	1207	288
E065	Watermelon	3.9	0.6	0.2	85	20
E068	Zizyphus (Ber)	9.4	1.3	0.35	204	49

Source: Longvah T, Ananthan R, Bhaskarachary K and Venkaiah K (2017). Indian Food Composition Tables, National Institute of Nutrition, (Indian Council of Medical Research), Department of Health Research, Ministry of Health and Family Welfare, Government of India, Hyderabad.

2 APPENDIX

Dietary Fiber in Common Foods (100 g of Edible Portion)

Food Code	Food Name	Total Dietary Fiber (TDF) (g)	Insoluble Dietary Fiber (IDF) (g)	Soluble Dietary Fiber (SDF) (g)
A. Cereals				
A003	Bajra	11.5	9.1	2.3
A005	Jowar	10.2	8.5	1.7
A006	Maize, Dry	11.2	11.3	0.9
A010	Ragi	11.1	9.5	1.7
A015	Rice	2.8	2.0	0.8
A019	Wheat flour	11.4	9.7	1.6
B. Pulses and Legumes				
B002	Bengal Gram, Whole	25.2	22.7	2.5
B001	Bengal Gram, Dhal	15.2	12.7	2.5
B003	Black Gram, Dhal	11.4	7.6	4.4
B004	Black Gram, Whole	20.4	15.5	5.0
B011	Green Gram, Whole	17.0	14.6	2.5
B010	Green Gram, Dhal	9.4	7.8	1.6
B014	Lentil, Whole	16.8	14.2	2.7
B013	Lentil, Dhal	10.4	8.6	1.8
B021	Red Gram, Dhal	9.1	6.7	2.4
B020	Rajmah	17.0	14.3	2.6
C. Green Leafy Vegetables				
C002	Amaranth	4.4	3.2	1.2
C017	Cabbage	2.8	1.9	0.9
C018	Colocasia, Green	5.6	4.3	1.3
C019	Drumstick	8.2	6.1	2.1
C020	Fenugreek	5.0	3.2	1.7
C031	Radish	1.9	1.2	0.6
C033	Spinach	2.4	1.5	0.9
F. Roots and Tubers				
F001	Beetroot	3.3	2.6	0.7
F003	Carrot	4.5	3.1	1.4
F006	Potato	1.7	1.1	0.6
F010	Radish	2.7	2.0	0.7
F013	Sweet Potato	4.0	2.6	1.4
D. Other Vegetables				
D005	Bitter Gourd	3.5	3.1	0.7
D007	Bottle Gourd	2.1	1.7	0.5
D010	Brinjal	3.6	2.4	1.2
D035	Broad Bean	8.6	6.6	2.0

Food Code	Food Name	Total Dietary Fiber (TDF) (g)	Insoluble Dietary Fiber (IDF) (g)	Soluble Dietary Fiber (SDF) (g)
D036	Cauliflower	3.7	2.7	1.0
D043	Cucumber	2.1	1.5	0.6
D058	Onion Stalks	5.2	3.8	1.5
D061	Peas, Green	6.3	5.0	1.3
H. Nuts and Oil Seeds				
H001	Almond	13.1	10.6	2.5
H006	Coconut, Dry	15.9	14.6	1.3
H011	Gingelly Seeds (Til)	17.0	13.5	3.6
H012	Groundnut	10.4	8.6	1.8
H014	Linseed (Flax Seed)	26.2	21.8	4.3
G. Condiments and Spices				
G024	Coriander	44.8	35.3	10.0
G025	Cumin Seeds	30.4	25.7	4.6
G026	Fenugreek	47.6	27.6	20.0
G022	Red Chilies, Dry	31.2	26.6	4.6
E. Fruits				
E049	Papaya	2.8	1.0	1.1
E001	Apple	2.6	1.4	1.2
E017	Dates, Dry	9.0	7.5	1.4
E028	Guava	8.6	7.1	1.5
E009	Banana	2.2	1.4	0.8
E051	Pear	4.5	4.0	0.5
E021	Amla (Gooseberry)	7.8	6.2	1.6

Source: Longvah T, Ananthan R, Bhaskarachary K and Venkaiah K (2017) Indian Food Composition Tables, National Institute of Nutrition, (Indian Council of Medical Research), Department of Health Research, Ministry of Health and Family Welfare, Government of India, Hyderabad.

APPENDIX 3

Energy Requirements of Indian Men and Women at Different Ages and Body Weights

Sex	Body weight (kg)	19–30 years				30–60 years				>60 years			
		BMR (kcal/day)	Sedentary work (kcal/day)	Moderate work (kcal/day)	Heavy work (kcal/d)	BMR (kcal/day)	Sedentary work (kcal/day)	Moderate work (kcal/day)	Heavy work (kcal/day)	BMR (kcal/day)	Sedentary Work (kcal/day)	Moderate work (kcal/day)	Heavy work (kcal/day)
Males	45	1235	1728	2222	2839	1251	1752	2253	2878	1003	1404	1805	2306
	50	1302	1823	2344	2996	1303	1824	2346	2997	1055	1478	1900	2427
	55	1370	1919	2467	3152	1355	1897	2439	3116	1108	1551	1995	2549
	60	1438	2014	2589	3308	1407	1969	2532	3235	1161	1625	2089	2670
	65	1506	2109	2711	3465	1458	2042	2625	3354	1213	1699	2184	2791
	70	1574	2204	2834	3621	1510	2114	2718	3473	1266	1772	2279	2912
	75	1642	2299	2956	3777	1562	2187	2812	3592	1319	1846	2374	3033
Females	40	982	1374	1767	2258	1064	1490	1916	2448	930	1303	1675	2140
	45	1049	1468	1888	2412	1101	1542	1982	2533	972	1361	1749	2235
	50	1116	1563	2009	2567	1138	1593	2048	2618	1013	1419	1824	2331
	55	1184	1657	2130	2722	1175	1645	2115	2702	1055	1477	1898	2426
	60	1251	1751	2252	2877	1212	1696	2181	2787	1096	1535	1973	2521
	65	1318	1846	2373	3032	1249	1748	2247	2872	1138	1593	2048	2616
	70	1386	1940	2494	3187	1285	1800	2314	2957	1179	1650	2122	2711

Sources: Nutrient Requirements of Indians, Recommended Dietary Allowances, Estimated Average Requirements, A Report of the Expert Group, 2020, Indian Council of Medical Research, National Institute of Nutrition, Department of Health Research, Ministry of Health and Family Welfare, Government of India.

APPENDIX 4

Summary of Estimated Average Requirements (EAR) for Indians–2020

Age group		Category of work	Body weight (kg)	Energy (**) (kcal/day)	Fats/Oils (visible) (#) (g/day)	Protein (g/day)	CHO (g/day)	Calcium (mg/day)	Magnesium (mg/day)	Iron (mg/day)	Zinc (mg/day)	Iodine (µg/day)	Thiamine (mg/day)	Riboflavin (mg/day)	Niacin (mg/day)	Vit B6 (mg/day)	Folate (µg/day)	Vit B12 (µg/day)	Vit C (mg/day)	Vit A (µg/day)	Vit D (IU/day)
Men		Sedentary	65	2110	25	42.9	100	800	320	11	14.0	95	1.2	1.6	12	1.6	250	2	65	460	400
		Moderate		2710	30								1.5	2.1	15	2.1					
		Heavy		3470	40								1.9	2.7	19	2.6					
		Sedentary	55	1660	20	36.3	100	800	270	15	11.0	95	1.1	1.6	9	1.6	180	2	55	390	400
		Moderate		2130	25								1.4	2.0	12	1.6					
		Heavy		2720	30								1.8	2.6	15	2.1					
Women		Pregnant woman	55 +10	+350	30	+7.6 (2nd trimester) +17.6 (3rd trimester)	135	800	320	32	12.0	180	1.6	2.3	+2	1.9	480	+0.2	+10	406	400
		Lactation 0-6 m	-	+600		+13.6	155	1000	270	16	12.0	200	1.7	2.5	+4	+0.22	280	+0.8	+40	720	400
		Lactation 7-12 m		+520	30	+10.6	155						1.7	2.4	+4	+0.16	280				
Infants		0-6 m*	5.8	550	-	6.7	-	-	-	-	-	130	-	-	-	-	-	-	-	-	-
		6-12m	8.5	670	25	8.8	-	-	-	2	2.0	-	0.6	0.8	-	0.5	71	1	-	170	-
Children		1-3y	11.7	1010	25	9.2	100	400	111	6	2.5	65	0.6	0.8	6	0.8	90	1	22	180	400
		4-6y	18.3	1360	25	12.8	100	450	131	8	3.7	80	0.8	1.1	8	1.0	111	1	27	240	400
		7-9y	25.3	1700	30	19.0	100	500	178	10	4.9	80	1.0	1.3	10	1.3	142	2	36	290	400
Boys		10-12y	34.9	2220	35	26.2	100	650	223	12	7.0	100	1.3	1.7	12	1.7	180	2	45	360	400
Girls		10-12y	36.4	2060	45	26.6	100	650	214	16	7.1	100	1.2	1.6	12	1.6	186	2	44	370	400
Boys		13-15y	50.5	2860	50	36.4	100	800	294	15	11.9	100	1.6	2.2	16	2.2	238	2	60	430	400
Girls		13-15y	49.6	2400	35	34.7	100	800	270	17	10.7	100	1.3	1.9	13	1.8	204	2	55	420	400
Boys		16-18y	64.4	3320	40	45.1	100	850	338	18	14.7	100	1.9	2.5	19	2.5	286	2	69	480	400
Girls		16-18y	55.7	2500	35	37.3	100	850	279	18	11.8	100	1.4	1.9	14	1.9	223	2	57	400	400

* Adequate intake (AI).
** There is no RDA for energy, the EAR for energy. The EAR is equivalent to the estimated energy requirement (EER).
# Visible fat requirement is in proportion to EER.

APPENDIX 5

Glycemic Index and Glycemic Load of Some Commonly Consumed Foods and Food Preparations

Food Items	Weight of the Food (g)	Glycemic Index (GI)	Glycemic Load (GL)
Apple	120	36	5
Pineapple	120	51	8
Pear	120	38	4
Papaya	120	60	17
Mango	120	60	9
Kiwi	120	47	6
Banana	120	48	11
Orange	120	45	5
Apricot (dried)	120	32	10
Watermelon	150	73	4
Bajra	75	49	25
Whole wheat	50	30	11
Barley	150	48	20
Maize	30	59	8
Green peas	80	54	4
Rajmah	150	19	6
Cooked food preparations			
Poori potato masala	150	82	34
Rice (boiled)	150	43	16
Brown rice (boiled)	280	35	3
Dal fry	150	24	3
Rice puttu channa dal curry	250	79	58
Pongal cooked in pressure cooker	250	90	47
Idli (white rice)	50	86	12
Idli (brown rice)	50	68	4
Dosa (parboiled rice)	250	77	40
Ragi dosa*	182	50	40
Rava dosa*	216	68	54
Moong dosa*	265	63	47
Onion sambhar	150	24	2
Wheat chapati with lauki and tomato	60	66	21

Food Items	Weight of the Food (g)	Glycemic Index (GI)	Glycemic Load (GL)
Wheat chapati with moong dal	200	81	41
Potato (steamed)	150	65	18
Potato (fry)	150	73	20
Mix vegetables	150	58	4
Samosa	100	58	4
Masala vada	30	10	1
Plain biscuit	1 (5g)	85	3
Beverages			
Coffee with milk and sugar	150 ml	60	8

*Sathiya V, Chithra R. Nutritive Value, Glycemic Index and Glycemic Load of Selected Dosa Varieties. International Journal of Health Sciences and Research. 2019;9(3): 215-9.

Source: Atkinson FS, Foster-Powell K, Brand-Miller JC. International tables of glycemic index and glycemic load values: 2008. Diabetes Care. 2008;31(12):2281-3.

Vaidya R, Mohan V, Bai MR, Vasudevan S. Glycemic Index of Indian Cereal Staple Foods and their Relationship to Diabetes and Metabolic Syndrome. Madras Diabetes Research Foundation, Dr Mohan's Diabetes Specialties Centre, WHO Collaborating Centre for Non-Communicable Diseases, and International Diabetes Federation (IDF) Centre of Education, Gopalapuram, Chennai, India. Chapter 25 in Watson RR, Preedy VR And Zibadi S (Eds). Wheat and rice in disease prevention and health, benefits, risks and mechanisms of whole grains in health promotion, Academic Press 2014: 333-346.

Bajaj M (2018) Diet Metrics, Handbook of Food Exchanges. Notionpress.com:57-58.

Index

Page numbers followed by *f* refer to figure and *t* refer to table, respectively.

A

Abelmoschus esculentus 498
Absorption 74, 90, 113
Acacia
   senegal 32
   seyal 32
Accelerometers 127
Acesulfame-K 43
Acetylcholine 169
   formation of 185
Achlorhydria 343
Achras sapota 500
Acid 258
   base balance 203, 206, 208, 240, 258, 259, 261, 263
      disorders in 262
      maintenance of 48, 261
      production 208
      rain 203
Acidosis 258, 262
   metabolic 262
   respiratory 262
Acne vulgaris 177
Acquired immune deficiency syndrome 402
Actinidia sinensis 501
Activated protein C 165
Acute mountain sickness 470
Addison's disease 205
Adductor pollicis muscle
   study of 416
   thickness 416
Adenosine triphosphate 117, 118*f*, 169
Adipocytes 132
Adipocytokines 136
Adipokines 136
Adiponectin 136
Adipose
   derived stem cells 156
   tissue 86, 132
      formation of 21
Adrenal
   cortex 132
   medulla 132
Advanced glycation end-products 526
Aegle marmelos 500
Aerobic exercises 458
A-inositol phosphoglycans 186
Air displacement plethysmography 140, 399
Alanine 69
   aminotransferase 539
Albumin 50, 401, 402
Aldosterone 246, 255
Alkaline phosphatase 219, 539
Alkalosis 258, 262
   metabolic 262
   respiratory 262
Allium
   cepa 494, 496
   sativum 494
Alpha-amylase inhibitors 490
Alpha-linolenic acid 97, 98, 100, 108
Alpha-melanocyte-stimulating hormone 132
Alpha-tocopherol transfer protein 163
Alternate healthy eating index 290
Aluminum 550
Alzheimer's disease 88, 164, 169, 228
Amaranthus cruentus 494
American Academy of Pediatrics 166
American Diabetes Association 40, 137, 293, 298, 493
American Heart Association 460, 491
American Society for Parenteral and Enteral Nutrition 390
Amine oxidase 225
Amino acid 46, 46*t*, 52, 53, 63, 66, 71
   basic structure of 52*f*
   categories of 53*t*
   classification of 52, 52*f*
   conditionally indispensable 53
   essential 52, 53, 67
   food sources of 71*t*
   functions of 66
   glucogenic 52
   ketogenic 52
   metabolism 167, 180, 184
   nonessential 52, 53, 68
   nonproteinogenic 53, 71
   number of 46, 64
   pool 61, 61*f*
   requirements 71*t*
   score 63
   total essential 71
Amino peptidases 74
Ammonia buffer 260, 261
Amorphophallus paeoniifolius 493
Amylase rich food 25, 330, 328, 546
Amylin 133
Amylopectin 29, 29*t*
Amylose 29, 29*t*
Anacardium occidentale 505
Ananas comosus 501
Androgens 87
Android 144
Androstenedione 87
Anemia 59, 364*t*, 400
   classification of 361
   clinical features of 365
   consequences of 365
   hypochromic 227
   indicators of 364
   macrocytic 183, 362
   megaloblastic 183, 362, 402
   microcytic 362
   normocytic normochromic 362
   nutritional 348, 361, 361*f*, 362*t*
   pernicious 183, 362
   prevalence of 365, 365*t*
   prevention of 365
   severe 353
   stages of 213, 213*f*
   treatment of 365
Anemia Mukt Bharat 431, 440
Anganwadi centers 442
Animal
   foods 510
   proteins 56
Annapoorna Scheme 443
Annona cherimola 500
Anorexia 353
   nervosa 133
Anterior pituitary gland 132
Anthocyanidins 454
Anthocyanins 454
Anthropometry
   advantages of 394*t*
   functional 394
   limitations of 394*t*
   physical 394
   uses of 140
Antiatherogenic effects 90
Antibodies 47
   formation of 177
Anticancer activity 90
Anticariogenic effects 65
Anti-inflammatory effect 65
Antiketogenic effect 22
Antilipemic effect 65
Antinutritional factors 490*t*
   reduction of 545
Antioxidant 172, 474
   activity 162
   defense 226
   dietary 468
   effect 65
   function 222
Antithrombotic effect 65
Antyodya Anna Yojana 441
Apigenin 453

Apium graveolens 496
Apolipoproteins 83
Apoproteins 84
Appetite 129
    test, criteria for 354t
Arachidonic acid 79, 97-99, 332
Arachis hypogea 505
Arginine 70, 71
Arsenic 234
    deficiency of 235
    functions of 235
Arthritis 160
Artocar pusaltilis 503
Artocarpus heterophyllus 503
Ascites 254
Ascorbic acid 166, 167
Asparagine 71
Asparagus officinalis 499
Aspartame 43
Aspartate 71
    aminotransferase 539
Aspartic acid 70, 71
Asthma 160
Atherosclerosis 66
Atmosphere packaging, modified 552
Atomic energy regulatory board 440
Australian Nutrition Screening Initiative 418
Autoimmune diseases 35, 160
Avena sativa 486

B

Bacillus thuringiensis 435
Bariatic surgery 227
Basal metabolic rate 121, 125, 128, 270
    estimation of 123
    factors affecting 122
Basal metabolism 120
Basic and advanced carb counting, methods of 301t
B-cells 153
B-complex vitamins 166
Behavior
    modification 382
    problems 372
Benincasa hispida 498
Beriberi 169, 171
    infantile 171
    wet 171
Bertholletia excels 506
Beta vulgaris 493, 496
Beta-carotene
    chemical structure of 150f
    content 154
Beta-glucan soluble fiber 32, 36
Betaine 316
Beverages 285, 286, 554
    types of 468
Bhabha Atomic Research Center 440
Biaxially oriented polypropylene 553
Bicarbonate 250, 251
    buffer 260
    ions 34
Bile acids, component of 88
Binge eating 133, 134

Bioactive compounds 450
Biochemical
    indicators 399
    parameters 401
Bioelectrical impedance analysis 137
Bioflavonoids 169
Biofortification 432
Biological compounds, component of 197
Biotechnology 434
Biotin 166, 184
    deficient intake of 184
    excessive intake of 184
    food sources of 184
    functions of 184, 235
Bisdemethoxycurcumin 454
Black and white vision 152
Blood 83, 473
    brain barrier 88
    cell synthesis 178
    clot, formation of 164
    coagulation of 48, 226
    glucose level 374, 377
        modifies 36
    lipids profile 85t
    pH, regulation of 219
    pressure
        high 381
        maintenance of 203
        reduce high 381
        systolic 380
    sugar
        changes 465
        levels 36, 376t
        hormonal control of 376
    tests, factors influencing interpretation of 400f
    volume 309, 310
        maintenance of 203
Blurred vision 250
B-monooxygenase 225
Body
    build 144
    building foods 280
    composition 122, 134, 134f, 135f, 342, 398, 461
        assessment models of 138f
        changes in 323
    fat 136
        mass 145
    fluids 251, 473
        balance, regulation of 48
        changes in 343
        components of 241
        distribution of 241f
    functions 117
    mass index 13, 136, 140, 141f, 367, 368, 562
    organs 350
    parts of 410
    size 122
    surface area 122
    temperature 122
    thermal insulation of 79
    types 143
    water, total amount of 241, 351

    weight 116, 141, 144, 241, 274, 275, 395, 562
        assessment of 144
        deviations in 145
        regulation, theory for 142
Bone 473
    bank 193
    formation of 157, 164
    health, poor 35
    marrow iron 408
    mass 338
        density 161
    mineral
        accelerated loss of 227
        density 195
    mineralization 198, 219
Boron
    deficiency of 236
    excess intake of 236
Brain 132, 226, 350
    amygdala in 132
    development 185, 231, 338
        effect on 352
    functions 209, 219
    lipids, component of 88
    swelling of 250
Branched chain amino acids 67
Brassica
    campestris 495
    oleracea italica 496, 497
    rapa 494, 496
Breastfeeding 321
Broca's index 144
Broiling 537
Brown adipose tissue 143
Buchanania latifolia 506
Buffers 258, 261
    system 198, 260, 260f
    types of 260
Bulimia nervosa 133
Butanoic acid 94
Butter 513, 554
Butylated hydroxyanisole 92, 431
Butylated hydroxytoluene 93, 431
Butyric acid 94

C

Cadmium 236
Caffeic acid 170
Calcidiol 156
Calcitriol 156
Calcium 193, 250, 251, 257, 315, 316, 334, 339, 381, 431, 474, 563
    absorption 157, 195
        factors affecting 195f
    deficiency 196, 383
    excessive intake of 197
    food sources of 196, 196f
    functions of 193
    high 114
    iodate 430
    signaling 175
    status 408
    supplements 196
Camellia sinensis 519

Canadian Nutrition Screening Tool 418
Cancer 160
Canola oil 515
Capillary blood pressure 246
Capric acid 94
Caproic acid 94
Caprylic acid 94
Capsaicinoids 454
Capsicum annuum 498
Caramelization 526
Carbohydrate 4, 21-23, 33, 34, 119*f*, 274, 287, 325, 380, 469, 470, 557
   absorption of 43, 44*f*
   changes in 351
   classification of 22, 22*t*
   counting 301, 380
   digestion of 43, 44*f*
   excessive intake of 35
   food sources of 34
   functions of 21
   group 298
   loading 465
   metabolism 169, 178, 184, 206, 231, 232
   non-digestible 36
   non-glycemic 23
   role of 464
Carbon 4
   atom 94, 97
   dioxide, dense phase 549
   source of 21
Carbonic acid 259, 261, 262
Carbonic anhydrases 219
Carboxymethylcellulose 31
Carboxypeptidase 74, 219
Cardioprotective Mediterranean Diet Index 291
Cardiovascular disease 96, 158, 293, 381
Cardiovascular system 226
Carica papaya 500
Carnitine 188
   deficiency of 188
   food sources of 188
   synthesis of 167
Carotenes 452
   dioxygenase 151
Carotenoids 149, 150, 154*t*, 451, 451*t*
   absorption of 151*f*
   amount of 151
   factors affecting absorption of 151
   groups of 451*f*
   types of 151
Carya illinoensis 505
Caseinophosphopeptides 65
Catabolic index 404
Catch-up growth 335
Catechin 453
Cell
   differentiation 48, 153, 158
   division 219
   energy consuming activities of 118
   membrane 48, 194, 203
      component of 197
      structural component of 88
      structural integrity of 185
   proliferation 200
   signaling 49, 153, 173, 185, 194
Cellular retinoic acid-binding protein 153
Cellulose 31, 36, 151
Celtic salt 205
Central nervous system 171
   myelination of 323
   noradrenergic neurons of 132
   specific neurons of 132
Cephalin 82
Cereals 285, 482, 487, 552, 559, 560
   exchanges 295, 295*f*, 295*t*
   products 552
      ready-to-use 488
   proteins 54
   non-gluten 483*f*
Cerebrosides 82
Ceruloplasmin 225
Cheilosis 173
Chemical
   buffer systems 260
   energy 116
   score 63
Chenopodium
   album 495
   quinoa 488
Chertow formula 242
Chitin 37
Chitosan 37
Chloramphenicol 183
Chloride 208, 250, 251, 256
   deficiency of 208
   excessive intake of 208
   food sources of 208
   functions of 208
Chlorine 207, 208
Chlorogenic acid 170
Cholecalciferol 156
Cholecystokinin 113, 132
Cholesterol 80, 84, 87, 88, 89
   chemical structure of 88*f*
   synthesis of 177
Cholestyramine 183
Choline 185, 316
   deficient intake of 186
   excessive intake of 186
   food sources of 186
   functions of 185
   precursor of 316
Chromium 232
   deficiency of 233
   excessive intake of 233
   food sources of 233
   functions of 232
Chromoproteins 51
Chronic energy deficiency 13, 108
Chronic mountain sickness 470
Chylomicrons 84
Chymotrypsinogen 74
Cicer arietinum 496
Cimetidine 183
Circulatory system 226, 343
Citric acid cycle 172
Citrulline 72
Citrullus vulgaris 499
Citrus
   aurantiifolia 502
   aurantium 502
   fruits 502
   reticulata 502
   sinensis 502
   X paradisi 502
Climate 122
Coagulation 48, 528
Cobalt 236
Cocoa 519
Cocos nucifera 506
Codex alimentarius
   Codex 437
   Commission 35
Colchicine 183
Cold plasma 549
Collagen 50
   synthesis 166
Colloidal osmotic pressure 253
Colocasia esculenta 493, 496
Color vision 152
Colostrum 322
Coma 250
Community food banks 443
Complementary foods
   consistency of 328
   frequency of intake of 328
Complex lipids, component of 185
Comprehensive National Nutrition Survey 13
Computed tomography 139
Condiments 516, 518, 561
Confusion 250
Connective tissue, formation of 226, 231
Convulsions 250, 353
Copper 169, 225, 315, 362, 384
   deficiency of 227
   excessive of 227
   food sources of 226
   functions of 226
   recommended intake of 226
   status 409
Coriandrum sativum 495
Corn
   flour 485
   oil 486, 514
   syrup 486
Cornea, vascularization of 173
Coronary artery disease 529
Corticotropin-releasing hormone 132
Cortisol 87, 132
COVID-19 434
   infection 351
   pandemic 421, 422
Cramps 250
C-reactive protein 58, 165, 368, 400, 401
Creatinine height index 403
Cretinism 360
Crohn's disease 158, 224
Cryptoxanthin 154
Cucumis
   melo 499
   sativa 497
Cucurbita moschata 498, 505

Curcuminoids 454
Cushing's syndrome 86
Cyanogenic glycosides 490
Cyclamates 43
Cysteine 69, 71
Cytochrome-C oxidase 225

D

Daucus carota 493
Daytime sleepiness, excessive 160
Deamination 61
Decanoic acid 94
Defense against free radicals 219, 231
Dehydration 247, 541, 542
    causes of 247
    clinical signs of 248, 249*f*
    effects of 541
    levels of 248*f*
    prevention of 249
Dehydroascorbic acid 166
Dementia 175
Demethoxycurcumin 454
Denaturation 527
Dental caries 35, 372
Deoxyribonucleic acid 21
    replication and repair 210
    transcription 233
Depression 35
Dermatitis 175
Detoxification 22, 167, 210
Development 153, 173, 180, 215
    principles of 305
Deworming 367
Dextrin 30
Dextrinization 527
Diabetes 86, 160, 373
    causes of 377
    complications of 378
    diagnostic criteria for 376
    dietary management of 378
    mellitus
        gestational 318, 374, 375
        insulin-dependent 374
        non-insulin dependent 316, 374
    types of 374, 374*t*
Diacetyl 526
Diarrhea 175, 247, 355
Diet 263, 282
    balanced 282
    planning 282
    quality index 290
    recall using multiple-pass method 412
    record 412
Dietary
    carbohydrate 23
        nutritional groupings of 23*t*
    deficiency 160
    diversification 356, 357
    fiber 35, 39, 274, 560
        food sources of 40
        functions of 36
        health benefits of 36
        total 40*f*, 560
    folate equivalents 180
    guidelines 107, 273, 277, 318, 321, 340, 342, 345
    iron, forms of 211*f*
    requirement 55
    supplements 456
        Health and Education Act 448, 456
        side effects of 457
        uses of 457
    vitamin D
        absorption of 160
        digestion of 160
Dietetics 3
Digestible indispensable amino acid score 63, 330
Digestion 72, 113, 219
Digestive system 343
Dihydroxycholecalciferol 156
Diiodothyronine 359
Dipeptidase 74
Dipeptide 46
Direct Benefit Transfer Program 442
Disaccharides 22, 25, 44
Docosahexaenoic acid 97-101, 178, 325, 332, 333, 510
Docosanoic acid 94
Dopamine 225
Double bond
    configuration of 91, 92
    position of 91
Double-fortified salt 431
Down's syndrome 228
Drugs 183
    detoxification of 177
Drum drying 541
Dry baking 538
Dry beriberi 171
Dry heat methods 534
Dry mouth 245
Dual energy X-ray absorptiometry 139, 368
Dual fortification 431
Dubois body surface chart 122
Duodenum 44

E

Eating
    disorders 133
    habits 369
    patterns 369
Ectomorph 143, 144
Edema 48, 57, 254
    peripheral 254
    pulmonary 254
Egg 509
    exchange 297
    proteins 54
    shell 509
    white 509
    yolk 509
Eicosanoic acid 94
Eicosanoids 102
    derivatives of 103*t*
    formation of 103*f*
    source of 79
Eicosapentaenoic acid 97, 98, 100, 178, 510

Elastin 50
Electrolytes 240, 241, 250, 251, 255, 261, 324, 332, 336, 469, 471
    balance 203, 206, 208, 250, 251, 254, 461
        hormonal control of 254
    buffer 260
    concentration of 246
    role of 468
Electron transport chain 118, 119, 172
Eleusine coracana 488
Elevated blood triglyceride levels 35
Embryonic period 308
Emotions 11
Employment Guarantee Scheme 422
Endocrine
    factors 369
    functions 320
Endomorph 143
Endopeptidases 74
Endorphins 132
Energy 56, 116, 311, 320, 324, 325, 332, 333, 336, 339, 341, 463, 470, 557, 563
    balance 116, 120, 120*f*
        negative 120
        positive 120
    concentrated source of 78
    currency for 117
    density 130, 289*t*
    expenditure 120, 461
        estimation of 125
        total 124, 125, 128
    food sources of 557
    forms of 117
    generating pathways 118
    generation of 119*f*, 176
    intake 120, 129
    malnutrition 348
    metabolism 116, 117, 197, 200, 209, 215, 226
    nutrients 172
    potential 116
    release 172
    requirements 127, 128, 312*f*, 562
    rich foods 280
    spent 125
    storage form of 21
Enzymatic theory 142
Enzymes 47
    activation of 208, 231
    cofactor for 206, 210
    component of 209
    copper dependent 225
    enhanced activity of 545
    synthesis of 231
Epicatechin 453
Epicatechin-3-gallate 453
Epinephrine 84, 376, 377
Epithelial cells 355
Epithelial tissue 152, 226
Epoxyeicosatrienoic acids 99
Eriobotrya japonica 503
Eriodictyol 454
Erucic acid 97, 105
Erythritol 26, 27

Index | 571

Erythrocyte
    protoporphyrin 408
    transaminases 405
    transketolase activity 170, 404
Escherichia coli 66, 325
Esters 526
Estradiol 87
Estrogens 87
Estrone 87
Ethanolic fermentation 544
Ethylene
    oxide polymers 32
    vinyl acetate 553
European Nutraceutical Association 448
Excretory system 343
Exercises 135, 345, 457-459
    balance 459
    cardiac 459
    cool-down 459
    flexibility 459
    isometric 458
    isotonic 458
    resistance 459
    strength-building 458
    types of 458, 458*f*
    warm-up 459
Exotic oils 516
Expressed maternal milk 322
Extracellular buffers 260
Extracellular fluids 48, 193, 194, 241, 242, 250, 251*t*, 253, 255, 332, 351
    electrolytes of 253
Extrusion 547
Eye 355

F

Fagopyrum esculentum 487
Famotidine 183
Farnesol 80
Fast proteins 54
Fat 4, 77, 78, 108, 274, 287, 316, 320, 324, 325, 332, 334, 336, 339, 341, 471, 512, 554, 557, 563
    abdominal 368
    absorption of 113
    analogs 110
    buffer 260
    cell theory 142
    classification of 79
    digestion of 113
    essential 136
    excessive consumption of 108
    exchanges 298
    extenders 110
    food sources of 107
    free mass 135, 241
    functions of 78
    group 299
    hydrogenated 105
    insufficient intake of 108
    metabolism of 169, 184
    mimetics 110
        carbohydrate-based 112
        protein-based 112
    mobilization of 86
    presence of 42
    replacers 110
        carbohydrate-based 110
        cellulose-based 112
        lipids-based 110
        protein-based 110, 111
    role of 467
    soluble vitamins 149
    storage of 136
    subcutaneous 136, 368
    substitutes 110
    synthesis of 177
    utilization, impaired 86
Fatty acid 78, 91, 94, 95, 97, 101, 316
    beta-oxidation of 86
    binding protein 113
    classification of 93, 94*f*
    composition 108*t*
    essential 79, 86, 91, 97, 98, 102, 103, 163, 326
    kind of 114
    metabolism 210
    nomenclature systems of 93, 93*t*
    production of 184
    saturated 91-93, 94*t*, 107
    unsaturated 96, 97*t*
Fatty liver 59, 186
    disease, nonalcoholic 160, 227
Feces 244
Feeding, complementary 327, 329*t*
Fermentation 543
Ferric iron 211*f*
Ferritin, serum 364, 408
Ferulic acid 454
Fetal
    development 307
    growth 315
    nutrition 310
    period 308
Fever, high 353
Fiber, types of 37
Fibrin 50
Ficus carica 500
Fin fish 510
Fish 509
Fitness, level of 125
Flavanones 453
Flavin adenine dinucleotide 21, 172
Flavones 453
Flavonoids 453, 453*t*
Flavonols 453
Flavoprotein 51
Flaxseed oil 515
Fluid 332
    balance 246, 246*f*
Fluoride 229, 384, 431
    excessive intake of 229
    food sources of 229
Fluorine 228
    functions of 228
    overload 230
Fluorosis 229
Folate 166, 275, 563
    deficiency 181, 402
    excessive intake of 181
Folic acid 179, 313, 316, 362, 404
    functions of 180
    total 181, 181*t*
Follicle stimulating hormone 49
Food 1, 2, 62, 420, 447
    access 420
    acidity level of 42
    Adulteration Act, prevention of 361
    and Agricultural Organization 17, 79, 266, 267, 421, 440
    and Drug Administration 43
    and nutrition security analysis 421
    based approach 356, 357, 366
    carbohydrate content of 41
    choice of 5, 329
        factors of 6*f*
    cholesterol content of 89*t*
    classification, Nova system of 16
    composition of 42, 369
    composition tables 281
        limitations of 282
        uses of 281
    cravings 369
    derived biologically active peptides 64
    diary 412
    different types of 473, 473*t*, 552
    eat variety of 278
    economics, factors affecting 10
    energy density of 130
    exchanges 293-295
        importance of 294
    formula 331*f*
    fortification 432
        resource centre 366
    frequency questionnaire 413
    functions of 2, 3*f*, 280*t*
    genetically modified 436
    glycemic index of 41
    groups 279, 280
        uses of 279
    guide 276
        pyramid 273
    habits 18
    high-glycemic 41
    insecurity, range of 422*f*
    intake, short-term regulation of 130*f*
    irradiation 438, 440, 543
        functions of 439
    liquid 243
    low-glycemic 40
    macronutrient composition of 130
    matrix 151
    natural form of 473
    nutritious 2
    packaging, types of 551
    physical state of 130
    preparation 330
    preservative 204
    processing 529
        and packaging, nutritional implications of 523
        techniques 151, 533*f*
        stages of 530*f*
    products 524*t*
        development and food labeling 272

proteins 54, 63f
pyramid 276f
radiation, effect of 439
ready-to-serve 489
Safety and Standards Authority of India 2, 456, 550
security 420, 424
    allowance rules 442
    dimensions of 423, 423f
    four components of 420f
sight of 129
smell of 129
solid 243
sources 180, 182, 235, 451
supplements 456
thermic effect of 124
utilization of 420, 424
weight of 564
Fortification 356, 357, 360, 366, 428
    evolution of 428
    limitations of 432
    methods of 429
Frailty 344
Free fatty acids 376
Free foods 300, 300t
Free radicals, excessive production of 462
Free thiamine 404
Freeze-dried food 473
Fresh food 473
Frozen food 473
Fructans 23
Fructooligosaccharides 24, 28
Fructose 23, 24
Fruits 499, 554, 559, 561
    exchange 297, 298t
Functional tests 399t
Fusarium moniliforme 503

G

Galactogogues 321
Galactopoiesis 319
Galactose 25
Galanin 132
Gallic acid 454
Gamma-aminobutyric acid 70, 132, 169
    receptors 219
Gamma-glutamyl carboxypeptidase 219
Gamma-linolenic acid 97-99
Ganglioside 83
Gas chromatography-combustion isotope ratio mass spectrometry 407
Gastric acid inhibitors 183
Gastrointestinal hormones 131
Gastrointestinal system, changes in 323
Gastrointestinal tract 350, 363
Gel formation 528
Gelatinization 526
Gelation 527, 528
Gene
    expression 48, 98, 153, 157, 184, 219, 477
    revolution 1
Genetic
    deficiency 234
    Engineering Appraisal Committee 437

factors 369
    mutations 378
Genistein 454
Genome 477
Genomics 477
Geriatric Nutritional Risk Index 418
Geriatric population 418
Germination 544
Ghrelin 130, 132
Global Food Security Index 420
Global Hunger Index 425
Global Nutrition Report 17
Global subjective assessment 415
Globular protein 50
Globulin 50
Glomerular filtration rate 60, 343
Glossitis 173
Glucagon 132, 376, 377
Glucocorticoids 87, 319, 376, 377
Glucose 21, 23
    intolerance 316
    tolerance factor 232
    transporter 47
Glutamate 70, 132
Glutamic acid 70
Glutamine 70, 71
Glutathione 172
    disulfide 172
    peroxidase 59, 223
Glutelins 50
Gluten cereals 483f
Glycans 21
Glycemic
    carbohydrates 23
    glucose 42
    impact 42
    index 40, 41, 564
    load 41, 564
    responses, factors affecting 42
Glycerolipids 80
Glycerophospholipid 80
    structure of 83f
Glycine 68, 71
Glycitein 454
Glycogen 33
    stores 461
Glycogenesis 24
Glycolipids 77, 81, 82
Glycolysis 118
Glycomacropeptide 65
Glycoproteins 51
Glycosphingolipid, structure of 83f
Goiter 359
    detection of 361
    stages of 360f
Goitrogens 490
Gonadal steroids 87
Gonadotropin-releasing hormone 64
Good nutrition 11, 12
    characteristics of 12t
Grain
    legumes 557
    structure 482
Green leafy vegetables 297t, 494, 494t, 560
Greenhouse gases 6

Grewia asiatica 503
Growth 47, 135, 153, 173, 178, 180, 182, 215, 219, 232, 305
    characteristics of 305
    different stages of 305f
    hormone 47, 84, 146, 319, 351, 377
        deficiency 86
    retardation 59, 355
    velocity 417
Gums 32
    types of 32t
Gynoid 144

H

Hamwi's equation 144
Head circumference 397
Headaches 250
Health 1, 18
    benefits 22, 90
    check up 443
    conditions 378
    education and awareness activities 361
    stages of 392
    state of 130, 389
    status 7, 55
    supplements 456
Healthy eating index 289, 290
Heart 182
    diseases, coronary 92, 107
    rate monitoring 127
    transfer, medium of 78
Height, alternative indicators for 416
Helianthus annuus 506
Helicobacter pylori infection 213, 363
Hemagglutinins 490
Hematocrit value 364
Hematopoiesis 361
Hematopoietic nutrients 362t
Heme iron 211, 212
Hemicelluloses 31
Hemochromatosis
    primary 214
    secondary 214
Hemoglobin 261, 401
    formation of 177
    synthesis 362f
Hephaestin 225
Herbs 516, 517, 518
    addition of 382
Hesperidin 454
Hexadecanoic acid 94
Hexa-fluoro-silicate acid 431
Hexanoic acid 94
High energy
    bonds 117
    compound 117
    phosphate bond 197
High fat sugar and salt 11
High formiminoglutamic acid 402
High plasma sodium level 256
High-density lipoprotein 48, 84, 85
    cholesterol levels 35
High-fructose corn syrup 24, 486, 512
Himalayan pink salt 205
Histamine 2-receptor antagonists 183

Histidine 68, 71
    load test 405
Histones 50
Home fortification 432, 433
Homeostasis 205, 240, 245
Homeostatic model assessment 97
Homocysteine 183, 394
Hordeum vulgare 487
Hormone 47, 74, 132, 178
    adrenocorticotropic 84, 319
    affecting food intake 130, 132*t*
    antidiuretic 246, 252, 255
    buffer 260
    levels 310
        changes in 351
    parathyroid 156, 193, 197, 255, 257, 383
    precursor of 79
    synthesis of 88
Hot air bed drying 541
Human genome 477
Human growth, phases of 306*f*
Human milk
    bank 322
    characteristics of 324, 325
    composition of 324
Human nutrition 3
Hum-Weyers formula 241
Hunger 129
Huntington's disease 88
Hydrochloric acid 72, 259
Hydrogen
    ions 260
        sources of 259
    selenide 225
Hydrogenated starch hydrolysate 26, 27
Hydrogenation 95
Hydrolytic rancidity 528
Hydrostatic weighing 139
Hydroxycholecalciferol 156
Hydroxycinnamic acid 454
Hydroxypropyl methylcellulose 36
Hypercalcemia 197, 257
Hyperchloremia 256
Hyperglycemia 376
Hyperinsulinemia 86, 374
Hyperkalemia 207, 256, 257
Hypernatremia 205, 256
Hyperphosphatemia 257
Hypertension 158, 160, 316, 380, 381
    causes of 381
Hypertonic dehydration
    signs of 248*t*
    symptoms of 248*t*
Hypertonic solution 253
Hypocalcemia 257
Hypochloremia 256
Hypoglycemia 353, 376, 379
Hypokalemia 257
Hypomagnesemia 258
Hyponatremia 205, 256
Hypophosphatemia 257
Hypotensive effects 65
Hypothalamus 132
Hypothermia 353
Hypothyroidism 86

Hypotonic dehydration
    signs of 248*t*
    symptoms of 248*t*
Hypotonic solution 253
Hypoxia inducible factor 1 168

I

Immune
    dysregulation 474
    function 222
    memory, development of 323
    response 208
    system 79, 158, 226, 343, 355
Immunity 152, 210, 219
    protective nutrients for 352*f*
Immunization 443
Impaired glucose tolerance 158, 375
Indian Academy of Pediatrics 354, 373
Indian Council of Medical Research 33, 105, 267, 273, 281, 358
Indian Dietetic Association 293, 294
Indian Food Composition Tables 281
Indian Research Fund Association 281
Infant feeding practices, guidelines for 330
Infant Health and Development Program 417
Infection 349
Inflammation 35
Inflammatory bowel disease 158, 455
Inositol 186
    excessive intake of 187
    food sources of 187
    functions of 187
    phosphoglycans 186
Insoluble dietary fiber 560
Insulin 131, 376
    growth factor 312, 401
    resistance 35, 316, 375
Insulinoma 86
Integrated child development services 271, 390, 441, 442
Intensity 125
Interactive computer and web-based technologies 414
Interleukins 100
Intermediate-density lipoproteins 84
International Atomic Energy Agency 440, 543
International Conference on Electronics Packaging 552
International Fund for Agricultural Development 421
International Scientific Association for Probiotics and Prebiotics 455
Interstitial fluid 242, 253, 254
    role of 253
Intestinal cells 132
Intestine, small 113
Intracellular fluids 48, 241, 242, 250, 251*t*, 255
    electrolytes of 253
Intrauterine growth retardation 155, 309, 312, 315, 355
Intravascular fluid 242

Inulin 30
Iodate compounds 430
Iodide 430
Iodine 214, 274, 313*f*, 314, 316, 430, 563
    content 430, 430*t*
    deficiency disorder 192, 217, 348, 358, 359*f*
        causes of 358
        consequences of 359
        control of 360
        prevalence of 360*t*
        prevention of 360
    excessive intake of 217
    food sources of 215
    functions of 215
    inadequate utilization of 358
Ion transport 200
Iron 169, 209, 274, 314, 316, 334, 339, 408, 430, 474, 563
    absorption 167
        factors affecting 212*f*
    containing enzymes 210
    deficiency 212, 363
        anemia 363
        serum ferritin concentration indicative of 365*t*
    excessive intake of 214
    food sources of 212, 212*f*
    fortification 430*t*
    functions of 209
    homeostasis 210
    loss of 363
    low body stores of 363, 364
    metabolism 226
    nonheme 211, 212
    poor absorption of 363
    rich foods, low-dietary intake of 363
    serum 408
    storage of 210
    supplements 366
    transport 210
Irradiation 438
    food for 439*t*
Islet amyloid polypeptide 133
Isoflavones 384
Isoflavonoids 454
Isoleucine 68, 71
Isomalt 26, 27
Isomaltase 44
Isotonic dehydration
    signs of 248*t*
    symptoms of 248*t*
Isotonic solution 253

J

Jaivik bharat 438
Juglans regia 505

K

Kangaroo care 332
Keratin 50
Keshan disease 224
Ketoacids 259
Ketone bodies 22
Ketonic rancidity 529

Kidney 261, 262, 350
    functions 310
        maturation of 323
        role of 246, 246f, 261
Kinetic energy 116
Kishori Shakti Yojana 443
Kosher salt 205
Krebs' cycle 184
Kwashiorkor 352
    features of 352t

L

Lactase 44
Lactating breast structure 319f
Lactation 122, 319, 319f
    advantages of 320
    factors affecting 320
    stages of 319
Lactic acid 259
    fermentation 544
Lactitol 26, 27
Lactobacillus
    bifidus 326
    lactis 181
Lactogenesis 319
Lactones 526
Lactose, intolerance 25
Lactuca sativa 495
Lagenaria siceraria 498
Lansoprazole 183
Large bowel function 36
Lathyrogens 490
Lauric acid 94
L-carnitine supplementation 189
Lead 238
Lean
    body mass 122, 135, 332, 461
    soft tissue 135
Lecithin 82
Lectins 490
Legumes 489, 560
Lepidium sativum 505
Leptin 131, 132, 136
Lethargy 353
Leucine 68, 71
Leukopenia 227
Leukotrienes 103, 104
Life insurance corporation tables,
    uses of 145
Lignans 454, 455
Lignins 37
Limonoids 451
Linoleic acid 97, 98, 108
    conjugated 104, 513
Linum usitatissimum 506
Lipids 4, 77, 78, 83, 85, 86, 119f, 310
    changes in 350
    classification of 79, 80f, 80t
    derived 86
    functions of 78
    metabolism 178, 184, 231, 233
    peroxidation 92, 529
        effect of 92
    simple 80
    structured 110, 111

Lipoic acid 189, 190
Lipopolysaccharide 33
Lipoproteins 48, 51, 77, 81, 83-85
    components of 79
    composition of 84t
    lipase 84, 142
    lipids content of 84f
    role of 84t
Lipoyl carrier protein 189
Liver 85, 350
    role of 75
Long chain fatty acids 91, 94, 96, 112, 324
    absorption of 114f
    digestion of 114f
Low birth weight 317
    babies, nutrition for 331
Low plasma sodium level 256
Low-density
    lipoprotein 48, 79, 84, 85, 162, 455, 505
    polyethylene 553
Lower respiratory tract infection 353
Low-serum retinol, prevalence of 356t
Luffa acutangula 498
Lungs 244, 261
    maturation of 323
    role of 261
Lutein 154, 452
Luteolin 453
Lycopene 154, 452
Lycopersicon esculentum 497
Lysine 67, 71, 545
    content 67
    score 67
Lysyl oxidase 225

M

Macadamia integrifolia 506
Macronutrient 4
Macrophages 153
Magnesium 199, 250, 251, 258, 274, 315,
    381, 563
    deficiency of 201, 383
    excessive intake of 202
    food sources of 200, 201f
    functions of 200
    ion 258
    status 409
Magnetic resonance
    imaging 139, 368
    tomography 139
Mahatma Gandhi National Rural
    Employment Guarantee Program
    443
Maillard reaction 525
Malabsorption syndrome 151
Malaria eradication 367
Malnutrition 11, 348
    factors influencing 15t
    impact of 16f
    micronutrients-related 12
    moderate acute 353, 398
    universal screening tool 415, 418
Maltase 44
Maltitol 26, 27
Maltodextrin 28, 112

Maltooligosaccharides 28
Maltose 25
Malus sylvestris 499
Manganese 230, 384
    deficiency of 231
    excessive intake of 232
    food sources of 231
    functions of 231
    recommended acceptable intake
        for 231
Mangifera indica 503
Mannitol 26
Mannose 24
    binding
        lectin 24
        protein 24
Marasmus 352
    features of 352t
Margarine 513
Marine food exchange 296t
Mastication 130
Maternal tissues, development of 310
Mature red blood cells, formation of 180
Meal 282
    planning 282, 283, 294
        aims of 283
        steps in 283
Mean cell volume 362
Mean corpuscular
    hemoglobin concentration 362
    volume 362
Meat 299, 510, 554
    analogs 511
    exchange 296t
    products 554
    substitutes 299
Medical nutrition therapy 375
Mediterranean diet
    quality index 291
    score 290
Mediterranean dietary pattern adherence
    index 291
Medium-chain
    fatty acids 91, 94, 96, 112
    triglycerides 217
Melanin-concentrating hormone 132
Membrane potential, maintenance of 206
Menkes' syndrome 227
Mental
    development, poor 59
    disturbances 344
Mentha arvensis 495
Metabolic rate 121, 343
Metabolic syndrome 378
Metabolomics 477
Metal transport protein 1 211
Metalloenzymes, constituent of 231
Metalloproteins 51
    constituent of 226
Metallothioneins 226
Metformin 183
Methionine 67, 71
Methylation 180
Methylhistidine 404
Methylmalonic acid 394

Methylsulfonylmethane 203
Microcytic hypochromic anemia 179
Microencapsulation 476
Micronutrients 4, 56, 313, 336, 406, 406*t*
   status of 351
Mid-day meal scheme 271, 441
Mid-upper arm circumference 397, 397*t*, 353
   assessment criteria for 398*t*
   measurement of 354*t*
Milk 506, 553
   exchanges 296, 296*t*
   pasteurization for 546
   products 285, 506, 507*t*, 553
   proteins 54
Millets 482, 488, 557
Milliequivalent 263
Mineralocorticoids 87
Minerals 5, 192, 320, 324, 325, 332, 339, 342, 408, 471, 545
   classification of 192
   fertilization 432
   role of 467
Mini nutritional assessment 415, 418
Mixed triglyceride 91
Mobile-based technologies 414
Moist heat cooking methods 532, 533*t*
Molybdenum 233
   deficiency of 234
   excess intake of 234
   food sources of 234
   functions of 233
Momordica charantia 498
Monoiodothyronine 359
Monomeric units 36
Monosaccharides 22, 23
Monounsaturated fatty acid 91, 92, 96, 107, 505
Mood 130
Moringa oleifera 495
Mother's milk, advantages of 325
Motion, energy of 116
Mouth 113
Mucopolysaccharides 33
Mucoproteins 51
Murraya koenigii 495
Musa paradisiaca 500
Muscle 473
   activity 206
   contraction 194, 200
   endurance 213
   excitability 203
   proteins 54
   relaxation 194, 200
   strength 343, 395
   wasting 58
Musculoskeletal structure 47
Myelin sheath 169
   formation of 172
Myristic acid 94

N

N-acetylglucosamine 80
N-acetylneuraminic acid 83
Nanoemulsions 475
Nanosensor 475
Nanotechnology 474
   potential uses of 475
Naringenin 454
National Crechè Scheme 442
National Family Health Survey 13, 360
National Food Security
   Act 440, 441, 442
   Mission 441, 444
National Goiter Control Programme 360
National Horticulture Mission 444
National Institute of Nutrition 105, 273, 281, 293
National Institution for Transforming India 444, 357
National Iodine Deficiency Disorders Control Programme 360
National Nutrition Mission 440, 442, 444
National Nutrition Monitoring Bureau 39, 425, 482
National Nutrition Programme 357
National Nutrition Strategy 440
National Nutritional Anaemia Prophylaxis Programme 366, 367
National Old Age Pension Scheme 443
National Rural Health Mission 444
National Sample Survey Organization 425
National Urban Health Mission 444
Natural killer cells 153
Neomycin 183
Nephrolithiasis, animal protein-induced 60*f*
Nerve
   fibers 79
   impulse, transmission of 48, 208
   transmission 177, 194
Nervous system 132, 170, 182, 226, 344, 350
Net dietary protein energy ratio 62
Net protein
   ratio 63
   utilization 62
Neural tube defects 318
Neurotransmitters 47, 59, 133
   formation of 178
Neutropenia 227
Neutrophils 153
Newtonian data 394
Niacin 166, 174, 275, 405, 563
   deficiency of 175
   excessive intake of 176
   food sources of 175
   formation of 178
   functions of 174
Nickel 236
Nicotinamide adenine dinucleotide 21, 235
   phosphate 169, 174
Niemann-Pick type C disease 88
Night blindness 356*t*
Nitrogen
   balance 61, 404
      negative 61
      positive 61
   metabolism 231
Nitrous oxide 183
Nixtamalization 485
Non-cellulosic polymers 31
Non-communicable diseases 39, 106, 460, 478
Non-glyceride components 90
Non-oxidant functions 162
Nonprotein molecule 50
Non-starch polysaccharides 23, 29*f*, 31
Nonsteroidal anti-inflammatory drugs 179
Norepinephrine 132
Nuclear energy 116
Nucleoproteins 51
Nutrient 3, 203
   absorption of 310
   bioavailability of 271
   classification of 4, 4*f*
   composition 281*t*
   contribution of 280*t*
   deficiency 362, 410*t*
   density 288
      uses of 289
   functions of 4
   ingestion of 461
   intake 136
   losses 530*f*
   metabolism of 219
   requirements 341
   rich foods 289
   role of 316*t*
Nutrigenetics 476
Nutrigenomics 476
Nutrition 1-3, 18, 304, 469, 471
   and health education 356, 357, 443
   assessment 391
   education 360, 367
   factors affecting 344
   poor 12, 12*t*
   rehabilitation centres 354
   role of 468
   screening 390, 390*t*, 391
   security 424, 425
   supplementary 442
   total parenteral 234
Nutritional assessment 389, 390, 390*t*, 391, 395*t*, 417
   components of 393*t*
   dietary methods of 411*f*
   methods of 393
Nutritional deficiencies 345
Nutritional deficits, impact of 315
Nutritional genetic modification 432
Nutritional imbalance 372
Nutritional quality
   calculation of index of 289
   index of 289
Nutritional requirements 311, 320, 323, 333, 335, 339, 344, 474
Nutritional risk
   index 415
   screening 415, 418
Nutritional screening 518
Nutritional status 122, 389
   assessment of 353, 389
   classification of 353*t*, 397*t*
   continuum of 392*f*
Nuts 504, 554, 558, 561
   exchanges 297, 298*t*

O

Obesity 35, 160, 318, 367, 368, 372, 373
    adulthood 372
    childhood 371-373
    factors affecting 369
    hyperplastic 142
    hypertrophic 142
    morbid 368
    severe 368
Obsessive compulsive disorder 160
Obstructive sleep apnea 160
Octadecanoic acid 94
Octanoic acid 94
Ohmic heating 548
Oils 77, 78, 108, 512, 554, 563
    classification of 79
    excessive consumption of 108
    food sources of 107
    insufficient intake of 108
Oleic acid 80, 97
Oligopeptide 46
Oligosaccharides 22, 28
    nondigestible 23
Omega-3 fatty acids, functions of 100
Omega-3 index 102
Omeprazole 183
Oncotic pressure 48, 253, 254
Onion tears 203
Opioid effects 66
Optimal complementary feeding 321
Optimal nutritional status 389
Oral rehydration solution 249
Orange carotenoids 451
Organ functions, changes in 350
Organic acid 251
Organic foods 437
Ornithine 72
Oryza sativa 484
Osmolality 245, 246
Osmolarity 246, 252
Osmole 252
Osmolytes 252
Osmoreceptors 246
Osmosis 252
Osmotic force 252
Osteomalacia 161
Osteoporosis 161, 382
    causes of 383
    control of 385
    prevention of 385
    risk factors for 382
    symptoms of 383
Overnutrition 12, 16
Overweight 35, 367, 368, 372
    factors affecting 369
Oxidation 119
Oxidative phosphorylation 119
Oxidative rancidity 528
    stages of 529f
Oxidative stress 162, 462
Oxygen
    radical absorbance capacity 501
    transport 209
Oxyhemoglobin 261

Oxyntomodulin 132
Oxytocin 319f

P

Packed food 285
Palmitic acid 94
Palmitoleic acid 97
Pancreas 132, 350
Pancreatic polypeptide 132
Pantothenic acid 166, 176
    deficient intake of 177
    excessive intake of 177
    food sources of 177
    functions of 176
Para amino benzoic acid 166, 179, 187
Parasitic infection 151
Parathormone 157
Paresthesia 171
Parkinson's disease 169, 179
Pasteurization 546
P-coumaric acid 454
Peak bone mass 194
Pectic polysaccharides 31
Pectin 39, 151
Pedometers 127
Pelargonidin 454
Pennisetum glaucum 488
Pepsinogen 74
Peptidases 219
Peptides 63, 64
    biological significance of 64t
Periodontal disease 158
Personal digital assistant 411, 414
Pesticides, uses of 19
Peucedanum graveolens 496
Phenolic acids 452, 454
Phenotype 477
Phenylalanine 67, 71
Phenylketonuria 67
Phoenix dactylifera 504
Phosphate 250, 251
    buffer 260, 261
    ions 197
Phosphatidylcholine 80
Phosphatidylinositol 187
Phospholipids 77, 81, 82, 84
Phosphoproteins 51, 198
Phosphoric acid 259
Phosphorus 197, 257
    deficient intake of 199
    excess of 383
    excessive consumption of 199
    food sources of 198, 199f
    functions of 197
    levels, regulation of 198
Phosphorylation 198
Photosynthesis 21
Physalis peruviana 501
Physical activity level 128
Phytochemicals 5, 450
    classification of 450f
Phytoestrogens 454
Phytosterols 88
Pineal gland 229
P-inositol phosphoglycans 186

Pinus gerardiana 506
Pistacia vera 505
Pisum sativum var arvense 497
Placenta, functions of 309
Plant sterol 151
Plasma 242
    ascorbate concentration 405
    folate, normal range of 404t
    iron 408
    lipoprotein production 86
    proteins 47, 261, 310
Plasminogen activator inhibitor 136
Plasmodium
    falciparum 213, 367
    vivax 367
Pollution 19
Polycyclic aromatic hydrocarbon 537
Polycystic ovarian syndrome 35, 86, 193, 375, 378
Polydextrose 38, 43, 112
Polyethylene terephthalate 553
Polyglycitol 27
Polyketides 80
Polymerization, degree of 26, 29
Polymers 22
Polymorphism 477
Polyols 23
Polypeptide 46
Polyphenols 452
Polysaccharides 22, 29
    starch based 29f
Polyunsaturated fatty acid 91, 79, 92, 97, 154, 510
Polyvinyl chloride 539, 553
Polyvinylpyrrolidone 32
Portulaca oleracea 497
Potassium 204t, 205, 250, 251, 256, 381
    deficiency symptoms of 206
    excessive intake of 207
    food sources of 206, 207f
    functions of 206
    imbalance
        causes of 257t
        manifestation of 257t
    iodate 430
    iodide 430
    ion 256
    recommended intake of 206
Potential renal acid load 263
Poultry 510, 511
Pradhan Mantri Matru Vandana Yojana 442
Prealbumin 402
Prebiotics 455
Pregnancy 122, 307, 317, 318
Pre-menstrual syndrome 99
Prenol lipids 80
Pressure
    cooking 534
    hydrostatic 254
Preterm babies, nutrition for 332
Probiotics 455
Processing foods, advantages of 524f
Progesterone 87
Progestogen 87

Prognostic hospital index 415
Prognostic nutritional index 415
Prolactin, role of 319f
Prolamins 50
Proline 70, 71
Prostacyclin 103
Prostaglandin, formation of 103f
Prosthetic group 50
Protamines 50
Protective foods 280
Protein 4, 46, 46t, 47, 48, 49, 53, 84, 119f, 251, 261, 274, 287, 311, 316, 320, 324, 325, 332, 334, 336, 339, 341, 348, 383, 403, 469, 471, 557, 563
   after enzymatic action, final product of 74
   agouti-related 132
   changes in 350
   classification of 49, 49t
   complementary 54
   complete 53, 54
   concentration of 246
   conjugated 50
   deficiency of 47
   derived 50, 51
   dietary 56
   digestibility 62
      corrected amino acid score 63, 63f, 312
      values 62t
   digestion of 72
   efficiency ratio 56, 62
   energy malnutrition 75, 349, 402
      causes of 349t
      control of 354
      effects of 349
      etiology of 349
      prevention of 354
   excessive intake of 59
   external 51
   food sources of 56
   functions of 47
   homeostasis 60, 61, 61f
   incomplete 53, 54
   internal 51
   metabolism 169, 178
   modification 210
   molecular structure of 51
   molecule 50
   nonheme 209
   primary derived 51
   quality, assessment methods for 62
   quality, evaluation of 61
   reference 53
   role of 466
   safe level of 71
   secondary derived 51
   secreted 51
   serum 403t
   simple 50
   slow 54
   source 62, 67
   sparing action 22
   status 394, 402
   status, assessment of 401t
   synthesis 206
   synthesis of 200
   total 71
   transmembrane 51
   transport 47
   turnover 61
   types of 49, 54t
Proteome 60
Proton-pump inhibitors 183
Prunus
   armeniaca 502
   avium 503
   domestica 503
   dulcis 504
   persica 499, 503
Pseudo-cereals 487
Psidium guajava 500
Psyllium husk 36
Pteroylglutamic acid 179
Puberty 338
Public distribution system 271, 272, 361, 422, 425, 440, 442
Pulsed electric fields 548
Pulses 285, 489, 560
   protein 54
Punica granatum 500
Pure water depletion 247
Pyridoxal phosphate 177, 178
Pyridoxamine phosphate 177
Pyridoxine 166, 177, 275
   phosphate 177

Q

Quercetin 453

R

Radiant energy 116
Radiation 438
   uses of 19
Rajasic foods 481t
Rajiv Gandhi Drinking Water Mission 444
Rajiv Gandhi Scheme for Empowerment of Adolescent Girls 443
Rajsik foods 481
Rancidity 92, 528
Ranitidine 183
Raphanus sativus 493, 496
Rapidly digestible starch 30
Rashtriya Krishi Vikas Yojana 444
Rashtriya Poshan Abhiyan 444
Rat acrodynia 177
Recommended dietary allowance 33, 154, 215, 265-269, 442
   basis of 269
   calcium 195
   carbohydrates 33
   chloride 208
   dietary fiber 39
   energy 274t, 275t
   evolution of 266
   fats 105
   fluoride 229
   folate 180
   iron 212
   limitations of 272
   magnesium 200
   niacin 175
   oils 105
   pantothenic acid 177
   phosphorus 198
   protein 55
   pyridoxine 179
   riboflavin 173
   selenium 223
   sulfur 202
   thiamine 170
   vitamin 275t
      A 154
      B12 182
      C 168
      D 158
      E 163
      K 165
   zinc 220
Red blood
   cell 47, 153, 361, 362
      formation of 173, 183
   corpuscles 362
Red carotenoids 451
Renal disease, end-stage 207
Respiratory infection 227
Restlessness 250
Restoration 427
Resveratrol 454
Reticulocyte hemoglobin 408
Retinal 150
Retinaldehyde 150
Retinoic acid 150
   receptor 154
Retinoids 150
Retinol 149, 150
   activity 154
   binding protein 48, 151, 402
Retrogradation 527
Rheumatoid arthritis 158, 177
Ribes nigrum 504
Riboflavin 166, 172, 173, 275, 316, 362, 405
   deficiency of 173, 174
   food sources of 173, 173t
   functions of 172
Ribonucleic acid 21
Rice bran hemicellulose, modified 31
Rickets 161
Rock salt 205
Roots 492, 557, 560
Rubus idaeus 501

S

Saccharides 22
Saccharin 43
Saccharolipids 80
S-adenosylmethionine 235, 477
Sago exchange 296
Salmonella paratyphii 504
Salt replacers 204
Sampurna Gramin Rozgar Yojna 443
Saponins 451, 490
Sarcopenia 58, 343
Saturation, degree of 91
Satvic foods 481, 481t

Schilling test 394
Scleroproteins 50
Sclerosis, multiple 158
Sea salt 205
Seafoods 509
Secale cereale 487
Secretion, source of 74
Selenium 222, 431
    deficiency of 224
    excess intake of 225
    food sources of 223, 224f
    functions of 222
Selenoproteins 223, 223t
Sensible water loss 244
Sensitivity 392
Serine 69
Serotonin 132
    formation of 175
Sesamum indicum 505
Set point theory 142
Severe acute malnutrition 353, 354, 398
    diagnosis of 354
    integrated management of 354
Sex hormones
    female 87
    male 87
Sexually transmitted diseases 443
Shell fish 510
Shock absorber 79
Short nutritional assessment questionnaire 418
Short-chain
    carbohydrates 22
    fatty acids 94, 37, 91, 95, 129, 455
Silicon 236
Single nucleotide polymorphism 477
Sirtuins 175
Skeletal structure, formation of 193
Skin 244
    diseases 160
    health 167
    lesion 353
    type 160
Skinfold caliper 137
Skinfold measurement 137, 398
Sleep 122
    disorders 160
Small gestational age 317
Smith-Lemli-Opitz syndrome 88
Sodium 203, 204t, 250, 251, 255, 474
    deficiency of 205
    food sources of 204
    functions of 203
    high 384
    imbalance 255
        causes of 256t
        manifestation of 256t
    iodate 430
    iodide 430
    recommended intake of 204
Solanum
    melongena 498
    tuberosum 492
Soluble dietary fiber 560
Soluble transferrin receptors 408

Sorbitol 26
Sorghum vulgare 488
Sound energy 116
Space food, types of 472
Spheroprotein 50
Sphingolipids 77, 80, 82
    structure of 83f
Sphingomyelin 82
Sphingosine 80, 82
Spices 516, 561
Spinacia oleracea 495
Sports 458
    classification of 463t
    different levels of 464t
    nutrition 457, 463
    types of 458t
Sportsmen
    carbohydrate foods for 465
    protein requirements of 466t
Stanols 89
Starch 29, 29f, 44
    modified 30
    resistant 39, 38
    slowly digestible 30
    source of 29
    types of 30t
Static tests 399, 399t
Steam baking 538
Stearic acid 94
Sterilization 546
Steroid hormone 87, 87t
Sterols 77, 86, 89
    basic structure of 87f
    lipids 80
Stevioside 43
Stilbenes 454, 455
Stomach 113, 132
Streptococcus mutans 65
Stress 11, 123
    different types of 462
    management 167
    metabolic 462
    physical 462
    psychological 463
Sucralose 43
Sucrose 25, 43t
    fatty acid esters 111
Sugar 22, 511
    alcohols 23, 26, 129
    craving 35
    exchange 298
    substitutes 43
    types of 512t
Sulfate 250, 251
Sulfur 202
    deficiency of 202
    food sources of 202
    functions of 202
    spring 203
    toxicity 202
Sulfuric acid 259
Superoxide dismutase 93, 225, 226, 231
Supports vitamin metabolism 173
Sustainable development goal 1, 420, 421
Swarna Jayanti Gram Swarozgar Yojna 443

Synbiotics 456
Syzygium cumini 504

T

Tamasic foods 481, 481t
Tannins 454, 490
Targeted public distribution system 440, 441
Taurine 71
T-cells 153
Terpenes 451
Terpenoids 451
Tertiary butyl hydroquinone 92
Testosterone 87
Tetracosanoic acid 94
Tetrahydrofolate 179
Therapeutic food, ready-to-use 354
Thermal energy 116
Thermogenesis 124
    diet-induced 120, 124
    theory of 143
Thermostabilized food 473
Thiamine 169, 170, 275, 404, 563
    deficiency of 170
    excessive intake of 172
    food sources of 170
    functions of 169
    pyrophosphate 169, 404
Thirst 245
Threonine 68, 71
Thrombin 48
Thromboxanes 103
Thyroid
    hormone, formation of 215, 222
    peroxidase 359
    stimulating hormone 210, 215-218, 319
Thyrotropin-releasing hormone 64
Thyroxine-binding
    albumin 358
    globulin 358
    prealbumin 358
Tin 550
Tissue building 173
Tooth
    decay 36
    enamel, formation of 228
Total iron-binding capacity 402, 408
Toxic overload 86
Toxicity 235
Trace elements 208
Transcellular fluid 242
Trans-fatty acid 105
Transferrin 402
    saturation 408
Triacylglycerol 77, 80, 86
Tricarboxylic acid cycle 66
Triceps skinfold measurement, method of 398
Triglycerides 77, 78, 81, 84, 86
Trigonellafoenum graecum 495
Trimethyl amine 510
Tripeptide 46
Triticum aestivum 483
Trypsin inhibitor 490
Trypsinogen 74

Tryptophan 67, 71
Tubers 492, 557, 560
Tumor necrosis factor 136, 351
Twenty four-hour recall method 412
Tyrosinase 225
Tyrosine 69, 71

U

Ultra-high temperature 526, 546
Ultrasound 140
    uses of 548
Ultratrace elements 234
Ultraviolet B 159
Unconsciousness 353
Undernutrition 11, 12
    reasons for 13, 14f
Underweight 12
United Nations Children's Fund 421
United States Public Health Service 293
Universal Salt Iodization Program 360
Upper gastrointestinal tract 73f
Urea 401
    excretion 404
Urinary creatinine 403
Urinary iodine concentration 217, 218
Urinary thiamine 404, 404t
Urinary tract infection 355, 501
Urinary urea excretion 404
Urine 244

V

Vaccinium
    corymbosum 501
    macrocarpon 501
Vacuum packaging 552
Valine 68, 71
Vanadium 237
Vanaspati 515
Vascular endothelial growth factor 31
Vegetable 285, 492, 554
    exchanges 297
    oils 514
    proteins 56
Very long chain fatty acids 91, 94, 96
Very low-density lipoprotein 84, 186
Vigna unguiculata 496
Visceral fat 136, 368
Vision 152
Visual cycle 152f
Vitamin 4, 149, 320, 324, 325, 332, 339, 341, 411, 471
    A 149, 151, 275, 313f, 314, 316, 362, 405, 431
        absorption of 151f
        different compounds of 150f
        excessive intake of 155
        food sources of 154
        functions of 152
        oral prophylactic dose of 356t
        rich foods 357
        supplementation 356
    A deficiency 155, 348, 355, 357
        causes of 355
        consequences of 355
        control of 356
        diagnosis of 355
        prevalence of 355
        prevention of 356, 357
    B complex 166
    B1 166
    B12 166, 181, 275, 313, 362, 405, 406
        activation of 231
        deficiency of 182, 183
        dietary deficiency of 182
        excessive intake of 183
        functions of 182
        interactions 183
        laboratory tests for 406t
    B2 166, 172, 314
    B3 166, 174
    B5 166
    B6 166, 177, 178, 179, 314, 316, 362, 405
        deficiency of 179
        excessive intake of 179
        food sources of 179
        functions of 178
    B9 166
    C 166-169, 275, 314, 316, 362, 405
        content 168
        deficiency 168
        excessive intake of 168
        food sources of 168, 168t
        functions of 166, 167t
        synthesis of 545
    classification of 149, 149f
    D 149, 156, 157, 160, 275, 314, 316, 407, 431, 474
        deficiency of 159, 160
        excessive intake of 161
        forms of 156
        functions of 157
        metabolite ratio 407
        receptors 157
        sources of 159
        supplementation 160
        synthesis of 156f
    E 92, 149, 161, 162, 169, 314, 362, 407
        deficiency of 163
        excessive intake of 163
        food sources of 163
        forms of 162
        functions of 162
    fat-soluble 79, 405
    K 149, 164, 314, 383, 407
        deficiency of 165
        excessive intake of 166
        food sources of 165
        functions of 164
    K1 165
    K2, role of 165
    role of 467
    water-soluble 149, 166, 172, 404
Vitis viifera 504
Vomiting 247
    intractable 353

W

Waist circumference 141
    cut off values for 369t
Waist-height ratio 141
Waist-hip ratio 141, 368
Water 5, 203, 240, 461, 469, 474
    balance 243
        regulation of 244
    buffer 260
    electrolytes 471
    fluoridation of 229
    functions of 240f
    imbalance 247
    intake 243, 243t
    intoxication 250
        symptoms of 250
    output 243
        routes of 244
    role of 468
Waxes 81
Weight
    alternative indicators for 416
    bearing exercises 459
    gain 465
        gestational 309
        total 309t
Wernicke-Korsakoff
    encephalopathy 171
    syndrome 171
Wheat products 483t
White adipose tissue 143
White blood cells 178, 208
Wilson's disease 228
Wolff-Chaikoff effect 218
Womb, fetal changes in 315
World Food Programme 421
World Health Organization 18, 266, 267, 421
Wound healing, delayed 58

X

Xanthophylls 154
Xerophthalmia, classification of 356t
Xylitol 26

Y

Yellow carotenoids 451
Yoga 458
    practice 382

Z

Zeaxanthin 154, 452
Zinc 218, 274, 315, 316, 339, 384, 563
    deficiency 155, 221, 351
    excessive intake of 221
    fingers 220, 220f
    food sources of 220, 220f
    functions of 219
    homeostasis 219
    protoporphyrin 402, 408
    status 409
Ziziphus jujuba 504
Z-score 396

EU GSPR Authorised Reprsentative
Logos Europe, 9 rue Nicolas Poussin
1700, La Rochelle, France
Phone: +33 (0) 6 67 93 73 78
E-mail: contact@logoseurope.eu

www.ingramcontent.com/pod-product-compliance
Ingram Content Group UK Ltd.
Pitfield, Milton Keynes, MK11 3LW, UK
UKHW050430150426
5217IPUK00019B/1325